ALREADY REGISTERED?

1. Log in at expertconsult.com
2. Scratch off your Activation Code below
3. Enter it into the "Add a Title" box
4. Click "Activate Now"
5. Click the title under "My Titles"

FIRST-TIME USER?

1. *REGISTER*
   - Click "Register Now" at expertconsult.com
   - Fill in your user information and click "Continue"
2. *ACTIVATE YOUR BOOK*
   - Scratch off your Activation Code below
   - Enter it into the "Enter Activation Code" box
   - Click "Activate Now"
   - Click the title under "My Titles"

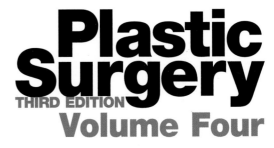

Plastic Surgery
THIRD EDITION
Volume Four
Lower Extremity, Trunk and Burns

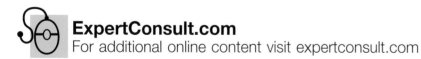

ExpertConsult.com
For additional online content visit expertconsult.com

Content Strategists: Sue Hodgson, Belinda Kuhn
Content Development Specialists: Poppy Garraway, Louise Cook, Alexandra Mortimer
Content Coordinators: Emma Cole, Trinity Hutton, Sam Crowe
Project Managers: Caroline Jones, Cheryl Brant
Design: Stewart Larking, Miles Hitchen
Illustration Manager: Jennifer Rose
Illustrator: Antbits
Marketing Manager: Helena Mutak
Technical Copyeditors: Darren Smith, Colin Woon
Video Reviewers: Leigh Jansen, James Saunders
Artwork Reviewer: Priya Chadha

Plastic Surgery

THIRD EDITION

Volume Four

Lower Extremity, Trunk and Burns

Editor in Chief

Peter C. Neligan
MB, FRCS(I), FRCSC, FACS
Professor of Surgery
Department of Surgery, Division of Plastic
Surgery
University of Washington
Seattle, WA, USA

Volume Editor

David H. Song
MD, MBA, FACS
Cynthia Chow Professor of Surgery
Chief, Section of Plastic and Reconstructive Surgery
Vice-Chairman, Department of Surgery
The University of Chicago Medicine & Biological
Sciences
Chicago, IL, USA

Video Editor

Allen L. Van Beek
MD, FACS
Adjunct Professor
University Minnesota School of Medicine
Division Plastic Surgery
Minneapolis, MN, USA

ELSEVIER
SAUNDERS

London, New York, Oxford, St Louis, Sydney, Toronto

ELSEVIER
SAUNDERS

SAUNDERS an imprint of Elsevier Inc

First edition 1990
Second edition 2006
Third edition 2013

Notices

Knowledge and best practice in this field are constantly changing. As new research and experience broaden our understanding, changes in research methods, professional practices, or medical treatment may become necessary.

Practitioners and researchers must always rely on their own experience and knowledge in evaluating and using any information, methods, compounds, or experiments described herein. In using such information or methods they should be mindful of their own safety and the safety of others, including parties for whom they have a professional responsibility.

With respect to any drug or pharmaceutical products identified, readers are advised to check the most current information provided (i) on procedures featured or (ii) by the manufacturer of each product to be administered, to verify the recommended dose or formula, the method and duration of administration, and contraindications. It is the responsibility of practitioners, relying on their own experience and knowledge of their patients, to make diagnoses, to determine dosages and the best treatment for each individual patient, and to take all appropriate safety precautions.

To the fullest extent of the law, neither the Publisher nor the authors, contributors, or editors, assume any liability for any injury and/or damage to persons or property as a matter of products liability, negligence or otherwise, or from any use or operation of any methods, products, instructions, or ideas contained in the material herein.

Volume 4 ISBN: 978-1-4557-1055-3
Volume 4 Ebook ISBN: 978-1-4557-4048-2
6 volume set ISBN: 978-1-4377-1733-4

ELSEVIER your source for books, journals and multimedia in the health sciences
www.elsevierhealth.com

Working together to grow
libraries in developing countries

www.elsevier.com | www.bookaid.org | www.sabre.org

ELSEVIER   BOOK AID International   Sabre Foundation

The publisher's policy is to use paper manufactured from sustainable forests

Printed in China
Last digit is the print number: 9 8 7 6 5 4 3 2 1

Contents

Volume Four: Lower Extremity, Trunk and Burns

David Song

Volume Five: Breast

James C. Grotting

Volume Six: Hand and Upper Extremity
James Chang

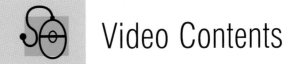

Video Contents

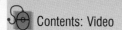

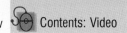

Foreword

In many ways, a textbook defines a particular discipline, and this is especially true in the evolution of modern plastic surgery. The publication of Zeis's *Handbuch der Plastischen Chirurgie* in 1838 popularized the name of the specialty but von Graefe in his monograph *Rhinoplastik*, published in 1818, had first used the title "plastic". At the turn of the last century, Nélaton and Ombredanne compiled what was available in the nineteenth century literature and published in Paris a two volume text in 1904 and 1907. A pivotal book, published across the Atlantic, was that of Vilray Blair, entitled *Surgery and Diseases of the Jaws* (1912). It was, however, limited to a specific anatomic region of the human body, but it became an important handbook for the military surgeons of World War I. Gillies' classic *Plastic Surgery of the Face* (1920) was also limited to a single anatomic region and recapitulated his remarkable and pioneering World War I experience with reconstructive plastic surgery of the face. Davis' textbook, *Plastic Surgery: Its Principles and Practice* (1919), was probably the first comprehensive definition of this young specialty with its emphasis on plastic surgery as ranging from the "top of the head to the soles of the feet." Fomon's *The Surgery of Injury and Plastic Repair* (1939) reviewed all of the plastic surgery techniques available at that time, and it also served as a handbook for the military surgeons of World War II. Kazanjian and Converse's *The Surgical Treatment of Facial Injuries* (1949) was a review of the former's lifetime experience as a plastic surgeon, and the junior author's World War II experience. The comprehensive plastic surgery text entitled *Plastic and Reconstructive Surgery*, published in 1948 by Padgett and Stephenson, was modeled more on the 1919 Davis text.

The lineage of the Neligan text began with the publication of Converse's five volume *Reconstructive Plastic Surgery* in 1964. Unlike his co-authored book with Kazanjian 15 years earlier, Converse undertook a comprehensive view of plastic surgery as the specialty existed in mid-20th century. Chapters were also devoted to pertinent anatomy, research and the role of relevant specialties like anesthesiology and radiology. It immediately became the bible of the specialty. He followed up with a second edition published in 1977, and I was the Assistant Editor. The second edition had grown from five to seven volumes (3970 pages) because the specialty had also grown. I edited the 1990 edition which had grown to eight volumes and 5556 pages; the hand section was edited by J. William Littler and James W. May. I changed the name of the text from *Reconstructive Plastic Surgery* to *Plastic Surgery* because in my mind I could not fathom the distinction between both titles. To the mother of a child with cleft lip, the surgery

is "cosmetic," and many of the facelift procedures at that time were truly reconstructive because of the multiple layers at which the facial soft tissues were being readjusted. The late Steve Mathes edited the 2006 edition in eight volumes. He changed the format somewhat and V.R. Hentz was the hand editor. At that time, the text had grown to more than 7000 pages.

The education of the plastic surgeon and the reference material that is critically needed are no longer limited to the printed page or what is described in modern parlance as "hard copy". Certainly, Gutenberg's invention of movable type printing around 1439 allowed publication and distribution of the classic texts of Vesalius (*Fabrica*, 1543) and Tagliacozzi (*De Curtorum Chirurgia Per Insitionem* (1597) and for many years, this was the only medium in which surgeons could be educated. However, by the nineteenth century, travel had become easier with the development of reliable railroads and oceangoing ships, and surgeons conscientiously visited different surgical centers and attended organized meetings. The American College of Surgeons after World War II pioneered the use of operating room movies, and this was followed by videos. The development of the internet has, however, placed almost all information at the fingertips of surgeons around the world with computer access. In turn, we now have virtual surgery education in which the student or surgeon sitting at a computer is interactive with a software program containing animations, intraoperative videos with sound overlay, and access to the world literature on a particular subject. We are rapidly progressing from the bound book of the Gutenberg era to the currently ubiquitous hand held device or tablet for the mastery of surgical/knowledge.

The Neligan text continues this grand tradition of surgical education by bringing the reader into the modern communications world. In line with advances of the electronic era, there is extra online content such as relevant history, complete reference lists and videos. The book is also available as an e-book. It has been a monumental task, consuming hours of work by the editor and all of its participants. The "text" still defines the specialty of plastic surgery. Moreover, it ensures that a new generation of plastic surgeons will have access to all that is known. They, in turn, will not only carry this information into the future but will also build on it. Kudos to Peter Neligan and his colleagues for continuing the chronicle of the plastic surgery saga that has been evolving over two millennia.

Joseph G. McCarthy, MD
2012

I have always loved textbooks. When I first started my training I was introduced to Converse's *Reconstructive Plastic Surgery*, then in its second edition. I was over-awed by the breadth of the specialty and the expertise contained within its pages. As a young plastic surgeon in practice I bought the first edition of this book, *Plastic Surgery*, edited by Dr. Joseph McCarthy and found it an invaluable resource to which I constantly referred. I was proud to be asked to contribute a chapter to the second edition, edited by Dr. Stephen Mathes and never thought that I would one day be given the responsibility for editing the next edition of the book. I consider this to be the definitive text on our specialty so I took that responsibility very seriously. The result is a very changed book from the previous edition, reflecting changes in the specialty, changes in presentation styles and changes in how textbooks are used.

In preparation for the task, I read the previous edition from cover to cover and tried to identify where major changes could occur. Inevitably in a text this size, there is some repetition and overlap. So the first job was to identify where the repetition and overlap occurred and try to eliminate it. This allowed me to condense some of the material and, along with some other changes, enabled me to reduce the number of volumes from 8 to 6. Reading the text led me to another realization. That is that the breadth of the specialty, impressive when I was first introduced to it, is even more impressive now, 30 years later and it continues to evolve. For this reason I quickly realized that in order to do this project justice, I could not do it on my own. My solution was to recruit volume editors for each of the major areas of practice as well as a video editor for the procedural videos. Drs. Gurtner, Warren, Rodriguez, Losee, Song, Grotting, Chang and Van Beek have done an outstanding job and this book truly represents a team effort.

Publishing is at a crossroads. The digital age has made information much more immediate, much more easy to access and much more flexible in how it is presented. We have tried to reflect that in this edition. The first big change is that everything is in color. All the illustrations have been re-drawn and the vast majority of patient photographs are in color. Chapters on anatomy have been highlighted with a red tone to make them easier to find as have pediatric chapters which have been highlighted in green. Reflecting on the way I personally use textbooks, I realized that while I like access to references, I rarely read the list of references at the end of a chapter. When I do though, I frequently pull some papers to read. So you will notice that we have kept the most important references in the printed text but we have moved the rest to the web. However, this has allowed us to greatly enhance the usefulness of the references. All the references are hyperlinked to PubMed and expertconsult facilitates a search across all volumes. Furthermore, while every chapter has a section devoted to the history of the topic, this is again something I like to be able to access but rarely have the leisure to read. That section in each of the chapters has also been moved to the web. This not only relieved the pressure on space in the printed text but also allowed us to give the authors more freedom in presenting the history of the topic. As well, there are extra illustrations in the web version that we simply could not accommodate in the printed version. The web edition of the book is therefore more complete than the printed version and owning the book, automatically gets one access to the web. A mouse icon has been added to the text to mark where further content is available online. In this digital age, video has become a very important way to impart knowledge. More than 160 procedural videos contributed by leading experts around the world accompany these volumes. These videos cover the full scope of our specialty. This text is also available as an e-Book.

This book then is very different from its predecessors. It is a reflection of a changing age in communication. However I will be extremely pleased if it fulfils its task of defining the current state of knowledge of the specialty as its predecessors did.

Peter C. Neligan, MB, FRCS(I), FRCSC, FACS
2012

List of Contributors

Neta Adler, MD
Senior Surgeon
Department of Plastic and Reconstructive
Surgery
Hadassah University Hospital
Jerusalem, Israel
*Volume 3, Chapter 40 Congenital melanocytic
nevi*

Ahmed M. Afifi, MD
Assistant Professor of Plastic Surgery
University of Winsconsin
Madison, WI, USA
Associate Professor of Plastic Surgery
Cairo University
Cairo, Egypt
*Volume 3, Chapter 1 Anatomy of the head and
neck*

Maryam Afshar, MD
Post Doctoral Fellow
Department of Surgery (Plastic and
Reconstructive Surgery)
Stanford University School of Medicine
Stanford, CA, USA
*Volume 3, Chapter 22 Embryology of the
craniofacial complex*

Jamil Ahmad, MD, FRCSC
Staff Plastic Surgeon
The Plastic Surgery Clinic
Mississauga, ON, Canada
*Volume 2, Chapter 18 Open technique
rhinoplasty*
*Volume 5, Chapter 8.3 Superior or medial
pedicle*

Hee Chang Ahn, MD, PhD
Professor
Department of Plastic and Reconstructive
Surgery
Hanyang University Hospital, School of
Medicine
Seoul, South Korea
Volume 6, Chapter 22 Ischemia of the hand
*Volume 6, Video 22.01 Radial artery periarterial
sympathectomy*
*Volume 6, Video 22.02 Ulnar artery periarterial
sympathectomy*
*Volume 6, Video 22.03 Digital artery periarterial
sympathectomy*

Tae-Joo Ahn, MD
Jeong-Won Aesthetic Plastic Surgical Clinic
Seoul, South Korea
*Volume 2, Video 10.01 Eyelidplasty non-
incisional method*
Volume 2, Video 10.02 Incisional method

Lisa E. Airan, MD
Assistant Clinical Professor
Department of Dermatology
Mount Sinai Hospital
Aesthetic Dermatologist
Private Practice
New York, NY, USA
Volume 2, Chapter 4 Soft-tissue fillers

Sammy Al-Benna, MD, PhD
Specialist in Plastic and Aesthetic Surgery
Department of Plastic Surgery
Burn Centre, Hand Centre, Operative
Reference Centre for Soft Tissue Sarcoma
BG University Hospital Bergmannsheil, Ruhr
University Bochum
Bochum, North Rhine-Westphalia, Germany
*Volume 4, Chapter 18 Acute management of
burn/electrical injuries*

Amy K. Alderman, MD, MPH
Private Practice
Atlanta, GA, USA
*Volume 1, Chapter 10 Evidence-based medicine
and health services research in plastic surgery*

Robert J. Allen, MD
Clinical Professor of Plastic Surgery
Department of Plastic Surgery
New York University Medical Centre
Charleston, SC, USA
*Volume 5, Chapter 18 The deep inferior
epigastric artery perforator (DIEAP) flap*
*Volume 5, Chapter 19 Alternative flaps for breast
reconstruction*
*Volume 5, Video 18.02 DIEP flap breast
reconstruction*

Mohammed M. Al Kahtani, MD, FRCSC
Clinical Fellow
Division of Plastic Surgery
Department of Surgery
University of Alberta
Edmonton, AB, Canada
*Volume 1, Chapter 33 Facial prosthetics in
plastic surgery*

Faisal Al-Mufarrej, MB, BCh
Chief Resident in Plastic Surgery
Division of Plastic Surgery
Department of Surgery
Mayo Clinic
Rochester, MN, USA
*Volume 6, Chapter 20 Osteoarthritis in the hand
and wrist*

Gary J. Alter, MD
Assistant Clinical Professor
Division of Plastic Surgery
University of Califronia at Los Angeles School
of Medicine
Los Angeles, CA, USA
Volume 2, Chapter 31 Aesthetic genital surgery

Al Aly, MD, FACS
Director of Aesthetic Surgery
Professor of Plastic Surgery
Aesthetic and Plastic Surgery Institute
University of California
Irvine, CA, USA
Volume 2, Chapter 27 Lower bodylifts

Khalid Al-Zahrani, MD, SSC-PLAST
Assistant Professor
Consultant Plastic Surgeon
King Khalid University Hospital
King Saud University
Riyadh, Saudi Arabia
Volume 2, Chapter 27 Lower bodylifts

Kenneth W. Anderson, MD
Marietta Facial Plastic Surgery & Aesthetics
Center
Mareitta, GA, USA
Volume 2, Video 23.04 FUE FOX procedure

Alice Andrews, PhD
Instructor
The Dartmouth Institute for Health Policy and
Clinical Practice
Lebanon, NH, USA
*Volume 5, Chapter 12 Patient-centered health
communication*

Louis C. Argenta, MD
Professor of Plastic and Reconstructive Surgery
Department of Plastic Surgery
Wake Forest Medical Center
Winston Salem, NC, USA
*Volume 1, Chapter 27 Principles and applications
of tissue expansion*

Charlotte E. Ariyan, MD, PhD
Surgical Oncologist
Gastric and Mixed Tumor Service
Memorial Sloan-Kettering Cancer Center
New York, NY, USA
Volume 3, Chapter 14 Salivary gland tumors

Stephan Ariyan, MD, MBA
Clinical Professor of Surgery
Plastic Surgery
Otolaryngology Yale University School of
Medicine Associate Chief
Department of Surgery
Yale New Haven Hospital Director
Yale Cancer Center Melanoma Program
New Haven, CT, USA
Volume 1, Chapter 31 Melanoma
Volume 3, Chapter 14 Salivary gland tumors

Bryan S. Armijo, MD
Plastic Surgery Chief Resident
Department of Plastic and Reconstructive
Surgery
Case Western Reserve/University Hospitals
Cleveland, OH, USA
*Volume 2, Chapter 20 Airway issues and the
deviated nose*

Eric Arnaud, MD
Chirurgie Plastique et Esthétique
Chirurgie Plastique Crânio-faciale
Unité de chirurgie crânio-faciale du
departement de neurochirurgie
Hôpital Necker Enfants Malades
Paris, France
Volume 3, Chapter 32 Orbital hypertelorism

Christopher E. Attinger, MD
Chief, Division of Wound Healing
Department of Plastic Surgery
Georgetown University Hospital
Georgetown, WA, USA
Volume 4, Chapter 8 Foot reconstruction

Tomer Avraham, MD
Resident, Plastic Surgery
Institute of Reconstructive Plastic Surgery
NYU Medical Center
New York, NY, USA
*Volume 1, Chapter 12 Principles of cancer
management*

Kodi K. Azari, MD, FACS
Associate Professor of Orthopaedic Surgery
Plastic Surgery Chief
Section of Reconstructive Transplantation
Department of Orthopaedic Surgery and
Surgery
David Geffen School of Medicine at UCLA
Los Angeles, CA, USA
*Volume 6, Chapter 15 Benign and malignant
tumors of the hand*

Sérgio Fernando Dantas de Azevedo, MD
Member
Brazilian Society of Plastic Surgery
Volunteer Professor of Plastic Surgery
Department of Plastic Surgery
Federal University of Pernambuco
Permambuco, Brazil
*Volume 2, Chapter 26 Lipoabdominoplasty
Volume 2, Video 26.01 Lipobdominoplasty
(including secondary lipo)*

Daniel C. Baker, MD
Professor of Surgery
Insitiue of Reconstructive Plastic Surgery
New York University Medical Center
Department of Plastic Surgery
New York, NY, USA
*Volume 2, Chapter 11.5 Facelift: Lateral
SMASectomy*

Steven B. Baker, MD, DDS, FACS
Associate Professor and Program Director
Co-director Inova Hospital for Children
Craniofacial Clinic
Department of Plastic Surgery
Georgetown University Hospital
Georgetown, WA, USA
*Volume 3, Chapter 30 Cleft and craniofacial
orthognathic surgery*

Karim Bakri, MD, MRCS
Chief Resident
Division of Plastic Surgery
Mayo Clinic
Rochester, MN, USA
*Volume 6, Chapter 20 Osteoarthritis in the hand
and wrist*

Carla Baldrighi, MD
Staff Surgeon
Reconstructive Microsurgery Unit
Azienda Ospedaliera Universitaria Careggi
Florence, Italy
*Volume 6, Chapter 30 Growth considerations in
pediatric upper extremity trauma and
reconstruction
Volume 6, Video 30.01 Epiphyseal transplant
harvesting technique*

Jonathan Bank, MD
Resident, Section of Plastic and Reconstructive
Surgery
Department of Surgery
Pritzker School of Medicine
University of Chicago Medical Center
Chicago, IL, USA
*Volume 4, Chapter 12 Abdominal wall
reconstruction*

A. Sina Bari, MD
Chief Resident
Division of Plastic and Reconstructive Surgery
Stanford University Hospital and Clinics
Stanford, CA, USA
*Volume 1, Chapter 16 Scar prevention,
treatment, and revision*

Scott P. Bartlett, MD
Professor of Surgery
Peter Randall Endowed Chair in Pediatric
Plastic Surgery
Childrens Hospital of Philadelphia, University of
Philadelphia
Philadelphia, PA, USA
*Volume 3, Chapter 34 Nonsyndromic
craniosynostosis*

Fritz E. Barton, Jr., MD
Clinical Professor
Department of Plastic Surgery
University of Texas Southwestern Medical
Center
Dallas, TX, USA
*Volume 2, Chapter 11.7 Facelift: SMAS with skin
attached – the "high SMAS" technique
Volume 2, Video 11.07.01 The High SMAS
technique with septal reset*

Bruce S. Bauer, MD, FACS, FAAP
Director of Pediatric Plastic Surgery, Clinical
Professor of Surgery
Northshore University Healthsystem
University of Chicago, Pritzker School of
Medicine, Highland Park Hospital
Chicago, IL, USA
*Volume 3, Chapter 40 Congenital melanocytic
nevi*

Ruediger G.H. Baumeister, MD, PhD
Professor of Surgery Emeritus
Consultant in Lymphology
Ludwig Maximilians University
Munich, Germany
*Volume 4, Chapter 3 Lymphatic reconstruction of
the extremities*

Leslie Baumann, MD
CEO
Baumann Cosmetic and Research Institute
Miami, FL, USA
*Volume 2, Chapter 2 Non surgical skin care and
rejuvenation*

Adriane L. Baylis, PhD
Speech Scientist
Section of Plastic and Reconstructive Surgery
Nationwide Children's Hospital
Columbus, OH, USA
*Volume 3, Chapter 28 Velopharyngeal
dysfunction
Volume 3, Video 28 Velopharyngeal
incompetence (1-3)*

Elisabeth Beahm, MD, FACS
Professor
Department of Plastic Surgery
University of Texas MD Anderson Cancer
Center
Houston, TX, USA
*Volume 5, Chapter 10 Breast cancer: Diagnosis
therapy and oncoplastic techniques
Volume 5, Video 10.01 Breast cancer: diagnosis
and therapy*

Michael L. Bentz, MD, FAAP, FACS
Professor of Surgery Pediatrics and
Neurosurgery Chairman
Chairman of Clinical Affairs
Department of Surgery
Division of Plastic Surgery Vice
University of Wisconsin School of Medicine and
Public Health
Madison, WI, USA
Volume 3, Chapter 42 Pediatric tumors

Aaron Berger, MD, PhD
Resident
Division of Plastic Surgery, Department of
Surgery
Stanford University Medical Center
Palo Alto, CA, USA
Volume 1, Chapter 31 Melanoma

Pietro Berrino, MD
Teaching Professor
University of Milan
Director
Chirurgia Plastica Genova SRL
Genoa, Italy
Volume 5, Chapter 23 Poland's syndrome

Valeria Berrino, MS
In Training
Chirurgia Plastica Genova SRL
Genoa, Italy
Volume 5, Chapter 23 Poland's syndrome

Miles G. Berry, MS, FRCS(Plast)
Consultant Plastic and Aesthetic Surgeon
Institute of Cosmetic and Reconstructive
Surgery
London, UK
*Volume 2, Chapter 11.3 Facelift: Platysma-SMAS
plication*
*Volume 2, Video 11.03.01 Facelift – Platysma
SMAS plication*

Robert M. Bernstein, MD, FAAD
Associate Clinical Professor
Department of Dermatology
College of Physicians and Surgeons
Columbia University
Director
Private Practice
Bernstein Medical Center for Hair Restoration
New York, NY, USA
Volume 2, Video 23.04 FUE FOX procedure
*Volume 2, Video 23.02 Follicular unit hair
transplantation*

Michael Bezuhly, MD, MSc, SM, FRCSC
Assistant Professor
Department of Surgery, Division of Plastic and
Reconstructive Surgery
IWK Health Centre, Dalhousie University
Halifax, NS, Canada
*Volume 6, Chapter 23 Nerve entrapment
syndromes*
*Volume 6, Video 23.01-04 Carpal tunnel and
cubital tunnel releases in the same patient in one
procedure with field sterility – local anaesthetic
and surgery*

Sean M. Bidic, MD, MFA, FAAP, FACS
Private Practice
American Surgical Arts
Vineland, NJ, USA
Volume 6, Chapter 16 Infections of the hand

Phillip N. Blondeel, MD, PhD, FCCP
Professor of Plastic Surgery
Department of Plastic and Reconstructive
Surgery
University Hospital Gent
Gent, Belgium
*Volume 5, Chapter 18 The deep inferior
epigastric artery perforator (DIEAP) Flap*
*Volume 5, Chapter 19 Alternative flaps for breast
reconstruction*
*Volume 5, Video 18.02 DIEP flap breast
reconstruction*

Sean G. Boutros, MD
Assistant Professor of Surgery
Weill Cornell Medical College (Houston)
Clinical Instructor
University of Texas School of Medicine
(Houston)
Houston Plastic and Craniofacial Surgery
Houston, TX, USA
*Volume 3, Video 7.02 Reconstruction of
acquired ear deformities*

Lorenzo Borghese, MD
Plastic Surgeon
General Surgeon
Department of Plastic and Maxillo Facial
Surgery
Director of International Cooperation South
East Asia
Pediatric Hospital "Bambino Gesu'"
Rome, Italy
*Volume 4, Chapter 19 Extremity burn
reconstruction*
*Volume 4, Video 19.01 Extremity burn
reconstruction*

Trevor M. Born, MD, FRCSC
Lecturer
Division of Plastic and Reconstructive Surgery
The University of Toronto
Toronto, Ontario, Canada
Attending Physician
Lenox Hill Hospital
New York, NY, USA
Volume 2, Chapter 4 Soft-tissue fillers

Gregory H. Borschel, MD, FAAP, FACS
Assistant Professor
University of Toronto Division of Plastic and
Reconstructive Surgery
Assistant Professor
Institute of Biomaterials and Biomedical
Engineering
Associate Scientist
The SickKids Research Institute
The Hospital for Sick Children
Toronto, ON, Canada
*Volume 6, Chapter 35 Free functioning muscle
transfer in the upper extremity*

Kirsty U. Boyd, MD, FRCSC
Clinical Fellow – Hand Surgery
Department of Surgery – Division of Plastic
Surgery
Washington University School of Medicine
St. Louis, MO, USA
*Volume 1, Chapter 22 Repair and grafting of
peripheral nerve*
Volume 6, Chapter 33 Nerve transfers

James P. Bradley, MD
Professor of Plastic and Reconstructive Surgery
Department of Surgery
University of California, Los Angeles David
Geffen School of Medicine
Los Angeles, CA, USA
Volume 3, Chapter 33 Craniofacial clefts

Burton D. Brent, MD
Private Practice
Woodside, CA, USA
Volume 3, Chapter 7 Reconstruction of the ear

Mitchell H. Brown, MD, Med, FRCSC
Associate Professor of Plastic Surgery
Department of Surgery
University of Toronto
Toronto, ON, Canada
*Volume 5, Chapter 3 Secondary breast
augmentation*

Samantha A. Brugmann, PHD
Postdoctoral Fellow
Department of Surgery
Stanford University
Stanford, CA, USA
*Volume 3, Chapter 22 Embryology of the
craniofacial complex*

Terrence W. Bruner, MD, MBA
Private Practice
Greenville, SC, USA
Volume 2, Chapter 28 Buttock augmentation
Volume 2, Video 28.01 Buttock augmentation

Todd E. Burdette, MD
Staff Plastic Surgeon
Concord Plastic Surgery
Concord Hospital Medical Group
Concord, NH, USA
*Volume 1, Chapter 36 Robotics, simulation, and
telemedicine in plastic surgery*

Renee M. Burke, MD
Attending Plastic Surgeon
Department of Plastic Surgery
St. Alexius Medical Center
Hoffman Estates, IL, USA
*Volume 3, Chapter 8 Acquired cranial and facial
bone deformities*
*Volume 3, Video 8.01 Removal of venous
malformation enveloping intraconal optic nerve*

Charles E. Butler, MD, FACS
Professor, Department of Plastic Surgery
The University of Texas MD Anderson Cancer
Center
Houston, TX, USA
Volume 1, Chapter 32 Implants and biomaterials

**Peter E. M. Butler, MD, FRCSI, FRCS,
FRCS(Plast)**
Consultant Plastic Surgeon
Honorary Senior Lecturer
Royal Free Hospital
London, UK
*Volume 1, Chapter 34 Transplantation in plastic
surgery*

Yilin Cao, MD
Director, Department of Plastic and
Reconstructive Surgery
Shanghai 9th People's Hospital
Vice-Dean
Shanghai Jiao Tong University Medical School
Shanghai, The People's Republic of China
*Volume 1, Chapter 18 Tissue graft, tissue repair,
and regeneration*
*Volume 1, Chapter 20 Repair, grafting, and
engineering of cartilage*

Joseph F. Capella, MD, FACS
Chief, Post-Bariatric Body Contouring
Division of Plastic Surgery
Hackensack University Medical Center
Hackensack, NJ, USA
Volume 2, Chapter 29 Upper limb contouring
Volume 2, Video 29.01 Upper limb contouring

Brian T. Carlsen, MD
Assistant Professor of Plastic Surgery
Department of Surgery
Mayo Clinic
Rochester, MN, USA
*Volume 6, Chapter 20 Osteoarthritis in the hand
and wrist*

Robert C. Cartotto, MD, FRCS(C)
Attending Surgeon
Ross Tilley Burn Centre
Health Sciences Centre
Toronto, ON, Canada
*Volume 4, Chapter 23 Management of patients
with exfoliative disorders, epidermolysis bullosa,
and TEN*

Giuseppe Catanuto, MD, PhD
Research Fellow
The School of Oncological Reconstructive
Surgery
Milan, Italy
*Volume 5, Chapter 14 Expander/implant breast
reconstructions*
*Volume 5, Video 14.01 Mastectomy and
expander insertion: first stage*
*Volume 5, Video 14.02 Mastectomy and
expander insertion: second stage*

Peter Ceulemans, MD
Assistant Professor
Department of Plastic Surgery
Ghent University Hospital
Ghent, Belgium
*Volume 4, Chapter 13 Reconstruction of male
genital defects*

Rodney K. Chan, MD
Staff Plastic and Reconstructive Surgeon
Burn Center
United States Army Institute of Surgical
Research
Fort Sam
Houston, TX, USA
*Volume 3, Chapter 19 Secondary facial
reconstruction*

David W. Chang, MD, FACS
Professor
Department of Plastic Surgery
MD. Anderson Centre
Houston, TX, USA
*Volume 4, Chapter 3 Lymphatic reconstruction of
the extremities*
*Volume 4, Video 3.01 Lymphatico-venous
anastomosis*
*Volume 6, Chapter 15 Benign and malignant
tumors of the hand*

Edward I. Chang, MD
Assistant Professor
Department of Plastic Surgery
The University of Texas M.D. Anderson Cancer
Center
Houston, TX, USA
*Volume 3, Chapter 17 Carcinoma of the upper
aerodigestive tract*

James Chang, MD
Professor and Chief
Division of Plastic and Reconstructive Surgery
Stanford University Medical Center
Stanford, CA, USA
*Volume 6, Introduction: Plastic surgery
contributions to hand surgery*
*Volume 6, Chapter 1 Anatomy and biomechanics
of the hand*
Volume 6, Video 11.01 Hand replantation
Volume 6, Video 12.01 Debridement technique
*Volume 6, Video 19.01 Extensor tendon rupture
and end-side tendon transfer*
*Volume 6, Video 29.01 Addendum pediatric
trigger thumb release*

Robert A. Chase, MD
Holman Professor of Surgery – Emeritus
Stanford University Medical Center
Stanford, CA, USA
*Volume 6, Chapter 1 Anatomy and biomechanics
of the hand*

Constance M. Chen, MD, MPH
Plastic and Reconstructive Surgeon
Division of Plastic and Reconstructive Surgery
Lenox Hill Hospital
New York, NY, USA
Volume 3, Chapter 9 Midface reconstruction

Philip Kuo-Ting Chen, MD
Director
Department of Plastic and Reconstructive
Surgery
Chang Gung Memorial Hospital and Chang
Gung University
Taipei, Taiwan, The People's Republic of China
Volume 3, Chapter 23 Repair of unilateral cleft lip

Yu-Ray Chen, MD
Professor of Surgery
Department of Plastic and Reconstructive
Surgery
Chang Gung Memorial Hospital
Chang Gung University
Tao-Yuan, Taiwan, The People's Republic of
China
*Volume 3, Chapter 15 Tumors of the facial
skeleton: Fibrous dysplasia*

Ming-Huei Cheng, MD, MBA, FACS
Professor and Chief, Division of Reconstructive
Microsurgery
Department of Plastic and Reconstructive
Surgery
Chang Gung Memorial Hospital
Chang Gung Medical College
Chang Gung University
Taoyuan, Taiwan, The People's Republic of
China
*Volume 3, Chapter 12 Oral cavity, tongue, and
mandibular reconstructions*
*Volume 3, Video 12.02 Ulnar forearm flap for
buccal reconstruction*

You-Wei Cheong, MBBS, MS
Consultant Plastic Surgeon
Department of Surgery
Faculty of Medicine and Health Sciences,
University of Putra Malaysia
Selangor, Malaysia
*Volume 3, Chapter 15 Tumors of the facial
skeleton: Fibrous dysplasia*

Armando Chiari Jr., MD, PhD
Adjunct Professor
Department of Surgery
School of Medicine of the Federal University of
Minas Gerais
Belo Horzonti, Minas Gerais, Brazil
*Volume 5, Chapter 8.5 The L short scar
mammaplasty*

Ernest S. Chiu, MD, FACS
Associate Professor of Plastic Surgery
Department of Plastic Surgery
New York University
New York
USA
*Volume 2, Chapter 9 Secondary blepharoplasty:
Techniques*

Hong-Lim Choi, MD, PhD
Jeong-Won Aesthetic Plastic Surgical Clinic
Seoul, South Korea
Volume 2, Video 10.01 Eyelidplasty non-incisional method
Volume 2, Video 10.02 Incisional method

Jong Woo Choi, MD, PhD
Associate Professor
Department of Plastic and Reconstructive
Surgery
Asan Medical Center
Ulsan University
College of Medicine
Seoul, South Korea
Volume 2, Chapter 10 Asian facial cosmetic surgery

**Alphonsus K. Chong, MBBS, MRCS,
MMed(Orth), FAMS(Hand Surgery)**
Consultant Hand Surgeon
Department of Hand and Reconstructive
Microsurgery
National University Hospital
Assistant Professor
Department of Orthopaedic Surgery
Yong Loo Lin School of Medicine
National University of Singapore
Singapore
Volume 6, Chapter 3 Diagnostic imaging of the hand and wrist
Volume 6, Video 3.01 Diagnostic imaging of the hand and wrist – Scaphoid lunate dislocation

David Chwei-Chin Chuang, MD
Senior Consultant, Ex-President, Professor
Department of Plastic Surgery
Chang Gung University Hospital
Tao-Yuan, Taiwan, The People's Republic of
China
Volume 6, Chapter 36 Brachial plexus injuries-adult and pediatric
Volume 6, Video 36.01-02 Brachial plexus injuries

Kevin C. Chung, MD, MS
Charles B. G. de Nancrede, MD Professor
Section of Plastic Surgery, Department of
Surgery
Assistant Dean for Faculty Affairs
University of Michigan Medical School
Ann Arbor, MI, USA
Volume 6, Chapter 8 Fractures and dislocations of the carpus and distal radius
Volume 6, Chapter 19 Rheumatologic conditions of the hand and wrist
Volume 6, Video 8.01 Scaphoid fixation
Volume 6, Video 19.01 Silicone MCP arthroplasty

Juan A. Clavero, MD, PhD
Radiologist Consultant
Radiology Department
Clínica Creu Blanca
Barcelona, Spain
Volume 5, Chapter 13 Imaging in reconstructive breast surgery

Mark W. Clemens, MD
Assistant Professor
Department of Plastic Surgery
Anderson Cancer Center University of Texas
Houston, TX, USA
Volume 4, Chapter 8 Foot reconstruction
Volume 5, Chapter 15 Latissimus dorsi flap breast reconstruction
Volume 5, Video 15.01 Latissimus dorsi flap technique

Steven R. Cohen, MD
Senior Clinical Research Fellow, Clinical
Professor
Plastic Surgery
University of California
San Diego, CA
Director
Craniofacial Surgery
Rady Children's Hospital, Private Practice,
FACES+ Plastic Surgery, Skin and Laser Center
La Jolla, CA, USA
Volume 2, Chapter 5 Facial skin resurfacing

Sydney R. Coleman, MD
Clinical Assistant Professor
Department of Plastic Surgery
New York University Medical Center
New York, NY, USA
Volume 2, Chapter 14 Structural fat grafting
Volume 2, Video 14.01 Structural fat grafting of the face

John Joseph Coleman III, MD
James E. Bennett Professor of Surgery,
Department of Dermatology and Cutaneuous
Surgery
University of Miami Miller School of Medicine
Miami, FA
Chief of Plastic Surgery
Department of Surgery
Indiana University School of Medicine
Indianapolis, IN, USA
Volume 3, Chapter 16 Tumors of the lips, oral cavity, oropharynx, and mandible

Lawrence B. Colen, MD
Associate Professor of Surgery
Eastern Virginia Medical School
Norfolk, VA, USA
Volume 4, Chapter 8 Foot reconstruction

E. Dale Collins Vidal, MD, MS
Chief
Section of Plastic Surgery
Dartmouth-Hitchcock Medical Center
Professor of Surgery
Dartmouth Medical School
Director of the Center for Informed Choice
The Dartmouth Institute (TDI) for Health Policy
and Clinical Practice
Hanover, NH, USA
Volume 1, Chapter 10 Evidence-based medicine and health services research in plastic surgery
Volume 5, Chapter 12 Patient-centered health communication

Shannon Colohan, MD, FRCSC
Clinical Instructor, Plastic Surgery
Department of Plastic Surgery
University of Texas Southwestern Medical
Center
Dallas, TX, USA
Volume 4, Chapter 2 Management of lower extremity trauma

Mark B. Constantian, MD, FACS
Active Staff
Saint Joseph Hospital
Nashua, NH (private practice)
Assistant Clinical Professor of Plastic Surgery
Division of Plastic Surgery
Department of Surgery
University of Wisconsin
Madison, WI, USA
Volume 2, Chapter 19 Closed technique rhinoplasty

Peter G. Cordeiro, MD, FACS
Chief
Plastic and Reconstructive Surgery
Memorial Sloan-Kettering Cancer Center
Professor of Surgery
Weill Cornell Medical College
New York, NY, USA
Volume 3, Chapter 9 Midface reconstruction
Volume 4, Chapter 14 Reconstruction of acquired vaginal defects

Christopher Cox, MD
Chief Resident
Department of Orthopaedic Surgery
Stanford University Medical School
Stanford, CA, USA
Volume 6, Chapter 5 Principles of internal fixation as applied to the hand and wrist
Volume 6, Video 5.01 Dynamic compression plating and lag screw technique

Albert Cram, MD
Professor Emeritus
University of Iowa
Iowa City Plastic Surgery
Coralville, IO, USA
Volume 2, Chapter 27 Lower bodylifts

Catherine Curtin, MD
Assistant Professor
Department of Surgery Division of Plastic
Stanford University
Stanford, CA, USA
*Volume 6, Chapter 37 Restoration of upper
extremity function*
*Volume 6, Video 37.01 1 Stage grasp IC 6 short
term*
*Volume 6, Video 37.02 2 Stage grasp release
outcome*

Lars B. Dahlin, MD, PhD
Professor and Consultant
Department of Clinical Sciences, Malmö-Hand
Surgery
University of Lund
Malmö, Sweden
*Volume 6, Chapter 32 Peripheral nerve injuries of
the upper extremity*
Volume 6, Video 32.01 Digital Nerve Suture
Volume 6, Video 32.02 Median Nerve Suture

Dai M. Davies, FRCS
Consultant and Institute Director
Institute of Cosmetic and Reconstructive
Surgery
London, UK
*Volume 2, Chapter 11.3 Facelift: Platysma-SMAS
plication*
*Volume 2, Video 11.03.01 Platysma SMAS
plication*

**Michael R. Davis, MD, FACS, LtCol,
USAF, MC**
Chief
Reconstructive Surgery and Regenerative
Medicine
Plastic and Reconstructive Surgeon
San Antonio Military Medical Center
Houston, TX, USA
*Volume 5, Chapter 1 Anatomy for plastic surgery
of the breast*

Jorge I. De La Torre, MD
Professor and Chief
Division of Plastic Surgery
University of Alabama at Birmingham
Birmingham, AL, USA
*Volume 5, Chapter 1 Anatomy for plastic surgery
of the breast*

A. Lee Dellon, MD, PhD
Professor of Plastic Surgery
Professor of Neurosurgery
Johns Hopkins University
Baltimore, MD, USA
*Volume 4, Chapter 6 Diagnosis and treatment of
painful neuroma and of nerve compression in the
lower extremity*
*Volume 4, Video 6.01 Diagnosis and treatment
of painful neuroma and of nerve compression in
the lower extremity*

Sara R. Dickie, MD
Resident, Section of Plastic and Reconstructive
Surgery
Department of Surgery
University of Chicago Medical Center
Chicago, IL, USA
*Volume 4, Chapter 9 Comprehensive trunk
anatomy*

Joseph J. Disa, MD, FACS
Attending Surgeon
Plastic and Reconstructive Surgery in the
Department of Surgery
Memorial Sloan Kettering Cancer Center
New York, NY, USA
Volume 3, Chapter 9 Midface reconstruction
*Volume 4, Chapter 14 Reconstruction of
acquired vaginal defects*

Risal Djohan, MD
Head of Regional Medical Practice
Department of Plastic Surgery
Cleveland Clinic
Cleveland, OH, USA
*Volume 3, Chapter 1 Anatomy of the head and
neck*

Erin Donaldson, MS
Instructor
Department of Otolaryngology
New York Medical College
Valhalla, NY, USA
*Volume 1, Chapter 36 Robotics, simulation, and
telemedicine in plastic surgery*

Amir H. Dorafshar, MBChB
Assistant Professor
Department of Plastic and Reconstructive
surgery
John Hopkins Medical Institute
John Hopkins Outpatient Center
Baltimore, MD, USA
Volume 3, Chapter 3 Facial fractures

Ivica Ducic, MD, PhD
Professor – Plastic Surgery
Director – Peripheral Nerve Surgery Institute
Department of Plastic Surgery
Georgetown University Hospital
Washington, DC, USA
*Volume 6, Chapter 23 Complex regional pain
syndrome in the upper extremity*

Gregory A. Dumanian, MD, FACS
Chief of Plastic Surgery
Division of Plastic Surgery, Department of
Surgery
Northwestern Feinberg School of Medicine
Chicago, IL, USA
*Volume 4, Chapter 11 Reconstruction of the soft
tissues of the back*
*Volume 6, Chapter 40 Treatment of the upper
extremity amputee*
*Volume 6, Video 40.01 Targeted muscle
reinnervation in the transhumeral amputee –
Surgical technique and guidelines for restoring
intuitive neural control*

William W. Dzwierzynski, MD
Professor and Program Director
Department of Plastic Surgery
Medical College of Wisconsin
Milwaukee, WI, USA
*Volume 6, Chapter 11 Replantation and
revascularization*

L. Franklyn Elliott, MD
Assistant Clinical Professor
Emory Section of Plastic Surgery
Emory University
Atlanta, GA, USA
*Volume 5, Chapter 16 The bilateral pedicled
TRAM flap*
*Volume 5, Video 16.01 Pedicle TRAM breast
reconstruction*

Marco Ellis, MD
Chief Resident
Division of Plastic Surgery
Northwestern Memorial Hospital
Northwestern University, Feinberg School of
Medicine
Chicago, IL, USA
Volume 2, Chapter 8 Blepharoplasty
Volume 2, Video 8.01 Periorbital rejuvenation

Dino Elyassnia, MD
Associate Plastic Surgeon
Marten Clinic of Plastic Surgery
San Francisco, CA, USA
*Volume 2, Chapter 12 Secondary deformities
and the secondary facelift*

Surak Eo, MD, PhD
Chief, Associate Professor
Plastic and Reconstructive Surgery
DongGuk University Medical Center
DongGuk University Graduate School of
Medicine
Gyeonggi-do, South Korea
*Volume 6, Video 34.01 EIP to EPL tendon
transfer*

Elof Eriksson, MD, PhD
Chief
Department of Plastic Surgery
Joseph E. Murray Professor of Plastic and
Reconstructive Surgery
Brigham and Women's Hospital
Boston, MA, USA
*Volume 1, Chapter 11 Genetics and prenatal
diagnosis*

Simon Farnebo, MD, PhD
Consultant Hand Surgeon
Department of Plastic Surgery, Hand Surgery
and Burns
Institution of Clinical and Experimental
Medicine, University of Linköping
Linköping, Sweden
*Volume 6, Chapter 32 Peripheral nerve injuries of
the upper extremity*
Volume 6, Video 32.01 Digital Nerve Suture
Volume 6, Video 32.02 Median Nerve Suture

Jeffrey A. Fearon, MD
Director
The Craniofacial Center
Medical City Children's Hospital
Dallas, TX, USA
Volume 3, Chapter 35 Syndromic craniosynostosis

John M. Felder III, MD
Resident Physician
Department of Plastic Surgery
Georgetown University Hospital
Washington, DC, USA
Volume 6, Chapter 23 Complex regional pain syndrome in the upper extremity

Evan M. Feldman, MD
Chief Resident
Division of Plastic Surgery
Baylor College of Medicine
Houston, TX, USA
Volume 3, Chapter 29 Secondary deformities of the cleft lip, nose, and palate
Volume 3, Video 29.01 Complete takedown
Volume 3, Video 29.02 Abbé flap
Volume 3, Video 29.03 Thick lip and buccal sulcus deformities
Volume 3, Video 29.04 Alveolar bone grafting
Volume 3, Video 29.05 Definitive rhinoplasty

Julius Few Jr., MD
Director
The Few Institute for Aesthetic Plastic Surgery
Clinical Associate
Division of Plastic Surgery
University of Chicago
Chicago, IL, USA
Volume 2, Chapter 8 Blepharoplasty
Volume 2, Video 8.01 Periorbital rejuvenation

Alvaro A. Figueroa, DDS, MS
Director
Rush Craniofacial Center
Rush University Medical Center
Chicago, IL, USA
Volume 3, Chapter 27 Orthodontics in cleft lip and palate management

Neil A. Fine, MD
Associate Professor of Clinical Surgery
Department of Surgery
Northwestern University
Chicago, IL, USA
Volume 5, Chapter 5 Endoscopic approaches to the breast
Volume 5, Video 5.01 Endoscopic transaxillary breast augmentation
Volume 5, Video 5.02 Endoscopic approaches to the breast
Volume 5, Video 11.02 Partial breast reconstruction with a latissimus D

Joel S. Fish, MD, MSc, FRCSC
Medical Director Burn Program
Department of Surgery, University of Toronto,
Division of Plastic and Reconstructive Surgery
Hospital for Sick Children
Toronto, ON, Canada
Volume 4, Chapter 23 Management of patients with exfoliative disorders, epidermolysis bullosa, and TEN

David M. Fisher, MB, BCh, FRCSC, FACS
Medical Director, Cleft Lip and Palate Program
Division of Plastic and Reconstructive Surgery
The Hospital for Sick Children
Toronto, ON, Canada
Volume 3, Video 23.02 Unilateral cleft lip repair – anatomic subunit approximation technique

Jack Fisher, MD
Department of Plastic Surgery
Vanderbilt University
Nashville, TN, USA
Volume 2, Chapter 23 Hair restoration
Volume 5, Chapter 8.1 Reduction mammaplasty
Volume 5, Chapter 8.2 Inferior pedicle breast reduction

James W. Fletcher, MD, FACS
Chief Hand Surgery
Department Plastic and Hand Surgery
Regions Hospital
Assistant Prof. U MN Dept of Surgery and Dept Orthopedics
St. Paul, MN, USA
Volume 6, Video 20.01 Ligament reconstruction tendon interposition arthroplasty of the thumb CMC joint

Joshua Fosnot, MD
Resident
Division of Plastic Surgery
The University of Pennsylvania Health System
Philadelphia, PA, USA
Volume 5, Chapter 17 Free TRAM breast reconstruction
Volume 5, Video 17.01 The muscle sparing free TRAM flap

Ida K. Fox, MD
Assistant Professor of Plastic Surgery
Department of Surgery
Washington University School of Medicine
Saint Louis, MO, USA
Volume 6, Chapter 33 Nerve transfers
Volume 6, Video 33.01 Nerve transfers

Ryan C. Frank, MD, FRCSC
Attending Surgeon
Plastic and Craniofacial Surgery
Alberta Children's Hospital
University of Calgary
Calgary, AB, Canada
Volume 2, Chapter 5 Facial skin resurfacing

Gary L. Freed, MD
Assistant Professor Plastic Surgery
Dartmouth-Hitchcock Medical Center
Lebanon, NH, USA
Volume 5, Chapter 12 Patient-centered health communication

Jeffrey B. Friedrich, MD
Assistant Professor of Surgery, Orthopedics and Urology (Adjunct)
Department of Surgery, Division of Plastic Surgery
University of Washington
Seattle, WA, USA
Volume 6, Chapter 13 Thumb reconstruction (non microsurgical)

Allen Gabriel, MD
Assitant Professor
Department of Plastic Surgery
Loma Linda University Medical Center
Chief of Plastic Surgery
Southwest Washington Medical Center
Vancouver, WA, USA
Volume 5, Chapter 2 Breast augmentation
Volume 5, Chapter 4 Current concepts in revisionary breast surgery
Volume 5, Video 4.01 Current concepts in revisionary breast surgery

Günter Germann, MD, PhD
Professor of Plastic Surgery
Clinic for Plastic and Reconstructive Surgery
Heidelberg University Hospital
Heidelberg, Germany
Volume 6, Chapter 10 Extensor tendon injuries and reconstruction

Goetz A. Giessler, MD, PhD
Plastic Surgeon, Hand Surgeon, Associate Professor of Plastic Surgery, Fellow of the European Board of Plastic Reconstructive and Aesthetic Surgery
BG Trauma Center Murnau
Murnau am Staffelsee, Germany
Volume 4, Chapter 4 Lower extremity sarcoma reconstruction
Volume 4, Video 4.01 Management of lower extremity sarcoma reconstruction

Jesse A. Goldstein, MD
Chief Resident
Department of Plastic Surgery
Georgetown University Hospital
Washington, DC, USA
Volume 3, Chapter 30 Cleft and craniofacial orthognathic surgery

Vijay S. Gorantla, MD, PhD
Associate Professor of Surgery
Department of Surgery, Division of Plastic and
Reconstructive Surgery
University of Pittsburgh Medical Center
Administrative Medical Director
Pittsburgh Reconstructive Transplantation
Program
Pittsburgh, PA, USA
*Volume 6, Chapter 38 Upper extremity
composite allotransplantation*
*Volume 6, Video 38.01 Upper extremity
composite allotransplantation*

Arun K. Gosain, MD
DeWayne Richey Professor and Vice Chair
Department of Plastic Surgery
University Hospitals Case Medical Center
Chief, Pediatric Plastic Surgery
Rainbow Babies and Children's Hospital
Cleveland, OH, USA
Volume 3, Chapter 38 Pierre Robin sequence

Lawrence J. Gottlieb, MD, FACS
Professor of Surgery
Director of Burn and Complex Wound Center
Director of Reconstructive Microsurgery
Fellowship
Section of Plastic and Reconstructive Surgery
Department of Surgery
University of Chicago
Chicago, IL, USA
*Volume 3, Chapter 41 Pediatric chest and trunk
defects*

Barry H. Grayson, DDS
Associate Professor of Surgery (Craniofacial
Orthodontics)
New York University Langone Medical Centre
Institute of Reconstructive Plastic Surgery
New York, NY, USA
Volume 3, Chapter 36 Craniofacial microsomia
Volume 3, Video 24.01 Repair of bilateral cleft lip

Arin K. Greene, MD, MMSc
Associate Professor of Surgery
Department of Plastic and Oral Surgery
Children's Hospital Boston
Harvard Medical School
Boston, MA, USA
Volume 1, Chapter 29 Vascular anomalies

James C. Grotting, MD, FACS
Clinical Professor of Plastic Surgery
University of Alabama at Birmingham;
The University of Wisconsin, Madison, WI;
Grotting and Cohn Plastic Surgery
Birmingham, AL, USA
Volume 5, Chapter 7 Mastopexy
Volume 5, Chapter 8.7 Sculpted pillar vertical
*Volume 5, Video 8.7.01 Marking the sculpted
pillar breast reduction*
Volume 5, Video 8.7.02 Breast reduction surgery

Ronald P. Gruber, MD
Associate Adjunct Clinical Professor
Division of Plastic and Reconstructive Surgery
Stanford University
Associate Clinical Professor
Division of Plastic and Reconstructive Surgery
University of California, San Francisco
San Francisco, CA, USA
Volume 2, Chapter 21 Secondary rhinoplasty

**Mohan S. Gundeti, MB, MCh, FEBU,
FRCS, FEAPU**
Associate Professor of Urology in Surgery and
Pediatrics, Director Pediatric Urology, Director
Centre for Pediatric Robotics and Minimal
Invasive Surgery
University of Chicago and Pritzker Medical
School Comer Children's Hospital
Chicago, IL, USA
*Volume 3, Chapter 44 Reconstruction of
urogenital defects: Congenital*
*Volume 3, Video 44.01 First stage hypospadias
repair with free inner preputial graft*
*Volume 3, Video 44.02 Second stage
hypospadias repair with tunica vaginalis flap*

Eyal Gur, MD
Head
Department of Plastic and Reconstructive
Surgery
The Tel Aviv Sourasky Medical Center
The Tel Aviv University School of Medicine
Tel Aviv, Israel
Volume 3, Chapter 11 Facial paralysis
Volume 3, Video 11.01 Facial paralysis

Geoffrey C. Gurtner, MD, FACS
Professor and Associate Chairman
Stanford University Department of Surgery
Stanford, CA, USA
*Volume 1, Chapter 13 Stem cells and
regenerative medecine*
*Volume 1, Chapter 35 Technology innovation in
plastic surgery*

Bahman Guyuron, MD
Kiehn-DesPrez Professor and Chairman
Department of Plastic Surgery
Case Western Reserve University School of
Medicine
Cleveland, OH, USA
*Volume 2, Chapter 20 Airway issues and the
deviated nose*
*Volume 3, Chapter 21 Surgical management of
migraine headaches*
Volume 2, Video 3.02 Botulinum toxin

Steven C. Haase, MD
Clinical Associate Professor
Department of Surgery, Section of Plastic
Surgery
University of Michigan Health
Ann Arbor, MI, USA
*Volume 6, Chapter 8 Fractures and dislocations
of the carpus and distal radius*

Robert S. Haber, MD, FAAD, FAAP
Assistant Professor, Dermatology and
Pediatrics
Case Western Reserve University School of
Medicine
Director
University Hair Transplant Center
Cleveland, OH, USA
*Volume 2, Video 23.08 Strip harvesting the
haber spreader*

Florian Hackl, MD
Research Fellow
Division of Plastic Surgery
Brigham and Women's Hospital
Harvard Medical School
Boston, MA, USA
*Volume 1, Chapter 11 Genetics and prenatal
diagnosis*

Phillip C. Haeck, MD
Private Practice
Seattle, WA, USA
*Volume 1, Chapter 4 The role of ethics in plastic
surgery*

Bruce Halperin, MD
Adjunct Associate Clinical Professor of
Anesthesia
Department of Anesthesia
Stanford University School of Medicine
Palo Alto, CA, USA
*Volume 1, Chapter 8 Patient safety in plastic
surgery*

Moustapha Hamdi, MD, PhD
Professor and Chairman of Plastic and
Reconstructive Surgery
Department of Plastic Surgery
Brussels University Hospital
Brussels, Belgium
*Volume 5, Chapter 21 Local flaps in partial
breast reconstruction*

Warren C. Hammert, MD
Associate Professor of Orthopaedic and
Plastic Surgery
Department of Orthopaedic Surgery
University of Rochester Medical Center
Rochester, NY, USA
*Volume 6, Chapter 7 Hand fractures and joint
injuries*

Dennis C. Hammond, MD
Clinical Assistant Professor
Department of Surgery
Michigan State University College of Human
Medicine
East Lansing
Associate Program Director
Plastic and Reconstructive Surgery
Grand Rapids Medical Education and Research
Center for Health Professions
Grand Rapids, MI, USA
*Volume 5, Chapter 8.4 Short scar periareolar
inferior pedicle reduction (SPAIR) mammaplasty*
Volume 5, Video 8.4.01 Spair technique

Scott L. Hansen, MD, FACS
Assistant Professor of Plastic and
Reconstructive Surgery
Chief, Hand and Microvascular Surgery
University of California, San Francisco
Chief, Plastic and Reconstructive Surgery
San Francisco General Hospital
San Francisco, CA, USA
*Volume 1, Chapter 24 Flap classification and
applications*

James A. Harris, MD
Cosmetic Surgeon
Private Practice
Hasson & Wong Aesthetic Surgery
Vancouver, BC, Canada
Volume 2, Video 23.05 FUE Harris safe system

Isaac Harvey, MD
Clinical Fellow
Department of Paediatric Plastic and
Reconstructive Surgery
Hospital for Sick Kids
Toronto, ON, Canada
*Volume 6, Chapter 35 Free functional muscle
transfers in the upper extremity*

Victor Hasson, MD
Cosmetic Surgeon
Private Practice
Hasson & Wong Aesthetic Surgery
Vancouver, BC, Canada
*Volume 2, Video 23.07 Perpendicular angle
grafting technique*

Theresa A Hegge, MD, MPH
Resident of Plastic Surgery
Division of Plastic Surgery
Southern Illinois University
Springfield, IL, USA
*Volume 6, Chapter 6 Nail and fingertip
reconstruction*

Jill A. Helms, DDS, PhD
Division of Plastic and Reconstructive Surgery
Department of Surgery
School of Medicine
Stanford University
Stanford, CA, USA
*Volume 3, Chapter 22 Embryology of the
craniofacial complex*

Ginard I. Henry, MD
Assistant Professor of Surgery
Section of Plastic Surgery
University of Chicago Medical Center
Chicago, IL, USA
*Volume 4, Chapter 1 Comprehensive lower
extremity anatomy, embryology, surgical exposure*

Vincent R. Hentz, MD
Emeritus Professor of Surgery and Orthopedic
Surgery (by courtesy)
Stanford University
Stanford, CA, USA
*Volume 6, Chapter 1 Anatomy and biomechanics
of the hand*
*Volume 6, Chapter 37 Restoration of upper
extremity function in tetraplegia*
*Volume 6, Video 37.01 1 Stage grasp IC 6 short
term*
*Volume 6, Video 37.02 2 Stage grasp release
outcome*

**Rebecca L. von der Heyde, PhD,
OTR/L, CHT**
Associate Professor
Program in Occupational Therapy
Maryville University
St. Louis, MO, USA
Volume 6, Chapter 39 Hand therapy
*Volume 6, Video 39.01 Hand therapy
Goniometric measurement*
Volume 6, Video 39.02 Threshold testing
*Volume 6, Video 39.03 Fabrication of a
synergistic splint*

Kent K. Higdon, MD
Former Aesthetic Fellow
Grotting and Cohn Plastic Surgery;
Current Assistant Professor
Vanderbilt University
Nashville, TN, USA
Volume 5, Chapter 7 Mastopexy
Volume 5, Chapter 8.1 Reduction mammaplasty
*Volume 5, Chapter 8.7 Sculpted pillar vertical
mammaplasty*

John Hijjawi, MD, FACS
Assistant Professor
Department of Plastic Surgery, Department of
General Surgery
Medical College of Wisconsin
Milwaukee, WI, USA
*Volume 4, Chapter 20 Cold and chemical injury
to the upper extremity*

Jonay Hill, MD
Clinical Assistant Professor
Anesthesiology Department
Anesthesia and Critical Care
Stanford University School of Medicine
Stanford, CA, USA
*Volume 6, Chapter 4 Anesthesia for upper
extremity surgery*

Piet Hoebeke, MD, PhD
Full Senior Professor of Paediatric Urology
Department of Urology
Ghent University Hospital
Ghent, Belgium
*Volume 4, Chapter 13 Reconstruction of male
genital defects*
*Volume 4, Video 13.01 Complete and partial
penile reconstruction*

William Y. Hoffman, MD
Professor and Chief
Division of Plastic and Reconstructive Surgery
University of California, San Francisco
San Francisco, CA, USA
Volume 3, Chapter 25 Cleft palate

Larry H. Hollier Jr., MD, FACS
Professor and Program Director
Division of Plastic Surgery
Baylor College of Medicine and Texas
Children's Hospital
Houston, TX, USA
*Volume 3, Chapter 29 Secondary deformities of
the cleft lip, nose, and palate*
Volume 3, Video 29.01 Complete takedown
Volume 3, Video 29.02 Abbé flap
*Volume 3, Video 29.03 Thick lip and buccal
sulcus deformities*
Volume 3, Video 29.04 Alveolar bone grafting
Volume 3, Video 29.05 Definitive rhinoplasty

Joon Pio Hong, MD, PhD, MMM
Chief and Associate Professor
Department of Plastic Surgery
Asian Medical Center University of Ulsan
School of Medicine
Seoul, Korea
*Volume 4, Chapter 5 Reconstructive surgery:
Lower extremity coverage*

Richard A. Hopper, MD, MS
Chief
Division of Pediatric Plastic Surgery
University of Washingtion
Surgical Director
Craniofacial Center
Seattle Childrens Hospital
Associate Professor
Division of Plastic Surgery
Seattle, WA, USA
Volume 3, Chapter 26 Alveolar clefts
Volume 3, Chapter 36 Craniofacial microsomia

Philippe Houtmeyers, MD
Resident
Plastic Surgery
Ghent University Hospital
Ghent, Belgium
*Volume 4, Chapter 13 Reconstruction of male
genital defects*
*Volume 4, Video 13.01 Complete and partial
penile reconstruction*

Steven E.R. Hovius, MD, PhD
Head
Department of Plastic, Reconstructive and
Hand Surgery
ErasmusmMC
University Medical Center
Rotterdam, The Netherlands
*Volume 6, Chapter 28 Congenital hand IV
disorders of differentiation and duplication*

Michael A. Howard, MD
Clinical Assistant Professor of Surgery
Division of Plastic Surgery
University of Chicago, Pritzker School of
Medicine
Northbrook, IL, USA
*Volume 4, Chapter 9 Comprehensive trunk
anatomy*

Jung-Ju Huang, MD
Assistant Professor
Division of Microsurgery
Plastic and Reconstructive Surgery
Chang Gung Memorial Hospital
Taoyuan, Taiwan, The People's Republic of
China
*Volume 3, Chapter 12 Oral cavity, tongue, and
mandibular reconstructions*
*Volume 3, Video 12.01 Fibula
osteoseptocutaneous flap for composite
mandibular reconstruction*
*Volume 3, Video 12.02 Ulnar forearm flap for
buccal reconstruction*

C. Scott Hultman, MD, MBA, FACS
Ethel and James Valone Distinguished
Professor of Surgery
Division of Plastic Surgery
University of North Carolina
Chapel Hill, NC, USA
*Volume 1, Chapter 5 Business principles for
plastic surgeons*

Leung-Kim Hung, MChOrtho (Liv)
Professor
Department of Orthopaedics and Traumatology
Faculty of Medicine
The Chinese University of Hong Kong
Hong Kong, The People's Republic of China
*Volume 6, Chapter 29 Congenital hand V
disorders of overgrowth, undergrowth, and
generalized skeletal deformities*

Gazi Hussain, MBBS, FRACS
Clinical Senior Lecturer
Macquarie Cosmetic and Plastic Surgery
Macquarie University
Sydney, Australia
Volume 3, Chapter 11 Facial paralysis

Marco Innocenti, MD
Director Reconstructive Microsurgery
Department of Oncology
Careggi University Hospital
Florence, Italy
*Volume 6, Chapter 30 Growth considerations in
pediatric upper extremity trauma and
reconstruction*
*Volume 6, Video 30.01 Epiphyseal transplant
harvesting technique*

Clyde H. Ishii, MD, FACS
Assistant Clinical Professor of Surgery
John A. Burns School of Medicine
Chief, Department of Plastic Surgery
Shriners Hospital
Honolulu Unit
Honolulu, HI, USA
*Volume 2, Chapter 10 Asian facial cosmetic
surgery*

Jonathan S. Jacobs, DMD, MD
Associate Professor of Clinical Plastic Surgery
Eastern Virginia Medical School
Norfolk, VA, USA
*Volume 2, Chapter 16 Anthropometry,
cephalometry, and orthognathic surgery*
*Volume 2, Video 16.01 Anthropometry,
cephalometry, and orthognathic surgery*

Jordan M.S. Jacobs, MD
Craniofacial Fellow
Department of Plastic Surgery
New York University Langone Medical Center
New York, NY, USA
*Volume 2, Chapter 16 Anthropometry,
cephalometry, and orthognathic surgery*
*Volume 2, Video 16.01 Anthropometry,
cephalometry, and orthognathic surgery*

**Ian T. Jackson, MD, DSc(Hon), FRCS,
FACS, FRACS (Hon)**
Emeritus Surgeon
Surgical Services Administration
William Beaumont Hospitals
Royal Oak, MI, USA
*Volume 3, Chapter 18 Local flaps for facial
coverage*

Oksana Jackson, MD
Assistant Professor of Surgery
Division of Plastic Surgery
University of Pennsylvania School of Medicine
Clinical Associate
The Children's Hospital of Philadelphia
Philadelphia, PA, USA
Volume 3, Chapter 43 Conjoined twins

Jeffrey E. Janis, MD, FACS
Associate Professor
Program Director
Department of Plastic Surgery
University of Texas Southwestern Medical
Center
Chief of Plastic Surgery
Chief of Wound Care
President-Elect
Medical Staff
Parkland Health and Hospital System
Dallas, TX, USA
Volume 4, Chapter 16 Pressure sores

Leila Jazayeri, MD
Resident
Stanford University Plastic and Reconstructive
Surgery
Stanford, CA, USA
*Volume 1, Chapter 35 Technology innovation in
plastic surgery*

Elizabeth B. Jelks, MD
Private Practice
Jelks Medical
New York, NY, USA
*Volume 2, Chapter 9 Secondary blepharoplasty:
Techniques*

Glenn W. Jelks, MD
Associate Professor
Department of Ophthalmology
Department of Plastic Surgery
New York University School of Medicine
New York, NY, USA
*Volume 2, Chapter 9 Secondary blepharoplasty:
Techniques*

Mark Laurence Jewell, MD
Assistant Clinical Professor of Plastic Surgery
Oregon Health Science University
Jewell Plastic Surgery Center
Eugene, OR, USA
*Volume 2, Chapter 11.4 Facelift: Facial
rejuvenation with loop sutures, the MACS lift and
its derivatives*

Andreas Jokuszies, MD
Consultant Plastic, Aesthetic and Hand
Surgeon
Department of Plastic, Hand and
Reconstructive Surgery
Hanover Medical School
Hanover, Germany
*Volume 1, Chapter 15 Skin wound healing:
Repair biology, wound, and scar treatment*

Neil F. Jones, MD, FRCS
Chief of Hand Surgery
University of California Medical Center
Professor of Orthopedic Surgery
Professor of Plastic and Reconstructive Surgery
University of California Irvine
Irvine, CA, USA
Volume 6, Chapter 22 Ischemia of the hand
*Volume 6, Chapter 34 Tendon transfers in the
upper extremity*
*Volume 6, Video 34.01 EIP to EPL tendon
transfer*

David M. Kahn, MD
Clinical Associate Professor of Plastic Surgery
Department of Surgery
Stanford University School of Medicine
Stanford, CA, USA
Volume 2, Chapter 21 Secondary rhinoplasty

Ryosuke Kakinoki, MD, PhD
Associate Professor
Chief of the Hand Surgery and Microsurgery
Unit
Department of Orthopedic Surgery and
Rehabilitation Medicine
Graduate School of Medicine
Kyoto University
Kyoto, Japan
*Volume 6, Chapter 2 Examination of the upper
extremity*
*Volume 2, Video 2.01-2.17 Examination of the
upper extremity*

Alex Kane, MD
Associate Professor of Surgery
Washington University School of Medicine
St. Louis, WO, USA
Volume 3, Chapter 23 Repair of unilateral cleft lip

Gabrielle M. Kane, MBBCh, EdD, FRCPC
Medical Director, Associate Professor
Department of Radiation Oncology
Associate Professor
Department of Medical Education and
Biomedical Informatics
University of Washington School of Medicine
Seattle, WA, USA
*Volume 1, Chapter 28 Therapeutic radiation:
Principles, effects, and complications*

Michael A. C. Kane, MD
Attending Surgeon Manhattan Eye, Ear and
Throat Institute
Department of Plastic Surgery
New York, NY, USA
Volume 2, Chapter 3 Botulinum toxin (BoNT-A)

Dennis S. Kao, MD
Hand Fellow
Department of Plastic Surgery
Medical College of Wisconsin
Milwaukee, WI, USA
*Volume 4, Chapter 20 Cold and chemical injury
to the upper extremity*

Sahil Kapur, MD
Resident, Plastic and Reconstructive Surgery
Department of Surgery, Division of Plastic and
Reconstructive Surgery
University of Wisconsin
Madison, WI, USA
Volume 3, Chapter 42 Pediatric tumors

Leila Kasrai, MD, MPH, FRCSC
Head, Division of Plastic Surgery
St Joseph's Hospital
Toronto, ON, Canada
Volume 2, Video 22.01 Setback otoplasty

Abdullah E. Kattan, MBBS, FRCS(C)
Clinical Fellow
Division of Plastic Surgery
Department of Surgery
University of Toronto
Toronto, ON, Canada
*Volume 4, Chapter 23 Management of patients
with exfoliative disorders, epidermolysis bullosa,
and TEN*

David L. Kaufman, MD, FACS
Private Practice Plastic Surgery
Aesthetic Artistry Surgical and Medical Center
Folsom, CA, USA
Volume 2, Chapter 21 Secondary rhinoplasty

Lindsay B. Katona, BA
Research Associate
Thayer School of Engineering
Dartmouth College
Hanover, NH, USA
*Volume 1, Chapter 36 Robotics, simulation, and
telemedicine in plastic surgery*

Henry K. Kawamoto, Jr., MD, DDS
Clinical Professor
Division of Plastic Surgery
University of California at Los Angeles
Los Angeles, CA, USA
Volume 3, Chapter 33 Craniofacial clefts

Jeffrey M. Kenkel, MD, FACS
Professor and Vice-Chairman
Rod J Rohrich MD Distinguished Professorship
in Wound Healing and Plastic Surgery
Department of Plastic Surgery
Southwestern Medical School
Director
Clinical Center for Cosmetic Laser Treatment
Dallas, TX, USA
*Volume 2, Chapter 24 Liposuction: A
comprehensive review of techniques and safety*

Carolyn L. Kerrigan, MD, MSc
Professor of Surgery
Section of Plastic Surgery
Dartmouth Hitchcock Medical Center
Lebanon, NH, USA
*Volume 1, Chapter 10 Evidence-based medicine
and health services research in plastic surgery*

Marwan R. Khalifeh, MD
Instructor of Plastic Surgery
Department of Plastic Surgery
Johns Hopkins University School of Medicine
Washington, DC, USA
*Volume 4, Chapter 12 Abdominal wall
reconstruction*

Jae-Hoon Kim, MD
April 31 Aesthetic Plastic Surgical Clinic
Seoul, South Korea
*Volume 2, Video 10.03 Secondary rhinoplasty:
septal extension graft and costal cartilage strut
fixed with K-wire*

**Timothy W. King, MD, PhD, MSBE,
FACS, FAAP**
Assistant Professor of Surgery and Pediatrics
Director of Research
Division of Plastic Surgery, Department of
Surgery
University of Wisconsin School of Medicine and
Public Health
Madison, WI, USA
Volume 1, Chapter 32 Implants and biomaterials

Brian M. Kinney, MD, FACS, MSME
Clinical Assistant Professor of Plastic Surgery
University of Southern California School of
Medicine
Los Angeles, CA, USA
*Volume 1, Chapter 7 Photography in plastic
surgery*

Richard E. Kirschner, MD
Chief, Section of Plastic and Reconstructive
Surgery
Director, Ambulatory Surgical Services
Director, Cleft Lip and Palate Center
Co-Director Nationwide Children's Hospital
Professor of Surgery and Pediatrics
Senior Vice Chair, Department of Plastic Surgery
The Ohio State University College of Medicine
Columbus, OH, USA
Volume 3, Chapter 28 Velopharyngeal dysfunction
*Volume 3, Video 28.01-28.03 Velopharyngeal
incompetence*

Elizabeth Kiwanuka, MD
Division of Plastic Surgery
Brigham and Women's Hospital
Harvard Medical School
Boston, MA, USA
*Volume 1, Chapter 11 Genetics and prenatal
diagnosis*

Grant M. Kleiber, MD
Plastic Surgery Resident
Section of Plastic and Reconstructive Surgery
University of Chicago Medical Center
Chicago, IL, USA
*Volume 4, Chapter 1 Comprehensive lower
extremity anatomy, embryology, surgical exposure*

Mathew B. Klein, MD, MS
David and Nancy Auth-Washington Research
Foundation Endowed Chair for Restorative
Burn Surgery
Division of Plastic Surgery
University of Washington
Program Director and Associate Professor
Division of Plastic Surgery
Harborview Medical Center
Seattle, WA, USA
Volume 4, Chapter 22 Reconstructive burn surgery

Kyung S Koh, MD, PhD
Professor of Plastic Surgery
Asan Medical Center, University of Ulsan
School of Medicine
Seoul, Korea
*Volume 2, Chapter 10 Asian facial cosmetic
surgery*

John C. Koshy, MD
Postdoctoral Research Fellow
Division of Plastic Surgery
Baylor College of Medicine
Houston, TX, USA
*Volume 3, Chapter 29 Secondary deformities of
the cleft lip, nose, and palate*
Volume 3, Video 29.01 Complete takedown
Volume 3, Video 29.02 Abbé flap
*Volume 3, Video 29.03 Thick lip and buccal
sulcus deformities*
Volume 3, Video 29.04 Alveolar bone grafting
Volume 3, Video 29.05 Definitive rhinoplasty

Evan Kowalski, BS
Section of Plastic Surgery
University of Michigan Health System
Ann Arbor, MI, USA
Volume 6, Video 19.02 Silicone MCP arthroplasty

Stephen J. Kovach, MD
Assistant Professor of Surgery
Division of Plastic and Reconstructive Surgery
University of Pennsylvannia Health System
Assistant Professor of Surgery
Department of Orthopaedic Surgery
University of Pennsylvannia Health System
Philadelphia, PA, USA
Volume 4, Chapter 7 Skeletal reconstruction

Steven J. Kronowitz, MD, FACS
Professor, Department of Plastic Surgery
MD Anderson Cancer Center
The University of Texas
Houston, TX, USA
*Volume 1, Chapter 28 Therapeutic radiation
principles, effects, and complications*

Todd A. Kuiken, MD, PhD
Director
Center for Bionic Medicine
Rehabilitation Institute of Chicago
Professor
Department of PMandR
Fienberg School of Medicine
Northwestern University
Chicago, IL, USA
*Volume 6, Chapter 40 Treatment of the upper
extremity amputee*
*Volume 6, Video 40.01 Targeted muscle
reinnervation in the transhumeral amputee*

Michael E. Kupferman, MD
Assistant Professor
Department of Head and Neck Surgery
Division of Surgery
The University of Texas MD Anderson Cancer
Center
Houston, TX, USA
*Volume 3, Chapter 17 Carcinoma of the upper
aerodigestive tract*

Robert Kwon, MD
Plastic Surgeon
Regional Plastic Surgery Center
Richardson, TX, USA
Volume 4, Chapter 16 Pressure sores

**Eugenia J. Kyriopoulos, MD, MSc, PhD,
FEBOPRAS**
Attending Plastic Surgeon
Department of Plastic Surgery and Burn Center
Athens General Hospital "G. Gennimatas"
Athens, Greece
*Volume 5, Chapter 21 Local flaps in partial
breast reconstruction*

Donald Lalonde, BSC, MD, MSc, FRCSC
Professor Surgery
Division of Plastic Surgery
Saint John Campus of Dalhousie University
Saint John, NB, Canada
*Volume 6, Chapter 24 Nerve entrapment
syndromes*
*Volume 6, Video 24.01 Carpal tunnel and cubital
tunnel releases*

Wee Leon Lam, MB, ChB, M Phil, FRCS
Microsurgery Fellow
Department of Plastic and Reconstructive
Surgery
Chang Gung Memorial Hospital
Taipei, Taiwan, The People's Republic of China
*Volume 6, Chapter 14 Thumb and finger
reconstruction – microsurgical techniques*
Volume 6, Video 14.01 Trimmed great toe
Volume 6, Video 14.02 Second toe for index
*Volume 6, Video 14.03 Combined second and
third toe for metacarpal hand*

Julie E. Lang, MD, FACS
Assistant Professor of Surgery
Department of surgery
Director of Breast Surgical Oncology
University of Arizona
Tucson, AZ, USA
*Volume 5, Chapter 10 Breast cancer: Diagnosis
therapy and oncoplastic techniques*
*Volume 5, Video 10.01 Breast cancer: diagnosis
and therapy*

Patrick Lang, MD
Plastic Surgery Resident
University of California
San Francisco, CA, USA
*Volume 1, Chapter 24 Flap classification and
applications*

Claude-Jean Langevin, MD, DMD
Assistant Professor University of Central Florida
Department of Surgery MD Anderson Cancer
Center
Plastic and Reconstructive Surgeon
University of Central Florida
Orlando, FL, USA
Volume 2, Chapter 13 Neck rejuvenation

Laurent Lantieri, MD
Department of Plastic Surgery
Hôpital Européen Georges Pompidou
Assistance Publique Hôpitaux de Paris
Paris Descartes University
Paris, France
Volume 3, Chapter 20 Facial transplant
Volume 3, Video 20.1 and 20.2 Facial transplant

Michael C. Large, MD
Urology Resident
Department of Surgery, Division of Urology
University of Chicago Hospitals
Chicago, IL, USA
*Volume 3, Chapter 44 Reconstruction of
urogenital defects: Congenital*
*Volume 3, Video 44.01 First stage hypospadias
repair with free inner preputial graft*
*Volume 3, Video 44.02 Second stage
hypospadias repair with tunica vaginalis flap*

Don LaRossa, MD
Emeritus Professor of Surgery
Division of Plastic and Reconstructive Surgery
Perelman School of Medicine
University of Pennsylvania
Philadelphia, PA, USA
Volume 3, Chapter 43 Conjoined twins

Caroline Leclercq, MD
Consultant Hand Surgeon
Institut de la Main
Paris, France
*Volume 6, Chapter 17 Management of
Dupuytren's disease*

Justine C. Lee, MD, PhD
Chief Resident
Section of Plastic and Reconstructive Surgery
Department
University of Chicago Medical Center
Chicago, IL, USA
*Volume 3, Chapter 41 Pediatric chest and trunk
defects*

W. P. Andrew Lee, MD
The Milton T. Edgerton, MD, Professor and
Chairman
Department of Plastic and Reconstructive
Surgery
Johns Hopkins University School of Medicine
Baltimore, MD, USA
*Volume 1, Chapter 34 Transplantation in plastic
surgery*
*Volume 6, Chapter 38 Upper extremity
composite allotransplantation*
*Volume 6, Video 38.01 Upper extremity
composite tissue allotransplantation*

Valerie Lemaine, MD, MPH, FRCSC
Assistant Professor of Plastic Surgery
Department of Surgery
Division of Plastic Surgery
Mayo Clinic
Rochester, MN, USA
*Volume 1, Chapter 10 Evidence-based medicine
and health services research in plastic surgery*

**Ping-Chung Leung, SBS, OBE, JP, MBBS,
MS, DSc, Hon DSocSc, FRACS, FRCS,
FHKCOS, FHKAM (ORTH)**
Professor Emeritus
Orthopaedics and Traumatology
The Chinese University of Hong Kong
Hong Kong, The People's Republic of China
*Volume 6, Chapter 29 Congenital hand V
disorders of overgrowth, undergrowth, and
generalized skeletal deformities*

Benjamin Levi, MD
Post Doctoral Research Fellow
Division of Plastic and Reconstructive Surgery
Stanford University
Stanford, CA
House Officer
Division of Plastic and Reconstructive Surgery
University of Michigan
Ann Arbor, MI, USA
*Volume 1, Chapter 13 Stem cells and
regenerative medicine*

L. Scott Levin, MD, FACS
Chairman of Orthopedic Surgery
Department of Orthopaedic Surgery
University of Pennsylvania School of Medicine
Philadelphia, PA, USA
Volume 4, Chapter 7 Skeletal reconstruction

Bradley Limmer, MD
Assistant Clinical Professor
Department of Internal Medicine
Division of Dermatology
Associate Clinical Professor
Department of Plastic and Reconstructive
Surgery
Surgeon, Private Practice
Limmer Clinic
San Antonio, TX, USA
*Volume 2, Video 23.02 Follicular unit hair
transplantation*

Bobby L. Limmer, MD
Professor of Dermatology
University of Texas
Surgeon, Private Practice
Limmer Clinic
San Antonio, TX, USA
*Volume 2, Video 23.02 Follicular unit hair
transplantation*

Frank Lista, MD, FRCSC
Medical Director
Burn Program
The Plastic Surgery Clinic
Mississauga, ON, Canada
*Volume 5, Chapter 8.3 Superior or medial
pedicle*

Wei Liu, MD, PhD
Professor of Plastic Surgery
Associate Director of National Tissue
Engineering Research Center
Department of Plastic and Reconstructive
Surgery
Shanghai 9th People's Hospital
Shanghai Jiao Tong University School of
Medcine
Shanghai, The People's Republic of China
*Volume 1, Chapter 18 Tissue graft, tissue repair,
and regeneration*
*Volume 1, Chapter 20 Repair, grafting, and
engineering of cartilage*

Michelle B. Locke, MBChB, MD
Honourary Lecturer
University of Auckland Department of Surgery
Auckland City Hospital Support Building
Grafton, Auckland, New Zealand
*Volume 2, Chapter 1 Managing the cosmetic
patient*

Sarah A. Long, BA
Research Associate
Thayer School of Engineering
Dartmouth College
San Mateo, CA, USA
*Volume 1, Chapter 36 Robotics, simulation, and
telemedicine in plastic surgery*

Michael T. Longaker, MD, MBA, FACS
Deane P. and Louise Mitchell Professor and
Vice Chair
Department of Surgery
Stanford University
Stanford, CA, USA
*Volume 1, Chapter 13 Stem cells and
regenerative medicine*

Peter Lorenz, MD
Chief of Pediatric Plastic Surgery, Director
Craniofacial Surgery Fellowship
Department of Surgery, Division of Plastic
Surgery
Stanford University School of Medicine
Stanford, CA, USA
*Volume 1, Chapter 16 Scar prevention,
treatment, and revision*

Joseph E. Losee, MD, FACS, FAAP
Professor of Surgery and Pediatrics
Chief, Division Pediatric Plastic Surgery
Children's Hospital of Pittsburgh
University of Pittsburgh Medical Center
Pittsburgh, PA, USA
Volume 3, Chapter 31 Pediatric facial fractures

Albert Losken, MD, FACS
Associate Professor Program Director
Emory Division of Plastic and Reconstructive
Surgery
Emory University School of Medicine
Atlanta, GA, USA
*Volume 5, Chapter 11 The oncoplastic approach
to partial breast reconstruction*

Maria M. LoTempio, MD
Assistant Professor in Plastic Surgery
Medical University of South Carolina
Charleston, SC
Adjunct Assistant Professor in Plastic Surgery
New York Eye and Ear Infirmary
New York, NY, USA
*Volume 5, Chapter 19 Alternative flaps for breast
reconstruction*

Otway Louie, MD
Assistant Professor
Division of Plastic and Reconstructive Surgery
Department of Surgery
University of Washington Medical Center
Seattle, WA, USA
Volume 4, Chapter 17 Perineal reconstruction

David W. Low, MD
Professor of Surgery
Division of Plastic Surgery
University of Pennsylvania School of Medicine
Clinical Associate
The Children's Hospital of Philadelphia
Philadelphia, PA, USA
Volume 3, Chapter 43 Conjoined twins

Nicholas Lumen, MD, PhD
Assistant Professor of Urology
Urology
Ghent University Hospital
Ghent, Belgium
*Volume 4, Chapter 13 Reconstruction of male
genital defects*
*Volume 4, Video 13.01 Complete and partial
penile reconstruction*

Antonio Luiz de Vasconcellos Macedo, MD
General Surgery
Director of Robotic Surgery
President of Oncology
Board of Albert Einstein Hospital
Sao Paulo, Brazil
*Volume 5, Chapter 20 Omentum reconstruction
of the breast*

Gustavo R. Machado, MD
University of California Irvine Medical Center
Department of Orthopaedic Surgery, Orange,
CA, USA
*Volume 6, Video 34.01 EIP to EPL tendon
transfer*

Susan E. Mackinnon, MD
Sydney M. Shoenberg, Jr. and Robert H.
Shoenberg Professor
Department of Surgery, Division of Plastic and
Reconstructive Surgery
Washington University School of Medicine
St. Louis, MO, USA
*Volume 1, Chapter 22 Repair and grafting of
peripheral nerve*
Volume 6, Chapter 33 Nerve transfers
Volume 6, Video 33.01 Nerve transfers

Ralph T. Manktelow, BA, MD, FRCS(C)
Professor
Department of Surgery
University of Toronto
Toronto, ON, Canada
Volume 3, Chapter 11 Facial paralysis

Paul N. Manson, MD
Professor of Plastic Surgery
University of Maryland Shock Trauma Unit
University of Maryland and Johns Hopkins
Schools of Medicine
Baltimore, MD, USA
Volume 3, Chapter 3 Facial fractures

Daniel Marchac, MD
Professor
Plastic, Reconstructive and Aesthetic
College of Medicine of Paris Hospitals
Paris, France
Volume 3, Chapter 32 Orbital hypertelorism

Malcom W. Marks, MD
Professor and Chairman
Department of Plastic Surgery
Wake Forest University School of Medicine
Winston-Salem, NC, USA
*Volume 1, Chapter 27 Principles and applications
of tissue expansion*

Timothy J. Marten, MD, FACS
Founder and Director
Marten Clinic of Plastic Surgery
Medical Director
San Francisco Center for the Surgical Arts
San Francisco, CA, USA
*Volume 2, Chapter 12 Secondary deformities
and the secondary facelift*

Mario Marzola, MBBS
Private Practice
Norwood, SA, Australia
Volume 2, Video 23.01 Donor closure tricophytic technique

Alessandro Masellis, MD
Plastic Surgeon
Department of Plastic Surgery and Burn
Therapy
Ospedale Civico ARNAS Palermo
Palermo, Italy
Volume 4, Chapter 19 Extremity burn reconstruction

Michele Masellis, MD, PhD
Plastic Surgeon
Former Chief
Professor Emeritus
Department of Plastic Surgery and Burn Unit
ARNAS Civico Hospital
Palermo, Italy
Volume 4, Chapter 19 Extremity burn reconstruction

Jaume Masia, MD, PhD
Professor and Chief
Plastic Surgery Department
Hospital de la Santa Creu i Sant Pau
Universidad Autónoma de Barcelona
Barcelona, Spain
Volume 5, Chapter 13 Imaging in reconstructive breast surgery

David W. Mathes, MD
Associate Professor of Surgery
Department of Surgery, Division of Plastic and
Reconstructive Surgery
University of Washington School of Medicine
Chief of Plastic Surgery
Puget Sound Veterans Affairs Hospital
Seattle, WA, USA
Volume 1, Chapter 34 Transplantation in plastic surgery

Evan Matros, MD
Assistant Attending Surgeon
Department of Surgery
Memorial Sloan-Kettering Cancer Center
Assistant Professor of Surgery (Plastic)
Weill Cornell University Medical Center
New York, NY, USA
Volume 1, Chapter 12 Principles of cancer management

G. Patrick Maxwell, MD, FACS
Clinical Professor of Surgery
Department of Plastic Surgery
Loma Linda University Medical Center
Loma Linda, CA, USA
Volume 5, Chapter 2 Breast augmentation
Volume 5, Chapter 4 Current concepts in revisionary breast surgery

Isabella C. Mazzola
Milan, Italy
Volume 1, Chapter 2 History of reconstructive and aesthetic surgery

Riccardo F. Mazzola, MD
Professor of Plastic Surgery
Postgraduate School Plastic Surgery
Maxillo-Facial and Otolaryngolog
Department of Specialistic Surgical Science
School of Medicine
University of Milan
Milan, Italy
Volume 1, Chapter 2 History of reconstructive and aesthetic surgery

Steven J. McCabe, MD, MSc
Assistant Professor
Department of Bioinformatics and Biostatistics
University of Louisville School of Public Health
and Information Sciences
Louisville, KY, USA
Volume 6, Chapter 18 Occupational hand disorders

Joseph G. McCarthy, MD
Lawrence D. Bell Professor of Plastic Surgery,
Director Institute of Reconstructive Plastic
Surgery and Chair
Department of Plastic Surgery
New York University Langone Medical Center
New York, NY, USA
Volume 3, Chapter 36 Craniofacial microsomia

Mary H. McGrath, MD, MPH
Plastic Surgeon
Division of Plastic Surgery
University of California San Francisco
San Francisco, CA, USA
Volume 1, Chapter 3 Psychological aspects of plastic surgery

Kai Megerle, MD
Research Fellow
Division of Plastic and Reconstructive Surgery
Stanford Medical Center
Stanford, CA, USA
Volume 6, Chapter 10 Extensor tendon injuries

Babak J. Mehrara, MD, FACS
Associate Member, Associate Professor of
Surgery (Plastic)
Memorial Sloan-Kettering Cancer Center
Weil Cornell University Medical Center
New York, NY, USA
Volume 1, Chapter 12 Principles of cancer management

Bryan Mendelson, FRCSE, FRACS, FACS
Private Plastic Surgeon
The Centre for Facial Plastic Surgery
Melbourne, Australia
Volume 2, Chapter 6 Anatomy of the aging face

Constantino G. Mendieta, MD, FACS
Private Practice
Miami, FL, USA
Volume 2, Chapter 28 Buttock augmentation
Volume 2, Video 28.01 Buttock augmentation

Frederick J. Menick, MD
Private Practitioner
Tucson, AZ, USA
Volume 3, Chapter 6 Aesthetic nasal reconstruction
Volume 3, Video 6.01 Aesthetic reconstruction of the nose – The 3-stage folded forehead flap for cover and lining,
Volume 3, Video 6.02 Aesthetic reconstruction of the nose-First stage transfer and intermediate operation

Ursula Mirastschijski, MD, PhD
Assistant Professor
Department of Plastic, Hand and
Reconstructive Surgery, Burn Center Lower
Saxony, Replantation Center
Hannover Medical School
Hannover, Germany
Volume 1, Chapter 15 Skin wound healing: Repair biology, wound, and scar treatment

Takayuki Miura, MD
Emeritus Professor of Orthopedic Surgery
Department of Orthopedic Surgery
Nagoya University School of Medicine
Nagoya, Japan
Volume 6, Chapter 29 Congenital hand V: Disorders of overgrowth, undergrowth, and generalized skeletal deformities

Fernando Molina, MD
Professor of Plastic, Aesthetic and
Reconstructive Surgery
Reconstructive and Plastic Surgery
Hospital General "Dr. Manuel Gea Gonzalez"
Universidad Nacional Autonoma de Mexico
Mexico City, Mexico
Volume 3, Chapter 39 Treacher-Collins syndrome

Stan Monstrey, MD, PhD
Professor in Plastic Surgery
Department of Plastic Surgery
Ghent University Hospital
Ghent, Belgium
Volume 4, Chapter 13 Reconstruction of male genital defects
Volume 4, Video 13.01 Complete and partial penile reconstruction

Steven L. Moran, MD
Professor and Chair of Plastic Surgery
Division of Plastic Surgery, Division of Hand
and Microsurgery
Professor of Orthopedics
Rochester, MN, USA
Volume 6, Chapter 20 Management of osteoarthritis of the hand and wrist

Luis Humberto Uribe Morelli, MD
Resident of Plastic Surgery
Unisanta Plastic Surgery Department
Sao Paulo, Brazil
Volume 2, Chapter 26 Lipoabdominoplasty
Volume 2, Video 26.01 Lipobdominoplasty
(including secondary lipo)

Robert J. Morin, MD
Plastic Surgeon and Craniofacial Surgeon
Department of Plastic Surgery
Hackensack University Medical Center
Hackensack, NJ
New York Eye and Ear Infirmary
New York, NY, USA
Volume 3, Chapter 8 Acquired cranial and facial
bone deformities

Steven F. Morris, MD, MSc, FRCS(C)
Professor of Surgery
Professor of Anatomy and Neurobiology
Dalhousie University
Halifax, NS, Canada
Volume 1, Chapter 23 Vascular territories

**Colin Myles Morrison, MSc (Hons),
FRCSI (Plast)**
Consultant Plastic Surgeon
Department of Plastic and Reconstructive
Surgery
St. Vincent's University Hospital
Dublin, Ireland
Volume 2, Chapter 13 Neck rejuvenation
Volume 5, Chapter 18 The deep inferior
epigastric artery perforator (DIEAP) flap

Wayne A. Morrison, MBBS, MD, FRACS
Director
O'Brien Institute
Professorial Fellow
Department of Surgery
St Vincent's Hospital
University of Melbourne
Plastic Surgeon
St Vincent's Hospital
Melbourne, Australia
Volume 1, Chapter 19 Tissue engineering

Robyn Mosher, MS
Medical Editor/Project Manager
Thayer School of Engineering (contract)
Dartmouth College
Norwich, VT, USA
Volume 1, Chapter 36 Robotics, simulation, and
telemedicine in plastic surgery

Dimitrios Motakis, MD, PhD, FRCSC
Plastic and Reconstructive Surgeon
Private Practice
University Lecturer
Department of Surgery
University of Toronto
Toronto, ON, Canada
Volume 2, Chapter 4 Soft-tissue fillers

A. Aldo Mottura, MD, PhD
Associate Professor of Surgery
School of Medicine
National University of Córdoba
Cordoba, Argentina
Volume 1, Chapter 9 Local anesthetics in plastic
surgery

Hunter R. Moyer, MD
Fellow
Department of Plastic and Reconstructive
Surgery
Emory University, Atlanta, GA, USA
Volume 5, Chapter 16 The bilateral Pedicled
TRAM flap

Gustavo Muchado, MD
Plastic surgeon
Division of Plastic and Reconstructive Surgery
and Department of Orthopaedic Surgery
University of California Irvine Medical Center
Orange, CA, USA
Volume 6, Video 34.01 EIP to EPL tendon
transfer

Reid V. Mueller, MD
Associate Professor
Division of Plastic and Reconstructive Surgery
Oregon Health and Science University
Portland, OR, USA
Volume 3, Chapter 2 Facial trauma: soft tissue
injuries

John B. Mulliken, MD
Director, Craniofacial Centre
Department of Plastic and Oral Surgery
Children's Hospital
Boston, MA, USA
Volume 1, Chapter 29 Vascular anomalies
Volume 3, Chapter 24 Repair of bilateral cleft lip

Egle Muti, MD
Associate Professor of Plastic Reconstructive
and Aesthetic Surgery
Department of Plastic Surgery
University of Turin School of Medicine
Turin, Italy
Volume 5, Chapter 23.1 Congenital anomalies of
the breast
Volume 5, Video 23.01.01 Congenital anomalies
of the breast: An example of tuberous breast
type 1 corrected with glandular flap type 1

Maurice Y. Nahabedian, MD
Associate Professor Plastic Surgery
Department of Plastic Surgery
Georgetown University and Johns Hopkins
University
Northwest, WA, USA
Volume 5, Chapter 22 Reconstruction of the
nipple-areola complex
Volume 5, Video 11.01 Partial breast
reconstruction using reduction mammaplasty
Volume 5, Video 11.03 Partial breast
reconstruction with a pedicle TRAM

Foad Nahai, MD, FACS
Clinical Professor of Plastic Surgery
Department of Surgery
Emory University School of Medicine
Atlanta, GA, USA
Volume 2, Chapter 1 Managing the cosmetic
patient

Fabio X. Nahas, MD, PhD
Associate Professor
Division of Plastic Surgery
Federal University of São Paulo
São Paulo, Brazil
Volume 2, Video 24.01 Liposculpture

**Deepak Narayan, MS, FRCS (Eng),
FRCS (Edin)**
Associate Professor of Surgery
Yale University School of Medicine
Chief
Plastic Surgery
VA Medical Center
West Haven, CT, USA
Volume 3, Chapter 14 Salivary gland tumors

Maurizio B. Nava, MD
Chief of Plastic Surgery Unit
Istituto Nazionale dei Tumori
Milano, Italy
Volume 5, Chapter 14 Expander/implant
reconstruction of the breast
Volume 5, Video 14.01 Mastectomy and
expander insertion: first stage
Volume 5, Video 14.02 Mastectomy and
expander insertion: second stage

Carmen Navarro, MD
Plastic Surgery Consultant
Plastic Surgery Department
Hospital de la Santa Creu i Sant Pau
Universidad Autónoma de Barcelona
Barcelona, Spain
Volume 5, Chapter 13 Imaging in reconstructive
breast surgery

**Peter C. Neligan, MB, FRCS(I), FRCSC,
FACS**
Professor of Surgery
Department of Surgery, Division of Plastic
Surgery
University of Washington
Seattle, WA, USA
Volume 1, Chapter 1 Plastic surgery and
innovation in medicine
Volume 1, Chapter 25 Flap pathophysiology and
pharmacology
Volume 3, Chapter 10 Cheek and lip
reconstruction
Volume 4, Chapter 3 Lymphatic reconstruction of
the extremities
Volume 3, Video 11.01-03 (1) Facial paralysis (2)
cross fact graft, (3) gracilis harvest
Volume 3, Video 18.01 Facial artery perforator
flap
Volume 4, Video 3.02 Charles Procedure
Volume 5, Video 18.01 SIEA
Volume 5, Video 19.01-19.03 Alternative free
flaps

Jonas A Nelson, MD
Integrated General/Plastic Surgery Resident
Department of Surgery
Division of Plastic Surgery
Perelman School of Medicine
University of Pennsylvania
Philadelphia, PA, USA
Volume 5, Video 17.01 The muscle sparing free TRAM flap

David T. Netscher, MD
Clinical Professor
Division of Plastic Surgery
Baylor College of Medicine
Houston, TX, USA
Volume 6, Chapter 21 The stiff hand and the spastic hand

Michael W. Neumeister, MD
Professor and Chairman
Division of Plastic Surgery
SIU School of Medicine
Springfield, IL, USA
Volume 6, Chapter 6 Nail and fingertip reconstruction

M. Samuel Noordhoff, MD, FACS
Emeritus Superintendent
Chang Gung Memorial Hospitals
Taipei, Taiwan, The People's Republic of China
Volume 3, Chapter 23 Repair of unilateral cleft lip

Christine B. Novak, PT, PhD
Research Associate
Hand Program, Division of Plastic and Reconstructive Surgery
University Health Network, University of Toronto
Toronto, ON, Canada
Volume 6, Chapter 39 Hand therapy

Daniel Nowinski, MD, PhD
Director
Department of Plastic and Maxillofacial Surgery
Uppsala Craniofacial Center
Uppsala University Hospital
Uppsala, Sweden
Volume 1, Chapter 11 Genetics and prenatal diagnosis

Scott Oates, MD
Professor
Department of Plastic Surgery
The University of Texas MD Anderson Cancer Center
Houston, TX, USA
Volume 6, Chapter 15 Benign and malignant tumors of the hand

Kerby Oberg, MD, PhD
Associate Professor
Department of Pathology and Human Anatomy
Loma Linda University School of Medicine
Loma Linda, CA, USA
Volume 6, Chapter 25 Congenital hand 1: embryology, classification, and principles

James P. O'Brien, MD, FRCSC
Associate Professor of Surgery
Dalhousie University
Halifax Nova Scotia
Clinical Associate Professor of Surgery
Memorial University
St. John's Newfoundland
Vice President Research
Innovation and Development
Horizon Health Network
New Brunswick, NB, Canada
Volume 6, Chapter 24 Nerve entrapment syndromes

Andrea J. O'Connor, BE(Hons), PhD
Associate Professor of Chemical and Biomolecular Engineering
Department of Chemical and Biomolecular Engineering
University of Melbourne
Melbourne, VIC, Australia
Volume 1, Chapter 19 Tissue engineering

Rei Ogawa, MD, PhD
Associate Professor
Department of Plastic
Reconstructive and Aesthetic Surgery Nippon Medical School
Tokyo, Japan
Volume 1, Chapter 30 Benign and malignant nonmelanocytic tumors of the skin and soft tissue

Dennis P. Orgill, MD, PhD
Professor of Surgery
Division of Plastic Surgery, Brigham and Women's Hospital
Harvard Medical School
Boston, MA, USA
Volume 1, Chapter 17 Skin graft

Cho Y. Pang, PhD
Senior Scientist
Research Institute
The Hospital for Sick Children
Professor
Departments of Surgery/Physiology
University of Toronto
Toronto, ON, Canada
Volume 1, Chapter 25 Flap pathophysiology and pharmacology

Ketan M. Patel, MD
Resident Physician
Department of Plastic Surgery
Georgetown University Hospital
Washington DC, USA
Volume 5, Chapter 22 Reconstruction of the nipple-areola complex

William C. Pederson, MD, FACS
President and Fellowship Director
The Hand Center of San Antonio
Adjunct Professor of Surgery
The University of Texas Health Science Center at San Antonio
San Antonio, TX, USA
Volume 6, Chapter 12 Reconstructive surgery of the mutilated hand

José Abel de la Peña Salcedo, MD
Secretario Nacional
Federación Iberolatinoamericana de Cirugía Plástica, Estética y Reconstructiva
Director del Instituto de Cirugia Plastica, S.C.
Hospital Angeles de las Lomas
Col.Valle de las Palmas
Huixquilucan, Edo de Mexico, Mexico
Volume 2, Chapter 28 Buttock augmentation
Volume 2, Video 28.01 Buttock augmentation

Angela Pennati, MD
Assistant Plastic Surgeon
Unit of Plastic Surgery
Istituto Nazionale dei Tumori
Milano, Italy
Volume 5, Chapter 14 Expander/implant breast reconstructions
Volume 5, Video 14.01 Mastectomy and expander insertion: first stage
Volume 5, Video 14.02 Mastectomy and expander insertion: second stage

Joel E. Pessa, MD
Clinical Associate Professor of Plastic Surgery
UTSW Medical School
Dallas, TX
Hand and Microsurgery Fellow
Christine M. Kleinert Hand and Microsurgery
Louisville, KY, USA
Volume 2, Chapter 17 Nasal analysis and anatomy

Walter Peters, MD, PhD, FRCSC
Professor of Surgery
Department of Plastic Surgery
University of Toronto
Toronto, ON, Canada
Volume 5, Chapter 6 Iatrogenic disorders following breast surgery

Giorgio Pietramaggiori, MD, PhD
Plastic Surgery Resident
Department of Plastic and Reconstructive Surgery
University Hospital of Lausanne
Lausanne, Switzerland
Volume 1, Chapter 17 Skin graft

John W. Polley, MD
Professor and Chairman
Rush University Medical Center
Department of Plastic and Reconstructive Surgery
John W. Curtin – Chair
Co-Director, Rush Craniofacial Center
Chicago, IL, USA
Volume 3, Chapter 27 Orthodontics in cleft lip and palate management

Bohdan Pomahac, MD
Assistant Professor
Harvard Medical School
Director
Plastic Surgery Transplantation
Medical Director
Burn Center
Division of Plastic Surgery
Brigham and Women's Hospital
Boston, MA, USA
Volume 1, Chapter 11 Genetics and prenatal diagnosis

Julian J. Pribaz, MD
Professor of Surgery Harvard Medical School
Division of Plastic Surgery
Brigham and Women's Hospital
Boston, MA, USA
Volume 3, Chapter 19 Secondary facial reconstruction

Andrea L. Pusic, MD, MHS, FRCSC
Associate Attending Surgeon
Department of Plastic and Reconstructive
Memorial Sloan-Kettering Cancer Center
New York, NY, USA
Volume 1, Chapter 10 Evidence-based medicine and health services research in plastic surgery
Volume 4, Chapter 14 Reconstruction of acquired vaginal defects

Oscar M. Ramirez, MD, FACS
Adjunct Clinical Faculty
Plastic Surgery Division
Cleveland Clinic Florida
Boca Raton, FL, USA
Volume 2, Chapter 11.8 Facelift: Subperiosteal facelift
Volume 2, Video 11.08.01 Facelift: Subperiosteal mid facelift endoscopic temporo-midface

William R. Rassman, MD
Director
Private Practice
New Hair Institution
Los Angeles, CA, USA
Volume 2, Video 23.04 FUE FOX procedure

Russell R. Reid, MD, PhD
Assistant Professor of Surgery, Bernard Sarnat Scholar
Section of Plastic and Reconstructive Surgery
University of Chicago
Chicago, IL, USA
Volume 1, Chapter 21 Repair and grafting of bone
Volume 3, Chapter 41 Pediatric chest and trunk defects

Neal R. Reisman, MD, JD
Chief of Plastic Surgery, Clinical Professor
Plastic Surgery
St. Luke's Episcopal Hospital
Baylor College of Medicine
Houston, TX, USA
Volume 1, Chapter 6 Medico-legal issues in plastic surgery

Dominique Renier, MD, PhD
Pediatric Neurosurgeon
Service de Neurochirurgie Pédiatrique
Hôpital Necker-Enfants Malades
Paris, France
Volume 3, Chapter 32 Orbital hypertelorism

Dirk F. Richter, MD, PhD
Clinical Director
Department of Plastic Surgery
Dreifaltigkeits-Hospital Wesseling
Wesseling, Germany
Volume 2, Chapter 25 Abdominoplasty procedures
Volume 2, Video 25.01 Abdominoplasty

Thomas L. Roberts III, FACS
Plastic Surgery Center of the Carolinas
Spartanburg, SC, USA
Volume 2, Chapter 28 Buttock augmentation
Volume 2, Video 28.01 Buttock augmentation

Federico Di Rocco, MD, PhD
Pediatric Neurosurgery
Hôpital Necker Enfants Malades
Paris, France
Volume 3, Chapter 32 Orbital hypertelorism

Natalie Roche, MD
Associate Professor
Department of Plastic Surgery
Ghent University Hospital
Ghent, Belgium
Volume 4, Chapter 13 Reconstruction of male genital defects
Volume 4, Video 13.01 Complete and partial penile reconstruction

Eduardo D. Rodriguez, MD, DDS
Chief, Plastic Reconstructive and Maxillofacial Surgery, R Adams Cowley Shock Trauma Center
Professor of Surgery
University of Maryland School of Medicine
Baltimore, MD, USA
Volume 3, Chapter 3 Facial fractures

Thomas E. Rohrer, MD
Director, Mohs Surgery
SkinCare Physicians of Chestnut Hill
Clinical Associate Professor
Department of Dermatology
Boston University
Boston, MA, USA
Volume 2, Video 5.02 Facial resurfacing

Rod J. Rohrich, MD, FACS
Professor and Chairman Crystal Charity Ball
Distinguished Chair in Plastic Surgery
Department of Plastic Surgery
Professor and Chairman Betty and Warren
Woodward Chair in Plastic and Reconstructive Surgery
University of Texas Southwestern Medical Center at Dallas
Dallas, TX, USA
Volume 2, Chapter 17 Nasal analysis and anatomy
Volume 2, Chapter 18 Open technique rhinoplasty

Joseph M. Rosen, MD
Professor of Surgery
Division of Plastic Surgery, Department of Surgery
Dartmouth-Hitchcock Medical Center
Lyme, NH, USA
Volume 1, Chapter 36 Robotics, simulation, and telemedicine in plastic surgery

E. Victor Ross, MD
Director of Laser and Cosmetic Dermatology
Scripps Clinic
San Diego, CA, USA
Volume 2, Chapter 5 Facial skin resurfacing

Michelle C. Roughton, MD
Chief Resident
Section of Plastic and Reconstructive Surgery
University of Chicago Medical Center
Chicago, IL, USA
Volume 4, Chapter 10 Reconstruction of the chest

Sashwati Roy, PhD
Associate Professor of Surgery
Department of Surgery
The Ohio State University Medical Center
Columbus, OH, USA
Volume 1, Chapter 14 Wound healing

J. Peter Rubin, MD, FACS
Chief of Plastic Surgery
Director, Life After Weight Loss Body Contouring Program
University of Pittsburgh
Pittsburgh, PA, USA
Volume 2, Chapter 30 Post-bariatric reconstruction
Volume 2, Video 30.01 Post bariatric reconstruction – bodylift procedure
Volume 5, Chapter 25 Contouring of the arms, breast, upper trunk, and male chest in the massive weight loss patient
Volume 5, Video 25.01 Brachioplasty part 1: contouring of the arms
Volume 5, Video 25.02 Bracioplasty part 2: contouring of the arms

Alesia P. Saboeiro, MD
Attending Physician
Private Practice
New York, NY, USA
Volume 2, Chapter 14 Structural fat grafting
Volume 2, Video 14.01 Structural fat grafting of the face

Justin M. Sacks, MD
Assistant Professor
Department of Plastic and Reconstructive Surgery
The Johns Hopkins University School of Medicine
Baltimore, MD, USA
Volume 3, Chapter 17 Carcinoma of the upper aerodigestive tract
Volume 6, Chapter 15 Benign and malignant tumors of the hand

Hakim K. Said, MD
Assistant Professor of Surgery
Division of Plastic Surgery
University of Washington
Seattle, WA, USA
Volume 4, Chapter 17 Perineal reconstruction

Michel Saint-Cyr, MD, FRCSC
Associate Professor Plastic Surgery
Department of Plastic Surgery
University of Texas Southwestern Medical Center
Dallas, TX, USA
Volume 4, Chapter 2 Management of lower extremity trauma
Volume 4, Video 2.01 Alternative flap harvest

Cristianna Bonneto Saldanha, MD
Resident
General Surgery Department
Santa Casa of Santos Hospital
São Paulo, Brazil
Volume 2, Chapter 26 Lipoabdominoplasty
Volume 2, Video 26.01 Lipobdominoplasty (including secondary lipo)

Osvaldo Ribeiro Saldanha, MD
Chairman of Plastic Surgery
Unisanta
Santos
Past President of the Brazilian Society of Plastic Surgery (SBCP)
International Associate Editor of Plastic and Reconstructive Surgery
São Paulo, Brazil
Volume 2, Chapter 26 Lipoabdominoplasty
Volume 2, Video 26.01 Lipobdominoplasty (including secondary lipo)

Osvaldo Ribeiro Saldanha Filho, MD
São Paulo, Brazil
Volume 2, Chapter 26 Lipoabdominoplasty
Volume 2, Video 26.01 Lipobdominoplasty (including secondary lipo)

Douglas M. Sammer, MD
Assistant Professor of Plastic Surgery
Department of Plastic Surgery
University of Texas Southwestern Medical Center
Dallas, TX, USA
Volume 6, Chapter 19 Rheumatologic conditions of the hand and wrist

Joao Carlos Sampaio Goes, MD, PhD
Director Instituto Brasileiro Controle Cancer
Chairman
Department Plastic Surgery and Mastology of IBCC
Sao Paulo, Brazil
Volume 5, Chapter 8.6 Periareolar technique with mesh support
Volume 5, Chapter 20 Omentum reconstruction of the breast

Michael Sauerbier, MD, PhD
Chairman and Professor
Department for Plastic, Hand and Reconstructive Surgery
Cooperation Hospital for Plastic Surgery of the University Hospital Frankfurt
Academic Hospital University of Frankfurt a. Main
Frankfurt, Germany
Volume 4, Chapter 4 Lower extremity sarcoma reconstruction
Volume 4, Video 4.01 Management of lower extremity sarcoma reconstruction

Hani Sbitany, MD
Plastic and Reconstructive Surgery
Assistant Professor of Surgery
University of California
San Francisco, CA, USA
Volume 1, Chapter 24 Flap classification and applications

Tim Schaub, MD
Private Practice
Arizona Center for Hand Surgery, PC
Phoenix, AZ, USA
Volume 6, Chapter 16 Infections of the hand

Loren S. Schechter, MD, FACS
Assistant Professor of Surgery
Chief, Division of Plastic Surgery
Chicago Medical School
Chicago, IL, USA
Volume 4, Chapter 15 Surgery for gender identity disorder

Stephen A. Schendel, MD
Professor Emeritus of Surgery and Clinical Adjunct Professor of Neurosurgery
Department of Surgery and Neurosurgery
Stanford University Medical Center
Stanford, CA, USA
Volume 3, Chapter 4 TMJ dysfunction and obstructive sleep apnea

Saja S. Scherer-Pietramaggiori, MD
Plastic Surgery Resident
Department of Plastic and Reconstructive Surgery
University Hospital of Lausanne
Lausanne, Switzerland
Volume 1, Chapter 17 Skin graft

Clark F. Schierle, MD, PhD
Vice President
Aesthetic and Reconstructive Plastic Surgery
Northwestern Plastic Surgery Associates
Chicaho, IL, USA
Volume 5, Chapter 5 Endoscopic approaches to the breast

Stefan S. Schneeberger, MD
Visiting Associate Professor of Surgery
Department of Plastic Surgery
Johns Hopkins Medical University
Baltimore, MD, USA
Associate Professor of Surgery
Center for Operative Medicine
Department for Viszeral
Transplant and Thoracic Surgery
Innsbruck Medical University
Innsbruck, Austria
Volume 6, Chapter 38 Upper extremity composite allotransplantation

Iris A. Seitz, MD, PhD
Director of Research and International Collaboration
University Plastic Surgery
Rosalind Franklin University
Clinical Instructor of Surgery
Chicago Medical School
University Plastic Surgery, affiliated with Chicago Medical School, Rosalind Franklin University
Morton Grove, IL, USA
Volume 1, Chapter 21 Repair and grafting of bone

Chandan K. Sen, PhD, FACSM, FACN
Professor and Vice Chairman (Research) of Surgery
Department of Surgery
The Ohio State University Medical Center
Associate Dean
Translational and Applied Research
College of Medicine
Executive Director
OSU Comprehensive Wound Center
Columbus, OH, USA
Volume 1, Chapter 14 Wound healing

Subhro K. Sen, MD
Clinical Assistant Professor
Division of Plastic and Reconstructive Surgery
Robert A. Chase Hand and Upper Limb
Center, Stanford University Medical Center
Palo Alto, CA, USA
Volume 1, Chapter 14 Wound healing
Volume 6, Chapter 4 Anesthesia for upper
extremity surgery
Volume 6, Video 4.01 Anesthesia for upper
extremity surgery

Joseph M. Serletti, MD, FACS
Henry Royster – William Maul Measey
Professor of Surgery and Chief
Division of Plastic Surgery
Vice Chair (Finance)
Department of Surgery
University of Pennsylvania
Philadelphia, PA, USA
Volume 5, Chapter 17 Free TRAM breast
reconstruction
Volume 5, Video 17.01 The muscle sparing free
TRAM flap

Randolph Sherman, MD
Vice Chair
Department of Surgery
Cedars-Sinai Medical Center
Los Angeles, CA, USA
Volume 6, Chapter 12 Reconstructive surgery of
the mutilated hand

Kenneth C. Shestak, MD
Professor of Plastic Surgery
Division of Plastic Surgery
University of Pittsburgh
Pittsburgh, PA, USA
Volume 5, Chapter 9 Revision surgery following
breast reduction and mastopexy
Volume 5, Video 7.01 Circum areola mastopexy

Lester Silver, MD, MS
Professor of Surgery
Department of Surgery/Division of Plastic
Surgery
Mount Sinai School of Medicine
New York, NY, USA
Volume 3, Chapter 37 Hemifacial atrophy

Navin K. Singh, MD, MSc
Assistant Professor of Plastic Surgery
Department of Plastic Surgery
Johns Hopkins University School of Medicine
Washington, DC, USA
Volume 4, Chapter 12 Abdominal wall
reconstruction

Vanila M. Singh, MD
Clinical Associate Professor
Stanford University Medical Center
Department of Anesthesiology and Pain
Management
Stanford, CA, USA
Volume 6, Chapter 4 Anesthesia for upper
extremity surgery

Carla Skytta, DO
Resident
Department of Surgery
Doctors Hospital
Columbus, OH, USA
Volume 3, Chapter 5 Scalp and forehead
reconstruction

Darren M. Smith, MD
Resident
Division of Plastic Surgery
University of Pittsburgh Medical Center
Pittsburgh, PA, USA
Volume 3, Chapter 31 Pediatric facial fractures

**Gill Smith, MB, BCh, FRCS(Ed),
FRCS(Plast)**
Consultant Hand, Plastic and Reconstructive
Surgeon
Great Ormond Street Hospital
London, UK
Volume 6, Chapter 26 Congenital hand II Failure
of formation (transverse and longitudinal arrest)

Paul Smith, MBBS, FRCS
Honorary Consultant Plastic Surgeon
Great Ormond Street Hospital London, UK
Volume 6, Chapter 26 Congenital hand II Failure
of formation (transverse and longitudinal arrest)

Laura Snell, MSc, MD, FRCSC
Assistant Professor
Division of Plastic Surgery
University of Toronto
Toronto, ON, Canada
Volume 4, Chapter 14 Reconstruction of
acquired vaginal defects

Nicole Z. Sommer, MD
Assistant Professor of Plastic Surgery
Southern Illinois University School of Medicine
Springfield, IL, USA
Volume 6, Chapter 6 Nail and fingertip
reconstruction

David H. Song, MD, MBA, FACS
Cynthia Chow Professor of Surgery
Chief, Section of Plastic and Reconstructive
Surgery
Vice-Chairman, Department of Surgery
The University of Chicago Medicine & Biological
Sciences
Chicago, IL, USA
Volume 4, Chapter 10 Reconstruction of the
chest

Andrea Spano, MD
Senior Assistant Plastic Surgeon
Unit of Plastic Surgery
Istituto Nazionale dei Tumori
Milano, Italy
Volume 5, Chapter 14 Expander/implant breast
reconstructions
Volume 5, Video 14.01 Mastectomy and
expander insertion: first stage
Volume 5, Video 14.02 Mastectomy and
expander insertion: second stage

Scott L. Spear, MD, FACS
Professor and Chairman
Department of Plastic Surgery
Georgetown University Hospital
Georgetown, WA, USA
Volume 5, Chapter 15 Latissimus dorsi flap
breast reconstruction
Volume 5, Chapter 26 Fat grafting to the breast
Volume 5, Video 15.01 Latissimus dorsi flap
technique

Robert J. Spence, MD
Director
National Burn Reconstruction Center
Good Samaritan Hospital
Baltimore, MD, USA
Volume 4, Chapter 21 Management of facial
burns
Volume 4, Video 21.01 Management of the
burned face intra-dermal skin closure
Volume 4, Video 21.02 Management of the
burned face full-thickness skin graft defatting
technique

Samuel Stal, MD, FACS
Professor and Chief
Division of Plastic Surgery, Baylor College of
Medicine and Texas Children's Hospital
Houston, TX, USA
Volume 3, Chapter 29 Secondary deformities of
the cleft lip, nose, and palate
Volume 3, Video 29.01 Complete takedown
Volume 3, Video 29.02 Abbé flap
Volume 3, Video 29.03 Thick lip and buccal
sulcus deformities
Volume 3, Video 29.04 Alveolar bone grafting
Volume 3, Video 29.05 Definitive rhinoplasty

Derek M. Steinbacher, MD, DMD
Assistant Professor
Plastic and Carniomaxillofacial Surgery
Yale University, School of Medicine
New Haven, CT, USA
Volume 3, Chapter 34 Nonsyndromic
craniosynostosis

Douglas S. Steinbrech, MD, FACS
Gotham Plastic Surgery
New York, NY, USA
Volume 2, Chapter 9 Secondary blepharoplasty:
Techniques

Lars Steinstraesser, MD
Heisenberg-Professor for Molecular Oncology
and Wound Healing
Department of Plastic and Reconstructive
Surgery, Burn Center
BG University Hospital Bergmannsheil, Ruhr
University
Bochum, North Rhine-Westphalia, Germany
Volume 4, Chapter 18 Acute management of
burn/electrical injuries

Phillip J. Stephan, MD
Clinical Instructor
Department of Plastic Surgery
University of Texas Southwestern
Wichita Falls, TX, USA
Volume 2, Chapter 24 Liposuction: A comprehensive review of techniques and safety

Laurie A. Stevens, MD
Associate Clinical Professor of Psychiatry
Columbia University College of Physicians and Surgeons
New York, NY, USA
Volume 1, Chapter 3 Psychological aspects of plastic surgery

Alexander Stoff, MD, PhD
Senior Fellow
Department of Plastic Surgery
Dreifaltigkeits-Hospital Wesseling
Wesseling, Germany
Volume 2, Chapter 25 Abdominoplasty procedures
Volume 2, Video 25.01 Abdominoplasty

Dowling B. Stough, MD
Medical Director
The Dermatology Clinic
Clinical Assistant Professor
Department of Dermatology
University of Arkansas for Medical Sciences
Little Rock, AR, USA
Volume 2, Video 23.09 Tension donor dissection

James M. Stuzin, MD
Associate Professor of Surgery (Plastic)
Voluntary
University of Miami Leonard M. Miller School of Medicine
Miami, FL, USA
Volume 2, Chapter 11.6 Facelift: The extended SMAS technique in facial rejuvenation
Volume 2, Video 11.06.01 Facelift – Extended SMAS technique in facial shaping

John D. Symbas, MD
Plastic and Reconstructive Surgeon
Private Practice
Marietta Plastic Surgery
Marietta, GA, USA
Volume 5, Chapter 16 The bilateral pedicled TRAM flap
Volume 5, Video 16.01 Pedicle TRAM breast reconstruction

Amir Taghinia, MD
Instructor in Surgery
Harvard Medical School
Staff Surgeon
Department of Plastic and Oral Surgery
Children's Hospital
Boston, MA, USA
Volume 6, Chapter 27 Congenital hand III disorders of formation – thumb hypoplasia
Volume 6, Video 27.01 Congenital hand III disorders of formation – thumb hypoplasia
Volume 6, Video 31.01 Vascular anomalies of the upper extremity

David M.K. Tan, MBBS
Consultant
Department of Hand and Reconstructive Microsurgery
National University Hospital
Yong Loo Lin School of Medicine
National University Singapore
Kent Ridge, Singapore
Volume 6, Chapter 3 Diagnostic imaging of the hand and wrist
Volume 6, Video 3.01 Diagnostic imaging of the hand and wrist – Scaphoid lunate dislocation

Jin Bo Tang, MD
Professor and Chair
Department of Hand Surgery
Chair
The Hand Surgery Research Center
Affiliated Hospital of Nantong University
Nantong, The People's Republic of China
Volume 6, Chapter 9 Flexor tendon injuries and reconstruction
Volume 6, Video 9.01 Flexor tendon injuries and reconstruction – Partial venting of the A2 pulley
Volume 6, Video 9.02 Flexor tendon injuries and reconstruction – Making a 6-strand repair
Volume 6, Video 9.03 Complete flexor-extension without bowstringing

Daniel I. Taub, DDS, MD
Assistant Professor
Oral and Maxillofacial Surgery
Thomas Jefferson University Hospital
Philadelphia, PA, USA
Volume 2, Chapter 16 Anthropometry, cephalometry, and orthognathic surgery
Volume 2, Video 16.01 Anthropometry, cephalometry, and orthognathic surgery

Peter J. Taub, MD, FACS, FAAP
Associate Professor, Surgery and Pediatrics
Division of Plastic and Reconstructive Surgery
Mount Sinai School of Medicine
New York, NY, USA
Volume 3, Chapter 37 Hemifacial atrophy

Sherilyn Keng Lin Tay, MBChB, MRCS, MSc
Microsurgical Fellow
Department of Plastic Surgery
Chang Gung Memorial Hospital
Taoyuan, Taiwan, The People's Republic of China
Specialist Registrar
Department of Reconstructive and Plastic Surgery
St George's Hospital
London, UK
Volume 1, Chapter 26 Principles and techniques of microvascular surgery

G. Ian Taylor, AO, MBBS, MD, MD (HonBrodeaux), FRACS, FRCS (Eng), FRCS (Hon Edinburgh), FRCSI (Hon), FRSC (Hon Canada), FACS (Hon)
Professor
Deparment of Plastic Surgery
Royal Melbourne Hospital
Professor
Department of Anatomy
University of Melbourne
Melbourne, Australia
Volume 1, Chapter 23 Vascular territories

Oren M. Tepper, MD
Assistant Professor
Plastic and Reconstructive Surgery
Montefiore Medical Center
Albert Einstein College of Medicine
New York, NY, USA
Volume 3, Chapter 36 Craniofacial microsomia

Chad M. Teven, BS
Research Associate
Section of Plastic and Reconstructive Surgery
University of Chicago
Chicago, IL, USA
Volume 1, Chapter 21 Repair and grafting of bone

Brinda Thimmappa, MD
Adjunct Assistant Professor
Department of Plastic and Reconstructive Surgery
Loma Linda Medical Center
Loma Linda, CA
Plastic Surgeon
Division of Plastic and Maxillofacial Surgery
Southwest Washington Medical Center
Vancouver, WA, USA
Volume 3, Chapter 4 TMJ dysfunction and obstructive sleep apnea

Johan Thorfinn, MD, PhD
Senior Consultant of Plastic Surgery, Burn Unit
Co-Director
Department of Plastic Surgery, Hand Surgery, and Burns
Linköping University Hospital
Linköping, Sweden
Volume 6, Chapter 32 Peripheral nerve injuries of the upper extremity
Volume 6, Video 32.01-02 Peripheral nerve injuries (1) Digital Nerve Suture (2) Median Nerve Suture

Charles H. Thorne, MD
Associate Professor of Plastic Surgery
Department of Plastic Surgery
NYU School of Medicine
New York, NY, USA
Volume 2, Chapter 22 Otoplasty

Michael Tonkin, MBBS, MD, FRACS (Orth), FRCS Ed Orth
Professor of Hand Surgery
Department of Hand Surgery and Peripheral
Nerve Surgery
Royal North Shore Hospital
The Childrens Hospital at Westmead
University of Sydney Medical School
Sydney, Australia
*Volume 6, Chapter 25 Congenital hand 1
Principles, embryology, and classification
Volume 6, Chapter 29 Congenital hand V
Disorders of Overgrowth, Undergrowth, and
Generalized Skeletal Deformities (addendum)*

Patrick L Tonnard, MD
Coupure Centrum Voor Plastische Chirurgie
Ghent, Belgium
*Volume 2, Video 11.04.01 Loop sutures MACS
facelift*

Kathryn S. Torok, MD
Assistant Professor
Division of Pediatric Rheumatology
Department of Pediatrics
Univeristy of Pittsburgh School of Medicine
Childrens Hospital of Pittsburgh
Pittsburgh, PA, USA
Volume 3, Chapter 37 Hemifacial atrophy

Ali Totonchi, MD
Assistant Professor of Surgery
Division of Plastic Surgery
MetroHealth Medical Center
Case Western Reserve University
Cleveland, OH, USA
*Volume 3, Chapter 21 Surgical management of
migraine headaches*

Jonathan W. Toy, MD
Body Contouring Fellow
Division of Plastic and Reconstructive Surgery
University of Pittsburgh
University of Pittsburgh Medical Center Suite
Pittsburg, PA, USA
*Volume 2, Chapter 30 Post-bariatric
reconstruction
Volume 5, Chapter 25 Contouring of the arms,
breast, upper trunk, and male chest in the
massive weight loss patient*

Matthew J. Trovato, MD
Dallas Plastic Surgery Institute
Dallas, TX, USA
*Volume 2, Chapter 29 Upper limb contouring
Volume 2, Video 29.01 Upper limb contouring*

Anthony P. Tufaro, DDS, MD, FACS
Associate Professor of Surgery and Oncology
Departments of Plastic Surgery and Oncology
Johns Hopkins University
Baltimore, MD, USA
*Volume 3, Chapter 16 Tumors of the lips, oral
cavity, oropharynx, and mandible*

Joseph Upton III, MD
Clinical Professor of Surgery
Department of Plastic Surgery
Children's Hospital Boston
Shriner's Burn Hospital Boston
Beth Israel Deaconess Hospital
Harvard Medical School
Boston, MA, USA
*Volume 6, Chapter 27 Congenital hand III
disorders of formation – thumb hypoplasia
Volume 6, Chapter 31 Vascular anomalies of the
upper extremity
Volume 6, Video 27.01 Congenital hand III
disorders of formation – thumb hypoplasia
Volume 6, Video 31.01 Vascular anomalies of
the upper extremity*

Walter Unger, MD
Clinical Professor
Department of Dermatology
Mount Sinai School of Medicine
New York, NY
Associate Professor (Dermatology)
University of Toronto
Private Practice
New York, NY, USA
Toronto, ON, Canada
Volume 2, Video 23.06 Hair transplantation

Francisco Valero-Cuevas, PhD
Director
Brain-Body Dynamics Laboratory
Professor of Biomedical Engineering
Professor of Biokinesiology and Physical
Therapy
By courtesy Professor of Computer Science
and Aerospace and Mechanical Engineering
The University of Southern California
Los Angeles, CA, USA
*Volume 6, Chapter 1 Anatomy and biomechanics
of the hand*

Allen L. Van Beek, MD, FACS
Adjunct Professor
University Minnesota School of Medicine
Division Plastic Surgery
Minneapolis, MN, USA
*Volume 2, Video 3.01 Botulinum toxin
Volume 2, Video 4.01 Soft tissue fillers
Volume 2, Video 5.01 Chemical peel
Volume 2, Video 18.01 Open technique
rhinoplasty*

Nicholas B. Vedder
Professor of Surgery and Orthopaedics
Chief of Plastic Surgery Vice Chair, Department
of Surgery
University of Washington
Seattle, WA, USA
*Volume 6, Chapter 13 Thumb reconstruction:
non microsurgical techniques*

Valentina Visintini Cividin, MD
Assistant Plastic Surgeon
Unit of Plastic Surgery
Istituto Nazionale dei Tumori
Milano, Italy
*Volume 5, Chapter 14 Expander/implant
reconstruction of the breast
Volume 5, Video 14.01 Mastectomy and
expander insertion: first stage
Volume 5, Video 14.02 Mastectomy and
expander insertion: second stage*

Peter M. Vogt, MD, PhD
Professor and Chairman
Department of Plastic Hand and Reconstructive
Surgery
Hannover Medical School
Hannover, Germany
*Volume 1, Chapter 15 Skin wound healing:
Repair biology, wound, and scar treatment*

Richard J. Warren, MD, FRCSC
Clinical Professor
Division of Plastic Surgery
University of British Columbia
Vancouver, BC, Canada
*Volume 2, Chapter 7 Forehead rejuvenation
Volume 2, Chapter 11.1 Facelift: Principles
Volume 2, Chapter 11.2 Facelift: Introduction to
deep tissue techniques
Volume 2, Video 7.01 Modified Lateral Brow Lift
Volume 2, Video 11.1.01 Parotid masseteric
fascia
Volume 2, Video 11.1.02 Anterior incision
Volume 2, Video 11.1.03 Posterior Incision
Volume 2, Video 11.1.04 Facelift skin flap
Volume 2, Video 11.1.05 Facial fat injection*

Andrew J. Watt, MD
Plastic Surgeon
Department of Surgery
Division of Plastic and Reconstructive Surgery
Stanford University Medical Center
Stanford University Hospital and Clinics
Palo Alto, CA, USA
*Volume 6, Chapter 17 Management of
Dupuytren's disease
Volume 6, Video 17.01 Management of
Dupuytren's disease*

Simeon H. Wall, Jr., MD, FACS
Private Practice
The Wall Center for Plastic Surgery
Gratis Faculty
Division of Plastic Surgery
Department of Surgery
LSU Health Sciences Center at Shreveport
Shreveport, LA, USA
Volume 2, Chapter 21 Secondary rhinoplasty

Derrick C. Wan, MD
Assistant Professor
Department of Surgery
Stanford University School of Medicine
Stanford, CA, USA
*Volume 1, Chapter 13 Stem cells and
regenerative medicine*

Renata V. Weber, MD
Assistant Professor Surgery (Plastics)
Division of Plastic and Reconstructive Surgery
Albert Einstein College of Medicine
Bronx, NY, USA
Volume 1, Chapter 22 Repair and grafting of peripheral nerve

Fu Chan Wei, MD
Professor
Department of Plastic Surgery
Chang Gung Memorial Hospital
Taoyuan, Taiwan, The People's Republic of China
Volume 1, Chapter 26 Principles and techniques of microvascular surgery
Volume 6, Chapter 14 Thumb and finger reconstruction – microsurgical techniques
Volume 6, Video 14.01 Trimmed great toe
Volume 6, Video 14.02 Second toe for index
Volume 6, Video 14.03 Combined second and third toe for metacarpal hand

Mark D. Wells, MD, FRCS, FACS
Clinical Assistant Professor of Surgery
The Ohio State University
Columbus, OH, USA
Volume 3, Chapter 5 Scalp and forehead reconstruction

Gordon H. Wilkes, MD
Clinical Professor and Divisional Director
Division of Plastic Surgery
University of Alberta Faculty of Medicine
Alberta, AB, Canada
Volume 1, Chapter 33 Facial prosthetics in plastic surgery

Henry Wilson, MD, FACS
Attending Plastic Surgeon
Private Practice
Plastic Surgery Associates
Lynchburg, VA, USA
Volume 5, Chapter 26 Fat grafting to the breast

Scott Woehrle, MS, BS
Physician Assistant
Department of Plastic Surgery
Jospeh Capella Plastic Surgery
Ramsey, NJ, USA
Volume 2, Chapter 29 Upper limb contouring
Volume 2, Video 29.01 Upper limb contouring

Johan F. Wolfaardt, BDS, MDent (Prosthodontics), PhD
Professor
Division of Otolaryngology-Head and Neck Surgery
Department of Surgery
Faculty of Medicine and Dentistry
Director of Clinics and International Relations
Institute for Reconstructive Sciences in Medicine
University of Alberta
Covenant Health Group
Alberta Health Services
Alberta, AB, Canada
Volume 1, Chapter 33 Facial prosthetics in plastic surgery

S. Anthony Wolfe, MD
Chief
Division of Plastic Surgery
Miami Children's Hospital
Miami, FL, USA
Volume 3, Chapter 8 Acquired cranial and facial bone deformities
Volume 3, Video 8.01 Removal of venous malformation enveloping intraconal optic nerve

Chin-Ho Wong, MBBS, MRCS, MMed (Surg), FAMS (Plast. Surg)
Consultant
Department of Plastic Reconstructive and Aesthetic Surgery
Singapore General Hospital
Singapore
Volume 2, Chapter 6 Anatomy of the aging face

Victor W. Wong, MD
Postdoctoral Research Fellow
Department of Surgery
Stanford University
Stanford, CA, USA
Volume 1, Chapter 13 Stem cells and regenerative medecine

Jeffrey Yao, MD
Assistant Professor
Department of Orthopaedic Surgery
Stanford University Medical Center
Palo Alto, CA, USA
Volume 6, Chapter 5 Principles of internal fixation as applied to the hand and wrist

Akira Yamada, MD
Assistant Professor
Department of Plastic and Reconstructive Surgery
Osaka Medical College
Osaka, Japan
Volume 3, Video 7.01 Microtia: auricular reconstruction

Michael J. Yaremchuk, MD, FACS
Chief of Craniofacial Surgery-Massachusetts General Hospital
Program Director-Plastic Surgery Training Program
Massachusetts General Hospital
Professor of Surgery
Harvard Medical School
Boston, MA, USA
Volume 2, Chapter 15 Skeletal augmentation
Volume 2, Video 15.01 Midface skeletal augmentation and rejuvenation

David M. Young, MD
Professor of Plastic Surgery
Department of Surgery
University of California
San Francisco, CA, USA
Volume 1, Chapter 24 Flap classification and applications

Peirong Yu, MD
Professor
Department of Plastic Surgery
The University of Texas M.D. Anderson Cancer Center
Houston, TX, USA
Volume 3, Chapter 13 Hypopharyngeal, esophageal, and neck reconstruction
Volume 3, Video 13.01 Reconstruction of pharyngoesophageal defects with the anterolateral thigh flap

James E. Zins, MD
Chairman
Department of Plastic Surgery
Dermatology and Plastic Surgery Institute
Cleveland Clinic
Cleveland, OH, USA
Volume 2, Chapter 13 Neck rejuvenation

Christopher G. Zochowski, MD
Chief Resident
Department of Plastic and Reconstructive Surgery
Case Western Reserve University
Cleveland, OH, USA
Volume 3, Chapter 38 Pierre Robin sequence

Elvin G. Zook, MD
Professor Emeritus
Division of Plastic Surgery
Southern Illinois University School of Medicine
Springfield, IL, USA
Volume 6, Chapter 6 Nail and fingertip reconstruction

Ronald M. Zuker, MD, FRCSC, FACS, FRCSEd(Hon)
Staff Plastic Surgeon
The Hospital for Sick Children
Professor of Surgery
Department of Surgery
The University of Toronto
Toronto, ON, Canada
Volume 3, Chapter 11 Facial paralysis

Acknowledgments

Editing a textbook such as this is an exciting, if daunting job. Only at the end of the project, over 4 years later, does one realize how much work it entailed and how many people helped make it happen. Sue Hodgson was the Commissioning Editor who trusted me to undertake this. Together, over several weekends in Seattle and countless e-mails and phone calls, we planned the format of this edition and laid the groundwork for a planning meeting in Chicago that included the volume editors and the Elsevier team with whom we have worked. I thank Drs. Gurtner, Warren, Rodriguez, Losee, Song, Grotting, Chang and Van Beek for tirelessly ensuring that each volume was as good as it could possibly be.

I had a weekly call with the Elsevier team as well as several visits to the offices in London. I will miss working with them. Louise Cook, Alexandra Mortimer and Poppy Garraway have been professional, thorough, and most of all, fun to work with. Emma Cole and Sam Crowe helped enormously with video content. Sadly, Sue Hodgson has left Elsevier, however Belinda Kuhn ably filled her shoes and ensured that we kept to our timeline, didn't lose momentum, and that the final product was something we would all be proud of.

Several residents helped, in focus groups to define format and style as well as specifically engaging in the editing process. I thank Darren Smith and Colin Woon for their help as technical copyeditors. Thanks to James Saunders and Leigh Jansen for reviewing video content and thanks also to Donnie Buck for all of his help with the electronic content. Of course we edited the book, we didn't write it. The writers were our contributing authors, all of whom engaged with enthusiasm. I thank them for defining Plastic Surgery, the book and the specialty.

Finally, I would like to thank my residents and fellows, who challenge me and make work fun. My partners in the Division of Plastic Surgery at the University of Washington, under the leadership of Nick Vedder, are a constant source of support and encouragement and I thank them. Finally, my family, Kate and David and most of all, my wife Gabrielle are unwavering in their love and support and I will never be able to thank them enough.

Peter C. Neligan, MB, FRCS(I), FRCSC, FACS
2012

I'd like to thank all the authors for their commitment to producing this volume, my colleagues and residents at the University of Chicago Medical Center who work tirelessly to advance Plastic Surgery, my parents who first inspired me to seek knowledge and most importantly my wife Janie and my daughters Olivia, Ava and Ella without whom this and all work loses meaning and significance for me.

David H. Song, MD, MBA, FACS
2012

Dedicated to the memory of Stephen J. Mathes

1

Comprehensive lower extremity anatomy

Ginard I. Henry and Grant M. Kleiber

SYNOPSIS

▪ The reconstructive surgeon who embarks on surgery on the lower extremity must be well acquainted with its complex anatomy.

▪ The essence of reconstructive surgery is using one's thorough knowledge of the nuances of the anatomical structures to enable borrowing from one or more structures to reconstruct the loss of others.

▪ This chapter aspires to provide a comprehensive review of the anatomical structures from the hip through to the plantar surface of the foot in order to provide the basis of mastery of lower-extremity reconstruction.

▪ The components of the lower extremity vary widely in regard to the redundancy of tissue, density of distinct structures, and function as one travels from proximal to distal regions. It is for this reason that the anatomical depiction of the lower extremity is divided into discussion of the thigh, knee, lower leg, and foot. Each of these structures differs greatly from each other. However, many reconstructive tasks bridge and cross these regions.

▪ Even though present in discrete sections, the anatomy of the lower extremity should be viewed as an interconnected and interrelated unit.

Embryology

The first recognizable sign of lower limb growth in the human embryo occurs during the third week of life. The initial limb development begins along the ventrolateral surface. Slow outgrowth of the apical epidermal ridge continues into the fifth week when a small flattened foot plate develops. The foot plate begins development straight with no dorsiflexion and the plantar surface pointed toward the head. Skeletogenesis occurs in the tibial/fibular region while the foot plate begins to rotate laterally (the right foot plate clockwise and the left counterclockwise). By the sixth week, digital rays appear and

external notching occurs. Through the sixth to the eighth week chondrification progresses throughout the future bony structures and the lower limb elongates.

The transition from the embryonic to the fetal period occurs during the eighth week. At this point, the phalanges, metatarsals, tarsals, malleoli, tibia, fibula, and femur are all present. Between the third and ninth month the foot dorsiflexes and pronates, and the thigh internally rotates. During this time period, lower limb structures are recognizable. The soft tissues further develop and bones begin to ossify. The first signs of detectable ossification begin in the foot, specifically in the distal phalanges and metatarsal shaft. The intervening proximal and middle phalanges follow. Tarsal bones begin ossification in the fifth month beginning with the talus and the cuboid. Ossification of the remaining regions of the lower extremity continues throughout the rest of gestation.

The lower extremity vascular anatomy of the embryo differs from the adult primarily by the development and transient presence of the sciatic artery (also called the axis or ischiadic artery). This artery arises from the umbilical artery and is separate from the femoral artery as it courses inferiorly along the posterior surface of the thigh, knee, and leg and is a major contributor to lower extremity vascular supply in early fetal development. The femoral artery passes along the anterior side of the thigh and branches into the primitive posterior tibial and peroneal artery and an anterior tibial artery. As the fetus grows, the femoral artery increases in size and the sciatic artery becomes attenuated. In normal development the sciatic artery involutes during the eighth week of gestation and its remnants contribute to the formation of the inferior gluteal, deep femoral, popliteal, and peroneal vessels **(Fig. 1.1)**. However, in 0.025–0.04% of the population a sciatic artery persists throughout fetal development and into adulthood. A persistent sciatic artery can lead to aneurysm formation, thrombosis, and embolization. Although it is a rare anomaly, failure to recognize a persistent sciatic artery can lead to inappropriate assumptions of vascular patterns to common lower extremity flaps.

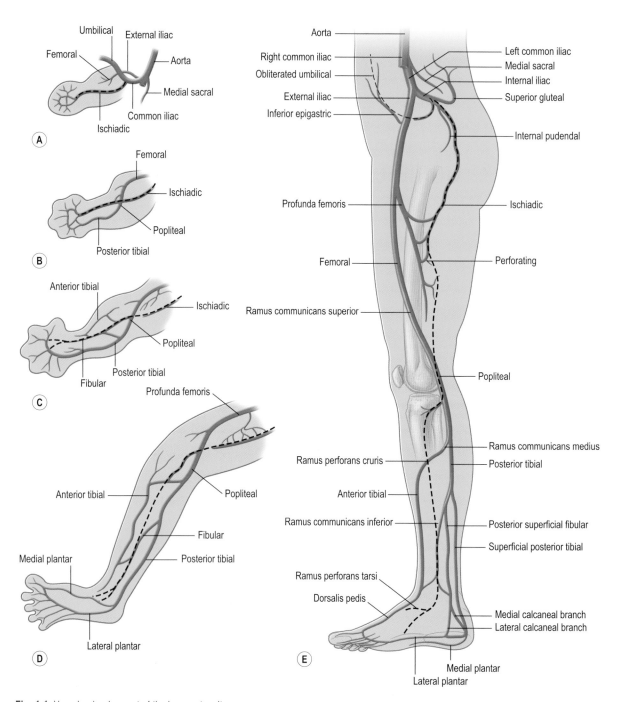

Fig. 1.1 Vascular development of the lower extremity.

The gluteal region

Gluteal skeletal structure

The pelvis consists of the two paired hip bones and the midline sacrum, articulating together at the two sacroiliac joints. The hip bones are formed by the fusion of the ilium, pubis, and ischium. These three bony regions of the pelvis coalesce to form the acetabulum *(Fig. 1.2)*. The complex bony structure of the pelvis serves to cradle the abdominal organs

during upright ambulation, and the large thick bony prominences of the pelvis serve as muscle attachments for the muscles of the hip and thigh. Dense ligaments reinforce the pelvis and distribute the numerous opposing forces acting on it. The sacrospinous ligament runs from the sacrum to the ischial spine, bounding the greater sciatic foramen. The sacrotuberous ligament attaches the sacrum to the ischial tuberosity and encloses the lesser sciatic foramen. Running from the anterior superior iliac spine to the pubic tubercle is the inguinal ligament. Most of the muscles of the thigh originate from the bony pelvis *(Fig. 1.3)*. The action of the multiple

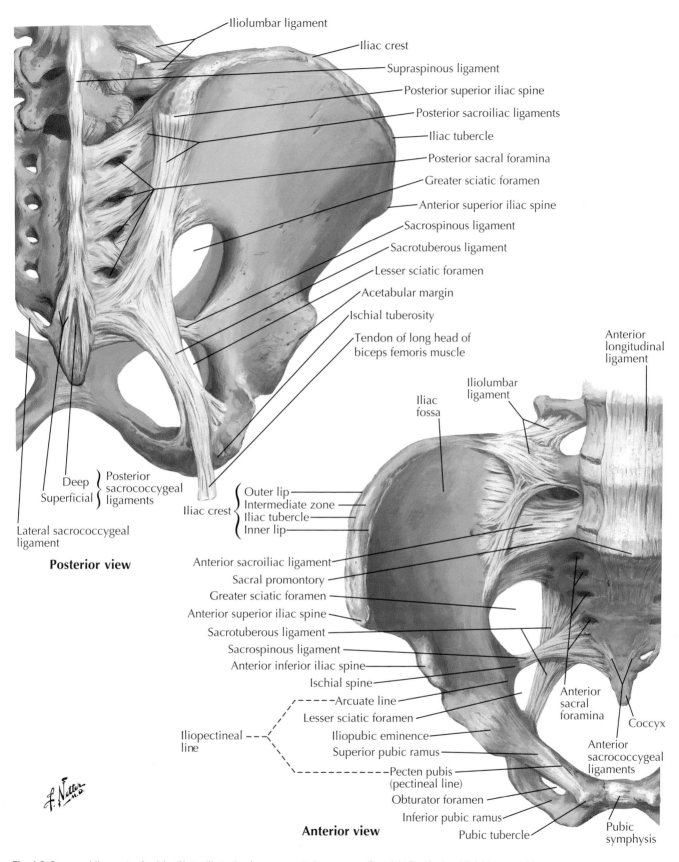

Iliolumbar ligament

Iliac crest

Supraspinous ligament

Posterior superior iliac spine

Posterior sacroiliac ligaments

Iliac tubercle

Posterior sacral foramina

Greater sciatic foramen

Anterior superior iliac spine

Sacrospinous ligament

Sacrotuberous ligament

Lesser sciatic foramen

Acetabular margin

Ischial tuberosity

Tendon of long head of biceps femoris muscle

Deep
Superficial } Posterior sacrococcygeal ligaments

Iliac crest {

Lateral sacrococcygeal ligament

Posterior view

Anterior longitudinal ligament

Iliolumbar ligament

Iliac fossa

Outer lip
Intermediate zone
Iliac tubercle
Inner lip

Anterior sacroiliac ligament

Sacral promontory

Greater sciatic foramen

Anterior superior iliac spine

Sacrotuberous ligament

Sacrospinous ligament

Anterior inferior iliac spine

Ischial spine

Arcuate line

Lesser sciatic foramen

Iliopectineal line

Iliopubic eminence

Superior pubic ramus

Pecten pubis (pectineal line)

Obturator foramen

Inferior pubic ramus

Pubic tubercle

Anterior sacral foramina

Coccyx

Anterior sacrococcygeal ligaments

Pubic symphysis

Anterior view

Fig. 1.2 Bones and ligaments of pelvis. (Netter illustration from www.netterimages.com. Copyright Elsevier Inc. All rights reserved.)

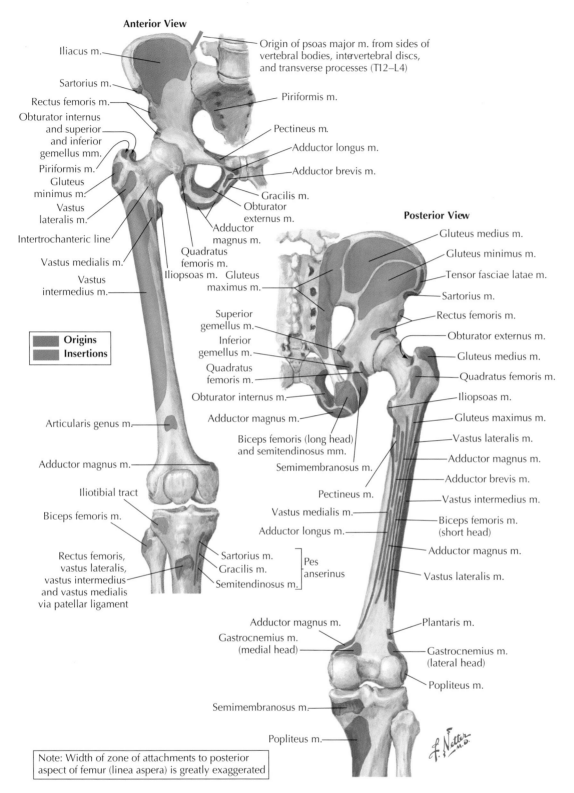

Anterior View

Iliacus m.

Origin of psoas major m. from sides of vertebral bodies, intervertebral discs, and transverse processes (T12–L4)

Sartorius m.

Rectus femoris m.

Piriformis m.

Obturator internus and superior and inferior gemellus mm.

Pectineus m.

Adductor longus m.

Piriformis m.

Adductor brevis m.

Gluteus minimus m.

Gracilis m.

Vastus lateralis m.

Obturator externus m.

Intertrochanteric line

Adductor magnus m.

Vastus medialis m.

Quadratus femoris m.

Vastus intermedius m.

Iliopsoas m.   Gluteus maximus m.

Posterior View

Gluteus medius m.

Gluteus minimus m.

Tensor fasciae latae m.

Sartorius m.

Rectus femoris m.

Superior gemellus m.

Obturator externus m.

Inferior gemellus m.

Gluteus medius m.

Quadratus femoris m.

Quadratus femoris m.

Obturator internus m.

Iliopsoas m.

Articularis genus m.

Adductor magnus m.

Gluteus maximus m.

Adductor magnus m.

Biceps femoris (long head) and semitendinosus mm.

Vastus lateralis m.

Adductor magnus m.

Semimembranosus m.

Adductor brevis m.

Iliotibial tract

Vastus intermedius m.

Biceps femoris m.

Pectineus m.

Biceps femoris m. (short head)

Rectus femoris, vastus lateralis, vastus intermedius and vastus medialis via patellar ligament

Vastus medialis m.

Adductor longus m.

Adductor magnus m.

Sartorius m.

Gracilis m.

Pes anserinus

Vastus lateralis m.

Semitendinosus m.

Adductor magnus m.

Plantaris m.

Gastrocnemius m. (medial head)

Gastrocnemius m. (lateral head)

Popliteus m.

Semimembranosus m.

Popliteus m.

☐ Origins
☐ Insertions

Note: Width of zone of attachments to posterior aspect of femur (linea aspera) is greatly exaggerated

Fig. 1.3 Bony attachments of buttock and thigh muscles. (Netter illustration from www.netterimages.com.)

flexors, extensors, and internal and external rotators on the hip joint serves to stabilize and position the torso during the complex process of ambulation.

Gluteal fascial anatomy

The fascial system of the gluteal region and the lower extremity contains various permutations of a nearly continuous superficial fascial and a deep fascial layer. The superficial system is located within the subcutaneous fat, usually as a dividing layer where superficial veins and nerves traverse to reach the overlying skin. The superficial layers are thinner than the deep layer, which becomes thinner with age to a point where its presence is described as variable. The deep fascial layer is thicker and frequently can be seen as a dual-layered fibrous band. It usually lies directly over the underlying limb musculature and its proper fascia.

The superficial fascia of the gluteal region is continuous with that over the low back and continues inferiorly into the proximal thigh. The deep fascia covering the gluteal muscles varies in thickness. Over the maximus it is thin, but over the anterior two-thirds of the medius it forms the thick, strong gluteal aponeurosis. This is attached to the lateral border of the iliac crest superiorly, and splits anteriorly to enclose tensor fasciae latae and posteriorly to enclose gluteus maximus.

Muscles of the buttocks

The gluteus maximus is the largest muscle in the body and lies most superficially in the gluteal region, originating from the posterior gluteal line of the ilium and the dorsal portion of the sacrum *(Fig. 1.4)*. The superficial fibers coalesce into a thick tendinous expansion which contributes to the iliotibial band of the fascia lata, while the deep fibers insert on the gluteal tuberosity of the femur. The gluteus maximus acts as a hip extensor when the hip is in a flexed position. When the lower extremity is fixed in position – as in standing – the gluteus maximus dorsally rotates the pelvis and torso. The vascular supply is primarily derived from the inferior gluteal vessels, which supply the inferior two-thirds of the muscle. The superior gluteal vessels supply the superior portion and the first perforator branch of the femoral profunda contributes to the vascular supply of the muscle laterally. For ease of description, the Mathes–Nahai classification system is used when discussing the vascular supply to muscle in this chapter *(Table 1.1)*. The vascular supply of gluteus maximus with two dominant pedicles (superior and inferior gluteal arteries) is considered to be type III.

Innervation to the gluteus maximus is provided by the inferior gluteal nerve. Underneath the gluteus maximus lie three bursae: the trochanteric, the gluteofemoral, and occasionally the ischiofemoral bursae, which allow frictionless movement over its underlying structures. The gluteus medius, situated immediately deep to the gluteus maximus, arises from the outer surface of the iliac wing and inserts on the greater trochanter of the femur. It is innervated by the superior gluteal nerve and functions to abduct the hip and medially rotate the femur. Blood supply to this muscle is from the deep branch of the superior gluteal artery and from the trochanteric connection.

Table 1.1 Mathes–Nahai classification system for muscle vascular supply

Muscle vascular supply type	Description
I	Single vascular pedicle
II	Dominant vascular pedicle and one or more minor pedicles
III	Two dominant pedicles
IV	Segmental vascular pedicles
V	Single dominant vascular pedicle and secondary segmental pedicles

The gluteus minimus lies deep to the gluteus medius and arises from the outer surface of the ilium. Its fibers join the aponeurosis of the gluteus medius to insert on the greater trochanter, and the two muscles function together to abduct the hip. The gluteus minimus is innervated by the superior gluteal nerve and receives blood supply from the superior gluteal artery and trochanteric connection. Several small muscles arise from the medial pelvis and insert on the greater trochanter of the femur, functioning collectively to rotate the hip externally. These muscles include piriformis, superior and inferior gemellus, quadratus femoris, obturator internus, and obturator externus.

Gluteal vasculature

The superior gluteal artery is the last branch of the posterior trunk of the internal iliac artery. It exits the pelvis through the greater sciatic foramen superior to the piriformis, dividing into two branches *(Fig. 1.5)*. The deep branch runs deep to the gluteus medius, dividing into superior and inferior branches. The superior branch travels laterally to the anterior superior iliac spine and connects with the ascending branch of the lateral circumflex femoral and the deep circumflex iliac. The inferior branch supplies the gluteus medius and minimus, and later joins with the lateral circumflex femoral. The superficial branch of the superior gluteal artery pierces the gluteus maximus, connecting intramuscularly with branches of the inferior gluteal artery, and sending musculocutaneous perforators to the overlying skin. The inferior gluteal artery branches from the anterior trunk of the internal iliac and exits the pelvis through the greater sciatic foramen below the piriformis. It runs deep to the gluteus maximus, supplying it and its overlying skin with musculocutaneous perforators. The artery continues down the posterior thigh, connecting with the perforating branches to supply the skin.

Gluteal innervation

The posterior cutaneous nerve of the thigh exits the pelvis with the inferior gluteal vessels *(Fig. 1.5)*. Several branches will curl around the inferior border of the gluteus maximus and run superiorly to innervate the overlying skin of the buttocks, while the posterior cutaneous nerve continues to descend down the posterior thigh deep to the fascia lata,

Superficial dissection

Deeper dissection

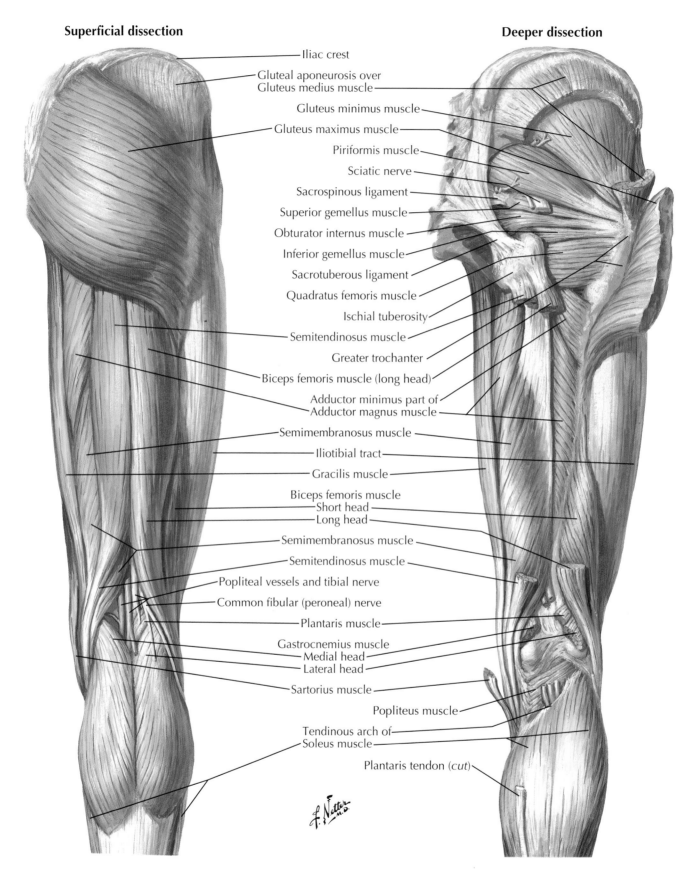

Iliac crest
Gluteal aponeurosis over
Gluteus medius muscle
Gluteus minimus muscle
Gluteus maximus muscle
Piriformis muscle
Sciatic nerve
Sacrospinous ligament
Superior gemellus muscle
Obturator internus muscle
Inferior gemellus muscle
Sacrotuberous ligament
Quadratus femoris muscle
Ischial tuberosity
Semitendinosus muscle
Greater trochanter
Biceps femoris muscle (long head)
Adductor minimus part of
Adductor magnus muscle
Semimembranosus muscle
Iliotibial tract
Gracilis muscle
Biceps femoris muscle
Short head
Long head
Semimembranosus muscle
Semitendinosus muscle
Popliteal vessels and tibial nerve
Common fibular (peroneal) nerve
Plantaris muscle
Gastrocnemius muscle
Medial head
Lateral head
Sartorius muscle
Popliteus muscle
Tendinous arch of
Soleus muscle
Plantaris tendon (*cut*)

Fig. 1.4 Muscles of hip and thigh: posterior views. (Netter illustration from www.netterimages.com. Copyright Elsevier Inc. All rights reserved.)

Deep dissection

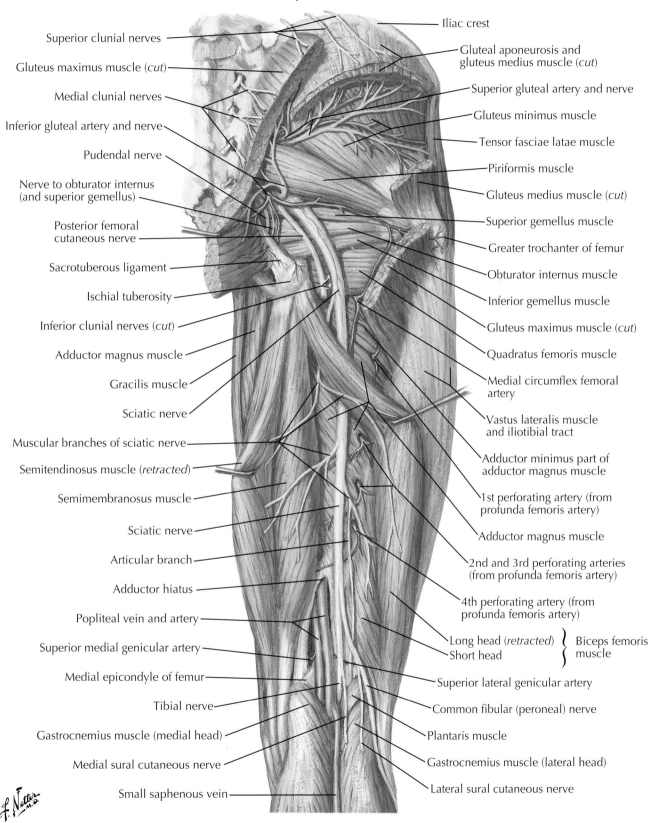

Superior clunial nerves

Gluteus maximus muscle (*cut*)

Medial clunial nerves

Inferior gluteal artery and nerve

Pudendal nerve

Nerve to obturator internus (and superior gemellus)

Posterior femoral cutaneous nerve

Sacrotuberous ligament

Ischial tuberosity

Inferior clunial nerves (*cut*)

Adductor magnus muscle

Gracilis muscle

Sciatic nerve

Muscular branches of sciatic nerve

Semitendinosus muscle (*retracted*)

Semimembranosus muscle

Sciatic nerve

Articular branch

Adductor hiatus

Popliteal vein and artery

Superior medial genicular artery

Medial epicondyle of femur

Tibial nerve

Gastrocnemius muscle (medial head)

Medial sural cutaneous nerve

Small saphenous vein

Iliac crest

Gluteal aponeurosis and gluteus medius muscle (*cut*)

Superior gluteal artery and nerve

Gluteus minimus muscle

Tensor fasciae latae muscle

Piriformis muscle

Gluteus medius muscle (*cut*)

Superior gemellus muscle

Greater trochanter of femur

Obturator internus muscle

Inferior gemellus muscle

Gluteus maximus muscle (*cut*)

Quadratus femoris muscle

Medial circumflex femoral artery

Vastus lateralis muscle and iliotibial tract

Adductor minimus part of adductor magnus muscle

1st perforating artery (from profunda femoris artery)

Adductor magnus muscle

2nd and 3rd perforating arteries (from profunda femoris artery)

4th perforating artery (from profunda femoris artery)

Long head (*retracted*)
Short head } Biceps femoris muscle

Superior lateral genicular artery

Common fibular (peroneal) nerve

Plantaris muscle

Gastrocnemius muscle (lateral head)

Lateral sural cutaneous nerve

Fig. 1.5 Arteries and nerves of thigh: deep dissection (posterior view). (Netter illustration from www.netterimages.com. Copyright Elsevier Inc. All rights reserved.)

sending segmental cutaneous branches to the skin of the posterior thigh. The gluteal muscles are innervated by the superior and inferior gluteal nerves. The superior gluteal nerve runs with the superior gluteal artery and divides into superior and inferior branches, which course respectively with the superior and inferior branches of the deep superior gluteal artery, supplying the gluteus medius and minimus. The inferior branch runs laterally to also innervate the tensor fascia latae. The inferior gluteal nerve runs with the inferior gluteal artery, exiting the pelvis below the piriformis and entering the gluteus maximus.

The thigh

The thigh serves a dual function of aid in truncal support and positioning of the knee in space; both processes are critical to ambulation. In the thigh, these functions are usually enacted by multiple muscles that perform in a redundant fashion. The muscles of the thigh are some of the largest in the body and their corresponding fasciocutaneous coverage is also large and relatively redundant. Thorough knowledge of the thigh anatomy is a key component that allows for exploitation of these redundancies. These attributes of the thigh allow it to be a generous source of harvest tissue for local, regional, and distant reconstructive surgical options.

Thigh skeletal structure

The thigh region is generally defined as the cylindrical proximal portion of the lower extremity that extends from the infragluteal crease and the inguinal ligament distally to the tibiofemoral joint. Most anterior thigh musculature originates from the pelvic bone and therefore the bony structure's interrelation between the pelvis and the femur is a principal anatomic foundation.

The femoral head articulates with the pelvic acetabulum to form the only true ball-and-socket joint in the body, allowing for stability under load as well as smooth multiplanar movement. A dense ligamentous capsule surrounds the hip joint circumferentially, extending from around the pelvic acetabulum to encase the femoral head and insert on the femoral neck (*Fig. 1.6*). The ligaments of the hip joint are the iliofemoral, pubofemoral, ischiofemoral, transverse acetabular and the ligamentum teres. As the hip moves, so do the capsular ligaments. The ligaments are reinforced with capsular thickenings which wind and unwind, tightening around the hip, affecting stability, excursion, and joint capacity.

The pelvic bone serves as the principal base for the thigh musculature. Eleven out of the 17 muscles of the thigh originate from the pelvis. Two bony prominences emanate from the femoral neck at about 90° from each other – the greater and lesser trochanters. These femoral prominences primarily serve as insertion sites for hip actors (*Fig. 1.3*). The greater trochanter receives insertions from the quadratus femoris, gluteus medius, obturator externus, piriformis, obturator internus, and gemellus muscles. The lesser trochanter is the insertion target for the iliopsoas muscle. The action of multiple flexors, extensors, and internal and external rotators on the hip joint serves to stabilize and position the torso during the complex process of ambulation.

The vascular supply of the femoral bone arises from multiple sources. The femoral head and neck are encircled by an arterial-connecting arcade contributed by the medial and lateral circumflex arteries with lesser contribution by the superior and inferior gluteal vessels. These vessels piece the hip joint synovial capsule and form a subsynovial intra-articular ring. The femoral shaft has multiple nutrient foramina via which branches from the second perforating artery from the profunda femoris (*Fig. 1.7*) enter and deliver endosteal blood supply. These foramina usually run along the linea aspera (Latin for "rough line") on the posterior surface of the femur in the middle one-third of the femoral shaft. Periosteal vascularity along the femur receives vascular input from either the perforating branches of the profunda or directly from the profunda femoris. The distal metaphyseal region of the femur also has multiple vascular foramina that are derived from the genicular arterial system.

This genicular system, based on the superficial femoral artery, is the anatomical basis for the clinically relevant medial femoral periosteal bone flap. Using the descending genicular artery (a medial branch of the superficial femoral artery) as a pedicle, periosteum, cortical and cancellous bone can be harvested from the medial femur as a vascularized flap. Usually used as a free flap (with or without an associated skin paddle off the saphenous artery), the medial femoral periosteal bone flap is utilized as an effective treatment for recalcitrant bony nonunions of the clavicle, humerus, tibia, and radius (*Fig. 1.8*).

Thigh fascial composition

Like the abdomen, the thigh has a superficial and deep fascial system. The superficial fascia lies within the subcutaneous fat of the thigh encircling the entire structure. Superficial vessels and nerves pass along and pierce this fascia as they travel from their deeper tributaries and surface to the superficial skin targets. The thickness of the fascia varies throughout the thigh but thickens proximally in the inguinal region. At the inguinal ligament the superficial fascia fuses with the deep thigh fascia.

The deep fascia structure of the lower extremity is a tough, well-vascularized fibrous tissue that lies beneath the superficial fascia and all the subcutaneous fat. This fibrous structure encircles and constrains the thigh musculature in a near-complete sheath, often found to be dual layers. The deep fascia of the thigh has been referred to and described by several different names, making the terminology somewhat confusing. The deep fascia of the thigh is also called investing fascia of the thigh; the fascia lata (*lata*, Latin for wide or broad); or, even more confusingly, the "thick layer of the superficial fascia." The deep fascia of the thigh attaches posteriorly to the sacrum and coccyx, anteriorly to the inguinal ligament, and laterally to the iliac crest. At the inguinal ligament, where the superficial fascia joins the deep fascia, lies the fossa ovalis. The fossa ovalis is an opening in both fascial layers through which the great saphenous vein, superficial branches of the femoral artery, and lymphatics pass through, transitioning between the deep and the superficial layers of

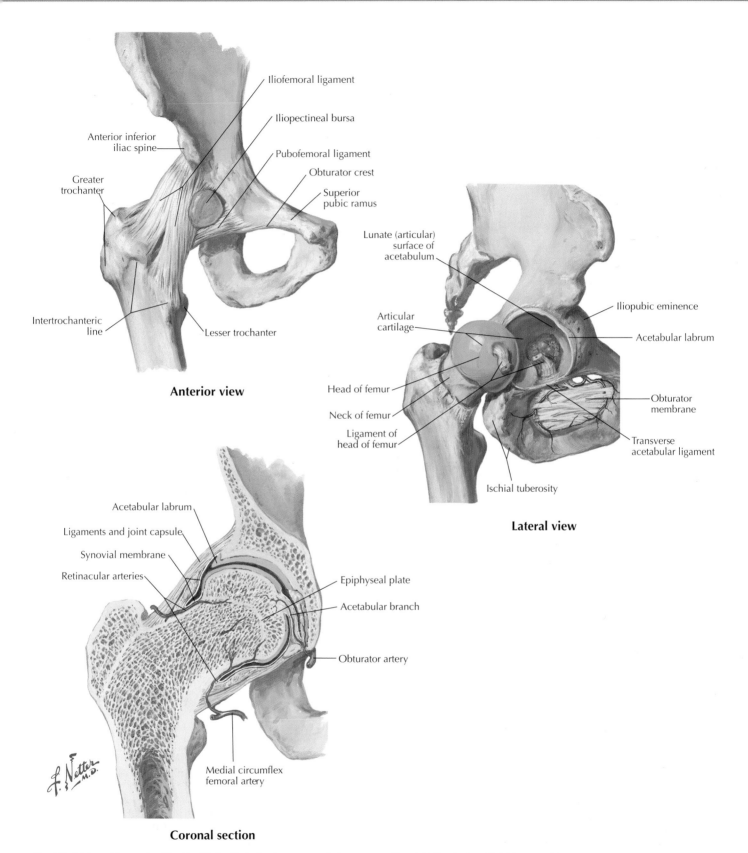

Anterior view

- Iliofemoral ligament
- Iliopectineal bursa
- Anterior inferior iliac spine
- Pubofemoral ligament
- Obturator crest
- Superior pubic ramus
- Greater trochanter
- Intertrochanteric line
- Lesser trochanter

Lateral view

- Lunate (articular) surface of acetabulum
- Articular cartilage
- Iliopubic eminence
- Acetabular labrum
- Head of femur
- Neck of femur
- Ligament of head of femur
- Obturator membrane
- Transverse acetabular ligament
- Ischial tuberosity

Coronal section

- Acetabular labrum
- Ligaments and joint capsule
- Synovial membrane
- Retinacular arteries
- Epiphyseal plate
- Acetabular branch
- Obturator artery
- Medial circumflex femoral artery

Fig. 1.6 Joints and ligaments of the hip. (Netter illustration from www.netterimages.com. Copyright Elsevier Inc. All rights reserved.)

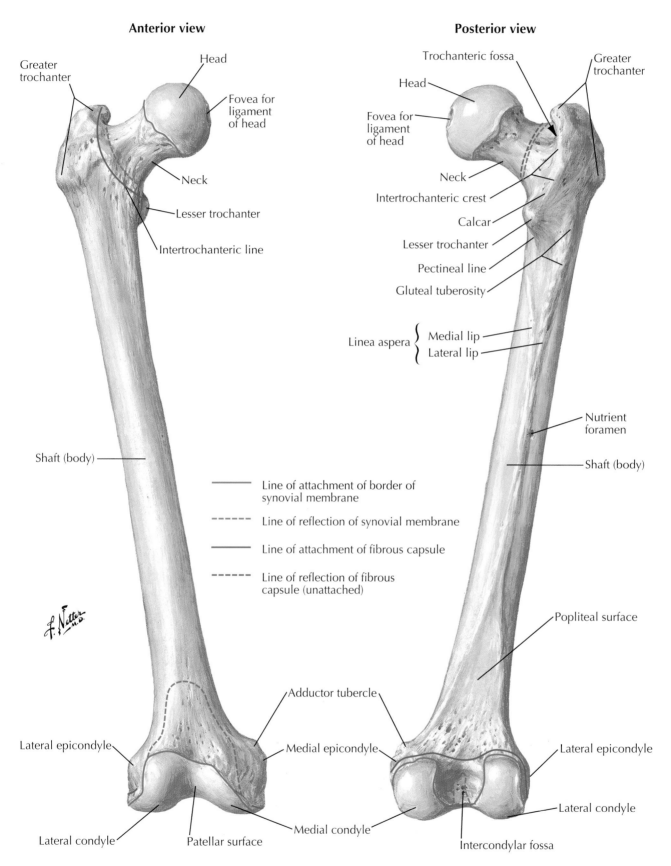

Anterior view

Greater trochanter

Head

Fovea for ligament of head

Neck

Lesser trochanter

Intertrochanteric line

Shaft (body)

——— Line of attachment of border of synovial membrane

- - - - Line of reflection of synovial membrane

——— Line of attachment of fibrous capsule

- - - - Line of reflection of fibrous capsule (unattached)

Lateral epicondyle

Adductor tubercle

Medial epicondyle

Lateral condyle

Medial condyle

Patellar surface

Posterior view

Trochanteric fossa

Greater trochanter

Head

Fovea for ligament of head

Neck

Intertrochanteric crest

Calcar

Lesser trochanter

Pectineal line

Gluteal tuberosity

Linea aspera { Medial lip / Lateral lip

Nutrient foramen

Shaft (body)

Popliteal surface

Lateral epicondyle

Lateral condyle

Intercondylar fossa

Fig. 1.7 Osteology of the femur. (Netter illustration from www.netterimages.com. Copyright Elsevier Inc. All rights reserved.)

There are three functional compartments of the thigh: anterior, posterior, and medial. The anterior compartment contains the knee extensor muscles; the posterior compartment is comprised of knee flexors; and the medial compartment retains the hip adductors *(Fig. 1.11)*. The medial and lateral intermuscular septa travel from the fascia lata to attach to the femur on the linea aspera along its posterior aspect. These septa then divide the anterior compartment from the posterior compartments and partition the thigh musculature according to knee function. Only the anterior and posterior compartments have definite fascial boundaries. The medial (adductor) compartment is not a true anatomical compartment as it has no defined intermuscular septa separating it. The muscles of the adductor compartment – gracilis, pectineus, adductor longus, adductor brevis, and adductor magnus – form a functional compartment in the proximal aspect of the thigh.

Thigh musculature

There are 17 muscles that have origins in, insertions to, or course through the region of the thigh. The iliacus and the psoas major originate from the lumbar vertebral column and insert on the lesser trochanter together. They are commonly considered as one functional unit – the iliopsoas – and are powerful hip flexors.

The three compartments of the thigh are a well-organized way to approach the thigh musculature *(Table 1.2)*. The anterior thigh compartment contains the sartorius, articularis genu, and quadriceps femoris, comprised of the rectus femoris, vastus lateralis, intermedius, and medialis *(Table 1.3)*. These muscles are the primary knee flexors. All of the anterior-compartment musculature is monoarticular functioning, with the exception of the sartorius and the rectus femoris, which crosses both the hip joint and the knee joint. These muscles are therefore biarticular muscles and flex both the hip and knee joints.

The sartorius muscle is the most superficial muscle of the thigh. It obliquely crosses the anterior thigh from superolateral to medial inferior. The proximal end of the sartorius makes up one of the three limbs of the femoral triangle. The medial border of the sartorius makes up the lateral side; the medial border of the adductor longus makes up the medial side of the triangle; and the inguinal ligament makes up the superior limb *(Fig. 1.12)*. The femoral triangle denotes the region where the femoral artery, nerve, and vein are transiently uncovered superficially by muscle in the proximal thigh. Here, all three structures radiate multiple branches in multiple directions to supply the vasculature and innervation to the groin region, lower abdomen, and proximal thigh. As the femoral artery, vein, and nerve descend distally in the thigh, they dive under the adductor longus and then proceed to the adductor canal. At the distal end of the sartorius, the muscle inserts on the proximal, medial surface of the tibia. The sartorius inserts in this region above the gracilis, which then inserts above the semitendinosus *(Fig. 1.13)*. This three-muscle insertion point forms the pes anserinus (a Latin derivation for "duck's foot") which is so named because of the three-toed pattern of the duck's foot. The sartorius' superficial and femoral triangle proximity location makes it an ideal candidate for muscle transposition coverage over proximal thigh wounds with femoral vessel exposure. It has a type IV

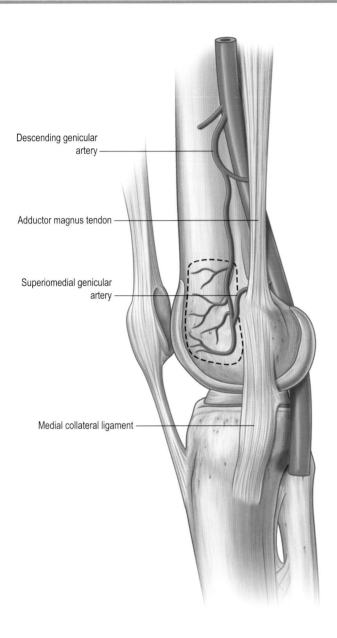

Fig. 1.8 The medial femoral periosteal bone flap.

Descending genicular artery

Adductor magnus tendon

Superiomedial genicular artery

Medial collateral ligament

the thigh *(Fig. 1.9)*. This opening is covered by a membranous layer of the superficial fascia called the cribriform fascia (derived from the Latin *cribrum* or sieve). A thickening of the fibrous tissues is present on the lateral aspect of the deep fascia (fascia lata) which is called the iliotibial band or tract *(Fig. 1.10)*. The iliotibial band is proximally attached to the tensor fascia latae muscle and together this myofascial unit aids in maintaining knee extension.

Septa pass from the deep fascial sheath to the bones within, confining the functional muscle groups within osteofascial compartments. The fascia functions as additional areas of attachment to the muscles and as a partition of similarly functioning musculature which augments their efficiency. In addition to separating musculature, fascial planes also provide pathways for vessel perforators to travel from deeper vasculature to the overlying skin they supply.

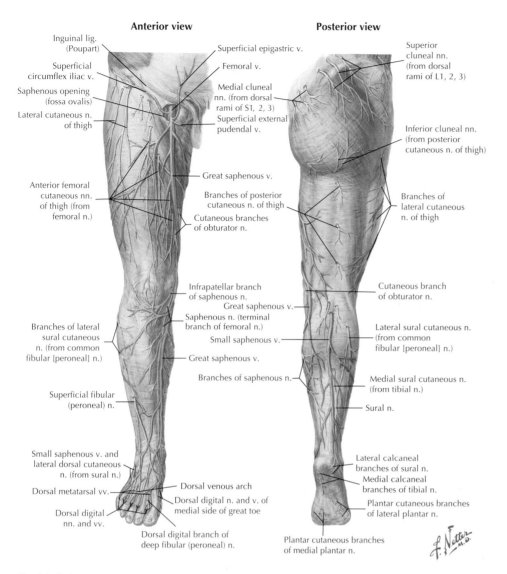

Anterior view   **Posterior view**

Inguinal lig. (Poupart)

Superficial circumflex iliac v.

Saphenous opening (fossa ovalis)

Lateral cutaneous n. of thigh

Anterior femoral cutaneous nn. of thigh (from femoral n.)

Branches of lateral sural cutaneous n. (from common fibular [peroneal] n.)

Superficial fibular (peroneal) n.

Small saphenous v. and lateral dorsal cutaneous n. (from sural n.)

Dorsal metatarsal vv.

Dorsal digital nn. and vv.

Dorsal digital branch of deep fibular (peroneal) n.

Superficial epigastric v.

Femoral v.

Medial cluneal nn. (from dorsal rami of S1, 2, 3)

Superficial external pudendal v.

Great saphenous v.

Branches of posterior cutaneous n. of thigh

Cutaneous branches of obturator n.

Infrapatellar branch of saphenous n.

Great saphenous v.

Saphenous n. (terminal branch of femoral n.)

Small saphenous v.

Great saphenous v.

Branches of saphenous n.

Dorsal venous arch

Dorsal digital n. and v. of medial side of great toe

Superior cluneal nn. (from dorsal rami of L1, 2, 3)

Inferior cluneal nn. (from posterior cutaneous n. of thigh)

Branches of lateral cutaneous n. of thigh

Cutaneous branch of obturator n.

Lateral sural cutaneous n. (from common fibular [peroneal] n.)

Medial sural cutaneous n. (from tibial n.)

Sural n.

Lateral calcaneal branches of sural n.

Medial calcaneal branches of tibial n.

Plantar cutaneous branches of lateral plantar n.

Plantar cutaneous branches of medial plantar n.

Fig. 1.9 Surface anatomy: superficial veins and nerves. (Netter illustration from www.netterimages.com. Copyright Elsevier Inc. All rights reserved.)

segmental blood supply but there exist more dominant segmental pedicles which allow for adequate vascular pivot points. In addition, partial sartorius muscle transfer can be effectively utilized to ensure vascular supply and close complex proximal thigh wounds.

The quadriceps muscles act as a unit through the patella and the patellar tendon to extend the lower leg at the knee. Knee extension is critical in human ambulation and upright posture maintenance. The redundancy in the function of these four muscles ensures this ability. However, removal of one or a portion of one of the quadriceps muscles can usually be tolerated with appropriate centralization techniques of the remaining musculature and with adequate physical therapy. This recovery potential is a primary factor in the ability to use the vascular type II rectus femoris muscle for regional and distant reconstructions. The dominant pedicle from the descending branch of the lateral circumflex artery allows for wide transposition of the rectus femoris muscle or musculocutaneous flap without sacrificing knee function after centralizing the remaining knee flexors.

The posterior compartment musculature is comprised of the knee flexion muscles, colloquially known as the hamstrings (termed referring to the posterior thigh culinary cut of the hog – ham) *(Table 1.4)*. The three muscles of this compartment facilitate knee flexion. The biceps – as its name denotes – has two heads, each with a slightly different origin and action. All three of these muscles span the posterior knee, with the tendons of the semitendinosus and semimembranosus traveling medially and forming one border of the popliteal fossa and the biceps femoris tendon traveling laterally and forming the other border *(Fig. 1.14)*.

The adductor compartment houses the adductor magnus, brevis, and longus, as well as the gracilis and pectineus *(Figs 1.15 and 1.16 and Table 1.5)*. All five muscles cross the hip joint but only one – the gracilis – crosses the knee. The gracilis is also the most superficial muscle of the adductor compartment. It begins from its origin on the pubic bone as a flat, broad muscle that tapers down into a narrow tendon that inserts into the pes anserinus. Because of its superficial location, its muscle vascular supply type II, and an associated

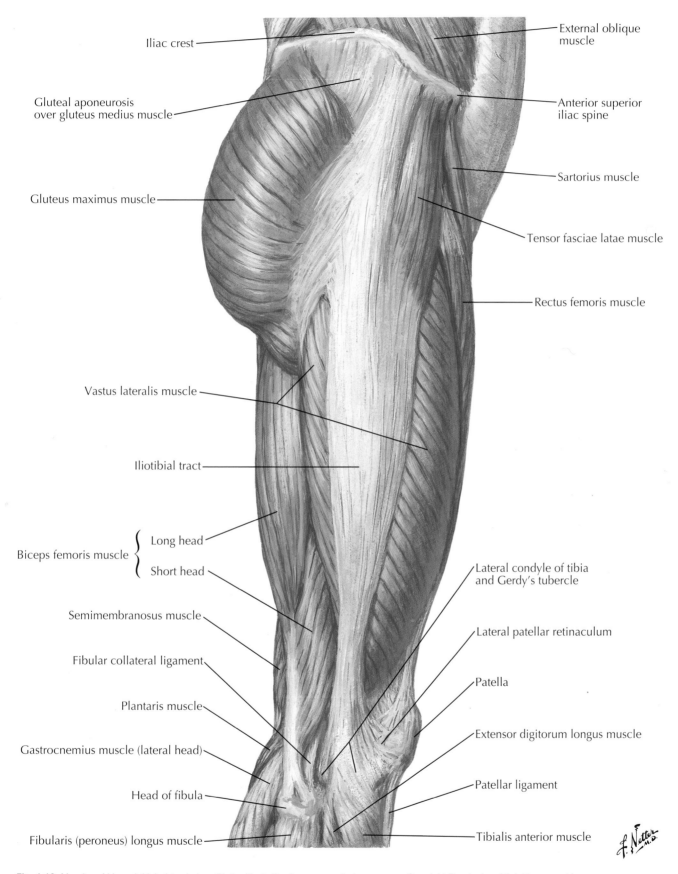

Iliac crest

External oblique muscle

Gluteal aponeurosis over gluteus medius muscle

Anterior superior iliac spine

Sartorius muscle

Gluteus maximus muscle

Tensor fasciae latae muscle

Rectus femoris muscle

Vastus lateralis muscle

Iliotibial tract

Biceps femoris muscle { Long head

Short head

Lateral condyle of tibia and Gerdy's tubercle

Lateral patellar retinaculum

Semimembranosus muscle

Fibular collateral ligament

Patella

Plantaris muscle

Extensor digitorum longus muscle

Gastrocnemius muscle (lateral head)

Head of fibula

Patellar ligament

Fibularis (peroneus) longus muscle

Tibialis anterior muscle

Fig. 1.10 Muscles of hip and thigh: lateral view. (Netter illustration from www.netterimages.com. Copyright Elsevier Inc. All rights reserved.)

Thigh: Serial Cross Sections

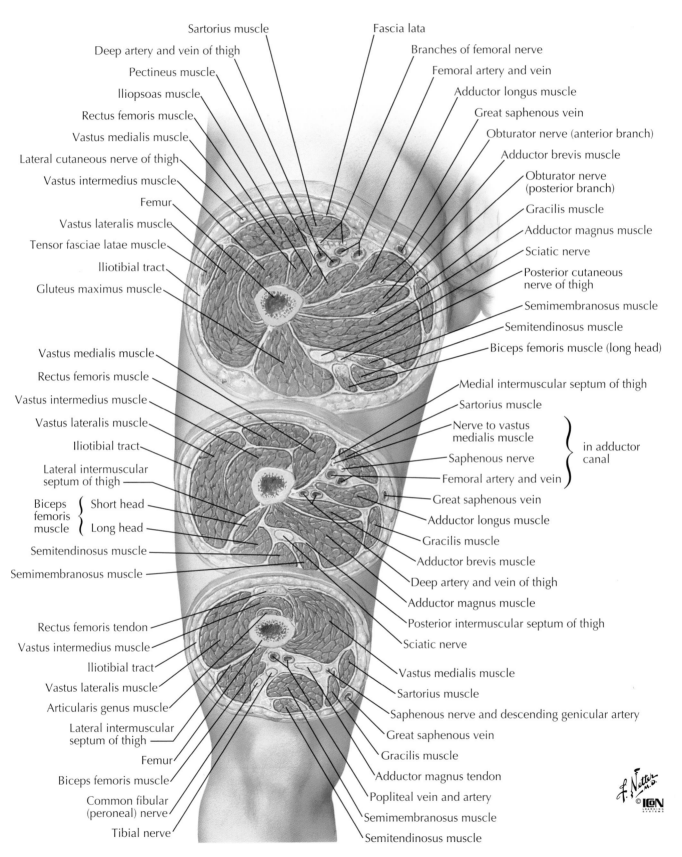

Fig. 1.11 Thigh: serial cross-sections. (Netter illustration from www.netterimages.com. Copyright Elsevier Inc. All rights reserved.)

Table 1.2 Thigh musculature

		Muscle	Origin	Insertion	Function	Blood supply	Flap blood supply type	Innervation
Hip-related	1	**Iliacus**	Pelvis – iliac fossa	Lesser trochanter of femur – inferior edge	Hip flexion and internal rotation	–	–	Femoral nerve – intra-abdominal
	2	**Psaos major**	Thoracic and lumbar spine (T12-L5)	Lesser trochanter of femur – middle region	Hip flexion and internal rotation	–	–	Lumbar spinal nerves
Anterior compartment	3	**Sartorius**	Anterior superior iliac spine (ASIS)	Medial, proximal tibia (pes anserinus)	Flexes, abducts, and external rotates thigh at hip; flexes, internally rotates leg at knee	Multiple branches for the superficial femoral artery	Segmental (type IV)	Femoral nerve (anterior division)
	4	**Rectus femoris**	ASIS and ilium	Quadriceps tendon–patella tendon–tibial tuberosity	Hip flexion and knee extension	Descending branch of LCFA (dominant); ascending branch of LCFA (minor), muscular branch of superficial femoral artery (minor)	One dominant and minor pedicles (type II)	Femoral nerve (posterior division)
	5	**Vastus lateralis**	Shaft of femur – upper intertrochanteric line, base of greater trochanter, lateral linea aspera, lateral supracondylar ridge, and lateral intermuscular septum	Quadriceps tendon–patella tendon–tibial tuberosity (lateral aspect)	Knee extension	Descending branch of LCFA (dominant); transverse branch of LCFA (minor), posterior branches of produnda femoris (minor), branch of superior genicular artery (minor)	One dominant and minor pedicles (type II)	Femoral nerve (posterior division)

Table 1.2 Continued

		Muscle	Origin	Insertion	Function	Blood supply	Flap blood supply type	Innervation
	6	**Vastus medialis**	Shaft of femur – lower intertrochanteric line, spiral line, medial linea aspera and medial intermuscular septum	Quadriceps tendon–patella tendon–tibial tuberosity	Knee extension, patellar stabilization	Branch of superficial femoral artery (dominant); distal branches of the superficial femoral artery (minor), branches of descending genicular artery (minor)	One dominant and minor pedicles (type II)	Femoral nerve (posterior division)
	7	**Vastus intermedialis**	Shaft of femur – inferior one-third	Quadriceps tendon–patella tendon–tibial tuberosity	Knee extension	Lateral direct branch from the profunda femoris (dominant); medial direct branch from the profunda femoris (minor)	One dominant and minor pedicles (type II)	Femoral nerve (posterior division)
	8	**Articularis genu**	Femur – anterior, distal surface of shaft	Apex of suprapatellar bursa	Retracts bursa as knee extends	Direct branch of profunda femoris	–	Femoral nerve (posterior division)
Posterior compartment	9	**Biceps femoris**	Long head: ischial tuberosity – posterior surface Short head: linea aspera – middle third and lateral supracondylar ridge of femur	Lateral condyle of tibia & head of fibula	Long head: extends knee Both heads: flexes and laterally rotates knee	Long head: first perforating branch of profunda femoris (dominant); inferior gluteal artery branch (minor), second perforating branch of profunda (minor); short head: second or third perforating branch of profunda (dominant); superior lateral genicular artery (minor)	One dominant and minor pedicles (type II)	Long head: tibial nerve Short head: common peroneal nerve
	10	**Semitendinosus**	Ischial tuberosity – medial surface	Medial, proximal tibia (pes anserinus) – below gracilis insertion	Extends hip, flexes, and medially rotates the knee	First perforating branch of profunda femoris (dominant); inferior gluteal artery branch (minor), second or third perforating branch of profunda (minor), superficial femoral	One dominant and minor pedicles (type II)	Tibial nerve

Compartment	#	Muscle	Origin	Insertion	Action	Arterial supply	Pedicle	Nerve
	11	Semimembranosus	Ischial tuberosity – lateral surface	Medial condyle	Extends hip, flexes, and medially rotates the knee	First perforating branch of profunda femoris (dominant); muscular branch of inferior gluteal artery (minor), descending branch of MCFA, inferior medial genicular artery	One dominant and minor pedicles (type II)	Sciatic nerve
Adductor compartment	12	Adductor magnus	Pubic bone – ischiopubic ramus	Femoral shaft, inferior – lower gluteal line and linea aspera	Hip adduction, internal hip rotation	Branches from the obturator, profunda femoris, and superficial femoral arteries	–	Obturator nerve (posterior division)
	13	Adductor longus	Pubic bone – pubic tubercle	Femur – inferior aspect of linea aspera	Hip adduction, internal hip rotation	Branch from profunda femoris (artery to the adductors); branches from MCFA, distal branch from the superficial femoral artery	–	Obturator nerve (anterior division)
	14	Adductor brevis	Pubic bone – superior and inferior ramus	Femur – superior aspect of linea aspera	Hip adduction	Variable – branch of profunda femoris versus branch from MCFA; obturator artery	–	Obturator nerve (anterior division)
	15	Gracilis	Pubic bone – ischiopubic ramus	Medial, proximal tibia (pes anserinus), below the sartorius	Hip adduction, knee flexion, and internal rotation	Ascending branch of MCFA (dominant); 1-2 branches from the superficial femoral artery	One dominant and minor pedicles (type II)	Obturator nerve (anterior division)
	16	Pectineus	Pubic bone	Proximal femur – below the lesser trochanter	Hip adduction, knee flexion, and internal rotation	Branches from the MCFA, common femoral, and obturator arteries	–	Femoral nerve (anterior division)
Extracompartmental	17	Tensor fascia latae	Iliac crest	Iliotibial tract–lateral tibia condyle (anterior surface)	Maintains knee extension (assists gluteus maximus) and hip abduction	Ascending branch of the LCFA	One dominant artery (type I)	Superior gluteal nerve

LCFA, lateral circumflex femoral artery; MCFA, medial circumflex femoral artery.

Superficial dissections

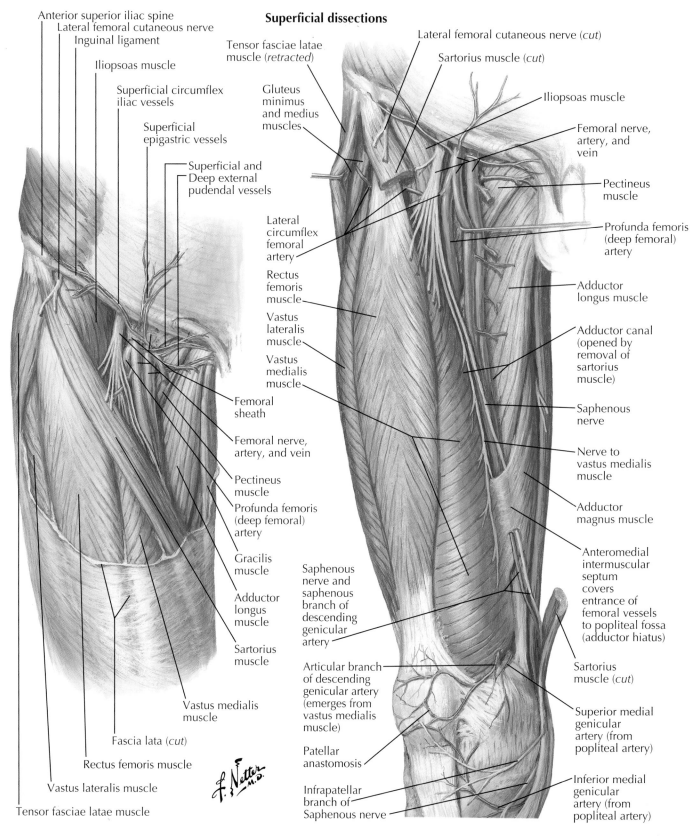

Anterior superior iliac spine
Lateral femoral cutaneous nerve
Inguinal ligament
Iliopsoas muscle
Superficial circumflex iliac vessels
Superficial epigastric vessels
Superficial and Deep external pudendal vessels
Tensor fasciae latae muscle (*retracted*)
Gluteus minimus and medius muscles
Lateral circumflex femoral artery
Rectus femoris muscle
Vastus lateralis muscle
Vastus medialis muscle
Femoral sheath
Femoral nerve, artery, and vein
Pectineus muscle
Profunda femoris (deep femoral) artery
Gracilis muscle
Adductor longus muscle
Sartorius muscle
Vastus medialis muscle
Fascia lata (*cut*)
Rectus femoris muscle
Vastus lateralis muscle
Tensor fasciae latae muscle

Saphenous nerve and saphenous branch of descending genicular artery
Articular branch of descending genicular artery (emerges from vastus medialis muscle)
Patellar anastomosis
Infrapatellar branch of Saphenous nerve

Lateral femoral cutaneous nerve (*cut*)
Sartorius muscle (*cut*)
Iliopsoas muscle
Femoral nerve, artery, and vein
Pectineus muscle
Profunda femoris (deep femoral) artery
Adductor longus muscle
Adductor canal (opened by removal of sartorius muscle)
Saphenous nerve
Nerve to vastus medialis muscle
Adductor magnus muscle
Anteromedial intermuscular septum covers entrance of femoral vessels to popliteal fossa (adductor hiatus)
Sartorius muscle (*cut*)
Superior medial genicular artery (from popliteal artery)
Inferior medial genicular artery (from popliteal artery)

Fig. 1.12 Arteries and nerves of thigh: anterior views. (Netter illustration from www.netterimages.com. Copyright Elsevier Inc. All rights reserved.)

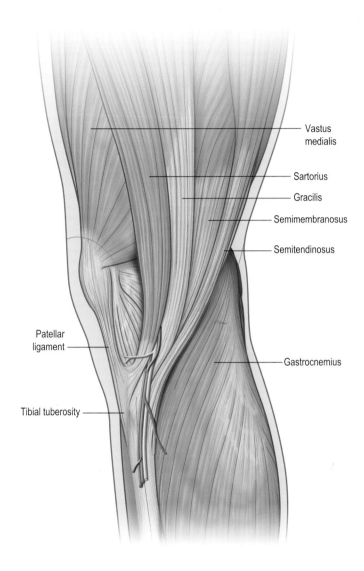

Fig. 1.13 Pes anserinus.

Table 1.3 Anterior thigh compartment musculature

Muscle	Function
Sartorius	Flexes, abducts, and external rotation of thigh at hip
	Flexes and internally rotates leg at knee
Rectus femoris	Hip flexion and knee extension
Vastus lateralis	Knee extension
Vastus medialis	Knee extension, patellar stabilization
Vastus intermedialis	Knee extension
Articularis genu	Retracts bursa as knee extends

Table 1.4 Posterior thigh compartment musculature

Muscle	Function
Biceps femoris	Long head: extends knee
	Both heads: flexes and laterally rotates knee
Semitendinosus	Extends hip, flexes and medially rotates the knee
Semimembranosus	Extends hip, flexes and medially rotates the knee

Table 1.5 Adductor compartment musculature

Muscle	Function
Adductor magnus	Hip adduction, internal hip rotation
Adductor longus	Hip adduction, internal hip rotation
Adductor brevis	Hip adduction
Gracilis	Hip adduction, knee flexion, and internal rotation
Pectineus	Hip flexion, adduction, and internal rotation

vascular branch that leads to the overlying skin, the gracilis is a frequent choice for a muscle or musculocutaneous flap. Due to their position and musculature structure, the remainder of the adductor muscles do not lend themselves easily for flap transposition.

The tensor fascia latae is not classically designated in the previously described compartments but included in the discussion of the thigh because of its intimate relation to thigh musculature and it utility in thigh reconstructive options. The tensor fascia latae lies on the proximal lateral aspect of the thigh originating from the iliac crest. As it descends distally, it is enveloped by the two layers of the iliotibial band of the fascia lata *(Figs 1.10 and 1.12)*. The tensor fascia latae muscle usually ends in the first third of the thigh but can extend down to the lateral femoral condyle. Its blood supply is from the ascending branch off the lateral circumflex femoral arterial system. This allows the muscle and fascia to be included with other flaps based off the same system if such a composite reconstruction is required. Also, with dissection to the branch to the source lateral circumflex femoral vessels, the tensor fascia latae with its long iliotibial band can be used to reconstruct other fascial defects in nearby regions such as the abdomen.

Thigh vasculature

The primary blood supply to the entire lower extremity is the femoral artery, passing beneath the inguinal ligament into the femoral canal *(Fig. 1.17)*. It courses with the femoral vein through the femoral sheath, a short canal composed of continuation of the transversalis fascia anteriorly and the iliac fascia posteriorly. These fascial layers fuse with the vascular adventitia approximately 4 cm inferior to the inguinal ligament. The femoral artery crosses beneath the sartorius muscle

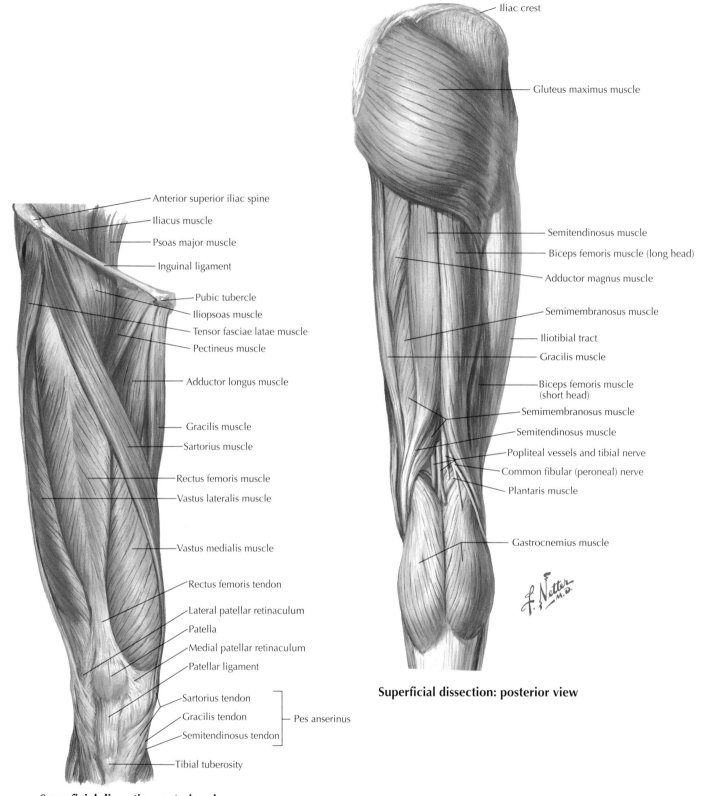

Superficial dissection: anterior view

Superficial dissection: posterior view

Fig. 1.14 Muscles of the thigh. (Netter illustration from www.netterimages.com. Copyright Elsevier Inc. All rights reserved.)

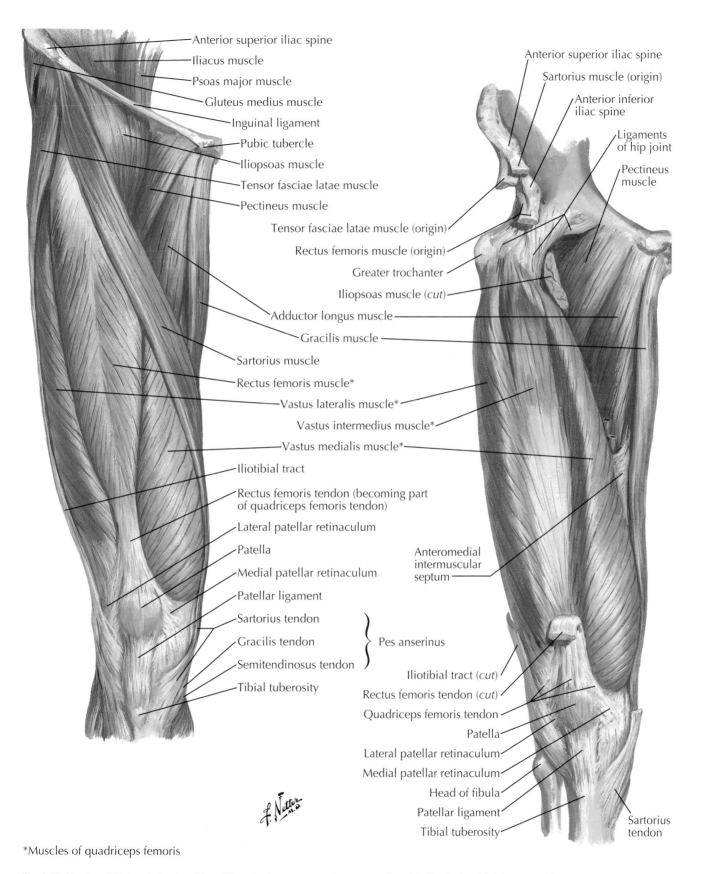

Anterior superior iliac spine
Iliacus muscle
Psoas major muscle
Gluteus medius muscle
Inguinal ligament
Pubic tubercle
Iliopsoas muscle
Tensor fasciae latae muscle
Pectineus muscle
Tensor fasciae latae muscle (origin)
Rectus femoris muscle (origin)
Greater trochanter
Iliopsoas muscle (*cut*)
Adductor longus muscle
Gracilis muscle
Sartorius muscle
Rectus femoris muscle*
Vastus lateralis muscle*
Vastus intermedius muscle*
Vastus medialis muscle*
Iliotibial tract
Rectus femoris tendon (becoming part
of quadriceps femoris tendon)
Lateral patellar retinaculum
Patella
Medial patellar retinaculum
Patellar ligament
Sartorius tendon
Gracilis tendon   } Pes anserinus
Semitendinosus tendon
Tibial tuberosity

Anterior superior iliac spine
Sartorius muscle (origin)
Anterior inferior
iliac spine
Ligaments
of hip joint
Pectineus
muscle

Anteromedial
intermuscular
septum

Iliotibial tract (*cut*)
Rectus femoris tendon (*cut*)
Quadriceps femoris tendon
Patella
Lateral patellar retinaculum
Medial patellar retinaculum
Head of fibula
Patellar ligament
Tibial tuberosity
Sartorius
tendon

*Muscles of quadriceps femoris

Fig. 1.15 Muscles of thigh: anterior view. (Netter illustration from www.netterimages.com. Copyright Elsevier Inc. All rights reserved.)

Muscles of Hip and Thigh

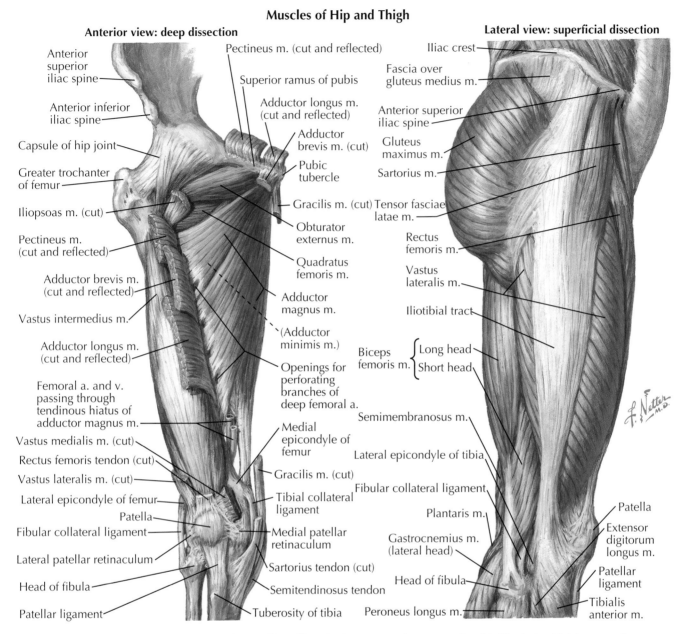

Fig. 1.16 Muscles of the thigh, deep dissection: anterior view. (Netter illustration from www.netterimages.com. Copyright Elsevier Inc. All rights reserved.)

and enters Hunter's canal, a fibromuscular canal bounded laterally by the vastus medialis, inferiorly by the adductor longus and magnus, and anteromedially by the sartorius. The femoral artery exits Hunter's canal through the adductor hiatus, entering the popliteal fossa, at which point its name changes to the popliteal artery.

In the proximal thigh, the femoral artery bifurcates 4 cm inferior to the inguinal ligament into the profunda femoris (also called the deep femoral artery) and the superficial femoral artery. Although there is some debate over the terminology of the femoral artery's origin and distal progression, it is usually described as follows: the external iliac artery becomes the femoral artery after it crosses the inguinal

ligament, then the femoral artery branches into the profunda femoris and the superficial femoral artery. The profunda femoris usually branches from the posterolateral aspect of the femoral artery then passes deep to the adductor longus muscle, between the insertions of the lateral and medial intermuscular septa, and runs posterior to the linea aspera of the femur (*Figs 1.11 and 1.18*).

Profunda femoris

In the thigh, the profunda femoris is the predominant blood supply source. There are some important contributions to thigh musculature by the superficial femoral artery (the

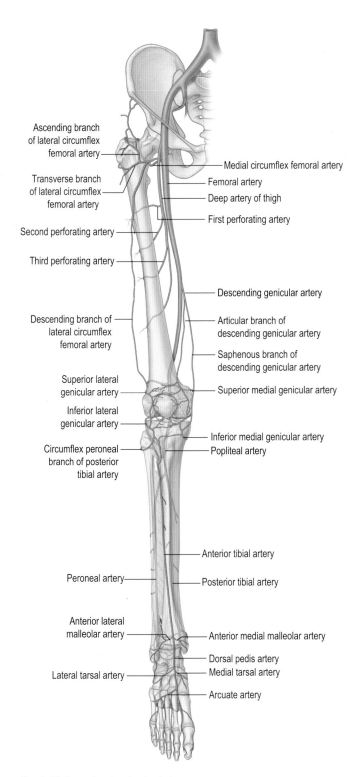

Ascending branch
of lateral circumflex
femoral artery

Transverse branch
of lateral circumflex
femoral artery

Second perforating artery

Third perforating artery

Descending branch of
lateral circumflex
femoral artery

Superior lateral
genicular artery

Inferior lateral
genicular artery

Circumflex peroneal
branch of posterior
tibial artery

Peroneal artery

Anterior lateral
malleolar artery

Lateral tarsal artery

Medial circumflex femoral artery

Femoral artery

Deep artery of thigh

First perforating artery

Descending genicular artery

Articular branch of
descending genicular artery

Saphenous branch of
descending genicular artery

Superior medial genicular artery

Inferior medial genicular artery

Popliteal artery

Anterior tibial artery

Posterior tibial artery

Anterior medial malleolar artery

Dorsal pedis artery
Medial tarsal artery

Arcuate artery

Fig. 1.17 Femoral and profunda arteries.

adductors, sartorius, and the vastus medialis) but the main vascular distribution for the three thigh compartment arises from the profunda femoris. The majority of the pedicles to thigh musculature arise in the proximal two-thirds of the thigh from the six major branches of the profunda femoris: the lateral and medial circumflex arteries and four perforating arteries *(Fig. 1.18)*.

Lateral circumflex femoral arterial system

The lateral circumflex femoral arterial system is particularly relevant to the reconstructive surgeon due to the number of harvest tissue options that have been developed based on it. The traditional description of the lateral circumflex femoral artery is as the second major branch of the profunda femoris that winds superolaterally and divides into three branches at the lateral border of the femoral triangle, namely, the ascending, transverse, and descending branch *(Fig. 1.19)*. The ascending branch travels along the intertrochanteric line, supplying the greater trochanter, the tensor fascia latae, anterior iliac crest, and the skin overlying the hip before connecting with the superior gluteal and deep circumflex iliac vessels. The transverse branch passes through the vastus lateralis and curls posteriorly around the femur, joining with the medial circumflex. The descending branch usually travels in the intermuscular septum between the vastus intermedius and the overlying rectus femoris. From these branches, cutaneous perforators either travel through the musculature (musculocutaneous perforators) or between the musculature along the intervening fibrous septa (septocutaneous perforators).

There is great variability in the lateral circumflex femoral artery system and the traditional description of the location of the vessels and their courses does not always hold. Greater than 20% of persons have the take-off of the lateral circumflex femoral artery in a different location from the profunda femoris. It can arise from the femoral artery itself (16%), present as a split artery traveling from the femoral artery and the profunda femoris separately (3%), from a common origin for the profunda femoris and the medial circumflex femoral artery (MCFA) (5%), from the MCFA itself (5%), or separate branches of the lateral circumflex femoral artery can develop from multiple other sites (4%).

The number, size, position, and course of the cutaneous perforators that emanate from the lateral circumflex femoral artery are also variable but still follow generalized patterns which are used to exploit this versatile arterial system. The most common pattern of lateral circumflex femoral artery limbs is three arterial branches: (1) ascending; (2) transverse (also termed oblique); and (3) descending. The position and take-off of these branches can also demonstrate great variability.

In spite of this multiplicity of anatomic variations, this system provides a robust interconnected blood supply to skin, muscle, fascia, and bone. This can be exploited for a plethora of flap compositions in a variety of orientations. In the particularly complex wound, the harvest of lateral circumflex femoral artery system can be designed to encompass composite flaps with multiple tissue types. If the lateral circumflex femoral artery system is properly dissected, a composite flap or rectus femoris, anterolateral skin and fascia, tensor fascia latae muscle, and iliac crest bone can be fashioned *(Fig. 1.20)*.

Medial circumflex femoral arterial system

The MCFA is typically the first major thigh-supplying branch off the femoral artery. The MCFA emerges from the medial and posterior aspect of the profunda, and winds around the medial side of the femur. It then passes between the pectineus and psoas major, and then between the obturator externus

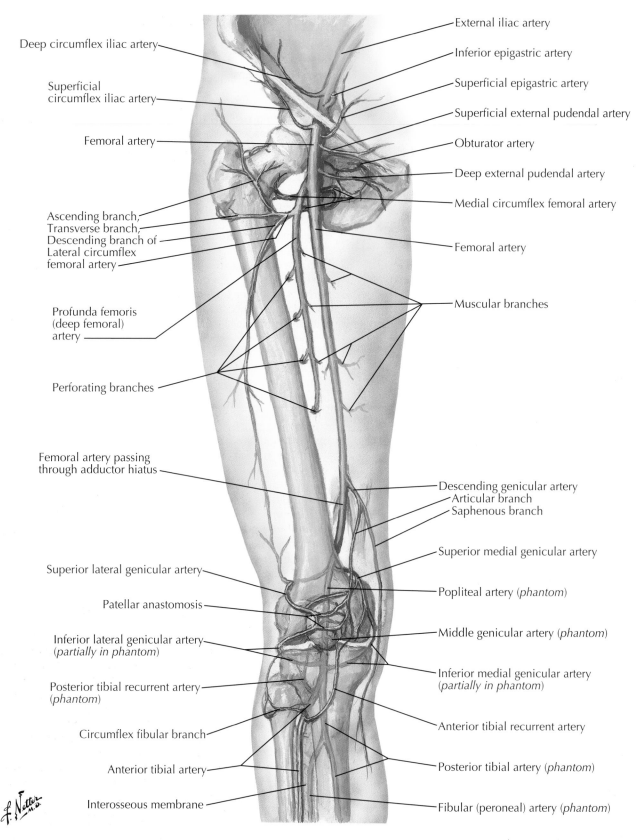

Deep circumflex iliac artery

Superficial circumflex iliac artery

Femoral artery

Ascending branch,
Transverse branch,
Descending branch of
Lateral circumflex
femoral artery

Profunda femoris
(deep femoral)
artery

Perforating branches

Femoral artery passing
through adductor hiatus

Superior lateral genicular artery

Patellar anastomosis

Inferior lateral genicular artery
(partially in phantom)

Posterior tibial recurrent artery
(phantom)

Circumflex fibular branch

Anterior tibial artery

Interosseous membrane

External iliac artery

Inferior epigastric artery

Superficial epigastric artery

Superficial external pudendal artery

Obturator artery

Deep external pudendal artery

Medial circumflex femoral artery

Femoral artery

Muscular branches

Descending genicular artery
Articular branch
Saphenous branch

Superior medial genicular artery

Popliteal artery (phantom)

Middle genicular artery (phantom)

Inferior medial genicular artery
(partially in phantom)

Anterior tibial recurrent artery

Posterior tibial artery (phantom)

Fibular (peroneal) artery (phantom)

Fig. 1.18 Arteries of thigh and knee: schema. (Netter illustration from www.netterimages.com. Copyright Elsevier Inc. All rights reserved.)

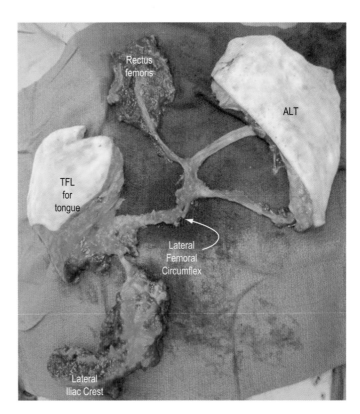

Fig. 1.20 Lateral circumflex femoral artery system. (Courtesy of Lawrence Gottlieb.)

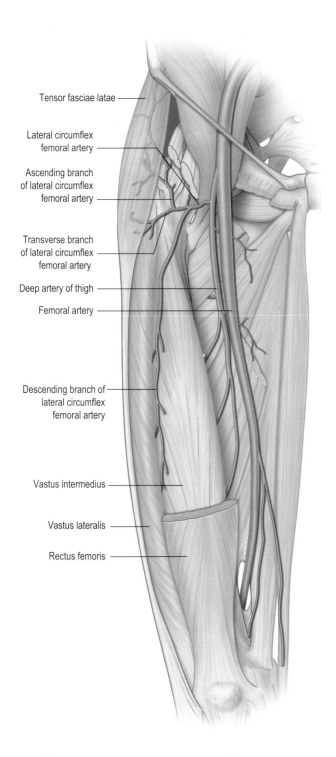

Fig. 1.19 Lateral circumflex femoral artery (LCFA). TFL, tensor fascia lata.

and the adductor brevis to supply the adductor compartment *(Fig. 1.21)*. As the artery passes between the quadratus femoris and the adductor magnus it splits into descending and transverse branches. The transverse branch passes posteriorly to the femur and joins the transverse branch of the lateral circumflex and the inferior gluteal artery, known as the cruciate

connection. The descending branch of the MCFA branches into several muscular branches to supply the gracilis muscle in most cases. The MCFA system mirrors the lateral circumflex femoral artery as a nexus of branches that supply multiple different muscles and cutaneous regions but branches of the MCFA are smaller than those of the lateral circumflex femoral artery.

Profunda femoris perforating branches

There are typically four perforating branches (counting the terminal extent as one branch) of the profunda femoris that arise distal to the circumflex arteries. Their name is derived from the course of the vessels traveling posteriorly near the linea aspera of the femur. These vessels perforate the tendon of the adductor magnus under small tendinous arches to supply the posterior thigh. The first perforating branches emerge from the profunda femoris above the adductor brevis, the second from in front of the adductor, and the third immediately below it. The distal aspect of the profunda becomes the fourth perforator *(Fig. 1.21)*. The first perforating branch supplies the adductor brevis, adductor magnus, biceps femoris, and gluteus maximus. The second perforating branch is larger than the first and divides into an ascending and descending branch. These branches supply the entire posterior-compartment muscles and are the source for the nutrient endosteal blood supply to the femoral bone. The third and fourth perforating branches also supply the posterior femoral muscles and join with branches of the MCFA and the popliteal artery.

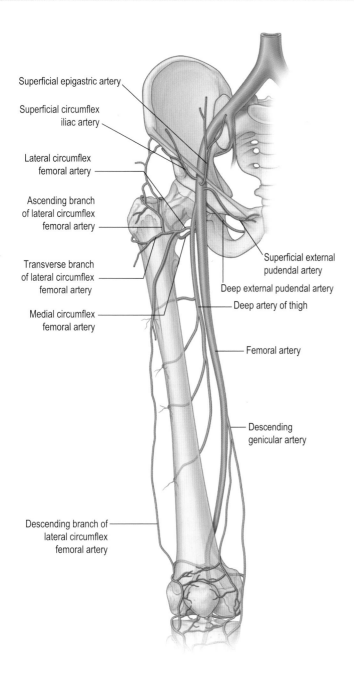

Superficial epigastric artery

Superficial circumflex
iliac artery

Lateral circumflex
femoral artery

Ascending branch
of lateral circumflex
femoral artery

Transverse branch
of lateral circumflex
femoral artery

Medial circumflex
femoral artery

Superficial external
pudendal artery

Deep external pudendal artery

Deep artery of thigh

Femoral artery

Descending
genicular artery

Descending branch of
lateral circumflex
femoral artery

Fig. 1.21 Profunda femoris perforating branches.

Innervation of the thigh

Motor innervation

The nerve supply of the compartments in the thigh follows a "one compartment, one nerve" pattern. The femoral nerve supplies the anterior compartment, the obturator nerve supplies the medial compartment, and the sciatic nerve supplies the musculature of the posterior compartment. Innervation to the thigh is derived originally from the lumbar and sacral plexuses. The femoral nerve, arising from the L2–L4 nerve

roots, passes beneath the inguinal ligament and splits into anterior and posterior divisions around the lateral femoral circumflex artery *(Fig. 1.22)*. The anterior division supplies muscular innervation to the sartorius and gives off the intermediate and medial cutaneous nerves of the thigh. The posterior division of the femoral nerve provides motor innervation to the quadriceps, sensory fibers to the knee joint, and also gives rise to the saphenous nerve. The obturator nerve, also arising from the L2–L4 spinal roots, enters the thigh through the obturator foramen and splits into anterior and posterior branches. The anterior branch of the obturator nerve provides motor innervation to the adductor longus brevis and gracilis, and sensory innervation to the hip joint, and communicates with the saphenous nerve to innervate the medial leg. The posterior branch of the obturator nerve innervates the adductor magnus and occasionally brevis, and supplies sensory innervation to a portion of the knee joint capsule. The sciatic nerve is the largest nerve in the body, arising from the L4–S3 nerve roots and entering the thigh through the sciatic foramen inferior to the piriformis *(Fig. 1.23)*. It divides into its two major components, the tibial and the common peroneal nerve, at a variable point within the thigh. The tibial nerve supplies all hamstring muscles with the exception of the short head of the biceps femoris, which is innervated by the common peroneal nerve.

Cutaneous innervation

The cutaneous innervation of the thigh is shared by two pure cutaneous nerves directly branching from the lumbosacral plexus (lateral and posterior femoral cutaneous nerves) and cutaneous branches from two mixed nerves (femoral and obturator) *(Figs 1.22–1.24)*. The lateral femoral cutaneous nerve arises from the dorsal branches of the second and third lumbar rami. It travels from intra-abdominal and behind the descending colon to exit to the thigh underneath or through the inguinal ligament. The lateral femoral cutaneous nerve divides into an anterior and posterior branch. The anterior branch pierces the fascia lata and becomes superficial ~10 cm below the anterior superior iliac spine. The posterior branch pierces the fascia lata more superiorly than the anterior branch. The posterior branch supplies the cutaneous region around the greater trochanter and midthigh. The anterior branch supplies the anterolateral skin of the thigh down to the knee.

The posterior femoral cutaneous nerve arises from the first and second sacral rami. It leaves the pelvis via the greater sciatic foramen and descends distally under the gluteus maximus with the inferior gluteal vessels. It travels down the thigh superficial to the long head of the biceps femoris but still under the fascia lata. It pierces the deep fascia behind the knee and continues down to the midcalf where its terminal branches communicate and contribute to the sural nerve. The posterior femoral cutaneous nerve supplies the majority of the posterior thigh skin via branches that pierce the fascia lata to travel superficially. The skin over the popliteal fossa is also supplied by the posterior femoral cutaneous nerve.

The femoral nerve course has been described previously. Its anterior division supplies the medial superior and inferior thigh skin by way of the intermediate cutaneous and medial cutaneous nerve of the thigh. The obturator nerve arises from the second to fourth lumbar rami. It exits the pelvis, initially

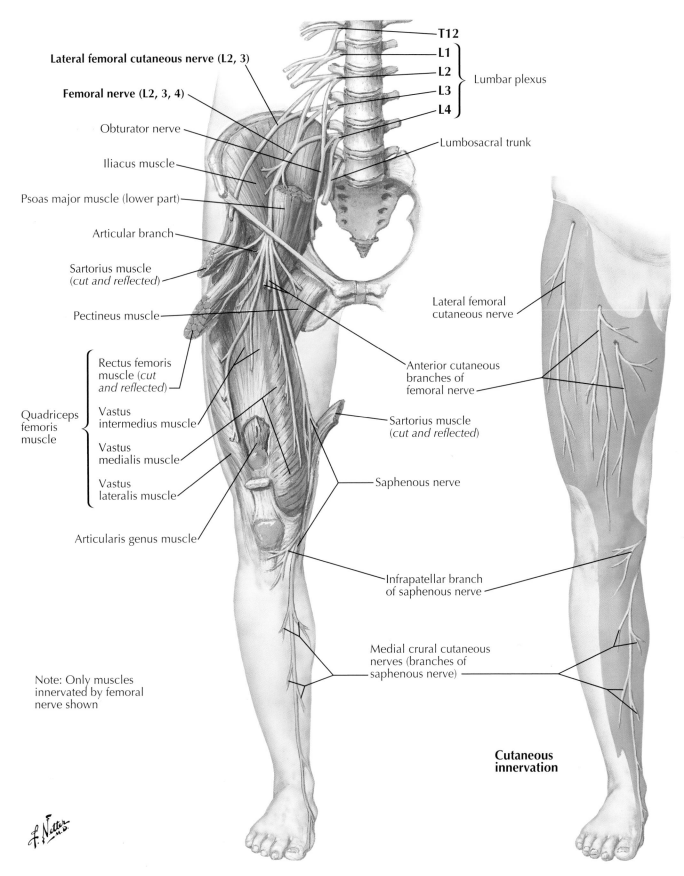

Lateral femoral cutaneous nerve (L2, 3)

Femoral nerve (L2, 3, 4)

Obturator nerve

Iliacus muscle

Psoas major muscle (lower part)

Articular branch

Sartorius muscle
(*cut and reflected*)

Pectineus muscle

Rectus femoris
muscle (*cut
and reflected*)

Quadriceps
femoris
muscle

Vastus
intermedius muscle

Vastus
medialis muscle

Vastus
lateralis muscle

Articularis genus muscle

Note: Only muscles
innervated by femoral
nerve shown

T12

L1

L2

L3

L4

Lumbar plexus

Lumbosacral trunk

Lateral femoral
cutaneous nerve

Anterior cutaneous
branches of
femoral nerve

Sartorius muscle
(*cut and reflected*)

Saphenous nerve

Infrapatellar branch
of saphenous nerve

Medial crural cutaneous
nerves (branches of
saphenous nerve)

**Cutaneous
innervation**

Fig. 1.22 Femoral nerve and lateral cutaneous femoral nerves. (Netter illustration from www.netterimages.com. Copyright Elsevier Inc. All rights reserved.)

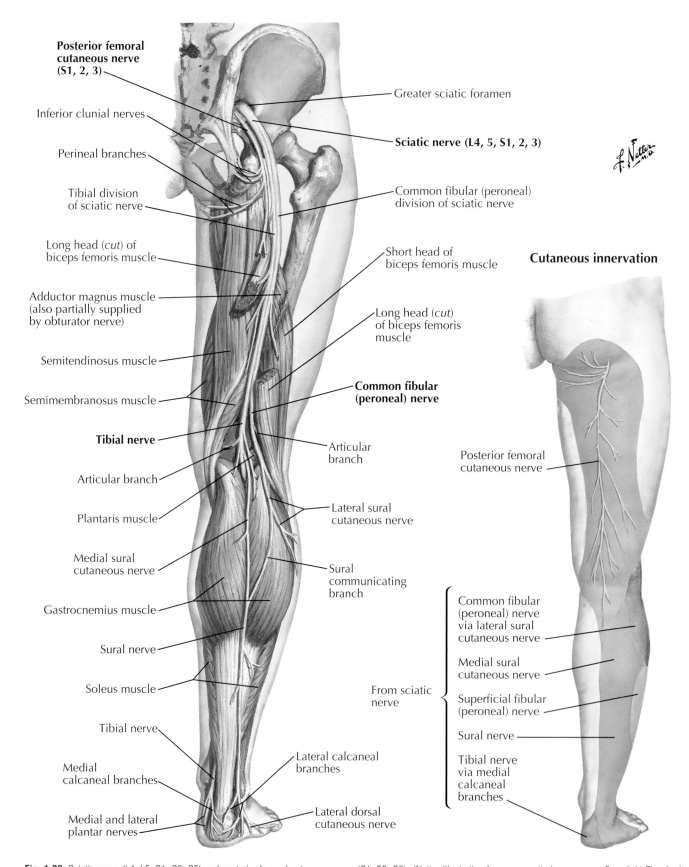

Posterior femoral cutaneous nerve (S1, 2, 3)

Inferior clunial nerves

Perineal branches

Tibial division of sciatic nerve

Long head (cut) of biceps femoris muscle

Adductor magnus muscle (also partially supplied by obturator nerve)

Semitendinosus muscle

Semimembranosus muscle

Tibial nerve

Articular branch

Plantaris muscle

Medial sural cutaneous nerve

Gastrocnemius muscle

Sural nerve

Soleus muscle

Tibial nerve

Medial calcaneal branches

Medial and lateral plantar nerves

Greater sciatic foramen

Sciatic nerve (L4, 5, S1, 2, 3)

Common fibular (peroneal) division of sciatic nerve

Short head of biceps femoris muscle

Long head (cut) of biceps femoris muscle

Common fibular (peroneal) nerve

Articular branch

Lateral sural cutaneous nerve

Sural communicating branch

Lateral calcaneal branches

Lateral dorsal cutaneous nerve

Cutaneous innervation

Posterior femoral cutaneous nerve

From sciatic nerve

Common fibular (peroneal) nerve via lateral sural cutaneous nerve

Medial sural cutaneous nerve

Superficial fibular (peroneal) nerve

Sural nerve

Tibial nerve via medial calcaneal branches

F. Netter m.d.

Fig. 1.23 Sciatic nerve (L4, L5; S1, S2, S3) and posterior femoral cutaneous nerve (S1, S2, S3). (Netter illustration from www.netterimages.com. Copyright Elsevier Inc. All rights reserved.)

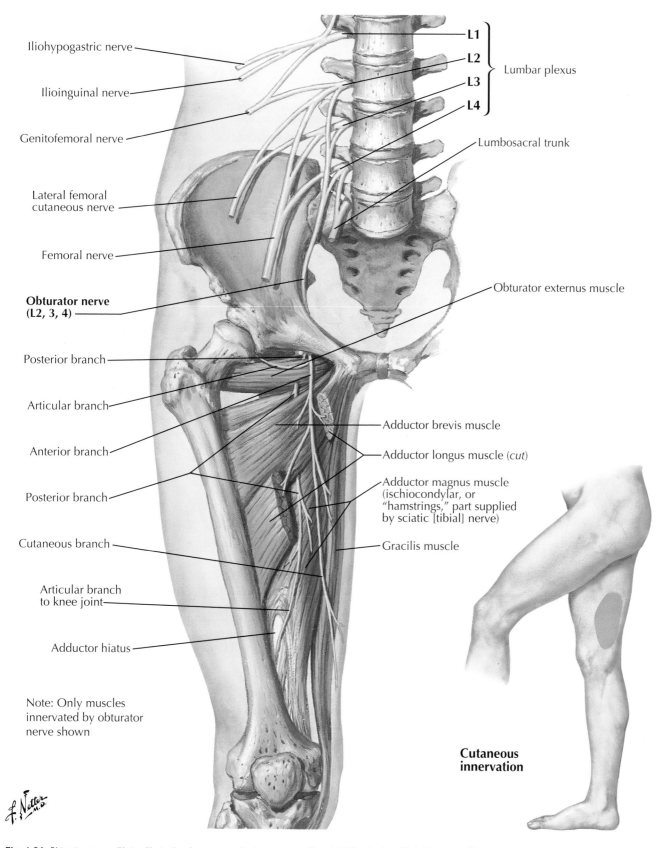

Iliohypogastric nerve

Ilioinguinal nerve

Genitofemoral nerve

Lateral femoral cutaneous nerve

Femoral nerve

Obturator nerve (L2, 3, 4)

Posterior branch

Articular branch

Anterior branch

Posterior branch

Cutaneous branch

Articular branch to knee joint

Adductor hiatus

Note: Only muscles innervated by obturator nerve shown

L1
L2
L3
L4
Lumbar plexus

Lumbosacral trunk

Obturator externus muscle

Adductor brevis muscle

Adductor longus muscle (*cut*)

Adductor magnus muscle (ischiocondylar, or "hamstrings," part supplied by sciatic [tibial] nerve)

Gracilis muscle

Cutaneous innervation

Fig. 1.24 Obturator nerve. (Netter illustration from www.netterimages.com. Copyright Elsevier Inc. All rights reserved.)

descending within the psoas major then finally through the obturator foramen, anterosuperior to the obturator vessels. It branches into an anterior and posterior division. The branches off the anterior division give cutaneous innervation to the inferomedial thigh *(Fig. 1.24)*.

The leg

As the lower extremity extends from the thigh to the leg, the anatomic structures narrow significantly and switch from primarily hip and knee function to ankle and foot movement. The knee and the ankle are the apices of the conical construction of the thigh and the leg which encompass the termini of their musculotendinous structures. As one travels distally on the leg, the tissues become more compact and intricate. The amount of redundant soft tissue that was present in the thigh is not available in the leg; there is also less redundancy of similar functioning muscles. These issues make the leg more of a target of tissue reconstruction rather than the source of harvest tissue.

Knee and leg skeletal structure

Knee skeletal structure

The knee is the largest synovial joint in the body. It is such, because it is comprised of the largest long bone of the body (femur) and the largest sesamoid bone (patella). The quadriceps tendon is invested in the patella. The tendons of the vastus lateralis, vastus medialis, vastus intermedialis, and rectus femoris all come to a confluence at the superior surface of the patella. Even though they join together to form the quadriceps tendon, each has a slightly specific location of insertion on the patella. The quadriceps tendon extensor system has fibers that envelop the patella and help form the patellar tendon which courses distally to insert on the tibial tuberosity *(Fig. 1.25)*. The primary functional role of the patella is to assist in knee extension. The patella augments the leverage of the quadriceps extensor system by increasing the moment arm of its line of pull. The presence of the patella amplifies the extensor force by 30%.

The knee is comprised of two joints, the patellofemoral and the tibiofemoral joint. The patellofemoral joint assists in producing leg flexion and extension at the tibiofemoral joint. In addition to flexion and extension, varying degrees of active medial to lateral rotation are possible at the knee. The tibiofemoral joint is a bicompartmental synovial joint whose stability and range of motion are governed by a complex interplay between the bony anatomy and its soft-tissue constraints. The femoral condyles, their articular surfaces on the tibia, and the intercondylar regions are all uniquely and asymmetrically shaped. This gives the knee lateral translocation and rotational movement beyond any hinge joint. The soft-tissue elements of the knee restrain excess motion but allow for wide latitude in mobility, as well as supporting and cushioning the weight-bearing bony components. The medial (tibial) collateral, lateral (fibular) collateral ligament, posterior cruciate, anterior cruciate, popliteofibular, transverse, coronary, and tibiofibular ligaments all work in cooperation with the muscular attachments to provide knee joint stability *(Fig. 1.26)*. The medial and lateral menisci are semilunar cartilaginous structures arranged in crescentic laminae that deepen the articulation surface on the tibia that receives the femoral condyles *(Fig. 1.27)*. The menisci are connected to the surrounding peripheral ligament structures and further stabilize the knee as well as buttress the femoral weight-bearing load *(Fig. 1.27)*.

Even though it is not a direct component of the knee, the tibiofibular joint contributes to leg operation. The main functions of the proximal tibiofibular joint are distributing torsional stresses applied to the ankle during bending movements, and resisting tensile forces creating with weight-bearing. Although not a significant contributor to weight-bearing, the tibiofibular joint accepts one-sixth of the axial load of the leg.

The terminal insertion of the knee-extending quadriceps muscle is the tibial tuberosity. The quadriceps muscles coalesce to the quadriceps tendon, encircle the patella, and then insert on the smooth proximal region of the tibial tuberosity as the patellar tendon. The tibial tuberosity is a small, raised triangular area where the anterior condylar surfaces merge. The pull of the quadriceps is lateral to the midline movement of the patellofemoral joint; this is due to the medial location of the tibia in relation to the femur.

The shafts of both the tibia and the fibula form triangular-type shapes when viewed from a cross-section cut. The apex of the tibia is oriented anteriorly with a smooth curvilinear medial surface and a shelf-like lateral surface that brackets the lateral compartment musculature. The triangular apex of the fibula is oriented lateral and 90° to that of the tibia. The interosseous membrane crosses the leg in the anterior one-third area and is attached between the interosseous crests of the tibia and the fibula *(Fig. 1.28)*.

Leg skeletal structure

The vascular supply to the tibia and fibula is provided from multiple sources. The tibia receives major endosteal vascularity through the proximal nutrient foramen that lies near the soleal line. The soleal line is an obliquely oriented bony ridge in the posterior superior aspect of the tibia, coursing from the tibia articulation with the fibula inferiorly to the medial edge of the tibia at the border between its middle and upper thirds. This ridge is the insertion site of the popliteus and the origin of the soleus, flexor digitorum longus, and tibialis posterior muscles *(Fig. 1.29)*. The endosteal blood supply to the tibia enters this area after branching off the posterior tibial artery as it exits the popliteal fossa. Alternatively, this tibial nutritive branch may also stem from the popliteal bifurcation of the anterior tibial artery and the tibioperoneal trunk. The periosteal supply to the tibial shaft arises from multiple segmental branches directly from the anterior tibial artery and from perforating branches from the surrounding musculature. The distal domain of the tibia is supplied by branches from the connection around the ankle between the peroneal and posterior tibial vessels.

The fibula receives its endosteal blood supply for the shaft region from a branch of the peroneal artery that enters the bone through a nutrient foramen in the middle one-third of the shaft with most of the foramen positioned at the midpoint of the bone. Most commonly there is only one nutrient vessel but less than 10% of the population may have two or more.

Knee Joint

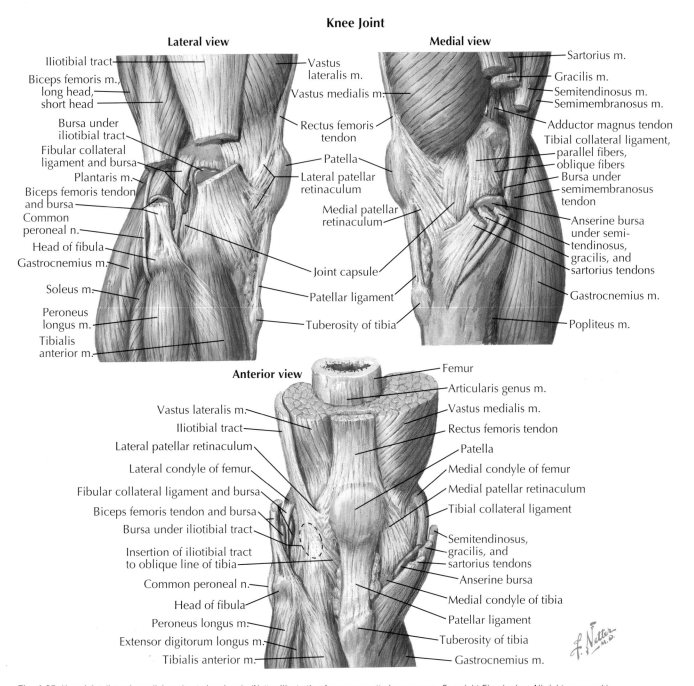

Lateral view

Iliotibial tract
Biceps femoris m., long head, short head
Bursa under iliotibial tract
Fibular collateral ligament and bursa
Plantaris m.
Biceps femoris tendon and bursa
Common peroneal n.
Head of fibula
Gastrocnemius m.
Soleus m.
Peroneus longus m.
Tibialis anterior m.

Vastus lateralis m.
Vastus medialis m.
Rectus femoris tendon
Patella
Lateral patellar retinaculum
Medial patellar retinaculum
Joint capsule
Patellar ligament
Tuberosity of tibia

Medial view

Sartorius m.
Gracilis m.
Semitendinosus m.
Semimembranosus m.
Adductor magnus tendon
Tibial collateral ligament, parallel fibers, oblique fibers
Bursa under semimembranosus tendon
Anserine bursa under semitendinosus, gracilis, and sartorius tendons
Gastrocnemius m.
Popliteus m.

Anterior view

Vastus lateralis m.
Iliotibial tract
Lateral patellar retinaculum
Lateral condyle of femur
Fibular collateral ligament and bursa
Biceps femoris tendon and bursa
Bursa under iliotibial tract
Insertion of iliotibial tract to oblique line of tibia
Common peroneal n.
Head of fibula
Peroneus longus m.
Extensor digitorum longus m.
Tibialis anterior m.

Femur
Articularis genus m.
Vastus medialis m.
Rectus femoris tendon
Patella
Medial condyle of femur
Medial patellar retinaculum
Tibial collateral ligament
Semitendinosus, gracilis, and sartorius tendons
Anserine bursa
Medial condyle of tibia
Patellar ligament
Tuberosity of tibia
Gastrocnemius m.

Fig. 1.25 Knee joint (lateral, medial, and anterior views). (Netter illustration from www.netterimages.com. Copyright Elsevier Inc. All rights reserved.)

Right knee in flexion: anterior view

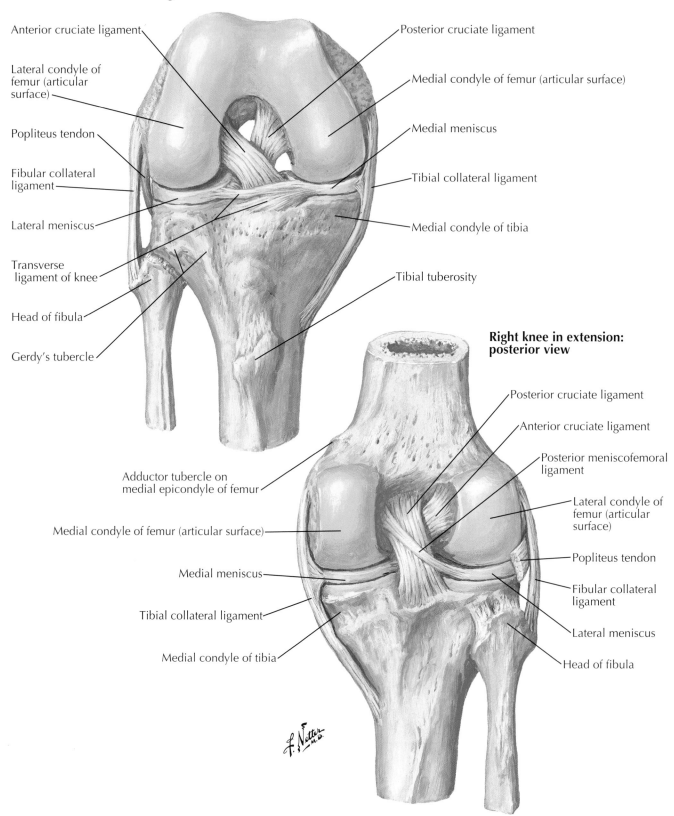

Anterior cruciate ligament

Lateral condyle of femur (articular surface)

Popliteus tendon

Fibular collateral ligament

Lateral meniscus

Transverse ligament of knee

Head of fibula

Gerdy's tubercle

Posterior cruciate ligament

Medial condyle of femur (articular surface)

Medial meniscus

Tibial collateral ligament

Medial condyle of tibia

Tibial tuberosity

Right knee in extension: posterior view

Adductor tubercle on medial epicondyle of femur

Medial condyle of femur (articular surface)

Medial meniscus

Tibial collateral ligament

Medial condyle of tibia

Posterior cruciate ligament

Anterior cruciate ligament

Posterior meniscofemoral ligament

Lateral condyle of femur (articular surface)

Popliteus tendon

Fibular collateral ligament

Lateral meniscus

Head of fibula

Fig. 1.26 Knee: cruciate and collateral ligaments. (Netter illustration from www.netterimages.com. Copyright Elsevier Inc. All rights reserved.)

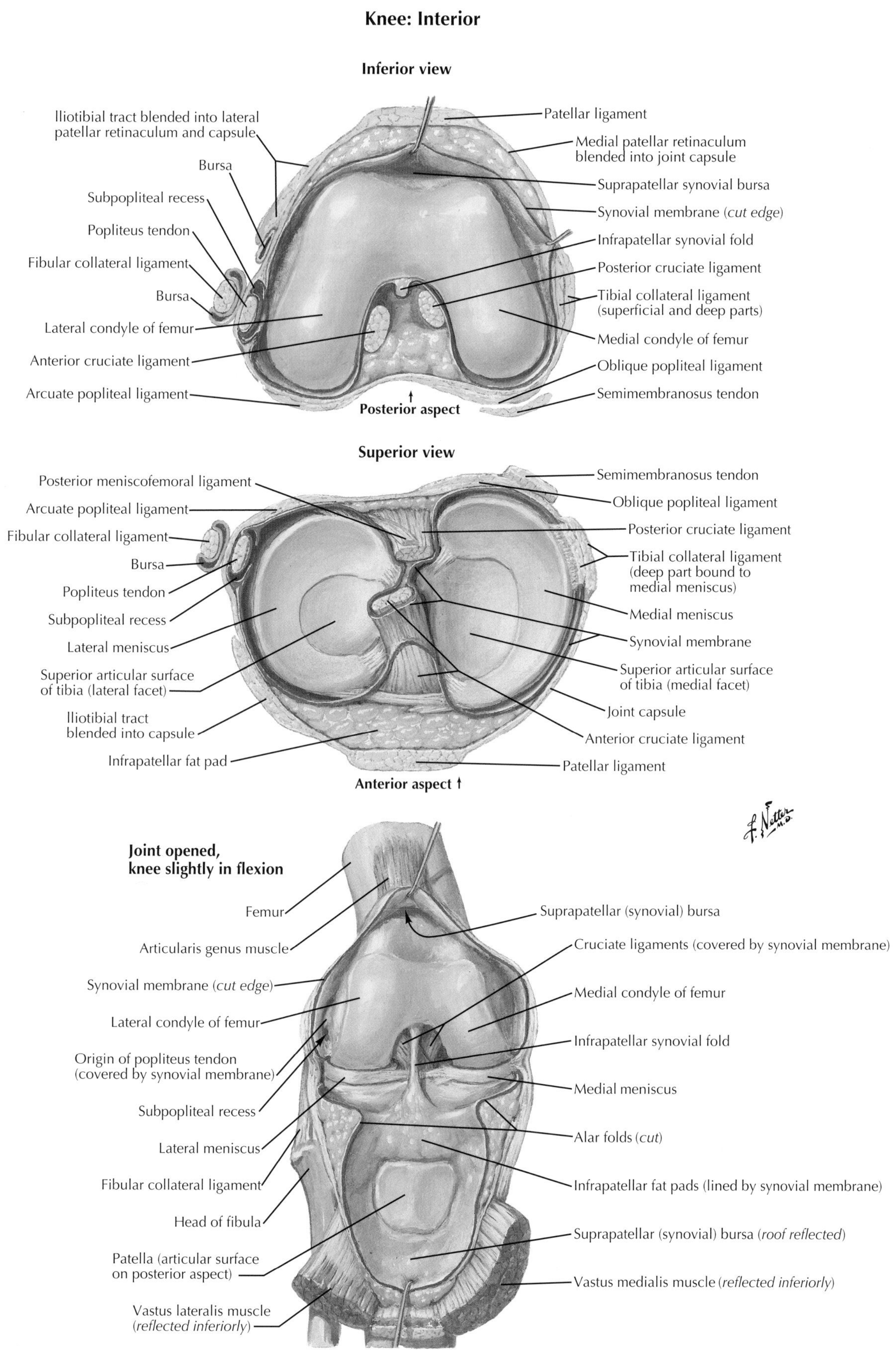

Knee: Interior

Inferior view

Iliotibial tract blended into lateral patellar retinaculum and capsule

Bursa

Subpopliteal recess

Popliteus tendon

Fibular collateral ligament

Bursa

Lateral condyle of femur

Anterior cruciate ligament

Arcuate popliteal ligament

Patellar ligament

Medial patellar retinaculum blended into joint capsule

Suprapatellar synovial bursa

Synovial membrane (*cut edge*)

Infrapatellar synovial fold

Posterior cruciate ligament

Tibial collateral ligament (superficial and deep parts)

Medial condyle of femur

Oblique popliteal ligament

Semimembranosus tendon

Posterior aspect ↑

Superior view

Posterior meniscofemoral ligament

Arcuate popliteal ligament

Fibular collateral ligament

Bursa

Popliteus tendon

Subpopliteal recess

Lateral meniscus

Superior articular surface of tibia (lateral facet)

Iliotibial tract blended into capsule

Infrapatellar fat pad

Semimembranosus tendon

Oblique popliteal ligament

Posterior cruciate ligament

Tibial collateral ligament (deep part bound to medial meniscus)

Medial meniscus

Synovial membrane

Superior articular surface of tibia (medial facet)

Joint capsule

Anterior cruciate ligament

Patellar ligament

Anterior aspect ↑

Joint opened, knee slightly in flexion

Femur

Articularis genus muscle

Synovial membrane (*cut edge*)

Lateral condyle of femur

Origin of popliteus tendon (covered by synovial membrane)

Subpopliteal recess

Lateral meniscus

Fibular collateral ligament

Head of fibula

Patella (articular surface on posterior aspect)

Vastus lateralis muscle (*reflected inferiorly*)

Suprapatellar (synovial) bursa

Cruciate ligaments (covered by synovial membrane)

Medial condyle of femur

Infrapatellar synovial fold

Medial meniscus

Alar folds (*cut*)

Infrapatellar fat pads (lined by synovial membrane)

Suprapatellar (synovial) bursa (*roof reflected*)

Vastus medialis muscle (*reflected inferiorly*)

Fig. 1.27 Knee: interior (interior, superior, and anterior views). (Netter illustration from www.netterimages.com. Copyright Elsevier Inc. All rights reserved.)

Anterior view with ligament attachments

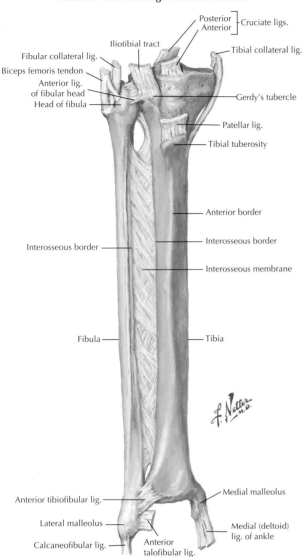

Fig. 1.28 Tibia and fibula. (Netter illustration from www.netterimages.com. Copyright Elsevier Inc. All rights reserved.)

The nutritive branch enters the fibula on the posteromedial surface, posterior to the interosseous membrane. The fibula also receives a periosteal blood supply from multiple branches from the peroneal artery. The fibular head receives a separate blood supply. The anterior tibial artery gives off recurrent branches and both the inferior lateral genicular arteries may supply the fibular head and neck. The distal metaphyseal region of the fibula is supplied by the ankle connection between the peroneal and posterior tibial vessels similar to the distal tibia.

Leg fascial composition

The fascial structure of the leg is in continuation with the fascial system of the thigh, which in turn is contiguous with some of the major fascial components of the abdomen. The superficial fascia of the leg lies within the subcutaneous

tissue. It is often present in two or more layers of areolar tissue but the layers can also be densely adherent and appear as one. Within these layers lie the superficial vessels and nerves. In the leg, the great and lesser saphenous veins and the sural and saphenous nerve travel along the superficial fascia (*Fig. 1.30*).

Deep fascia of the leg

The deep fascia of the leg (also called the investing fascia or fascia cruris) encircles and constrains the whole leg musculature. The deep fascia is actually a continuation of the fascia lata of the thigh and receives fascia expansions from the tendons of the extensor and flexor knee muscle retinacula. The deep fascia varies in thickness in different regions and is closely attached to the tissue structures just beneath it. Proximally, it is attached to the patellar tendon, tibial tuberosity and condyles, and the head of the fibula. On the posterior aspect of the leg, the deep fascia is thickened by transverse fibers over the popliteal fossa and is termed the popliteal fascia. In this region, the lesser saphenous vein and the sural nerve penetrate the fascia from superficial to deep as they travel from distal in the subcutaneous space to deep between the muscular heads of the gastrocnemius (*Fig. 1.9*). The medial aspect is adherent to the tibial periosteum. The anterior portion of the deep fascia thickens and fuses with the muscular fascia of the tibialis anterior and the extensor digitorum longus; laterally it covers the peroneus longus. In the posterior leg, the deep fascia thins as it courses over the fascia of the gastrocnemius and the soleus.

Interosseous membrane

The interosseous membrane of the leg (also called the middle tibiofibular ligament) is a band of dense fibrous fibers oriented obliquely that extends between the interosseous crests of the tibia and the fibula (*Fig. 1.30*). It separates the anterior (ankle dorsiflexion) compartment from the posterior (ankle plantarflexion) compartment. The muscles which lie directly on the membrane (anteriorly – tibialis anterior, extensor hallucis longus; posteriorly – tibialis posterior, flexor hallucis longus) use the membrane as a muscular origin site. At the superior aspect of the interosseous membrane is an oval aperture that allows for passage of the anterior tibial vessels traveling from the popliteal bifurcation in the popliteal fossa to the anterior leg. At the inferior edge of the interosseous membrane there is another opening that allows for the passage for perforating branches from the distal peroneal artery. The inferiormost aspect of the interosseous ligament contributes to the interosseous (tibiofibular) ligament. This interosseous ligament is a distinct structure which helps restrain tibiofibular articulation but allows for slight translational movement at the proximal ankle.

Lower leg compartments

When viewing the leg in cross-section, the deep fascia creates a peripheral circle of limiting fibrous tissue with the fibula, tibia, and interosseous membrane as an off-centered, central axis (*Fig. 1.30*). Intermuscular septa radiate from this central axis to the investing deep fascia and divide the leg musculature into compartments. These compartments organize

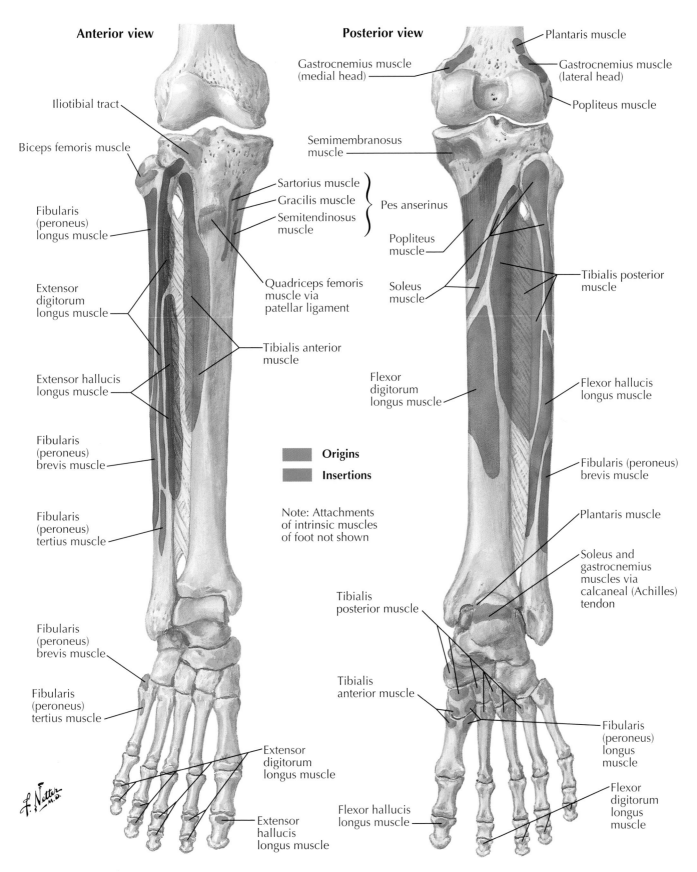

Anterior view

Iliotibial tract

Biceps femoris muscle

Fibularis (peroneus) longus muscle

Extensor digitorum longus muscle

Extensor hallucis longus muscle

Fibularis (peroneus) brevis muscle

Fibularis (peroneus) tertius muscle

Fibularis (peroneus) brevis muscle

Fibularis (peroneus) tertius muscle

Extensor digitorum longus muscle

Extensor hallucis longus muscle

Sartorius muscle
Gracilis muscle
Semitendinosus muscle

} Pes anserinus

Quadriceps femoris muscle via patellar ligament

Tibialis anterior muscle

Origins

Insertions

Note: Attachments of intrinsic muscles of foot not shown

Posterior view

Plantaris muscle

Gastrocnemius muscle (medial head)

Gastrocnemius muscle (lateral head)

Popliteus muscle

Semimembranosus muscle

Popliteus muscle

Soleus muscle

Tibialis posterior muscle

Flexor digitorum longus muscle

Flexor hallucis longus muscle

Fibularis (peroneus) brevis muscle

Plantaris muscle

Soleus and gastrocnemius muscles via calcaneal (Achilles) tendon

Tibialis posterior muscle

Tibialis anterior muscle

Fibularis (peroneus) longus muscle

Flexor digitorum longus muscle

Flexor hallucis longus muscle

Fig. 1.29 Bony attachments of muscles of leg. (Netter illustration from www.netterimages.com. Copyright Elsevier Inc. All rights reserved.)

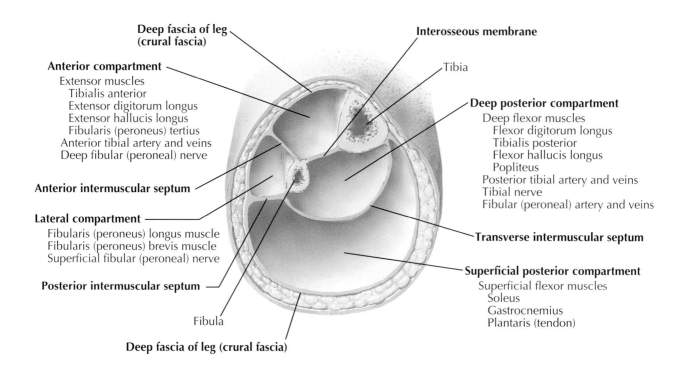

Deep fascia of leg
(crural fascia)

Interosseous membrane

Anterior compartment
  Extensor muscles
    Tibialis anterior
    Extensor digitorum longus
    Extensor hallucis longus
    Fibularis (peroneus) tertius
  Anterior tibial artery and veins
  Deep fibular (peroneal) nerve

Tibia

Deep posterior compartment
  Deep flexor muscles
    Flexor digitorum longus
    Tibialis posterior
    Flexor hallucis longus
    Popliteus
  Posterior tibial artery and veins
  Tibial nerve
  Fibular (peroneal) artery and veins

Anterior intermuscular septum

Lateral compartment
  Fibularis (peroneus) longus muscle
  Fibularis (peroneus) brevis muscle
  Superficial fibular (peroneal) nerve

Transverse intermuscular septum

Superficial posterior compartment
  Superficial flexor muscles
    Soleus
    Gastrocnemius
    Plantaris (tendon)

Posterior intermuscular septum

Fibula

Deep fascia of leg (crural fascia)

Cross section just above middle of leg

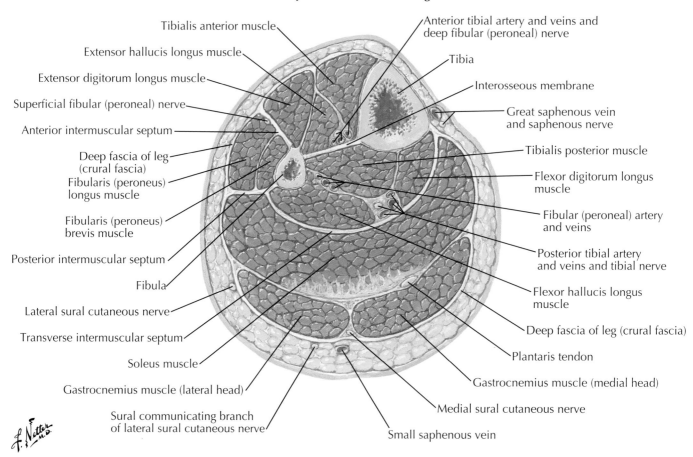

Tibialis anterior muscle

Anterior tibial artery and veins and
deep fibular (peroneal) nerve

Extensor hallucis longus muscle

Tibia

Extensor digitorum longus muscle

Interosseous membrane

Superficial fibular (peroneal) nerve

Great saphenous vein
and saphenous nerve

Anterior intermuscular septum

Deep fascia of leg
(crural fascia)

Tibialis posterior muscle

Fibularis (peroneus)
longus muscle

Flexor digitorum longus
muscle

Fibularis (peroneus)
brevis muscle

Fibular (peroneal) artery
and veins

Posterior intermuscular septum

Posterior tibial artery
and veins and tibial nerve

Fibula

Flexor hallucis longus
muscle

Lateral sural cutaneous nerve

Deep fascia of leg (crural fascia)

Transverse intermuscular septum

Plantaris tendon

Soleus muscle

Gastrocnemius muscle (medial head)

Gastrocnemius muscle (lateral head)

Medial sural cutaneous nerve

Sural communicating branch
of lateral sural cutaneous nerve

Small saphenous vein

Fig. 1.30 Leg: cross-sections and fascial compartments. (Netter illustration from www.netterimages.com. Copyright Elsevier Inc. All rights reserved.)

the lower extremity musculature into similarly functioning groups. The intervening fascia bands also give the muscles increased attachment surfaces and aid in contractile activity.

These intermuscular septa divide the leg into anterior, lateral, and posterior osteofascial compartments. The anterior muscle compartment is cradled by the tibial lateral surface medially and the interosseous membrane as its floor. The roof of the anterior compartment is the deep fascia of the leg and the lateral wall is the intermuscular septum that divides the anterior compartment from the lateral compartment. The lateral compartment, therefore, is located just lateral to the anterior compartment; its floor is the anterior surface of the fibula, the roof is the investing fascia of the leg, and the other wall is the intermuscular septum dividing the lateral from the posterior compartment. The posterior compartment is the largest of the three major osteofascial compartments and lies below the interosseous membrane. The posterior compartment has two subdivisions. The transverse intermuscular septum creates a division line from the lateral deep fascia wall to the medial deep fascia wall separating the posterior compartment into the deep and superficial layers. The superficial layer is then the only compartment that does not have a bony component. The medial surface of the tibia is bare with no muscular peripheral coverage and therefore there is no medial compartment (*Fig. 1.30*).

Compartment syndrome

The functional advantage of osteofascial compartment organization can turn to a clinical liability when the intracompartment volume is pathologically expanded against its minimally expansive fascial borders. Trauma, infection, and intravenous extravasation of liquids can increase compartmental volume through edema, inflammation, and/or direct volume addition. As the volume of a compartment increases, so does the intracompartmental pressure due to the rigid nature of the fascial boundaries. As extravascular, intercompartmental pressure rises above capillary and arterial filling pressure, perfusion and vascular inflow decreases or fails. Tissue ischemia and eventually necrosis of the structures within the compartment ensue. An understanding of the location and architecture of the compartments is essential to adequately treating and preventing compartment syndrome. Because the investing fascia of the leg is thickest on the anterior surface, the anterior compartment is the least expansile of the four major compartments of the leg. The posterior aspect of the investing fascia of the leg is the more pliable; therefore the superficial posterior compartment is much more expansile and slightly less at risk for compartment syndrome than its deeper compatriot.

Leg musculature

Anterior compartment

There are 14 muscles in the lower leg. All muscles except for the popliteus cause range of motion at the ankle, foot, or toes. The composition of the compartments of the leg follows a congruent order. The muscular components of each compartment share similar functions at the ankle and foot (*Table 1.6*). The anterior compartment (extensor compartment) is comprised of the four muscles (tibialis anterior, extensor digitorum longus, extensor hallucis longus, and peroneus tertius), one major artery (anterior tibial), and one major mixed nerve (deep peroneal) (*Figs 1.31 and 1.32*). These muscles of the anterior compartment are responsible for ankle, foot, and toe dorsiflexion (*Table 1.7*). The tibialis anterior is the most superficial muscle in the compartment and originates from lateral tibial condyle, the proximal two-thirds of the tibial shaft, and the interosseous membrane (*Fig. 1.29*). It overlies the anterior tibial vessels and the deep peroneal nerve in the proximal leg. The tibialis anterior proceeds distally and its tendon passes through the medial compartments of the superior and inferior foot extensor retinacula and inserts in the inferomedial surface of the medial cuneiform and the base of the first metacarpal bone (*Fig. 1.33*). Its specific mechanism of action is foot dorsiflexion and inversion. The tibialis receives its blood supply from the anterior tibial artery, usually in branches organized in two columns. These columns give off 8–12 branches and therefore the blood supply to the tibialis anterior muscle is classified as segmental. The extensor digitorum longus lies lateral to the tibialis anterior in the anterior compartment. Its origin is positioned similarly to the tibialis anterior (lateral tibial condyle, the proximal two-thirds of the tibial shaft, and the interosseous membrane). The extensor digitorum longus travels distally in the lateral aspect of the ankle and transitions to tendon at around the same point as the tibialis anterior. It divides into four slips that proceed to the second through fifth toes. Similar to the extensor digitorum in the hand, the extensor digitorum longus has multiple insertion points at the metatarsophalangeal joint and the extensor system of the toes on the dorsal proximal phalanx. The extensor digitorum longus extends the toes, dorsiflexes synergistically with the tibialis anterior and extensor hallucis, as well as everts the foot. It has a segmental blood supply from the anterior tibial artery similar to that of the anterior tibialis. The extensor hallucis longus has the same origin as the extensor digitorum longus but inserts on the base of the distal phalanx of the first toe. Its mechanism of action is dorsiflexion of the first toe and foot. Like all muscles in the anterior compartment, its blood supply is segmental from the anterior tibial artery. This then limits the mobility and arc of rotation of anterior-compartment muscles flaps. The peroneus tertius (also called the fibularis tertius – "third" peroneus or fibula-related muscle) is a muscle unique to the human species. Along with the popliteus, it is the shortest muscle in the leg. The peroneus tertius originates on the distal third of the fibula, below both the peroneus longus and brevis. The peroneus tertius inserts on the base of the fifth metatarsal bone. Its mechanism of action is to work in collaboration with the other muscles of the anterior compartment to dorsiflex and evert the foot, especially during the swing phase of gait. All the muscles of the anterior compartment are innervated by the deep peroneal nerve.

Lateral compartment

The lateral compartment is comprised of only two muscles – the peroneus longus and brevis (*Fig. 1.31 and Table 1.8*). They both originate from and are anatomically related to the fibula – the meaning of the word "peroneus." The peroneus longus

Text continued on page 43

Table 1.6 Leg musculature

	Muscle	Origin	Insertion	Function	Muscle	Blood supply	Flap blood supply type	Innervation
Anterior compartment	1 Tibialis anterior	Shaft of tibia and interosseous membrane	Medial cuneiform and base of first metatarsal	Foot dorsiflexion and inversion	Tibialis anterior	Anterior tibial	Segmental (IV)	Deep peroneal nerve
	2 Extensor digitorum longus	Shaft of fibula and interosseous membrane	Extensor expansion of lateral four toes	Foot and II-V toe dorsiflexion and foot eversion	Extensor digitorum longus	Anterior tibial	Segmental (IV)	Deep peroneal nerve
	3 Extensor hallucis longus	Shaft of fibula and interosseous membrane	Base of distal phalanx of big toe	First-toe dorsiflexion	Extensor hallucis longus	Anterior tibial	Segmental (IV)	Deep peroneal nerve
	4 Peroneus tertius	Shaft of fibula and interosseous membrane	Base of fifth metatarsal bone	Dorsiflexes (extends) foot; everts foot at subtalar and transverse tarsal joints	Peroneus tertius	Anterior tibial	Segmental (IV)	Deep peroneal nerve
Lateral compartment	5 Peroneus longus	Shaft of fibula	Base of first metatarsal and medial cuneiform	Plantarflexes foot; everts foot at subtalar and transverse tarsal joints; supports lateral longitudinal and transverse arches of foot	Peroneus longus	Peroneal	Dominant pedicle and minor pedicle(s) (II)	Superficial peroneal nerve
	6 Peroneus brevis	Shaft of fibula	Base of fifth metatarsal bone	Plantarflexes foot; everts foot at subtalar and transverse tarsal joints; supports lateral longitudinal arch	Peroneus brevis	Peroneal	Dominant pedicle and minor pedicle(s) (II)	Superficial peroneal nerve
Superficial posterior compartment	7 Medial gatrocnemius	Medial femoral condyle	Calcaneum via achilles tendon	Plantarflexes foot; flexes leg	Medial gatrocnemius	Posterior tibial	One vascular pedicle (I)	Tibial nerve

		Origin	Insertion	Action		Blood supply	Vascular pattern	Nerve
8	Lateral gastrocnemius	Lateral femoral condyle	Calcaneum via achilles tendon	Plantarflexes foot; flexes leg	Lateral gastrocnemius	Posterior tibial	One vascular pedicle (I)	Tibial nerve
9	Plantaris	Lateral supracondylar ridge of femur	Calcaneum	Plantarflexes foot; flexes leg	Plantaris	Posterior tibial	Segmental (IV)	Tibial nerve
10	Soleus	Shafts of tibia and fibula	Calcaneum via achilles tendon	Foot plantarflexion	Soleus	Posterior tibial	Dominant pedicles and minor pedicle (II)	Tibial nerve
Deep posterior compartment								
11	Popliteus	Lateral condyle of femur	Shaft of medial tibia	Flexes leg; unlocks full extension of knee by laterally rotating femur on tibia	Popliteus	Medial and lateral genicular arteries	Segmental (IV)	Tibial nerve
12	Flexor digitorum longus	Shaft of tibia	Distal phalanges of lateral four toes	Flexes distal phalanges of lateral four toes; plantarflexes foot; supports medial and lateral longitudinal arches of foot	Flexor digitorum longus	Posterior tibial branches	Segmental (IV)	Tibial nerve
13	Flexor hallucis longus	Shaft of fibula	Base of distal phalanx of big toe	Flexes distal phalanx of big toe; plantarflexes foot; supports medial longitudinal arch	Flexor hallucis longus	Peroneal branches	Segmental (IV)	Tibial nerve
14	Tibialis posterior	Shafts of tibia and fibula and interosseous membrane	Tuberosity of navicular bone and the medial cuneiform	Plantarflexes foot; inverts foot at subtalar and transverse tarsal joints; supports medial longitudinal arch of foot	Tibialis posterior	Posterior tibial and peroneal	Segmental (IV)	Tibial nerve

Muscles of Leg (Superficial Dissection): Anterior View

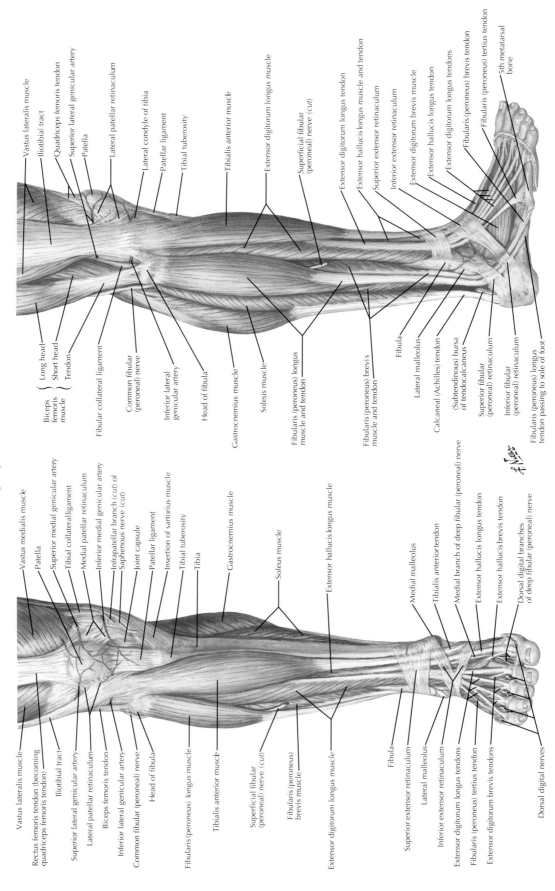

Vastus lateralis muscle
Iliotibial tract
Quadriceps femoris tendon
Superior lateral genicular artery
Patella
Lateral patellar retinaculum
Lateral condyle of tibia
Patellar ligament
Tibial tuberosity
Tibialis anterior muscle
Extensor digitorum longus muscle
Superficial fibular (peroneal) nerve (cut)
Extensor digitorum longus tendon
Extensor hallucis longus muscle and tendon
Superior extensor retinaculum
Inferior extensor retinaculum
Extensor digitorum brevis muscle
Extensor hallucis longus tendon
Extensor digitorum longus tendons
Fibularis (peroneus) brevis tendon
Fibularis (peroneus) tertius tendon
5th metatarsal bone

Biceps femoris muscle { Long head, Short head, Tendon }
Fibular collateral ligament
Common fibular (peroneal) nerve
Inferior lateral genicular artery
Head of fibula
Gastrocnemius muscle
Soleus muscle
Fibularis (peroneus) longus muscle and tendon
Fibularis (peroneus) brevis muscle and tendon
Fibula
Lateral malleolus
Calcaneal (Achilles) tendon
(Subtendinous) bursa of tendocalcaneus
Superior fibular (peroneal) retinaculum
Inferior fibular (peroneal) retinaculum
Fibularis (peroneus) longus tendon passing to sole of foot

Vastus medialis muscle
Patella
Superior medial genicular artery
Tibial collateral ligament
Medial patellar retinaculum
Inferior medial genicular artery
Infrapatellar branch (cut) of Saphenous nerve (cut)
Joint capsule
Patellar ligament
Insertion of sartorius muscle
Tibial tuberosity
Tibia
Gastrocnemius muscle
Soleus muscle
Extensor hallucis longus muscle

Vastus lateralis muscle
Rectus femoris tendon (becoming quadriceps femoris tendon)
Iliotibial tract
Superior lateral genicular artery
Lateral patellar retinaculum
Biceps femoris tendon
Inferior lateral genicular artery
Common fibular (peroneal) nerve
Head of fibula
Fibularis (peroneus) longus muscle
Tibialis anterior muscle
Superficial fibular (peroneal) nerve (cut)
Fibularis (peroneus) brevis muscle
Extensor digitorum longus muscle
Medial malleolus
Tibialis anterior tendon
Medial branch of deep fibular (peroneal) nerve
Extensor hallucis longus tendon
Extensor hallucis brevis tendon
Dorsal digital branches of deep fibular (peroneal) nerve
Fibula
Lateral malleolus
Inferior extensor retinaculum
Superior extensor retinaculum
Extensor digitorum longus tendons
Fibularis (peroneus) tertius tendon
Extensor digitorum brevis tendons
Dorsal digital nerves

Fig. 1.31 Muscles of leg (superficial dissection): anterior view. (Netter illustration from www.netterimages.com. Copyright Elsevier Inc. All rights reserved.)

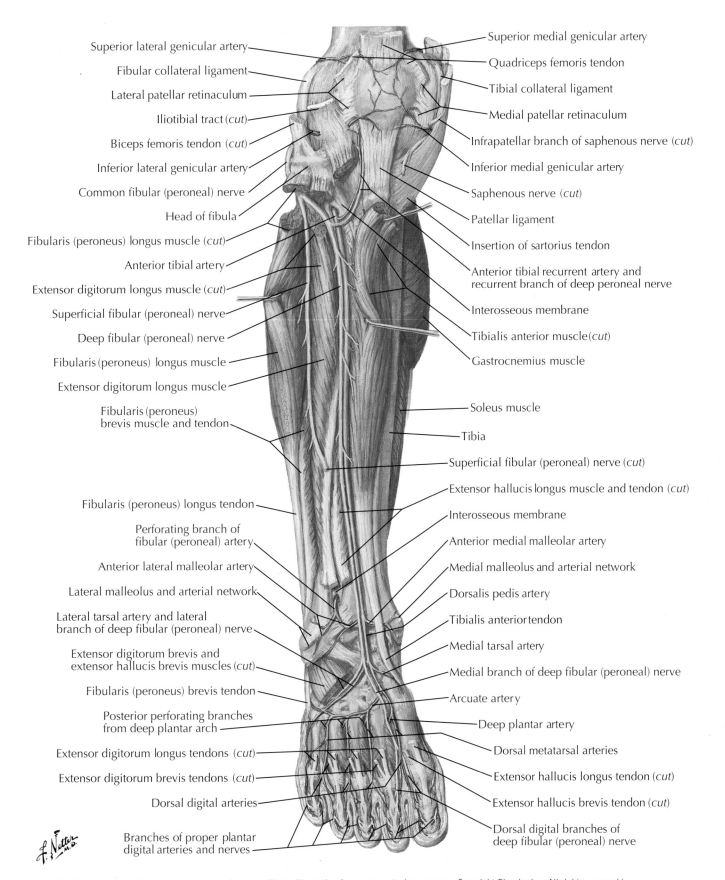

Superior lateral genicular artery

Fibular collateral ligament

Lateral patellar retinaculum

Iliotibial tract (cut)

Biceps femoris tendon (cut)

Inferior lateral genicular artery

Common fibular (peroneal) nerve

Head of fibula

Fibularis (peroneus) longus muscle (cut)

Anterior tibial artery

Extensor digitorum longus muscle (cut)

Superficial fibular (peroneal) nerve

Deep fibular (peroneal) nerve

Fibularis (peroneus) longus muscle

Extensor digitorum longus muscle

Fibularis (peroneus) brevis muscle and tendon

Fibularis (peroneus) longus tendon

Perforating branch of fibular (peroneal) artery

Anterior lateral malleolar artery

Lateral malleolus and arterial network

Lateral tarsal artery and lateral branch of deep fibular (peroneal) nerve

Extensor digitorum brevis and extensor hallucis brevis muscles (cut)

Fibularis (peroneus) brevis tendon

Posterior perforating branches from deep plantar arch

Extensor digitorum longus tendons (cut)

Extensor digitorum brevis tendons (cut)

Dorsal digital arteries

Branches of proper plantar digital arteries and nerves

Superior medial genicular artery

Quadriceps femoris tendon

Tibial collateral ligament

Medial patellar retinaculum

Infrapatellar branch of saphenous nerve (cut)

Inferior medial genicular artery

Saphenous nerve (cut)

Patellar ligament

Insertion of sartorius tendon

Anterior tibial recurrent artery and recurrent branch of deep peroneal nerve

Interosseous membrane

Tibialis anterior muscle(cut)

Gastrocnemius muscle

Soleus muscle

Tibia

Superficial fibular (peroneal) nerve (cut)

Extensor hallucis longus muscle and tendon (cut)

Interosseous membrane

Anterior medial malleolar artery

Medial malleolus and arterial network

Dorsalis pedis artery

Tibialis anterior tendon

Medial tarsal artery

Medial branch of deep fibular (peroneal) nerve

Arcuate artery

Deep plantar artery

Dorsal metatarsal arteries

Extensor hallucis longus tendon (cut)

Extensor hallucis brevis tendon (cut)

Dorsal digital branches of deep fibular (peroneal) nerve

Fig. 1.32 Muscles of leg (deep dissection): anterior view. (Netter illustration from www.netterimages.com. Copyright Elsevier Inc. All rights reserved.)

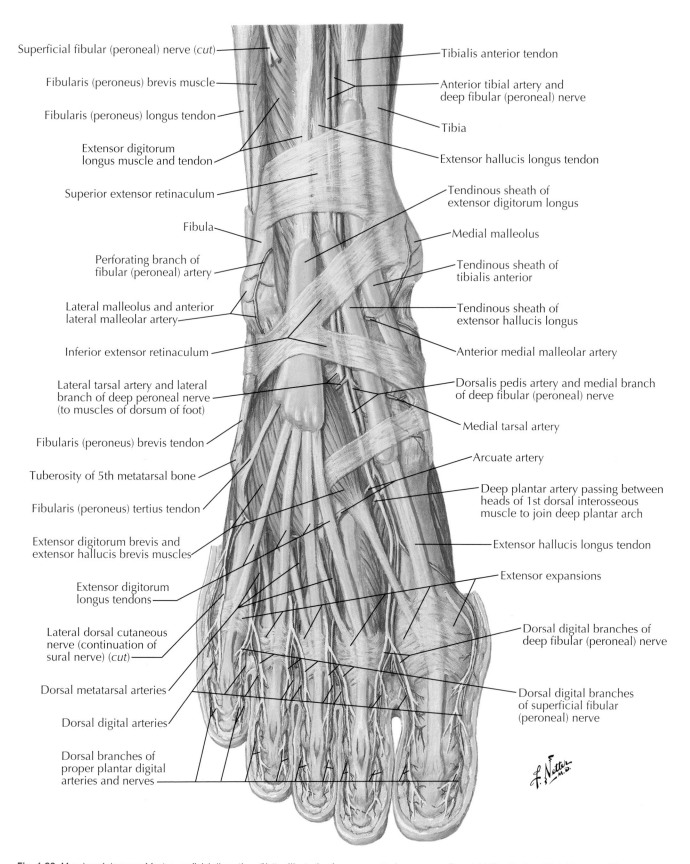

Superficial fibular (peroneal) nerve (*cut*)

Fibularis (peroneus) brevis muscle

Fibularis (peroneus) longus tendon

Extensor digitorum longus muscle and tendon

Superior extensor retinaculum

Fibula

Perforating branch of fibular (peroneal) artery

Lateral malleolus and anterior lateral malleolar artery

Inferior extensor retinaculum

Lateral tarsal artery and lateral branch of deep peroneal nerve (to muscles of dorsum of foot)

Fibularis (peroneus) brevis tendon

Tuberosity of 5th metatarsal bone

Fibularis (peroneus) tertius tendon

Extensor digitorum brevis and extensor hallucis brevis muscles

Extensor digitorum longus tendons

Lateral dorsal cutaneous nerve (continuation of sural nerve) (*cut*)

Dorsal metatarsal arteries

Dorsal digital arteries

Dorsal branches of proper plantar digital arteries and nerves

Tibialis anterior tendon

Anterior tibial artery and deep fibular (peroneal) nerve

Tibia

Extensor hallucis longus tendon

Tendinous sheath of extensor digitorum longus

Medial malleolus

Tendinous sheath of tibialis anterior

Tendinous sheath of extensor hallucis longus

Anterior medial malleolar artery

Dorsalis pedis artery and medial branch of deep fibular (peroneal) nerve

Medial tarsal artery

Arcuate artery

Deep plantar artery passing between heads of 1st dorsal interosseous muscle to join deep plantar arch

Extensor hallucis longus tendon

Extensor expansions

Dorsal digital branches of deep fibular (peroneal) nerve

Dorsal digital branches of superficial fibular (peroneal) nerve

Fig. 1.33 Muscles of dorsum of foot: superficial dissection. (Netter illustration from www.netterimages.com. Copyright Elsevier Inc. All rights reserved.)

Table 1.7 Anterior leg compartment musculature

Tibialis anterior
Extensor digitorum longus
Extensor hallucis longus
Peroneus tertius

Table 1.8 Lateral leg compartment musculature

Peroneus longus
Peroneus brevis

Table 1.9 Posterior leg compartment – superficial layer musculature

Medial gastrocnemius
Lateral gastrocnemius
Soleus
Plantaris

is the more superficial of the two and has a more superior origin on the fibula than the brevis *(Table 1.6)*. Both muscles convert to tendinous structures at the ankle and course in a groove behind the lateral malleolus. They then travel on the plantar surface of the foot to their insertions *(Fig. 1.34)*. The peroneus brevis inserts on the plantar surface of the base of the fifth metatarsal. The peroneus longus crosses the foot traveling beneath the midsole musculature to insert on the plantar surface of the base of the first metatarsal. Both muscles work together to evert and plantarflex the foot. The blood supply for both muscles is the same with the major pedicle branching from the peroneal artery in the proximal one-third and a distal minor branch coming off the anterior tibial artery in the distal two-thirds of the muscles (Mathes–Nahai muscle supply classification type II). There is no major vessel within the lateral compartment so both pedicles must traverse the intermuscular septa to reach their target muscles. Both the peroneus longus and brevis are innervated by the superficial branch of the peroneal nerve.

Posterior compartment – superficial layer

The posterior compartment is the largest compartment of the leg and is divided into deep and superficial layers by the deep transverse fascia. The superficial group contains four plantar-flexion muscles – medial and lateral gastrocnemius, soleus, and plantaris *(Fig. 1.35 and Table 1.9)*. The gastrocnemius and plantaris muscles originate on the femur and insert on the calcaneus *(Table 1.6)*. Therefore, these muscles cause activity on both the knee (flexion) and ankle joints (plantarflexion). The medial head gastrocnemius is larger and longer than the lateral head. The mass of the medial can be up to twice as great as that of the lateral. The proximal aspect of the gastrocnemius defines the inferior border of the popliteal fossa (the superior border is marked by the terminus of the biceps femoris, semitendinous, and semimembranosus). The lateral head overlies the biceps femoris and the medial head overlies the semimembranosus. The muscle mass of the gastrocnemius

extends to midcalf and transitions to its tendinous component more proximally than the soleus muscle.

Of note, in 10–30% of individuals, a sesamoid bone can be present in the proximal tendon of the lateral head of the gastrocnemius. Located behind the femoral condyle, this sesamoid body is called the fabella (Latin for little bean) and can be either fibrocartilaginous or bony. When seen on knee radiographs, the fabella can mistakenly be identified as a foreign body or an osteophyte.

Each head of the gastrocnemius is supplied by a sural branch off the popliteal artery. The medial sural artery always arises more proximally from the popliteal artery than the lateral, usually at the level of the tibiofemoral joint line. Each sural artery enters the deep surface of the gastrocnemius at about the level of the middle of the popliteal fossa. These muscles follow a single major pedicle vascular supply pattern (type I) but also have some small connecting vessels between the muscle heads. The sural artery enters each head paired with a motor branch for the tibial nerve. The plantaris muscle is a small, expendable muscle that lies between the gastrocnemius muscles superficially and the soleus deep. It is often resected and used as a source for tendon grafting, but can be absent in 10% of the population. It provides minimal activity at the ankle in a similar fashion to the gastrocnemius. The fourth muscle of the superficial posterior compartment is the soleus. It is a broad flat muscle that works synergistically with the other muscles of the compartment to plantarflex the foot. It originates from the proximal one-third of the tibia and posterior aspect of fibula head. On the tibia, the soleus has an aponeurotic origin along an obliquely oriented bony ridge of the proximal tibia, referred to as the soleal line (sometimes, popliteal line). Superior to this line is the origin of the popliteus. In the proximal calf, the gastrocnemius overlies the soleus. However, distal to the midcalf, the muscle belly of the soleus is still thick and wide and continues much more distally than the gastrocnemius until its musculotendinous transition and its tendinous insertion into the Achilles. The tendons of the gastrocnemius, soleus, and plantaris coalesce to create the broad, thick Achilles tendon which inserts into the posterior calcaneus. The soleus has a type II blood supply with three major dominant pedicles feeding it. It receives dominant pedicles from the popliteal, peroneal, and posterior tibial arteries. Proximally, near the soleal origin, the popliteal artery issues out two branches to the soleus; just below the tibioperoneal bifurcation, the peroneal artery contributes two branches; and the posterior tibial artery delivers two major pedicle branches in the proximal one-third of soleus. Additionally, there are minor pedicles that flow as segmental branches from the posterior tibial artery in the distal one-third of the leg. Because of the multiple different vascular supplies, basing an entire soleus muscle flap off one or two closely related pedicles usually results in some ischemia of the muscle area most distant from the arterial inflow. Of note, the superficial posterior compartment musculature is important to the "muscle pump" of venous return. There is an intramuscular venous plexus within the soleus that is important for adequate lower extremity venous return, especially when the individual maintains the upright position. The gastrocnemius muscles and the tight deep fascia of the leg both contribute to the deep venous system's return physiology. Consequently, most distal (calf) deep venous thromboses are seen in either the soleus or gastrocnemius.

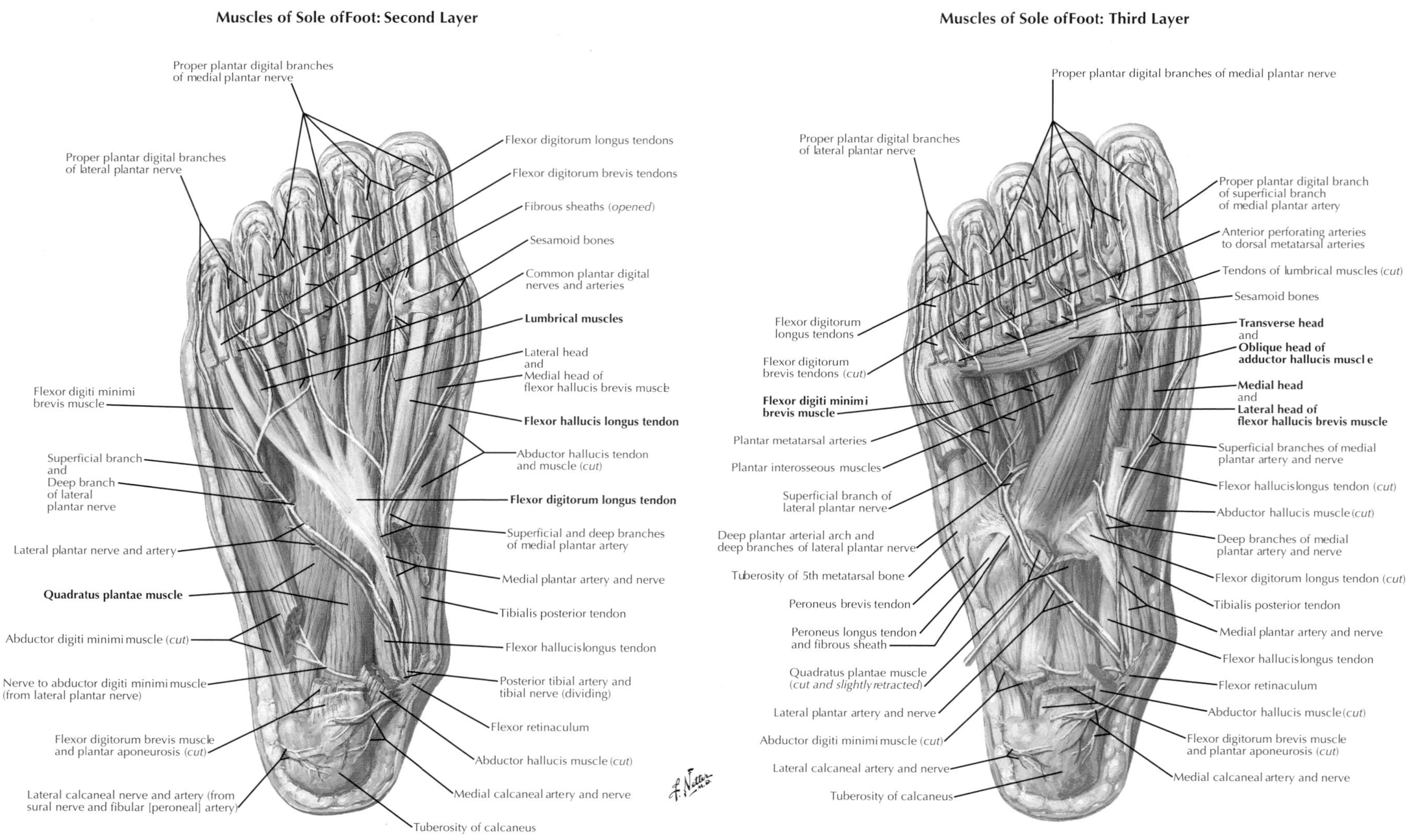

Muscles of Sole of Foot: Third Layer

Proper plantar digital branches of medial plantar nerve

Proper plantar digital branch of superficial branch of medial plantar artery

Anterior perforating arteries to dorsal metatarsal arteries

Tendons of lumbrical muscles (cut)

Sesamoid bones

Transverse head and **Oblique head of adductor hallucis muscle**

Medial head and **Lateral head of flexor hallucis brevis muscle**

Superficial branches of medial plantar artery and nerve

Flexor hallucis longus tendon (cut)

Abductor hallucis muscle (cut)

Deep branches of medial plantar artery and nerve

Flexor digitorum longus tendon (cut)

Tibialis posterior tendon

Medial plantar artery and nerve

Flexor hallucis longus tendon

Flexor retinaculum

Abductor hallucis muscle (cut)

Flexor digitorum brevis muscle and plantar aponeurosis (cut)

Medial calcaneal artery and nerve

Proper plantar digital branches of lateral plantar nerve

Flexor digitorum longus tendons

Flexor digitorum brevis tendons (cut)

Flexor digiti minimi brevis muscle

Plantar metatarsal arteries

Plantar interosseous muscles

Superficial branch of lateral plantar nerve

Deep plantar arterial arch and deep branches of lateral plantar nerve

Tuberosity of 5th metatarsal bone

Peroneus brevis tendon

Peroneus longus tendon and fibrous sheath

Quadratus plantae muscle (cut and slightly retracted)

Lateral plantar artery and nerve

Abductor digiti minimi muscle (cut)

Lateral calcaneal artery and nerve

Tuberosity of calcaneus

Muscles of Sole of Foot: Second Layer

Proper plantar digital branches of medial plantar nerve

Flexor digitorum longus tendons

Flexor digitorum brevis tendons

Fibrous sheaths (opened)

Sesamoid bones

Common plantar digital nerves and arteries

Lumbrical muscles

Lateral head and Medial head of flexor hallucis brevis muscle

Flexor hallucis longus tendon

Abductor hallucis tendon and muscle (cut)

Flexor digitorum longus tendon

Superficial and deep branches of medial plantar artery

Medial plantar artery and nerve

Tibialis posterior tendon

Flexor hallucis longus tendon

Posterior tibial artery and tibial nerve (dividing)

Flexor retinaculum

Abductor hallucis muscle (cut)

Medial calcaneal artery and nerve

Tuberosity of calcaneus

Proper plantar digital branches of lateral plantar nerve

Flexor digiti minimi brevis muscle

Superficial branch and Deep branch of lateral plantar nerve

Lateral plantar nerve and artery

Quadratus plantae muscle

Abductor digiti minimi muscle (cut)

Nerve to abductor digiti minimi muscle (from lateral plantar nerve)

Flexor digitorum brevis muscle and plantar aponeurosis (cut)

Lateral calcaneal nerve and artery (from sural nerve and fibular [peroneal] artery)

Fig. 1.34 Muscles of sole of foot: second layer. (Netter illustration from www.netterimages.com. Copyright Elsevier Inc. All rights reserved.)

Anterior view with ligament attachments

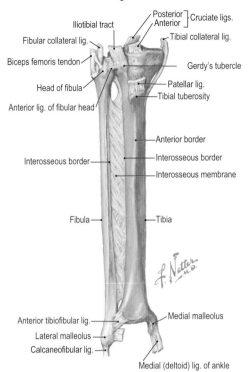

Fig. 1.35 Muscles of leg (intermediate dissection): posterior view. (Netter illustration from www.netterimages.com. Copyright Elsevier Inc. All rights reserved.)

Posterior compartment – deep layer

The deep posterior compartment (or deep flexor group) is comprised of four muscles – popliteus, flexor digitorum longus, flexor hallucis longus, and tibialis posterior *(Table 1.10; see also Table 1.6)*. These muscles lie below the deep transverse fascia and have a varied array of function, including knee flexion, toe flexion, and foot plantarflexion *(Fig. 1.36)*. The popliteus is a flat muscle that travels obliquely across the popliteal fossa from its origin on the posterior aspect of the lateral femoral condyle to the posterior aspect of the proximal tibial shaft. The popliteus is characterized as the muscle that "unlocks" the knee joint from full extension. It rotates the tibia medially on the femur to allow the beginning of knee flexion. The flexor digitorum longus and the flexor hallucis longus have similar attachments and functions. Both originate in the middle one-third of the leg, with the flexor digitorum longus originating from the tibia and the flexor hallucis longus originating from the fibula. The flexor digitorum longus descends down the leg and its tendon courses posterior to the medial malleolus and across the sole of the foot to insert to the plantar surfaces of the base of the distal phalanges. The flexor hallucis longus travels from the fibular origin down to the ankle with most of the muscle belly uniquely still present at the calcaneal level. It crosses the sole of the foot under the flexor digitorum longus to insert into the base of the plantar surface of the first-toe distal phalanx. Slips of tendons pass between and cause multiple interconnections among the flexor digitorum longus and the flexor hallucis longus. This allows a coordinated flexion of toes to maintain

Table 1.10 Posterior leg compartment – deep layer musculature
Popliteus
Flexor digitorum longus
Flexor hallucis longus
Tibialis posterior

their pads in firm contact with the ground, which improves balance and stability. The blood supply for the flexor digitorum longus comes from multiple segmental branches of the posterior tibial artery. The flexor hallucis longus, with its origin off the fibula, is supplied by the peroneal artery via multiple segmental branches. The tibialis posterior is the deepest muscle of the posterior compartment. Its origin lies adjacent to the proximal and mid one-third of the interosseous membrane and the surrounding tibia and fibula. As the tibialis posterior progresses to the musculotendinous junction, it courses behind the medial malleolus with the flexor digitorum longus and crosses the plantar surface of the foot beneath the flexor retinaculum. The tendon of the tibialis posterior inserts into the navicular and the medial cuneiform. Its blood supply is provided by multiple branches of the posterior tibial artery. The tibial nerve innervates the tibialis posterior. Because of its deep location and highly segmental blood supply the posterior tibialis is not a common flap choice.

Leg vasculature

The entire vascularity of the leg emanates from the popliteal artery *(Fig. 1.37)*. The popliteal artery is an extension of the femoral artery after it exits the adductor (Hunter's) canal and crosses the popliteal fossa. Just before it enters the fossa, it gives off multiple genicular branches which form a rich vascular plexus that wraps anteriorly around the knee. The superior genicular arteries connect with descending branches from the lateral circumflex femoral artery and branch directly off the superficial femoral artery *(Fig. 1.18)*. As the popliteal artery exits the popliteal fossa at the distal edge of the popliteus, it produces its first terminal branch, the anterior tibial artery.

The anterior tibial artery passes between the heads of the tibialis posterior and penetrates through the oval aperture in the superior aspect of the interosseous membrane. It then enters the anterior compartment where it supplies all its musculature. The anterior tibial artery descends along the anterior surface of interosseous membrane until it reaches the ankle. At the ankle, the anterior tibial artery is positioned midway between the lateral and medial malleoli on the anterior surface of the ankle and enters the foot as the dorsalis pedis artery *(Fig. 1.17)*.

In the knee, after the anterior tibial artery branches from the popliteal artery, there is usually a short segment of vessel that continues distally for a small distance, then divides into the peroneal and posterior tibial vessels. This tibioperoneal trunk may be present, but in a few cases the peroneal and posterior tibial artery can arise directly from the popliteal vessel, creating a true trifurcation with the anterior tibial artery. The posterior tibial and peroneal arteries split from the popliteal artery distal to the popliteus muscle *(Fig. 1.38)*. Both

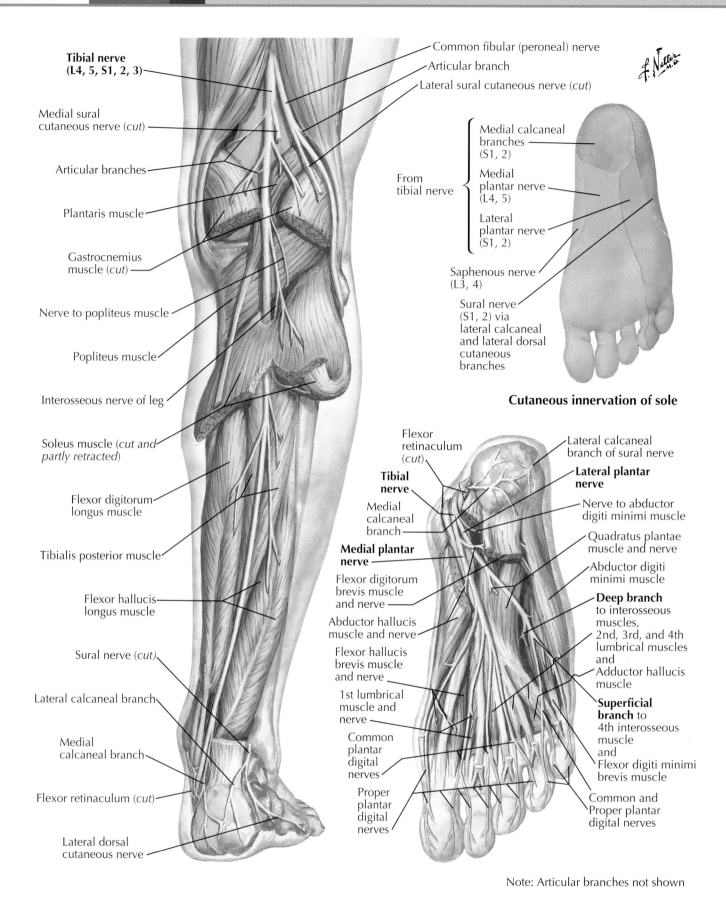

Tibial nerve (L4, 5, S1, 2, 3)

Medial sural cutaneous nerve (*cut*)

Articular branches

Plantaris muscle

Gastrocnemius muscle (*cut*)

Nerve to popliteus muscle

Popliteus muscle

Interosseous nerve of leg

Soleus muscle (*cut and partly retracted*)

Flexor digitorum longus muscle

Tibialis posterior muscle

Flexor hallucis longus muscle

Sural nerve (*cut*)

Lateral calcaneal branch

Medial calcaneal branch

Flexor retinaculum (*cut*)

Lateral dorsal cutaneous nerve

Common fibular (peroneal) nerve

Articular branch

Lateral sural cutaneous nerve (*cut*)

From tibial nerve {
Medial calcaneal branches (S1, 2)

Medial plantar nerve (L4, 5)

Lateral plantar nerve (S1, 2)
}

Saphenous nerve (L3, 4)

Sural nerve (S1, 2) via lateral calcaneal and lateral dorsal cutaneous branches

Cutaneous innervation of sole

Flexor retinaculum (*cut*)

Lateral calcaneal branch of sural nerve

Tibial nerve

Medial calcaneal branch

Lateral plantar nerve

Nerve to abductor digiti minimi muscle

Medial plantar nerve

Quadratus plantae muscle and nerve

Flexor digitorum brevis muscle and nerve

Abductor digiti minimi muscle

Abductor hallucis muscle and nerve

Deep branch to interosseous muscles, 2nd, 3rd, and 4th lumbrical muscles and Adductor hallucis muscle

Flexor hallucis brevis muscle and nerve

1st lumbrical muscle and nerve

Superficial branch to 4th interosseous muscle and Flexor digiti minimi brevis muscle

Common plantar digital nerves

Proper plantar digital nerves

Common and Proper plantar digital nerves

Note: Articular branches not shown

Fig. 1.36 Tibial nerve. (Netter illustration from www.netterimages.com. Copyright Elsevier Inc. All rights reserved.)

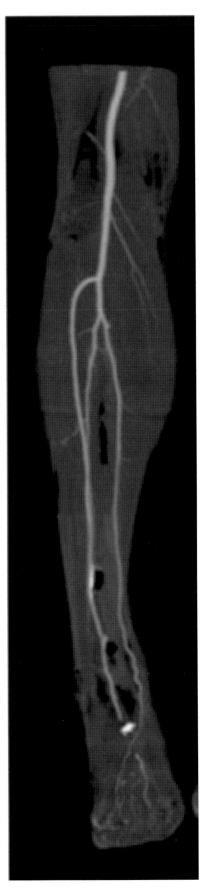

Fig. 1.37 The popliteal artery.

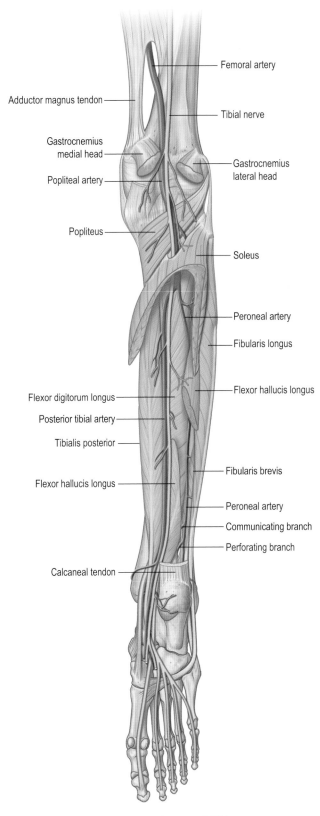

Adductor magnus tendon

Gastrocnemius medial head

Popliteal artery

Popliteus

Flexor digitorum longus

Posterior tibial artery

Tibialis posterior

Flexor hallucis longus

Calcaneal tendon

Femoral artery

Tibial nerve

Gastrocnemius lateral head

Soleus

Peroneal artery

Fibularis longus

Flexor hallucis longus

Fibularis brevis

Peroneal artery

Communicating branch

Perforating branch

Fig. 1.38 Posterior tibial and peroneal artery and tibial nerve.

arteries remain in the deep layer of the posterior compartment with the peroneal artery traveling deeper and laterally, closely related to the fibula. The posterior tibial artery descends down the leg, initially slightly more superficial than the peroneal artery, and then courses deeper to just under the deep transverse fascia. As it progresses distally, it becomes more superficially located until it is only covered by skin and subcutaneous fat as it traverses the ankle posterior to the medial malleolus. The tibial nerve runs with the posterior artery in the posterior calf. Approximately five fasciocutaneous perforators emerge between the flexor digitorum longus and the soleus to pass through the deep fascia to the skin (*Figs 1.39 and 1.40*). As the posterior tibial artery rounds the medial malleolus, it divides into its terminal branches – the medial and lateral plantar arteries.

Leg nerve anatomy

Lower leg nerve topography

Leg innervation is derived almost entirely from the tibial and peroneal branches of the sciatic nerve. The sciatic nerve bifurcates into the tibial and common peroneal nerves in the popliteal fossa. The tibial nerve continues down the deep posterior compartment running alongside the posterior tibial artery (*Fig. 1.36*). It innervates all the musculature of both the deep and superficial posterior compartments. The tibial nerve accompanies the descent of the posterior tibial artery to the ankle and they course together behind the medial malleolus under the flexor retinaculum. As the tibial nerve leaves the ankle and enters the plantar surface of the foot it bifurcates into the medial and lateral plantar nerves.

In the popliteal fossa, the common peroneal nerve branches off laterally from the sciatic nerve and then passes from the posterior to the lateral aspect of the leg (*Fig. 1.36*). It curves lateral to the fibular neck, deep to the peroneus longus muscle and divides into superficial and deep peroneal nerves (*Fig. 1.41*). The superficial peroneal nerve travels distally down the leg between the peronei and the extensor digitorum longus. In the proximal two-thirds of the leg, it gives off its motor innervation to the muscles of the lateral compartment. As the superficial peroneal nerve continues inferiorly to the distal one-third of the leg, it runs superficially to pierce the deep leg fascia to enter the subcutaneous space. Here it bifurcates into medial and lateral branches which provide innervation to the skin of the lower leg and foot.

The deep peroneal nerve begins its course splitting from the common peroneal nerve between the fibula and the proximal part of the peroneus longus. It crosses medially from the lateral leg compartment to the deep aspect of the anterior compartment. There, it travels down the leg in front of the interosseous membrane, behind the extensor digitorum longus. It descends to the ankle alongside the anterior tibial artery and sends terminal branches into the foot joints and dorsal skin.

Lower leg motor innervation

The motor innervation of the leg muscles follows a "one compartment, one nerve" principle. All the muscles within each compartment of the leg are innervated by a single nerve. The muscles of the anterior compartment are innervated by the deep peroneal nerve (*Table 1.11*); the lateral compartment muscles are innervated by the superficial peroneal nerve (*Table 1.12*); the muscles of the posterior compartment (both superficial and deep layers) are innervated by the tibial nerve (*Table 1.13*).

Lower leg cutaneous innervation

Cutaneous innervation of the leg is shared by branches of the major mixed nerves of the lower extremity (femoral and sciatic nerves) and the posterior cutaneous nerve of the thigh (*Figs 1.22 and 1.23*). The nerves that innervate the skin surfaces of the knee and leg are: saphenous, posterior femoral cutaneous, common peroneal, superficial peroneal, medial sural, and sural nerves.

The saphenous nerve branches from the femoral nerve in the distal one-third of the thigh. It travels along the adductor canal for a distance then exits medial to the sartorius muscle. It passes medially and underneath the sartorius then heads superficial between the sartorius and gracilis. Here, the saphenous nerves pierces the fascia lata and enters the subcutaneous space. As it descends inferiorly, it gives off an infrapatellar branch that innervates the medial knee and medial crural branches that supply the entire medial leg.

The posterior femoral cutaneous nerve is a pure sensory nerve that branches directly from the sacral plexus in the gluteal region. It descends beneath the gluteus maximus with the inferior gluteal artery. The posterior femoral cutaneous nerve runs subfascially until the middle of the thigh where it pierces the fascia lata and transitions to the subcutaneous space. Here, it sends off multiple branches to the posterior thigh but continues distally to innervate the posterior knee where it also forms communicating branches with the sural nerve.

The course of the common peroneal nerve in the proximal leg has previously been discussed. As it curves lateral to the fibula neck the common peroneal nerve gives off cutaneous branches that innervate the lateral knee skin. Beneath the

Table 1.11 **Muscles innervated by the deep peroneal nerve**

Tibialis anterior
Extensor hallucis longus
Extensor digitorum longus
Peroneus tertius

Table 1.12 **Muscles innervated by the superficial peroneal nerve**

Peroneus longus
Peroneus brevis

Table 1.13 **Muscles innervated by the tibial nerve**

Superficial layer	Deep layer
Medial gastrocnemius	Popliteus
Lateral gastrocnemius	Flexor digitorum longus
Soleus	Flexor hallucis longus
Plantaris	Tibialis posterior

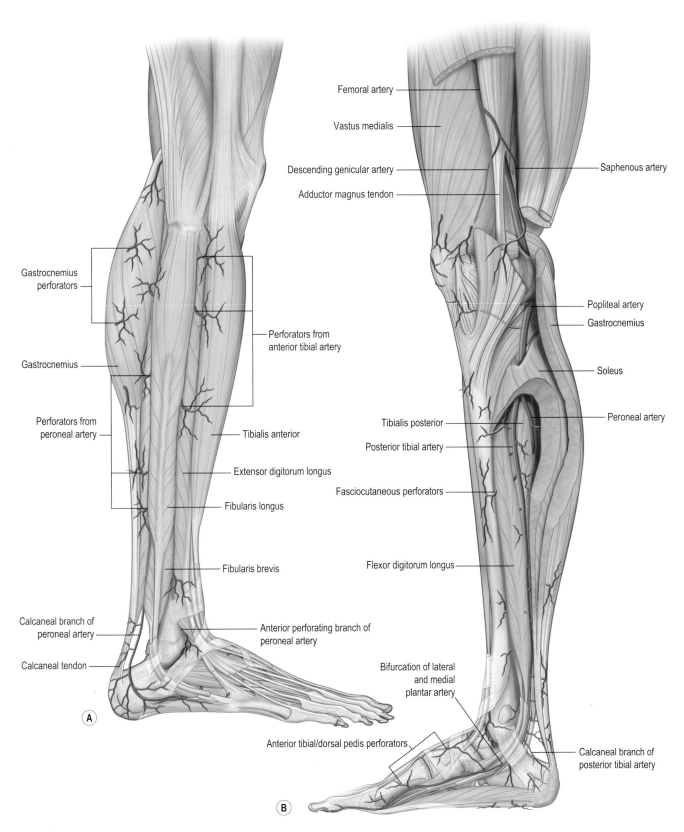

Fig. 1.39 Leg vasculature.

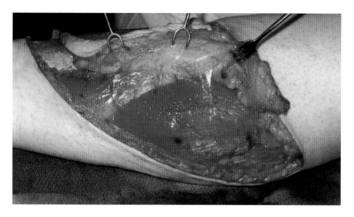

Fig. 1.40 Fasciocutaneous perforators.

peroneus longus muscle the common peroneal nerve divides into superficial and deep peroneal nerves *(Fig. 1.41)*.

The superficial peroneal nerve is responsible for the cutaneous nerve supply for the middle one-third area of the lateral leg *(Fig. 1.41)*. As it travels down the leg in the lateral compartment musculature if gives off cutaneous branches that innervate this area. The superficial peroneal nerve cutaneous innervation continues distally to the anterior ankle. Both the superficial and the deep peroneal branches exit the ankle into the foot to give dorsal cutaneous innervation. In the dorsal foot, the deep peroneal nerve courses below the superior extensor retinaculum; the superficial peroneal nerve passes above the retinaculum in the subcutaneous space. The majority of the dorsal foot innervation is supplied by the peroneal nerve. The deep peroneal nerve has only one small, unique area of cutaneous innervation in the entire lower extremity – the first webspace, medial side of the second toe, and lateral side of the great-toe dorsum *(Fig. 1.41)*. The cutaneous innervation of the lateral side of the dorsum of the foot is also provided by the sural nerve via the lateral dorsal cutaneous branch.

The sural nerve system is an intercommunicating complex of nerve branches that travel between the common peroneal and the tibial nerves. The terminology becomes somewhat confusing as the nomenclature for some branches is not uniform. Suffice to say, the term "sural" means calf and these branches serve the cutaneous regions of the remainder of the leg. There is a medial sural branch from the tibial that supplies the medial posterior portion of the leg and a lateral sural nerve from the common peroneal nerve that supplies the lateral posterior portion of the leg. The sural nerve is composed of several different possible intercommunicating cutaneous branches of the leg. The branches coalesce in the proximal leg and form the sural nerve. The sural nerve pierces the deep fascia of the leg at the inferior edge of the gastrocnemius head median raphe. It travels down the leg in the subcutaneous space with the lesser saphenous vein. It innervates the distal one-third of the leg skin.

The sural nerve is of specific clinical importance since it is a common nerve harvested as a nerve graft. The sural nerve is easily located posterior to the lateral malleolus, possesses a relatively small number of branches, and its removal yields a tolerable anesthetic defect in the lateral lower leg and foot. These reasons make the use of the sural nerve graft very

appealing for nerve reconstruction, especially in the upper extremity.

The ankle and foot

The ankle and foot are the fulcrum of the positioning forces of the entire upright human body. This is a highly functional area with thin soft-tissue coverage over highly complex and compact osteoligamentous structures. Adequate ambulation and balance rely on a proper interplay between proprioception through skin coverage and sensation; musculotendinous performance; and bony alignment. Proficient reconstruction of the ankle and foot requires a thorough understanding and a focus on maintaining these essential anatomic interactions.

Ankle and foot skeletal structure

There are 28 major bones in the human foot. The bony arrangement produces an intricate and intercalated system, reinforced by the surrounding ligament system that supports the entire weight of the body. The ankle is the region of transition from the leg to the foot and orientation of bones and muscles from vertical to horizontal.

Ankle

The ankle is comprised of two joints: (1) the articulation between the distal surfaces of the fibula (lateral malleolus) and tibia (medial malleolus) to the superior aspect of the talus; and (2) the subtalar joint – the articulation of the inferior aspect of the talus to the superior aspect of the calcaneus and four bones: (1) lateral malleolus; (2) medial malleolus; (3) talus; (4) calcaneus *(Fig. 1.42)*. Strong ligaments support this structure throughout its multiplanar movement. The anterior and posterior inferior tibiofibular ligaments, the interosseous ligament, and the interosseous membrane act synergistically to stabilize the joint. The ankle is has been described as hinge (i.e., ginglymus) or a mortise type of synovial joint. Both the hinge and the mortise imply a more rigid limited motion, but this conceptually belies that, in addition to plantarflexion–dorsiflexion, rotation and inversion–eversion movements occur at the ankle.

Foot

The ankle and foot are analogous to the hand in many ways. Similar to how the carpal bones are organized into a proximal and distal row, so too are the tarsal bones. The talus and calcaneus make up the proximal row in the foot, while the medial, intermediate, and lateral cuneiforms and the cuboid comprised the distal row. The navicular is the sole nonanalogous element in the foot as it is interspersed between the talus and the cuneiform, although one can see some analogous shape and position features with the scaphoid. The bones of the toes are very similar to the hand with the second through fifth toes consisting of metatarsal, proximal, middle, and distal phalanges. The first toe – like the thumb – is only three bones long and does not contain a middle phalanx *(Fig. 1.43)*.

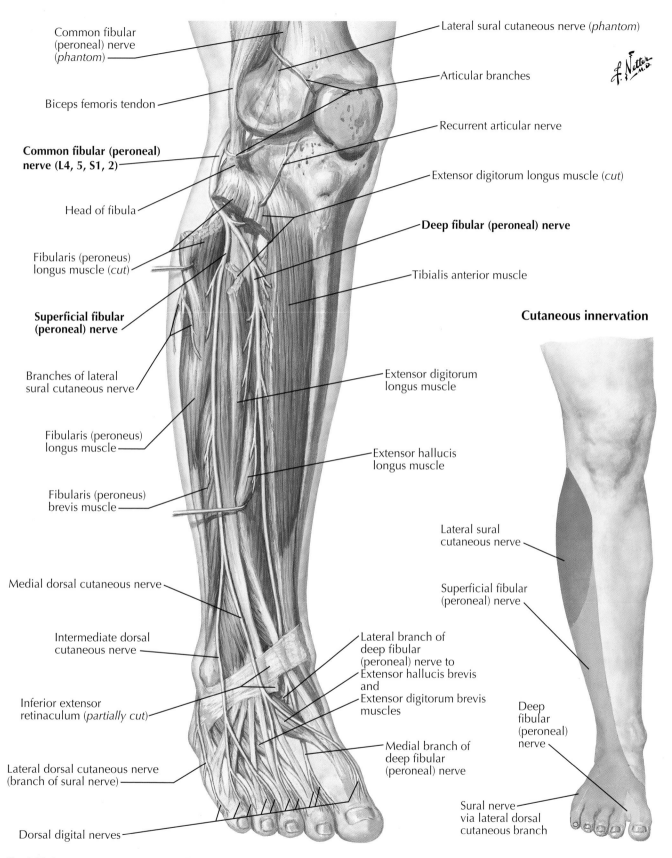

Common fibular (peroneal) nerve (*phantom*)

Biceps femoris tendon

Common fibular (peroneal) nerve (L4, 5, S1, 2)

Head of fibula

Fibularis (peroneus) longus muscle (*cut*)

Superficial fibular (peroneal) nerve

Branches of lateral sural cutaneous nerve

Fibularis (peroneus) longus muscle

Fibularis (peroneus) brevis muscle

Medial dorsal cutaneous nerve

Intermediate dorsal cutaneous nerve

Inferior extensor retinaculum (*partially cut*)

Lateral dorsal cutaneous nerve (branch of sural nerve)

Dorsal digital nerves

Lateral sural cutaneous nerve (*phantom*)

Articular branches

Recurrent articular nerve

Extensor digitorum longus muscle (*cut*)

Deep fibular (peroneal) nerve

Tibialis anterior muscle

Extensor digitorum longus muscle

Extensor hallucis longus muscle

Lateral branch of deep fibular (peroneal) nerve to Extensor hallucis brevis and Extensor digitorum brevis muscles

Medial branch of deep fibular (peroneal) nerve

Cutaneous innervation

Lateral sural cutaneous nerve

Superficial fibular (peroneal) nerve

Deep fibular (peroneal) nerve

Sural nerve via lateral dorsal cutaneous branch

Fig. 1.41 Common fibular (peroneal) nerve. (Netter illustration from www.netterimages.com. Copyright Elsevier Inc. All rights reserved.)

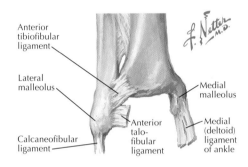

Medial view

Posterior view with ligaments

Fig. 1.42 Ankle joints. (Netter illustration from www.netterimages.com. Copyright Elsevier Inc. All rights reserved.)

Table 1.14 Structures restrained by the extensor retinaculum
Anterior tibial vessels
Deep peroneal nerve
Tibialis anterior tendon
Extensor hallucis longus
Extensor digitorum longus
Peroneus tertius

Table 1.15 Structures restrained by the flexor retinaculum
Posterior tibial vessels
Tibial nerve
Tibialis posterior tendon
Flexor digitorum longus tendon
Flexor hallucis longus tendon

Ankle and foot fascial composition

In the ankle and foot, the wide, encompassing fascial system that was present in the thigh and leg gives way to the formation of discrete retinacular bands of deep fascia that group tendons and prevent bowstringing. These bands create an important separation of functional units in a compact space and provide fulcrum points for gliding and levering of musculotendinous action.

The foot and ankle contain three major fascial retinacula: (1) the extensor retinacula are located on the dorsum of the foot; (2) the flexor retinaculum is located on the medial ankle; and (3) the peroneal retinaculum is located on the lateral ankle. Each retains similar functioning tendons. The sole of the foot also contains multiple fascial divisions extending from the tarsals and metatarsal to the plantar skin.

Extensor retinacula

There are two fascial retinacular bands that hold down the tendons of the dorsiflexion musculature of the ankle and foot – the superior and inferior extensor retinaculum. The superior extensor retinaculum dorsally restricts the tendons of the tibialis anterior, extensor hallucis longus, extensor digitorum longus, and the peroneus tertius at the level of the tibiofibular joint. This retinaculum is attached laterally to the distal end of the anterior border of the fibula and medially to the anterior

border of the tibia just above the prominence of the lateral and medial malleoli (*Fig. 1.33*). The anterior tibial vessels and the deep peroneal nerve course below the superior extensor retinaculum; the superficial peroneal nerve passes above the retinaculum in the subcutaneous space.

The inferior extensor retinaculum is a Y-shaped fascial band whose stem originates laterally on the superior surface of the calcaneus. The medial side of the retinaculum splits into two bands that separate different tendons and insert in two distinct locations. The proximal band encircles the extensor hallucis longus and tibialis anterior tendons and inserts on the medial malleolus. The distal band wraps around the instep of the foot and inserts on to the plantar aponeurosis (*Fig. 1.44*). This retinaculum retains the peroneus tertius, the extensor digitorum longus, the anterior tibial vessels, deep peroneal nerve, and the extensor hallucis longus (*Table 1.14*).

Flexor retinaculum

The flexor retinaculum (also called the laciniate ligament) is a medial ankle-located fascial band that restricts bowstringing of the plantar-flexing tendons traveling from the leg to the foot behind the medial malleolus (*Fig. 1.44*). The retinaculum is attached anterosuperiorly to the medial malleolus and fans out wide posteroinferiorly to the calcaneus and plantar aponeurosis. The flexor retinaculum retains the tendons of the flexor digitorum longus, flexor hallucis longus, and the tibialis posterior, the posterior tibial vessels, and the tibial nerve (*Table 1.15*). The tendons are usually located anteriorly and the neurovascular structures posteriorly.

An osteoligamentous passageway is created by the flexor retinaculum superficially and the talus and calcaneus deep. This structure is also called the tarsal tunnel and is analogous in many ways to the carpal tunnel of the hand. Both tunnels contain flexor tendons and a mixed motor and sensory nerve that gives supply to intrinsic muscles and the glabrous skin of the distal extremity. A significant similarity is the inelasticity of both osteoligamentous tunnels. There is very little pliancy in the ligament roofs of both tunnels and none in the bony floor. If the tunnel space is compromised by an intrinsic etiology (e.g., a space-occupying lesion (ganglion, lipoma, nerve or nerve sheath tumor, or varicose veins), swelling, inflammation of tendon sheaths) nerve compression can

Bones of Foot

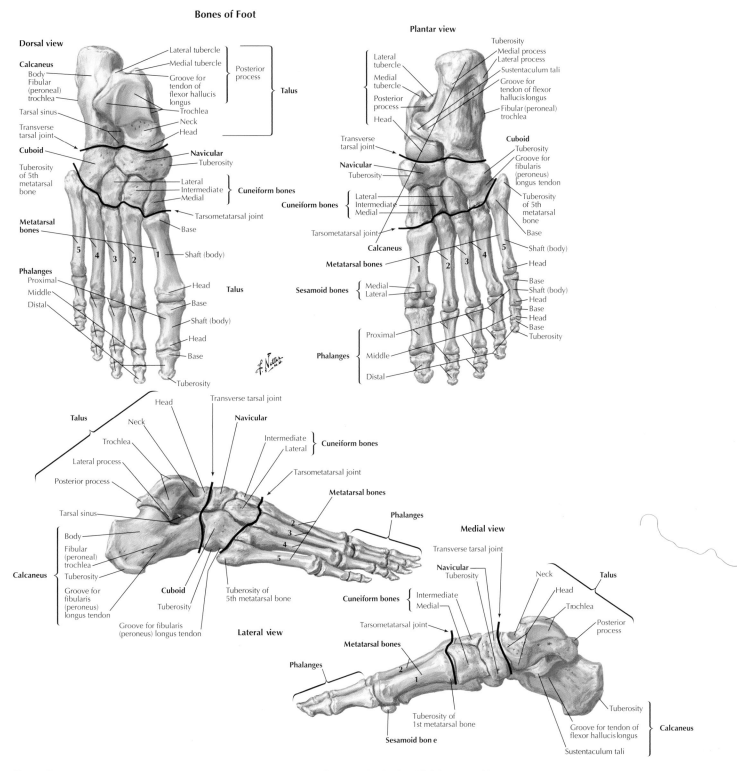

Fig. 1.43 Bones of the foot. (Netter illustration from www.netterimages.com. Copyright Elsevier Inc. All rights reserved.)

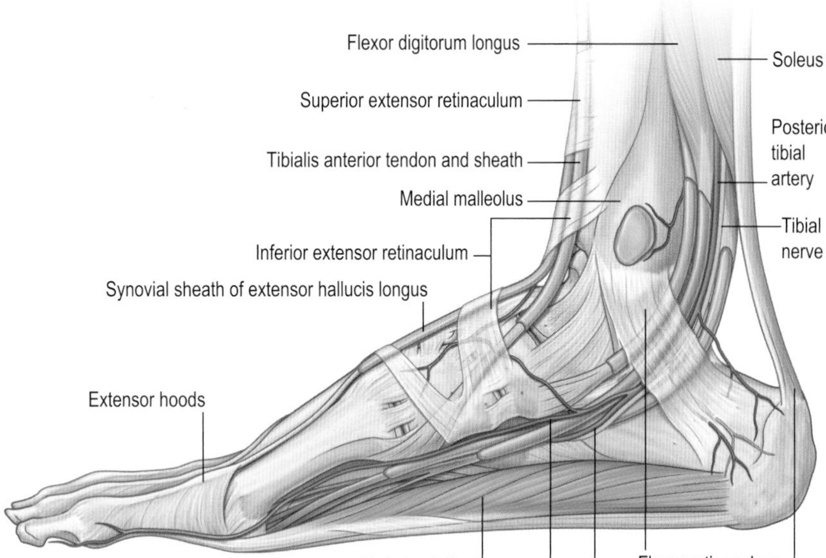

Flexor digitorum longus

Superior extensor retinaculum

Tibialis anterior tendon and sheath

Medial malleolus

Inferior extensor retinaculum

Synovial sheath of extensor hallucis longus

Extensor hoods

Soleus

Posterior tibial artery

Tibial nerve

Abductor hallucis

Medial plantar artery

Lateral plantar artery

Flexor retinaculum

Calcaneal tendon

Fig. 1.44 Fascial components of foot.

Table 1.16 Structures restrained by the peroneal retinaculum
Peroneus longus tendon
Peroneus brevis tendon

result. Bony prominences and exostoses may also contribute extrinsic pressures to cause disorder.

In the tarsal tunnel, if sufficient pressure is applied to the tibial nerve, local ischemia occurs and causes nerve conduction dysfunction. Similar to carpal tunnel syndrome, patients can experience paresthesias and dysesthesias; demonstrate a positive Tinel's sign at the tarsal tunnel; and demonstrate an abnormal nerve conduction study.

Peroneal retinaculum

On the lateral aspect of the ankle, the tendons of the peroneus longus and brevis are held in position by a dual-positioned fascial band – the peroneal retinaculum. The superior peroneal retinaculum extends from the posterior surface of the lateral malleolus to the calcaneus *(Fig. 1.44)*. The inferior peroneal retinaculum retains the tendons by attaching from the inferolateral surface of the calcaneus and inserting on the superior surface of the calcaneus. The inferior peroneal retinaculum shares its insertion on the superior calcaneus with the origin of the inferior extensor retinaculum. As the retinaculum crosses the peroneal tendons, it sends a septal fascia band to the peroneal trohclea, separating them. Damage to this fascial sheath causes peroneal muscular function instability.

The peroneal retinaculum retains only two structures: the peroneus longus tendon and the peroneus brevis tendon *(Table 1.16)*. The peroneal artery is not retained by the peroneal retinaculum whose course travels in the same area as the retinaculum but superficial to it. As the peroneal artery passes

distally from the leg to the foot, it exits from the deep region of the ankle to pass superficial to the peroneal retinaculum and provides vascular supply to the calcaneal and lateral malleolar regions of the ankle via multiple branches *(Fig. 1.44)*.

Plantar fascia

The plantar fascia (also called the plantar aponeurosis) is a thick fibrous band which constrains the intrinsic structures of the foot deeper to it and serves the fixed base for the densely adherent glabrous skin superficial to it. It is analogous to the palmar fascia of the hand in providing a stable base for overlying skin to resist shear forces and to facilitate ambulation. In the multilayered sole of the foot, the plantar fascia is the first defined structure beneath the subcutaneous fat. Proximally the plantar fascia is attached to the calcaneus and distally it divides into five slips which are joined by transverse fibers and then insert to the dermis beyond the metatarsal heads via retinacula cutis skin ligaments *(Fig. 1.45)*. It is joined at a right angle, just distal to the metatarsal heads, by the transverse metatarsal ligament. The plantar fascia is not uniform in its consistency; it is strongest and thickest centrally and thins laterally and distally.

Fascial compartment of foot

There are five major fascial compartments of the foot *(Table 1.17)*. These fascial compartments divide the foot musculature in functional units that facilitate efficient action. There are four separate plantar compartments bounded by intermuscular septa connecting the underlying bony components to the deep fascia of the foot and one dorsal foot compartment which is consider essentially as a single, multilayered compartment *(Fig. 1.46)*. For clinical reconstruction application, the medial and dorsal plantar compartments are the most

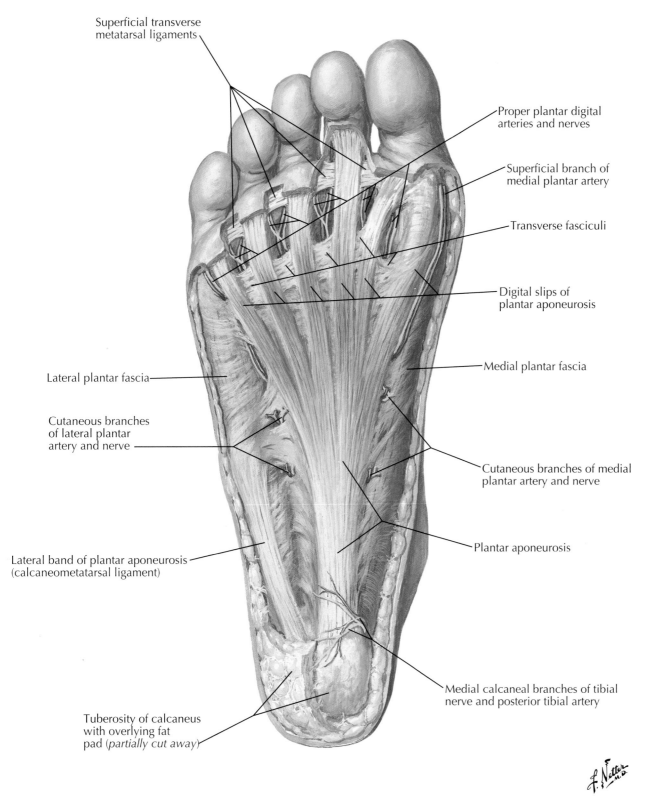

Superficial transverse
metatarsal ligaments

Proper plantar digital
arteries and nerves

Superficial branch of
medial plantar artery

Transverse fasciculi

Digital slips of
plantar aponeurosis

Medial plantar fascia

Lateral plantar fascia

Cutaneous branches
of lateral plantar
artery and nerve

Cutaneous branches of medial
plantar artery and nerve

Lateral band of plantar aponeurosis
(calcaneometatarsal ligament)

Plantar aponeurosis

Medial calcaneal branches of tibial
nerve and posterior tibial artery

Tuberosity of calcaneus
with overlying fat
pad (*partially cut away*)

Fig. 1.45 Sole of foot: superficial dissection. (Netter illustration from www.netterimages.com. Copyright Elsevier Inc. All rights reserved.)

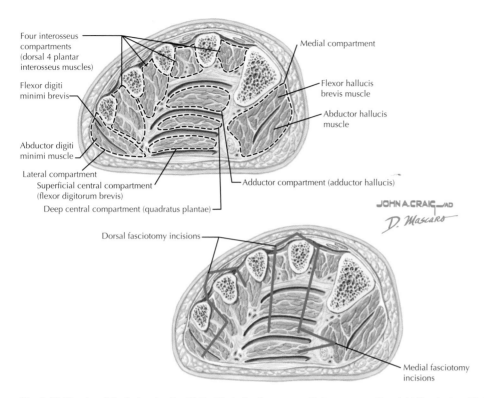

Fig. 1.46 Muscles of the foot and ankle. (Netter illustration from www.netterimages.com. Copyright Elsevier Inc. All rights reserved.)

Table 1.17 Fascial compartments of the foot	
Plantar	
Medial compartment	Contains abductor hallucis and flexor hallucis brevis
Central compartment	Contains flexor digitorum brevis, lumbricals, flexor accessorius, and adductor hallucis
Lateral compartment	Contains abductor digiti minimi and flexor digit minimi brevis
Interosseous compartment	Contains the seven interossei
Dorsal compartment	Although several fascial layers in dorsum, effectively there is one dorsal compartment

compartment does not have the plantar fascia overlying it. However, proximally the calcaneometatarsal ligament overlies the lateral plantar compartment.

Similar to the leg, conditions that cause increased intracompartmental pressure can lead quickly to compartment syndrome of the foot. Release of the surrounding fascial attachments is essential to avoid tissue ischemia and necrosis. Crush injuries, calcaneal fractures, and tarsometatarsal joint dislocations are the most common causes for foot compartment syndrome.

Foot musculature

The foot and ankle are acted upon by both extrinsic and intrinsic musculature. The extrinsic muscles all originate from proximal to the foot and have been described in the leg section. These muscles act on both the ankle and the toes. The intrinsic muscles of the foot originate and insert within the foot and act primarily on the toes. Their secondary function is to maintain posture balance through stabilization of the osteocartilaginous architecture of the foot.

The plantar muscles of the foot can be thought of as organized by layers from sole of the foot progressing deep to the bony structures *(Table 1.18)*. The first layer consists of muscles found just beneath the plantar aponeurosis – the flexor digitorum brevis, the abductor hallucis, and the abductor digiti minimi *(Fig. 1.47)*. These muscles extend from calcaneus to toes and create a functional group that assists in maintaining foot concavity. All three have been described as local muscle for pedicled reconstruction of the regional and ankle; all are Mathes–Nahai vascular supply type I muscles. The flexor digitorum brevis achieves vascular supply from branches of

significant. They contain the more useful intrinsic muscles that can be transposed for flap coverage. The remaining plantar compartments house smaller, deeper muscles with less transfer utility.

The medial plantar compartment contains two intrinsic muscles which act on the great toe – the abductor hallucis and the flexor hallucis brevis. The compartment lies beneath the medial border of the plantar aponeurosis and contains the most medial branches of the medial plantar artery and nerve *(Fig. 1.47)*.

The lateral plantar compartment contains two intrinsic muscles on the lateral foot which act on the small toe – abductor digiti minimi and flexor digiti minimi. Due to the medial orientation of the plantar fascia *(Fig. 1.47)*, the

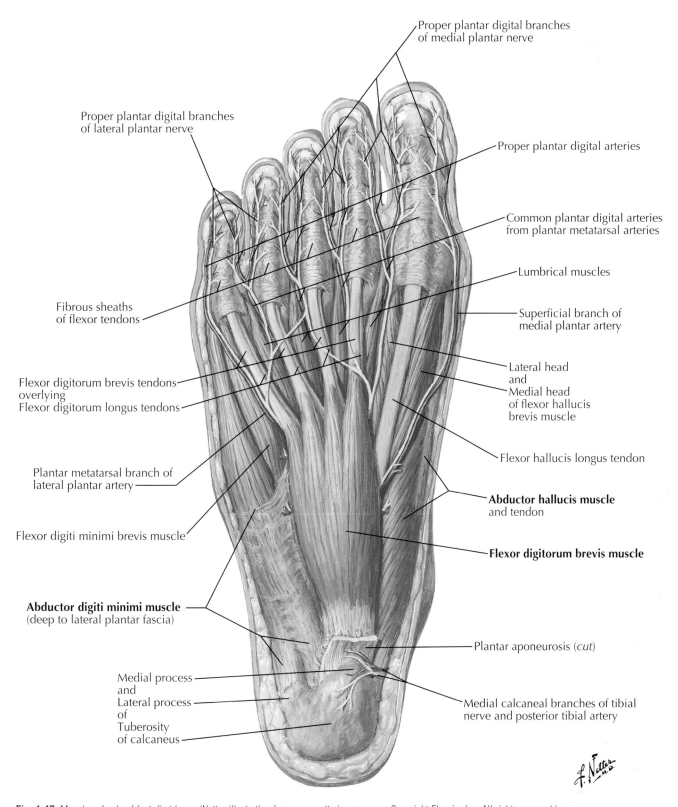

Proper plantar digital branches
of medial plantar nerve

Proper plantar digital branches
of lateral plantar nerve

Proper plantar digital arteries

Common plantar digital arteries
from plantar metatarsal arteries

Lumbrical muscles

Fibrous sheaths
of flexor tendons

Superficial branch of
medial plantar artery

Flexor digitorum brevis tendons
overlying
Flexor digitorum longus tendons

Lateral head
and
Medial head
of flexor hallucis
brevis muscle

Flexor hallucis longus tendon

Plantar metatarsal branch of
lateral plantar artery

Abductor hallucis muscle
and tendon

Flexor digiti minimi brevis muscle

Flexor digitorum brevis muscle

Abductor digiti minimi muscle
(deep to lateral plantar fascia)

Plantar aponeurosis (*cut*)

Medial process
and
Lateral process
of
Tuberosity
of calcaneus

Medial calcaneal branches of tibial
nerve and posterior tibial artery

Fig. 1.47 Muscles of sole of foot: first layer. (Netter illustration from www.netterimages.com. Copyright Elsevier Inc. All rights reserved.)

Table 1.18 Muscles of the foot

Plantar musculature		
First layer	Abductor hallucis Flexor digitorum brevis Abductor digiti minimi	All three extend from calcaneus to toes and create a functional group that assists in maintaining foot concavity
Second layer	Flexor digitorum accessorius Lumbrical muscles	Injury to the motor supply branch for the tibial nerve to the lumbricals can cause clawing of the toes
Third layer	Flexor hallucis brevis Adductor hallucis Flexor digiti minimi brevis	Highly interrelated musculature that contributes in the maintenance of the longitudinal plantar arch
Fourth layer (interosseous compartment)	Dorsal interossei Plantar interossei	The adduction–abduction activity of the interossei is based through the axis of the second toe (dissimilar from the third finger in the hand). Therefore the second toe is the least mobile of the metatarsophalangeal joints. Tendons of the tibialis posterior and the peroneus longus are considered part of the fourth layer
Dorsal musculature	Extensor digitorum brevis	Additional extensor of toes, if it is cut or the extensor digitorum longus the toes still extend and do not impede ambulation. Useful muscle flap for small skin defects and as joint interposition to prevent fusion (e.g., calcaneonavicular bar). Major vascular pedicle from dorsalis pedis perforator and minor pedicle from peroneal artery perforator
	Extensor hallucis brevis	Closely associated with the extensor digitorum brevis and sometimes considered variant slip of the extensor digitorum brevis

the posterior tibial artery and vein via the medial and lateral plantar arteries on its proximal deep surface. The abductor hallucis is supplied by a dominant pedicle on its deep surface and by a branch of the medial plantar artery in the proximal foot. The abductor digiti minimi muscle receives its dominant pedicle from a lateral branch of the proximal lateral plantar artery.

The first layer for the plantar foot is separated from the second layer by the tendons of the extrinsic muscles of the flexor digitorum longus and the flexor hallucis longus. Also, the medial and lateral plantar artery and nerve divide from the posterior tibial artery and the tibial nerve in this intermediary plane *(Fig. 1.34)*.

The second layer consists of the flexor digitorum accessories (also called the quadratus plantae muscle) and the lumbrical muscles of the foot. The quadratus plantae is one of the few muscles of the foot that does not have an analogous structure in the hand. It has two heads extending from the medial and lateral border of the calcaneus. It inserts into the tendon of the flexor digitorum longus and aids in plantarflexion of the second to fifth toes. The lumbricals of the foot mirror those of the hand in their unique attribute of both originating and inserting on tendons. They are four muscles that arise from the medial side of the flexor digitorum longus and insert on the extensor system of the second through fifth phalanges *(Fig. 1.34)*. The foot lumbricals follow the same course as those of the hand, and flex the metatarsophalangeal joints and extend the interphalangeal joints.

The third layer consists of the flexor hallucis brevis, the adductor hallucis, and flexor digiti minimi brevis phalanges

(Fig. 1.34). These form a small, deep intrinsic musculature that contributes in the maintenance of the longitudinal plantar arch and participates in the stabilization of intrinsic foot osteoligamentous intercalation and balance.

The fourth layer is the interosseous compartment which contains both the plantar and the dorsal interossei. The three plantar interosseous muscles adduct the toes. The four dorsal interosseous muscles abduct the toes. The adduction–abduction activity of the interossei is based through the axis of the second toe (dissimilar from the third finger in the hand). Therefore the second toe is the least mobile of the metarsophalangeal joints. Tendons of the tibialis posterior and the peroneus longus are considered part of the fourth layer.

The dorsum of the foot contains two muscles – the extensor digitorum brevis and extensor hallucis brevis *(Fig. 1.33)*. These muscles perform accessory toe extension function to the extrinsic toe extensors. The loss of these muscles does not significantly affect toe extension nor impede ambulation. The extensor digitorum brevis extends the second through fifth toes while the extensor hallucis brevis extends the great toe. The extensor digitorum brevis receives its blood supply from the lateral tarsal artery, a branch off the dorsalis pedis. The extensor digitorum brevis is a useful muscle flap for small skin defects of the foot and ankle *(Fig. 1.48)*. Also it can be used as joint interposition to prevent fusion in nearby tarsal joints (e.g., calcaneonavicular bar). Closely associated with the extensor digitorum brevis is the extensor hallucis brevis. It is a small, variable muscle that is sometimes considered a variant slip of the extensor digitorum brevis.

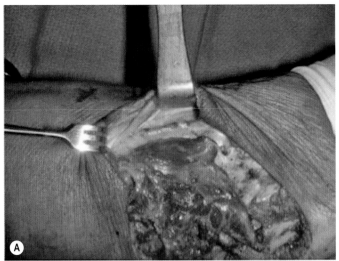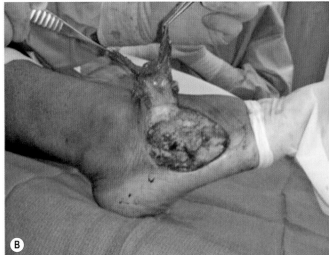

Fig. 1.48 (A, B) Extensor digitorum brevis muscle flap.

Foot and ankle vasculature

The foot and ankle receive their blood supply from three main proximal sources: the dorsalis pedis, the terminal branches of the posterior tibial artery, and the terminal branches of the peroneal artery.

Dorsalis pedis

The dorsalis pedis artery is a direct extension from the anterior tibial artery and is the major vascular supply for the dorsum of the foot. It passes from underneath the extensor retinaculum and travels underneath the extensor digitorum brevis. The dorsalis pedis artery passes between the tendons of the extensor hallucis longus medially and the extensor digitorum longus laterally. As it crosses over the tarsus and continues over the space between the first and second metatarsal, it give off a major terminal branch that dives deep between the first intermetatarsal space and joins the lateral plantar artery to complete the plantar arterial arch *(Fig. 1.49)*. This branching is significant because it provides communication between the dorsal foot circulation primarily supplied by the dorsalis pedis with the plantar circulation supplied by the posterior tibial artery (via the lateral and medial plantar arteries). Another major terminal branch from the dorsalis pedis is the first dorsal metatarsal artery that courses distally and supplies the dorsal skin of the first and second toes.

In the midforefoot, the dorsalis pedis (and variably the first dorsal metatarsal artery) gives off septocutaneous branches that supply the dorsal skin of the medial two-thirds of the foot. This area of skin can be harvested with the dorsalis pedis artery as a fasciocutaneous dorsalis pedis flap.

Posterior tibial artery – medial and lateral plantar arteries

The posterior tibial artery runs beneath the flexor retinaculum and splits in the medial and lateral plantar artery as it enters the sole of the foot in between the first and second layers *(Fig. 1.36)*. The bifurcation occurs under the abductor hallucis muscle and both the lateral and medial plantar arteries arborize to give branches to the toes. The medial plantar artery has a smaller caliber than that of the lateral. It runs along the medial side of the foot and contributes to the plantar digital arteries of the first through third toes. The lateral plantar artery is analogous to the ulnar artery in the hand and similarly is the dominant blood supply for the plantar arterial arch *(Fig. 1.36)*. At the first intermetatarsal space, a perforating branch from the dorsalis pedis dives from the dorsal side of the foot to the plantar surface and connects with the plantar arterial arch via the lateral plantar artery. Together the dorsalis pedis branch and the lateral plantar arch feed the toes through metatarsal branches. These branches in turn join with branches from the medial plantar artery to complete the connecting blood supply to the toes.

Peroneal arterial branches

The peroneal artery contribution in the distal lower extremity is primarily to the ankle blood supply *(Fig. 1.50)*. The terminal branches of the peroneal artery join with the lateral malleolar and calcaneal branches of the posterior tibial artery system at the posterior ankle and heel. The peroneal artery usually ends its contribution to the lower extremity at the calcaneus *(Fig. 1.51)*. However, the size and extent of the peroneal arterial system are in inverse proportion to the other arteries of the ankle and foot. Depending on the size and perfusion

Dorsal view

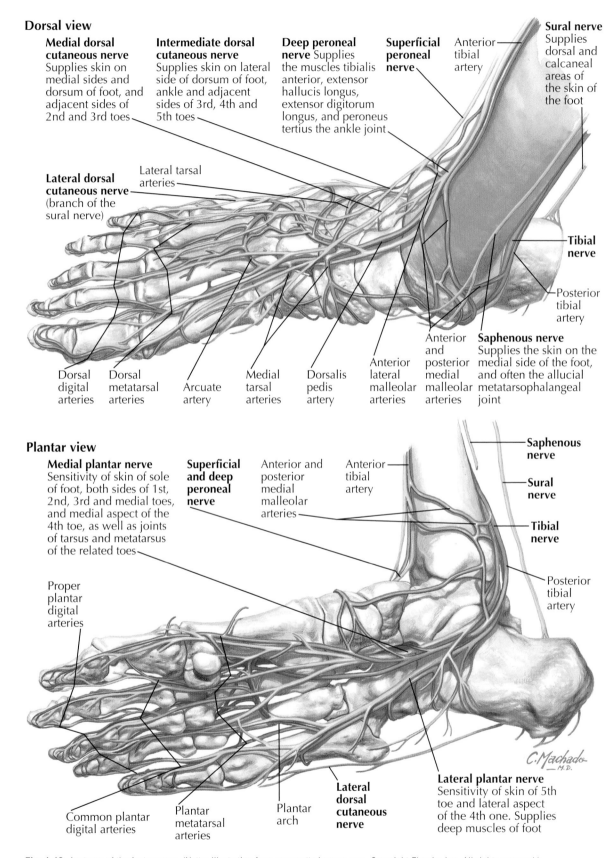

Medial dorsal cutaneous nerve
Supplies skin on medial sides and dorsum of foot, and adjacent sides of 2nd and 3rd toes

Intermediate dorsal cutaneous nerve
Supplies skin on lateral side of dorsum of foot, ankle and adjacent sides of 3rd, 4th and 5th toes

Deep peroneal nerve Supplies the muscles tibialis anterior, extensor hallucis longus, extensor digitorum longus, and peroneus tertius the ankle joint

Superficial peroneal nerve

Anterior tibial artery

Sural nerve
Supplies dorsal and calcaneal areas of the skin of the foot

Lateral dorsal cutaneous nerve (branch of the sural nerve)

Lateral tarsal arteries

Tibial nerve

Posterior tibial artery

Dorsal digital arteries

Dorsal metatarsal arteries

Arcuate artery

Medial tarsal arteries

Dorsalis pedis artery

Anterior lateral malleolar arteries

Anterior and posterior medial malleolar arteries

Saphenous nerve
Supplies the skin on the medial side of the foot, and often the allucial metatarsophalangeal joint

Plantar view

Medial plantar nerve
Sensitivity of skin of sole of foot, both sides of 1st, 2nd, 3rd and medial toes, and medial aspect of the 4th toe, as well as joints of tarsus and metatarsus of the related toes

Superficial and deep peroneal nerve

Anterior and posterior medial malleolar arteries

Anterior tibial artery

Saphenous nerve

Sural nerve

Tibial nerve

Posterior tibial artery

Proper plantar digital arteries

Common plantar digital arteries

Plantar metatarsal arteries

Plantar arch

Lateral dorsal cutaneous nerve

Lateral plantar nerve
Sensitivity of skin of 5th toe and lateral aspect of the 4th one. Supplies deep muscles of foot

C. Machado —M.D.

Fig. 1.49 Anatomy of the foot: nerves. (Netter illustration from www.netterimages.com. Copyright Elsevier Inc. All rights reserved.)

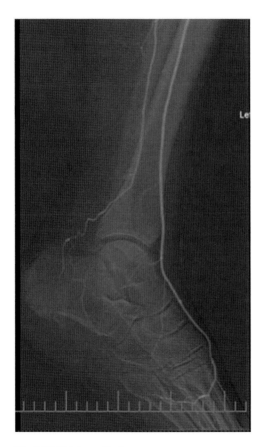

Fig. 1.50 The peroneal artery.

from the posterior tibial artery and anterior tibial artery systems, the peroneal artery system can be seen expanded to augment the foot and ankle vascular supply.

Ankle and foot nerve anatomy

Foot cutaneous innervation

The cutaneous innervation of the foot is shared by the superficial peroneal, the deep peroneal, saphenous, sural and tibial terminal branches (medial calcaneal, medial plantar, and lateral plantar) nerves *(Figs 1.36 and 1.41)*. Innervation from the sural, saphenous, deep and superficial peroneal nerves represents the dorsal, medial and lateral surface of the foot and the posterior ankle. Anatomical descriptions are discussed in the leg section, above. The remaining foot innervation is the plantar surface.

The cutaneous sensation of the sole of the foot is primarily the domain of the tibial nerve and its branches – medial calcaneal, medial plantar, and lateral plantar. The other additional nerve supply comes from the sural and saphenous nerves. The proximal, lateral edge of the foot is supplied by branches from the sural nerve – lateral calcaneal nerve; the proximal, medial edge of the foot is supplied by the saphenous nerve *(Fig. 1.36)*.

Foot motor innervation

The motor supply to the intrinsic muscle of the foot comes from the same nerves as the cutaneous innervation and is organized similarly. The dorsal muscles of the extensor hallucis brevis and the extensor digitorum brevis are innervated by the deep peroneal nerve. All the intrinsic muscles of the plantar surface are innervated by the tibial nerve via the medial and lateral plantar nerves.

The medial and lateral plantar nerves follow the course of the corresponding medial and lateral plantar arteries. The medial plantar artery follows an innervation pattern similar to the median nerve. The muscles to the first toe (abductor hallucis, flexor digitorum brevis, flexor hallucis brevis, and first lumbrical) and the medial plantar cutaneous region, including the first through third toes, are supplied by the medial plantar artery. The lateral plantar nerve mirrors the ulnar nerve as it innervates the deep muscles (interossei, second through fourth lumbricals, adductor hallucis, flexor digitorum brevis and flexor digitorum accessorius, and abductor digiti minimi) and the lateral side of the plantar skin, including the fourth and fifth toes.

Conclusion

It is incumbent to surgeons reconstructing the lower extremity to have a proficient knowledge of the relevant areas of operation. The anatomy is dense and complex and we have attempted to provide the reader with a comprehensive (but by no means exhaustive) study of the critical structures. This chapter's goal is to provide a hopefully valuable resource that be used throughout an entire career to learn, relearn, and review the lower extremity anatomy. With a thorough anatomical knowledge base, the reconstructive options of the following chapters will be easily understood and readers possibly stimulated into developing new reconstructive options themselves.

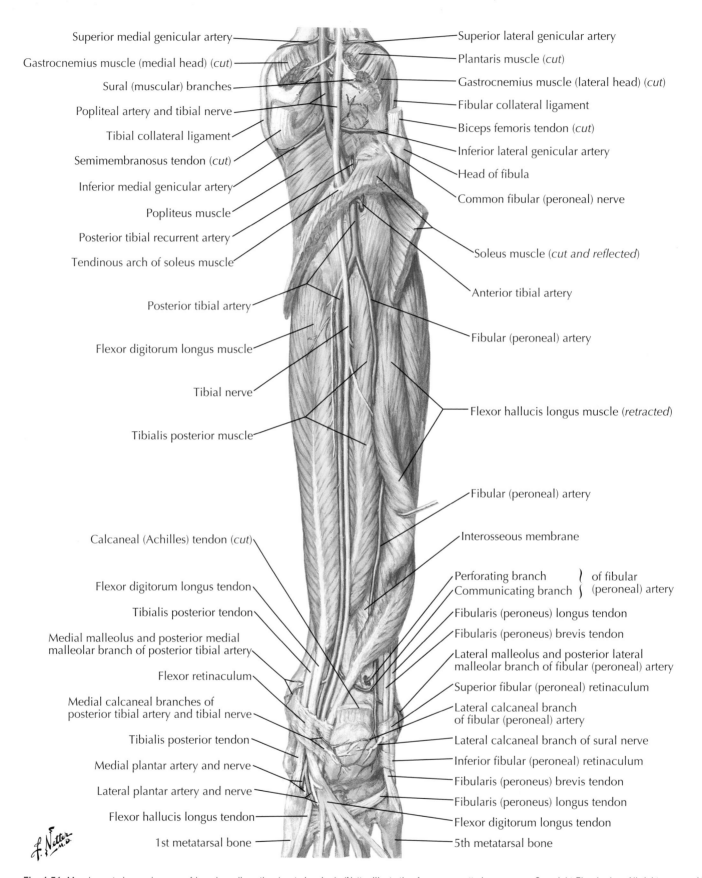

Superior medial genicular artery

Gastrocnemius muscle (medial head) (*cut*)

Sural (muscular) branches

Popliteal artery and tibial nerve

Tibial collateral ligament

Semimembranosus tendon (*cut*)

Inferior medial genicular artery

Popliteus muscle

Posterior tibial recurrent artery

Tendinous arch of soleus muscle

Posterior tibial artery

Flexor digitorum longus muscle

Tibial nerve

Tibialis posterior muscle

Calcaneal (Achilles) tendon (*cut*)

Flexor digitorum longus tendon

Tibialis posterior tendon

Medial malleolus and posterior medial malleolar branch of posterior tibial artery

Flexor retinaculum

Medial calcaneal branches of posterior tibial artery and tibial nerve

Tibialis posterior tendon

Medial plantar artery and nerve

Lateral plantar artery and nerve

Flexor hallucis longus tendon

1st metatarsal bone

Superior lateral genicular artery

Plantaris muscle (*cut*)

Gastrocnemius muscle (lateral head) (*cut*)

Fibular collateral ligament

Biceps femoris tendon (*cut*)

Inferior lateral genicular artery

Head of fibula

Common fibular (peroneal) nerve

Soleus muscle (*cut and reflected*)

Anterior tibial artery

Fibular (peroneal) artery

Flexor hallucis longus muscle (*retracted*)

Fibular (peroneal) artery

Interosseous membrane

Perforating branch } of fibular
Communicating branch ∫ (peroneal) artery

Fibularis (peroneus) longus tendon

Fibularis (peroneus) brevis tendon

Lateral malleolus and posterior lateral malleolar branch of fibular (peroneal) artery

Superior fibular (peroneal) retinaculum

Lateral calcaneal branch of fibular (peroneal) artery

Lateral calcaneal branch of sural nerve

Inferior fibular (peroneal) retinaculum

Fibularis (peroneus) brevis tendon

Fibularis (peroneus) longus tendon

Flexor digitorum longus tendon

5th metatarsal bone

Fig. 1.51 Muscles, arteries, and nerves of leg: deep dissection (posterior view). (Netter illustration from www.netterimages.com. Copyright Elsevier Inc. All rights reserved.)

2

Management of lower extremity trauma

Shannon Colohan and Michel Saint-Cyr

SYNOPSIS

- Lower extremity trauma is common, and often associated with other injuries.
- An Advanced Trauma Life Support (ATLS) approach is required in order to evaluate a patient with lower extremity injuries properly.
- Initial management includes fracture reduction to reduce bleeding, and appropriate radiologic investigations.
- External fixation is useful in the temporization of complex fractures until definitive fixation can be achieved.
- Evidence-based practice with regard to antibiotics, anticoagulation, and timing of reconstruction is recommended.
- A multidisciplinary approach is required in the acute and rehabilitative phases of a patient with lower extremity trauma.

Access the Historical Perspective section online at
http://www.expertconsult.com

Introduction

Major injuries are a significant cause of death and disability worldwide. Injuries are among the leading causes of death in the US, with unintentional injuries as the fifth leading cause of death in all ages.[1] During the years 1999–2007 unintentional injuries were the leading cause of death for those aged 1–44 years, and the third leading cause of death in those aged 45–54 years.[2] In the most recent National Vital Statistics Report (2007), motor vehicle collisions (MVCs) were responsible for 23% of injury-related deaths.[3] The World Health Organization ranked MVCs as the ninth leading cause of disability-adjusted life years, and predicted an increase in ranking to third by 2030.[4] According to the National Trauma Bank's Annual Report (2009),[5] the greatest number of incidents occur between the ages of 25 and 34 years, with a case-fatality rate of 3.70. The highest case-fatality rate occurred in those >85 years

of age (7.72). Males have a higher case fatality rate beyond age 15.

The majority of our trauma systems were designed following experience gained in military combat. This has been further modified and improved with the development of standardized trauma protocols such as those published by ATLS, and the establishment of scoring systems such as the Glasgow Coma Scale (GCS), Injury Severity Scale (ISS), and Trauma and Injury Severity Score (TRISS). Furthermore, scoring systems specific to lower extremity trauma have been developed, and include: the Mangled Extremity Severity Score (MESS), Limb Salvage Index (LSI), Predictive Salvage Index (PSI), the Hanover Fracture Scale-97 (HFS-97), and finally the Nerve injury, Ischemia, Soft-tissue Injury, Skeletal Injury, Shock, and Age of patient score (NISSSA).

The management of a patient with lower extremity trauma involves a multidisciplinary approach. Following the initial provision of emergent trauma care and evaluation by orthopedic and general surgery/vascular surgery colleagues, the plastic surgeon is often involved in the management of extremity coverage and reconstruction of both salvaged and amputated limbs. This is often done in conjunction with orthopedics, thus emphasizing Levin's concept of the "ortho-plastic approach."[6] The current literature is constantly evolving to reflect changes in practice regarding the criteria for limb salvage, timing of reconstruction, and appropriate supportive and adjunctive patient care.

Basic science and disease process

The body's response to trauma is a complex orchestration of inflammatory and immune responses. There is an interplay between those mediators produced at the site of injury (e.g., cytokines, growth factors, nitric oxide, and platelet-activating factors) and the activation of local and systemic polymorpho-nuclear neutrophils, lymphocytes, and macrophages.[16] The changes in hemodynamics, immune and metabolic responses following trauma are largely due to the effects of cytokines.

Cytokines act through specific cellular receptors, and activate intracellular signaling pathways that regulate gene transcription.

The amplitude of the inflammatory response is often related to the severity of the injury. In addition to the initial response to the trauma, a secondary response, or secondary hit phenomenon, occurs with further interventions, including surgical management of fractures and reconstruction.[17–19] There has been increasing focus on methods of avoiding or decreasing the effect of this second hit.

Those patients who succumb to their injury in the third peak of the trimodal distribution (days to weeks postinjury) may be victims of a hyperactive inflammatory response that leads to systemic inflammatory response syndrome, acute respiratory distress syndrome, and ultimately, multiple-organ failure syndrome.

Diagnosis and patient presentation

Lower extremity trauma is often seen in the setting of polytrauma, emphasizing the need to follow protocols during the assessment and management of these patients. Vigilance to rule out other injury is important, as complex lower-extremity injuries can be a significant form of distracting injury. Death due to trauma is often described as having a trimodal distribution.[20] Immediate death is attributed to central nervous system etiologies, including severe brain injury and high spinal cord injury, or major vessel/cardiac injury. Salvage of these patients is rare, emphasizing the need for prevention of such injuries. The second peak occurs within minutes to hours, and deaths are comprised of subdural/epidural hematomas, hemopneumothorax, intra-abdominal major-organ lacerations, pelvic fracture, and hemorrhage from multiple combined injuries. Finally, the third peak occurs within days to weeks, and is due to sepsis or multiple-organ failure, pulmonary embolism, and unrecoverable head injury.

The assessment of the patient with lower extremity trauma starts with triage, to insure that the patient is treated in the appropriate facility capable of managing the injuries. The ultimate goal is to provide timely care (in the "golden hour") to minimize secondary injury. In patients presenting with lower-extremity injuries associated life-threatening injuries may be present in 10–17%.[21] It is therefore paramount to use a protocol-based assessment of the patient such as the ATLS algorithm. Beginning with the primary survey, the airway is maintained or secured while providing cervical spine control, followed by assessment of breathing. Once this is complete, a circulatory exam is carried out, ensuring proper end-organ perfusion and peripheral circulation, as well as control of bleeding. The appropriate monitors are placed, two large-bore intravenous lines are inserted for fluid resuscitation, and a Foley catheter is inserted once a proper rectal/genitourinary screening exam is complete. Any areas of obvious hemorrhage are compressed, and splints or pelvic binders are placed to stabilize orthopedic injuries. Following this, a screening neurological exam is performed to assess the patient's level of consciousness *(Table 2.1)*, cranial nerve function, presence of lateralizing signs, and peripheral nerve exam, including documentation of motor/sensory levels. If it can be safely done,

Table 2.1 **Glasgow Coma Scale**

Eye opening	Spontaneously	4
	To speech	3
	To pain	2
	None	1
Verbal response	Oriented	5
	Confused	4
	Inappropriate	3
	Incomprehensible	2
	None	1
	None – intubated	1T
Motor response	Obeys commands	6
	Localizes to pain	5
	Withdraws from pain	4
	Flexion to pain (decorticate)	3
	Extension to pain (decerebrate)	2
	None	1
Maximum score		15
Minimum score		3 (3T if intubated)

the neurological exam is especially important to perform prior to analgesia, sedating medications, or intubation. Finally, head-to-toe examination of the patient is done in a manner that exposes the patient while preventing hypothermia. Once the primary survey is complete, a secondary survey is carried out, and appropriate radiologic and laboratory investigations are ordered. These may include, but are not limited to: cervical spine, chest and pelvic X-rays, diagnostic peritoneal lavage, or focused assessment sonograph trauma ultrasound for suspected intra-abdominal injuries; computed tomography (CT) scan or angiography; specific extremity X-rays; and laboratory tests, including hematologic and chemistry profiles, arterial blood gas, cross-match, and toxicology screen.

Concerning lower extremity injuries, it is not only important to assess the injury, but also to be aware of its associated complications, including significant bleeding from long-bone injuries, rhabdomyolysis from crush injury, fat embolization, and acute compartment syndrome. In the initial management of these injuries, splinting helps to control blood loss and reduce pain. During the secondary survey, an appropriate history helps determine the mechanism of injury and anticipated degree of injury. The physical examination of the lower extremity includes examination of the skin, neurological status, circulatory status, and skeletal or ligamentous injury. The degree of soft-tissue damage and contamination is important, as these patients will often require prophylactic broad-spectrum antibiotic coverage and tetanus immunization if not

Table 2.2 Tetanus prophylaxis Immunization schedule

History of tetanus immunization	Tetanus-prone wound		Nontetanus-prone wound	
	TD	TIG	TD	TIG
Unknown or <3 doses	Yes	Yes	Yes	No
≥3 doses	No*	No	No†	No

TD, tetanus/diphtheria vaccine; TIG, tetanus immune globulin.
*Yes, if >5 years since last booster.
†Yes, if >10 years since last booster.

Table 2.3 Classification of lower extremity injury

System	Grade	Details
Gustilo	I	Wound <1 cm Simple fracture, no comminution
	II	Wound >1 cm Minimal soft-tissue damage Moderate comminution/contamination
	III	Extensive soft-tissue damage, comminuted fracture, unstable
	IIIA	Adequate soft-tissue coverage
	IIIB	Extensive soft-tissue loss with periosteal stripping and exposed bone
	IIIC	Arterial injury requiring repair
Byrd	Type I	Wound <2 cm Low-energy causing spiral or oblique fracture pattern.
	Type II	Wound >2 cm, contusion of skin/muscle Moderate-energy force causing comminuted or displaced fracture
	Type III	Extensive skin loss and devitalized muscle High-energy force causing significantly displaced fracture with severe comminution, segmental fracture, or bone defect
	Type IV	Degloving or associated vascular injury requiring repair Extensive energy forces with type III fracture pattern

up to date *(Table 2.2)*. Neurological examination should include sensory, motor function, and deep tendon reflexes. Assessment of posterior tibial nerve function can be particularly important in guiding decisions regarding limb salvage. Any circulatory compromise suggests possible arterial injury. Initial management should include fracture reduction, and if pulses are still not restored, appropriate angiographic studies should be sought along with consultation of an orthopedic or vascular surgery colleague. Vascular injury should be suspected in cases of active hemorrhage, expanding or pulsatile hematoma, thrill/bruit over wound, absent distal pulses, or distal ischemic manifestations (the five "P's": pain, pallor, paralysis, paresthesia, poikilothermy).[22] Ischemic time should be estimated for any amputated or vascular-compromised segments. X-rays should be obtained of all areas of suspected injury, including the joint above and below the injury site.

Several grading systems exist to classify lower extremity trauma. The systems most commonly used are the Gustilo and the Byrd systems, in which tibial fractures are classified based on the size of the wound, amount of soft-tissue injury, bony injury, and presence of vascular injury *(Table 2.3)*.[23,24]

Patient selection

When managing the patient with complex lower extremity trauma, it is important to recognize that futile attempts at limb salvage may be associated with physical, mental, social, and financial implications.[25] Despite advances in microsurgical reconstruction, bony regeneration, and infection control, many patients undergo a number of surgeries only to have eventual amputation. It is important to try and identify such patients at the outset, and provide the patient with the best option that maximizes function and recovery.

Amputation versus salvage

The establishment of the MESS by Johansen *et al.* in 1990 was the first effort to produce a set of guidelines that would help a physician to decide between salvage and amputation.[26] This score relied on four criteria: (1) skeletal/soft-tissue injury; (2) limb ischemia; (3) shock; and (4) patient age *(Table 2.4)*. A score of 7 or greater was used as the cutoff point in favor of amputation. Unfortunately, even with this tool there was still debate over definitive criteria for amputation, and this led to the recent multicenter study entitled the Lower Extremity Assessment Project (LEAP), carried out at eight level I trauma centers in the US. This study looked prospectively at patients with traumatic amputations of the lower leg, Gustilo III (A–C) injuries, lower leg devascularizing injuries, major soft-tissue injuries of the lower leg, open pilon fractures (grade III) and ankle fractures (grade IIIB), and severe open hindfoot and midfoot injuries with degloving and nerve injury.[27] The goal of the study was to define the characteristics of the individuals sustaining lower extremity trauma. A total of 601 patients were enrolled, and the patient demographic was primarily male (77%), Caucasian (72%), and young (71% between 20 and 45 years old). The results demonstrated that the patients who sustained a high degree of extremity trauma had several disadvantages prior to their injury (social, economic, personality), and that quality of life and functional outcome data seemed more related to these than to the injury.

A subset of the LEAP studies assessed several available clinical decision-making scores relating to injury severity. These include MESS, LSI, PSI, NISSSA score, and HFS-97. When applying these scores to the open tibial fracture group, MESS, PSI, and LSI demonstrated high specificity (91%, 87%, 97% respectively) but low sensitivity (46% each).[28] Specificity is important to insure that a minimal number of salvageable limbs are incorrectly assigned to amputation, and sensitivity is important to guard against delay in amputation for limbs that are not salvageable. Discrimination was moderately good in assessing salvage versus amputation of the limb. Overall, the analysis did not validate the clinical utility of any of the lower extremity injury severity scores, and advised for their cautious application when making decisions regarding limb salvage. Additionally, these scores are not predictive of functional recovery in patients who undergo successful limb reconstruction, as shown by Ly et al.[29]

Unfortunately, despite a number of studies, there are still no definite criteria for amputation. Several proposed criteria have since been refuted following proper outcome studies. For example, it is a widely held belief that tibial nerve injury or absence of plantar foot sensation is an indication for amputation. However, in a study by Bosse et al.[30] examining functional outcomes of patients with severe lower extremity injuries, they found that more than half of the patients who initially presented with an insensate foot that underwent salvage regained sensation by 2 years. The authors concluded that initial plantar sensation was not prognostic of long-term plantar sensation status or functional outcome, and that this should therefore not be a criterion in limb salvage algorithms.

Risk factors that may contribute to or predict the need for amputation include[22]:

- Gustilo IIIC tibial injuries
- sciatic or tibial nerve injury
- prolonged ischemia (>4–6 hours)/muscle necrosis
- crush or destructive soft-tissue injury
- significant wound contamination
- multiple/severely comminuted fractures; segmental bone loss
- old age or severe comorbidity

Table 2.4 Mangled Extremity Severity Score (MESS) criteria		
Variable		**Points**
A	**Skeletal/soft-tissue injury**	
	Low-energy (stab, simple fracture, civilian gunshot wound)	1
	Medium-energy (open/multiple fractures, dislocation)	2
	High-energy (close-range shotgun, military gunshot wound, crush)	3
	Very-high-energy (above + gross contamination)	4
B	**Limb ischemia***	
	Pulse reduced or absent; perfusion normal	1
	Pulseless, paresthesias, diminished capillary refill	2
	Cool, paralyzed, insensate, numb	3
C	**Shock**	
	Systolic blood pressure always >90 mmHg	1
	Transient hypotension	2
	Persistent hypotension	3
D	**Age**	
	<30 years	1
	30–50 years	2
	>50 years	3
	Maximum score possible	16
	Threshold score for amputation	7
*Score doubled for ischemia time >6 hours.		

- apparent futility of revascularization or failed revascularization.

In addition to these risk factors, several prognostic factors for limb salvage have been identified.[22] These include: mechanism of injury, anatomy of injury (e.g., popliteal artery injury has worst prognosis), presence of associated injuries, age and physiologic health of the patient, and clinical presentation (e.g., shock, limb ischemia). The environmental circumstance may also play a role in determining salvage, with higher amputation rates in combat zones, austere environments, and multicasualty events.

Treatment and surgical techniques

Timing of treatment

There is no debate that a patient with complex trauma should undergo thorough irrigation of open fractures and debridement of devitalized tissue. This is considered to be of paramount importance for the prevention of infection. It is commonly taught that the standard of care is to take patients to the operating room within 6 hours of injury.[31,32] This timeframe is not supported by evidence, and was recently addressed in a subgroup analysis of the LEAP study. Among those patients who developed major infections, significant factors included bone loss >2 cm and Gustilo-type IIIC fractures. Factors such as degree of nerve/muscle damage, size of skin defect, injury severity score, and surgeon's assessment of the degree of contamination were nonpredictive of infection. Regarding their treatment, patients who were managed with intramedullary (IM) nail had a lower incidence of infection compared with those who were externally fixated or treated with plate/screw fixation. There was no significant difference in terms of mean time to debridement between patients who developed infection and those who did not. Time from initial debridement to eventual soft-tissue coverage was also not a risk factor for infection. Multivariate regression showed that patients with delayed admission to a primary trauma center (>2 hours postinjury) or delayed transfer from an outside institution to primary trauma center resulted in higher rates of infection.[33] It is unclear whether delay in admission to a trauma center was in fact a surrogate marker indicative of a higher degree of injury.

With regard to the timing of reconstruction of lower-extremity trauma, most believe that early reconstruction leads to better outcome. This follows the study by Godina[34] in which the timing of microsurgical reconstruction was analyzed with respect to flap failure, infection, bone-healing time, length of hospital stay, and number of operative procedures. This study stratified patients into three groups of repair: (1) within 72 hours; (2) between 72 hours and 3 months; and (3) beyond 3 months postinjury. The study concluded that reconstruction within 72 hours showed the best outcomes for all analyzed factors. Those reconstructed between 72 hours and 3 months postinjury had the highest flap failure rates and highest rates of infection. Those reconstructed beyond 3 months had the longest time to bone healing, and the greatest number of operations *(Table 2.5)*. Criticisms of

Godina's study include the fact that the initial 100 patients in the series were treated in a delayed fashion with average operative times of 6–8 hours, whereas those subsequently treated in an immediate fashion (when microsurgical experience was improved) had shorter operative times.[35] Patients were also not randomized to their treatment regimes, had variable reconstruction (i.e., different flap choices), and upper/lower extremity reconstruction outcomes were pooled. There have been several subsequent studies on this topic – and the results have varied from indifference to favoritism of immediate reconstruction.[23,35–39] Again, the majority of these have been retrospective reviews, where patients were not randomized to treatment, with nonstandardized reconstructive options.

Finally, it is important to recognize that immediate reconstruction is not an option for every patient – and relies on a surgeon capable of performing single-stage debridement and immediate reconstruction, a stable patient without other life-threatening injuries.[40] In this case, serial debridement and possibly the use of wound vacuum-assisted closure dressings may be optimal.

Fracture management

The initial orthopedic management of an open lower extremity fracture has traditionally involved external fixation, in an effort to avoid implantation of metal in a contaminated field. Recently, more orthopedic surgeons are choosing to fixate fractures acutely using IM nails, or even plates and screws using a technique called minimally invasive plate osteosynthesis.[40] The safety of an unreamed IM nail is thought to be equivalent to external fixation with respect to union, delayed union, deep infection, and chronic osteomyelitis.[41] Use of external fixators may be associated with pin tract infection, and may interfere with access for microvascular reconstruction.

Vascular injury

True vascular injury in the setting of lower extremity trauma is rare. Most definitive signs of vascular compromise can be attributed to soft-tissue and bone bleeding, traction of intact arteries with pulse loss (i.e., due to displaced fractures), or compartment syndrome. However, it is prudent to rule out vascular injury, and therefore liberal use of imaging should be carried out in the presence of hard signs. Traditionally, the arteriogram was the gold standard in the diagnosis of vascular injuries. Although it is accurate in diagnosing vascular injury, it has several disadvantages, including cost, duration of procedure, and potential delay to repair, and need for a specialized team to perform it.[42] There is also an associated risk of morbidity in the form of contrast allergy and percutaneous vascular access-related complications. The advent of CT angiography (CTA) has helped to provide rapid diagnosis of vascular injury with lower morbidity. It also enables multiple parts of the body to be assessed. CT angiographic signs of arterial injury include active extravasation of contrast material, pseudoaneurysm formation, abrupt narrowing of an artery, loss of opacification of an arterial segment, and arteriovenous fistula formation.[42] Studies comparing CTA and

Table 2.5 Godina's results on the timing of microsurgical repair			
	Early (<72 hours)	Delayed (72 hours– 3 months)	Late (>3 months)
Number of patients	134	167	231
Free flap failures	0.75%	12%	22%
Postoperative infection	1.5%	17.5%	6%
Bone healing time (average)	6.8 months	12.3 months	29 months
Time in hospital (average)	27 days	130 days	256 days
Number of surgeries (average)	1.3	4.1	7.8

conventional angiography have demonstrated a high sensitivity and specificity of CTA for arterial injury that was confirmed with conventional angiography. There is also a significant cost saving – in one institution savings exceeded $13 000 per patient when performing CTA alone.[43]

There is no doubt that "time is muscle," and prompt repair of any vascular injury should be carried out. Permanent ischemic injury may occur anywhere from 2 to 12 hours postinjury according to the literature. This wide range may be due to variation in injury mechanism, presence of collateral flow, and level of injury.[44] The decision to perform a definitive vascular repair in the setting of lower extremity trauma depends on the clinical circumstances. There are some situations in which the patient is best served with temporary intraluminal shunting following distal thrombectomy and heparinization. These include: unstable fractures, gross contamination of the wound bed, soft-tissue deficits that would lead to an exposed reconstruction/repair, unstable patient, unavailable resources/surgical expertise in vascular repair, and coincident life-threatening injury.[22]

In combined injuries involving bone and vascular disruption, the operative sequence of repair has been debated. In one systematic review, survival of the extremity was directly related to ischemic time, with a steep increase in incidence beyond 3–4 hours of ischemic time.[45] Those favoring immediate vascular repair believe that the reversal of ischemia is most important, whereas those favoring skeletal fixation prior to vascular repair argue that stabilization of the bony fragments first will avoid disruption of a vascular repair during bony manipulation. There have been several reports of fracture fixation following vascular repair, with no disruption of the repair.[46–48] A meta-analysis comparing the outcomes of surgical sequence in 14 published studies did not demonstrate a clear difference between groups regarding incidence of subsequent amputation.[49]

Reconstructive options

In patients with lower extremity trauma, it is important to consider all options for reconstruction, and choose that which is most reliable or will provide the best functional outcome. The reconstructive ladder is often considered, but in major lower extremity trauma where soft-tissue damage is extensive and the zone of injury is wide, local options are often eliminated, emphasizing the need for free flap coverage. When choosing a reconstructive option, consideration is given to the size and location of the defect, functional needs (i.e., innervated flap), zone of injury, proposed location of vascular anastomosis for free flap reconstruction, and accordingly the length of vascular pedicle required to achieve this. Consideration should also be given to the need for future operative interventions (e.g., tendon reconstruction, bony reconstruction), and flap choice should consider ease of re-elevation. Regardless of flap options chosen for reconstruction, adequate debridement of all nonviable tissue is imperative. High-energy trauma can result in significant soft-tissue destruction with a need for extensive debridement of nonviable tissue (*Fig. 2.1*).

The following is a brief overview of flap options that will be described in more detail in subsequent chapters on lower-extremity reconstruction.

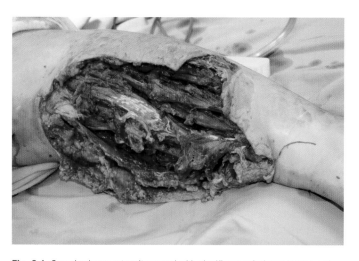

Fig. 2.1 Complex lower extremity wound with significant soft-tissue trauma and devitalization. This wound will require extensive debridement of nonviable skin, muscle, and bone prior to flap coverage in order to prevent infection.

Local flaps

There are a variety of local flap options available in lower-extremity reconstruction. Based on anatomical and angiographic studies, local flaps may be safely performed when based on known perforators. Local flaps are advantageous as they offer a viable reconstructive option with shorter operative times and less complexity.[50] They also provide tissue that is similar in composition to the area of the defect. Patients should be screened for comorbidities that would compromise vascular supply of the lower extremity, and have an appropriate vascular exam with or without investigations performed. A number of local flap options are discussed in the following sections on perforator flaps and muscle-based flaps.

Perforator flaps

The lower extremity is an anatomic region rich in vascular perforators available for harvest (*Figs 2.2 and 2.3*). These have been mapped out in extensive detail through cadaveric injection studies and angiographic investigations. In the gluteal region, the majority of the perforators are musculocutaneous, and arise from the superior and inferior gluteal arteries, with minor contributions from the iliolumbar artery and internal pudendal artery. These are the basis for commonly used gluteal perforator flaps including the superior and inferior gluteal artery perforator flaps.

In the hip and thigh region there are a combination of musculocutaneous and septocutaneous perforators from six source arteries originating from the common femoral artery.[51] The anteromedial thigh is supplied by femoral artery perforators and superficial femoral artery perforators that supply the anteromedial thigh perforator flap. The anterolateral thigh (ALT) is primarily supplied by the lateral circumflex femoral artery (ascending, transverse, and descending branches). These perforators supply the tensor fasciae latae perforator flap, and the ALT (*Figs 2.4 and 2.5*). Just superior to this is the superficial circumflex iliac artery, which provides perforators to the free superficial circumflex iliac artery perforator flap,

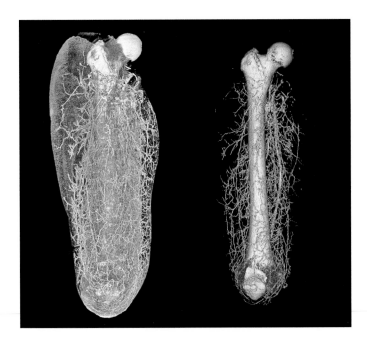

Fig. 2.2 Computed tomography angiography of perforators of the thigh demonstrating a rich density of available cutaneous perforators for flap design and harvest.

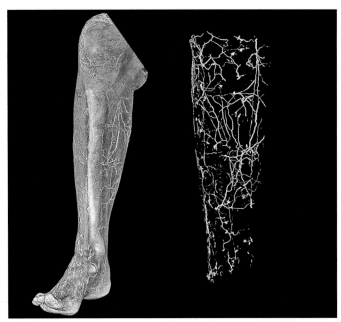

Fig. 2.3 Computed tomography angiography of perforators of the leg, demonstrating a rich density of available cutaneous perforators for flap design and harvest.

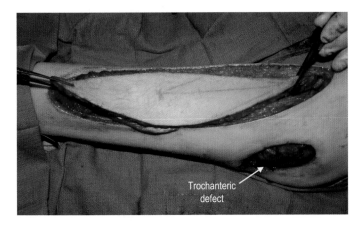

Fig. 2.4 Twenty-year-old paraplegic with a trochanteric pressure wound following debridement. There was a lack of available flap options in the posterior and lateral thigh regions, therefore a pedicle anterolateral thigh flap was used for coverage. Ample laxity was found in the anterior thigh region.

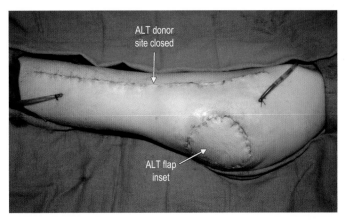

Fig. 2.5 Anterolatoral thigh flap tunneled and inset with primary closure of the donor site.

and contributes to the groin flap. Perforators from the medial circumflex femoral, profunda femoris, and popliteal arteries supply the posteromedial thigh. The posterolateral thigh is supplied by the profunda femoris and inferior gluteal arteries. Inferiorly, the medial and lateral superior genicular arteries supply the region around the knee, and are a source of local perforator flaps in knee reconstruction *(Figs 2.6, 2.7)*.

Surrounding the knee are musculocutaneous perforators from the femoral artery, as well as several septocutaneous branches including the descending genicular artery, medial/lateral superior genicular arteries, medial/lateral inferior genicular arteries, anterior tibial recurrent artery, and popliteal artery cutaneous branch[51] *(Figs 2.8–2.10)*. The saphenous artery is a superficial branch of the descending genicular artery, arising medially with the saphenous nerve and vein,

and is the basis of the saphenous perforator flap, which may incorporate the nerve to create an innervated flap. Posteriorly, the sural arteries (medial/lateral) arise from the popliteal trunk, and may be a source of local perforator flap, including the more reliable medial sural artery perforator flap.

Within the leg, perforators arise from the posterior tibial artery, anterior tibial artery, and peroneal artery. The posterior tibial perforator flap incorporates perforators (4–5 on average) arise in the intermuscular septum between the soleus and flexor digitorum longus. The anterior tibial perforator flap is based on perforators that occur in two rows – one from the tibialis anterior muscle or between the tibialis anterior and extensor hallucis longus, and the second from the anteromedial septum between the peroneus tertius and peroneus brevis muscles[51] *(Fig. 2.11)* The peroneal artery perforator flap is

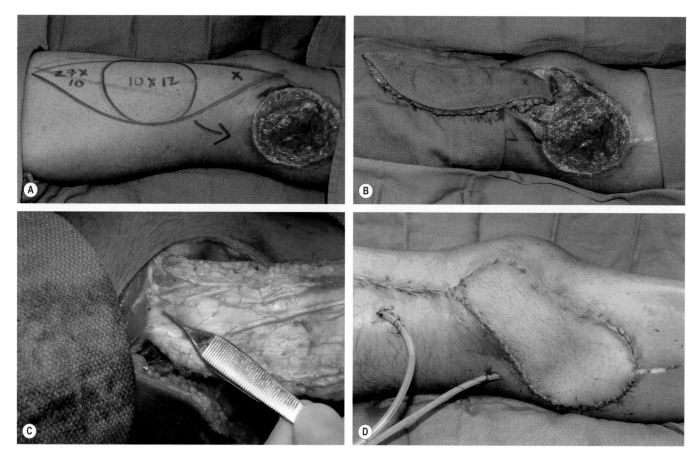

Fig. 2.6 Exposed popliteal arterial vein graft used to revascularize the lower extremity following a gunshot wound to the proximal leg. **(A)** The design of a lateral superior genicular artery pedicle perforator flap with the long axis of the flap designed parallel to the long axis of the thigh. **(B)** The pedicle perforator flap harvested based on a single lateral superior genicular artery perforator. **(C)** The perforator following subfascial harvest of the flap. **(D)** Flap inset with no tension and primary closure of the donor site.

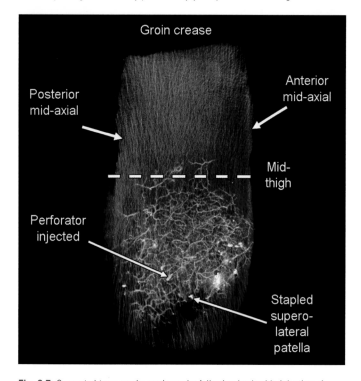

Fig. 2.7 Computed tomography angiography following lead oxide injection of a single lateral superior genicular artery perforator. Perfusion is seen to extend proximally up to the midthigh region and to the anterior and posterior mid axial lines bilaterally.

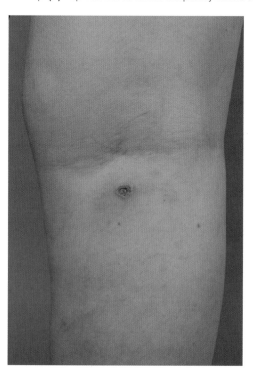

Fig. 2.8 A 54-year-old female with a melanoma in the left posterior knee region.

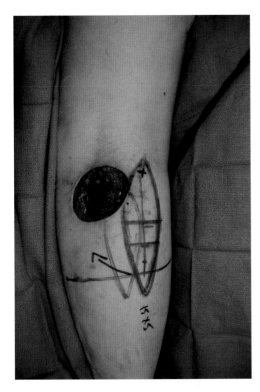

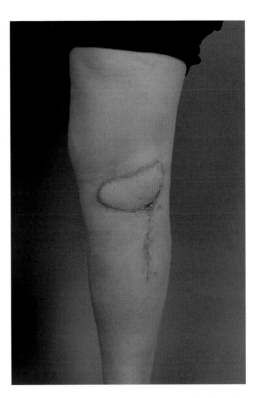

Fig. 2.9 The remaining defect following wide local resection was covered with a 15 × 5 cm freestyle pedicle perforator flap designed along the long axis of the leg and distal to the popliteal fossa.

Fig. 2.10 Two weeks postoperatively with well-perfused flap and stable wound coverage. Minor delayed healing of the donor site went on to heal uneventfully.

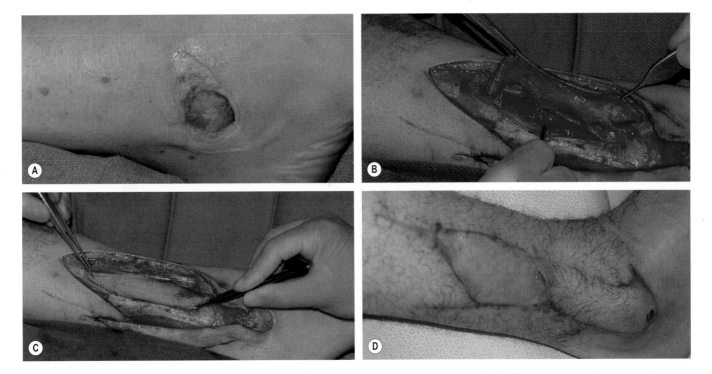

Fig. 2.11 (A–D) Lateral malleolus wound covered with an anterior tibial artery pedicle perforator flap, which was rotated 180° ("propeller" flap) to reach the defect.

comprised of perforators that emerge distally in the postero-lateral septum between the peroneus longus and soleus muscles *(Figs 2.12–2.15)*.

In the foot, the terminal branches of the anterior tibial, posterior tibial, and peroneal arteries are another source of perforator flaps. These include the lateral calcaneal artery perforator flap (the terminal branch of the peroneal artery), and medial plantar artery-based perforator flaps (medialis pedis flap, instep flap, abductor hallucis muscle flap) *(Fig. 2.16)*.

Muscle-based flaps

In the thigh, a number of local muscles may be used to reconstruct defects. These include the gracilis flap, based on the ascending branch of the medial circumflex femoral artery. As a local flap, this is commonly used to reconstruct the groin, perineum, and ischium. The sartorius flap is based on the superficial femoral artery (type IV vascular supply), may be used to cover groin defects and exposed femoral vessels, and is rarely used as an inferiorly based flap to cover small knee defects. The anterior thigh musculature may provide coverage of the inferior abdomen, groin and perineum, and ischium, and includes the rectus femoris flap (based on profunda femoris artery), the vastus lateralis (descending branch of lateral circumflex femoral artery (LCFA)), and vastus medialis (superficial femoral artery) flaps. Laterally, the tensor fasciae latae flap (ascending branch of LCFA) may be used for similar applications, and may additionally reach the trochanteric region and sacrum for pressure sore reconstruction. Posteriorly, the biceps femoris flap (profunda femoris) is used primarily for pressure sore reconstruction.

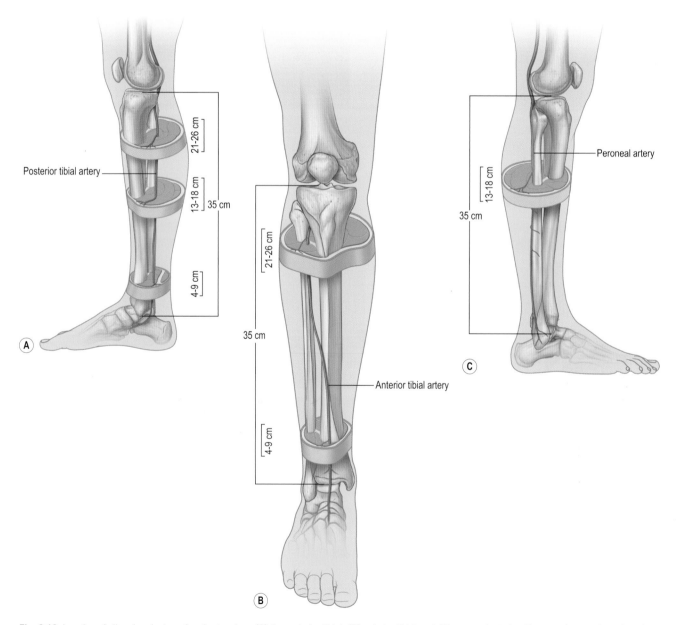

Fig. 2.12 Location of all major clusters of perforators from **(A)** the posterior tibial, **(B)** anterior tibial, and **(C)** peroneal arteries. These perforator cluster locations can help in the design and planning of local pedicle perforator flaps in the lower extremity.

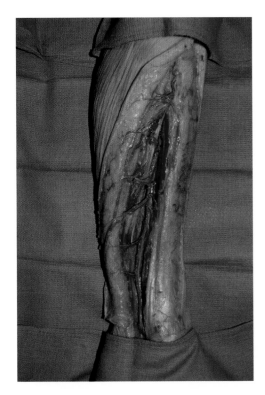

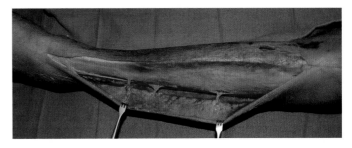

Fig. 2.15 Cadaver dissection showing peroneal artery perforators.

Fig. 2.13 Cadaver dissection of the leg with arterial red latex injection and venous blue latex injection of the posterior tibial artery (PTA) and vein respectively. Perforators of the posterior tibial artery are shown with their associated venae comitantes. Perforators from the PTA are among the largest in the lower extremity and can form the basis for various local pedicle perforator flaps for anterior tibial and lateral coverage in the distal third of the leg.

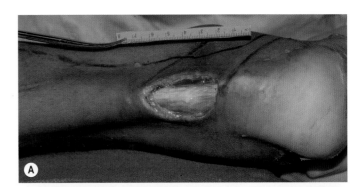

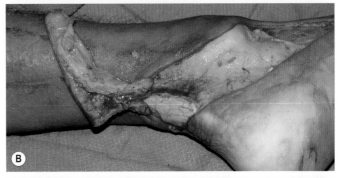

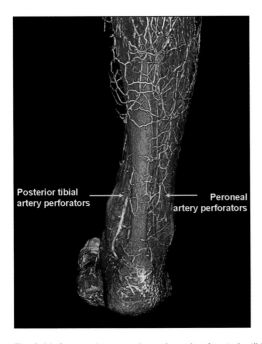

Fig. 2.14 Computed tomography angiography of posterior tibial artery and peroneal artery perforators of the leg demonstrating a rich density of available cutaneous perforators for local flap design and harvest.

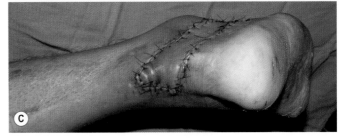

Fig. 2.16 **(A)** A 4-cm defect with exposure of the Achilles tendon following wound debridement. **(B)** Harvest of a calcaneal artery flap for Achilles tendon coverage. **(C)** Achilles coverage and flap inset following transfer.

In the lower leg, the most commonly used muscular flaps include the gastrocnemius and soleus muscle flaps. The gastrocnemius muscle has medial and lateral heads, based on the medial and lateral sural arteries, respectively. The medial head is most commonly used as it is longer and has better reach. This is used primarily in knee and upper-third leg coverage *(Figs 2.17, 2.18)*. The soleus flap is based on branches from the popliteal artery, posterior tibial artery, and peroneal artery. Distally, segmental branches from the posterior tibial artery allow for a reverse soleus flap. A number of other

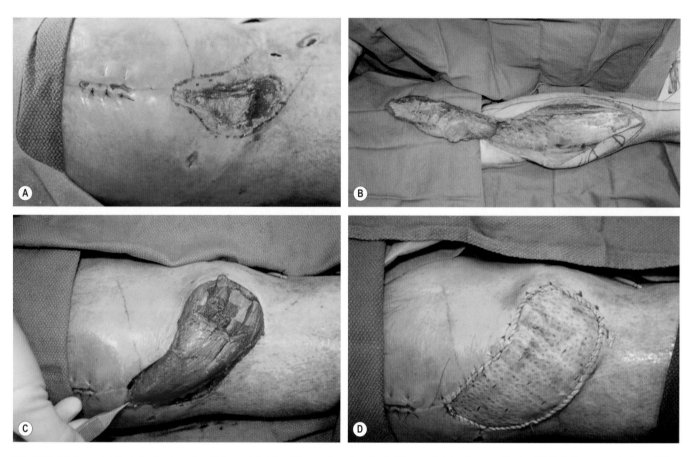

Fig. 2.17 (A) Exposed left patellar tendon with soft-tissue defect in a 56-year-old male patient with an underlying knee prosthesis. **(B)** Posterior approach via a midline incision for harvest of a medial gastrocnemius muscle flap. The posterior and anterior surface of the muscle fascia can be scored to achieve greater length and the muscle origin can also be detached for the same purpose. **(C)** Wound was debrided and defect covered with a tunneled pedicle medial gastrocnemius muscle flap. Tunnel must be adequately released so that no pressure is exerted on the muscle and its pedicle. **(D)** Final flap inset and coverage with a split-thickness skin graft.

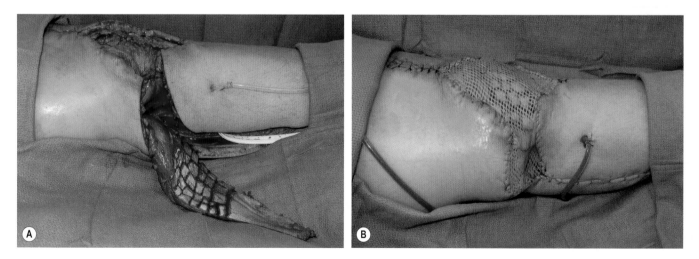

Fig. 2.18 (A) Alternatively, an anterior approach can be used to harvest a gastrocnemius flap for knee defects and this avoids any positional changes. Posterior and anterior muscle fascia scoring are also performed in order to maximize muscle length. The tendinous portion of the muscle can also be used to anchor the flap and provide additional well-vascularized tissue. **(B)** Final flap inset and split-thickness skin grafting with complete wound coverage.

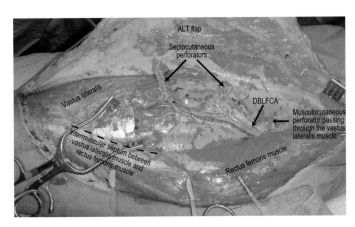

Fig. 2.19 Anterolateral thigh flap harvest showing perforators originating from the descending branch of the lateral circumflex femoral artery (DBLCFA). The DBLCFA is seen coursing between the vastus lateralis laterally and the rectus femoris medially. Once the rectus femoris muscle has been dissected and retracted medially all perforators from the DBLCFA become easily visible. The most direct and least intramuscular perforator is then selected for flap harvest.

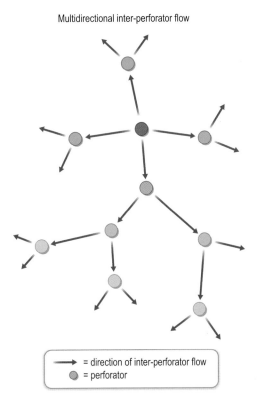

Fig. 2.20 Interperforator flow allows communication with multiple adjacent perforators via direct and indirect linking vessels.

smaller muscle-based flaps have been described (extensor hallucis longus, flexor hallucis longus, extensor digitorum longus, flexor digitorum longus, peroneus brevis/longus flaps), but these flaps provide minimal bulk and often suboptimal coverage in larger defects.

The foot is a source of several small local muscular flaps, including the abductor digiti minimi flap, abductor hallucis flap, and flexor digitorum brevis flap.

Fascial-based flaps

In the thigh, the ALT flap has become a workhorse flap, and is used primarily as a free flap. This flap is based on the descending branch of the LCFA, which arises from the profunda femoris artery. This flap is described as having three cutaneous perforators – A, B, and C – that lie along a line marked from the anterior superior iliac spine to the superolateral patella.[52] These perforators may have a septocutaneous course between the vastus lateralis and rectus femoris, or a musculocutaneous course through the vastus lateralis. Dissection may course either suprafascially or subfascially. An extended ALT flap has been described which incorporates distal linking vessels between the LCFA, common femoral, and superficial femoral arteries[53] *(Figs 2.19–2.22)*. Additionally, the reverse ALT flap has also been described as a distally based pedicled flap in lower extremity reconstruction.[54] Consideration may be given to supercharging this flap through anastomosis of the proximal LCFA to leg donor vessels (e.g., anterior tibial) if vascularity is questionable.[55]

In the leg, the sural artery flap and reverse sural artery flap provide coverage of the knee and calcaneal region, respectively. The sural artery flap is based on a direct cutaneous branch of the sural artery and lesser saphenous vein. The reverse sural artery flap is primarily based on septocutaneous perforators from the peroneal artery, and includes the lesser saphenous vein and median cutaneous sural nerve[56] *(Fig. 2.23)*. Venous congestion and partial flap ischemia are complications that can arise in the reverse sural artery flap, and may be overcome through a two-stage delay procedure, or through supercharging it[57,58] *(Fig. 2.24)*.

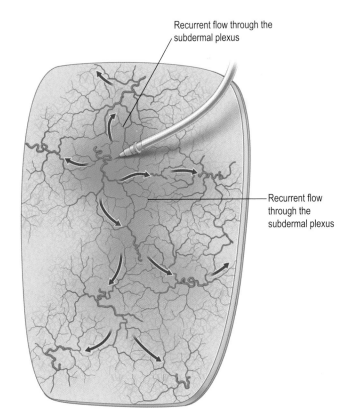

Fig. 2.21 A large (extended) anterolateral thigh flap can be harvested based on a single perforator. High arterial filling pressures from the selected perforator allow interperforator flow and increased flap vascular territory.

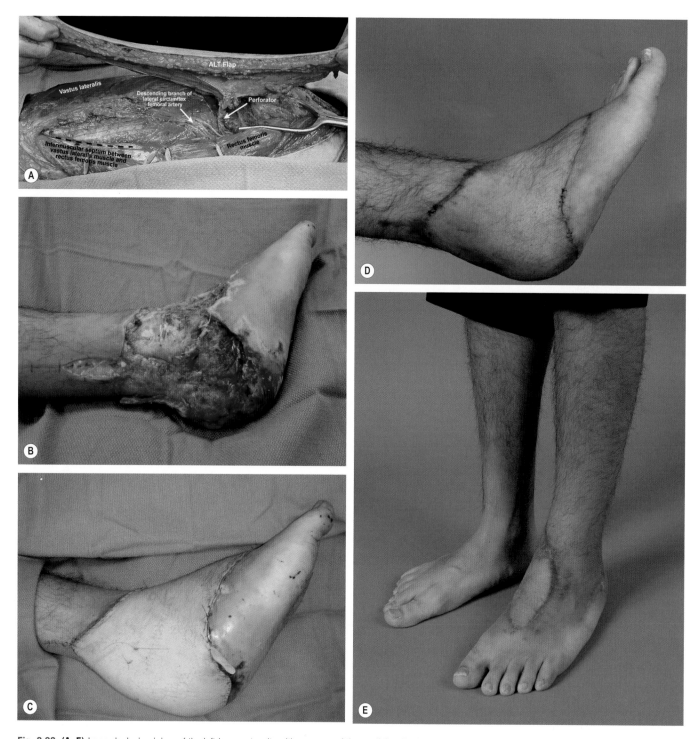

Fig. 2.22 (A–E) Large degloving injury of the left lower extremity with exposure of the medial malleolus, Achilles tendon, calcaneus, and extensor tendons. Following radical debridement, resurfacing was done with an extended anterolateral thigh (ALT) flap. The ALT flap was later liposuctioned for improved contour and the patient was able to wear his normal footwear and ambulate at his preinjury level.

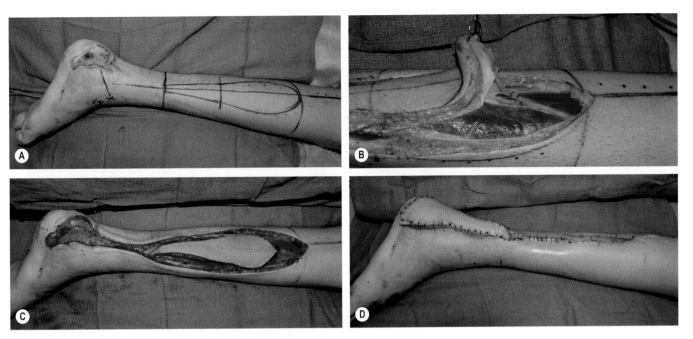

Fig. 2.23 (A) Left lower extremity defect with exposed Achilles tendon and calcaneus. Sural artery flap designed along a vertical axis centered from midpoint between the lateral malleolus and the Achilles tendon and the midpoint of the popliteal fossa. Maximal peroneal perforator density can be found within 8 cm of the lower transverse line. This location represents the proximal extent of the sural artery flap. The sural artery flap can safely extend three-quarters of the leg proximally. A delay procedure can be considered in patients with advanced age and medical comorbidities (e.g., diabetes) in order to maximize arterial perfusion and venous outflow. **(B)** Subfascial elevation of the sural artery flap from proximal to distal with early identification of the sural nerve and artery, which are incorporated into the flap. Note that this flap is principally based on peroneal perforators and can alternatively be harvested without sacrifice of the sural nerve. **(C)** Sural artery flap *in situ* following elevation and recipient site debridement. **(D)** Final flap inset without tension. Donor site is closed primarily with the addition of a split-thickness skin graft as needed. Liberal use of skin grafting should be done proximal to the flap base in order to minimize undue pressure on the perforators.

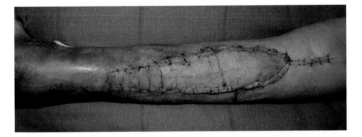

Fig. 2.24 Two weeks post surgical delay procedure of a sural artery flap in a diabetic 84-year-old patient. This delay procedure allows for a clear demarcation of flap viability. Note the proximal ischemic portion of the flap was discarded prior to definitive flap transfer.

Free tissue transfer – muscle

Larger defects of the lower extremity that require obliteration of dead space often warrant the use of a muscle-based free flap in combination with split-thickness skin graft. Commonly used muscles include the latissimus dorsi (thorocodorsal artery) *(Figs 2.25–2.27)*, rectus abdominis (deep inferior epigastric artery) *(Fig. 2.28)*, serratus anterior (lateral thoracic artery or branch to serratus from thoracodorsal artery), and free gracilis (ascending branch of medial circumflex artery) *(Figs 2.29–2.30)*. For small to moderate defects, muscle-sparing versions of the latissimus dorsi and rectus flaps can also provide an excellent option without sacrificing donor site function.

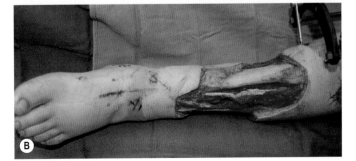

Fig. 2.25 (A) Complex left lower extremity defect with a comminuted fracture of the proximal tibia. **(B)** Defect following radical debridement and conversion of multiple wound units to a simpler single wound unit.

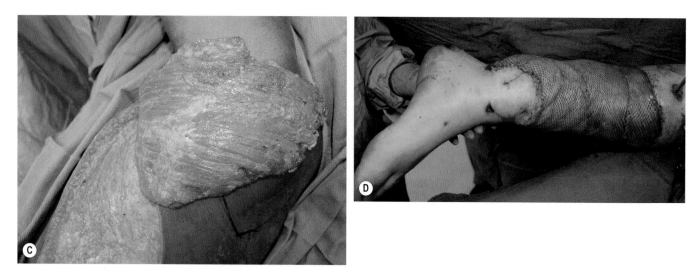

Fig. 2.25, cont'd (C) Free latissimus dorsi muscle flap harvested to provide coverage of a large surface area. This muscle flap also allows important deep space obliteration in cases involving comminuted fractures with complex three-dimensional wound defects. **(D)** Circumferential coverage of the lower extremity wound with a latissimus dorsi flap and split-thickness skin graft. Anastomosis was performed to the posterior tibial artery and vein distal to the zone of injury. Vessels distal to the zone of injury have the advantage of being more superficial, which facilitates vessel access and microsurgery.

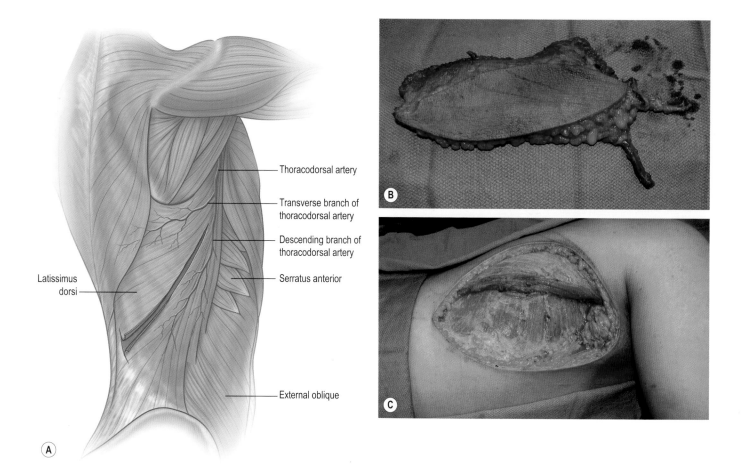

Fig. 2.26 (A) Alternatively, for smaller defects of the lower extremity, a free muscle-sparing latissimus dorsi (LD) flap can be used. This flap retains all of the advantages of its full LD counterpart without sacrificing donor muscle function. The muscle-sparing LD flap can be based on either the descending or transverse branch of the thoracodorsal artery and vein. **(B)** Muscle-sparing latissimus dorsi myocutaneous flap for lower extremity reconstruction. **(C)** Donor site following free muscle-sparing latissimus dorsi flap harvest. Note preservation of the anterior axillary line and majority of latissimus dorsi muscle.

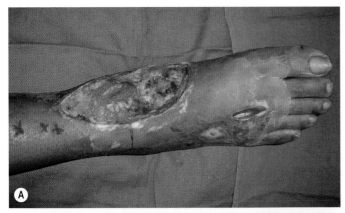

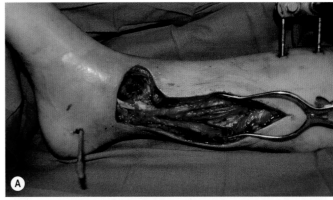

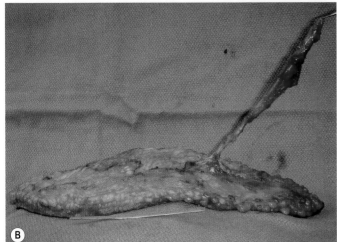

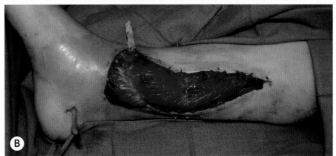

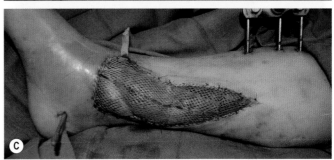

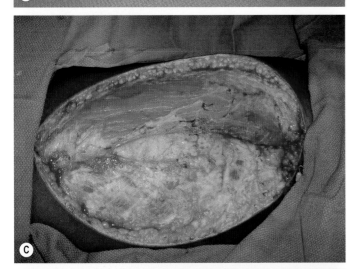

Fig. 2.28 (A) Right medial ankle defect with exposed medial malleolus and tendons. Radical debridement was performed and posterior tibial artery and vein were prepared as recipient vessels. Posterior tibial vessels are our recipient vessels of choice for medial and anteromedial defects. They provide large, dependable vessels that are usually well protected deep from the zone of injury. **(B)** Coverage of the medial ankle defect with a free muscle-sparing rectus flap. **(C)** Final inset and coverage with a split-thickness skin graft. Note that the external fixator can be temporarily dismantled for better vascular access and easier microsurgery.

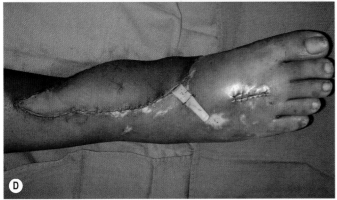

Fig. 2.27 (A) Right ankle wound with exposed medial malleolus and soft-tissue defect in a 45-year-old patient. **(B)** Thin thoracodorsal artery perforator flap harvested for resurfacing a medial ankle defect. **(C)** Thoracodorsal artery perforator flap donor site with preservation of entire latissimus dorsi muscle. Flap was based on a direct cutaneous branch, which followed the anterior border of the latissimus dorsi muscle. **(D)** Thoracodorsal artery perforator flap (8 × 20 cm) used to resurface the medial right ankle and malleolus.

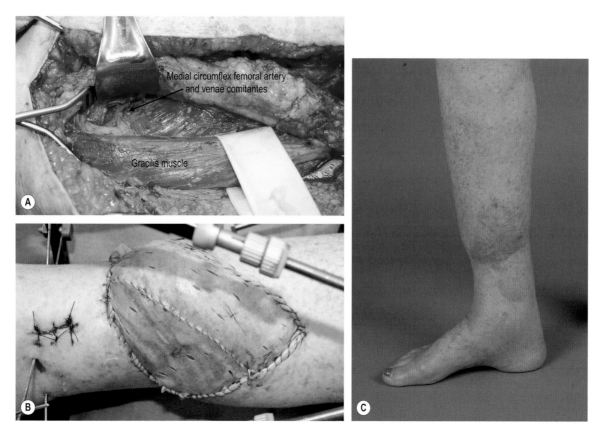

Fig. 2.29 (A) Dissection of a free gracilis flap with exposure of the medial circumflex femoral artery and venae comitantes. **(B)** Gracilis free flap inset with sheet split-thickness skin graft. **(C)** Final postoperative result after 1 year with low-profile contouring of the free gracilis flap. Note that this patient underwent minor debulking of the gracilis muscle at 6 months postoperatively. A dermatome was used for muscle debulking and also for split-thickness skin graft removal. The skin graft was recycled back on to the gracilis flap immediately following muscle shaving in order to avoid another skin graft donor site.

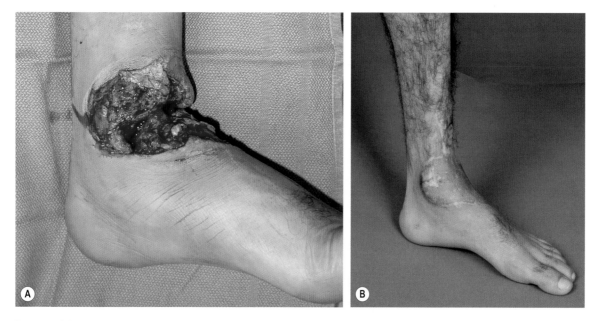

Fig. 2.30 (A) Exposed extensor tendons, left talus, distal tibia and fibula, with significant dead space. This open joint creates a complex three-dimensional defect, which can be effectively obliterated with an expendable free gracilis flap. **(B)** Postoperative result after 6 months with good contouring of the anterior ankle and minimal bulk. Denervated muscle atrophies significantly over time and contours well to its recipient site.

Free tissue transfer – fasciocutaneous

One of the most versatile and popular fasciocutaneous free flaps used in lower extremity reconstruction is the ALT. This can be converted into a sensate flap by incorporating the lateral femoral cutaneous nerve, which is useful in distal third and foot reconstruction where sensation is important. This flap is described above. The ALT flap can also be harvested as a thinner adipofascial flap which allows primary donor site closure. This flap variation can be very useful in patients who have an unsuitable ALT donor site due to excessive thickness *(Figs 2.31, 2.32)*.

Other fasciocutaneous flaps used in lower extremity reconstruction include the free radial forearm flap and the anteromedial thigh flap. The free radial forearm flap is based on the radial artery, which runs proximally between the brachioradialis and pronator teres. It can be made sensate through the incorporation of either the lateral or medial antebrachial cutaneous nerves. The anteromedial thigh flap is supplied by a septocutaneous branch of the LCFA, commonly arising between the medial border of the rectus femoris and the sartorius[59] *(Fig. 2.33)*. It provides a large skin paddle, with a well-hidden donor site. Additionally, it can be designed as a vascular flowthrough flap for combined soft-tissue/vascular reconstruction.

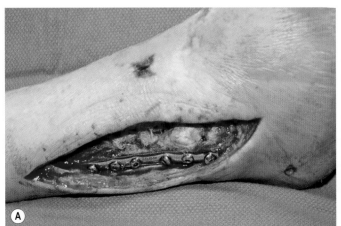

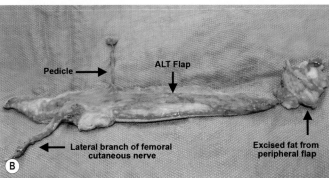

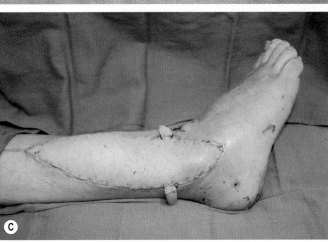

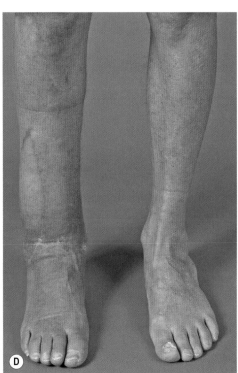

Fig. 2.31 (A–C) Right lateral ankle soft-tissue defect and exposed hardware resurfaced with a thinned and neurotized anterolateral thigh flap based on a lateral branch of the femoral cutaneous nerve. The periphery of the flap can also be thinned for better inset and less bulk. We do not recommend aggressive primary thinning of the anterolateral thigh flap and prefer to do this secondarily if necessary. **(D)** Postoperative results 6 months later with stable right-leg wound coverage and healed donor site.

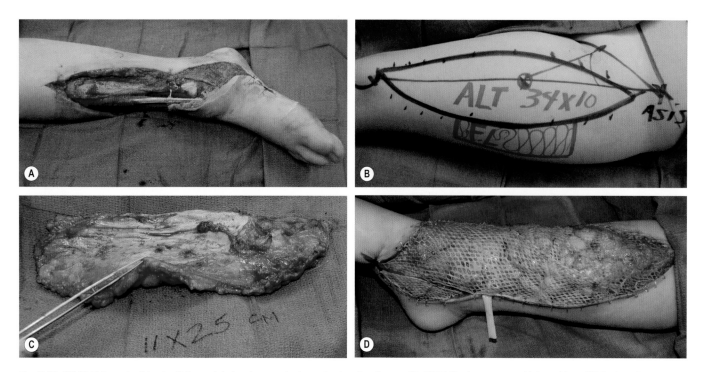

Fig. 2.32 (A) Right leg anterolateral soft-tissue defect and exposed extensor tendons in a 9-year-old child following a motor vehicle accident. **(B)** Design of a contralateral extended anterolateral thigh flap. **(C)** The anterolateral thigh (ALT) flap was converted into an adipofascial ALT flap in order to minimize bulk and maximize flap size while allowing primary donor site closure. A 25 × 11 cm adipofascial ALT flap was used for reconstruction and permitted entire wound coverage. **(D)** Adipofascial anterolateral thigh flap inset and coverage with a split-thickness skin graft. The posterior tibial artery and vein were used as reliable recipient vessels.

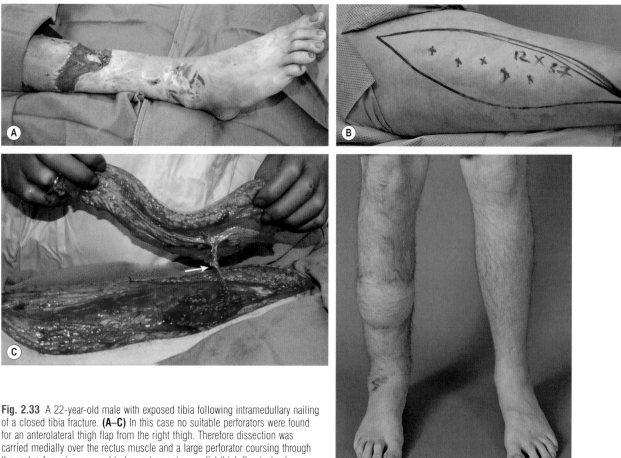

Fig. 2.33 A 22-year-old male with exposed tibia following intramedullary nailing of a closed tibia fracture. **(A–C)** In this case no suitable perforators were found for an anterolateral thigh flap from the right thigh. Therefore dissection was carried medially over the rectus muscle and a large perforator coursing through the rectus femoris was used to harvest an anteromedial thigh flap instead. **D** Postoperative results 6 months later with stable right-leg wound coverage and healed donor site.

Skeletal reconstruction

Options for bony reconstruction of the lower extremity include autogenous bone graft, vascularized bone transfer, and distraction osteogenesis, including the Ilizarov technique. Autogenous cancellous bone grafts are typically used to fill small defects in bone *(Fig. 2.34)*. While it is possible to bridge larger gaps (8–10 cm) with autogenous bone, it is not the favored approach. In this situation, the use of vascularized bone transfer or distraction techniques may be preferred. The most commonly employed vascularized bone flap is the free fibula flap, based on segmental and nutrient supply from the peroneal artery. Alternative flaps include the iliac crest vascularized bone flap (deep circumflex iliac artery), and the vascularized scapular flap (circumflex scapular artery). Bone flaps will hypertrophy over time, but this occurs over months to a few years. For defects over 10 cm, distraction osteogenesis is considered. This involves the division of cortical bone outside the zone of injury, preserving the medullary bone and blood supply. Pins are applied on either side of the bone ends, and a circumferential external distraction Ilizarov device is applied. Distraction starts 1 week later, with approximately 1 mm distraction carried out daily at the corticotomy sites. The process can take up to 1 year to allow adequate distraction followed by bony consolidation. It can be very arduous, with associated pin site infection and pain.

Negative-pressure wound therapy in lower extremity defects

As advances in wound care have evolved over the past decade, there is increasing reliance on their use in the management of complex soft-tissue wounds. In particular, the use of commercially available negative-pressure wound therapy (NPWT) devices is becoming more commonplace. It is thought that NPWT provides edema control and facilitation of wound closure via the application of soft-tissue macrostrain forces, stimulation of fibroblast proliferation and tissue granulation via macrostrain at a cellular level, limitation of destructive wound proteases, facilitation of bacterial clearance from the wound, and limitation of cross-contamination in a hospital environment.[60] DeFranzo et al.[61] used an NPWT system in 75 patients with exposed tendon, bone, or hardware, excluding those with frank osteomyelitis. All wounds underwent surgical debridement until viable tissues were present in the wound base, prior to the application of the NPWT device. The authors found that granulation tissue was often present by the second dressing change, with a reduction in wound edema and bacterial count. All patients achieved stable wound coverage via delayed primary closure, skin graft, or local flap, with no need for free tissue reconstruction. In their assessment of trends in lower extremity reconstruction, Parrett et al. (2009)[50] found that there was a trend down the reconstructive ladder, with a decreasing incidence of free flap reconstruction and more frequent use of NPWT devices. They stated that at their center the NPWT system was used in 50% of open fractures, and most Gustilo grade III tibial fractures, with closure being achieved through delayed primary, secondary, and skin graft methods. This is not only cost-effective, but may result in fewer complications related to long operative reconstructions, postoperative immobilization, and flap-related complications such as necrosis and flap loss. Additionally, the NPWT systems can be used in fasciotomy wounds and incisional edema management.[62]

Amputation

In the situation where amputation is indicated, or the trauma has resulted in a complete/near-complete amputation it is important to consider management of the amputation stump from a prosthetic standpoint. Preservation of length and creation of stable soft-tissue coverage are of paramount importance. If at all possible, maintaining a below-knee amputation length is important, as these are better tolerated from a prosthetic standpoint, and have much less energy demand for mobilization. In cases where there is inadequate soft-tissue coverage of a below-knee amputation bony stump, it is possible to use free flaps to maintain length. These can include musculocutaneous and fasciocutaneous options, similar to those discussed above. One can also consider the use of "spare parts" surgery, whereby portions of the amputated extremity (if intact/appropriate) can be used to reconstruct the remaining defect. Finally, if there is muscle coverage of the bony stump but no skin coverage, the use of skin grafts is appropriate to provide soft-tissue coverage.

Treatment of associated complications

Rhabdomyolysis

The concept of acute renal failure associated with crush injuries was first documented by Bywaters and Beal (1941). It was their observation that patients who had been buried for several hours (during the Blitzkrieg attacks in London) presented with swelling and anesthesia of their limbs, with progression to pallor, coldness, sweating, and unstable vital signs (shock). Eventually arterial pulses diminished and urine output dropped, coincident with an increase in albumin and dark brown casts within it. Patients subsequently developed hyperkalemia and renal failure, leading to an accelerated death.

The pathophysiology of rhabdomyolysis involves an injury to muscle resulting in myocyte injury resulting in sodium and calcium influx into the cytoplasm and potassium efflux into the extracellular fluid.[63] As a result of this myocyte injury, a

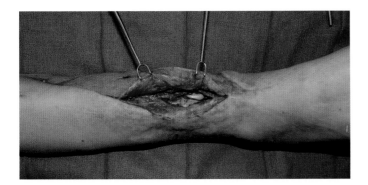

Fig. 2.34 Elevation of previous free muscle-sparing rectus muscle to medial distal third of right leg in order to remove methyl methacrylate and place definitive bone graft. Healed muscle flaps can be easily re-elevated during secondary procedures such as bone grafting or hardware removal.

large quantity of muscle enzymes and lactate dehydrogenase is released, in addition to an elevated creatine kinase. The diagnosis of rhabdomyolysis is supported by a positive urine dipstick for hemoglobin, in addition to laboratory confirmation of myoglobin and quantitative assessment. The severity of acute renal failure that ensues can be predicted by the presence of a urine myoglobin concentration >20 mg/L.[64] Renal failure associated with rhabdomyolysis has three main mechanisms: (1) tubular obstruction; (2) tubular damage by oxidant injury; and (3) vasoconstriction.[63]

In the treatment of rhabodmyolysis, the most important component is early volume replacement to help prevent the development of renal failure. Alkalinization of the urine using sodium bicarbonate (to a target pH 7.0) may be beneficial for myoglobin washout and the prevention of lipid peroxidation and renal vasoconstriction. The use of mannitol is more controversial, and may not be better than volume expansion alone.[65]

Fat embolization

Fat embolism is a rare entity, but occurs most commonly as a result of long-bone fractures and polytrauma. It may be related to movement of unstable fracture fragments or IM reaming during operative fixation. It is most common in young males aged 10–40 years, and is rare in children and the elderly. This may be related to the low fat content of bone marrow in children, and minimal trauma fractures that tend to occur in the elderly.[66]

Two theories regarding the pathophysiologic mechanism of fat embolism syndrome (FES) exist – the mechanical hypothesis and the biochemical hypothesis. The mechanical hypothesis postulates that an increase in IM pressure forces marrow particles, fat, or bone fragments into the circulation via the open venous sinusoids. This leads to obstruction of peripheral and lung microcirculation. This results in ventilation–perfusion mismatch, low partial pressure of oxygen, and low oxygen saturation. Cerebral and renal embolization may contribute to the symptoms. The biochemical theory postulates that physiochemical alteration occurs when fat globules are acted upon by lipoprotein lipase, resulting in the release of free fatty acids. This results in the release of toxic intermediates that can cause direct injury to pneumocytes and lung endothelial cells.[67]

FES is characterized by progressive respiratory insufficiency, deteriorating mental status, and petechial rash (major diagnostic criteria). Minor diagnostic criteria include pyrexia, tachycardia, retinal changes, jaundice, oliguria/anuria, thrombocytopenia, high erythrocyte sedimentation rate, and fat macroglobulinemia. According to Gurd and Wilson, the diagnosis of FES involves two major criteria, or one major plus four minor criteria plus fat microglobulinemia.[68] Typically, FES occurs within 24–72 hours of injury, and is largely a clinical diagnosis. Laboratory investigations may include an arterial blood gas to diagnose hypoxemia, and cytologic examination of urine, blood, or sputum looking for fat globules. Chest radiography may be normal in these patients, prompting investigation with chest CT or bronchoalveolar lavage looking for fat-laden macrophages.[69] Because of the lack of specific diagnostic criteria or investigations, the incidence of FES is likely underestimated.

Once FES is suspected, the management is largely supportive, and usually involves management of the hypoxemia.

Prophylactic measures in those considered at risk for FES are most important. These include early stabilization of long-bone/pelvic fractures, minimizing IM pressures during reaming, and irrigation of marrow prior to insertion of prostheses. Pharmacologic therapies have been disappointing, and despite initial interest in using steroids, there have not been any level 1 studies supporting their use.

Compartment syndrome

Compartment syndrome is a rare, but potentially devastating, complication of lower extremity trauma. Undiagnosed compartment syndrome can lead to nerve damage and muscle necrosis. Acute compartment syndrome involves a build-up of pressure within a nonelastic muscle compartment that is surrounded by fascia and bone. In the lower extremity there are four compartments: (1) anterior; (2) lateral; (3) superficial posterior; and (4) deep posterior. Compartment syndrome typically results from bleeding or edema within the compartment. Edema can create a barrier to perfusion, which results in hypoxia and acidosis. This is a self-perpetuating cycle, as this leads to further capillary permeability and fluid extravasation, worsening the edematous state.[70] The pathophysiology of compartment syndrome involves increasing interstitial pressure. This leads to increased intraluminal venous pressure in an effort to avoid vascular collapse. As a result, there is a decreased gradient between arterioles and veins, and capillary blood flow thus decreases and results in ischemia. The muscle undergoes ischemic scar formation, and necrosis leads to myoglobinemia.

The classic description of compartment syndrome was provided by Griffiths, in which he described the "four Ps" – pain, paresthesia, paresis, and pain with stretch.[71] This has been further expanded to "six Ps" with the addition of pulselessness and poikilothermia. Compartment syndrome is relatively uncommon, but should be anticipated in situations of high-velocity trauma, in patients on blood thinners, and with lower extremity vascular occlusion or disruption. Pain is the earliest and most sensitive clinical sign. Confirmation of the diagnosis can be achieved by measuring the intracompartmental pressure. The absolute threshold for fasciotomy has been debated, with some favoring pressures greater than 30 mmHg, and others looking at the difference between compartment pressure and mean arterial pressure (<30 mmHg below mean arterial pressure significant), or diastolic pressure (<30 mmHg below diastolic pressure significant).[70]

Following diagnosis, the treatment consists of urgent surgical decompression of all four compartments. Multiple approaches have been described, but the most common include release via a single lateral incision or combined anterolateral and posteromedial incisions. The single-incision approach involves an incision in line with the fibula extending from just distal to the head of fibula to 3–4 cm proximal to the lateral malleolus. Longitudinal fasciotomies of the anterior and lateral compartments are performed, followed by subcutaneous dissection posteriorly to access the superficial posterior compartment followed by the deep posterior compartment. In the two-incision technique, an anterolateral incision is placed between the tibial crest and fibula over the anterior intermuscular septum. Fasciotomies of the anterior and lateral compartments are carried out through this incision.

The posteromedial incision is placed 2 cm posterior to the posteromedial edge of the tibia. This allows access to the superficial posterior compartment, and, following division of the soleal bridge, the deep compartment can be accessed.

Postoperative care

Antibiotics

In 2009 the EAST practice management group published updated guidelines for antibiotic use in open fractures. Based on their literature review, they made several recommendations. These include level I recommendations: antibiotics with Gram-positive coverage to start at time of injury, with the addition of Gram-negative coverage in Gustilo grade III injuries. Also, high-dose penicillin should be added in the presence of fecal or possible clostridial contamination. They suggest that aminoglycosides do not offer an advantage over cephalosporin/aminoglycoside regimens, and they may have a detrimental effect on fracture healing. Level II recommendations include discontinuation of antibiotics within 24 hours of wound closure (grade I and II fractures) or 72 hours postinjury/24 hours post soft-tissue coverage in grade III fractures. A single dose of aminoglycoside is appropriate for grade II and III fractures.[72]

Anticoagulation

The risk of venous thromboembolism (VTE) is highest in patients who have sustained major trauma, with increased risk associated with spinal cord injury, lower extremity fractures, pelvic fractures, femoral central lines, age, immobility, and surgery.[49] Death from VTE is preventable, which is why the use of VTE protocols is on the rise. The prophylaxis of VTE is one of the goals of improved surgical care identified by the Surgical Care Improvement Project.[73]

Two of the commonly used anticoagulants include unfractionated heparin (UH) and low-molecular-weight heparin (LMWH). UH acts on antithrombin, catalyzing the reaction between antithrombin and thrombin (factor IIa) as well as factor Xa.[74] This inhibits the procoagulant activity of thrombin. LMWH is a depolymerized form of UH, and exerts its action via factor Xa, with less effect on antithrombin. Until recently, few studies existed comparing these drugs. One retrospective study comparing protocols involving both drugs found no difference in incidence of VTE or bleeding complications. Additionally, a three-times-daily UH routine was significantly cheaper to administer.[75]

Blood loss

Hemorrhage in the setting of lower extremity trauma is common, especially with long-bone or combined injuries. It may account for as much as 40% of trauma-related mortality, and is the second leading cause of death after injury.[76] As many as 30% of patients may require massive transfusion during the initial postinjury period. This is classified as transfusion of 10 or more units of packed red blood cells in the first 24 hours following injury.[77,78] Unfortunately, there is no ideal strategy for the management of posttraumatic hemorrhagic shock. The current trend is for control of bleeding via brief "damage control" surgeries, fluid resuscitation, and administration of blood products. In damage control surgery, there are four phases: (1) recognizing a patient who warrants the "damage control" approach; (2) salvage surgery for control of hemorrhage, contamination, and stabilization of long-bone and pelvic fractures; (3) intensive care unit management for restoration of physiologic and immunologic baseline functions; and (4) scheduled reconstructive surgeries for definitive management of the injury once the patient is stable enough.[79]

The threshold for starting blood transfusion is also debated. According to ATLS protocols, blood products should be considered in patients who are nonresponders or transient responders to fluid resuscitation, with estimated blood loss >30%. The original Transfusion Requirements In Critical Care trial looking at transfusion protocols provides a rough estimate of when to transfuse, suggesting that a restrictive approach (transfusing when hemoglobin <7 g/dL) may be safe.[80] However, this study population may not be equivalent to a patient involved in lower extremity trauma. It may be more accurate to follow base deficit and serum lactate in the assessment of bleeding and shock. Transfusion strategy also involves multiple components, including red blood cells, fresh frozen plasma, and platelets. The ratio of each varies significantly in the literature and is beyond the scope of this chapter. Finally, it is important to avoid other factors that may contribute to coagulopathy, such as hypothermia, and all attempts should be made to control any such preventable factors.

Outcomes, prognosis, and complications

Outcomes and prognosis

Functional outcomes

One of the biggest measures of reported functional recovery in patients sustaining lower extremity trauma is their return to work. Studies have demonstrated that at 1 year more than one-quarter of these patients have not returned to work. Butcher et al. tracked functional recovery long-term in those patients who do not return to work by 1 year.[81] Using the Sickness Impact Profile (SIP) questionnaire, they determined that return to work occurred in 72% of their patients by 12 months, and at 30 months 82% of the study group had returned to work. At 30 months, 64% of patients had no disability, 17% had mild disability, 12% had moderate disability, and 7% had severe disability. This study did not differentiate between those who underwent limb salvage and those with amputation.

Mackenzie et al.[82] examined functional outcomes in those patients who underwent amputation following trauma-related lower extremity injury. Study participants were part of the original LEAP cohort that had undergone amputation as a result of their injury. Patients were stratified according to level of amputation – above-knee, through-knee, and below-knee. At 24 months, patients with through-knee amputation had the highest SIP scores. There was a modest degree of disability among all patient groups. Overall, patients with through-knee amputation had worse outcomes with lower self-selected walking speed, ability to perform functional transfers, and ability to walk and stair-climb. There were no significant differences in SIP scores between those with below-knee and those with above-knee amputations.

Amputation versus salvage

A systematic review of outcomes and complications in patients undergoing reconstruction and amputation of grade IIIB and IIIC tibial injuries assessed 26 studies in the published literature.[83] It was found that hospital stay was longer in the amputation group (63.7 versus 56.9 days), but this was nonsignificant. Of those initially reconstructed, the pooled secondary amputation rate was 5.1% in type IIIB fractures, and 28.7% in type IIIC fractures. When regressed against the year of study publication, the secondary amputation rate decreased – likely due to improved operative technique and increasing incidence of successful salvage. The rate of osteomyelitis in limb salvage patients was variable, with a range of 4–56%. Complete flap loss was 5.8% (pooled result; range 0–15%). Overall, this study did not reveal a superior strategy in treating patients with lower limb-threatening injuries, as the outcomes were similar between groups.

Patient satisfaction

Very few studies have examined the differences between patient and physician perceptions in lower extremity trauma. The LEAP study looked at these perceptions in 463 patients with unilateral lower extremity injuries. Patient satisfaction was evaluated at 12 and 24 months postinjury via a structured clinical interview. Surgeons were asked to evaluate their satisfaction with the clinical recovery and cosmetic recovery of the lower extremity at the 24-month mark. The results demonstrated that there was poor agreement between the surgeons' and patients' perceptions of both overall and cosmetic outcomes.[84] Surgeons and patients differed particularly on the cosmetic outcome, with patients being less satisfied than their surgeons. Patients and surgeons were more likely to disagree regarding overall outcome if the injury severity score was greater than 17, a complication occurred that required hospital admission, if they were dissatisfied with their care, or failed to return to work at 1 year. Disagreement regarding cosmetic outcome was greater when patients were female, had sustained a traumatic amputation (patients were more satisfied in this group), or had complications requiring hospital admission, or unsatisfactory care. On the whole, 66% of patients were satisfied with their overall outcome at 2 years, and 34% were not satisfied.[85] No pre-existing patient factors were identified as predictive of this. The only factors that correlated with satisfaction were measures of physical function, psychological distress, clinical recovery, and return to work.

Cost-utility

There have been two large studies looking at cost-utility in lower extremity trauma. This is especially important as reconstructive endeavors are considered not only to be technically demanding and time-consuming, but they can be associated with a high risk of complications and rehabilitation time. It is important to justify this from a patient care and economic perspective. In 2007, Mackenzie et al.[86] conducted a multicenter study estimating the healthcare costs for 545 patients with unilateral limb-threatening lower extremity trauma. This was part of the original LEAP study. They found that, when costs associated with rehospitalization and post acute care were added to the initial cost of hospitalization, the 2-year overall cost was similar between salvage and amputation patients. However, when prosthesis-related costs were added, the amputation group had a much higher cost of treatment, with an initial $10 000 difference in cost, and projected lifetime cost that was three times higher ($509 275 versus $163 282) than the reconstruction group. In a study by Chung et al.,[87] a cost-utility analysis demonstrated that, independently of ongoing prosthetic-related needs and years of life remaining, amputation is more expensive overall. It was estimated that amputation results in $93 606–154 636 more overall cost to the 40-year-old patient when compared to a reconstructed patient. This study suggests that surgeons should select limb salvage more aggressively, in particular for patients where amputation is not clearly indicated.

Complications

Wound complications

The goal of reconstruction is to provide soft-tissue coverage that creates a closed wound, provides vascularized tissue, and prevents secondary complications of the injury, including late infection and nonunion. A subset of the LEAP study specifically examined wound complications as stratified by type of reconstruction. It was found that those reconstructed with free flaps were more likely to have multicompartment functional compromise in the leg with more severe soft-tissue injury. Despite this, there was no overall difference in complication rates between patients reconstructed with local rotational flaps versus those reconstructed with free tissue transfer. However, when patients were further stratified by underlying osseous injury, regression analysis demonstrated that this was an important predictor of wound complication. In patients with American Society for Internal Fixation–Orthopaedic Trauma Association type C osseous injury, those with rotational flap reconstruction were 4.3 times more likely to have a wound complication requiring operative intervention than those with free flap reconstruction.[88] Interestingly, there was not an increased rate of wound complications when the patients were stratified by time to reconstruction, suggesting that in this cohort, time to reconstruction was not an important predictor, as is suggested by Godina.[34]

Osteomyelitis

It has been shown that the tibia is the most common site of infected nonunion and chronic posttraumatic osteomyelitis.[89] This is associated with morbidity, and may be limb-threatening. In this regard, it is important to prevent the occurrence of osteomyelitis, and treat it early and aggressively. The LEAP study had an incidence of 7.7% of osteomyelitis, with 84% of these patients requiring operative intervention and hospitalization.[90]

It is thought that an aggregation of microbe colonies called "biofilm" is the key in the development and persistence of infection.[91] The most common organism in chronic osteomyelitis is *Staphylococcus aureus*, which may be combined with other pathogens, commonly including *Pseudomonas aeruginosa*.

Four anatomic types of osteomyelitis exist: (1) medullary (IM bone surface); (2) superficial (bone surface); (3) localized (full-thickness cortex extending into medullary canal); and (4) diffuse (circumferential bone involvement). Furthermore, the patient can be classified according to physiologic status: good systemic defenses (type A), systemic/local/combined deficiency in wound healing (type B), or severe local/systemic factors (type C). Infection may be clinically silent, emphasizing the need for a high index of suspicion. Diagnosis relies on clinical findings, laboratory tests (erythrocyte sedimentation rate, C-reactive protein), diagnostic imaging (X-ray, magnetic resonance imaging, technetium-99m bone scan), and, the gold standard, bone culture. The management of osteomyelitis includes debridement and antibiotics, in conjunction with fracture stabilization. It is necessary to remove all operative hardware, debride infected bony sequestra aggressively, and ream out the IM canal if rod fixation was used. It cannot be emphasized enough how important it is to perform extensive bony debridement until viable bone with punctate bleeding is achieved. It is possible to use local antibiotic therapy in the form of antibiotic-impregnated beads, placed in the defect site following debridement. Systemic antibiotic therapy should be broad initially, and tailored according to culture results. If internal fixation is removed and the fracture is not healed or in a state of nonunion, a temporary external fixator may be placed until the infection is eradicated. The secondary stages of reconstruction involve local or free tissue coverage (usually within 1 week of initial debridement), followed by management of bony defects or ununited fractures. Bone-grafting procedures are carried out once the soft-tissue envelope has healed and infection is under control, typically 6–8 weeks after soft-tissue coverage.

In some situations amputation may be required, including in those with extensive bone defects, poor soft-tissue coverage, neurovascular compromise of the extremity, anticipated poor function, and multiple comorbidities.[91]

Nonunion

In the LEAP study, nonunion was among the most common complications, with an incidence of 23.7%. Of these, 83% required operative intervention, and 72% required inpatient care.[90]

Chronic pain

It has long been suspected that chronic pain has been a complication of traumatic injury, but to date there has been little prospective evidence to document this. The LEAP study addressed chronic pain in a prospective cohort analysis of patients with severe lower extremity trauma. A total of 397 patients were followed for 7 years postdischarge from hospital, with a follow-up rate of 72%. Data were collected regarding injury and treatment characteristics, sociodemographics, and predictors of pain. Predictors included functional outcomes (ambulation, mobility, body care, communication), depression and anxiety scores, and pain intensity scores. This study demonstrated a high level of long-term chronic pain, with more than one-quarter of the study population reporting pain that interfered with daily activities, and 40% reporting clinically significant pain intensity.[92] The chronic pain levels in the study group were comparable to those of pain clinic back pain and headache populations. The multivariate analysis did not identify any predictors of pain relating to the injury and treatment, suggesting that the onset of chronic pain is independent of injury characteristics and surgical treatment decisions – supporting prior studies by Ashburn and Fine.[93] Protective factors included years of education and increased self-efficiency for return to usual major activities. Risk factors included alcohol use in the month prior to injury, symptoms of anxiety, depression, and sleep irregularities at 3 months postinjury, and, the strongest risk factor, intensity of acute pain at 3 months postinjury. Narcotic use at 3 months appeared to be protective as well, perhaps supporting the central sensitization theory for the development of chronic pain.

Secondary procedures

A variety of secondary procedures may be required following lower extremity reconstruction and limb salvage. These can fall into two broad categories: (1) secondary cosmetic procedures to improve the quality and appearance of the reconstruction (e.g., flap debulking); and (2) secondary functional procedures to finalize the reconstruction (e.g., delayed bone grafting).

Secondary cosmetic procedures

One of the most frequent secondary procedures required to improve the appearance of the reconstruction is flap debulking. For fasciocutaneous flap and perforator flaps we prefer to wait a minimum of 3 months, preferably 6 months, prior to any debulking procedures. Liposuction is the most common method of debulking. If excess skin requires excision, we usually perform this 3 months following liposuction in order not to compromise vascularity and limit skin excision to 50% or less of the flap circumference. Combined aggressive liposuction with flap skin excision should be avoided whenever possible in order to prevent complications. Several sessions of debulking may be required in certain flaps in order to provide the lowest profile resurfacing possible, for example, flaps for medial or lateral malleolus reconstruction (Figs 2.35–2.38).

For muscle flaps or myocutaneous flaps, debulking procedures can also be required but less frequently with free muscle flaps alone. Denervated muscle undergoes significant atrophy over time and provides excellent contouring for lower-extremity reconstruction. The skin paddle from a myocutaneous flap can also be removed as a split-thickness skin graft or thin full-thickness skin graft with a dermatome and then reused to cover the underlying muscle following excision of excess subcutaneous tissue. If required, the muscle can also be debulked and we prefer to use the dermatome for this to shave the muscle from superficial to deep, making sure to protect the pedicle at all times. For skin-grafted muscle flaps, a dermatome can also be used to remove the skin graft from the flap temporarily. The muscle is then debulked with progressive shaving using a dermatome and the skin graft is recycled to cover the muscle once debulking is completed. We prefer to use the tourniquet for all debulking procedures, perform meticulous hemostasis, and use a negative-pressure dressing to secure the skin graft following debulking (Fig. 2.29A and Figs 2.39, 2.40).

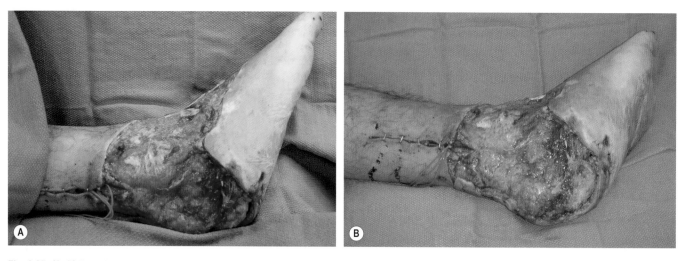

Fig. 2.35 (A, B) Extensive degloving injury following a motorcycle accident in a 24-year-old man, with exposure of the calcaneus, medial malleolus, and extensor tendons.

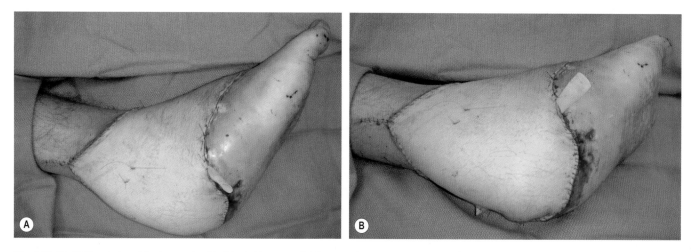

Fig. 2.36 (A, B) Resurfacing of the lower extremity defect with an extended free anterolateral thigh flap (384 cm^2).

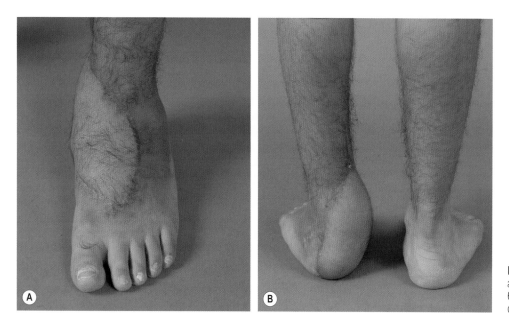

Fig. 2.37 (A, B) Appearance of the anterolateral thigh flap following liposuction at 6 months following the initial surgery. A total of 75 cc of lipoaspirate was removed.

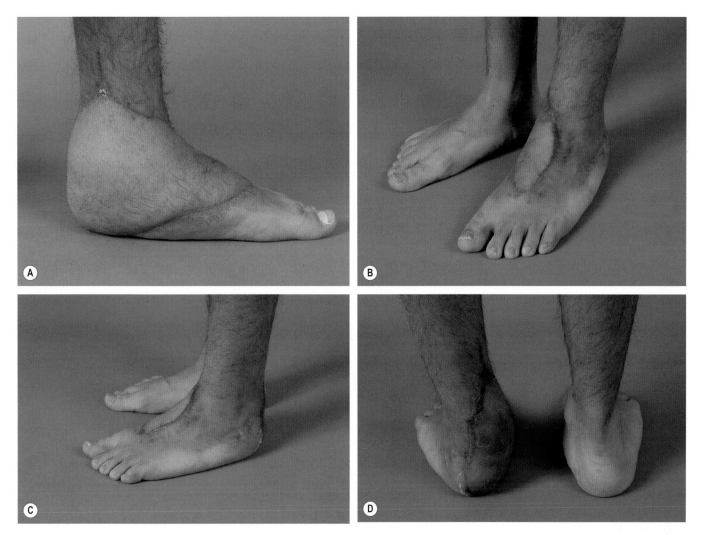

Fig. 2.38 (A–D) A second and final session of flap debulking was performed with liposuction. In this case the flap was aggressively liposuctioned, even in the area of the pedicle, to minimize bulk. If the peripheral flap incision is kept intact, then aggressive liposuction can be performed while maintaining adequate vascularity.

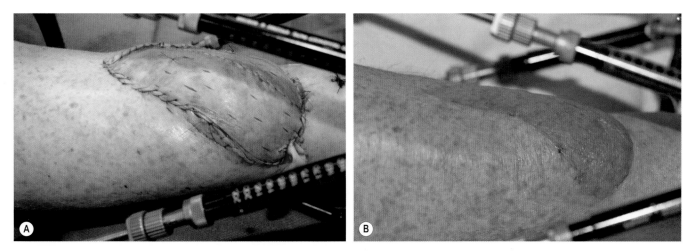

Fig. 2.39 (A,B) Coverage of lower extremity defect with a free gracilis flap and split-thickness skin graft.

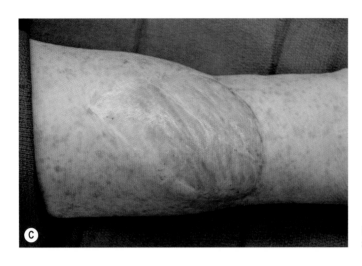

Fig. 2.39, cont'd (C) Appearance of the gracilis muscle flap at 3 months following surgery. Note significant muscle atrophy over time.

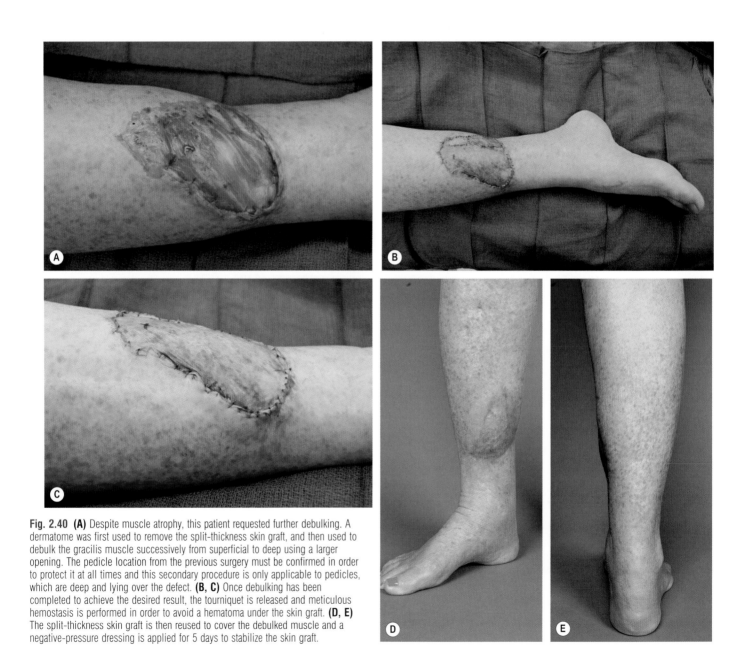

Fig. 2.40 (A) Despite muscle atrophy, this patient requested further debulking. A dermatome was first used to remove the split-thickness skin graft, and then used to debulk the gracilis muscle successively from superficial to deep using a larger opening. The pedicle location from the previous surgery must be confirmed in order to protect it at all times and this secondary procedure is only applicable to pedicles, which are deep and lying over the defect. **(B, C)** Once debulking has been completed to achieve the desired result, the tourniquet is released and meticulous hemostasis is performed in order to avoid a hematoma under the skin graft. **(D, E)** The split-thickness skin graft is then reused to cover the debulked muscle and a negative-pressure dressing is applied for 5 days to stabilize the skin graft.

Secondary functional procedures

Secondary procedures to restore function of the lower extremity are numerous and can include secondary bone grafting, hardware removal or replacement, tendon reconstruction, and nerve repair/grafting. For any anticipated orthopedic procedures, close collaboration with orthopedic surgery is important in order to re-elevate the flap for bone grafting safely, methyl methacrylate spacer removal, and for hardware removal/replacement. Muscle and skin flaps can be easily re-elevated, although skin flaps provide the greatest flexibility and ease for re-elevation, which is why we prefer to use them if secondary procedures are anticipated. The tourniquet is also used for secondary procedures and elevation of flaps.

Access the complete reference list online at **http://www.expertconsult.com**

6. Levin LS. The reconstructive ladder. An orthoplastic approach. *Orthop Clin North Am.* 1993;24(3):393–409.

17. Keel M, Trentz O. Pathophysiology of polytrauma. *Injury.* 2005;36(6):691–709.

22. Management of Complex Extremity Trauma. American College of Surgeons Committee on Trauma. Available from: http://www.facs.org/trauma/publications/traumaon.html. [Accessed August 1 1, 2010]

24. Gustilo RB, Mendoza RM, Williams DN. Problems in the management of type III (severe) open fractures: a new classification of type III open fractures. *J Trauma.* 1984;24(8):742–746.

27. Higgins TF, Klatt JB, Beals TC. Lower Extremity Assessment Project (LEAP)–the best available evidence on limb-threatening lower extremity trauma. *Orthop Clin North Am.* 2010;41(2):233–239.

An overview of the Lower Extremity Assessment Project (LEAP) protocol and substudy analyses. The inclusion criteria are reviewed, and objectives included. A total of 601 patients were enrolled and followed for a period of 44 months at eight centers. The LEAP study attempted to assess the characteristics of the patients sustaining lower extremity injury, environmental characteristics of the injury, physical and mental aspects of the injury, secondary medical issues arising from the injury, and functional status. It was found that social, economic, and personality disadvantages that existed prior to the injury play a large role in the functional and quality-of-life outcomes measured in the study. It was also found that the functional outcomes 2 years postinjury were similar between those undergoing limb salvage and those that underwent amputation.

29. Ly TV, Travison TG, Castillo RC, et al. Ability of lower-extremity injury severity scores to predict functional outcome after limb salvage. *J Bone Joint Surg Am.* 2008;90(8):1738–1743.

34. Godina M. Early microsurgical reconstruction of complex trauma of the extremities. *Plast Reconstr Surg.* 1986;78(3):285–292.

Landmark paper examining the timing of microsurgical reconstruction in extremity trauma. This study divided patients into three groups according to time of reconstruction: <72 hours, 72 hours–3 months, >3 months. Godina examined the incidence of flap failure, infection, bone-healing time, length of hospital stay, and number of operative procedures. He found that outcomes were the best in the group reconstructed within 72 hours. Those reconstructed between 72 hours and 3 months had the highest rate of infection, and those reconstructed >3 months postinjury had the longest bone-healing time and required the greatest number of operations.

40. Ong YS, Levin LS. Lower limb salvage in trauma. *Plast Reconstr Surg.* 2010;125(2):582–588.

An overview of the management of lower extremity trauma, including initial management, decision-making for salvage versus amputation, timing of reconstruction, and choice of flap. Also reviews outcomes of reconstruction, including flap failure, late complications, and function.

50. Parrett BM, Talbot SG, Pribaz JJ, et al. A review of local and regional flaps for distal leg reconstruction. *J Reconstr Microsurg.* 2009;25(7):445–455.

A thorough review of local and regional flap options available in distal leg reconstruction. Outlines the preoperative work-up, and provides an algorithmic approach to selecting the appropriate flap for reconstruction. Several flaps are reviewed in detail, including their indications, design, and surgical technique, and complications/pitfalls.

82. MacKenzie EJ, Bosse MJ, Castillo RC, et al. Functional outcomes following trauma-related lower-extremity amputation. *J Bone Joint Surg Am.* 2004;86-A(8):1636–1645.

A subset of the LEAP study, 161 patients who underwent above-the-ankle amputation following lower extremity trauma were followed prospectively for a total of 24 months. Outcomes included functional measures using the Sickness Inventory Profile (SIP), pain assessments, and degree of independence assessment. The SIP was not different between those amputated above versus below the knee. Physical function was affected by level of amputation, with walking speeds higher in the below-the-knee amputation patients.

3

Lymphatic reconstruction of the extremities

Ruediger G.H. Baumeister, David W. Chang, and Peter C. Neligan

SYNOPSIS

- In developed countries most cases of lymphedema are caused by a local obstruction of the lymphatic system after iatrogenic intervention.
- With the help of advanced microsurgery lymphatic vessels can be sutured and lymphatic bypasses can overcome blocked lymphatic and lymphovascular areas.
- Microsurgical lymphatic reconstruction is one step in the treatment algorithm. Initially, conventional treatment including physical therapy, exercises designed to mobilize tissue fluid, and compression should be instituted for 6 months. Thereafter the option of a direct reconstruction should be taken into consideration early. Resectional interventions are the very endpoint of the algorithm.
- Microsurgical lymphatic grafts have been shown to be effective by independent investigators in nuclear medicine – long-term significant improvement of lymphatic flow – and in radiology – long-term patent lymphatic grafts (more than 10 years) are found.
- After reconstruction secondary changes such as an increase in adipose and fibrous tissue may be treated using lipolymphosuction. Alternatively, localized resection may act as an adjunct to the bypass procedures.
- The ultimate goal of reconstruction using microsurgical grafting is to come as close as possible to the original status and to avoid additional ongoing treatment.

 Access the Historical Perspective section online at
http://www.expertconsult.com

Introduction

The lymphatic vascular system consists of a variety of lymphatic channels that appear as blind endings within the tissue, lymphatic precollectors, and finally lymphatic collectors which amount to a diameter of about 0.3 mm within the human thigh and are a similar size elsewhere in the body.

Lymphedema is a debilitating condition characterized by progressive indolent swelling in the soft tissues, usually involving the limbs but not infrequently also affecting the trunk, the genitalia and, less frequently, the head and neck. The swelling is initially caused by some failure of the lymphatic system to drain lymph fluid from the affected part, causing the area to become waterlogged. Subsequently, as the condition progresses, this is accompanied by increased adipose and fibrous tissue in the area, often accompanied by trophic skin changes, ulceration, and the propensity to develop soft-tissue infections. The lay term "elephantiasis" aptly describes the appearance of a chronically lymphedematous extremity.

Vascular surgery routinely deals with obstructions of the vascular system. These obstructions are dealt with using bypass techniques. With advances in microsurgical technique and instrumentation, the application of bypass techniques to the lymphatic system is now also possible.[1] Furthermore, just as parts of the vascular system can be used as grafts, e.g., vein grafts, segments of these lymphatic channels can also be used as grafts.[2,3] FIG 3.1–3.4 APPEARS ONLINE ONLY

Basic science/disease process

Lymphedema is characterized by an imbalance between the lymphatic load and the lymphatic transport capacity. The lymphatic load represents the amount of lymphoid fluid that has to be transported via the lymphatic system within a given time frame within a specific part of the body, e.g., an extremity. The lymphatic transport capacity on the other hand is the amount of lymphatic fluid that can be maximally transported by the lymphatic system. It is dependent on the number and functional status of the lymphatic vessels and the lymph nodes.[91] When the lymphatic load outstrips the transport capacity lymphedema results. This imbalance can have a number of causes, as already described, and may be congenital or acquired. As lymphedema progresses some changes occur in the tissues such that there is an increased amount of adipose tissue as well as fibrous tissue. Furthermore, the skin becomes thickened, firm, and unyielding and ultimately takes on an appearance similar to what one would imagine as elephant skin, hence the term "elephantiasis."

Classification and etiology of lymphedema

Lymphedema is classified as primary or secondary. Two types of primary lymphedema are recognized:

1. Type I (Nonne–Milroy): the familial congenital type is based on a vascular endothelial growth factor-receptor-3 mutation
2. Type II (Meige): can be seen as lymphedema praecox, arising during adolescence, and as lymphedema tarda, with an onset after the age of 35.

Reconstructive methods can only be applied in those cases where a localized atresia or obstruction of the lymphatic system is present.

Secondary lymphedema is due to acquired damage to the lymphatic system.

Globally, lymphedema caused by filariasis is the most common. Secondary lymphedema may also arise from infection, trauma, and malignancies influencing lymphatic flow. In western countries there is a predominance of lymphedema after surgical interventions, often combined with irradiation. Cases such as these, in which there is a localized blockade of the lymphatic draining system, are excellent candidates for reconstructive procedures.

Diagnosis/patient presentation

The clinical picture is characterized by increased tissue thickness and decreased tissue pliability.

The so-called Stemmer sign becomes positive. This means that on the dorsal side of the toe or of a finger the tissue cannot be lifted between the thumb and the index finger of the investigator in a normal way. The tissue becomes enlarged and thickened. The swelling in the lower extremity also affects the dorsum of the foot. This is important in order to differentiate between lymphedema and lipohypertrophy where the enlargement of the tissue ends at the level of the ankles. For further evaluation, a variety of technical procedures have been described.

Direct-contrast lymphography, using oily contrast medium and invasive administration via transected lymphatic vessels, was introduced by Kinmonth and greatly advanced our knowledge of the lymphatic system.[92] However, due to the invasiveness of the application (and injury to the lymphatic vessels and lymph nodes), it was found to cause worsening of lymphedema.

Indirect-contrast lymphography, using water-soluble contrast medium that is injected subepidermally, is unable to visualize lymphatic vessels to an extent comparable with direct lymphography and gained only limited use.[93] In primary lymphedema this technique might be used to

evaluate whether there are any lymphatic vessels present in the periphery and if so, if they might be able to transport lymph towards a proximally performed anastomosis.

First attempts to visualize lymphatic vessels with magnetic resonance imaging (MRI) using contrast medium administered subdermally are promising. This will prove useful for exact planning prior to reconstructive procedures as well as examining the patency of lymphatic grafts without damaging them.[94] For the detection of vascular lymphatic malformations, MRI is extremely valuable both with and without the use of contrast medium.

For routine procedures, the key diagnostic tool, aside from the clinical evaluation, is lymphoscintigraphy. It can be repeated and used for diagnostic as well as for follow-up purposes. It gives quite a good impression of the function and visualizes routes of lymphatic flow. Introducing the lymphatic transport index (TI), which summarizes the findings derived from the lymphoscintigraphic studies, allows for a semiquantitative evaluation of the lymphatic flow without the need for standardized physical movement on the part of the patient. It ranges from TI = 0 for an optimal lymphatic outflow to TI = 45 for no visible flow. Normal values are below 10. This transport index also provides a good basis for follow-up studies and can show lymphatic flow along the route of lymphatic grafts.[85,95]

Different approaches are described to improve exact quantification of lymphatic flow. When measuring regions of interest, it is critical to standardize the application of the radiopharmaceutical and the physical movements performed by the patient during the procedure.[96] The visualization of cutaneous lymphatic vessels using duplex sonography is controversial and is of limited value for surgeons. Another diagnostic tool that can be used is the subepidermal injection of Patent Blue dye. Normally, lymphatic transport is visualized in the superficial lymphatic collecting system. In pathologic situations, the so-called dermal back-flow leads to pooling of the contrast within the skin that results in a "cloud"-like appearance. Since allergic reactions have been reported, staining of lymphatic vessels with Patent Blue dye is generally performed during surgery under general anesthesia.

The use of indocyanine green, a fluorescent dye that is activated by a laser light source and imaged using near-infrared technology, is also proving to be a useful tool, particularly in the preoperative mapping of superficial lymphatics.

Patient selection

Nonsurgical therapy

The basic strategies for nonsurgical therapy consist of a combination of elevation of the extremities, exercises designed to optimize lymphatic flow, manual lymphatic drainage, and compression therapy. If a reconstructive procedure is being contemplated, conservative treatment should be performed first for a minimum of about 6 months because during this time period spontaneous regression of edema is possible. Compression therapy using pneumatic devices has also become popular. However there may be some concern, at least in theory, that the resulting elevation in pressure can damage the remaining lymphatic vessels. Diuretics do not have a place in the regular treatment protocol since removal of fluid may lead to enhanced fibrosis.

Patient selection for reconstruction

Surgery is generally not the primary approach in the treatment of lymphedema. However the results of medical treatment are sometimes transient and may disappear after about 6 months.

Within this period conservative treatment, as mentioned above, use of exercises, manual lymphatic drainage, and application of elastic stockings or compression garments are recommended. After this first treatment period the indication for surgery has to be evaluated and a decision made between physiologic reconstructive and diverting techniques on the one hand versus resectional or ablative procedures on the other. Secondary tissue changes such as increased adipose and fibrous tissue become more prevalent over time. For this reason, early reconstruction should be considered after the period of initial conservative treatment. For resectional surgical approaches the time is not crucial since the target is the surplus of tissue and not the improvement of lymphatic flow.

When recommending surgery it is important to consider the goals of treatment (Box 3.1) and to present the various options in that context. For example, if one is considering the use of lymphatic grafts, specific prerequisites have to be considered. The indication for this procedure is similar to the use of bypasses in other fields of vascular surgery where a localized interruption of the vascular system has to be treated. This is especially true after removal of lymph nodes and lymph vessels in the axillary, inguinal, or pelvic regions as well as in the medial aspect of the knee.

In primary lymphedema only regional lymphatic atresias may be treated by lymphatic grafting. According to the lymphographic findings of Kinmonth, unilateral lymphatic atresias can exist at the inguinal and pelvic region with normal lymphatic vessels distally.[92] This is a situation in which lymphatic transpositional grafts may be considered. The method of graft harvest is also crucial. As already mentioned, the ventromedial bundle of the lymphatics at the thigh consists of up to 16 lymphatic vessels that are running roughly parallel in the thigh. At the knee and in the inguinal region they are confluent and therefore only the region in between these endangered areas should be used for harvesting.

The length of the graft depends on the length of the thigh and amounts to about 20–30 cm. This length is sufficient to overcome the distance from the upper arm to the neck in cases of an axillary obstruction and the distance to the opposite thigh in cases of unilateral lymphedema of the lower extremities.

Box 3.1 **Goals of treatment**

Reduce swelling
- Debulking procedure
  - Excisional
  - Liposuction

Bypass lymphatic blockage
- Lymphaticovenular bypass
- Lymph node transfer
- Lymphatic graft

For maximal safety, any possible pre-existing lymphatic deficiency in the limb from which the grafts are being harvested must be excluded. There should be no prior history of edema in this leg. Lymphoscintigraphy has to show normal lymphatic transport. During surgery the behavior of lymphatic drainage after injection of Patent Blue (dye) should be normal and any evidence of persistent staining should be regarded as an indication of abnormal flow.

With respect to the affected extremities, prior to surgery, as far as possible lymphatic scintiscans should reveal the site of the obstruction and clarify the extent of the lymphatic disorder. In primary lymphedema especially, one should get additional information about the kind of lymphatic malformation by indirect lymphography using water-soluble contrast medium or nowadays preferably by MRI lymphography using gadolinium.

For resectional methods, advanced and incapacitating lymphedema is one of the prime indications for surgery.

Treatment/surgical technique

The history of the development of the various surgical strategies is described in the history segment of this chapter, which is available in the online version. Various surgical procedures have been used to treat lymphedema of the extremities, with varying degrees of success.[4–10] These operative strategies can be classified into two categories: ablative operations and physiological operations.

Ablative operations

Resection of dependent folds may contribute to the patient's comfort and can be done either in isolation, or as an adjunct to the physiologic procedures described below. Debulking procedures in which the lymphedematous tissue is resected while retaining the overlying skin is an option but is fraught with wound-healing problems. The first reported surgical procedure for lymphedema was published in 1912 by Charles, who described a procedure for scrotal lymphedema and its application to lower limb lymphedema.[5] The Charles procedure is an aggressive debulking surgery in which all overlying skin and soft tissue above the deep fascia in the lymphedematous area are resected. The resulting defect is covered by a skin graft harvested from the resected specimen (Fig. 3.1).[5] This procedure is now rarely performed but still has a role in the treatment of extreme lymphedema.

Although debulking operations are the simplest surgical approach to reducing the size of lymphedematous upper limbs, such operations result in extensive scarring and cause substantial morbidity. Therefore, these operations are no longer used except in extreme cases.

Liposuction, as a debulking procedure, is still practiced and Brorson and Svensson have reported good results and recommended liposuction as the preferred surgical procedure for treating lymphedema.[28] The rationale for this is not surprising since there is an acknowledged increase in the amount of adipose tissue in chronic lymphedema. Following debulking with liposuction, the patient must wear lifelong compression and failure to do so results in recurrence. Some argue that, while liposuction can be effective for initially reducing the volume of hypertrophic adipose tissue, it has a risk of damaging the residual lymphatic vessels and thus exacerbating the lymphedema.[29]

Physiological operations

Physiological operations are where new channels are created to improve lymphatic drainage. Various procedures have been attempted for draining lymph fluid trapped within the lymphedematous limb into other lymphatic basins or into the venous circulation. Current approaches include lymph node transplantation and lymphatic bypass operations.[30–33]

Lymphaticolymphatic bypass

Baumeister and colleagues[2,3] reported an approach to upper and lower extremity lymphedemas in which healthy lymphatic vessels from the medial thigh area are used as grafts (*Fig. 3.4*). Ho and colleagues[83] reported an approach for upper extremity lymphedema using a composite graft including the greater saphenous vein. Lymphatic vessels at each end of the graft are identified under the operating microscope and anastomosed to recipient lymphatic vessels in the neck and upper arm in accordance with the flow direction of the donor lymphatic vessels.

ideo
1,2

Postoperative patency of the lymphatic vessels within the graft can be verified using lymphoscintigraphy. In their series, Baumeister and Siuda demonstrated newly created lymph pathways as well as faster clearance of radioisotope in the postoperative as compared with the preoperative images.[79] In an early study the resulting volume reduction in the affected upper limb was maintained in patients for 3 years after the operation. However, the lymphatic graft operation leaves a long scar at the donor site and also has a risk of precipitating the development of lymphedema in the donor leg from which the lymphatic graft was harvested.

Campisi advocates using a vein interposition graft between the lymphatic vessel bundles above and below the site of lymphatic blockage to bypass the obstructed area (*Fig. 3.3*).[76] In this procedure, multiple lymphatic vessels are inserted into the distal cut end of a vein graft and secured by sutures, and lymphatic vessels in the supraclavicular area are anastomosed to the other end of the vein graft. However, despite the good results that Campisi has reported, other groups have not been able to produce consistent results.

Lymphatic vessel reconstruction: Baumeister technique

The lymphatic grafts are harvested from the patient's thigh where the ventromedial bundle contains up to 16 lymphatic vessels. About 1–4 lymphatic collectors are dissected in the medial area of the thigh and great care is taken to spare the lymphatic system where it narrows at the level of the knee and groin. In both these regions the lymphatic channels become confluent so that lymphedema is likely to result if these regions are breached. Often additional peripheral branches exist, which can be dissected as well in order to create a greater number of peripheral anastomoses.

For free transfers the grafts are ligated beneath the inguinal lymph nodes using 6-0 polyglactin 910 suture material. Distally, the grafts are transected proximal to the level of the knee. The distal ends are occluded either by placing a suture or by coagulation to avoid subsequent lymphatic leakage. The grafts can then be removed.

For upper limb lymphedema, resulting from interventions in the axilla, the grafts are interposed between ascending lymphatic vessels in the upper arm and lymphatic vessels or lymph nodes in the neck, and lympholymphatic anastomoses are performed at either end. To position the grafts between the sites of anastomosis, a tube drain is placed in the subcutaneous tissue between the incision in the upper arm and the neck. Subsequently, the grafts are pulled through the wet drain gently and without any friction. After removal of the tube the grafts remain in the subcutaneous tissue free of tension.

In the upper arm, the lymphatic vessels can be found mostly epifascially – if they are not present there, they may also be located subfascially in proximity to the vessels – and can best be found through an oblique incision made medially and superior to the route of the brachial vessels. The search for these vessels is performed under the microscope using a medium magnification. In the early stages of lymphedema the lymphatic vessels have a gray, shiny appearance and the lumen can be seen clearly after transection. As the lymphatic vessels undergo fibrosis in later stages of lymphedema it becomes more difficult to discriminate between small nerves and fibrous cords. In this case the final decision regarding potential use for grafting can only be made after transection of the structure.

In the area of the neck the wall of the lymphatic vessels is thinner than in the arms and legs. Here, injections of Patent Blue dye in the hair-bearing parietal area above the ear facilitate the search for appropriate vessels. If the lymphatic vessels stain appropriately, recognition is easy. However, suturing in this area is often difficult because of the collapsing thin-walled vessels. If this is the case, it is also possible to suture the grafts to lymph nodes. A superficial incision is made in the capsule of the node and the graft connected with approximately three single interrupted sutures.

In unilateral edema of the lower extremities the grafts remain attached to the inguinal lymph nodes. In such a transposition procedure, the grafts are dissected distally after double ligation and tunneled subcutaneously superior to the pubic symphysis to the contralateral side, where end-to-end lympholymphatic anastomoses are performed (*Fig. 3.5*). A wet tube drain placed in the subcutaneous tunnel aids in tension-free passing of the lymphatic graft. A tension-free anastomosing technique is used to anastomose the lymphatic vessels under the operating microscope using maximum magnification. Baumeister and Frick[81] advocate placement of the first suture on the side of the vessel opposite to the surgeon. Because of the fragility of the vessels, they are not turned over. A back-wall suture is placed and one or two further single stitches complete the anastomosis. The choice of suture material depends on the preference of the surgeon. Baumeister et al.,[3] for example, use absorbable polyglactin and found it to be superior to nonabsorbable material in their experimental studies. Currently 10-0 absorbable sutures (Polyglactin 910), armed with a BV 75-4 needle, are the finest absorbable materials available. Other authors use 11/0 or 12/0 nylon on a

50-μm needle for lympholymphatic or lymphaticovenular anastomoses.

Microvascular lymph node transfer

Becker and colleagues reported transplanting composite soft tissue, including inguinal lymph nodes, to the axilla and/or the elbow region in the lymphedematous limb.[68] Lin and colleagues transferred similar flaps to the wrist *(Fig. 3.6)*.[97] Microvascular lymph node transfer is expected to result in new lymphatic vessels sprouting from the transplanted lymph node to drain the region. However, no objective evidence has been demonstrated that lymphatic vessels actually regenerate from transferred nodes. Nevertheless, many groups are studying this issue and objective evidence is likely to be forthcoming.[98,99]

Lymphovenous bypass

Various lymphovenous anastomosis techniques have been described. A full description is available in the online version of this chapter.

Currently, one of the most popular treatments is the lymphovenous bypass operation, which is minimally invasive. Chang[100] reported early experience in using lymphaticovenular bypass in 20 patients with upper extremity lymphedema related to the treatment of breast cancer *(Fig. 3.7)*. The mean age of the patients was 54 years: 16 patients had received preoperative radiation therapy, and all patients had undergone axillary lymph node dissection. The mean duration of lymphedema was 4.8 years, and the mean volume differential of the lymphedematous arm compared with the unaffected arm was 34%. Evaluation included qualitative assessment and quantitative volumetric analysis before surgery and at 1, 3, 6, and 12 months after the procedure. Nineteen patients (95%) reported that their symptoms improved after surgery, and 13 patients had quantitative improvement. The mean reduction in volume differential was 29%, 36%, 39%, and 35% at 1, 3, 6, and 12 months, respectively *(Fig. 3.8)*.

Table 3.1 summarizes published results for lymphovenous bypass operations. Although the results cannot be directly compared because the methods of evaluation used were not uniform, it is notable that in some patients the volume of the lymphedematous limb was reduced substantially after the operation and this reduced volume was maintained for many years.[90]

Lymphovenous shunts

Anecdotal evidence suggests that lymphovenous shunt operations performed using microsurgical techniques are more effective in patients with early-stage lymphedema than in

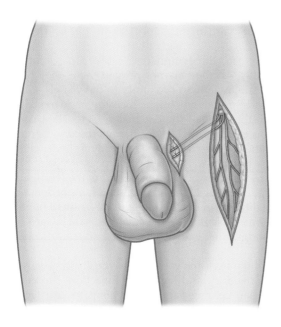

Fig. 3.5 Lymphatic grafting in unilateral edema of lower extremities. (Reproduced from Suami H, Chang DW. Overview of surgical treatments for breast cancer-related lymphedema. Plast Reconstr Surg 2010;126:1853–1863.)

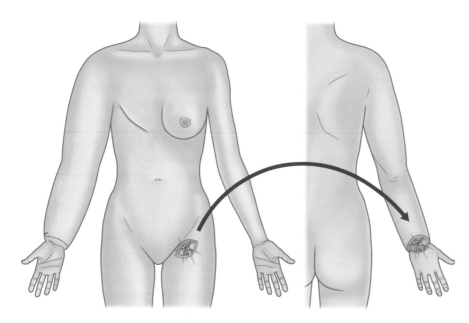

Fig. 3.6 The microvascular lymph node transfer procedure of Lin and colleagues.[86] A free vascularized flap, which includes the lymph nodes, is harvested from the inguinal region. The flap is transferred to the wrist with microvascular anastomoses. (Reproduced from Suami H, Chang DW. Overview of surgical treatments for breast cancer-related lymphedema. *Plast Reconstr Surg.* 2010;126:1853–1863.)

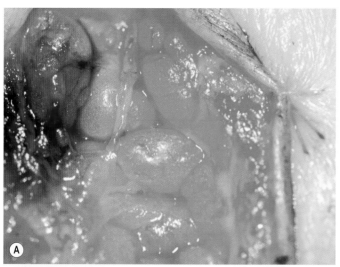

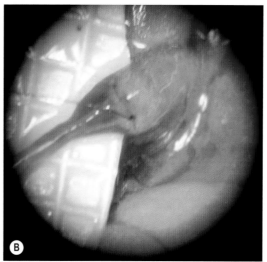

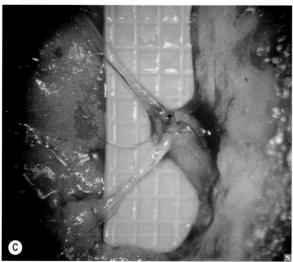

Fig. 3.7 (A) An example of lymphaticovenular bypass. Note the blue lymphozurin dye within the lymphatic vessel and the red blood within the venule. **(B)** Another example of lymphaticovenular bypass. A grid in the background measures 1 mm. **(C)** Two lymphatic vessels anastomosed to a venule. (Reproduced from Chang DW. Lymphaticovenular bypass for lymphedema management in breast cancer patients: a prospective study. *Plast Reconstr Surg.* 2010;126:752–758.)

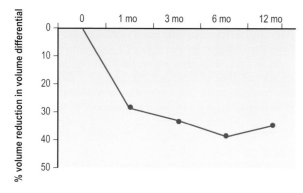

Fig. 3.8 Quantitative volumetric analysis at 1 month, 3 months, 6 months, and 1 year after bypass. (Reproduced from Chang DW. Lymphaticovenular bypass for lymphedema management in breast cancer patients: a prospective study. *Plast Reconstr Surg.* 2010;126:752–758.)

prophylactic surgery is controversial because lymphedema does not occur predictably.

Selecting functional lymphatic vessels is crucial for the success of the lymphovenous bypass operation. One recent advance in this area has been the use of fluorescence lymphography to image the lymphatic system during lymphovenous shunt operations and to diagnose the severity of lymphedema.[103–105] In this technique, an imaging system detects near-infrared light emitted by indocyanine green dye, which is injected into the affected limb. In the operating room, fluorescence lymphography allows surgeons to locate a functional lymphatic vessel for the lymphovenous shunt before making a skin incision. This technique allows for the prompt identification of the functional lymphatic vessels, and thus has the potential to improve the outcomes of lymphovenous bypass operations significantly *(Fig. 3.9)*.

Postoperative care

Following reconstruction by lymphatic grafting the extremities are elevated and elastic bandaging is continued. Additionally antibiotics are applied to prevent postoperative

those with late-stage lymphedema.[87] In fact, Boccardo and colleagues[101] and Nagase and colleagues[102] proposed that prophylactic lymphovenous bypass operations be performed to prevent the development of lymphedema. Although this concept may be feasible to retain function in lymphatic vessels,

Table 3.1 Lymphovenous shunt operations for breast cancer-related lymphedema

Year	First author	Surgical procedure	Number of patients	Type of measurement	Results	Follow-up	Additional treatment
1981	Fox[57]	End-to-side implantation	4	Volumetry	Improved: 2 Subjectively improved: 1 No change: 1	Not mentioned	Pneumatic pump, elastic compression
1988	Gloviczki[118]	End-to-end, end-to-side anastomoses	5	Circumference	Improved: 2 No change: 3	Not mentioned	Pneumatic pump, elastic compression
1990	O'Brien[86]	End-to-end anastomoses	46*	Circumference, volumetry	34% average reduction	6 months to 13.8 years†	Elevation and massage (soon after surgery)
1994	Flippetti[119]	End-to-side implantation	25	Circumference, lymphoscintigraphy	18 of 25 >50% improved: 3 <50% improved: 2 No change: 8	18 months	Not mentioned
1998	Yamamoto[10]	End-to-end implantation	5 (6 limbs)	Circumference	Improved: 6	9 months to 2.25 years	Not mentioned
2000	Koshima[90]	End-to-end anastomoses	12	Circumference	47.3% average reduction	11 months to 9 years	Elevation, elastic compression
2006	Campisi[120]	Shunts in both supraclavicular and deep lymphatics	194	Volumetry, lymphoscintigraphy	>75% improved: 73% 50-75% improved: 24% <25% improved: 3%*	Up to 15 years	Not mentioned

*Including other cases.
†Including lower limb cases.
(Reproduced from Suami H, Chang DW. Overview of surgical treatments for breast cancer–related lymphedema. Plast Reconstr Surg 2010;126:1853–1863.)

erysipelas. Long-term penicillin is given for 6 months. During that time period also elastic stockings are recommended. Thereafter the stockings are removed as the edema diminishes or disappears, otherwise additional therapy must be attempted and if necessary continued.

Outcomes, prognosis, and complications

Patients treated by lymphatic autografts have been followed using volume measurement, lymphoscintigraphy, indirect lymphography using water-soluble contrast medium, and MRI lymphography. The results were evaluated by volume estimation based on circumferential measurements along the limb in increments of 4 cm. Furthermore lymphatic outflow was measured semiquantitatively using the lymphatic transport index based on the findings of lymphoscintigraphic studies.[85]

Direct visualization of the grafts in patients was difficult because in lymphangiography using water-soluble contrast medium, the lymphatic vessels generally can be visualized only over short distances. However, in several patients patent grafts could be demonstrated more than 10 years after grafting with this technique.[80] Also with MRI lymphangiography, patent grafts have been proved more than 10 years after surgery.[106]

Baumeister and Frick reported on a series of 127 patients suffering from arm edema. In this cohort, a significant volume reduction was achieved from a mean of 3368 cm^3 preoperatively to a mean of 2567 cm^3 after 8–10 days ($P < 0.001$). At a mean follow-up period of 2.6 years the mean volume was 2625 cm^3 ($P < 0.001$). In a group of 8 patients with long-term follow-up of more than 10 years, the mean volume was reduced to 2273 cm^3, in contrast to a mean preoperative volume of 3004 cm^3 ($P < 0.001$).[81]

In another group of 81 adult patients with unilateral edema of the lower extremities, the mean preoperative volume of 13 098 cm^3 was reduced to a mean of 10 578 cm^3 ($P < 0.001$) at the time of hospital discharge. After a mean follow-up period of 1.7 years, the volume reduction was sustained, with a mean volume of 11 074 cm^3 ($P < 0.001$). In a subgroup of 12 patients with a further follow-up period of more than 4 years the volume was reduced to 10 692 cm^3 ($P < 0.001$).[81]

Despite these relatively large numbers, complications were relatively few. In the original group of patients, two developed erysipelas, there was one lymphocyst at the site of graft harvest, and one patient developed swelling of the lower leg secondary to venous thrombosis.

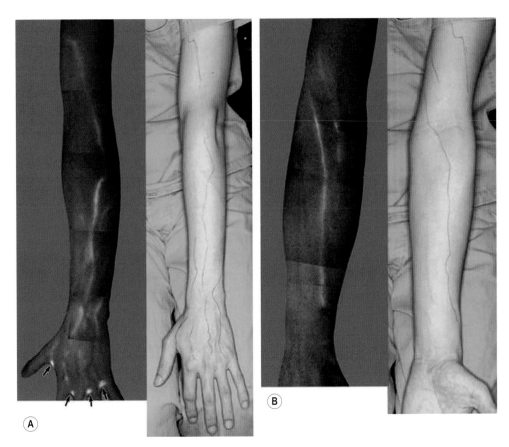

Fig. 3.9 (A, B) Indocyanine green (ICG) fluorescent lymphography images (black and white, montage from video images) of the normal upper limb, with photos of the limb (color). Arrows indicate the injection sites of ICG. (Reproduced from Suami H, Chang DW, Yamada K, et al. Use of indocyanine green fluorescent lymphography for evaluating dynamic lymphatic status. *Plast Reconstr Surg*. 2011;127:74e–76e.)

In another study, lymphoscintigraphic examinations were undertaken in 20 patients (12 upper, 8 lower extremities) with a follow-up period of 7 years. Seventeen of the 20 patients showed improved lymphatic outflow. In 5 patients, the patent grafts could be demonstrated directly by visualizing the routes of activity.[107]

Patent grafts could be demonstrated after more than 10 years with indirect lymphography as well as MRI lymphography.

Semiquantitative measurements of the lymphatic outflow were investigated by lymphoscintigraphy. In the group with the best clinical results. the flux of activity within the grafts could easily be seen showing normalization of the lymphatic outflow.

Secondary procedures following the reconstruction

Improvement of lymphatic outflow primarily affects the fluid retention component of the edema, which results clinically in a reduction of tenderness, softening of the tissues, and overall reduction in volume. If patients want a further reduction in volume in more severe cases, additional secondary procedures may be useful. Liposuction of the limb is theoretically minimally invasive, especially if the suction is performed in a longitudinal direction to protect the lymphatic vessels.[29] However direct excision of localized areas is also a good option and avoids the risk that liposuction may injure reconstructed lymphatic structures. Early experiences with these advanced stages of lymphedema show an additional significant reduction of volume after the suction. A continuous reduction of volume was possible also without further compression therapy, which means freedom of further treatment procedures can be reached.

Summary

Various surgical procedures have been attempted to treat lymphedema. However, whether and how to treat lymphedema surgically is still the subject of debate. Debulking operations have, for the most part, become less popular, and physiological lymphatic bypass operations have gained popularity.

However, the lymphatic bypass operation's effectiveness varies in reports, and its efficacy is difficult to evaluate because no standard protocol exists for measuring lymphedema. Numerous studies have provided information about lymphedema; however, most of the research data was obtained from clinical feedback, and basic research data on the etiology of lymphedema are limited. This lack of research data may be attributed to the features of the lymphatic system that make it difficult to study, such as its transparency and its fragility. However, advances are being made to address these difficulties. Several immunohistochemical markers are currently available to examine the lymphatic system histologically.[108–111] A new anatomical method for visualizing lymphatic vessels on radiographs has been developed in cadaveric specimens.[112–114] Several experimental animal models have also been developed for investigating lymphedema.[115–117] If these animal models are used with sound, evidence-based experimental methods, various surgical procedures can be evaluated to help develop definitive treatments for lymphedema.

Bonus images for this chapter can be found online at
http://www.expertconsult.com

Fig. 3.1 The Charles operation.[5] Skin and edematous soft tissue are excised, and split-thickness skin grafts are taken from the opposite thigh. The defect is covered by the skin grafts. (Reproduced from Suami H, Chang DW. Overview of surgical treatments for breast cancer-related lymphedema. *Plast Reconstr Surg.* 2010;126:1853–1863.)

Fig. 3.2 The Thompson operation. A long "hinge" skin flap is raised along the lateral aspect of the upper limb. The subcutaneous soft tissue and deep fascia are excised. The tip of the skin flap is de-epithelialized and embedded beside the neurovascular bundle. (Reproduced from Suami H, Chang DW. Overview of surgical treatments for breast cancer-related lymphedema. *Plast Reconstr Surg.* 2010;126:1853–1863.)

Fig. 3.3 The vein interposition graft procedure of Campisi.[76] A vein graft is harvested from the great or small saphenous vein or the anterior forearm. The vein graft is inserted between the lymphatic vessels above and below the site of lymphatic blockage.

Fig. 3.4 The lymphatic graft operation of Baumeister.[2,3] A lymphatic graft is harvested from the medial aspect of the thigh. The graft is inset subcutaneously, and lymphatic vessels at each end of the graft are anastomosed to recipient lymphatic vessels to create a lymphatic bypass route between the upper arm and neck. (Reproduced from Suami H, Chang DW. Overview of surgical treatments for breast cancer-related lymphedema. *Plast Reconstr Surg.* 2010;126:1853–1863.)

Access the complete references list online at http://www.expertconsult.com

18. Miller TA, Wyatt LE, Rudkin GH. Staged skin and subcutaneous excision for lymphedema: a favorable report of long-term results. *Plast Reconstr Surg.* 1998;102:1486.

51. Campisi C, Boccardo F, Tacchella M. Reconstructive microsurgery of lymph vessels: The personal method of lymphatic venous lymphatic (LVL) interpositioned grafted shunt. *Microsurgery.* 1995;16:161–166.
    Clinical observations in 64 patients affected by chronic obstructive lymphedema (either arm or leg) undergoing interposition autologous lymphatic-venous-lymphatic (LVL) anastomoses are reported. This microsurgical technique is an alternative to other lymphatic shunting methods, especially when venous dysfunction coexists in the same limb and, therefore, when direct lymphatic-venous anastomosis is accordingly inadequate. Preoperative diagnostic evaluation (including lymphatic and venous isotopic scintigraphy, Doppler venous flowmetrics, and pressure manometry) plays an essential role in assessing the conditions of both the lymphatic and venous systems and in establishing which microsurgical procedure, if any, is indicated. Our microsurgical technique consists of inserting suitably large and lengthy autologous venous grafts between lymphatic collectors above and below the site of obstruction to lymph

flow. The data show that, using this technique, both limb function and edema improved, and in all patients followed up for over 5 years edema regression was permanent.

81. Baumeister RGH, Frick A. The microsurgical lymph vessel transplantation. *Handchir Mikrochir Plast Chir.* 2003;35:201.

96. Weissleder H, Schuchhardt C. *Lymphedema: diagnosis and therapy.* Essen: Viavital; 2008.

107. Weiss M, Baumeister RGH, Tatsch K, Hahn K. Lymphoscintigraphy for non-invasive longterm follow-up for the functional outcome in patients with autologous lymph vessel transplantation. *Nuklearmedizin.* 1996;35:236–242.

118. Gloviczki P, Fisher J, Hollier LH, et al. Microsurgical lymphovenous anastomosis for treatment of lymphedema: a critical review. *J Vasc Surg.* 1988;7:647–652.

119. Filippetti M, Santoro E, Graziano F, et al. Modern therapeutic approaches to postmastectomy brachial lymphedema. *Microsurgery.* 1994;15:604–610.

120. Campisi C, Davini D, Bellini C, et al. Lymphatic microsurgery for the treatment of lymphedema. *Microsurgery.* 2006;26:65–69.

4

Lower extremity sarcoma reconstruction

Goetz A. Giessler and Michael Sauerbier

SYNOPSIS

- Any lesion in the lower extremity with a clinical history of pain, continuous growth, size over 5 cm or deep subfascial localization is suspicious of a sarcomatous malignancy and should be surgically biopsied according to established surgical rules.
- The single statistically proven modality of curing sarcomas and prolonging postsurgical lifespan remains surgical excision with wide margins, resulting in a postoperative R_0 status. To date, no other neoadjuvant or postoperative treatment modality can replace this approach. If wide margins cannot be achieved, adjuvant therapy is indicated for extremity preservation.
- Plastic surgical lower extremity sarcoma reconstruction, especially in bone sarcoma reconstruction, is the classical field of an interdisciplinary, multimodal approach, most commonly together with tumor and orthopedic surgeons, oncologic radiotherapists, and oncologists.
- Modern oncoplastic reconstructive surgery can provide adequate reconstructive options for almost any defect size and composition, so radical tumor excision can be combined with over 95% extremity preservation today.
- The plastic reconstructions in sarcoma-related limb-sparing surgery are often demanding and complex and consist of the full spectrum of plastic surgical options. They should be performed in specialized centers and specifically adapted to the patient and case profile.

 Access the Historical Perspective section online at
http://www.expertconsult.com

Introduction

Soft-tissue and bone sarcomas

Soft-tissue tumors are a highly heterogeneous group of about 100 different tumor entities that are classified histogenetically according to their main adult tissue component they resemble

most. The malignant subgroup of soft-tissue tumors is called sarcomas, which not only have the potential to grow locally invasive or even demonstrate destructive growth, but also have a variable risk of recurrence and metastatic potential. As the term "sarcoma" (derived from the Greek word σαρξ, *sarx* = meat) does not necessarily imply fast, expansive growth or metastasis, a further subclassification system into more aggressive sarcomas (high-grade, poorly differentiated) or less aggressive (low-grade, well-differentiated) types exists. Some lesions, like the atypical fibroxanthoma, are called "pseudosarcomas," as they demonstrate a benign clinical course but are histologically malignant. However, well-differentiated tumors usually show low-grade characteristics and vice versa.

Primary bone sarcomas are even less frequent than soft-tissue sarcomas, and most malignant osseous lesions are metastatic, especially in advanced age. Despite having a low incidence, bone sarcomas have a high significance for both patient and surgeon due to their impact on extremity function and overall mobility. Limb-preserving surgery after wide tumor resections frequently poses a real challenge for the reconstructive surgeon.

Sarcomas can occur in every part of the body, as they derive from mesodermic tissue like muscle, nerve, bone cartilage, blood vessels, or fat. The therapeutic mainstay for soft-tissue sarcomas is based on surgical excision whereas radiotherapy and, less so, chemotherapy are used as adjunct adjuvant therapeutic modalities. In primary osseous sarcomas neoadjuvant chemotherapy plays a more important role. The complexity of the surgical resection and the subsequent plastic surgical reconstruction differs considerably depending on the localization.

Like any oncologic discipline, sarcoma treatment is a typical field of modern interdisciplinary and multimodal therapy. Lower extremity sarcoma reconstruction, especially in bone sarcoma reconstruction, is also a fascinating field for an effective interaction between the surgical disciplines of oncologic, pediatric and podiatric surgeons, orthopedic surgeons and plastic reconstructive (micro-) surgeons.

Modern plastic reconstructive surgery can provide adequate reconstructive options for almost any defect size and composition, so considerations about defect size should not play a role in tumor excision. Over 95% of the extremities can be preserved after radical tumor excision today. The plastic reconstructive procedures are often demanding and complex and often encompass the full spectrum of plastic surgical options. These procedures may be best performed in specialized centers where individually adapted regimens to patient and case profiles may be optimized.

Sarcomas in the lower extremity

Sarcomas in the lower extremity are more common than in the upper limb (74 versus 26%) and represent the most common location of sarcomas in the body overall (45%).[1] Currently, they can be safely treated by extremity preservation in most cases, if properly performed according to the rules described in this chapter and in the pertinent current literature. In this context, several studies have now demonstrated that limb-sparing surgery is oncologically not inferior to amputation in the treatment of lower extremity sarcoma (see Outcomes, prognosis, and complications, below). While amputation was the keystone of previous surgical therapy several decades ago, it usually represents only an important last-line therapeutic modality today. The common misconceptions that amputations have a better outcome in both tumor safety and quality of life have both definitely been proven wrong.[2–4]

Sarcomas are rare and a "soft-tissue swelling" is often misinterpreted by both patient and physician because of this fact. This can considerably delay proper diagnosis. Still, tumor manifestations in the extremities are often detected slightly earlier than in the trunk, as the extremities are constantly under personal "visual" control in daily life. This may be even truer for tumors on the upper extremity than on the lower extremity.

Due to the highly functional anatomy of our extremities with vessels, nerves, tendons, bones, and muscles in close vicinity, even smaller tumors can represent a challenge to both the resecting tumor surgeon as well as the reconstructive plastic surgeon. Preservation of the lower extremity in sarcoma reconstruction differs from similar manifestations in the upper extremity[5] in several key points:

- Stability and weight-bearing capability are usually held in higher regard than functional mobility or range of motion in the lower extremity.
- Postoperative appearance is usually less important. In most urban cultures the reconstructed legs with their scars and possible voluminous flaps can easily be hidden in clothing and have a less important role in social interaction than the upper extremity (i.e., shaking hands).
- Weight-bearing demands are higher and atherosclerotic vessel damage and orthostatic venous pressure are more profound in the lower extremity: Both may play a major role in free tissue transfer.
- Nerve regeneration is less successful in the lower extremity at any age.
- Wound healing is slower and the risk of infectious complication is higher.

Basic science/disease process

Epidemiology soft-tissue sarcomas

Soft-tissue sarcomas are a rare disease entity with an incidence of 1:100000 in adults and 10–15% in children. This accounts for an incidence of about 10600 new cases in 2009 in the US, representing 1–2% of all malignancies (www.seer.cancer.gov). There is no overall significant gender predisposition and the overall median age at presentation is 50–60 years.

With about 45% of all sarcomas occurring in the lower extremity, 15% in the upper extremity, 10% in the head and neck region, 15% in the retroperitoneal space, and the remaining 15% in the abdomen and the chest wall,[6] the musculoskeletal system of the extremities and the abdominal and thoracic walls is the most common predilection site. Extremity sarcomas are most common in the thigh (50–60%).

While most cases of soft-tissue sarcomas are sporadic, there are some genetic and nongenetic risk factors, summarized in *Table 4.1*. Up to 60% of all soft-tissue sarcomas contain a somatic mutation of p53.[7] A detailed description of the various risk factors is beyond the scope of this chapter, but there are several strong associations to be mentioned: a history of radiation exposure accounts for up to 5.5% of all sarcomas. The risk is dose-dependent and the latency period between radiation and clinical tumor manifestation is around 5 years. Over 80% of radiation-associated sarcomas are high-grade types.[8] Neurofibromatosis type NF-1 is strongly associated with the cumulative lifetime risk of up to 13% for the occurrence of malignant peripheral nerve sheath tumors.

Table 4.1 Predisposing factors for soft-tissue sarcomas	
Genetic	Neurofibromatosis NF-1 (von Recklinghausen disease) Retinoblastoma Gardner's syndrome Werner's syndrome Bloom's syndrome Fumarate hydratase leiomyosarcoma syndrome Diamond–Blackfan anemia
Mechanical	Li–Fraumeni syndrome Postparturition
Chemical	Chronic irritation Polyvinylchloride Hemochromatosis Dioxin (TCDD): "Agent Orange"
Radiation	Arsenic Traumatic/accidental
Lymphedema	Posttherapeutic Parasitic (filariasis) Iatrogenic Stewart–Treves syndrome
Infectious (viral)	Congenital Kaposi sarcoma (human herpesvirus-8)

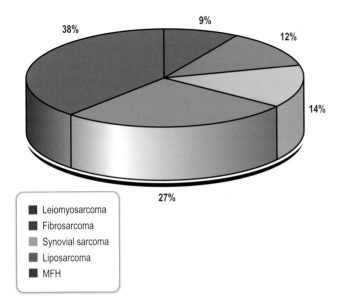

Fig. 4.1 Distribution of histopathologic types in extremity soft-tissue sarcomas. MFH, malignant fibrous histiocytoma. (Adapted from Weitz J, Antonescu CR, Brennan MF. Localized extremity soft tissue sarcoma: improved knowledge with unchanged survival over time. J Clin Oncol 2003;21:2719–2725.)

The sarcoma subtype is determined by light and electron microscopy, immunohistochemistry, and cytogenetic analysis. If it results in a tumor that cannot be designated accordingly, a descriptive evaluation is given for an "unclassified sarcoma." Obtaining reference pathologies for soft- and bone tissue sarcomas should be standard, as the rate of diagnostic agreement among specialists is below 75%.[9,10]

The most common histopathologic subtype distribution in extremities in the largest series in the literature is shown in *Figure 4.1*.

Bone sarcomas

About 2600 new primary bone sarcomas occur each year in the US (www.seer.cancer.gov). The overall median age at diagnosis is 39 years. Many predisposing factors for bone sarcomas are similar to those for soft-tissue sarcomas (retino-blastoma, Li–Fraumeni syndrome, radiation, and others) *(Table 4.1)*. Paget's disease, bone infarction, and fibrous dysplasia may also represent risk factors for bone sarcomas.

The most common type is the osteogenic sarcoma, which has a predilection for the metaphyses around the knee in about 50% of cases. It is the third most common cancer in the young (www.nhs.uk) with a second peak around age 60. The male-to-female ratio is almost 2:1 in large studies and for this specific tumor the median age at diagnosis is 17 years. Only 6.4% present initially with pathological fractures, whereas the majority are detected in the workup of a painful mass or swollen extremity.[11,12] It commonly arises in the medulla, but as a juxtacortical osteogenic sarcoma it arises from the external surface, most commonly the posterior aspect of the femur.

The spindle cell mesenchymal sarcoma group contains chondrosarcomas, intraosseous malignant fibrous histiocytomas, and fibrosarcomas. The tumors of this group only

have an incidence of about two-thirds of that of osteogenic sarcomas and primarily occur in an older population. Chondrosarcomas are slow-growing and relatively resistant to adjuvant therapy.

Ewing's sarcoma is classically located in the femur diaphyses in teenagers and only 20% occur in middle-aged adults. If extradiaphyseal, it is very common in the pelvis. It is the most common primary bone malignancy of the fibula. Ewing's sarcoma is very radiation-sensitive.

Tumor growth and metastasizing

Sarcomas in the extremity may spread locally by continuous expanding growth, irrespective of anatomical borders. In many cases it mistakingly seems that the tumor has developed a bordering capsule to surrounding "healthy tissue." However, this capsule is part of the tumor and soft-tissue satellite-like or intraosseous skip lesion tumor manifestations are beyond this capsule. This fact represents the main justification for a modern wide-resection concept in sarcoma surgery.

Hematogenic spread is most common in soft-tissue and bone sarcomas. For lower extremity tumors, the primary site for metastasis is the lung. Lymphatic metastases are present in less than 5% of all soft-tissue sarcomas (rhabdomyosarcoma, angiosarcoma, epithelioid-like sarcoma).[13,14]

Diagnosis/patient presentation/imaging

A detailed history and physical examination are the first initial and important steps to professional tumor surgery. In sarcomatous lesions, the patient often relates the tumor causally to an – often minor – traumatic event that brings the lesion to the patient's attention. Acute trauma, however, is not a proven predisposing factor for sarcoma development. Because of this, there is often a considerable time lag between this initial recognition and the first presentation of the lesion to a medical professional. Furthermore, the rationale of the lesion is often erratically misinterpreted and then causes a variety of inadequate treatments by both lays and physicians, further delaying proper diagnosis. The average duration of any symptoms before seeing a physician is 6 months in all soft-tissue sarcomas, but possibly shorter in extremity manifestation.[3] So in adults, lesions that: (1) have not disappeared after 4 weeks; (2) are located subfascially or in the popliteal or groin flexion creases; (3) continue to grow or are symptomatic (i.e., pain, paresthesias); or (4) are already larger than 5 cm on detection should generally be biopsied as they are highly suspicious for malignancy.

It is not unusual that sarcomas are found by physicians in the context of workup of a completely different medical problem (i.e., chronic venous insufficiency in the leg). Coincidental findings like articular pain and joint effusions are common, especially with osseous sarcomas, whereas clinically manifest neurovascular symptoms are relatively rare at initial presentation. Two-thirds of sarcoma patients present with a painless mass during their first clinical examination, and only one-third have current pain or have had a history of pain in the affected region.

The thorough physical examination is not only focused on the affected extremity but includes the complete body. The pertaining lymph node stations should be examined as well, even though lymphatic spread is uncommon in the majority of all sarcoma types. The general health status should be assessed and optimized by all relevant medical specialties. This is especially important in multimorbid patients with concomitant acute and chronic comorbidities in the context of planned operative procedures. Terminal illnesses and comorbidities have to be taken into consideration for the extent of both resection and reconstructive surgery.

Clinical assessment and staging of the patient must be completed by adequate imaging diagnostics for evaluating local and generalized tumor manifestations. Any imaging of the tumor region must be performed before surgical biopsy as the latter may confound the picture to a considerable extent.

Gadolinium contrast-enhanced MRI is currently the diagnostic mainstay to define exact tumor location, its relation to neighboring neurovascular structures and muscular compartments, to determine its homogeneity, integrity, vascularization, and its presumed main tissue component. MRI is specifically useful for detecting skip lesions. It allows three-dimensional planning of the resection and helps to assess the necessary reconstruction procedures preoperatively.

Modern spiral CT scans are indispensable for clarifying the detailed anatomy of osseous sarcomas, determining the effect on skeletal structures of neighboring soft-tissue tumors, and aiding in operative planning of these sarcomatous entities. Thoracic and abdominal CT scans are the diagnostics of choice for staging of high-grade sarcomas of the extremities and detect intrapulmonary and abdominal metastases. In recurrent disease, positron emission tomography (PET) CT can augment information about suspicious lesions in selected cases, though it is not accepted as a standard instrument for preoperative workup.[20–22]

CT angiography with three-dimensional reconstructions is a valuable tool to determine the overall vascular status of the affected leg, to reveal underlying generalized vessel disease and the vascularity of the tumor, and to show vascular displacements, collateral perfusion systems, vessel invasion, and tumor-related occlusion. It also provides valuable information about the feasibility of microvascular anastomoses and the presence of suitable recipient vessels, especially in elderly patients.

Plain X-ray films demonstrate specific periosteal or cortical signs, osteolyses and paraosseous calcifications in diaphyseal and metaphyseal bony lesions. Even today, a plain radiograph remains the diagnostic method of choice for primary bone sarcomas *(Fig. 4.2)*. A plain chest radiograph is still considered the standard for clinical staging in low-grade extremity lesions.

Ultrasound with or without contrast media is a cheap, fast, and painless adjunctive diagnostic measure which may be especially helpful in highly vascularized tumors. Ultrasound was often the diagnostic device of coincidental tumor findings but is also used for getting an initial overall picture of the lesion.

A ^{99m}Tc-pyrophosphate bone scan is essential to bone tumor staging and screening for multicentric disease or metastases.

A special laboratory workup for soft-tissue sarcomas does not exist, whereas elevated alkaline phosphatase and lactate

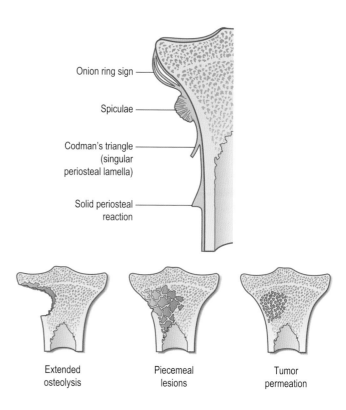

Onion ring sign

Spiculae

Codman's triangle (singular periosteal lamella)

Solid periosteal reaction

Extended osteolysis

Piecemeal lesions

Tumor permeation

Fig. 4.2 Typical radiologic features of malignant and benign primary osseous tumors.

dehydrogenase over 400 U/L are independent predictors of an unfavorable outcome in bone sarcomas.[23]

Patient profile/general considerations/ treatment planning

Patient profile

The goals of surgery in sarcoma reconstruction in the lower extremity depend on the individual case profile, which comprises personal factors and the available reconstructive options:

The most important personal factors that need to be taken into consideration are: age, size and weight, concomitant chronic diseases relevant to general health and operability, medications, social status, functional and aesthetic conceptions, previous operations and tissue quality of the affected extremity.

The pertinent reconstructive options that need to be discussed with the patient are the relevant operative methods according to the applicable steps of the reconstructive ladder, counterbalancing their advantages and disadvantages for the tumor stage, location, oncologic safety, and potential adjuvant procedures (i.e., irradiation).

General considerations

Above all, the prime goal should be an R_0 resection with tumor-free and adequately wide margins, which provides the best chance of complete surgical cure of the disease. This might create a considerable surgical defect and can imply major surgical reconstructive procedures for the patient. The extent of adequate wide tissue resection is almost never realized by the patient presenting with a palpable mass and has to be explained to him or her in detail.

If surgical cure is not possible, resection of as much tumor mass as possible (tumor debulking) is paramount (R_1/R_2), usually followed by adjuvant radiotheapy and, less frequently, chemotherapy according to the recommendations of a multidisciplinary tumor board. At this point, the reconstructive goal should aim for a functional lower extremity capable for full weight-bearing that appears as aesthetically as possible in the given case and circumstances. The surgical therapy should create a status for the patient to be integrated in social life, allowing him or her to wear normal clothing and having a closed skin envelope. In selected cases, creating a stable open chronic wound is the only remaining palliative option; however, it should be free of copious discharge and secretions and avoid any olfactory nuisance: For example, a stable open wound producing minimal drainage that can be treated by daily dressing changes at home may offer a higher quality of life than performing another resection and reconstructive effort that may force the patient to stay in the clinic during his or her last days.

Treatment planning

Each case should be discussed in a multidisciplinary tumor board with all relevant medical disciplines involved in the setup of a treatment plan (tumor surgeon, medical oncologist, orthopedic surgeon, plastic surgeon, internal medicine, psychologist, radiologist, oncologic radiotherapy specialist, prosthetic technician). For optimal planning and strategy development, all diagnostic procedures, the radiologic imaging and the definitive histology should already be present (see below).

The tumor board treatment recommendations are thoroughly explained to, and discussed with, the patient including all operative options (including amputation), neoadjuvant or adjuvant chemo- or radiotherapy. It is important for many patients to outline a timeframe of the various surgical or multimodal therapeutic options.

Finally, tumor staging is done according to the current staging systems for soft-tissue sarcomas. The American Joint Committee on Cancer (AJCC) system is designed for extremity sarcomas *(Table 4.2)* including most, but not all, histologic subtypes. Dermatofibrosarcoma protuberans and angiosarcoma, among others, are exempt from AJCC staging. For primary bone sarcomas like osteogenic sarcoma, the Muskuloskeletal Tumor Society staging system is used *(Table 4.3)*.

Surgery

To date, no other treatment modality provides better cure for sarcomas than adequate surgery. Oncological safety is paramount, but preservation of the leg or foot should be achieved

---

Table 4.2 American Joint Committee on Cancer staging system for soft-tissue sarcomas

Classification and staging	Characteristic
Primary tumor (T)	
T1	Tumor 5 cm or less in greatest dimension
T1a	Superficial tumor (in relation to investing fascia)
T1b	Deep tumor (visceral and retroperitoneal sarcomas are defined as deep tumors)
T2	Tumor larger than 5 cm in greatest dimension
T2a	Superficial tumor
T2b	Deep tumor
Regional lymph nodes (N)	
N0	No evidence of nodal metastasis
N1	Nodal metastasis present
Distant metastasis (M)	
M0	No distant metastasis
M1	Distant metastasis present
Grade (G)	
G1	Low-grade
G2 and G3	High-grade
Staging	
Stage I	Low-grade tumors, no evidence of regional nodes or distant metastases (T1a, T1b, T2a, T2b)
Stage II	High-grade, small tumors (T1a and b), and superficial, large tumors (T2a), no evidence of regional nodes or distal metastases
Stage III	High-grade, deep tumors larger than 5 cm (T2b), no evidence of regional nodes or distant metastases
Stage IV	Any tumor with regional nodes or distant metastases

(Reproduced from Papagelopoulos PJ, Mavrogenis AF, Mastorakos DP, *et al.* Current concepts for management of soft tissue sarcomas of the extremities. J Surg Orthop Adv 2008;17:204–215.)

Table 4.3 Muskuloskeletal Tumor Society staging system

Stage	Characteristic
IA	Low-grade, intracompartmental
IB	Low-grade, extracompartmental
IIA	High-grade, intracompartmental
IIB	High-grade, extracompartmental
IIIA	Low- or high-grade, intracompartental with metatases
IIIB	Low- or high-grade, extracompartental with metatases

(Reproduced from Papagelopoulos PJ, Mavrogenis AF, Mastorakos DP, *et al.* Current concepts for management of soft tissue sarcomas of the extremities. J Surg Orthop Adv 2008;17:204–215.)

to preserve patient integrity, which is usually possible. This avoids the need for prosthesis adaptation and use and prosthesis-related problems. Several considerations in sarcoma-related defect reconstruction need to be mentioned that differ from sarcoma-related surgery at the upper extremity: the capability for stable weight-bearing is more important than joint mobility in the lower extremity, whereas preservation or restoration of sensitivity is less important in the leg and foot than the arm or hand: While sensitivity should be preserved as far as possible, in selective cases, asensitive "stilt legs" are superior to amputations, especially in elderly patients who would have problems in adapting to prosthesis-handling. Not being able to preserve the main nerves and thereby sensitivity is not an indication for amputation by itself!

Radiotherapy

Radiotherapy is the primary adjunctive treatment method in sarcoma management today. Neoadjuvant radiation in large sarcomas uses external-beam irradiation, which helps in tumor shrinkage, thickening of the tumor capsule that facilitates adequate resection and the achievement of negative margins during wide resection, and reduces potential surgical tumor seeding. The disadvantages of preoperative irradiation are a higher rate of wound-healing complications compared to postoperative radiotherapy and the creation of necrotic tumor material for the pathologist.[2]

Intraoperative radiation comprises single-dose electron radiation and has its indications in the lower extremity for locations around the groin and foot. It is especially effective in increasing the tumor dose relative to the normal tissue dose. Its availability is limited even in modern tumor centers.

Postoperative irradiation is done with brachytherapy and electron beam therapy both used alone and in combination regimens. Brachytherapy is especially useful after resection of local recurrences in a previously irradiated field.

Chemotherapy

To date, any adjuvant or neoadjuvant chemotherapy for sarcomas should only be conducted in clinical studies (EORTC, COSS, EURO-Ewing). The various protocols are beyond the scope of this chapter and are changing rapidly. The reader is therefore advised to consult the pertinent most recent literature in that matter.

Isolated extremity perfusion or hyperthermia is currently indicated for patients who would otherwise require primary amputation. The precise selection criteria have not been clearly defined yet and valid comparisons to other approaches are lacking.[2]

Treatment/surgical resection techniques

Histological confirmation, grading, and subtyping of the presumed malignant sarcomatous tumor on the lower extremity must be achieved before the overall treatment strategy is planned in the tumor board and definitive, usually more extensive, surgery is initiated. However, not all known biopsy techniques are useful for a correct and safe diagnosis of a sarcoma.

Biopsy techniques

Fine-needle or core needle aspirations

These techniques gain only a very small amount of tissue, even in the hands of an experienced clinician. Although tissue aspiration with a 23-gauge needle usually harvests only a very small number of cells, the volume of tissue gained from a core-needle biopsy is slightly higher. Still, both methods have the disadvantage of not representing the tumor tissue components correctly, especially in larger tumors, which makes it very difficult for the histopathologist to find the exact diagnosis, perform the necessary number of different studies, and determine the correct grading. However, if combined with CT scan or ultrasound-guided needle placement, core biopsies may achieve a correct diagnosis in up to 90% of cases under optimal circumstances. Fine-needle aspirations only reach 56–72%.[24–26] Although single core biopsies may harvest too little tissue for an extensive pathological workup with several stainings and immunohistochemical diagnostics, they have the advantage of gathering tissue from different parts of the tumor to create a comprehensive picture.[26]

Both methods are atraumatic and only very rarely cause dangerous tumor cell-dissipating hematomas. In several institutions, core biopsies are reserved for surgically unresectable tumors (i.e., retroperitoneal lesions) to determine tissue type and guide an eventual neoadjuvant therapy,[3] while others use it as a prime diagnostic tissue-sampling method.[26]

In summary, fine-needle biopsies do not have a place in sarcoma diagnosis in lower extremities, and both core biopsy and open surgical biopsy are very operator-dependent: If poorly performed, the risk of getting an inadequate diagnostic sample or tumor seeding is high.[27,28]

Bone-forming lesions are very difficult to sample adequately percutaneously and open biopsies are preferable.[29]

Excisional biopsy

Excisional biopsies aim for the removal of all tumor tissue *in toto* with primary closure of the surrounding tissue and are therefore reserved for lesions less than 3–5 cm in diameter and epifascial location. As the definitive diagnosis is not known beforehand, no tissue margin of defined thickness is left with this procedure.

Any surgical biopsy on the lower extremity should be performed with a pressurized tourniquet (no exsanguination!) if tumor location permits. The bloodless field not only aids in exact and atraumatic safe dissection, but also inhibits possible tumor cell contamination during surgery.

Before incising the skin, it is absolutely necessary that the surgeon already imagines any secondary, definitive tumor resections and has possible muscle and tendon transfers and local flap options in mind. The biopsy incision should interfere as little as possible with these factors. Usually, a longitudinal incision as short as possible for an adequate exposure directly over the tumor is made, providing the shortest reasonable access route to the neoplasm.

The tumor should be excised in a no-touch/no-see technique including any pseudocapsule (if present) without opening it. Any "shelling out" of the tumor should not be performed, as in sarcomas this capsule is part of the tumor and its remaining walls contain tumor cells.

After the excision, it may be useful to mark the resection bed with titanium or vitallium microclips to make later excision easier, if malignancy was affirmed. Localization sutures are fixed to the tumor, and both instruments and gloves are changed.

Meticulous hemostasis and the placement of a closed suction drainage within the wound to prevent possible tumor seeding through a hematoma are paramount before a layered skin closure is done. The skin should be closed with single interrupted stitches or intracutaneous sutures. Mattress sutures or separate drainage perforations leave stitch marks too far away from the incision: as they all have to be excised in case of malignancy, this would enlarge the amount of tissue to be resected. A sterile circular compressive dressing is placed and the affected extremity is immobilized, especially in procedures close to joints. Temporary splinting for a few days assists well here.[3]

Incisional biopsy

The surgical resection of a representative part of the sarcoma is the gold standard in the diagnosis of extremity tumors for any lesions that are larger than 3–5 cm and in a subfascial location. This technique should only be performed by an experienced surgeon, as the gathering of a respective tissue specimen and the handling of the tissue are crucial to the success of the procedure. The advantages of getting adequate tissue for a full range of diagnostics greatly outweigh the disadvantages of opening the tumor and the potential of tumor cell seeding in the path of the access route.

Again, the procedure should be performed with a tourniquet, as detailed dissection is possible and intraoperative contamination of surrounding tissue areas during resection of the histologic specimen with potentially tumor cell containing blood is minimized.

The guidelines for the skin incision are practically the same as for the excisional biopsies, keeping any further operative options in mind. An incision parallel to the axis of the extremity is made. It should be as short as possible for an adequate exposure directly over the tumor providing the shortest reasonable access route to the neoplasm. The incision must not unnecessarily interfere with later procedures needed to cover the defect.

A properly conducted incision biopsy should harvest a relevant, at least $2 \times 1 \times 1$ cm, tissue block from all areas of the tumor, including the capsule. It is a common misconception to gain tissue only from the central portion, as this area often contains considerable amounts of necrotic tissue which is not adequate for pathology or makes definitive histological classification impossible. The tissue block removed should be manipulated as little as possible and should not come into contact with the wound edges of the surgical access route. Any instrument used to hold or manipulate the biopsy specimen must not be used for wound closure or retraction. After removal of the tumor block, localization sutures are tied on it and both instruments and gloves are changed.

Meticulous hemostasis and the placement of a closed suction drainage within the wound to prevent possible tumor seeding through a hematoma are paramount before a multi-layered skin closure is done. The skin should be closed with single interrupted stitches or intracutaneous sutures. Mattress sutures or separate drainage perforations leave stitch marks too far away from the incision: As they all have to be excised in case of malignancy, this would enlarge the amount of tissue to be resected. A sterile circular compressive dressing is placed and the affected extremity is immobilized, especially in procedures close to joints. Temporary splinting or an external fixator for a few days serves the purpose here.

When mounting an external fixator to the affected lower extremity at the time of biopsy, care must be taken not to interfere with the later resection margins for definitive tumor resection. Preoperative findings of intraosseous skip lesions in bone sarcomas must be taken into consideration in this context. A fixator pin must never be set into an area of later resection, or the pin tract has to be included in the resection specimen.

Both incisional and excisional biopsies are not intended to remove the tumor adequately according to oncologic rules. Therefore, temporary vacuum-assisted closure techniques should not be used and are rarely required anyway. Their angiogenetic potential and the risk of dissipation of tumor cell-containing wound secretions into the rest of the wound may negatively affect local oncologic safety. Larger studies are missing, however.

Reoperative biopsies and surgical revisions

Tumor centers frequently have to perform a surgical revision to confirm the diagnosis of sarcoma or to accomplish a correct surgical-oncological treatment. After previous attempts of inadequate biopsy or even after surgery that was intended to be definitive and curative, a reoperation is considered mandatory, if at least one of the following situations is present:

- Only inadequate tissue material for definitive histology was gained at the first operation.
- Previous resections have not been performed according to current oncological guidelines (see Case 4.2, below): suspicious hints indicating reoperation are incisions placed horizontally to the axis of the extremity opening up several muscle compartments, intact nerve function after resection of a malignant peripheral nerve sheath tumor or normal leg motor function after radical excision of extensor or flexor muscles.
- A clinically unsuspicious and presumably benign tumor was resected with the techniques of benign tumor surgery, but the postoperative histopathological workup showed an unexpected malignancy.
- A tumor was resected during nononcologic surgery and detected in the postoperative workup ("unplanned excision").
- The tumor surface was visible intraoperatively.
- Previous operating room (OR) reports describe an "easy shelling out from a capsule" but clinical and/or histological and/or radiographic workup confirms a highly suspicious lesion or malignancy. A sarcoma resection out of its pseudocapsule results in local recurrences in up to 90% of patients.[6]

Table 4.4 World Health Organization classification of tumor resection margins	
R_0	Resection with microscopically tumor-free specimen margins
R_1	Resection with microscopically tumor-positive specimen margins
R_2	Resection with macroscopically remaining tumor

- The patient presents with early local tumor recurrence, despite a "radical resection," as stated in the previous OR report.
- Previous OR reports state a "compartment resection" in the axilla or around the elbow, popliteal fossa, or groin (which is anatomically not possible).
- OR reports and pathological reports differ considerably in amount and integrity of the resected tumor.
- Any remaining tumor is present in any postoperative imaging (MRI).

In all these situations, at least an R_1 situation must be anticipated. The secondary resection should follow the exact principles of the surgical technique for definitive resection, described below. The previous tumor bed should not be opened or visualized at all. If macroscopically visible remaining tumor is encountered during surgery (R_2 situation), the secondary revisional surgery may at least reduce the situation into an R_1-situation *(Table 4.4)*. Following these revisional surgeries, radiotherapy is usually indicated for a reduction in the probability of local tumor recurrence.

Surgical technique for definitive resection

Soft-tissue sarcomas

As soon as the definitive histology is found and the tumor type, grading, and staging of the disease have been completed in the multidisciplinary workup, definitive surgery is initiated. If the tumor is deemed to be resectable and no neoadjuvant therapy was planned, the therapy of choice today is a wide excision with adequate margins. Before any definitive surgery is performed, the reconstructive strategy should be planned as meticulously as possible. It is necessary to inform the patient fully about the expected extent and length of the procedure and of possible donor sites of flaps, nerves, vessels, or skin grafts. Furthermore the anesthesiological risk and invasiveness of monitoring should be explained to the patient and planned accordingly with the anesthesiologist. Also, placement of vascular access routes and regional pain catheters is important. A well-planned patient positioning on the OR table can allow a simultaneous team approach of oncologic and plastic surgeons and save a considerable amount of operative time.

Definitive sarcoma resection with a curative approach should be performed in a bloodless field with a pneumatic tourniquet or even temporary occlusion of the iliac or femoral artery by vascular surgery techniques. This reduces not only the risk for potential hemorrhage-induced contamination of the field with tumor cells but blood loss in general and is mandatory for a detailed dissection.

The resection must include all previous skin incisions, all previous stitch marks, and drain sites with a margin of 4 cm of healthy skin around them. This margin is also true for any ulcerated tumor locations. If the previous incision was performed properly, it creates an elliptical defect along the longitudinal axis of the leg. The advantages of this orientation are the preservation of the remaining subdermal lymph vessels and ease in wound closure.

After adequate epifascial mobilization, the muscle fascia is opened and the sarcoma is resected with a no-touch/no-see technique leaving a cuff of macroscopically unaffected tissue of 2–5 cm around it. There are no conclusive studies about the exact margins in sarcoma surgery, but many centers currently recommend a margin of 2 cm from the deep surface of the tumor and 4–5 cm laterally.[2,3,24,30] Any palpable pseudocapsule of the tumor belongs to the tumor itself and should be resected but neither be opened nor seen at all, otherwise the procedure is regarded as a R_1 resection. The tumor should not be retracted or manipulated with sharp or pointed-tipped instruments and should be resected in continuity with the skin island containing the previous incision.

The aforementioned margins are often difficult to maintain in the periphery of the lower extremity. Under these circumstances, ray amputations may suffice to achieve comparable local recurrence rates (<10%) if combined with local deperiostation and tenosynovectomy.[3]

Vascular involvement

Relevant deep vascular structures that are not directly infiltrated or encased in the tumor can usually be treated by longitudinal opening of the vascular adventitia opposite the tumor and subsequent microsurgical stripping of the adventitia under loupe magnification en bloc with the tumor. Accompanying veins are usually ligated and included in this specimen if venous drainage of the extremity is still guaranteed in a different compartment. Preoperative MRI helps in finding this decision, otherwise the affected vessels have to be resected en bloc and replaced by a venous patch (less common), vein graft or, less commonly, by artificial vessel graft material (i.e., Gore-Tex®). Any arterial side branches that do not lead into the tumor should be evaluated as possible recipient vessels for microvascular tissue reconstruction and be preserved. Preservation of septal branches or muscular vessels that are outside the tumor resection area may lifeguard local or regional muscle and skin flaps that can aid in postoperative dead-space elimination and wound closure but also in simple primary wound healing. Extraneous vessel ligation should therefore be avoided.

If the superficial venous systems (great and lesser saphenous vein) are not included in the resected sarcoma specimen, they should be preserved together with their subcutaneous branches if possible. This prevents venous congestion if the deep venous systems close to the tumor must be resected as mentioned above, adding to the radicality and safety. While there should always be an adequate arterial perfusion of the lower extremity after tumor removal, only the main arteries are reconstructed immediately. Interpositional vein grafts for large-vein reconstruction in tumor patients have a higher risk of thrombotic failure than in traumatic cases and should be reserved for selected cases only.

Nerve involvement

The same dissection strategy applies to the main nerves in the lower extremity. Any affected epineural tissue or connective tissue around the nerve inside the safety margin around the tumor should be stripped or removed with careful microsurgical techniques. If only a few fascicles of an important main nerve trunk are adherent to the tumor, it is considered acceptable to resect these and leave the unaffected nerve bundles intact for some basic motor function and sensitivity. If a major nerve is encased completely, it must be resected and should be reconstructed primarily or secondarily.

Osseous involvement

For soft-tissue tumors in the lower extremity that are not primary osseous sarcomas and that grow close to bone, the appropriate treatment has to be guided by clinical judgment and preoperative MRI and CT scan. Real bony erosion is relatively rare, and periosteal stripping, decortication, and partial bone resection are reasonable methods to comply with safe margins according to the principles of wide resection. However, these procedures weaken the bone mechanically in an area where later adjuvant radiotherapy further weakens the bone in the beam, to an extent that may even cause spontaneous fractures. Together with systemically prevalent osteoporosis, this poses a considerable risk for spontaneous fractures.[3,31] Any resection of weight-bearing bones and joint segments should be carefully balanced against the complexity of reconstructing them. Frequently, the preservation of important skeletal structures permits quality of life to a degree that is well comparable to an acceptable oncological risk. Nevertheless, the full range of the plastic reconstructive operative armamentarium, including bone flaps, should be evaluated in providing the best outcome for the patient.

Primary osseous sarcomas

Primary osseous sarcomas may be diagnosed relatively accurately by plain radiographic imaging alone. The biopsy techniques are the same as in soft-tissue sarcomas, with the addition of opening up the bone cortex with a round burrhole under X-ray-assisted localization, gaining the biopsy and obtaining wound swabs for bacteria, fungi, and tuberculosis (differential diagnosis) and closing the hole with alloplastic hemostatic material.[29]

Wide surgical resection is also the treatment of choice for primary osseous sarcomas with comparable reconstructive demands later. Sometimes, the biopsy procedure may cause structural instability and external casts, splints, or external fixators are necessary. The method of choice for postresection leg stabilization should at best be determined before biopsy. If external fixators are planned for a definitive skeletal stabilization, the montage may already be applied during biopsy if the diagnosis is verified by a pathognomonic bone X-ray.

Specimen handling

If the resection is completed, the tumor and the tumor bed are photographed and the specimen is removed. It is extremely important to mark the decisive anatomical landmarks clearly and the topographical orientation of the tumor in its previous bed to allow unequivocal and exact determination of margins by the pathologist. Optimally, the examining histopathologist is present at this stage of the procedure. The surgeon has to ensure that any identifying orientation markings on the tumor are not shifted or torn off during transport.

Wound closure

Before wound closure, a meticulous hemostasis and the placement of sufficient closed suction drains are necessary. Skin closure should be done in a multilayered fashion, taking great care to approximate of the wound edges exactly in order to avoid any wound-healing disturbances that might hinder fast implementation of radiation therapy. Primary wound closure is dependent on the size of the tumor and the location in the leg. In the thigh, primary wound closure after wide resections is frequently possible, whereas around the knee and distally from it in the lower leg this is usually not feasible. The tumor resection bed should be narrowed by appropriate muscular and fascial sutures to prevent seroma and hematoma collection in it. Naturally, this usually only applies to tumor locations at the thigh or proximal lower leg.

Any wound closure must aim for a stable skin closure with only minor tension for fast primary wound healing and must avoid stretching of thinned-out, unsupported adipofascial skin flaps over empty wound cavities or bony protuberances. Wound closure must not be a trade-off to the appropriate radicality in tumor resection, especially in the context of modern plastic surgical reconstructive options.

It is often useful to immobilize the operated leg with a splint for postoperative handling, analgesia, and to aid in hemostasis. A sterile circular compressive dressing is placed as well. However, in case of a flap reconstruction, many surgeons defer from using this option because of the fear of compression forces on to the flap or the microvascular pedicle. An interim placement of external fixators is very useful in this context. They easily permit the bedside elevation of the operated extremity, especially in cases with free flaps that may not be dressed with circular bandages in the first postoperative days. External fixators may help in later daily wound care and in safe and fast flap healing, but may also be mounted in the proximal and distal metaphyses when a diaphyseal resection must be performed, or for interim stabilization until a surgical arthroplasty is healed or an orthopedic joint replacement is performed.

Depending on the patient and case profile, an immediate reconstruction may not be possible due to a variety of reasons. Cardiovascular instability, ventilation problems, a large blood loss, or unexpected surgical findings may render a continuation of the operation too dangerous, especially in patients with several comorbidities or advanced biological age. In these cases, temporary vacuum-assisted wound closure may be used until final reconstruction. There is no evidence in the literature that these angiogenesis-promoting subatmospheric-pressure devices have negative effects on oncological safety after a wide resection which was intended to remove all neoplastic tissue, including an appropriate safety margin.[32,33] This is in contrast to the situation after incisional or excisional biopsies where they are not recommended (see above).

Lymph node dissection

Less than 5% of all sarcomas spread in a lymphatic way. Therefore there is no indication for a standardized simultaneous dissection of the relevant lymph node areas (i.e., popliteal fossa/groin) if the region is not clearly involved clinically or radiographically. A lymph node dissection should always be performed, however, in sarcomatous tumor entities that are known for their lymphatic spread, like the rhabdomyosarcoma, angiosarcoma, and epithelioid-like sarcoma subtypes. If regional lymph node metastases are present, a radical lymphadenectomy significantly improves median survival.[13,14]

Indications for amputation

In selected cases, amputation of the leg must be considered the best option for the patient despite very detailed imaging techniques, modern oncological resection strategies, advanced sophisticated plastic reconstructions, and advances in radiologic and chemotherapeutic therapeutic regimens. Primary amputations for treatment of lower extremity sarcomas are necessary in less than 5% of all patients and in less than 15% in recurrences while demonstrating a comparable long-term survival.[2–4]

Amputations are chosen as an adequate primary therapy if significant medical comorbidities prevent the safe completion of a major tumor resection with immediate defect reconstruction. Usually these cases are very rare, and almost always the reconstruction can be deferred to a secondary operation. Modern advances in anesthesiology and intensive care medicine usually allow long procedures to be performed safely. The only exceptions where an immediate reconstruction must be performed are immediate revascularization procedures in cases with extensive main arterial involvement. Extensive lower limb reconstruction procedures also have to be balanced cautiously against amputation in para- or tetraplegic patients or patients with severe cerebral impairment who are bedridden for life.

If the tumor demonstrates transmetatarsal growth, penetrates the interosseus membrane in the lower leg, already shows locoregional dissemination – for example, with rhabdomyosarcomas – or the patient presents with a very large and extensively ulcerated tumor with circular leg involvement, an amputation may be inevitable. Primary multicomponent sarcomas in the proximal thigh may be treated best with an amputation as well as extensive tumor recurrences after all adjuvant or surgical modalities have been exhausted.

Uncontrollable chronic diseases that are not acceptable for major (microvascular) procedures or that render the preservation of the sarcoma-infested extremity useless can make an amputation inevitable. Examples are open ulcers because of chronic venous insufficiency or atherosclerotic occlusive disease in the same leg, an ipsilateral unrelated tumor, or a history of previous trauma with subsequent subclinical osteitis. The latter could reactivate in the context of major surgery or adjuvant therapy.

Furthermore, the predictable inability of reconstructing a stable extremity and/or wounds that are not suitable for safe conservative wound care and patient handling is an indication for amputation if the full reconstructive spectrum has been evaluated for leg salvage and a suitable solution was not found. This might include the unavailability of relevant donor sites for (microvascular) extremity reconstruction.

Lastly, patient preference in favor of amputation is very rare after thorough information about modern reconstructive possibilities but has to be respected in selected cases.

Reconstructive options for lower extremity preservation

Plastic surgical involvement in sarcoma treatment begins during tumor resection. Several examples that demand plastic surgical and microsurgical knowledge during skin incision, tissue dissection, and neurovascular preparation were mentioned above. In general, the plastic surgical reconstruction follows the reconstructive ladder with the lowest rung being the least invasive method (secondary healing) and the highest rung representing customized chimeric multicomponent free flaps. As in many other reconstructive problems, the best option for the individual patient must be chosen regardless of whether it is a more complicated surgery (reconstructive elevator).[34–36]

The following subsections demonstrate the vast diversity of plastic surgical methods, also found elsewhere in this book in detail. For sarcoma reconstruction, the surgeon must keep in mind that pre- or postoperative radiation or previous chemotherapy can spoil his or her success rate, especially in complicated microvascular reconstructions. The use of large recipient vessels outside the radiation field, supple soft-tissue closure, and as little foreign material as possible are proven ways for successful surgery.

Soft tissue

Soft-tissue coverage for sarcoma reconstruction must always be seen in the context of preoperative and adjuvant radiotherapy. The goals are obliteration of dead space, closure of large skin defects with tension-free wound closure, preservation of thin but viable skin edges by supporting them with voluminous muscle flaps, and to cushion exposed bony prominences around the tibia, joints, or amputation stumps.

Local and regional fasciocutaneous flaps are slightly superior to skin-grafted muscle transposition flaps (i.e., medial or lateral gastrocnemius head or peroneus brevis) in terms of fast wound healing and radiation resistance. They may be of limited availability after large tumor resection. Local perforator flaps are very useful for primary reconstructions. However if the area was irradiated, the perforators in the field are less reliable and extremely difficult to dissect due to fibrosis or because they are now very small and fragile. Furthermore, the skin quality and elasticity are inferior for donor site closure in secondary reconstructions with local flaps.

Useful pedicled regional flaps to cover defects in the thigh may be harvested from the deep inferior epigastric artery system of the lower abdomen (i.e., transverse rectus abdominus myocutaneous, vertical rectus abdominus myocutaneous (VRAM), deep inferior epigastric perforator, rectus abdominis muscle) or from the buttock area (superior gluteal artery perforator, inferior gluteal artery perforator). The latter may have a suitable rotation radius if isolated on the respective perforators (Case 4.3).

Microvascular free flaps from all over the body may be used for lower extremity reconstruction and are chosen according to the defect geometry and depth, location, and functional requirements. For secondary reconstructions, recipient vessels are rare or fragile, if the area was irradiated and a preoperative angiogram is warranted. Sensate flaps (i.e., lateral arm flap) should be considered for weight-bearing areas at the foot or on amputation stumps.

Neuromuscular unit

Resected main nerves can be microsurgically reconstructed with multiple cable grafts from the sural nerve or other donor sites according to the cross-section of the recipient nerve. Meticulous technique and the use of an operative microscope are paramount. In selected sarcoma resections, which include bone and nerves, the bone may be restabilized with shortening of the extremity. This scales down the soft-tissue defect, facilitates wound closure, and can make primary nerve coaptation possible.

Depending on the muscular units which have to be resected, muscle or tendon transfers may be performed primarily. Biceps tendon or posterior tibial transfers are the most common transfers in the lower extremity to reconstruct knee extension and foot elevation, respectively (Case 4.1). Tenodeses may preserve muscular power in partially resected

compartments (i.e., adductors) and allow muscular stabilization of joints. Of course, free functional muscle transfers (gracilis, gastrocnemius[37]) are very useful in young patients with high neuroregenerative potential as well.

Skeletal reconstruction

Reconstruction of the skeleton after resection of soft-tissue sarcomas involving bone secondarily and primary osseous sarcomas is the main interdisciplinary field of orthopedic and plastic surgeons. Expandable and nonexpandable tumor prostheses, Van Ness or Borggreve rotationplasty,[38] resection arthroplasties, distraction osteogenesis, segment transport, or total joint replacements commonly belong to orthopedic techniques. However, a combination of the above with pedicled or free vascularized bone may benefit the patient and augment the therapeutic armamentarium. Therefore, this "orthoplastic approach"[39] refers not only to posttraumatic reconstructions but is also a fruitful strategy for oncologic plastic surgery as well.

In selected cases, the variety of traditional techniques like fibula-pro-tibia transfer *(Fig. 4.3)* require microsurgical dissection of the pedicle or an orthopedic osteosynthesis in the metaphyseal area may benefit from additional vascularized bone from a composite flap to augment the construction. Very useful flaps here are the latissimus bone flap and the (para-)

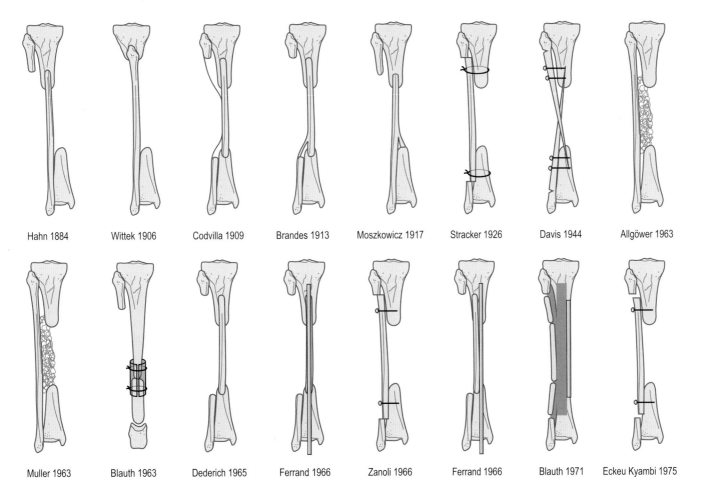

Hahn 1884   Wittek 1906   Codvilla 1909   Brandes 1913   Moszkowicz 1917   Stracker 1926   Davis 1944   Allgöwer 1963

Muller 1963   Blauth 1963   Dederich 1965   Ferrand 1966   Zanoli 1966   Ferrand 1966   Blauth 1971   Eckeu Kyambi 1975

Fig. 4.3 Historical overview of various fibula-pro-tibia techniques for lower leg reconstruction.

scapular bone flap with a lateral and/or medial scapular bone segment of up to 11 × 3 cm that provides coverage or filling of extensive soft-tissue defects or prosthetic material. For smaller defects around the foot, composite flaps like the osteo-fasciocutaneous lateral arm flap are useful.[40]

It is more difficult to reconstruct large defects of the long bones with autologous tissue in the lower than in the upper extremity.[41] This is due to the geometrical and size mismatch of the largest human bone flaps, that is free fibula and vascularized iliac crest based on the deep circumflex iliac artery. However, vascularized bone is a vital, dynamic, growing, infection-resistant and relatively radiation-resistant tissue. The various methods for single and double fibula reconstruction of extensive long bone defects in the lower extremity are discussed elsewhere in this book and apply to sarcoma reconstruction alike (Chapter 7).

In the context of adjuvant radiotherapy, avascular autologous or allogeneic bone grafts, with their high complication rate of fracture, infection, slow integration, and creeping substitution, should be used very carefully and only in selected cases. When using these grafts, special emphasis should be laid on ample vascularization of the surrounding soft-tissue bed and obliteration of any dead spaces around the bone. This optimizes creeping substitution of the avascular allograft and reduces the probability of graft exposure after radiation.

Combination techniques of an avascular structural allograft with a vascularized free fibula inside, described by Capanna,[42] offer promising results, especially for extensive skeletal defects in young tumor patients (Case 4.7).[43] This hotdog-like construct combines optimal vascularization of the vascularized autologous fibula with the structural stability of the geometrically matched allograft "shell." The osteosynthetic stabilization of this construct over the length of a long bone and in metaphyseal areas may be a compromise as the vascular pedicle and vascularization of the inner fibula must be preserved. Burring a trough into the allograft for guiding the peroneal pedicle through the allograft cortex to their recipient vessels has proven quite useful.[43,44]

Vascular surgery

Main arteries that need to be resected together with the tumor should be reconstructed immediately by interpositional vein grafts in the lower leg. Proximal to the knee, autologous vein grafts may be too small and alloplastic material may be considered alternatively for vessel replacement or extra-anatomical bypasses. It is paramount to ensure a good soft-tissue coverage for those materials to prevent exposure, which is easier to achieve in the thigh than in the lower leg.

In selected cases, a temporary arteriovenous loop connected to large-bore vessels proximal to the recipient area offers large-diameter vascular access for microvascular anastomosis distant to any previously scarred or irradiated area. For the proximal thigh and groin area, even the contralateral femoral vessels can be used as recipients for a cross-over graft.[45] If available, autologous vein grafts should be used for vessel reconstruction. In selected cases with tumor-related resection of main arteries, a simultaneous defect coverage and vessel reconstruction can be provided by flow-through flaps (i.e., anterolateral thigh, radial forearm, free fibula).

Due to the high rate of venous graft occlusion for vein reconstruction in oncologic patients, the procedure should be done only in selected cases.[46] One of the reasons for this might be the use of longer vein grafts in oncologic surgery than in trauma patients, who are more prone to thrombosis. Compared to trauma cases, venous outflow compromise by invasive tumor growth occurs slower and the dynamic nature of the lower leg venous system almost always allows the development of sufficient venous collaterals, if the affected deep veins are resected.

Complex approaches

For complex defects, free microvascular composite flaps from the subscapular, external iliac, or lateral circumflex femoral vessel systems provide large, multilobed transplants with a variety of different tissues for simultaneous soft-tissue and skeletal reconstruction. Chimeric flaps further expand this enormous variability (i.e., free fibula with anterolateral thigh flap).

In selected cases, where amputation or segment amputation is inevitable, the distal limb segments are viable and healthy. According to the spare-part principle of plastic surgery, the tissue may be transferred as a composite fillet flap either pedicled or free microvascular on to the amputation site, providing length and suitable tissue quality for coverage. Preservation or coaptation of the contained nerves may achieve a sensate flap of excellent quality and skin texture.

Postoperative care

Immediate postoperative care

A firm concept of postoperative care is very important following biopsies and definitive sarcoma resection and after any reconstructive surgical procedures, for a variety of reasons:

The postoperative protocol after incisional or excisional biopsies is focused on the prevention of hematoma and seroma formation and thereby possible tumor spread. While meticulous hemostasis and drainage placement are paramount, postoperative fluid collections in the resection bed and in tissue planes can be effectively prevented by bed rest, elevation of the affected lower extremity, and immobilization by external fixators or splints. Circular elastic bandaging and compressive dressings are also helpful.

Most reconstructive procedures in sarcoma surgery with larger lesions need defect closure with flaps of some kind. Lower extremities that were reconstructed with local, regional or free flaps need to be positioned in a slightly elevated position for 5–7 days to accommodate the circulation rearrangements in the flap tissue and to prevent early venous congestion in the transplanted tissue. Frequent flap perfusion monitoring is paramount in the first days and ensures immediate intervention if a pedicle thrombosis or hematoma occurs. Patients with neoadjuvant chemotherapy or preoperative intra-arterial perfusion are at high risk for vascular complications in this context.

Following this period of elevation, orthostatic "flap training" can be initiated by lowering the reconstructed extremity for 5 minutes t.i.d. associated with external compression by elastic bandaging. After this, the flap is clinically evaluated and the procedure can be extended in increments of 5–15 minutes daily over the next week until 1 hour is accumulated. This allows reasonable intervals for early gait training and mobilization by stage-adapted physiotherapy.

Compressive bandaging should be replaced by custom-fit compressive garments worn for at least 6 months in all soft-tissue flap reconstructions in the lower extremity except pure osseous flap reconstructions. Usually, garment-wearing is initiated when the sutures are removed and the wound is healed.

Postoperative weight-bearing is a question of the bony resection and reconstruction procedures that were performed, the hardware used for osteosynthesis, and the bone quality. The mobilization schedule should be determined exclusively by the operating surgeon. Serial roentgenograms or CT scans help to determine the bony healing and regained functional stability of the extremity.

Oncologic postoperative care and follow-up

Patients after sarcoma resection with adequate margins and R_0 situation need postoperative adjuvant radiation therapy under most circumstances, especially in tumors which are classified as high-grade (G_2/G_3). Only superficial, low-grade lesions with tumor-free wide margins may be treated with wide resection only. The radiation oncologists start with the therapy according to the appropriate treatment protocol established by the tumor board decision as soon as the wound is healed. If any unexpected oncologically relevant factors occurred during resection or reconstruction (inappropriate or positive margins, vessel invasions, histology), the new findings should be presented in the tumor board as the treatment plan needs to be revised accordingly. This is also true for any late follow-up findings that imply a change in the normal course of healing by emerging local recurrences or distant metastases.

The modalities or patient follow-up after completion of resection and possible adjuvant treatment are not clearly defined in the literature. The following investigations are well accepted in the current literature:

- Thoracic CT scan: distant metastases in lower extremity sarcomas almost exclusively occur through hematogenous spread into the lung with only a few exceptions (see above). It should be repeated every 3 months.
- Contrast-enhanced MRI of the primary tumor site every 3 months: it should always be evaluated by or together with the surgeons. MRI is also the diagnostic method of choice for evaluating lymphatic spread, if applicable. However, MRI criteria of tumor stability or progression may not correlate with the tumor status correctly.
- Serial radiographs of the primary tumor location at least every 6 months if the skeleton was affected by the primary tumor or included in resection or reconstruction. The osteointegration of prosthetic material, bony healing, bone grafts, or transplants is controlled more frequently in the postoperative period anyway. A CT scan should be performed if the information from the plain radiograph is insufficient or suspicious findings occur.
- New imaging techniques evaluating the metabolic activity of tumor material, like PET or PET CT or magnetic resonance spectroscopy (MRS), are promising. While this is a fast-developing field and the numbers of tracers are increasing, these methods are increasingly

accurate in controlling preoperative response to adjuvant therapy and postoperative follow-up. No commonly accepted follow-up schedule exists for sarcomas so far and patients should be integrated into suitable studies.

Secondary procedures

Early secondary procedures – soft tissue

After the initial tumor resection and extremity reconstruction are performed successfully and the wounds are healed, in the majority of cases plastic surgical therapy must continue during or after possible radiotherapy to optimize the overall result.

Despite adequate healing during the primary reconstructive phase, wound-healing disturbances, fistulas, and incision breakdowns may occur during the scheduled radiation cycles. If the initial soft-tissue closure was supple enough, early wound excision and secondary closure may suffice in minor cases. However, larger skin breakdowns may lead to exposure of functional structures like tendons, vessels, nerves, and bones, that need to be covered urgently to prevent radiation-induced osteitis, vessel thrombosis, or tissue necrosis. Local flap solutions are only possible, however, if the appropriate vessels are still intact, as mentioned before.

With the radiation cycles completed, many patients experience fibrosis, scar formation, contractures, and tendon adhesions. Early function-improving procedures include tenolyses, contracture and scar releases, serial excisions or tendon transfers that were not possible or justified primarily. It is often very difficult to evaluate during tumor resection if any remaining musculature or nerves fascicles will suffice for an adequate basic motor function. A typical example for a secondary procedure like this is the posterior tibial tendon transfer for a clinical dropfoot caused by a muscular or neural insufficiency of the peroneal compartment. Neuroma formation or nerve entrapments in irradiated and fibrotic tissue should be approached with desensitization and conservative therapy first but frequently may require early operative neurolyses.

Contour-improving procedures of bulky transferred tissue should be performed not earlier than 6 months to be less independent from the vascular pedicle. They follow standard plastic surgical debulking techniques like direct sequential flap excision, tangential subcutaneous thinning, tangential thinning, and secondary resurfacing with split- or full-thickness skin grafts in muscle flaps or aspiration lipectomy. The same timeframe applies to secondary procedures for forming amputation stumps. However, additive procedures on amputated legs like cushioning and stump-lengthening by local and free flaps or sensitization by transfer of neurotized transplants can be planned earlier than 6 months after the amputation.

Early secondary procedures – skeleton

As mentioned above, skeletal reconstruction and stabilization should be performed as completely as possible during the primary reconstructive stage. Usually, orthopedic prosthetic joint or long bone replacements do not need any secondary surgery if the initial montage demonstrated uneventful osteointegration. Prosthetic replacement is mostly used in primary osseous sarcomas with large skeletal defects after resection. However, infection, mechanical failure, and loosening are among the most common prosthetic complications in the context of radio- and chemotherapy. Major revision surgery is needed then, which is described in the pertinent orthopedic literature.

If plastic surgical reconstruction of the lower limb skeleton was performed by free autologous bone grafts, vascularized bone transplants, avascular allogeneic bone grafts, or combinations of the above, osseous healing is often slow in sarcoma patients, especially if the radiation field encompasses the zone of skeletal reconstruction. Therefore, augmentation of previously inserted bone transplants or revision of pseudarthroses with corticocancellous bone packing is necessary quite often – especially in nonvascularized grafts. At this stage, the osteosynthesis may also be changed to a more stable and definitive method if the primary one has failed.

The microvascular medial femoral condyle corticoperiosteal flap may be a useful tool to provide vascularity and osteogenic potential for recalcitrant pseudarthroses in a previously irradiated field.[47,48]

Sarcoma-related partial joint resections in the weight-bearing lower extremity may be critical. Painless function with an acceptable range of motion must be the reconstructive goal. Especially after partial joint resections or resection arthroplasties, the functional outcome often cannot be adequately assessed until complete mobilization of the patient has taken place. If joint salvage surgery was not successful primarily, resulting in an unstable or painful joint with a severely impaired range of motion, secondary arthroplasties, joint replacement surgery, or arthrodeses may be necessary.

If the limb-preserving surgery consisted of a shortening of the limb, secondary distraction osteogenesis for extremity length adaptation can now be performed with all the soft tissue healed and the radiation therapy completed. However, docking failures are more frequent in irradiated patients. Corticocancellous augmentation is then needed to achieve stability.

Late secondary procedures

The number of patients who are long-term survivors after successful sarcoma therapy in the lower extremity is constantly increasing. A considerable number of them need late secondary reconstructions or surgical corrections of their reconstructed leg. The plastic surgical therapy at this stage aims to correct the sequelae of the previous interdisciplinary plastic surgical, radiological, and orthopedic therapy. Though not life- or limb-saving anymore, these procedures are nevertheless important to help patients complete their personal and social coping after the disease and to improve their quality of life.

Because of functional and aesthetic reasons that began in the early secondary stage, scar releases and flap debulkings frequently need revisions for several years. Irradiation may leave a hard, constrictive, and fibrotic soft-tissue integument behind, which may be painful at rest and in motion or while wearing clothing and shoes. If postirradiation ulcers and unstable scars further deteriorate, the plastic surgeon must be aware of late local recurrences and secondary malignancies in the affected area. Excision of the lesions or the constricted, scarred skin and transfer of unimpaired, healthy tissue by local, regional, or free tissue transfer can improve the patient's quality of life considerably. Of course, any excised tissue from these areas must be evaluated histopathologically.

Peripheral neuropathies are less common after irradiation but more common after chemotherapy and may cause the patient disabling chronic pain. Frequently, the nerve is relatively healthy, but entrapped and fixed by surrounding dense, fibrotic, and irradiated tissue. Adequate therapy consists of careful neurolysis, rerouting, and wrapping of the nerve in well-vascularized tissue by microsurgical methods.

Late secondary procedures after implantation of major hardware, like modular prostheses or total joint replacements, may include hardware exchange due to wear, mechanical failure, or loosening.

Long-term sarcoma survivors with a previous lower limb amputation may experience stump problems like retracted soft tissue with insufficient soft-tissue coverage of the bone, skin folds that impair proper wear of the prosthesis, painful neuromas, and trophic skin changes. Many patients are very experienced with their prosthesis and ask for specific plastic surgical stump corrections. In selected cases, this might include microvascular free flap transfers, preferably with sensate flaps.

Outcomes, prognosis, and complications

Outcomes and prognosis

Several specialized evaluation scores do exist (Musculoskeletal Tumor Society (MSTS),[49] Toronto Extremity Salvage Score (TESS),[50] European Organization for Research and Treatment of Cancer (EORTC) Quality of Life Questionnaire (QLQ)-C30) which rate a various set of subjective and objective parameters of functionality, quality of life, emotional and social factors.[51,52]

Soft-tissue sarcomas

The current age-adjusted death rate for soft-tissue sarcomas is 1.3 per 100 000/year, based on data between 2001 and 2005.[1]

A large recent series from the Memorial Sloan Kettering Cancer Center of 1706 patients with primary and secondary soft-tissue sarcomas of the extremities with a mean follow-up of 55 months demonstrated a 5-year disease-specific actuarial survival of 85% in patients treated between 1997 and 2001. This number did not differ significantly from survival in the previously treated patients from this group. The same was true for the subset of high-risk patients in this group with a 61% 5-year disease-specific actuarial survival in treated cases between 1997 and 2001. This indicates that the prognosis of patients with extremity soft-tissue sarcomas has not changed over the last 20 years. Throughout this period, tumor depth, size, grade, margins, patient age, presentation status, location (proximal versus distal) and certain histopathologic subtypes remained significant prognostic factors (*Table 4.5*).[1]

Steinau *et al.*[3] report about 85 soft-tissue sarcomas in the lower extremity among 744 sarcoma patients between 1980

Table 4.5 Prognostic factors in soft-tissue sarcoma therapy

Factor	Distant recurrence-free survival	Local recurrence-free survival	Relapse-free survival	Disease-specific survival
Age >50 years	–	–	–	–
Recurrent sarcoma	–	–	–	–
Size >5 cm	–	–	–	–
Deep location	–			–
High-grade	–		–	–
Proximal position				–
Histology				
Fibrosarcoma		–		
Leiomyosarcoma	–		–	–
Positive microscopic margin	–	–		–
Time period of treatment				

Minus symbols indicate an independent adverse prognostic factor, and blank fields indicate a nonindependent prognostic factor.
(Adapted from Weitz J, Antonescu CR, Brennan MF. Localized extremity soft tissue sarcoma: improved knowledge with unchanged survival over time. J Clin Oncol 2003;21:2719–2725.)

and 1996. Mean age at presentation was 42.9 years (range 6–80 years), with 38 patients being previously operated elsewhere. Eighteen patients had 2–9 recurrences. Still, in 81 patients (95.3%) an R_0 resection with curative intention could be performed, whereas 4 patients underwent a palliative resection due to multilocular distant metastases. In 41/81 patients extensive tissue defects resulted after the resection and 17 local and 24 free flaps were needed for closure. Thirteen patients received a simultaneous tendon transfer with defect closure to improve their gait. In 18 patients with local skeletal infiltration, special plastic surgical bone reconstructions, conventional partial-foot amputations, or atypical hindfoot amputations were done. All of those patients received individualized orthopedic shoe and inlay adaptation and finally achieved a better gait both with and without these shoes and during sports activities than with comparable lower leg prostheses. In 2 patients, a transtibial amputation was inevitable. In this group of 85 patients, a mean survival of 132 months and a 5-year survival rate of 62% were found.[3]

The Finnish experience with 73 patients with lower limb soft-tissue sarcomas who received limb salvage surgery reports a 5-year local recurrence-free survival of 82%, a metastasis-free survival of 59%, a disease-free survival of 56%, and a disease-specific overall survival of 70% over a follow-up time of 65.9 months. Three-quarters of patients were able to walk normally or had only minor walking impairment. The authors emphasize that microsurgery is an essential part of modern tumor surgery.[53] Long-term survivors have a higher probability of experiencing both sequelae of their primary plastic surgical treatment (i.e., contractures, bulky flaps, unstable scars) and secondary malignomas (i.e., postradiation angiosarcomas).

A large study from an interdisciplinary sarcoma center in Germany had a mean follow-up of 36 months in 167 patients with extremity liposarcomas. Over this time, only 5 (3%) of the patients had to undergo amputation throughout this period. A clear margin R_0 resection could be achieved in 158 patients. The authors report an overall 79% 5-year survival,

though the study collective was biased in favor of extensive and previously operated cases due to the reference center status of the clinic. Patients with primary tumors had 90% 5-year survival and an overall number of 37 local recurrences was found. The myxoid liposarcoma was responsible for most recurrences. Patients with recurrent tumors had 69% 5-year survival.[30]

Bone sarcomas

The European Osteosarcoma Intergroup reports a 57% 5-year survival in a patient group of 202 patients with a 49–85% limb salvage rate. An important finding of this study was that patients having undergone limb salvage surgery with later local recurrence had a slightly better survival than primarily amputated patients (37% versus 31% at 5 years).[11,12] Marulanda et al. stated that for osteosarcoma patients there is no difference in survival between amputations and properly performed limb-salvaging procedures.[54]

Carty et al. reported their results after limb-sparing surgery of 20 intra-articular knee osteosarcoma patients and their reconstruction with endoprostheses. Evaluated with the MSTS and TESS scores, moderate to high function was achieved.[52]

A Norwegian study involving 118 patients with osteosarcomas or Ewing's sarcoma in the extremities evaluated the long-term functional outcome a minimum of 5 years after treatment. The function was evaluated with MSTS and TESS scores, while quality of life was assessed using the Short Form-36 (SF-36). The mean age at follow-up was 31 years (15–57 years) and the mean follow-up was for 13 years (6–22 years). A total of 67 patients (57%) initially had limb-sparing surgery, but four had a secondary amputation. The median MSTS score was 70% (17–100%) and the median TESS was 89% (43–100%). The amputees had a significantly lower MSTS score than those with limb-sparing surgery ($P < 0.001$), but there was no difference for the TESS. Tumor localization above knee level resulted in significantly lower MSTS and TESS scores. There were no significant differences in quality of life between amputees and those with limb-sparing surgery except in physical functioning. In multivariate analysis, amputation, tumor location above the knee and having muscular pain were associated with low physical function. Most of the bone tumor survivors managed well after adjustment to their physical limitations. A total of 105 patients were able to work and had an overall good quality of life.[55]

Complications – management of recurrent disease

If local tumor recurrences are present, they are usually found quite early if the patient is compliant with his or her follow-up protocol. In many cases, this implies a heavy psychological burden for the patient and careful and empathic communication and conjoint treatment planning are very important.

The surgical procedures in local recurrences do not differ in general from the initial tumor resection. However, previous surgery, flap transplantation with microvascular pedicles in a scarred and sometimes irradiated field, extra-anatomical nerve and vessel grafts do make the resection much more difficult this time. Even then, a local recurrent tumor

manifestation does not necessarily mean amputation. If local sarcoma recurrences can be re-excised and treated surgically, about two-thirds of patients have a long-term survival benefit.

Depending on the previous protocol and overall radiation dose, secondary radiation therapy (brachytherapy) after resection of local recurrences should be evaluated together with the oncologic radiation specialist.

Case 4.1

A 35-year-old male presented with a growing tumor and painless swelling in his right quadriceps muscle. The patient referred this to a blunt trauma while playing soccer 6 months ago. Ultrasound and contrast-enhanced MRI demonstrated a large intramuscular tumor suspicious for a liposarcoma *(Fig. 4.4A and B)*. Histology was verified with incision biopsy. Staging with abdominal and thoracic CT scan showed no distant metastases. The treatment protocol was discussed in the local tumor board and wide excision of the tumor was performed *(Fig. 4.4C)*. As four-fifths of the quadriceps muscle had to be resected *(Fig. 4.4D)*, a free functional musculocutaneous latissimus dorsi flap was

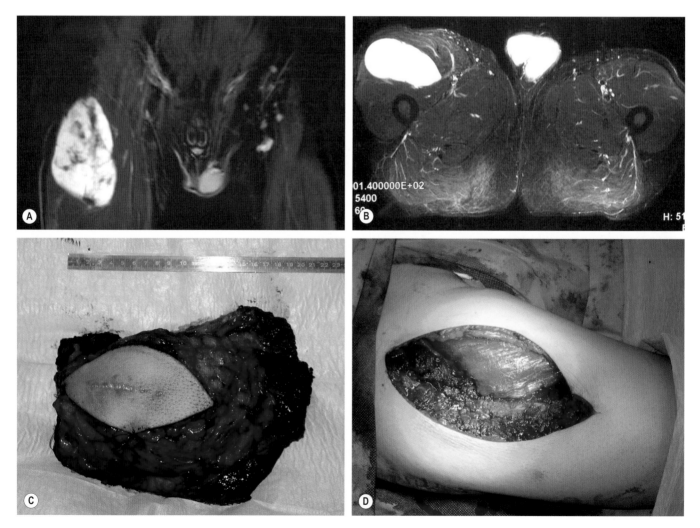

Fig. 4.4 (A, B) Contrast-enhanced magnetic resonance imaging demonstrating a large intramuscular tumor suspicious for a liposarcoma. **(C)** Tumor specimen after wide excision, including the incision biopsy scar. **(D)** The quadriceps muscle had to be resected subtotally.

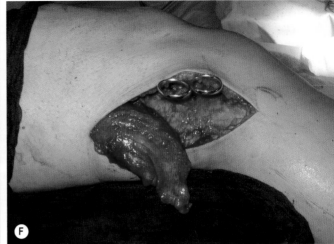

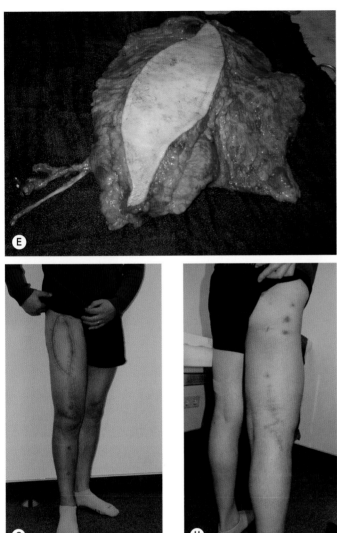

Fig. 4.4, cont'd (E) This free functional musculocutaneous latissimus dorsi flap was harvested and revascularized to local vessels. Nerve coaptation was done to a branch of the femoral nerve close to the groin that could be spared from the resection. **(F)** To assist leg function this pedicled biceps femoris flap was rerouted around the distal lateral femur and woven into the new latissimus–quadriceps–tendon extensor apparatus. **(G, H)** Clinical result 3 months after resection.

harvested *(Fig. 4.4E)* and connected to local vessels. Nerve coaptation was done to a branch of the femoral nerve close to the groin that could be spared from the resection. The muscle transplant was fixed at the anterior superior iliac spine and the remaining vastus medialis head and its tendon were woven into the quadriceps tendon and fixed securely with 1-0 nonresorbable sutures. To assist leg function until the latissimus muscle was reinnervated, we simultaneously also transferred a functional biceps femoris flap through a separate posterior incision *(Fig. 4.4F)* around the distal lateral femur and sutured it into the new latissimus–quadriceps–tendon extensor apparatus with an adequate pretension. The muscle bulk of the latissimus easily obliterated the space of the resected quadriceps muscle, while the skin island served for tension-free closure of the integument. For protection of the tendomuscular reconstructions, an external fixator across the knee was applied for 6 weeks. Healing was uneventful; the pathology showed clear and adequate margins (R_0). The fixator was removed in an outpatient procedure and physiotherapy began. Three months after the resection and simultaneous reconstruction procedure the patient showed an almost completely normal gait *(Fig. 4.4G, H)*.

Case 4.2

This 48-year-old male patient was referred to us with a horizontal (nononcological) incision of the right anterior lower leg *(Fig. 4.5A, B)* after a nononcological resection of a malignant fibrous histiocytoma, leaving positive margins (R_1) elsewhere. Reoperation with a wide excision (9×8 cm; *Fig. 4.5C, D*) was performed in our center and the defect closed with a pedicled medial gastrocnemius muscle flap *(Fig. 4.5E, F)* and split-thickness skin graft from the ipsilateral thigh. Histology now showed adequately wide and clear margins of this R_0 resection. Further healing was uneventful. Figure 4.5G–I demonstrate follow-up result at 3 months after flap transposition and defect closure.

Case 4.3

This 56-year-old male patient demonstrated a large intramuscular tumor highly suspicious of a soft-tissue sarcoma in the proximal left thigh close to the groin. His clinical complaints were swelling and pain for 6 months. MRI demonstrated close proximity to the superficial femoral vessels; however, the femoral nerve could not be identified on the MRI *(Fig. 4.6A, B)*. The incisional biopsy showed

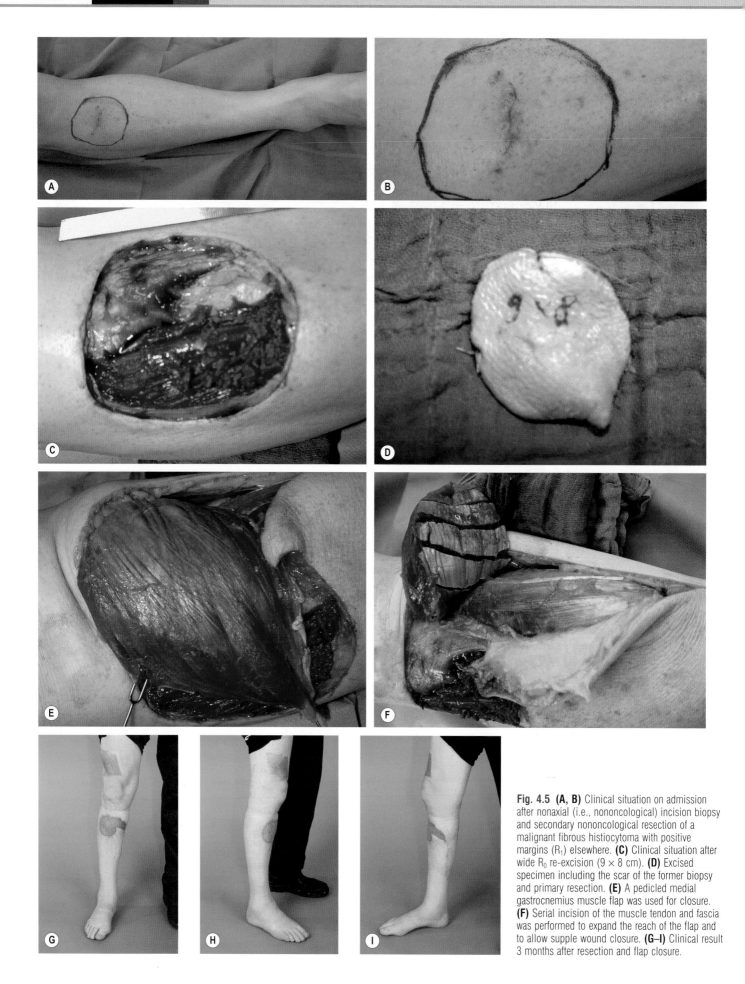

Fig. 4.5 (A, B) Clinical situation on admission after nonaxial (i.e., nononcological) incision biopsy and secondary nononcological resection of a malignant fibrous histiocytoma with positive margins (R_1) elsewhere. **(C)** Clinical situation after wide R_0 re-excision (9×8 cm). **(D)** Excised specimen including the scar of the former biopsy and primary resection. **(E)** A pedicled medial gastrocnemius muscle flap was used for closure. **(F)** Serial incision of the muscle tendon and fascia was performed to expand the reach of the flap and to allow supple wound closure. **(G–I)** Clinical result 3 months after resection and flap closure.

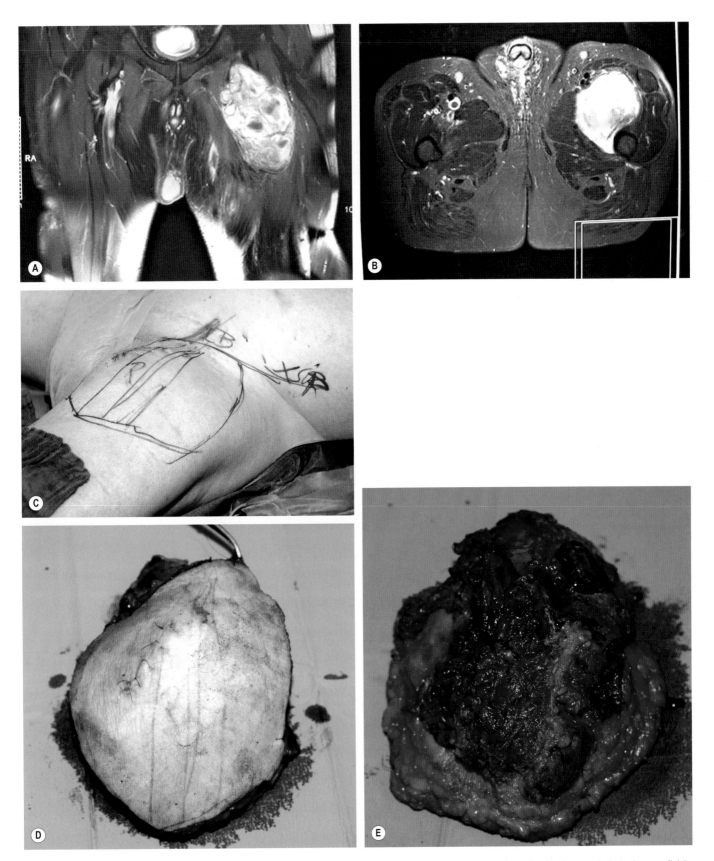

Fig. 4.6 (A, B) Large intramuscular tumor highly suspicious of a soft-tissue sarcoma in the proximal left thigh close to the groin with close proximity to the superficial femoral vessels; however, the femoral nerve could not be identified in the magnetic resonance imaging. **(C)** After the incisional biopsy, wide resection including most of the extensor muscles was planned. **(D, E)** Resection specimen 23 × 18 × 20 cm including the tumor.

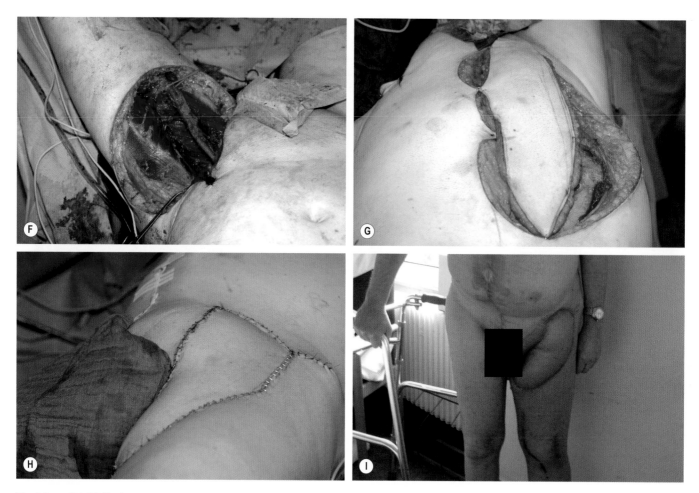

Fig. 4.6, cont'd (F) The femoral nerve was encased by tumor tissue and had to be resected according to oncologic principles. **(G)** A contralateral pedicled vertical musculocutaneous rectus abdominis muscle flap (30 × 18 cm) was harvested. **(H)** Flap closure of the defect. **(I)** Clinical picture 2 years after surgery.

a highly malignant synovial cell sarcoma (G₃). After preoperative planning in the tumor board, a wide resection including most of the extensor muscles *(Fig. 4.6C)* was performed according to oncological guidelines, yielding a 23 × 18 × 20 cm tissue specimen including the tumor *(Fig. 4.6D–F)*. The femoral nerve was encased by tumor tissue and had to be resected according to oncologic principles. From the contralateral abdomen, a pedicled VRAM flap (30 × 18 cm) was harvested and transferred into the defect *(Fig. 4.6G, H)*. Additionally, the biceps femoris as well as the semitendinosus muscles were transferred to the remnants of the patellar tendon to reconstruct knee extension. The postoperative course was uneventful, with the exception of a small wound dehiscence applicable for conservative local wound care at the midabdomen flap harvest site. The patient underwent radiation therapy as well as chemotherapy due to metastases in the lung. Two years postsurgery the patient was able to extend his leg and had no recurrence of the tumor or the metastases in the lung *(Fig. 4.6I)*.

Case 4.4

A 6 × 7 × 5 cm painless mass was detected in the right calf of this 31-year-old male patient. Contrast-enhanced MRI showed a lesion highly suspicious for a soft-tissue sarcoma. This diagnosis was confirmed by a longitudinal incision

biopsy according to oncologic guidelines and definitive tumor resection was planned *(Fig. 4.7A)*. The tumor resection was performed according to international standards for wide excision, leaving a cuff of tissue surrounding the tumor of at least 2 cm deep and at least 4 cm to the sides *(Fig. 4.7B, C)*. As the posterior tibial vessels and the tibial nerve were encased by the tumor, they had to be resected as well *(Fig. 4.7D)*. The tibial nerve was immediately reconstructed microsurgically by a free sural nerve harvested from the contralateral side *(Fig. 4.7E, F)*. The sural nerve was doubled as a cable graft to allow cross-sectional matching to the tibial nerve and was set in 180° to improve neurotization. The resection defect was controlled for a perfect hemostasis and drains were placed. As the tumor provided a "tissue expansion-like" stretching of the calf, the wound could easily be closed primarily without having relevant dead spaces or skin "tenting" over unsupported wound cavities *(Fig. 4.7G)*. Further follow-up showed uneventful healing and recurrence of sensation at the plantar side of the foot after 2-year follow-up.

Case 4.5

A 70-year-old female complained of a painless mass in the lower extremity *(Fig. 4.8A)*. The preoperative MRI showed a tumor in the posterior and lateral compartment which also

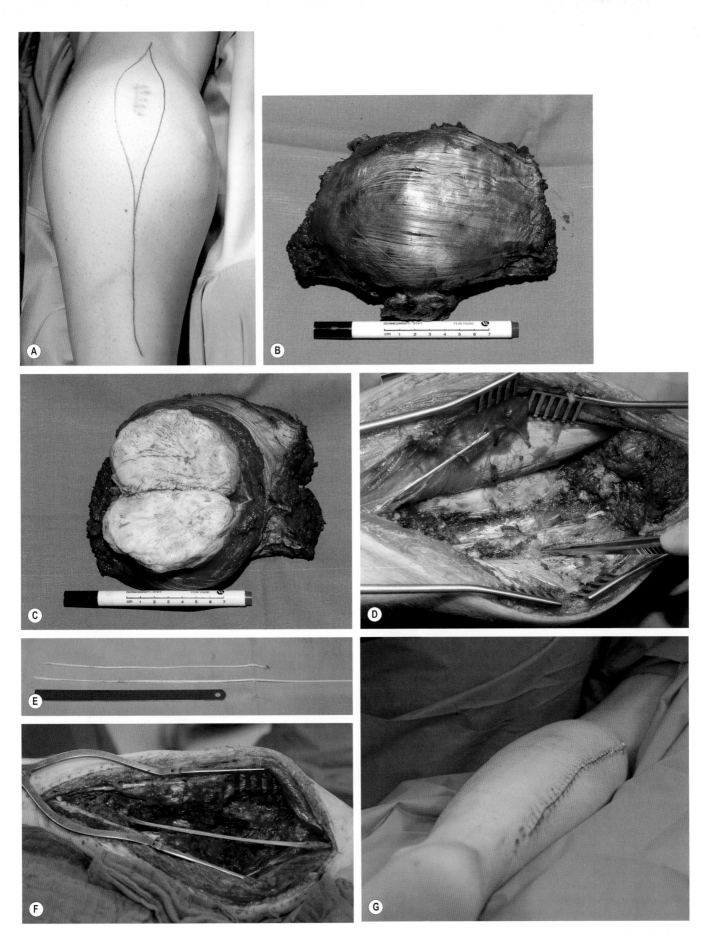

Fig. 4.7 **(A)** A 6 × 7 × 5 cm painless mass in the right calf suspicious for a soft-tissue sarcoma. A longitudinal incision biopsy according to oncologic guidelines and the definitive tumor resection were planned. **(B, C)** The tumor resection was performed according to international standards for wide excision, leaving a cuff of tissue surrounding the tumor of at least 2 cm deep and at least 4 cm to the sides. **(D)** Posterior tibial vessels and tibial nerve were encased and had to be resected as well. **(E, F)** The tibial nerve was immediately reconstructed microsurgically by a free sural nerve harvested from the contralateral side. The sural nerve was doubled as a cable graft to allow cross-sectional matching to the tibial nerve and was set in 180° to improve neurotization. **(G)** Postoperative view after primary closure without having relevant dead spaces or skin "tenting" over unsupported wound cavities.

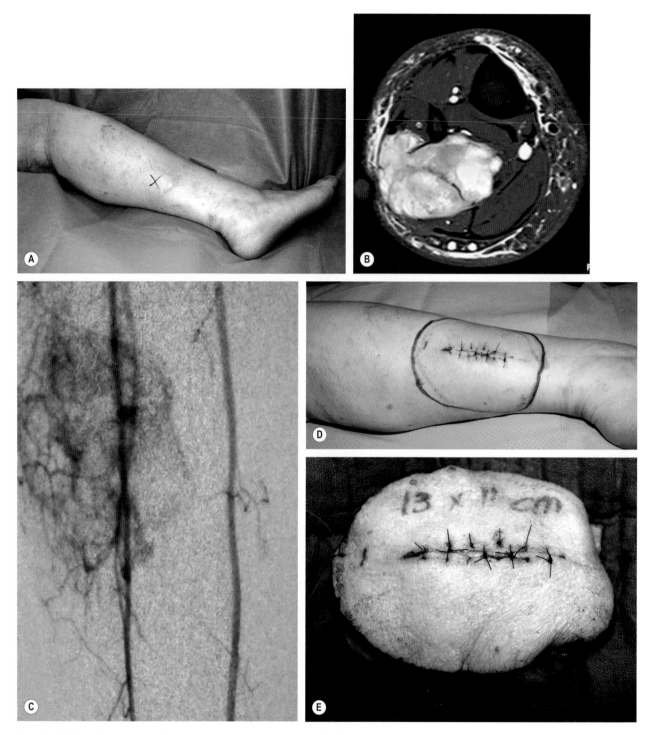

Fig. 4.8 (A) Clinical picture of a painless mass in the right lower extremity. **(B)** Preoperative magnetic resonance imaging showing a tumor in the posterior and lateral compartment also affecting the fibula. **(C)** Preoperative angiogram demonstrating a well-vascularized tumor including the peroneal vessels. **(D)** After an incisional biopsy, which demonstrated a liposarcoma G$_2$, the planned resection was outlined. **(E)** En bloc resected, 13 × 11-cm large specimen including a fibula segment.

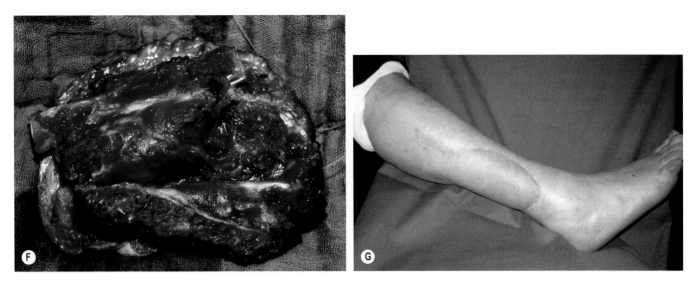

Fig. 4.8, cont'd (F) The tumor was not seen during surgery and covered well with muscle according to adequate tumor margins. **(G)** Clinical picture 2 years after free parascapular flap closure.

affected the fibula *(Fig. 4.8B)*. Due to the overall age and the amount of resection, which included the peroneal vessels, a preoperative angiogram was done demonstrating a well-vascularized tumor as well as appropriate vessels for a free tissue transplantation and limb perfusion (posterior tibial vessels: *Fig. 4.8C*). After an incisional biopsy, which demonstrated a liposarcoma G$_2$, the planned resection was outlined *(Fig. 4.8D)* and a 13 × 11 cm specimen resected en bloc including a fibular segment *(Fig. 4.8E, F)*. The defect was closed with a free fasciocutaneous parascapular flap and radiation therapy was initiated. Two years later, the patient was doing well without any metastases or local tumor recurrence *(Fig. 4.8G)*.

Case 4.6

Figure 4.9A shows the foot of a 51-year-old-female with a mass 5 × 5 cm at the dorsum of the right foot. Diagnostic MRI demonstrated a tumor which encased the extensor tendons of the first ray *(Fig. 4.9B)*. The incisional biopsy *(Fig. 4.9C)* confirmed a malignant fibrous histiocytoma (G$_2$). A wide excision, including the extensor tendons of the first ray, the dorsal half of the first and second metatarsal bone, as well as the capsule of the metatarsophalangeal joint 1, was performed *(Fig. 4.9D)*. Due to resulting instability of this joint of the first ray, an immediate arthrodesis was carried out and the defect covered with a free anterolateral thigh

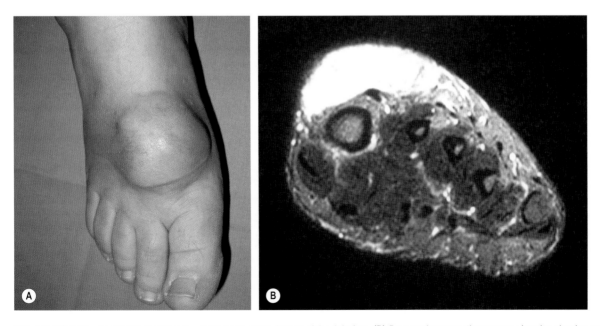

Fig. 4.9 (A) A 51-year-old-female with a 5 × 5 cm mass at the dorsum of the right foot. **(B)** Preoperative magnetic resonance imaging showing encasement of the extensor tendons of the first ray.

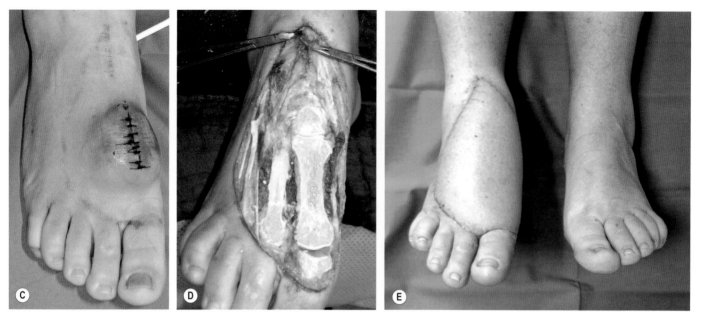

Fig. 4.9, cont'd (C) Clinical picture after incisional biopsy. **(D)** Clinical picture after wide excision including the extensor tendons of the first ray, the dorsal half of the first and second metatarsal bone as well as the capsule of the metatarsophalangeal joint 1. **(E)** One year after the operation and radiation.

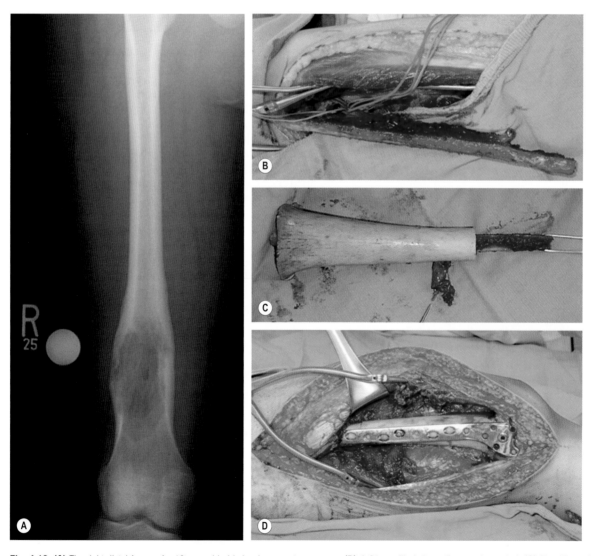

Fig. 4.10 (A) The right distal femur of a 12-year-old girl showing an osteosarcoma. **(B)** A 21-cm fibula bone flap was harvested. **(C)** The 15-cm long intercalary allograft and a vascularized fibula bone flap placed into the medullary canal of the allograft. **(D)** Fixation of the allograft with a 12-hole lateral locking plate. (Courtesy of Dr. David W. Chang, Department for Plastic Surgery, MD Anderson Cancer Center, Houston, TX.)

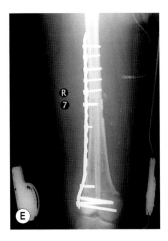
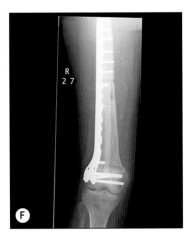
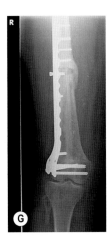

Fig. 4.10, cont'd (E) Postoperative radiograph. Proximally, 4 cm of vascularized fibula bone flap was inserted into the host femur diaphysis and distally, 2 cm of fibula flap was inserted into the host femur metaphysis. **(F)** Radiograph 5 months later, showing a small amount of callus formation and remodeling at the proximal and distal allograft–host junctions. **(G)** Radiograph after 11 months before progression to full weight-bearing.

perforator flap. One year after the operation and radiation therapy the patient was tumor-free and able to walk and exercise *(Fig. 4.9E)*.

Case 4.7

The patient was a 12-year-old girl with an osteosarcoma of the right distal femur *(Fig. 4.10A)*. She received four cycles of neoadjuvant chemotherapy consisting of doxorubicin and intra-arterial cisplatin. A total segment of 15 cm was then resected from the femur, with the distal transepiphyseal cut 3 cm proximal to the lateral joint line of the knee. A 21-cm fibula bone flap was harvested *(Fig. 4.10B)*. The bone defect was repaired with an intercalary allograft and a vascularized fibula bone flap placed into the medullary canal of the allograft *(Fig. 4.10C)*. The vascular pedicle of the fibula flap was brought out through a side hole burred into the allograft. The allograft was fixed to the native bone with a

12-hole lateral locking plate *(Fig. 4.10D)*. Proximally, 4 cm of vascularized fibula bone flap was inserted into the host femur, and distally, 2 cm of fibula flap was inserted into the host femur *(Fig. 4.10E)*. Microvascular anastomoses were performed end-to-end to branches of the femoral artery and vein.

Postoperatively, the patient received two additional cycles of chemotherapy. At 2 months, radiographs showed signs of healing with no complications, and touch weight-bearing was started. At 5 months, radiographs showed a small amount of callus formation and remodeling at the proximal and distal allograft-host junctions *(Fig. 4.10F)*. The patient was allowed partial weight-bearing on the leg with a limit of 10–20 lb (4.5–9 kg). Six months later, the patient progressed to full weight-bearing, with the restrictions of no running and no sports activity until full radiographic union *(Fig. 4.10G)*. (Case courtesy of David W Chang, MD, MD Anderson Cancer Center, Houston, TX.[43])

Access the complete references list online at http://www.expertconsult.com

1. Weitz J, Antonescu CR, Brennan MF. Localized extremity soft tissue sarcoma: improved knowledge with unchanged survival over time. *J Clin Oncol.* 2003;21:2719–2725.

   This comprehensive single institution overview analyses the risk factors of soft-tissue sarcoma treatment in 1261 patients.

3. Steinau HU, Homann HH, Drucke D, et al. [Resection method and functional restoration in soft tissue sarcomas of the extremities.] *Chirurg.* 2001;72:501–513.

6. Enzinger FM, Weiss SW. *Soft Tissue Tumors.* 3rd ed. St. Louis: Mosby; 1995.

   This comprehensive textbook still provides the basics of tumor biology and describes the vast majority of the soft-tissue tumors in great detail.

12. Grimer RJ, Taminiau AM, Cannon SR. Surgical outcomes in osteosarcoma. *J Bone Joint Surg Br.* 2002;84:395–400.

   This paper describes the outcomes of 202 patients treated in three different tumor centers of the European Osteosarcoma Intergoup. A very detailed paper which provides a comprehensive view of current osteosarcoma prognosis.

13. Fong Y, Coit DG, Woodruff JM, et al. Lymph node metastasis from soft tissue sarcoma in adults. Analysis of data from a prospective database of 1772 sarcoma patients. *Ann Surg.* 1993;217:72–77.

   This paper examines the natural history of lymph node metastasis in sarcomas and the utility of therapeutic lymphadenectomy in various tumor types. The data are based on a prospective sarcoma database including 1772 patients.

24. Tunn PU, Kettelhack C, Durr HR. Standardized approach to the treatment of adult soft tissue sarcoma of the extremities. *Recent Results Cancer Res.* 2009;179: 211–228.

26. Abraham JA, Baldini EH, Butrynski JE. Management of adult soft-tissue sarcoma of the extremities and trunk. *Expert Rev Anticancer Ther.* 2010;10:233–248.

   This recent paper summarizes the current treatment strategy in soft-tissue sarcomas seen from a single institution viewpoint but with a current and extensive reference list. It is more therapeutically oriented and serves well as an addendum and update to reference 3 above.

42. Capanna R, Campanacci DA, Belot N, et al. A new reconstructive technique for intercalary defects of long bones: the association of massive allograft with vascularized fibular autograft. Long-term results and comparison with alternative techniques. *Orthop Clin North Am.* 2007;38:51–60, vi.

46. Mahendra A, Gortzak Y, Ferguson PC, et al. Management of vascular involvement in extremity soft tissue sarcoma. *Recent Results Cancer Res.* 2009;179: 285–299.

53. Barner-Rasmussen I, Popov P, Bohling T, et al. Microvascular reconstruction after resection of soft tissue sarcoma of the leg. *Br J Surg.* 2009;96:482–489.

5

Reconstructive surgery: Lower extremity coverage

Joon Pio Hong

SYNOPSIS

- The reconstructive surgery for the lower extremity have evolved from a staged approach to proving best solutions for functional and cosmetic outcome.
- This chapter covers the classical approach with a gradual change of principle that advocates an one stage elevator approach.
- Special considerations should be given to overcome the complexity of lower extremity reconstruction, such as diabetes and chronic infection.
- Finally, introduction of perforator flaps, the use of multiple flaps by combination, and supermicrosurgery will help you design and widen the reconstructive choice for the lower extremity.

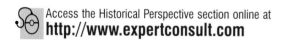

Access the Historical Perspective section online at
http://www.expertconsult.com

Introduction

Lower extremity reconstruction following severe trauma, cancer ablation and chronic infections remains to be challenging. The involvement of multiple structures from bone, muscle, vessel, nerve to skin makes it difficult to achieve the goals of lower extremity reconstruction where restoration of limb function, coverage for vital structures and satisfactory appearance is achieved.

In the recent years, the management of lower extremity has evolved with numerous new techniques and innovations and thus extremities are salvaged as to being amputated in the past. Introduction of vascularized bone grafting, Ilizarov lengthening, bone matrix, and growth factors to manage the bone defects along with new ideas for coverage like perforator flaps, propeller flaps, negative pressure therapy and increased knowledge for anatomy has led to successful management of lower extremity soft tissue and bone defects. If the extremity cannot be salvaged, the next goal would be to maintain

maximal functional length with good soft tissue coverage on the stump to bear the prosthesis for functional gait.

Extremity salvage is a long and complex process for the medical professionals as well as patients. Patients and family members must be educated and be included in the decision-making process and made aware of expected prognosis. Patient's motivation and compliance along with family's support will be critical during physical and psychological recovery.

Although early amputation and prosthetic treatment was thought to offer the potential of faster recovery and lower cost, recently reports have provided different views. A multi-center, prospective, observational study to determine the functional outcome of 569 patients with severe leg injuries resulting in reconstruction or amputation has provided information based on Sickness Impact Profile, a measure of self-reported health status.[1] Although reconstruction may be faced with more challenging process, the Lower Extremity Assessment Project, or LEAP study showed no significant difference in outcome at 2 years. Costs following amputation and salvage were also derived from data in a study that emerged from the Lower Extremity Assessment Project concluding that amputation is more expensive than salvage and amputation yields fewer life quality-adjusted life-years than salvage.[2] Other reports have shown similar findings where projected lifetime healthcare cost for amputation may be as high as three times.[3,4]

Treatment of salvage evolves as with the coverage strategy. But still this process can be long and complicated. Despite that normal function and appearance can be difficult to achieve, it may be warranted to support successful reconstruction leading to successful salvage of the extremity.

Principles

The primary goal of surgical reconstruction of the lower extremity wound is to restore or maintain function. Function is addressed through a well vascularized extremity, skeletal structure able to support gait and weight-bearing and innervated plantar surface to provide protective sensation. Without proper function, the value of reconstruction will be reduced significantly increasing emotional and financial burden to the patient.

An evaluation of the patient as a whole allows proper decisions to be made within regards to systemic conditions, socioeconomic status, and rehabilitative potential. Extremity injuries are best approached by teams of surgeons with knowledge of skeletal, vascular, neurologic and soft tissue anatomy. Although evaluations such as Mangled Extremity Severity Score (MESS), the Predictive Salvage Index, and the Limb Salvage Index can assist the team in making a decision for amputation, it must not be used as a sole criterion and the decision to amputate must be individualized for each patient.[19,25–28]

The value of autologous tissue

Whether acute or chronic, evaluation of lower extremity wounds and the eligibility for soft tissue reconstruction begins with vascular status evaluation. If clinical and diagnostic examination reveals inadequate perfusion and the value of reconstruction minimal, amputation should be individually decided. An amputated or avulsed tissue should never be disregarded, especially in acute traumas, unless severely contaminated or lacks vascular structure. Nothing can mimic the superiority of an autologous tissue and all tissues from amputated parts should be considered as potential donor tissues for reconstruction. The skin harvested from the degloved or amputated part can be utilized as biologic dressings to permanent skin grafts *(Fig. 5.1)*.[29] The leg length can be preserved using soft tissue distal form the zone of injury as fillet pedicled or free flaps.[30–33] Amputated bones can be banked or used as a flap to reconstruct the leg.[34,35]

The reconstructive elevator

Once the wound is evaluated to have good vascular supply, stable skeletal structures and a relatively clean wound, soft tissue coverage is then considered. The concept of reconstructive ladder was proposed to achieve wounds with adequate closure using a stepladder approach from simple to complex procedures *(Fig. 5.2A)*. Although still valued and widely taught, the reconstructive ladder comes from the concept of wound-closure ladder dating back beyond the era of modern reconstructive surgery.[36] In the era of modern reconstructive surgery, one must consider not only adequate closures but form and function. A skin graft after mastectomy can still provide coverage but a pedicled TRAM (Transverse Rectus Abdominis muscle) flap will provide superior results in addition to coverage. Now with introduction of DIEP (Deep Inferior Epigastric Perforator) flaps, the reconstructive ladder approach seems to show more flaws. Other techniques including tissue expansion, skin stretching and vacuum-assisted closure has made new changes in approaching reconstructive options. A simpler reconstructive option may not necessarily produce optimal results. This is especially true for lower extremity coverage, where consequences of inadequate coverage will lead to complications such as additional soft tissue

loss, osteomyelitis, functional loss, increased medical cost and even amputation. Thus to provide optimal form and function, we jump up and down the rungs of the ladder. The reconstructive elevator requires creative thoughts and considerations of multiple variables to achieve the best form and function rather than a sequential climb up the ladder *(Fig. 5.2B)*. This paradigm of thought does not eliminate the concept of reconstructive ladder but replaces it as a ladder of wound closure and makes its mark in the field where variety of advanced reconstructive procedures and techniques are not readily available. Based on the reconstructive elevator, method of reconstruction should be chosen based on procedures that results in optimal function as well as appearance.

Skin grafts and substitutes

Autologous skin grafts are used in variety of clinical situations. It can be full or partial thickness and requires a recipient bed that is well vascularized and free of bacterial contamination. The split-thickness grafts are usually used as the first line of treatment where wounds cannot be closed primarily or undue tension is suspected. In the extremity often with complex wounds; bone exposure and/or avascular beds, infected wounds, wound with dead space and poorly coagulated beds, skin grafts should be avoid. Autologous cultured keratinocytes can be used where split-thickness donor sites are limited. However, the use of cultured epithelial autograft has been hampered by reports that show it to be more susceptible to bacterial contamination, has a variable take rate, and is costly.[37]

A skin substitute is defined as a naturally occurring or synthetic bioengineered product that is used to replace the skin in a temporary, semi-permanent or permanent fashion.[38] Temporary epidermal replacements may be beneficial in superficial to mid-dermal depth wounds. In deeper wounds, dermal replacements are of primary importance. Bioengineered products for superficial wounds are porcine products such as EZ-derm and Mediskin (Brennen Medical-LLC, St Paul, MN), which helps to close the wound, decrease pain and improve rate of healing.[38] Biobrane (UDL Laboratories Inc, Rockford, Illinois) is a bilaminate skin substitute that is used temporarily. The outer layer is formed with thin silicone payer with pores that allow removal of exudates and penetration of antibiotics. The inner layer is composed of three dimensional nylon filament weave impregnated with type I collagen to adhere to the wound. Bioengineered products that are used for deep wounds are Allograft, Alloderm (Life Cell Corporation, Woodlans, TX), Integra (Integra Life Sciences, Plainsboro, NJ), and Apligraf (Organogenesis Inc, Canton, MA). The gold standard for temporary skin coverage is cadaver skin or allograft. Allograft is used to cover extensive partial- and full-thickness wounds. It prevents tissue dessication, decreases pain, insensible loss of water, electrolytes and protein, suppress the proliferation of bacteria, and decreases the hypermetabolic component of thermal injuries.[39,40] Alloderm is an acellular dermal matrix engineered from banked, human cadaver skin. It can also provide single stage reconstruction when used with a split-thickness skin graft.[41] Alloderm is known to improve functional and cosmetic results in deep burn wounds *(Fig. 5.3)*.[42] Integra is an acellular collagen matrix composed of type I bovine collagen

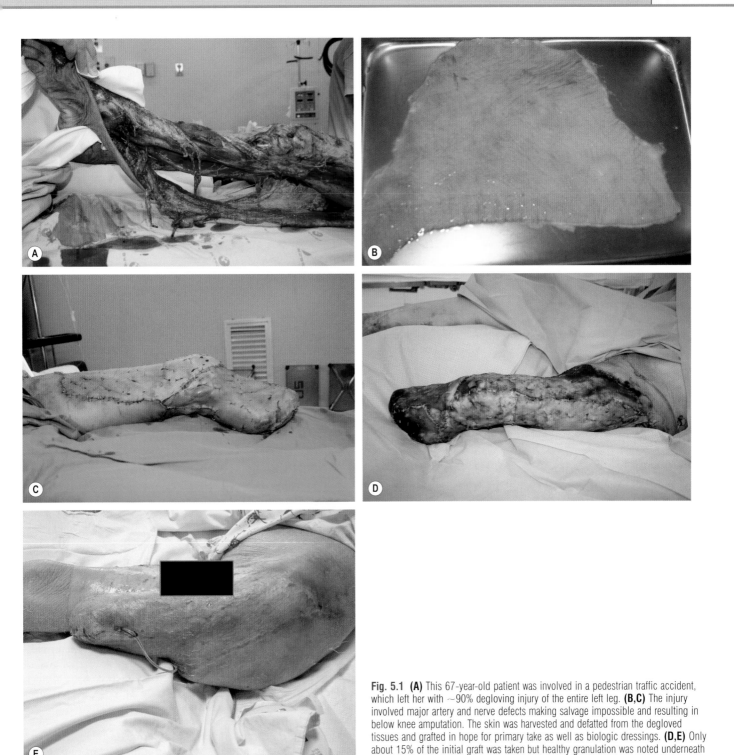

Fig. 5.1 (A) This 67-year-old patient was involved in a pedestrian traffic accident, which left her with ~90% degloving injury of the entire left leg. **(B,C)** The injury involved major artery and nerve defects making salvage impossible and resulting in below knee amputation. The skin was harvested and defatted from the degloved tissues and grafted in hope for primary take as well as biologic dressings. **(D,E)** Only about 15% of the initial graft was taken but healthy granulation was noted underneath the biologic dressing and made a favorable bed for secondary graft procedure.

cross-linked with chondroitin-6-sulfate and covered by a thin silicone layer that serves as an epidermis.[43] It is readily available and does not require a donor site and coverts open to closed wound and decreases metabolic demand on the patient. However, Integra must be used on clean wounds and requires a two-stage procedure later for the graft. Simultaneous use with negative wound pressure therapy may accelerate the vascularization. Apligraf is a bilaminate human epidermal and dermal analogue that can act as a permanent skin substitute. The epidermal layer is formed by human keratinocytes with a well differentiated stratum corneum. The dermal layer is formed with bovine type I collagen lattice impregnated with human fibroblasts from neonatal foreskin. Apligraf is not antigenic and the dermal layer incorporates into the wound bed. Apligraf has been shown to significantly decrease the time of venous ulcer healing compared to compression.[44]

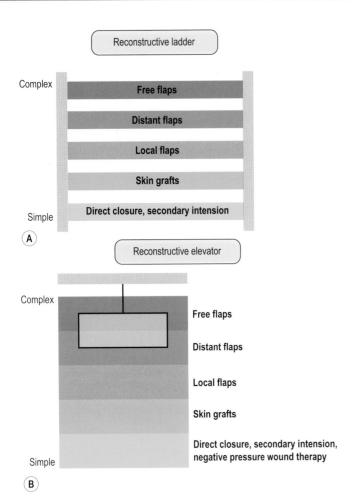

Fig. 5.2 The reconstructive elevator requires creative thoughts and considerations of multiple variables to achieve the best form and function rather than a sequential climb up the ladder. This paradigm of thought does not eliminate the concept of reconstructive ladder but replaces it as a ladder of wound closure and makes its mark in the field where variety of advanced reconstructive procedures and techniques are not readily available. Based on the reconstructive elevator, method of reconstruction should be chosen based on procedures that results in optimal function as well as appearance.

Approach by location (local flaps)

Thigh

The thigh can be divided into three parts: the proximal thigh, midthigh, and the distal thigh (supracondylar knee) regions.

The proximal thigh wounds can result from various causes such as complications from hip fractures, infected bypass vascular graft, after tumor resection, and trauma. The medial portion of the proximal thigh can be especially challenging due to location of vital structures and the likely formation of dead space. Local lower extremity muscle or myocutaneous flap options include using the flaps based from the lateral circumflex femoral artery such as tensor fascia lata, vastus lateralis, and rectus femoris flaps. Vertical rectus abdominis muscle or myocutaneous flap using the deep inferior epigastric artery can allow stable coverage of the proximal thigh. The gracilis muscle or myocutaneous flap based on the medial femoral circumflex artery may lack muscle bulk but is a good option when the dead space is not extensive. Now with

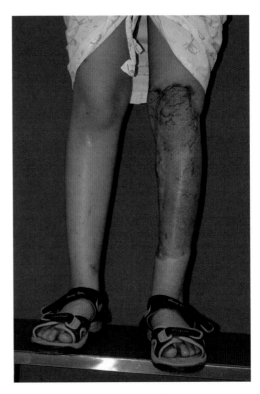

Fig. 5.3 A 10-year-old patient was seen 3 years after reconstruction of one-stage dermal allograft, an acellular dermal matrix engineered from banked human cadaver skin, and split thickness skin graft. The patient is seen to have good elasticity and acceptable cosmetic results.

increased knowledge of perforator and perforator based flaps, basically any perforator can be chosen as a source of vascular supply to the skin flap and be rotated to cover a defect.[45–47] When the use of local flaps is not feasible due to the complexity of the wound, free tissue transfer is indicated.

The midthigh wound, due to the anatomical character where femur is surrounded by a thick layer of soft tissue, rarely requires reconstruction using free tissue transfer and often is sufficiently reconstructed by skin graft or local flap. Local muscle or musculocutaneous flaps based on the lateral or medial femoral circumflex artery can be used when available. Also, any perforator can be chosen as a source of vascular supply to the skin flap and be rotated to cover a defect. However, if the patient has undergone massive resection or has special considerations such as postoperative radiation therapy, it may warrant free tissue coverage.

The wounds of the distal thigh (supracondylar knee) can be very difficult due to the limit of rotation from previously described local muscle or musculocutaneous flaps from the thigh. Pedicled medial gastrocnemius muscle or musculocutaneous flap from the lower leg can be extended to cover this region. However, extensive or complex defects may require free tissue transfer or coverage using a perforator based rotation/advancement skin flap *(Fig. 5.4)*.

Lower leg

The traditional planning for reconstruction of the lower extremity has been approached according to the location of the defect. Divided into thirds, gastrocnemius muscle flap for proximal third, soleus muscle flap for middle third and free

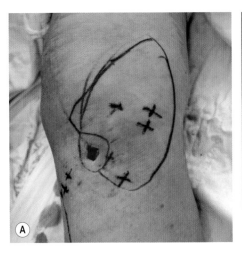
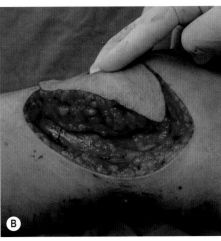
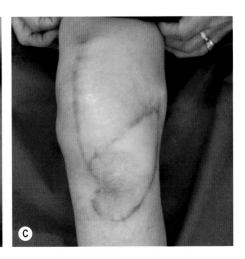

Fig. 5.4 **(A)** A 70-year-old patient is noted with chronic drainage after failed total knee replacement. **(B)** After complete debridement, a perforator based flap was elevated and advanced using a perforator (dissected until just beneath the fascia) with visible pulse. **(C)** Long-term follow-up shows no recurrence of any infections allowing her to undergo total knee replacement.

flap transfer for the distal third of the leg. Like the reconstructive ladder concept, this traditional approach can be useful but the surgeon must individualize each wound and choose the initial procedure that can yield the best chance of success and avoid morbidity.

Microvascular free tissue transfer

One must choose a proper surgical plan to achieve optimal function and cosmesis. Flaps are selected based on accessibility of local tissue and donor morbidity. Frequently in lower extremity trauma, due to the high energy impact, results in extensive and complex wounds. Workhorse for soft tissue coverage includes muscle or musculocutaneous flaps such as latissimus dorsi, rectus abdominis, and gracilis. The perforator flap, where a skin flap is based on a single or multiple perforators, such as the anterolateral thigh flap or thoracodorsal artery perforator flap have added on to the list.

Whichever flap you select, the guideline for lower extremity reconstruction using free flaps remains the same: anastomose the vessel outside the zone of injury, make end-to-side arterial anastomosis and end-to-side or end-to-end venous anastomosis, and reconstruct the soft tissues first and then restore the skeletal support.[48]

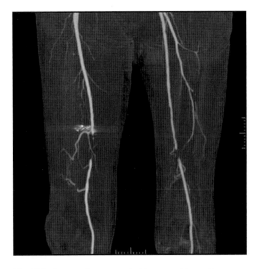

Fig. 5.5 Preoperative computed tomographic angiogram revealing collateral flows on bilateral femoral arteries for a patient with diabetes and poor pedal pulses. The use of CT angiography may obtain vascular information of the recipient region without the risk of complications. The preoperative is selectively recommended in patients who have loss of one or more peripheral pulses, a neurologic deficit secondary to the injury, or a compound fracture of the extremity that has undergone reduction and either external or internal fixation.

Treatment approach

Preoperative evaluation

The initial evaluation of the lower extremity wound involves visual and manual examination. An examination on the location, size, depth and character of the wound is made. Neurological evaluation well as vascular and skeletal evaluation is made to develop a plan for reconstruction. Also, presence of comorbidities including smoking, diabetes, obesity and peripheral vascular disease should be accounted for. The initial evaluation allows to assess the overall function and to consider possible outcome. One must not make the mistake

in addressing the wound locally but rather approach the patient as a whole and must also take into consideration of socioeconomic status, rehabilitative potential, patient's motivation and compliance.

After the decision is made to reconstruct the lower extremity, the first preoperative evaluation should start with vascular status. Physical examination of palpable pulse, color, capillary refill, and turgor of the extremity allows to assess initial status and Doppler examination can provide additional information.[49] The use of preoperative arteriography for lower extremity reconstruction is considered when physical/Doppler exam reveals inconclusive vascular status or chronic vascular disease is suspected *(Fig. 5.5)*. The use of computed tomographic angiography may obtain vascular information of the recipient region without the risk of complications from arterial puncture of the groin and also can provide vascular information of the donor flap facilitating the planning and the surgical procedure.[50–52] In association with prior injuries to the lower extremity, the routine preoperative use of angiogram is controversial.[24,49,50,53–55] It is selectively recommended in patients who have loss of one or more peripheral pulses, a neurologic deficit secondary to the injury, or a compound fracture of the extremity that has undergone reduction and either external or internal fixation.[54]

Nerve injuries that are irreversible may require special considerations. Peroneal nerve injuries results in foot drop and loss of sensation of the dorsum of the foot. Thus lifelong splinting or tendon transfers may be required. Complete loss of tibial nerve function results in loss of plantar flexion and is a absolute contraindication for reconstruction.[56] The loss of plantar sensation can be devastating and may hinder the need for reconstruction although is not an absolute contraindication.[57]

An algorithm of approach is outlined in *Figure 5.6*.

Primary limb amputation

A study by Lange describes absolute and relative indications for primary amputation of limbs with open tibial fractures.[56] Absolute indications include: anatomically complete disruption of the posterior tibial nerve in adults and crush injuries with warm ischemia time greater than 6 h. Relative indications include: serious associated polytrauma, severe ipsilateral foot trauma, and anticipated protracted course to obtain soft tissue coverage and tibial reconstruction.

In these cases where limb salvage is not possible, attempts should be made to salvage as much limb length as possible. Every effort should be made to save the functional knee joint as below-knee amputation results in far superior ambulatory outcome and up to 2–3 folds more full mobility compared to above knee amputation.[58] The energy consumption is far less for below-knee amputation and this allows these patients to walk significant daily distances, thus maintaining good quality of life.[59] Though the ideal stump length below the knee is more than 6 cm, any length of tibia should be preserved.[60]

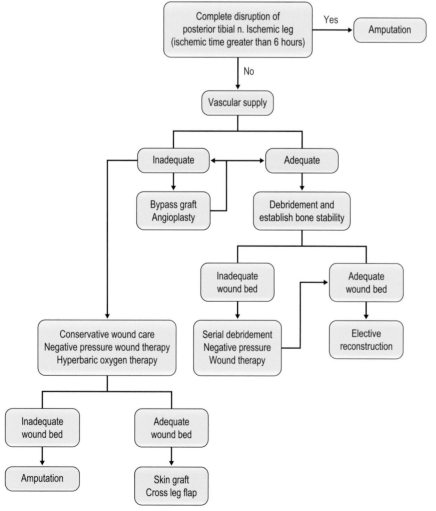

Fig. 5.6 Algorithm of approach for soft tissue reconstruction of lower extremity.

If adequate soft tissue exists, stump may be closed primarily and where local tissue is inadequate, microsurgery allows preserving maximal length of the stump. If the tissue distal to the amputation is usable, a fillet flap can be performed. Other flaps such as muscle, musculocutaneous, fasciocutaneous and perforator flaps can be used for microsurgical reconstruction and achieves the same goal as well. Muscle flaps may have a tendency to heal slowly and to shrink due to muscle atrophy, while skin flaps may provide better contour and sensibility.[61]

Debridement

Bony stability is first established using external or internal fixation devices. An external device is usually preferred if there is significant bone loss or bone devascularization and may facilitate coverage procedure. Debridement must cover devitalized soft tissue and bone and be performed until fresh bleeding is noted. Multiple stages of debridement may be needed to achieve adequate wound bed prior to soft tissue coverage.

The vacuum-assisted closure can be used to optimize the wound bed and minimize dressing changes until definitive reconstruction. It must be used with caution and in conjunction with serial debridement. It does not replace surgical debridement and should not be used in heavily contaminated wound with necrotic tissues. If a lower extremity wound is clean, bony stability is present, and no vital structures are exposed, application may be indicated.[54] This device facilitates dressing of the wound and often promotes healing.

Timing of reconstruction

Regardless of the degree of contamination and extent of injury when indicated for salvage, there is no need to delay definitive coverage provided that the general condition of the patient and the status of the wound allows it. General consensus favors early aggressive wound debridement and soft issue coverage. Byrd et al. described acute, subacute, and chronic phases of an open tibial fracture.[62] Ideally, the wound is covered in the first 5–6 days after injury at the acute phase of the wound. In severe Gustillo type IIIB and type IIIC injuries, free muscle transplantation obtained the best results. At 1–6 weeks the wound enters the subacute phase where wounds had higher tendency of infections and flap failures. Between 4 and 6 weeks, the wound enters the chronic phase and clear demarcation between viable and nonviable bone becomes apparent. Godina further demonstrated that radical debridement and coverage within 72 h results in best outcome where only 0.75% of flap fails, 1.5% are infected, and 6.8 months are needed for union of the bone.[11] The failure rate compared remarkable to 12% when reconstructed from day 3 to 3 months and 10% when reconstructed after 3 months of injury. Yaremchuk et al. recommended early coverage between days 7 and 14 after several debridements allowing better identification of zone of injury.[63] The common idea behind early intervention is that it minimizes the risk for increasing bacterial colonization and inflammation leading to complications. Acute coverage by day 5–7 is generally accepted as having a good prognosis in terms of decreased risk of infection, flap survival, and fracture healing.[11,24,62,63] If patient condition does not allow prolong surgical procedures, then the wound should be debrided as early as possible and maintain a clean and well vascularized recipient bed till conditions allow definitive reconstruction.[64]

Selection of recipient vessel

Many lower extremity wounds resulting from trauma are high-energy injuries with a substantial "zone of injury." This thrombogenic zone is known to extend beyond what is macroscopically evident, and failure to recognize the true extent of this zone is cited as a leading cause of microsurgical anastomotic failure. Within the zone, perivascular changes such as increased friability of vessels and increased perivascular scar tissue may lead to difficult dissection of recipient vessels and higher incidence of thrombosis after anastomosis.[65] How extensive is clinically very difficult to realize. Thus, Isenberg and Sherman demonstrated that clinical presentation of recipient vessel (vessel wall pliability and the quality of blood from transected end of vessel) was more important than the distance from the wound.[66] Park et al. also concluded that site of injury and vascular status of the lower extremity was the most important factor in choosing a recipient vessel.[67] This idea was further supported by successful anastomosis of perforator to perforator adjacent to or within zone of injury.[68] Based on these findings, one of the most important factors in selecting the recipient vessel may be the vascular quality itself.

Special considerations

Osteomyelitis

Osteomyelitis often follows severe open leg fractures with massive contamination or devascularized soft tissue and bone. Inadequate debridement or delayed coverage of the wound increases the chance for osteomyelitis and early debridement remains to be the key to prevention.[69] Osteomyelitis should be seen as a spectrum of disease and should be individualized and managed accordingly. Factors known to be of prognostic significance include the duration of infection, the extent of bony involvement, the presence of associated fracture or nonunion, and overall immune status of the patient.[70] The wound is composed of exposed bone, infected bone, devitalized bone, and scarred tissue surrounding the bone. These components have diminished vascular supply making antibiotics difficult to reach. Thus, to achieve the goal of infection control and the restoration of function, treatment principles for chronic osteomyelitis are debridement including the complete resection of involved bone, flap coverage with vascularized tissue, and brief course of antibiotic treatment (*Fig. 5.7*). Local method of antibiotic delivery can be used when complete debridement of bone is not possible. Although there have been controversy in selecting the type of flap for coverage, muscle have shown experimentally to have increased blood flow and antibiotics delivery, increased oxygen tension, increased phagocytic activity, and decreased bacterial counts in wounds reconstructed with muscle flaps than fasciocutaneous flaps.[71–73] Clinically, complete debridement and

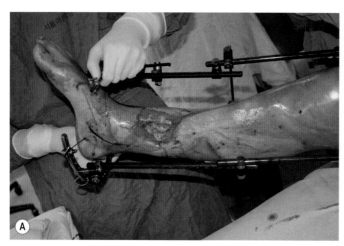
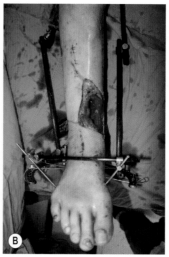
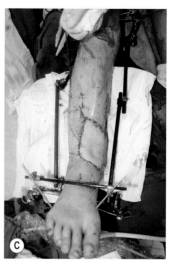

Fig. 5.7 **(A)** A patient with chronic osteomyelitis is noted with soft tissue defect. **(B)** Complete debridement including resection of the involved bone was performed. **(C)** Flap coverage with well vascularized anterolateral thigh flap combined with vastus lateralis muscle tissue was used with 6 weeks of antibiotic treatment.

obliteration of dead space are the most important steps to treat osteomyelitis and the type of flaps seems less crucial.[74,75] Bone defects can be managed with vascularized bone flap, secondary bone grafting, bone distraction lengthening or a combination of these techniques.

Not all chronic osteomyelitis can be salvaged. As with the indication for amputation, legs with nerves too damaged after osteomyelitis should not be salvaged. General and socioeconomic condition of the patient should also be considered and the patient should be offered the option of amputation and early rehabilitation.

Diabetes

Patients with diabetes require additional concerns from chronic renal failures, nutrition to blood sugar control. These multiple issues are best approached by a multidisciplinary team.[76–79] Patients will frequently have chronic bacterial colonization, osteomyelitis, complex wounds, bone deformity, local wound ischemia and vascular disease. The etiology behind these complicated wounds is from macrovascular angiopathy, bony deformities leading to pressure points, neuropathy, and poor metabolic control. When patients with diabetes are required to undergo reconstructive procedure of the extremity, vascular status must be evaluated to ensure success.[80,81] Any vascular problems must be addressed first and corrected. If not correctable, the surgeon may be faced with a high risk of failure. One must consider the probability of successful reconstruction, based on eliminating the underlying problems of the diabetic wound and also take into account long-term ambulation after reconstruction. In a retrospective study by Hong, only 71 patients out of 216 were deemed functionally salvageable using microsurgical approach and reported successful outcome in 66 patients (*Figs 5.8, 5.9*).[80] Large and composite diabetic wounds must be aggressively debrided including the necrotic bone and be covered with well-vascularized tissue.

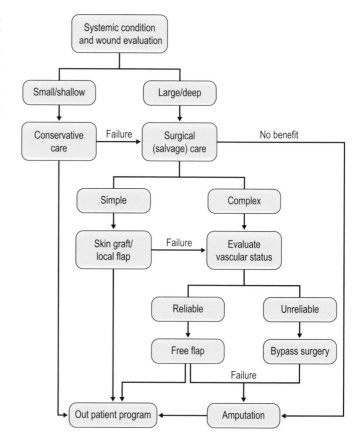

Fig. 5.8 Algorithm for diabetic foot reconstruction.

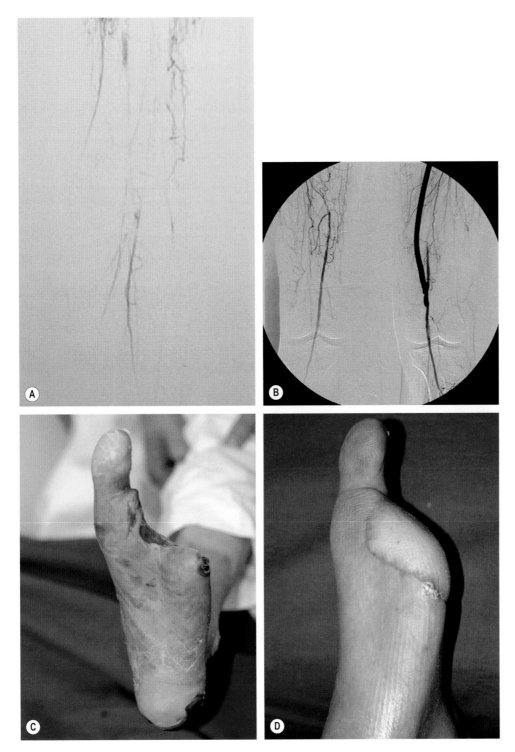

Fig. 5.9 A diabetic patient after partial amputation of the foot was noted with poorly healing stump. **(A,B)** The angiogram revealed poor flow to the lower leg and femoral-popliteal bypass was performed. **(C,D)** With improved circulation, the patient underwent reconstruction with anterolateral thigh perforator flap and salvaged his foot.

Coverage after tumor ablation

As with any reconstructive procedure, the aim of reconstruction after tumor ablation is to maintain quality of life by preserving function and achieving acceptable appearance. In addition, coverage must be able to withstand adjuvant therapy with radiation therapy and/or chemotherapy and play a role to achieve long-term local control of disease. Surgeons should have close cooperation with the oncologists and must acquire adequate knowledge of tumor characteristics, behavior, and adjuvant treatment to plan and choose the type of reconstructive procedure. Knowing that reconstruction is feasible allows the oncologic surgeon to achieve a comfortable and satisfactory excision margin and may lead to a better outcome. Skin grafts are always an option especially for very extensive defects where flap coverage is not available. But for wounds scheduled for postoperative radiation therapy or located over joints and high friction regions, skin graft should be avoided and be reconstructed with a durable flap.[82] Special consideration should be made to preoperative radiation therapy where skin would become fibrotic and ischemic around the cancer and thus will not allow local coverage. Regarding adjuvant chemotherapy, free flap procedures will not interfere with chemotherapy nor will chemotherapy have an impact on free flap survival.[83,84] Overall success rate was shown to be 96.6% in a series of 59 free flaps in 57 patients undergoing lower extremity reconstruction after tumor ablation, with 12% major and 7% minor complications.[83] Various flaps from omentum, muscle with skin graft, musculocutaneous, and perforator flaps can be used for reconstruction depending on location, size, depth, adjuvant therapy, function, and cosmetic appearance (*Fig. 5.10*).

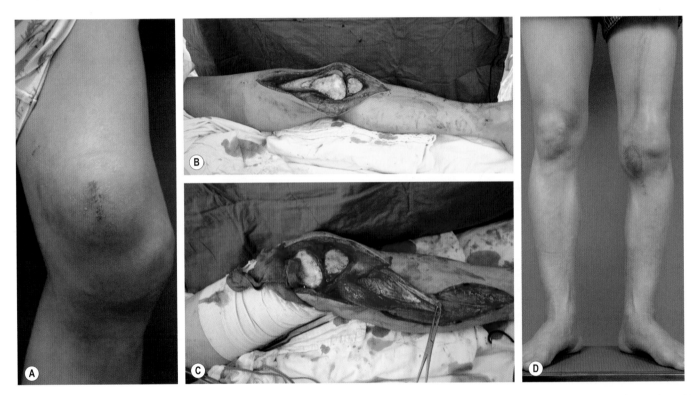

Fig. 5.10 **(A)** A patient with soft tissue sarcoma of the knee region was noted. **(B,C)** After wide excision including the bone, a hemi-gastrocnemius muscle was elevated to resurface the knee joint. **(D)** Long-term results shows good contour with acceptable function and appearance.

Exposed prosthesis

The traditional method to manage exposed hardware includes irrigation, debridement, antibiotics, and likely removal of hardware. However, several factors should be taken into account to manage exposed hardware before considering removal, which may set back the treatment plan. Factors such as location of the hardware, infection (type of bacteria and duration of infection), duration of exposure of hardware, and hardware loosening should be considered as important prognostic factors for successful management of exposed hardware.[85] In a retrospective review by Viol et al., they concluded that if hardware is clinically stable, time of exposure is less than 2 weeks, infection is controlled, and the location of the hardware is for bony consolidation, then it may increase the likelihood of salvage of hardware using surgical soft tissue coverage *(Fig. 5.11)*.[85]

Exposed vascular grafts present life- and limb-threatening complications. It should be managed with early debridement and muscle flap coverage to salvage the graft. Synthetic grafts can susceptible to bacteria colonization and should consider replacing with an autologous graft. Local muscle flaps such as gracilis, sartorius, and tensor fascia lata are very useful in providing adequate coverage for exposed groin synthetic vascular prosthesis. If the defect is extensive inferiorly based, a vertical rectus abdominis musculocutaneous flap can be considered. The management of exposed vascular grafts requires close cooperation with the vascular surgeon, aggressive debridement, and coverage with a well vascularized tissue.

Soft tissue expansion

The use of tissue expansion in the lower extremity has not been successful as in other areas of the body, such as the breast and scalp. The potential advantages of using expanded skin in the lower extremity include improved contour, coverage with like tissue, and improved aesthetic result. However, the use in lower extremity has been associated with high rate of infection and extrusion of the implant. Wound infection and dehiscence are the most common complications, but seroma, implant displacement, neurapraxia, hematoma, and contour defects can also occur. The technique can be reserved for unstable soft tissues or scars of moderate size. The implant is placed suprafascially in the subcutaneous pocket in the lower extremity and application on the ankle and foot region must be avoided. Transverse expansion has lower failure rate compared to longitudinal advancement. For avoidance of wound dehiscence, neurapraxia, and fat necrosis, expansion should proceed slowly, stopping before the onset of pain or, if it is measured before intraexpander pressure exceeds 40 mmHg.[86] Flap prefabrication with tissue expansion may have a role in select reconstructions of the lower extremity.[87]

Postoperative care

Monitoring

During the postoperative period, the patient as a whole and the flap should be closely monitored. It is especially important to monitor hemodynamic and pulmonary function as adequate hydration and oxygenation are critical to flap survival. Input and output of fluid should be monitored closely as distal perfusion is primarily effected by hypotensive episodes. Patients who have chronic renal failures and require assistance of dialysis often removes large volumes and can make fluid maintenance difficult. Limiting range of motion may be needed for flaps covering the joints as extension or flexion may increase the tension of the pedicle. Monitoring

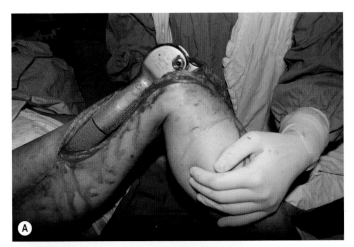

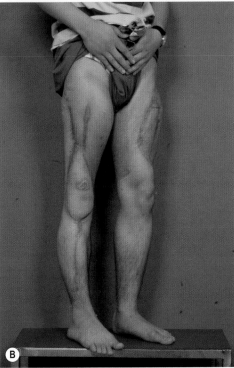

Fig. 5.11 A patient with total knee replacement after contraction of the knee due to traffic accident came with unstable skin and pending exposure of knee implant for 1 month. **(A)** The unstable region of the skin is completely debrided and irrigated. **(B)** Upon debridement there was no apparent signs of infection. A large anterolateral thigh perforator flap including the deep fascia was taken to resurface the exposed prothesis and shows stable recovery after 2 years.

flaps, especially free flaps in the first 24 h is essential due to the majority of thrombosis occurring at this time. According to Chen et al., up to 85% of the compromised flaps can be salvaged when the first sign of vascular compromise is clinically noted during the first 3 days after microsurgery.[88] There is no ideal method of flap monitoring but recent techniques such as tissue oxygen measurement, implantable Doppler device, laser Doppler flowmetry, and fluorescent dye injections may assist the judgment made from clinical evaluation which remains as the "golden standard" of monitoring. Emergent re-exploration should be performed once pedicle compromise is noted.

Management of flap complications

Although there are no clinical reviews that conclusively show any agents that increase flap survival rate, about 96% among surveyed 106 microsurgeons use some form of prophylactic antithrombotic treatment such as heparin, dextran, and aspirin or in combinations with other agents.[89–91] The routine use of dextran should be carefully approached due to allergic reaction and pulmonary edema but aspirin, heparin or low molecular weight heparin can be considered on a theoretical basis and related studies from different disciplines. Thrombolytics such as urokinase can be used when flow is not immediately re-established after pedicle rearrangement or revision anastomosis.[91] But no agent can replace the meticulous surgical technique and early diagnosis of flap compromise.

Leeches have a role in the postoperative care for a jeopardized flap. In cases of venous congestion, by injecting a salivary component called hirudin, which inhibits platelet aggregation and coagulation cascade, leeches can decongest by extracting blood directly and further by oozing after it detaches. The use of leeches for 5–7 days can sometimes help salvage the flaps that do not resolve, despite re-exploration of the venous flow.

Secondary operations

Bone grafts are usually placed 6 weeks later after soft tissue reconstruction to allow time for transferred tissue to settle in and sterilize the wound.[19] Cancellous autografts or vascularized bone transfers are can be chosen depending on length of the bone gap. Bone transfer mechanism can be an alternative to free bone transfer of bone defects longer than 6 cm.

To achieve optimal motion of tendons of the lower extremity, secondary tenolysis procedure may be needed. The risk for adhesion may increase when skin graft is performed over granulated tissue directly above the tendons and may warrant flap coverage.

The final stage to consider after reasonable functional recovery is appearance of the extremity. Patients after recovery frequently show scars, depression, bulky flaps, and donor site morbidities. Although complete restoration is nearly impossible, a reasonable endpoint should be set and efforts to minimize scars and achieve good contours should be made. Debulking by surgical excision or liposuction can improve the contour of the flap and fat grafts can be added to elevate depressed scars. Scar revision by z-plasties or expanders can help to alleviate scars not only physical but psychological.

Muscle/musculocutaneous flaps

Tensor fascia lata

The tensor fascia lata is a small, thin and short muscle with a long fascial extension from the iliotibial tract of the facia lata to the lateral aspect of the knee. The muscle originates anterior 5–8 cm of the external lip of the anterior superior iliac crest immediately behind sartorius. It inserts to the iliotibial tract. It abducts, medially rotates, and flexes the hip, acting to tighten the fascia lata and iliotibial tract but is an expendable muscle. Its flat shape, excellent length, and reliable type I circulation pattern (dominant pedicle is the ascending branch of the lateral femoral circumflex artery and venae comitantes) making it useful in many reconstructive scenarios, both as a pedicled flap for local and regional coverage and as a free, composite unit that incorporates skin, muscle, and iliac bone. Motor innervation is from the superior gluteal nerve entering the deep surface between the gluteus medius and gluteus maximus. Sensation is derived from T12 innervates the upper skin territory and the lateral femoral cutaneous nerve of the thigh (L2–3) innervates the lower skin.

When based on the dominant pedicle, located 8–10 cm below the anterior superior iliac spine, the anterior arc of location will reach the abdominal areas, groin, and perineum while the posterior arc can reach the greater trochanter, ischium, perineum, and sacrum *(Fig. 5.12).*[92,93] The flap can

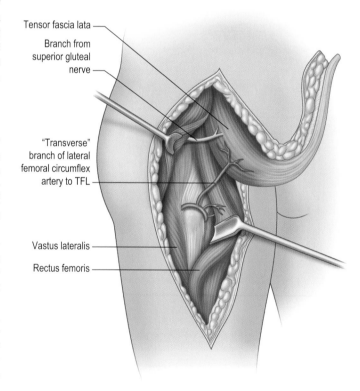

Tensor fascia lata

Branch from superior gluteal nerve

"Transverse" branch of lateral femoral circumflex artery to TFL

Vastus lateralis

Rectus femoris

Fig. 5.12 Tensor fascia lata flap elevation. When based on the dominant pedicle, located 8–10 cm below the anterior superior iliac spine, anterior arc of location will reach the abdominal areas, groin, and perineum while the posterior arc can reach the greater trochanter, ischium, perineum, and sacrum.

also be advanced superiorly as a V-Y flap to cover trochanteric wounds.[94] The skin overlying the muscle and fascia lata can be harvested as a unit with the flap and can extend to within 10 cm above the knee.

The marking begins by identifying the major landmarks; the anterior superior iliac spine, lateral condyle of femur, and the pubic tubercle. A line from the anterior superior iliac spine straight down the thigh to a point 10–12 cm above the knee joint, presents the anterior border of the flap and a parallel line 12–15 cm posterior to the first line is drawn straight down the thigh, curving anteriorly as it crosses posterior to the lateral epicondylar area to meet at the same point. The skin island can be designed within this long strip, according to the needs and distance to the recipient defect. The distal margin of the flap is entered, carrying the incision through the fascia lata and dissecting deep to the fascia lata and iliotibial tract. The pedicle is located approximately 10 cm below the anterior iliac spine along the line drawn. One must modify the flap when composite tissues are taken for reconstruction.

Rectus femoris

The rectus femoris is located superficially on the middle of the anterior thigh, extending between the ilium and patella. It is a central muscle of the quadriceps femoris extensor muscles group and acts to extend the leg at the knee. The muscle originates with two tendons, one from the anterior inferior iliac spine and one from the acetabulum. It inserts to the patella. It is a thigh flexor and a leg extensor important in stabilizing the weight-bearing knee, thus is not considered expendable. It has a type II pattern of circulation (the dominant pedicle is the descending branch of the lateral circumflex femoral artery with minor pedicles from the ascending branch of the same vessel as well as from muscle branches of the superficial femoral artery) and can reach to cover the inferior abdomen, groin, perineum and ischium.[95,96] Motor innervation is from the femoral nerve, and muscle branches enter adjacent to the dominant pedicle. This motor innervation and the adequate dimension of the flap allows it to be used as a functional muscle flap *(Fig. 5.13)*.[97] The intermediate anterior femoral cutaneous nerve (L2–3) provides sensation. The skin perforators are most reliable over the midanterior two-thirds of the muscle itself in the central strip up to 12 × 20 cm.

A longitudinal incision is marked from 3 cm below the anterior superior iliac spine to just above the superior margin of the patella. With the anterior thigh muscle contraction, the lateral border of the vastus medialis and the medial border of the vastus lateralis is visualized, creating a depression of skin. The tendon of the rectus femoris can be easily noted below the depression and above the patella. The skin island should be designed on the middle-third of the thigh as the majority of the perforators are located in this region. Incision at the distal edge of the skin island, along the axis allows the rectus femoris muscle to be identified and separated from the vastus medialis and lateralis. The skin island is then incised circumferentially down to the fascia of the muscle. The rectus is elevated from distal to proximal and from medial to lateral so that the pedicle and nerve can be identified and protected medially along the underside of the muscle. The dominant pedicle enters the posteromedial muscle at a variable distance of 7–10 cm below the symphysis pubis and care must be given

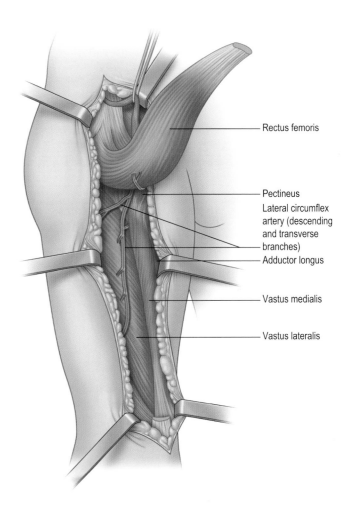

Fig. 5.13 Rectus femoris muscle flap elevation. It is a type II pattern of circulation (the dominant pedicle is the descending branch of the lateral circumflex femoral artery with minor pedicles from the ascending branch of the same vessel as well as from muscle branches of the superficial femoral artery) and can reach to cover the inferior abdomen, groin, perineum and ischium.

Labels in figure:
- Rectus femoris
- Pectineus
- Lateral circumflex artery (descending and transverse branches)
- Adductor longus
- Vastus medialis
- Vastus lateralis

to preserve the motor branches from the femoral nerve to the adjacent vastus lateralis and tensor fascia lata. The donor area should be repaired by careful suturing of the tendinous fascia of the vastus medialis and lateralis together above the patella in an effort to preserve full knee extension.

Biceps femoris

This large, well-vascularized posterior muscle of the mid and lateral thigh is useful for the coverage of ischial pressure sores. The muscle has two heads; the long head originates on the ischial tuberosity and the short head originates on the linea aspera of femur and both inserts to head of fibula. The long head extends the hip, and both heads flex the leg at the knee and thus is not expandable. The pattern of circulation is type II (the long head has dominant and minor pedicles from the first and second perforating branches of the profunda femoris artery, respectively, and the short head receives the second (or third) perforating branch of the profunda and a minor source from the lateral superior geniculate artery) and can be turned over to cover the ischial regions based on the

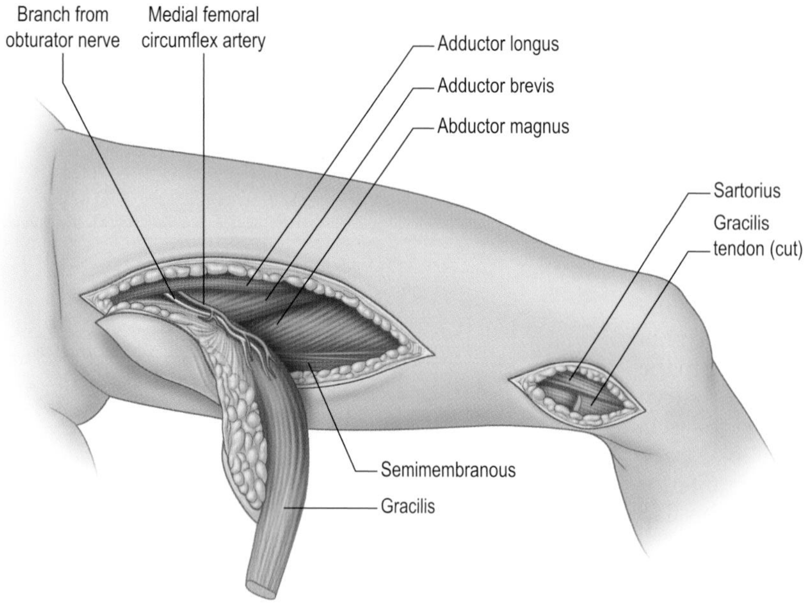

Fig. 5.14 Gracilis muscle flap elevation. It is a type II circulation pattern (the dominant pedicle is the terminal branch of the medial circumflex femoral artery and one or two minor pedicles arise as branches of the superficial femoral artery) and can reach to cover the abdomen, ischium, groin and perineum as a muscle or musculocutaneous flap.

dominant pedicle.[98] The long head derives its motor innervations from the tibial division of the sciatic nerve, the short head from the peroneal division of the sciatic nerve. The postcutaneous nerve of the thigh (S1–3) supplies the sensation.

The entire skin of the posterior thigh can be elevated and be advanced in V-Y fashion as musculocutaneous unit. The upper base of the skin flap is horizontally marked along the buttock crease and the apex just above the popliteal fossa. The relatively short pedicles make the flap unsuitable for wide rotation flaps but serve well in sliding the muscle proximally along the femur towards the pelvis. The medial thigh skin may also be left uncut, preserving skin as a rotation advancement modification of the flap.[99]

With the skin island isolated, the tendon is divided distally. The tendon is sectioned, and the dissection proceeds from the distal thigh towards the ischium, freeing the muscle on its deep aspect from the femur and from the adductor group of muscles medially, until enough mobility is attained so that the defect can easily be filled. The flap should be inset and sutured with the patient in a jack-knife position and the hips flexed to prevent dehiscence of the flap.

Gracilis

This is located on the medial thigh extending between the pubis and the medial knee. It is thin and flat muscle which lies between the adductor longus and sartorius muscle anteriorly and the semimembranous posteriorly. It originates on the pubic symphysis and inserts into the medial tibial condyle. The gracilis function is a thigh adductor but is expandable from the compensation made from abductor longus and magnus muscle. The muscle has a type II circulation pattern (the dominant pedicle is the terminal branch of the medial circumflex femoral artery and one or two minor pedicles arise as branches of the superficial femoral artery) and can reach to cover the abdomen, ischium, groin, and perineum as a muscle

or musculocutaneous flap *(Fig. 5.14)*. Motor innervation is from the anterior branch of the obturator nerve and enters the gracilis on its deep medial surface immediately superior to the entry of the dominant pedicle. The motor nerve allows gracilis to be used as a functional muscle flap for facial reanimation and upper extremity.[100] The sensory innervation is from the anterior femoral cutaneous nerve (L2–3), which provides sensation to the anteromedial thigh.[101]

When skin is harvested with the gracilis muscle, the flap is generally oriented longitudinally and centered over the proximal third of the muscle, where the majority of the musculocutaneous perforators are located. A proximal transversely oriented skin flap is optional and the bulky fat of the medial thigh makes this flap suitable for breast reconstruction.[102–104] The symphysis pubis and the medial condyle of the femur are major landmarks. The muscle extends the full length of the medial thigh and averages about 6 cm in width proximally and tapers to about 2–3 cm in the distal third of the muscle. Although the width may be narrow, the muscle can be fanned out to provide coverage over larger defects. With the patient in lithotomy position and slight extension of the knee will allows the gracilis to be seen and felt, and it tends to be more posterior than expected.

For muscle elevation, an incision is made 2–3 cm posterior to the line drawn connecting the symphysis pubis and medial condyle of the knee. The muscle is identified posterior to the adductor longus. If a skin flap is planned, the skin territory should be designed on the proximal part of the inner thigh. Usually, the dissection is easily approached by distal incision identifying the tendon of the gracilis posterior to the saphenous vein and the distal sartorius muscle. Tendinous insertion of semimembranous and semitendinosus muscle can be indentified posterior to the gracilis. Traction on the tendon will highlight the proximal outline of the muscle and allow accurate estimation of the location. This is an important step to minimize faulty elevation of the skin component, as the medial thigh is mobile and makes it easy to incorrectly predict the skin position over the muscle. Dissection of the anterior and posterior skin borders then proceed proximally, approximately half the length of the muscle, whereby the distal tendon is divided and the distal muscle elevated. During the elevation of the middle and distal third of the flap, one or two minor perforators from the superficial femoral artery will be identified and ligated. Retraction of the adductor longus muscle will expose the major pedicle passing over the deep adductor magnus, approximately 10 cm below the pubic symphysis.

Soleus

The soleus is a very broad, large bipenniform muscle lying deep to the gastrocnemius muscle. The muscle has two muscle bellies, medial and lateral, separated by a midline intramuscular septum in the distal half. The lateral belly originates from the posterior surface of the head of the fibula and posterior surface of the body of the fibula and the medial belly originated from the middle-third of the medial border of the tibia. Both bellies of the soleus inserts into the calcaneus bone through the Achilles tendon. It contributes to the plantar flexion of the foot. Soleus is expandable, taken that at least one head of gastrocnemius is intact with function. The pattern of circulation is type II (with dominant pedicles from the popliteal, posterior tibial and peroneal arteries and the minor pedicles rise from the posterior tibial and peroneal arteries supplying the distal medial and lateral bellies, respectively), and can cover the middle and lower-third of the leg (*Fig. 5.15A*). Motor nerve is derived from the posterior tibial and popliteal nerves.[105]

The arc of rotation for a proximally-based soleus flap after division of minor pedicles and elevation of the distal two-thirds of the muscle can cover the middle-third of the tibia. Hemisoleus flaps may improve the arc of rotation and preserve soleus function while sacrificing flap coverage area. The medial reversed hemisoleus pivots around the most superior distal minor perforator of the posterior tibial artery,

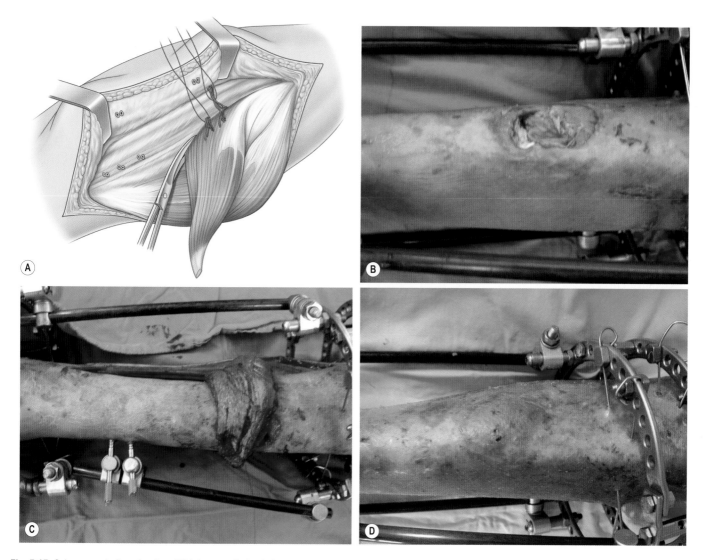

Fig. 5.15 Soleus muscle flap elevation. **(A)** It is a type II circulation pattern (with dominant pedicles from the popliteal, posterior tibial and peroneal arteries and the minor pedicles rises from posterior tibial and peroneal arteries supplying the distal medial and lateral bellies, respectively) and can cover the middle and lower-third of the leg. **(B–D)** A patient with chronic osteomyelitis of the middle-third of the tibia is reconstructed using a hemi-soleus flap.

approximately 7 cm above the malleolus; the lateral reversed hemisoleus has a tenuous blood supply through minor perforators from the peroneal and a shorter arc of rotation. The distal half of the muscle can be reversely transposed based on minor segment pedicles and cover the distal third of the leg.[106]

The medial border of the tibia is the landmark for medial exposure and the fibula itself is the landmark for lateral exposure. A line can be drawn 2 cm medial to the medial edge of tibia or laterally along the fibula. Subcutaneous neurovascular structures are identified and preserved, and the posterior compartment fascia is opened. The plane between the soleus and gastrocnemius is usually well-defined superiorly, but sharp scalpel dissection is needed to separate the tendons and maintain the gastrocnemius contributions to the Achilles tendon. For proximally based flaps, distal perforators are divided in the deep plane, and the tendon is divided distally. The dominant pedicle is usually located on the upper third of the muscle for both bellies of the soleus. Identification and dissection of the midline raphe allow a hemisoleus flap to be developed *(Fig. 5.15B–D)*.

Gastrocnemius

The gastrocnemius muscle is the most superficial muscle of the posterior calf and has two heads, medial and lateral, which form the distal boundary of the popliteal space. Each head can be used as a separate muscle or musculocutaneous unit, based on its own pedicle. The medial head originates from the medial condyle of the femur and the lateral from the lateral condyle of the femur and both heads insert to the calcaneus through the Achilles tendon. It contributes to the plantar flexion of the foot and either or both heads of the gastrocnemius are expandable if the soleus is intact. The pattern of circulation is type I (the medial muscle is supplied by the medial sural artery and the lateral muscle is supplied by the lateral sural artery) and provides reliable coverage to the upper third of the tibia, suprapatellar thigh, and knee regions *(Fig. 5.16)*. Both heads receive a minor source across the raphe that joins them as anastomotic vessels within the muscle substance. Motor innervation derives from branches of the tibial nerve. The sensation to the skin overlying the medial head is from the saphenous nerve and that to the lateral and distal skin overlying the lateral head is from the sural nerve.[107]

The arc of rotation of the medial head after complete elevation can cover the inferior thigh, knee, and upper third of the tibia. When origin of the muscle is divided, an extended arc of rotation by 5–8 cm can be achieved to extend to the upper part of the knee. The lateral head can be elevated to cover the suprapatellar region, knee and proximal third of the tibia. It also can be extended with the division of the muscle origin. Both heads can be inferiorly rotated, based on the vascular anastomosis across the raphe between the two muscle heads to reach the middle third of the leg. A skin paddle can be designed based on the perforating vessels with dimension of 10 × 15 cm for the medial and 8 × 12 cm for the lateral head. But the use of a skin paddle leaves an unsightly donor scar.

A line is drawn either 2 cm medial to the medial edge of the tibia or along the posterior midleg. If the muscle alone is employed, a midline posterior incision affords excellent access to both heads. During elevation, care is taken to protect the

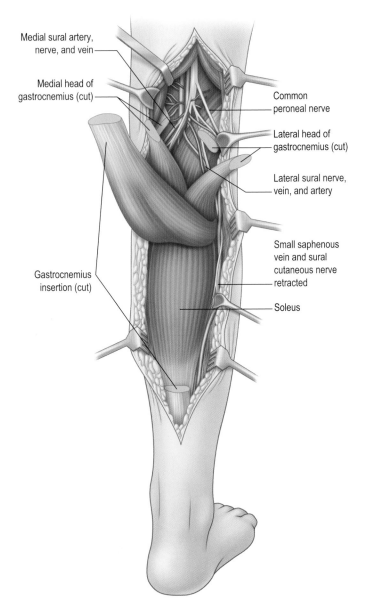

Fig. 5.16 Gastrocnemius flap elevation. It is a type I circulation pattern (the medial muscle is supplied by the medial sural artery and the lateral muscle is supplied by the lateral sural artery) and provides coverage to the upper-third of the tibia, suprapatellar thigh, and knee regions.

neurovascular structures, especially the more superficial saphenous and sural nerves. In the proximal third, medial surface of the medial head is easily separated from the soleus. The dissection starts at the medial edge of the gastrocnemius muscle and plantaris can be easily noted below the gastrocnemius and above the soleus. The midline muscular raphe is located, and with finger dissection, the underlying soleus muscle is separated from the gastrocnemius proximally and distally. The musculotendinous raphe is then separated sharply. Distally, the thick tendinous layer is sharply dissected free from the remaining calcaneal tendon. The transaction of the origin of the muscle allows increased freedom. If a tunnel is made over the lateral proximal leg, care must be given not to violate the deep peroneal nerve.

Fasciocutaneous/perforator flap

A perforator flap is defined as a flap based on a musculocutaneous perforating vessel that is directly visualized and dissected free of surrounding muscles and an adequate pedicle length is achieved.[108] This concept may be still confusing because the same flap can be a septocutaneous flap when it is based on vessel traveling intermuscular septum and becomes a perforator flap if the pedicel is from a direct musculocutaneous perforator. However, despite the confusion in nomenclature, this approach helps to achieve better accuracy by alleviating concerns of anatomic variations and minimizes donor site morbidity. This kind of flap that may be based on any perforator, "Freestyle free flap", allows the freedom of flap selection from anywhere of the body.[108] This principle is used in the local flaps as well where a flap can be rotated based on a single perforator to cover the defect as well as minimize donor site morbidity.[47] Although this is a very useful flap, it provides limited coverage. Further advancement by Koshima et al. where the flap and the pedicle is taken above the fascia as a perforator flap truly allows the donor site to have minimal morbidity.[109,110] But the anastomosis can be difficult with the vessel's diameter <1 mm, hence this technique is known as supermicrosurgery. Hong and Koshima have also stretched the boundary of microsurgery opening the possibility of using perforators as recipient vessels, and introduced the concept of "free style reconstruction".[111]

Since the basic approach may be similar, the septocutaneous and perforator flaps will be discussed together when necessary.

Groin/SCIP (superficial circumflex iliac perforator)

The groin flap may be elevated extending between the femoral vessels and the posterior iliac spine. This flap has been one of the early fasciocutaneous flaps introduced. The dominant pedicle is the superficial circumflex iliac artery, and venae comitantes and superficial circumflex iliac vein. Variation in anatomy with superior inferior epigastric artery have been reported but Harii and Ohmori conclude that either source can supply the flap efficiently (*Fig. 5.17*).[112] The pedicle is very short, i.e., up to only 3 cm. Koshima defined that the SCIP flap is different from groin flap in that it is nourished by only a perforator of the superficial circumflex iliac system (*Fig. 5.18*).[113] The T12 sensory innervations is at the lateral margin of the flap away from the pedicle, precluding use as a sensate flap.

The long axis of the flap is centered over a line parallel and 3 cm inferior to the inguinal ligament with a flap width of 6–10 cm. The flap can be used as a free or pedicled flap. For pedicled flaps, the dissection should proceed from lateral to medial and distal to proximal. Elevation in begun in a plane superficial to fascia lata and when the Sartorius muscle is visualized, the flap is elevated deep to the fascia and superficial to the muscle. The perforator flap is elevated suprafascially until a sizable perforator is located and is used either as pedicled or free flap.

The groin flap as a septocutaneous flap provides a large amount of skin and soft tissue and may need debulking where

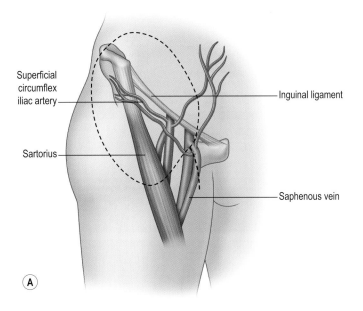

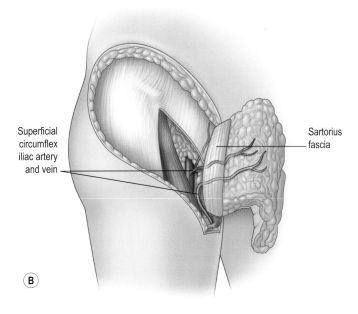

Fig. 5.17 Groin flap elevation. The dominant pedicle is the superficial circumflex iliac artery **(A)**, and venae comitantes and superficial circumflex iliac vein **(B)**.

excess tissue is not needed. However, the perforator flap allows elevation, with thin skin above the fascia. The donor site is well tolerated and well hidden, but the pale skin and frequent hair growth of the donor site make for a poor match, particularly with head and neck reconstructions.

Medial thigh/anteromedial perforator and gracilis perforator

The medial thigh skin is supplied by musculocutaneous as well as septocutaneous perforators. The medial thigh flap located at the midthigh, the dominant blood supply for this fasciocutaneous flap, is the anterior septocutaneous artery

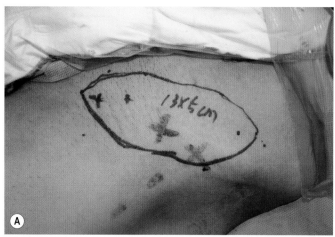

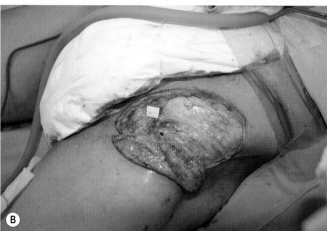

Fig. 5.18 The SCIP flap is nourished by only a perforator of the superficial circumflex iliac system. A large dimension of skin from the inguinal region can be sufficiently supplied by a single perforator.

and venae comitantes from the superficial femoral artery and vein at the apex of the femoral triangle *(Fig. 5.19).*[114] The coverage extends to the abdomen, groin, and perineum. The saphenous vein may be elevated with the flap for improved venous drainage. The sensory innervations are from medial anterior cutaneous nerve of the thigh (L2–3). When the flap is based more anteriorly, it is termed the anteromedial thigh flap and is based on a branch of the lateral femoral circumflex artery emerging from the lateral border of the sartorius. Minor pedicles are contributed by musculocutaneous perforating vessels of the sartorius and gracilis muscles. When the flap is moved proximally to the groin, a perforator from the gracilis muscle is found originating from the profunda femoris vessel or the medial femoral circumflex vessel. All these flaps can be elevated as a perforator-based flap and named a medial thigh perforator flap, anteromedial thigh perforator flap, and gracilis perforator (medial circumflex femoral artery perforator) flap, respectively.[115–118]

For the medial thigh septocutaneous flap, the dominant pedicle is typically located at the apex of the femoral triangle approximately 6–8 cm below the inguinal ligament and is bordered medially by the adductor longus and laterally by the sartorius. A proximal incision is made to locate the vessels at the apex of the femoral triangle. The remainder of the flap is then incised and elevated subfascially.

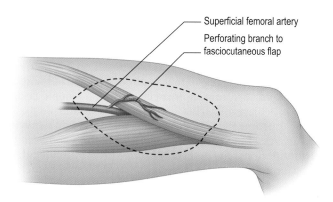

Fig. 5.19 The medial thigh flap located at the mid thigh. The dominant blood supply for this fasciocutaneous flap is the anterior septocutaneous artery and venae comitantes from the superficial femoral artery and vein at the apex of the femoral triangle.

Lateral thigh/profunda femoris perforator

The lateral thigh flap located along the lateral aspect of the thigh between the greater trochanter and the knee can be based on the three perforating branches of the profunda femoris *(Fig. 5.20).*[114] The first perforator arises just below the

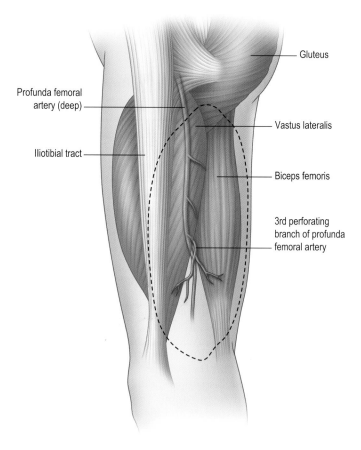

Fig. 5.20 The lateral thigh flap. It is located along the lateral aspect of the thigh between the greater trochanter and the knee can be based on the three perforating branches of the profunda femoris.

insertion of the gluteus maximus and flaps based on this perforator is used for proximally based flaps to reach the trochanteric and ischial areas. The third perforator arises between the vastus lateralis and biceps femoris muscles, midway between the greater trochanter and lateral condyle of the femur and the flaps based on the second or third perforator is for use as a microvascular transplantation because of the long pedicle. The flap is innervated from the lateral cutaneous nerve of the thigh (L2–3).

Anterolateral thigh perforator

The anterolateral thigh perforator flap is one of the most widely used perforator flaps. This flap was first reported as a fasciocutaneous flap by Baek and Song et al.[114,119] The skin can be elevated from a septocutaneous or musculocutaneous perforator. Numerous perforators are found along the region of intermuscular septum between the vastus lateralis and rectus femoris. These perforators usually drains into the descending branch of the lateral femoral circumflex artery then proximally to lateral circumflex artery then to the profunda femoris artery *(Fig. 5.21)*. When perforators are traced to the source vessel, it allows the pedicle to have long length and thicker diameter. Innervation of the anterolateral thigh region is from lateral femoral cutaneous nerve (L2–3). The perforator frequently dissected is usually located on the midpoint of the line drawn between anterior superior iliac spine and superior

lateral border of the patella. The perforator branches are identified with Doppler near the midpoint of this line. According to our clinical experience, about 90% of perforators are found within 3 cm diameter drawn at the midpoint of the line. The skin flap is designed to include the perforator and then elevated from the medial border. The flaps can be large as 35 × 25 cm, based on a single perforator.[120] The incision is made through the deep fascia and raised subfascially until the intermuscular septum between the rectus femoris and vastus lateralis muscle is reached. Now with increased knowledge of the perforator flap anatomy, flaps can be easily elevated suprafascially taking just a small cuff of fascia. At that point, the descending branch of the lateral femoral circumflex is explored along with the perforator to the skin flap. The flap can be harvested, either as a perforator flap including only the perforator branch to the skin or combined with the vastus lateralis muscle, as a musculocutaneous flap. The skin paddle may be defatted according to the need up to 3–4 mm thickness, except for the portion which the perforator branch enters *(Fig. 5.22)*. The motor branch of the femoral nerve running medial to the descending branch of the lateral circumflex femoral artery should be preserved. To elevate as a sensate flap, a branch of the lateral femoral cutaneous nerve should be included. The donor site can be primarily closed depending on the laxity of the skin.

Anterolateral thigh flap isolated on lateral branch of descending lateral femoral circumflex artery and lateral femoral cutaneous nerve

Fig. 5.21 The anterolateral thigh flap. Numerous perforators are found along the region of intermuscular septum between the vastus lateralis and rectus femoris. These perforators usually drains into the descending branch of the lateral femoral circumflex artery then proximally to lateral circumflex artery then to the profunda femoris artery.

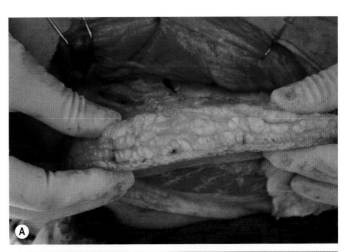

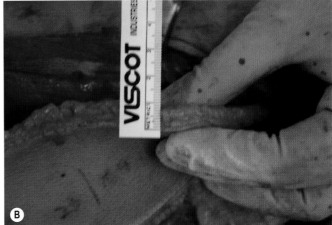

Fig. 5.22 (A,B) The deep fat portion of the anterolateral thigh can be debulked to obtain a thinner pliable flap.

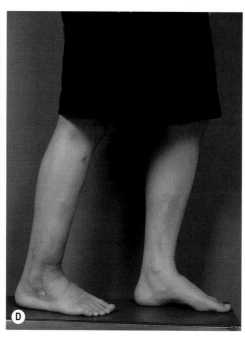

Fig. 5.22, cont'd (C,D) The patient with soft tissue defect of the ankle region is seen with excellent contour after reconstruction without further debulking.

Sural

The sural flap is located between the popliteal fossa and the midportion of the leg over the midline raphe between the two heads of the gastrocnemius muscle. It is one of the longest fasciocutaneous flap of the lower leg based on the direct cutaneous artery (sural artery branch) in the upper central calf and extending to the Achilles tendon distally.[121,122] The lesser saphenous vein provides venous drainage. It can cover defects of the knee, popliteal fossa, and upper-third of the leg. When used distally based on a reverse flow through anastomoses between the peroneal artery and the communicating vascular network of the medial sural nerve, it can reach difficult areas of defects in the lower leg and the ankle and heel region *(Fig. 5.23)*.[123] It is innervated by the medial sural cutaneous nerve (S1–2).

The flap is raised from distal to proximal, in the plane beneath the deep fascia and above the gastrocnemius muscles. The sural nerve and lesser saphenous vein are divided distally and elevated with the flap. The pedicle should be visualized and protected in the popliteal fossa, with continued dissection of the pedicle for free tissue harvesting. For free tissue transplantation, proximal superficial veins should be dissected and preserved for possible anastomosis because the venae comitantes are small.

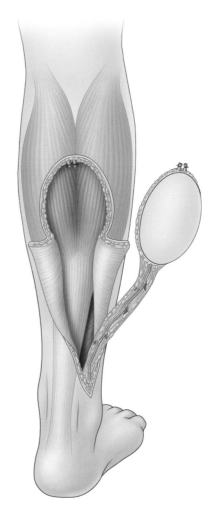

Fig. 5.23 The reverse sural artery flap is a fasciocutaneous flap based on the median superficial sural artery and its communication with the perforating branch of the peroneal artery situated in the region of the lateral malleolar gutter. Reverse flow is established after elevation of the flap and with division of the sural artery and the nerve proximally.

Tap (thoracodorsal artery perforator)

This flap was first described by Angrigiani et al.[124] The vascular territory lies on top of the latissimus dorsi muscle. The main perforators are located along the course of the descending branch of thoracodorsal artery or from the lateral branch. The most proximal perforator reaches the subcutaneous tissue in a point located 2 or 3 cm posterior to the lateral edge of the muscle and 8 cm below the posterior axillary fold.[125] The patient is positioned in a lateral decubitus position with the upper arm in 90° abduction and 90° flexion at the elbows. The lateral border of the latissimus is palpated and marked. Doppler can be useful to identify potential perforators for the flap. Most proximal perforators can be anticipated as mentioned above. Once perforators are identified, a flap can be designed based on the perforator. Although larger flap dimensions have been reported, flap dimensions under 255 cm² within its vascular territory should be safe from partial necrosis.[126] Incision is made from the anterointerior border of the flap allowing the identification of the anterior border of the latissimus dorsi muscle. The dissection is performed between the fat and deep fascia covering the muscle. This plane is easy to dissect as it is in a loose areolar plane. While dissecting for the perforator, care should be given when dissecting the proximal portion as direct cutaneous or perforators adjacent to the anterior borders are easily missed. After a suitable perforator is identified, the design of the flap, in accordance with the defect and pedicle, can be made. Perforators can be isolated or taken with a muscle cuff reaching down to the main pedicle. Total pedicle length depends on the location of perforator and the intramuscular course of the pedicle. Pedicle length can be acquired up to 14–18 cm (*Fig. 5.24*).

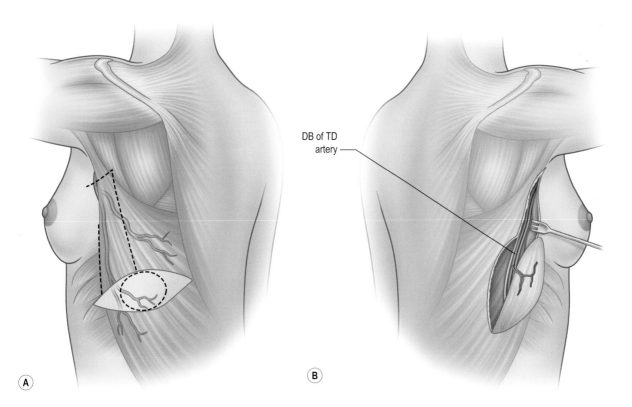

DB of TD
artery

(A)   (B)

Fig. 5.24 Thoracodorsal artery perforator flap. The main perforators are located along the course of descending branch (DB) of thoracodorsal (TD) artery or from the lateral branch. The most proximal perforator reaches the subcutaneous tissue in a point located 2 or 3 cm posterior to the lateral edge of the muscle and 8 cm below the posterior axillary fold.

Compound flaps

The complexity of reconstruction has changed from simple coverage to addressing the issue of function and cosmetics. Frequently, a simple flap can result in adequate reconstruction and may undergo several revisions until the final outcome becomes acceptable. A compound flap consists of multiple tissue components linked together in a manner that allows their simultaneous transfer.[127] These separate components can be maneuvered and placed in a three-dimensional manner to achieve an ideal one-stage reconstruction. Today, as complex and complicated defects are challenged, reconstruction using these compound flaps is becoming routine for these cases.

According to Hallock's classification, the subdivisions of compound flaps are those with a solitary source of vascularization and those with combinations of sources of vascularization (*Fig. 5.25*).[128] Those with a solitary source include composite flaps, defined as multiple tissue components, all served by the same single vascular supply, and thereby consisting of dependent parts. Those flaps with combinations of sources of vascularization include conjoined flaps and chimeric flaps. Conjoined flaps are defined as multiple flap territories, dependent because of some common physical junction, yet each retains its independent vascular supply. The chimeric flaps are defined as multiple flap territories, each with an independent vascular supply, and independent of any physical interconnection, except where linked by a common source vessel (*Fig. 5.26*).

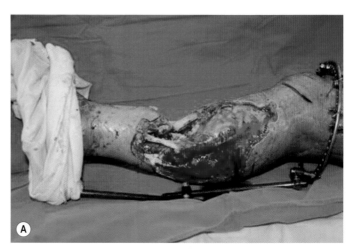

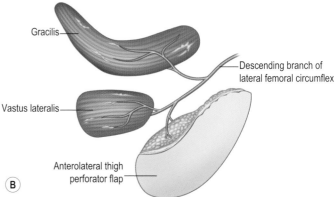

Gracilis

Vastus lateralis

Descending branch of lateral femoral circumflex

Anterolateral thigh perforator flap

B

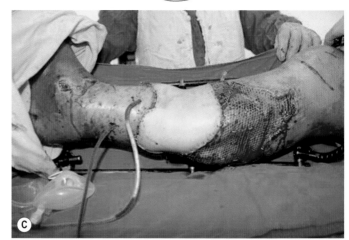

C

Fig. 5.26 The chimeric flaps defined as multiple flap territories, each with an independent vascular supply, and independent of any physical interconnection except where linked by a common source vessel. Example of complex extremity reconstruction is shown using a chimeric approach. The source vessel of the descending branch of the lateral femoral circumflex artery feeding the vastus lateralis and the anterolateral thigh perforator flap. A gracilis is connected using a branch from the source vessel.

Composite

Conjoined

Chimeric

Fig. 5.25 Classification of compound flaps.

Supermicrosurgery

The supermicrosurgery technique is defined as microsurgical anastomosis of vessels, with a diameter <0.8 mm.[109,129] This technique, although reported frequently on lymphaticovenous shunting to treat lymphedema and sporadically in soft tissue reconstruction with specific indications is relatively a new concept for lower extremity reconstruction.[129–132] For the lower extremity soft tissue reconstruction, one of the applications can be seen in the perforator-to-perforator anastomoses approach.[68,111] With an evident pulse on the perforating artery, it can be successfully used as a recipient vessel to supply a sizable flap. This approach will allow an increase in the selection of recipient pedicles. By using a perforator-to-perforator anastomosis approach, less time is consumed to secure the recipient vessel, to elevate the flap by taking just a short segment of the perforator pedicle, and minimizes any risk for major vessel injury or can utilize collateral circulation without apparent flow of major vessels while having acceptable flap survival (*Fig. 5.27*). Further, studies on physiology and anatomy will be needed to evaluate the extent of application.

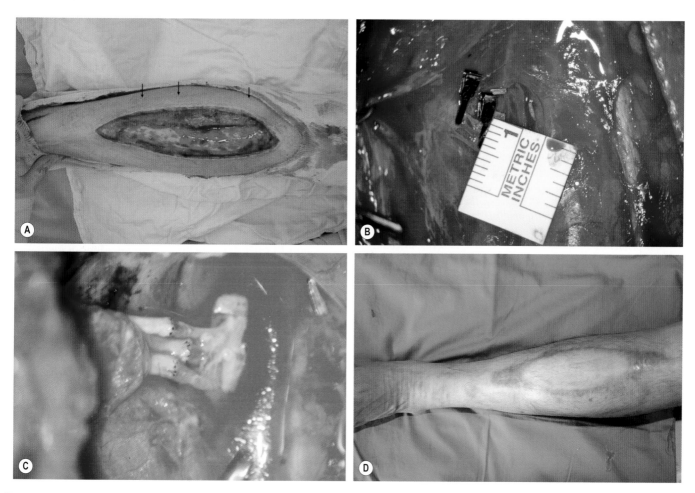

Fig. 5.27 (A) The application of supermicrosurgery (perforator to perforator anastomosis) on the lower extremity is shown. A patient with chronic osteomyelitis is seen after debridement. **(B)** A recipient perforator was located adjacent to the defect margin piercing the fascia with a good visual pulse. **(C)** After the elevation of anterolateral thigh with a short perforator pedicle segment, anastomosis is performed. **(D)** The flap is shown to have good contour without recurrence of infection.

Access the complete reference list online at **http://www.expertconsult.com**

1. Bosse MJ, MacKenzie EJ, Kellam JF, et al. An analysis of outcomes of reconstruction or amputation after leg-threatening injuries. *N Engl J Med*. 2002;347(24): 1924–1931.

   The authors from Carolinas Medical Center performed a multicenter, prospective, observational study of 569 patients with severe leg trauma and evaluated the sickness-impact profile, a multidimensional self-reported health status to determine the long-term outcomes after amputation or limb reconstruction. They report that at 2 years, there was no significant difference in scores for the Sickness Impact Profile between the amputation and reconstruction groups. They advise patients with limbs at high risk for amputation may undergo reconstruction and will have results in 2-year equivalent to those of amputation

2. Chung KC, Saddawi-Konefka D, Haase SC, et al. A cost-utility analysis of amputation versus salvage for Gustilo type IIIB and IIIC open tibial fractures. *Plast Reconstr Surg*. 2009;124(6):1965–1973.

   The authors from the University of Michigan Health System evaluated the cost following amputation and salvage using the data presented in a study from the Lower Extremity Assessment Project. The authors extracted relevant data on projected lifetime costs and analyzed them to include discounting and sensitivity analysis by considering patient age. They report amputation is more expensive than salvage, independently of varied ongoing prosthesis needs, discount rate, and patient age at presentation. Moreover, amputation yields fewer quality-adjusted life-years than salvage. Salvage is deemed the dominant, cost-saving strategy.

11. Godina M. Early microsurgical reconstruction of complex trauma of the extremities. *Plast Reconstr Surg*. 1986;78(3):285–292.

19. Ong YS, Levin LS. Lower limb salvage in trauma. *Plast Reconstr Surg*. 2010;125(2):582–588.

    The authors from the Duke University Medical center review the approach to lower limb salvage. They state that the primary goal of limb salvage is to restore or maintain function based on proper patient selection, timely reconstruction, and choosing the best procedure which should be individualized for each patient. Aggressive debridement and skeletal stabilization, followed by early reconstruction, are the current standard of practice and give better results than the more traditional approach of repeated debridements and delayed flap cover. For reconstruction, they state that free tissue transfer remains the best choice for large defects, but local fasciocutaneous flaps are a reasonable alternative for smaller defects and cases in which free flaps are deemed not suitable.

36. Gottlieb LJ, Krieger LM. From the reconstructive ladder to the reconstructive elevator. *Plast Reconstr Surg*. 1994;93(7):1503–1504.

56. Lange RH. Limb reconstruction versus amputation decision making in massive lower extremity trauma. *Clin Orthop Relat Res*. 1989;Jun(243):92–99.

    This study from the University of Wisconsin describes the absolute and relative indications for primary amputation of limbs with open tibial fractures. Absolute indications include: anatomically complete disruption of the posterior tibial nerve in adults and crush injuries with warm ischemia time greater than 6 h. Relative indications include: serious associated polytrauma, severe ipsilateral foot trauma, and anticipated protracted course to obtain soft tissue coverage and tibial reconstruction. However, he states that Individual patient variables, specific extremity injury characteristics, and associated injuries must all be weighed before a decision can be reached and further prospective studies are necessary before a well-defined protocol for primary amputation can be properly developed.

68. Hong JP. The use of supermicrosurgery in lower extremity reconstruction: the next step in evolution. *Plast Reconstr Surg*. 2009;123(1):230–235.

69. Kindsfater K, Jonassen EA. Osteomyelitis in grade II and III open tibia fractures with late debridement. *J Orthop Trauma*. 1995;9(2):121–127.

88. Chen KT, Mardini S, Chuang DC, et al. Timing of presentation of the first signs of vascular compromise dictates the salvage outcome of free flap transfers. *Plast Reconstr Surg*. 2007;120(1):187–195.

108. Wei FC, Celik N. Perforator flap entity. *Clin Plast Surg*. 2003;30(3):325–329.

    The authors from the Chang Gun Memorial hospital state the perforator flap is not a new concept in microsurgery but there is still confusion and that studies about the differences between these flaps and the conventional flaps, including donor site morbidity and long-term follow-ups, are increasing in literature. Better accuracy in reconstruction, including the use of only cutaneous tissue, minimization of the morbidity, and preserving the same survival rate in free flaps are reassurances to microsurgeons to perform perforator flaps. He believes that in the near future with refinements in the techniques and instruments, perforator flaps will be the first choice flap.

6

Diagnosis and treatment of painful neuroma and of nerve compression in the lower extremity

A. Lee Dellon

SYNOPSIS

- Neuroma pain is due to regenerating axon sprouts trapped in scar:
  - Nerve block will identify the peripheral nerve causing the pain
  - Remember that more than one peripheral nerve may be involved
  - A critical sensory nerve should be reconnected to its target
  - A noncritical sensory nerve should have the neuroma resected
  - It is OK to "lose your nerve": trade pain for anesthesia
  - The proximal end of resected nerve must be placed into "quiet place"
  - Implantation of sensory nerve into a normal muscle is evidence-based
  - Choose an appropriate muscle for the location of the peripheral nerve
  - Remember that the painful neuroma may be in a painful joint
  - Postoperative rehabilitation must include water walking and not massage.
- Chronic nerve compression is common in the lower extremity:
  - The most common site of entrapment is the distal tibial nerve
  - Next most common site is peroneal nerve at fibular neck
  - Next most common site is deep peroneal nerve at foot dorsum
  - Superficial peroneal nerve (SPN) can be entrapped too
  - Remember to look in both anterior and lateral compartment for SPN
  - Tarsal tunnel is not carpal tunnel, but analogous to the forearm
  - Must neurolyse medial and lateral plantar nerves distal to tarsal tunnel
  - Must neurolyse calcaneal nerve in its tunnel distal to tarsal tunnel
  - Postoperative rehab must include immediate ambulation.
- Standards of care
  - Use of tourniquet, loupe magnification, and bipolar coagulation.

Access the Historical Perspective section online at
http://www.expertconsult.com

Introduction

The lower extremity is clearly included within the scope of practice of the plastic surgeon from many points of view. As this volume attests, the lower extremity can be deformed congenitally and it can be injured, both requiring reconstruction. The reconstruction might even be considered aesthetic, in terms of those patients requesting calf implants or those requesting skin tightening following massive weight loss. Surely, loss of tissue after burns or high- or low-velocity ballistic injuries, with or without bone loss, is truly reconstructive in nature. Finally, the lower extremity is now considered an invaluable "bank" of all combinations of parts that can be used, through microsurgery, to reconstruct virtually all other body parts: intermetatarsophalangeal joint, second plus third toe, or great toe to reconstruct fingers and the thumb. The gracilis muscle can be used to reconstruct the facial smile or forearm flexor muscles, or the anterolateral thigh fasciocutaneous flap can be used to reconstruct soft-tissue defects from the orbit to the abdominal wall or the contralateral extremity.

With the exception of harvesting the sural nerve from the leg to use as a graft for various upper extremity nerve reconstructions, or for cross-facial nerve grafting, the peripheral nerve component of the lower extremity has been largely ignored. To be sure, orthopedic or podiatric foot and ankle surgery textbooks have an obligatory chapter on the tarsal tunnel syndrome and Morton's neuroma, but relatively little else. Mackinnon and Dellon, in 1989, attempted to apply those principles established for upper extremity peripheral nerve surgery to the lower extremity,[1] addressing, for example, the problems related to the tibial nerve at the level of the ankle, and the problems related to the peroneal nerve at the knee, leg, and foot level, as well as the problems with the sural nerve and the interdigital nerve.

The pathophysiology of chronic nerve compression and neuroma formation has been described, and approaches have been elucidated to diagnose these problems, clinically stage them, and surgically treat them. Over the past two decades, much more has been learned about lower extremity peripheral nerve problems, and it is the purpose of this chapter to introduce the evidence base now available to improve patient care. The continued failure of a patient to be treated successfully for a painful neuroma is most likely due to our failure to educate physicians about this relatively newly acquired knowledge. All medical and surgical disciplines that deal with these patients – plastic surgeons, pain management physicians, neurologists, neurosurgeons, and both the orthopedic and the podiatric foot and ankle surgeons – should be aware of these conditions and have an understanding of how they are best treated.

Basic science/disease process

The painful neuroma

Understanding, diagnosing, and treating a painful neuroma should no longer be a mystery or a problem. The response of the peripheral nerve to injury has been defined, the factors that thwart neural regeneration so that a neuroma does not form have been defined, and techniques to treat the painful neuroma have been developed.

A peripheral nerve is covered with a myelin sheath produced by a Schwann cell.

The cell body for a sensory neuron of the peripheral nervous system lies in a dorsal root ganglion and from the exit of this nerve from the vertebral foramen it is covered with Schwann cells *(Fig. 6.1)*. This is in contrast to the true cranial nerves with sensory function, like the optic and olfactory nerves, which are extensions of the central nervous system, and do not regenerate successfully to the distal target organ.[6] When a peripheral nerve is injured, for example by a complete transection, the distal portion of the nerve degenerates (Wallerian degeneration).[7] Since the Schwann cell is a single cell living along the length of the degenerating axon of the peripheral nerve, the Schwann cell remains alive. Ultimately, all that will remain of the nerve is the basement membrane that was elaborated by the Schwann cell. When the interaction between the axon and the Schwann cell is lost, the Schwann cell up-regulates and produces nerve growth factor.[8] The proximal end of the peripheral nerve will produce axon sprouts within 24 hours of the nerve transection, which will begin to regenerate distally. The sprouts are lured by the nerve growth factor, and will track preferentially along the basement membrane, for whose negatively charged laminin and type IV collagen the sprouts have an affinity *(Fig. 6.2)*.[9–11] The regeneration will proceed along the distal pathway towards the appropriate target end-organ.[12]

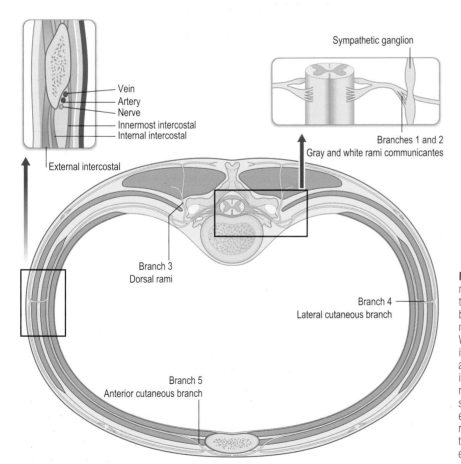

Vein
Artery
Nerve
Innermost intercostal
Internal intercostal
External intercostal

Sympathetic ganglion

Branches 1 and 2
Gray and white rami communicantes

Branch 3
Dorsal rami

Branch 4
Lateral cutaneous branch

Branch 5
Anterior cutaneous branch

Fig. 6.1 The spinal nerve is formed from a ventral (motor) root and a dorsal (sensory) root of the spinal cord. Note that the dorsal root is joined to dorsal ganglia that contain the cell bodies of the sensory neurons, whereas the cell bodies of the motor neurons are contained within the spinal cord itself. When the spinal nerve exits the vertebral foramen it becomes ensheathed by Schwann cells and is termed a peripheral nerve. This particular peripheral nerve is illustrated as arising from the thoracic spine region, in which region its sensory branches directly innervate the skin without formation of a plexus, as occurs for the lower extremity from the lumbosacral plexus. Note that the dorsal ramus of the spinal nerve can be entrapped in its passage to the lower back, causing symptoms of chronic nerve entrapment termed "notalgia paraesthetica."

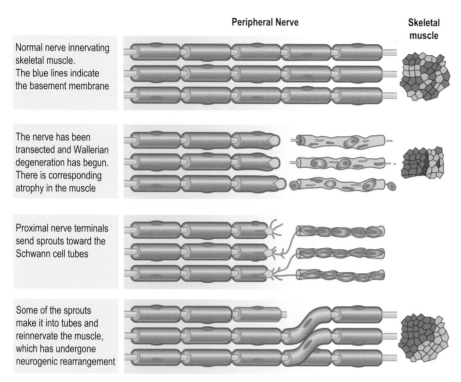

Peripheral Nerve

Skeletal muscle

Normal nerve innervating skeletal muscle. The blue lines indicate the basement membrane

The nerve has been transected and Wallerian degeneration has begun. There is corresponding atrophy in the muscle

Proximal nerve terminals send sprouts toward the Schwann cell tubes

Some of the sprouts make it into tubes and reinnervate the muscle, which has undergone neurogenic rearrangement

Fig. 6.2 **(A)** A transection injury to a peripheral nerve results in degeneration of the axon distal to the site of transection (wallerian degeneration). **(B)** The Schwann cells along this distal segment of the axon survive, up-regulate, and produce nerve growth factor, while the axons of the proximal segment produce sprouts for distal regeneration. **(C)** When neural regeneration proceeds unimpeded, the axons will return to their distal target organ, with the creation of an in-continuity neuroma. **(D)** When neural regeneration is impeded by scar tissue from the injury, distal regeneration does not occur and an end-bulb neuroma forms.

If this process is thwarted at the site of neural regeneration, a neuroma will form. A neuroma is a benign tumor created by axon sprouts becoming encased in collagen. A neuroma will become painful if it is located in an area that subjects these sprouts to stimulation. Such sites include locations that are superficial, next to joints, adherent to moving tendons, and subjacent to weight-bearing surfaces. The common denominator for all of these is tension. The tension causes the fibroblasts in the region of the axon sprouts to produce the collagen that results in the growth of the neuroma and the adherence of the neuroma to surrounding structures.[13]

Within this evolving mass of axon sprouts and fibroblasts, abnormal communications or synapse-like structures may form between nerves that normally do not communicate with each other. These are the source of ephaptic conduction, which has been shown to be the origin of pain signals from the small myelinated group A-delta and unmyelinated group C fibers. Spontaneous origin of signals from these pain and temperature fibers have been recorded by single-unit neurophysiologic techniques from neuromas of the radial sensory nerve in the baboon.[14] For example, that study found that 10% of more than 200 fibers that were studied had spontaneous activity in a 2-month neuroma, and this percentage increased to 18% in a 7-month neuroma, which was twice the activity found in the same-diameter intact (control) nerves. That study also demonstrated that the neuroma was mechanosensitive; just touching it generated signals, which did not occur from the control nerves. These findings provide the basis for the author's current treatment strategy that involves resecting the end-bulb neuroma, instead of the traditional approach that involved just moving the "mature end-bulb neuroma" to a new place that was "quiet."[15–17]

Chronic nerve compression

The pathophysiology of chronic nerve compression implies that the evaluation of nerve function must be based upon the knowledge that there will be a progressive loss of peripheral nerve function. Therefore, the diagnosis and treatment of chronic nerve compression are based upon an understanding of this pathophysiology. The structure and function of the peripheral nerve, and how these are altered with increasing degrees of pressure and with increasing lengths of time, have been investigated in rat, rabbit, and monkey animal models,[18–28] and many of these models have used the sciatic nerve. Therefore, the disease process is the same for the better-known upper extremity nerve compressions as it is for the lesser-known lower extremity peripheral nerve compressions.

A review of this literature indicates that if there is a constriction of greater than 20% placed upon the diameter of the peripheral nerve, then acute axonal degeneration will occur. If there is a pressure of greater than 20 mmHg applied to the peripheral nerve, there will be a decrease in blood flow. In the acute situation, these conditions produce pain. If this degree of compression comes on over a gradual period of time, and over a length of the peripheral nerve that is several times the diameter of the nerve, then the conditions produce chronic nerve compression. After about 2 months of compression by a silicone tube that does not constrict the diameter of the nerve, the first changes in the pathophysiology occur. These are a weakening of the tight junctions of the endothelial cells in the perineurium, and this results in serum entering the endoneurial space. This creates endoneurial edema. When this occurs in the relatively tight confines of the perineurium, there is an increase in pressure that will decrease blood flow. The conscious perception of this is paresthesia. At this point in time, the only clinical findings will be related to the cutaneous sensory threshold for touch, which will first become elevated for static two-point discrimination, or will manifest itself as a change in perception of vibratory stimuli applied with a tuning fork or a vibrometer.[29,30] These pathophysiologic concepts provide a basis for staging chronic nerve compression *(Tables 6.1–6.4)*.

After about 6 months of this degree of compression, the first histologic changes in myelin can be observed. This consists of thinning of the myelin. With progressive compression, there will be increasing loss of myelin, so that under slides in which a myelin stain has been used, it appears as if there has been a loss of the large myelinated, touch, fibers. They will not actually have begun to degenerate yet, as demonstrated by electron microscopy, in which the unmyelinated large fibers can be demonstrated still to be present. At this stage, the patient will have weakness in the motor system related to the muscles supplied by that nerve, and increasing numbness in the territory (fingers) related to the sensory supply of that nerve. Pinch and grip strength can be measured directly. There will be no atrophy, because without true loss of the motor axons, there will be no decrease in bulk of the muscles. At this stage of compression, the cutaneous pressure thresholds will be elevated increasingly for the quickly adapting fibers, measured either with vibrometry or with moving two-point discrimination with the Pressure-Specified Sensory Device (PSSD),[31] and for the slowly adapting fibers, measured with static two-point discrimination with the PSSD. Although no longitudinal study using the Semmes–Weinstein nylon monofilaments has been published in patients with chronic nerve compression,[33] the analogous measurement, made with the PSSD, which is one-point static touch, is still normal at this stage of compression.[12] Two-point discrimination, measured in millimeters, is still normal, because no nerve fibers have died. At this stage in chronic nerve compression, with myelin thinning, traditional electrodiagnostic testing may begin to detect increases in the distal sensory latency. Amplitudes will still be normal because no nerve fibers have died yet. In general, quantitative neurosensory testing is more

sensitive than traditional electrodiagnostic testing (nerve conduction study/electromyogram), so it is more likely to detect this stage of nerve compression. Neurosensory testing is less expensive than nerve conduction study/electromyogram, and will not cause the patient any pain.[34,35]

If either the length of time is increased for this degree of compression, or if the degree of compression increases, whether due to work, metabolic or rheumatologic disease, then neural degeneration occurs. As suggested in the preceding paragraph, this will be detected in the motor system by muscle wasting and in the sensory system by abnormal distance at which one from two points can be distinguished. Examples of these changes are given in *Table 6.2* for median nerve compression at the wrist, *Table 6.3* for ulnar nerve compression at the elbow, and *Table 6.4* for tibial nerve compression in the tarsal tunnel.[27,29] Using the PSSD, this change occurs first for static two-point discrimination and then for moving two-point discrimination. This was demonstrated in a retrospective analysis of patients with carpal and cubital tunnel syndrome. The one-point static touch measurement will become abnormal some time after the change in two-point discrimination distance, and is therefore a relatively

Table 6.1 Numerical grading scale for any peripheral nerve[32]

Grade	Description
0	Normal
1	Intermittent sensory symptoms
2	Increased sensorimotor threshold
3	Increased sensorimotor threshold
4	Increased sensorimotor threshold
5	Persistent sensory symptoms
6	Sensorimotor degeneration
7	Sensorimotor degeneration
8	Sensorimotor degeneration
9	Anesthesia
10	Muscle atrophy, severe

Table 6.2 Numerical grading scale for the median nerve at the wrist level[32]

Numerical score		Description of impairment
Sensory	Motor	
0	0	None
1		Paresthesia, intermittent
2		Abnormal pressure threshold (Pressure-Specifice Sensory Device)
		<45 years old: ≤3 mm, at 1.0–20 g/mm^2
		≥45 years old: ≤4 mm, at 2.2–20 g/mm^2
	3	Weakness, thenar muscles
4		Abnormal pressure threshold (Pressure-Specifice Sensory Device)
		<45 years old: ≤3 mm, at >20 g/mm^2
		≥45 years old: ≤4 mm, at 20 g/mm^2
5		Paresthesias, persistent
6		Abnormal innervation density (Pressure-Specifice Sensory Device)
		<45 years old: ≥4 mm < 8 mm, at any g/mm^2
		≥45 years old: ≥5 mm < 9 mm, at any g/mm^2
	7	Muscle wasting (1–2/4)
8		Abnormal innervation density (Pressure-Specifice Sensory Device)
		<45 years old: ≥8 mm, at any g/mm^2
		>45 years old: ≥9 mm, at any g/mm^2
9		Anesthesia
	10	Muscle wasting (3–4/4)

Table 6.3 Numerical grading scale for the ulnar nerve at the elbow level[32]

Numerical score		Description of impairment
Sensory	Motor	
0	0	None
1		Paresthesia, intermittent
	2	Weakness: pinch/grip (lb)
		Female: 10–14/26–39
		Male: 13–19/31–59
3		Abnormal pressure threshold (Pressure-Specified Sensory Device)
		<45 years old: ≤3 mm, at 1.0–20.0 g/mm^2
		≥45 years old: ≤4 mm, at 1.9–20.0 g/mm^2
	4	Weakness: Pinch/grip (lb)
		Female: 6–9/15–25
		Male: 6–12/15–30
5		Paresthesia, persistent
6		Abnormal innervation density (Pressure-Specified Sensory Device)
		<45 years old: ≥4 mm <8 mm, at any g/mm^2
		≥45 years old: ≥9 mm, at any g/mm^2
9		Anesthesia
	10	Muscle wasting (3–4/4)

Table 6.4 Numerical grading scale for the tibial nerve at ankle level

Numerical score		Description of impairment
Sensory	Motor	
0	0	None
1		Paresthesia, intermittent
2		Abnormal pressure threshold (Pressure-Specified Sensory Device)
		<45 years old: ≤5.6 mm, at 1.0–20 g/mm^2
		≥45 years old: ≤7.8 mm, at 2.2–20 g/mm^2
	3	Weakness, abductor hallucis
4		Abnormal pressure threshold (Pressure-Specified Sensory Device)
		<45 years old: ≤5.6 mm, at 20 g/mm^2
		≥45 years old: ≤7.8 mm, at 20 g/mm^2
5		Paresthesias, persistent
6		Abnormal innervation density (Pressure-Specified Sensory Device)
		<45 years old: ≥7 mm <10 mm, at any g/mm^2
		≥45 years old: ≥9 mm < 12 mm, at any g/mm^2
	7	Intrinsic muscle wasting, clawing (1–2/4)
8		Abnormal innervation density (Pressure-Specified Sensory Device)
		<45 years old: ≥11 mm, at any given g/mm^2
		≥45 years old: ≥15 mm, at any g/mm^2
9		Anesthesia
	10	Intrinsic muscle wasting, clawing (3–4/4)

insensitive tool for detecting the onset of this stage. Vibrometry and tuning fork use can identify this stage, but does not permit the therapist to identify correctly which nerve is being compressed without additional testing. It must be remembered that the vibratory stimulus travels as a wave, whereas the pressure stimulus remains localized to the applied test site.[23,24,31] For example, if the involved nerve is the tibial nerve, and the hallux pulp is tested, there may still be relatively preserved sensation mediated by the peroneal nerve. Testing of both the dorsum of the foot and hallux pulp and medial heel may permit distinction of which nerve is involved.

If there is some limitation on the gliding of the peripheral nerve through its site of anatomic narrowing, then, when the adjacent joint moves, there will an increase in tension along the length of the nerve which may manifest itself as a further increase in pressure upon the nerve. This limitation of gliding may come from some injury or anatomic variant that limits excursion of the nerves. This subject will be discussed in detail related to individual nerve compression syndromes.

Statistical evaluation of the results of the treatment of nerve compression has been difficult due to the failure of most reports to distinguish the degree of nerve compression among the patients in the study. An entire group of patients with nerve compression is usually described following surgery as having results that are excellent, good, fair, or poor. In comparing one published study to another, it would be helpful to be able to know the degree of severity of nerve compression in the patients being reported. It would be useful in a given study to know how patients with different degrees of nerve compression responded to the same operation. Even if this is recognized as a goal, without a numerical grading system the author is left only with the choice of indicating what percentage of people who had a mild degree of nerve compression improved, and what percentage of patients with a severe degree of nerve compression improved. With a numerical grading system, as outlined above, a unique number, representing the pathophysiologic condition of the compressed nerve as manifested by its functional impairment can be assigned to each patient, and these numbers can be treated statistically. Finally, treatment strategies and outcome analysis for the peripheral nerve can be analyzed mathematically. When this is done, it should be remembered to use nonparametric statistics.

Diagnosis/patient presentation

The painful neuroma

The patient with a painful neuroma will complain of an area of skin or a joint that causes pain either at rest, or, more commonly, when the part is touched or moved. When an area of pain relates to the territory of a peripheral nerve, and the patient has had an injury or an operation in that area, then consideration must be given to the presence of a painful neuroma of that peripheral nerve. In earlier times, this would have been called "causalgia," but today, if the pain persists for more than 6 months, it is termed "complex regional pain syndrome I." If movement of the ankle or knee creates pain, then consideration must be given to the presence of a neuroma of the nerve that innervates that joint. Anatomy books do not show nerves innervating joints, and this knowledge required cadaver dissections, which have been published for the knee (*Fig. 6.3 B and C*)[36] and for the ankle (*Fig. 6.3A*).[37] Clinical

approaches and results for the lower extremity were reviewed in 2009.[5] Beginning with the knee, and then extending this approach to the ankle, anatomical dissections were performed to identify joint innervation, With this knowledge routes for the administration of local anesthetic were identified. Demonstrating that pain relief is possible by anesthetic blockade in patients who failed traditional musculoskeletal approaches led to the creation of surgical approaches to resect involved nerve(s).

When pain is outside the territory of a single peripheral nerve, and the pain has been present for more than 6 months, and especially if there is an associated change in skin color or temperature, or sweating (sympathetic activity), this syndrome was called reflex sympathetic dystrophy. Today this is called complex regional pain syndrome II. This condition is usually managed by the anesthesia pain management doctor with lumbar sympathetic blocks, and neuropathic pain medication. Ultimately, an implanted spinal nerve stimulator (dorsal column stimulator) or a peripheral nerve stimulator may be implanted. There is often more than one peripheral

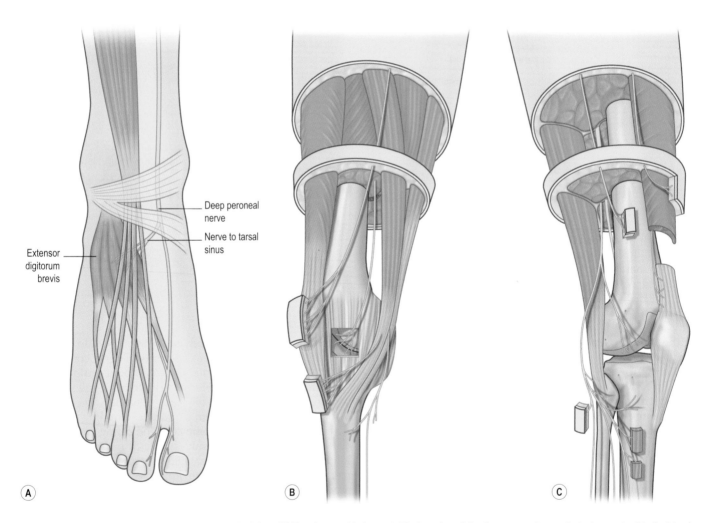

Extensor digitorum brevis

Deep peroneal nerve

Nerve to tarsal sinus

(A)   (B)   (C)

Fig. 6.3 Illustrations of the innervation of lower extremity joints. **(A)** The sinus tarsi is innervated by branches of the deep peroneal nerve that arise proximal to the lateral malleous, just before the branch to the extensor digitorum brevis. **(B)** The medial aspect of the knee joint is innervated by a branch of the femoral nerve. After the femoral nerve innervates the vastus medialis, at which point anatomy books show the nerve terminating, the nerve continues distally and past the end of the muscle to innervate the medial knee structures. **(C)** The lateral aspect of the knee joint is innervated by a branch of the sciatic nerve, which, after it innervates the posterior knee capsule, travels anterior, deep to the biceps tendon, and then innervates the lateral knee structures. The medial and lateral retinacular nerves likely overlap anteriorly, although this has not been proven. (Reproduced with permission from Dellon.com.)

nerve involved: there may be a true cutaneous neuroma, neuroma of the joint afferent, and nerve entrapment or a second peripheral nerve with a neuroma that accounts for the wide distribution of pain. This is a critical diagnostic concept, because it means that the nerve block should be applied to more than one nerve if a single nerve block has not been successful and that the block may also be necessary for the joint afferent. Furthermore, if this approach is successful, spinal stimulators will be unnecessary.

Motor function should be normal physiologically with the exception of two considerations. Firstly, if there is ankle pain, then the patient may not use muscles that cause ankle movement, leading to disuse atrophy of the muscles. Secondly, there is often wasting of the extensor digitorum brevis associated with ankle pain, since the nerve that innervates this muscle, the deep peroneal nerve, has been injured, usually with the stretch/traction associated with an inversion sprain.

Chronic nerve compression

The patient with chronic compression of a peripheral nerve will complain of numbness or paresthesias in the skin territory innervated by that nerve. The patient will complain of weakness in the muscles innervated by that nerve. If both the peroneal and tibial nerves have chronic compression at the same time, the patient will have numbness over the dorsal and plantar aspects of the foot and arising proximal to the ankle. This will give the same appearance as if the patient had a peripheral neuropathy, especially if the problem occurs in both legs. This type of situation occurs in patients who have sports injuries, or other injuries. As a contrast in etiology, but with the same clinical presentation, will be patients who do have a metabolic neuropathy, for example, those with diabetes, or chemotherapy-induced neuropathy, who have secondary chronic nerve compressions. These patients with present with a history of neuropathy, and frequently will not have been examined to identify the presence of a chronic nerve compression.[38] If the nerve compression is diagnosed and treated in such patients, they will frequently experience sensory recovery despite the presence of diabetic neuropathy.

The pathognomonic feature of chronic nerve compression on physical examination is the presence of a positive Hoffman–Tinel sign. With an understanding of the pathophysiology of chronic nerve compression (see above), it becomes clear that in the earliest stage there will be intermittent symptoms and there will be no physical findings present. This is often the situation with musicians, such as the pianist or violinist who complains of numbness in the little finger, from playing with the elbow bent, but has no Hoffman–Tinel sign over the ulnar nerve at the cubital tunnel. In the lower extremity, an analogous situation occurs with the soccer player whose leg may seem to give out, who has received many a blunt trauma to the outside of the knee or repeated ankle inversion sprains, and who has compression of the common peroneal nerve at the fibular neck. With further time and a greater degree of compression, axons will demyelinate and there will be an increase in the threshold required to produce a sensory response; a higher degree of vibration with the tuning fork, or a greater pressure required to discriminate one from two points touching the big-toe pulp with the PSSD while

two-point discrimination distance remains normal. In the motor system, this will correspond to weakness on manual muscle testing. At this point, the Hoffman–Tinel sign will become positive. With further time and degree of compression, axons will die, and there will be a decrease in two-point static touch discrimination (the distance before two points can be distinguished will increase), and muscle atrophy will occur. The Hoffman–Tinel sign will remain positive. With a very advanced degree of compression, the peripheral nerve seems to stop its attempt to remyelinate and regenerate, and the Hoffman–Tinel sign becomes negative. This variation in the presence of the Hoffman–Tinel sign over time is understandable in terms of progression of compression and changes within the peripheral nerve, and should not be interpreted as a failure of the Hoffman–Tinel sign to be a valuable clinical examination technique.[39,40]

Patient selection

The painful neuroma

Selection of the patient for surgical treatment of the painful neuroma begins after the first 6 months of pain. During the first 6 months of the patient's pain, management will usually be done by the primary care physician and/or the original treating surgeon, often in conjunction with a therapist. Most often, the patient will have tried opiates, nonsteroidal anti-inflammatory drugs, massage, ultrasound, and steroid injection. Once the pain has lasted 6 months, the patient enters the phase of chronic pain, and is now traditionally referred to a pain management physician. At this point, the patient will usually be tried on neuropathic pain medication, such as nortriptyline, Neurontin, Cymbalta, or Lyrica, and often a combination of these.

A nerve block is critical in patient selection. In the management of the patient with chronic pain, the pain management physician will often do a nerve block with or without cortisone to identify and treat the peripheral nerve believed to be the source of the pain. If the pain resolves for a few hours and then returns, this block was actually a diagnostic block. If the pain partially resolves, then perhaps more than one peripheral nerve is the source of the pain. If the block fails to resolve, then the local anesthetic failed to achieve its effect either due to the presence of a second involved nerve, or due to an anatomic variation in the peripheral nerve that was supposed to be blocked. If the block actually relieves pain for a prolonged period of time, then it was therapeutic, and it should be repeated by the pain management physician when or if the pain recurs. Failure of the repeat block to achieve pain relief signals an appropriate time for surgical intervention. A sequence of nerve blocks for a painful foot dorsum is given in *Figure 6.4*.

It is the goal of a nerve block to place the local anesthetic adjacent to, not into, the peripheral nerve. If the patient has immediate pain when the needle is inserted, and the pain radiates in the territory of that nerve, then the needle is in the nerve and you should not inject the anesthetic or you will cause a nerve injection injury. You should pull the needle slightly away and then inject. Success of the nerve block requires the patient to say that the pain is gone, and if

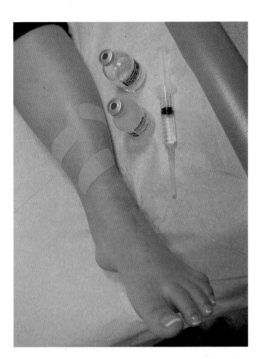

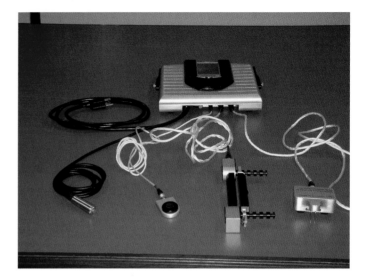

Fig. 6.5 The Pressure-Specified Sensory Device is shown with its components for grip and pinch strength, as well as the device with the two prongs, each of which is attached to a pressure transducer (silver attachment with prongs). The configuration shown is the PDA platform which is portable between offices. No needlestick or electrical stimulation is used. Once the patient perceives the stimulus correctly, a button is pushed by the patient, ending digital signal acquisition, and therefore this is a subjective test of sensibility. (With permission from Sensory Management Services, LLC, Towson, Maryland.)

Fig. 6.4 Sequence of nerve blocks to identify source of dorsal foot pain. The nerve block is done using sterile technique. After swabbing the skin with Betadine, a mixture is prepared that contains half 1% xylocaine and half 0.5 % bupivacaine, each without epinephrine, is prepared. This is injected first next to the saphenous nerve, proximal to the medial malleolus. This is for a painful tarsal tunnel incision, a crushed foot, or a painful bunion incision. Then the deep peroneal nerve is blocked next, above the ankle, between the extensor hallucis longus and the extensor digitorum communis tendons. At this level, the block will also denervate the sinus tarsi. If sinus tarsi pain is only partially eliminated, then you must block the sural nerve, posterior to the lateral malleolus (not shown) as this nerve contributes to sinus tarsi innervation in 25% of patients. Finally, the superficial peroneal nerve is blocked next. This can be done as shown here at the site of a positive Tinel sign, or just dorsolateral to the ankle joint. Following this the patient must attempt to walk, squat, and touch the top of the foot to determine the effect of the block on pain.

it is a cutaneous nerve, that the expected area of skin becomes numb.

Chronic nerve compression

Selection of the patient for surgical decompression of a peripheral nerve requires that at least four conditions are met:

1. the patient's symptoms fit with both the motor and sensory distribution of the given peripheral nerve

2. the impairment is documented by appropriate measurement of the motor and sensory function of that nerve

3. there is a positive Tinel sign at the known site of anatomic narrowing of that nerve

4. all possible nonoperative measures have been employed for 3 months without success in relieving the symptoms.

Note that it is not essential that an electrodiagnostic test be performed and it is not essential that the results of that test demonstrate chronic nerve compression. This is because, even where traditional nerve conduction and electromyography are best for the median nerve at the wrist, the false-negative rate is 33%, and in patients with diabetes, this type of testing

cannot be relied upon to identify the presence of a chronic nerve compression in the presence of an underlying neuropathy.[41] In the lower extremity, in a patient over the age of 55, the false-positive rate for the medial plantar and electromyogram of the medial plantar-innervated muscles is 50%, and therefore, in the adult even without neuropathy, this testing is prone to error. Since traditional testing cannot identify nerve compression in the presence of neuropathy at the wrist, it certainly cannot identify it reliably at the ankle. Therefore, the clinician must rely upon the presence of a positive Hoffman–Tinel sign to indicate the location of the chronic nerve compression.

Neurosensory testing with the PSSD is the most sensitive method to document sensibility in a piece of skin (*Fig. 6.5*). This has been documented to be valid and reliable for both the upper and lower extremity,[31,33,34,41–43] and to be essentially equivalent to the information obtained with traditional electrodiagnostic studies for the median nerve at the wrist in a level I study.[35] For the patient with heel pain, for example, the medial calcaneal nerve will have an abnormal pressure threshold with normal distance for distinguishing one-point from two-point static touch, with normal measurements for the medial plantar (hallux pulp) and normal measurements over the dorsum of the foot. When treatment for plantar fasciitis continues to fail after 3 months, and when the two-point static distance becomes abnormal, then it is appropriate to do a neurolysis of the calcaneal nerve. If the measurements for the hallux pulp are also abnormal, then tarsal tunnel syndrome is present. If the measurements for the dorsum of the foot are abnormal in addition to those for the tibial nerve, then the peroneal nerve is involved too. If the patient has back symptoms that radiate into the foot, then it is appropriate to obtain electrodiagnostic studies to be sure that there is not an L5 or L4 radiculopathy present.

Surgical technique

The painful neuroma (Box 6.1)

The common lower extremity neuromas of cutaneous nerves requiring surgical treatment are those of the SPN,[44] the deep peroneal nerve,[44] the saphenous nerve,[44] the sural nerve,[44] and the calcaneal nerve.[45] A Morton's neuroma is not a true neuroma, but a chronic nerve compression of an interdigital nerve caused by the intermetatarsal ligament, and the treatment is therefore neurolysis by division of the intermetatarsal ligament.[46] However, since most foot and ankle surgeons treat a Morton's neuroma by excision of the interdigital nerve, failure of that approach does create a true neuroma of an interdigital nerve, and this must be treated as a neuroma.[47,48] The most common lower extremity neuroma of a joint afferent is that of the deep peroneal nerve to the sinus tarsi (*Fig. 6.3A*),[37,49] followed by neuromas of the medial and lateral retinacular nerves to the knee joint (*Fig. 6.3B and C and Box 6.2*).[50,51]

A neuroma of the SPN is most often caused by surgical procedures about the lateral ankle, either during open reduction and internal fixation of a fracture/dislocation or during a lateral ankle stabilization procedure. The physical examination usually demonstrates a painful scar with radiation into the dorsum of the foot, either dorsomedial or dorsolateral, but not to the first webspace. The incision is centered on a vertical line that is about 10 cm proximal to the lateral malleolus (*Fig. 6.6*). Both the anterior and the lateral compartment must be opened since it has been demonstrated that about 25% of people will have a high division of this nerve, in either the anterior or both the anterior and the lateral compartment.[52] The branches of the SPN are injected proximally to shield the spinal cord from the pain signal associated with dividing this nerve. The nerve is cauterized distally to prevent bleeding. A

segment can be sent to pathology but this will be a normal nerve, since the neuroma itself, in the scar, is not resected. Implanting the nerve proximally is done into the deep portion of the extensor digitorum communis, the largest muscle. Be careful to prevent kinking of the nerve across the intermuscular septum. The best way to do this is to excise the septum proximally for about 3 cm, being sure to cauterize the septum as it contains blood vessels. The edges of the fasciotomy of the anterior and lateral compartment are also cauterized to prevent postoperative bleeding. A suture of the epineurium into the muscle is not necessary since there is plenty of nerve length and the proximal joint (the knee) is extended during this procedure. Bupivacaine is then injected into the muscle and skin edges and the wound is closed with 4-0 Monocryl interrupted intradermal sutures, and 5-0 interrupted and continuous sutures to the skin.

A neuroma of the deep peroneal nerve can be due to injury over the dorsum of the foot, or a stretch traction injury that causes problems with the nerve that innervates the sinus tarsi proximal to the ankle (*Fig. 6.3A*). In either situation, the surgical technique to resect the deep peroneal nerve is through an incision about 5 cm in length centered about 10 cm proximal to the lateral malleolus. Both the anterior and lateral compartments must be opened to gain access. A neurolysis of the SPN must be done to insure its safety. Then a dissection is done across the interosseous membrane, using the bipolar to lift the muscle origins from the membrane. The dissection continues until the tibia is reached. The retractor is then elevated and the neurovascular bundle is visualized. The deep peroneal nerve is dissected from the artery and vein. Bupivacaine is injected into the nerve proximally (*Fig. 6.6*). A 2.5-cm segment of the nerve is resected, cauterizing the nerve proximally and distally with the bipolar coagulator first. The nerve proximally does not have to be implanted formally into muscle since it is surrounded by muscle. Bupivacaine is then injected into the muscle and skin edges and the wound is closed with 4-0 Monocryl interrupted intradermal sutures, and 5-0 interrupted and continuous sutures of the skin.

A neuroma of the distal saphenous nerve is most often due to a previous surgical procedure, such as ankle arthroscopy, harvesting the saphenous vein, or a tarsal tunnel release. The incision for the neuroma resection must be proximal to the previous site of injury. Once the saphenous vein is identified, if it has not been harvested, you must explore both the sides of the vein, anteriorly and posteriorly for small (<1 mm) nerves. The saphenous nerve has often branched at this point to send the posterior branch into the region of the tarsal tunnel incision and the anterior branch into the region of the ankle arthroscopy. The nerves are each divided distally, dissected proximally, and a window opened into the fascia overlying the soleus muscle (*Fig. 6.7*). A tunnel is created into the muscle and the nerves are loosely implanted. Bupivacaine is then placed, and the skin closed as above.[53]

A neuroma of the sural nerve is due to previous surgery about the ankle, most often during procedures to tighten the ankle from repeated inversion sprains, but often to approaches used for open reduction and internal fixation of fractures. Somewhat more proximally, the nerve may have been injured during a sural nerve biopsy or excision of a skin lesion, or from a direct injury. The approach to the sural nerve must recognize that resecting the sural nerve in the leg, while technically easier, places the nerve at a location where shoes or

---

Box 6.1   Succesful treatment of the painful neuroma

Obtain complete relief of pain with a preoperative nerve block

Remember that more than one nerve may be involved

Remember that an afferent joint may be involved

Remember that part of the pain may be from a compressed nerve

Resect the painful neuroma

Implant the proximal end of the divided nerve into a normal muscle

---

Box 6.2   Implantation of proximal end of nerve into a muscle

The proximal divided end of a cutaneous nerve will attempt to regenerate distally

It has been demonstrated in nonhuman primates that a sensory nerve implanted into a normal muscle will not form a neuroma

Choose a relatively large muscle that is proximal to a joint

Choose a muscle with a relatively short excursion

Implant a relatively long and loose loop of nerve into that muscle

Do not suture the nerve into the muscle (suturing epineurium to fascia is OK)

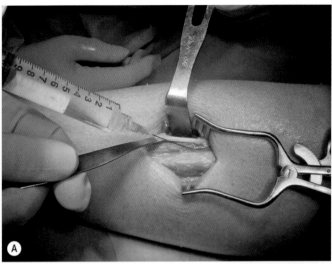

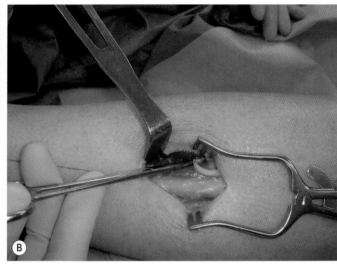

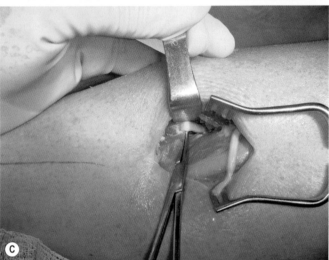

Fig. 6.6 Resection of the superficial peroneal nerve for a painful neuroma is done **(A)** at a distance of about 10 cm proximal to the lateral malleolus. Both the anterior and the lateral compartment must be opened, as shown here, since about 25% of people have a branch located in the anterior compartment. Note the nerve is blocked prior to dividing it to shield the spinal cord from the pain impulse. **(B)** The divided proximal end of the nerve is implanted into the underside of the extensor digitorum communis muscle, loosely, and without impinging upon the septum, a portion of which must always be resected to prevent recurrent pain. No suture is necessary. **(C)** Resection of the deep peroneal nerve requires a neurolysis of the superficial peroneal nerve and release of both the anterior and lateral compartments to prevent postoperative compartment pressure elevations related to the dissection. As is seen in this patient, sometimes this nerve and the superficial peroneal nerve must be resected in the same patient. The dissection proceeds along the interosseous membrane until the neurovascular bundle is identified against the tibia. The nerve is dissected as shown here, then injected, and a 3-cm section is resected, and the proximal end of the nerve allowed to drop back into the intermuscular space.

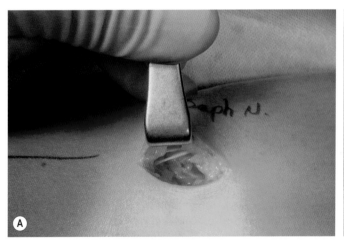

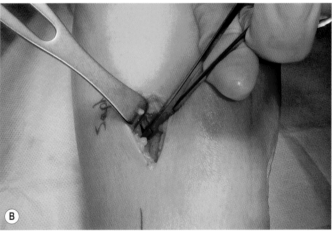

Fig. 6.7 The saphenous nerve innervates the skin of the proximal portion of the tarsal tunnel incision and can be the source of this scar hurting. Ankle arthroscopy can injure it as well. **(A)** The incision is made at the site of the Tinel sign, and either one or two small branches will be identified, most commonly one on each side of the saphenous nerve. Each must be resected, dissected proximally, and then **(B)** a window created in the soleus fascia and the proximal ends of the nerves implanted into this muscle.

boots will rub against the site into which the nerve is implanted, and if the nerve is implanted into the gastrocnemius muscle, then plantar flexion and extension may stimulate the nerve at the implantation site. From the experience of harvesting the sural nerve as a source of nerve graft material, there is considerable experience with leaving the proximal end of the nerve in the popliteal fossa. Therefore my preferred approach *(Fig. 6.8)* is to make an incision over the fibular neck, extending posteriorly into the popliteal fossa.

First the common peroneal nerve is identified beneath the fascia, then followed distally and a neurolysis completed by releasing the fascia of the peroneus muscle group and elevating these muscles to relase a fibrous band, found in about 20% of normals.[54] Then, having safely identified and protected this nerve, the dissection proceeds into the popliteal fossa deep to this fascia. There is great variability in the sural nerve anatomy.[55] At the ankle, this is actually the common sural nerve. If the commonest variation is present, there will be one large sural nerve present with two fascicles and an artery, having been formed from a short medial sural branch from the tibial nerve and a short lateral sural nerve from the common peroneal nerve. A nerve stimulator is used to prove this is not an anomalous motor branch to a gastrocnemius or foot flexor. Then bupivacaine is infiltrated into the nerve proximally under very little pressure so it is not forced proximally towards the sciatic nerve. The nerve is cauterized distally and proximally and the intervening 3-cm segment submitted to pathology, and the proximal end allowed to retract into the popliteal fossa proximal to the knee joint.

About 20% of the time, there will be a separate medial and a separate lateral sural nerve already present in the popliteal fossa, each going distally to join somewhere in the distal leg to form the common sural nerve. If the popliteal fossa exploration identifies a single fascicle, then you must continue the dissection into the medial part of the popliteal fossa to search for the second component. If the sural branches cannot be identified with certainty, then you must make an incision over the distal lateral leg, identify the common sural nerve, and gently put it under traction to identify the proximal components. In some patients, even after the proximal resection, there will still be some sensation and pain in the sural distribution. This is almost certainly due to the lateral sural nerve sending some axons along with the SPN. In this situation, there will be a posterior branch from the sural nerve that can be identified about 10 cm proximal to the ankle, and if pain is persistent after the proximal resection of the sural nerve, then a neurolysis of the SPN is indicated to identify and resect this branch.

A neuroma of the calcaneal nerve is due to an injury, most often during neurolysis of the tibial nerve during tarsal tunnel surgery or during an open or endoscopic plantar fasciotomy.[45] It is now appreciated that the posterior branch of the distal saphenous nerve innervates the part of the tarsal tunnel incision that is most proximal,[56] can be indentified as a distally radiating sign anterior and proximal to this incision, and can be relieved with a block of the distal saphenous nerve. Pain in the tarsal tunnel scar distal to this, or at the site of the medial plantar fasciotomy site, is due to a neuroma of one or more branches of the calcaneal nerve. This anatomy has been well defined.[57] For the most distal site of pain, this is a calcaneal branch that arises from the medial plantar nerve, crosses the vessels, and goes through the fascia of the abductor hallucis to enter the skin of the medial arch. This distal site is resected and gentle traction will reveal the fascicle giving origin to it as the most anterior fascicle of the medial plantar nerve within the tarsal tunnel. This fascicle can be divided and implanted into the flexor hallucis longus muscle, the most distal muscle in the leg *(Fig. 6.9)*. If the heel pain is more

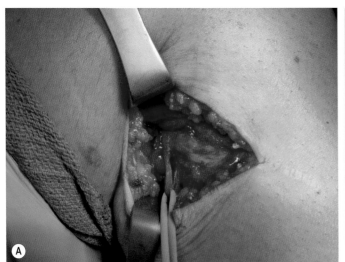
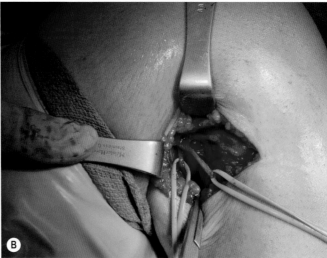

Fig. 6.8 The sural nerve ideally should be resected so its proximal end lies in the popliteal fossa. The sural nerve at the ankle is the common sural nerve. In the popliteal fossa there is one branch, the lateral sural nerve, arising from the common peroneal nerve and a second branch, the medial sural nerve, arising from the tibial nerve. **(A)** The common peroneal nerve is approached first, doing a neurolysis to protect it from harm. This large nerve is noted in the superior aspect of the incision. The incision has an extension into the popliteal fossa. The dissection goes beneath the deep fascia, and here the lateral sural nerve is usually found first, as seen in the vessel loop. **(B)** Two distinct fascicles should be identified, and a deeper dissection then demonstrates the medial sural nerve, show in the second vessel loop. If the two branches have joined quite proximally, there may be one large nerve with two fascicles and one artery. Intraoperative electrical stimulation should be done to be sure these are not aberrant motor fascicles.

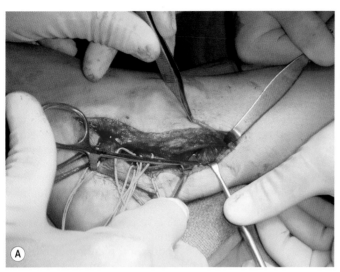 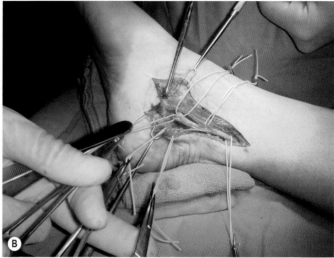

Fig. 6.9 The calcaneal nerve is resected whenever it has been injured by previous surgery, usually for plantar fasciitis, or in previous tarsal tunnel surgery. **(A)** There is often more than one calcaneal branch. Here there are branches related to the medial plantar nerve, held with vessel loops, and from the lateral plantar nerves, also held with vessel loops. The tibial nerve has had a neurolysis from the previous tarsal tunnel decompression scar. **(B)** The proximal end of the divided calcaneal nerve is ready to be implanted into the flexor hallucis longus muscle, just posterior to the tibial nerve.

proximal, then it is due to a neuroma of one or more of the traditionally depicted branches of the lateral plantar nerve, or even the tibial nerve, arising on the posterior aspect of the tibial or lateral plantar nerve. This nerve is identified, divided, and implanted into the flexor hallucis longus muscle. This often requires microdissection, intraneural neurolysis, in order to preserve the distal sensory and motor branches of the lateral plantar nerve.

A neuroma of the interdigital plantar nerve is a true neuroma. The so-called Morton's neuroma, on the other hand, is not a true neuroma. It is a compression caused by the inter-metatarsal ligament and the treatment is neurolysis by division of the intermetatarsal ligament.[46] If the Morton's neuroma is resected through the typical dorsal incision, and pain returns, then there is a true neuroma of this plantar interdigital nerve. If there has been an injury, due to a penetrating foreign body or fracture fixation, then there is a true neuroma. The treatment of the true neuroma is to identify the correct interdigital nerve through a plantar incision in the nonweight-bearing surface of the foot.[47,48] First, the plantar fascia is split longitudinally, and the flexor brevis muscle is dissected from this origin to permit inspection of both the medial and lateral plantar nerve as they exist the medial and lateral plantar tunnels. The branch to the medial side of the hallux and the branch to the lateral side of the fifth toe will not be seen as they originate more proximally. You must identify the branch to the first/second webspace and the fourth/fifth webspace and preserve these. The motor branches are identified with a nerve stimulator. The remaining branches, those to the second/third and third/fourth webspaces, can be resected if necessary depending upon the exact distal injury or previous surgery. These resected nerves then require microdissection, intraneural neurolysis, proximally until the point where they can be rotated and implanted into the arch of the foot without placing tension on the remaining intact nerves. These nerves must be implanted into the arch of the foot.

While it is hard to place a suture into the arch of the foot, this can be done and the epineurium of the resected nerves can be attached loosely to that suture. My current preferred technique is to use a mini- (not micro-) Mitek anchor *(Fig. 6.10)*. Remove the large suture that comes with it, and replace it with a 6-0 nylon. Suture the nerve loosely to the anchor, and then gently press the anchor into the fibrous structures of the arch. The nerve(s) are then suspended and covered with the plantar quadratus and the flexor brevis muscles. The plantar fascia is loosely closed with 4-0 Monocryl. The skin is closed with interrupted and continuous sutures of 4-0 nylon. Please note that about 75% of these patients also have tarsal tunnel syndrome, and this needs to be addressed at the same operation.[48]

A neuroma of the infrapatellar branch of the saphenous nerve is most often due to previous knee surgery with a midline incision. There is numbness over the lateral infrapatellar skin with a painful trigger over the insertion of the adductor muscles at Gerdy's tubercle. There can be two or three branches at this level. The surgical approach is through a longitudinal incision, identifying the branch or branches deep to the fascia, dissecting them proximally through their well-defined tunnel, injecting them with bupivacaine, dividing them distally after cauterization, and implanting them proximally within their tunnel into one of the adductor muscles. This is done "blindly" without actually seeing the muscle *(Fig. 6.11)*.[51]

A neuroma of the saphenous nerve in the adductor canal is rare. Most often the adductor canal must be opened to identify branches of the saphenous nerve at this level due to failure of more distal resections to resolve the pain problem. This is most often due to anomalous saphenous and obturator nerve branches. The nerves are first stimulated to be sure you are denervating part of the vastus medialis, and then the resected nerve has its proximal end implanted into the adductor magnus *(Fig. 6.12)*.

A neuroma of the innervation of the knee joint, the medial and/or lateral retinacular nerve is due to previous surgery, whether to reconstruct the ligaments, or endoscopy, or to total knee replacement. The innervation of the knee joint has been

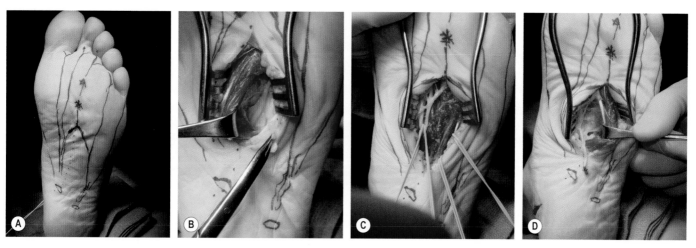

Fig. 6.10 True neuroma of the plantar interdigital nerve. **(A)** After resection of the nerve compression, incorrectly termed Morton's neuroma, a true neuroma will form. If it becomes symptomatic, it must be approached plantarly, and the presumed anatomy is drawn. **(B)** After making an incision on the nonweight-bearing skin, and incising the plantar fascia, the flexor brevis is retracted laterally to dissect the medial plantar nerve. **(C)** Then the lateral plantar nerve is dissected and the branches to the neuroma, in this case, one from each, are encircled with the vessel loop. **(D)** The divided nerves have been dissected proximally, brought into the wound and inserted on to a mini-Mitek metal suture to be implanted into the fibrous structures of the arch of the foot.

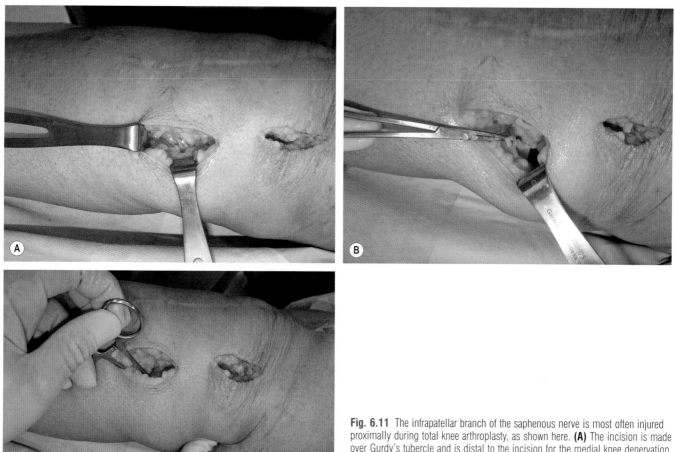

Fig. 6.11 The infrapatellar branch of the saphenous nerve is most often injured proximally during total knee arthroplasty, as shown here. **(A)** The incision is made over Gurdy's tubercle and is distal to the incision for the medial knee denervation (shown). While the leg is exsanguinated, the knee is left with some blood still present, and this helps identify the nerve adjacent to the vein. **(B)** The nerve is divided distally, cauterized to prevent bleeding from its end, and its tunnel is dissected. **(C)** The proximal end of the nerve is then pushed backwards into the tunnel with a clamp which is used to implant the nerve into an adductor muscle proximal to the knee joint.

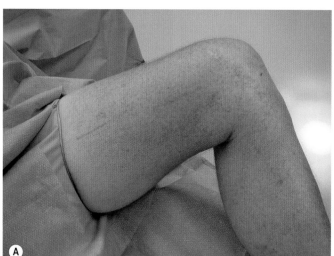

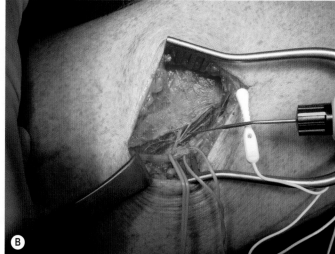

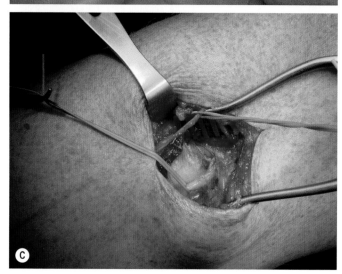

Fig. 6.12 The adductor canal should contain the saphenous nerve. Distal to the canal, this nerve divides into the infrapatellar and distal branches, but these divisions may exist within the canal already. **(A)** The incision for either decompression of the saphenous nerve or resection of the nerve is the same and is located at about the junction of the middle and distal third of the medial thigh at the site of the maximum tenderness. This patient had seven previous attempts to resect the infrapatellar branch at more distal sites. **(B)** A femoral nerve motor branch is often in the canal to the vastus medialis, and here electrical stimulation is used before resecting a nerve to be sure that just a sensory nerve is being resected. **(C)** Two distinct nerves are apparent in this patient. Each will be resected and implanted proximally into an adductor muscle.

described and is constant *(Fig. 6.3)*.[36] Depending upon the nerve block, these nerves, usually both of them, must be resected. If the patient has had a total knee arthroplasty, the implant is not exposed. Longitudinal incisions are made midmedial and midlateral. Medially *(Fig. 6.13)*, the medial retinaculum is opened and just distal to the vastus medialis, the medial retinacular nerve will be identified next to the recurrent geniculate vessels. The nerve is blocked proximally, cauterized distally, and then dissected proximally where its proximal end is implanted into the vastus medialis muscle. Laterally *(Fig. 6.14)*, the iliotibial tract is incised longtitudinally, at which location it has become the lateral retinacular, and, just distal to the vastus lateralis, and adjacent to the recurrent geniculate vessels is the lateral retinacular nerve. It is blocked proximally with bupivacaine, cauterized distally, dissected proximally to where it goes deep to the biceps femoris insertion, cauterized again, and resected under tension and dropped into the popliteal fossa, since it originates from the sciatic nerve.[5,50,51]

Chronic nerve compression *(Box 6.3)*

The diagnosis and treatment of lower extremity chronic nerve compression are the same as that for upper extremity chronic

---

Box 6.3 Successful neurolysis

Take time listening to patients' complaints: diagnosis often comes from the history

Document the sensory and motor exam for the peripheral nerves in question

Localize site of entrapment with your own physical diagnosis: use the Tinel sign

Remember that more than one nerve may be compressed in the same extremity

Remember that the same nerve can be compressed at more than one site along its path

Remember: an underlying systemic disease, a neuropathy, predisposes to compressions

External neurolysis separates the peripheral nerve from surrounding structures

Intraneural fibrosis, determined intraoperatively, requires intraneural neurolysis

Segmental blood flow can be disrupted: respect longitudinal blood flow of the nerve

Postoperative mobilization is a critical aspect of neurolysis

Don't become a wrapper!

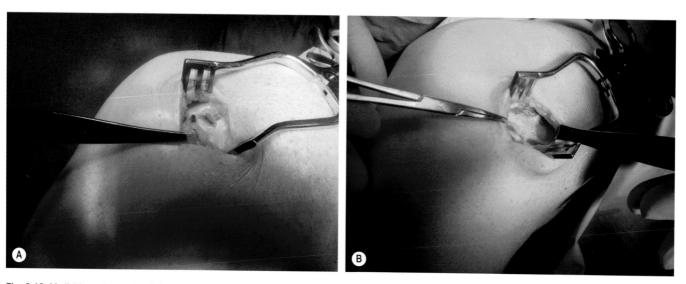

Fig. 6.13 Medial knee denervation **(A)** is approached through an incision just distal to the vastus medialis, where the medial retinaculum is opened. The medial retinacular nerve is adjacent to the recurrent geniculate vessels, which are visible because the knee region has not been exsanguinated by the tourniquet. **(B)** The medial retinacular nerve is dissected proximally from its origin beneath the vastus medialis muscle, and implanted deep into this muscle.

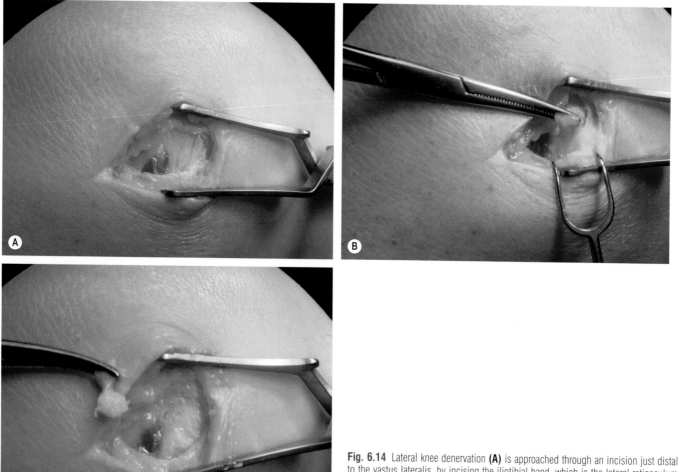

Fig. 6.14 Lateral knee denervation **(A)** is approached through an incision just distal to the vastus lateralis, by incising the iliotibial band, which is the lateral retinaculum. The lateral retinacular nerve is adjacent to the recurrent geniculate vessels, which are visible because the knee region has not been exsanguinated by the tourniquet. **(B)** The lateral retinacular nerve is dissected proximally from its origin beneath the biceps tendon and **(C)** is resected so it drops into the popliteal fossa.

Box 6.4 **New in neurolysis**

Intraoperative tibial nerve pressures have documented the necessity to decompress four medial ankle tunnels for the treatment of tarsal tunnel syndrome[58]

Superficial peroneal neurolysis requires fasciotomy of both anterior and lateral compartments: 25% of people have a branch in the anterior compartment,[52] and, rarely, it can be within the septum itself[61]

Deep peroneal neurolysis almost never requires release of the anterior tarsal tunnel

Common peroneal neurolysis potentially requires release of several structures[56]

In the diabetic, there can be multiple peripheral nerve entrapments in the same limb[38,41]

The proximal tibial nerve can be entrapped at the soleal sling – soleal sling syndrome[62,63]

---

nerve compression: only the anatomy differs. To begin treating patients with lower extremity peripheral nerve compression, it is advisable to review your anatomy, and to do a cadaver dissection.

The fact that many patients with chronic nerve compression syndromes are not referred is due to many issues, not least of which is an ignorance on the part of the primary care physician of the various nerve compressions and the symptoms associated with them. There is also a degree of ignorance to the fact that there are subspecialists who are interested in conditions of the peripheral nerve. Towards these ends, the American Society for Peripheral Nerve was begun in 1990, and includes surgeons from plastic surgery, orthopedic surgery, and neurosurgery. Compression of the tibial and peroneal nerves were among the first to be recognized.[1] The principles used to evaluate and treat these nerves were the same as those developed to treat the upper extremity nerves, and relied upon detailed neurosensory and motor evaluation, and careful attention to surgical technique. Without much change, the approach today should be the same as the approach recorded then.

The most common nerve entrapment is the tibial nerve and its branches at the tarsal tunnel region. The next most frequent is entrapment of the common peroneal nerve at the fibular neck. The third most common is the deep peroneal nerve over the dorsum of the foot. The fourth most common is the SPN. Interdigital plantar nerve compression may be treated more commonly than many of the above, but most of these are treated conservatively. Calcaneal nerve entrapment may be common, but often goes misdiagnosed as plantar fasciitis *(Box 6.4)*.

Decompression of the four medial ankle tunnels has been described in detail.[1,2,38,41] An incision is made proximal and posterior to the medial malleolus extending to the end of the tarsal tunnel. If there has been no previous injury, edema, or surgery, the deep fascia is thin and immediately subjacent is the thicker, but usually loose, flexor retinaculum, that used to be called the lancinate ligament. Once this has been divided the tarsal tunnel is officially released. If there is no space-occupying lesion, the surgery is done, and it is appreciated that not much has been decompressed. It is appropriate to elevate the tibial artery and veins from the tibial nerve, and

evaluate if there is intraneural fibrosis or not, if there is a high division of the tibial nerve or not, and the number of calcaneal nerves originating within the tarsal tunnel. It has been demonstrated now that the pressure within the tarsal tunnel of patients with neuropathy is not different than it is in the tarsal tunnel of cadavers.[58] The pressure here does increase with ankle plantar flexion and pronation, and this is no longer occurs after release of the flexor retinaculum. With the realization that the tarsal tunnel was analogous to the carpal tunnel in the human forearm, an operation was developed that decompressed the medial and lateral plantar tunnels and the calcaneal tunnel(s) and removed the septum that is between the medial and lateral plantar tunnels in order to create a larger volume for these nerves *(Fig. 6.15)*. To accomplish this in surgery, an incision is made towards the plantar aspect of the foot and comes proximal to join the incision for the tarsal tunnel release *(Fig. 6.16)*. Of course, these two incisions can be drawn and made at the same time, but it is important conceptually to appreciate that these distal tunnels are at the foot level, and the entrapment sites are not within the tarsal tunnel. The tarsal tunnel ends at the origin of the abductor hallucis. The fascia superficial to the abductor is incised, taking care not to injure the branch from the medial plantar nerve, often through this fascia, and into the skin of the medial arch. This little nerve remains unnamed, after its initial description.[54] The abductor muscle is then retracted to reveal its ligamentous origin, which forms the roof of the medial and lateral plantar tunnels. Each roof is incised. The septum between them is cauterized and then longitudinally released and excised. This septum is of variable size. Sometimes the medial, sometimes the lateral, and sometimes both plantar tunnels are small and constricting of the nerves within them. Intraoperative pressure measurements in patients with neuropathy demonstrate that these are the sites of elevated pressures, even with the ankle in the neutral position, and these pressures increase dramatically with plantar flexion and pronation. It is necessary to release each of these tunnels and excise the septum to get maximum reduction of these pressures.[58] If the patient has had complaints of heel pain, and has not responded to treatment for plantar fasciitis, it is likely that the source of heel pain is compression of the calcaneal nerve(s). Often there are more than one of these and more than one tunnel. Each must be decompressed to relieve the heel pain.

Neurolysis of the common peroneal nerve at the fibular head is well known[59] *(Fig. 6.17)*. However it is an operation that is usually deferred by orthopedic surgeons as their literature supports expectant waiting once a foot drop develops after a hip or knee procedure, or a sports injury. From a peripheral nerve perspective, the position can be defended to do the neurolysis at 3 months or sooner.[60] In addition to foot drop, neurolysis is indicated to relieve chronic pain related to this compression. The incision does not have to be longer than 4–5 cm in a normal-sized leg. The incision is oblique in case you must extend the surgery into the popliteal fossa or distally in the leg *(Fig. 6.18)*. There is sometimes a cutaneous nerve in this location, the lateral cutaneous nerve of the calf, and this should be preserved. The deep fascia, in the absence of trauma, will not be adherent to the common peroneal nerve. This nerve is white in the absence of glucose intolerance, in which case it is swollen and infiltrated by yellow fat, giving it almost the apperance of a lipoma. This is not a

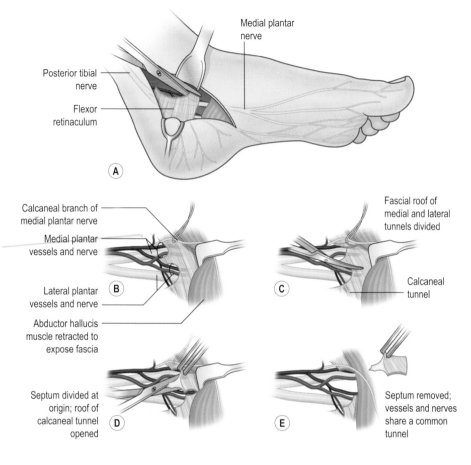

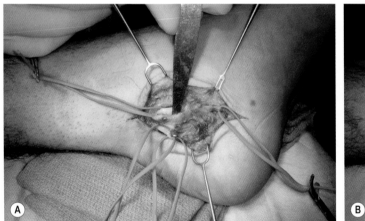

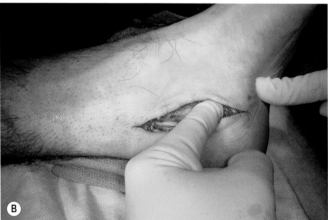

Fig. 6.15 Release of the four medial ankle tunnels. **(A)** The tarsal tunnel is opened. **(B)** The abductor hallucis is retracted, protecting the calcaneal branch from the medial plantar nerve to the arch. **(C)** The roof of the medial and the lateral plantar tunnels is incised. **(D)** The calcaneal tunnel is incised. **(E)** The septum between the medial and lateral plantar tunnels is excised. (Reproduced with permission from Dellon.com.)

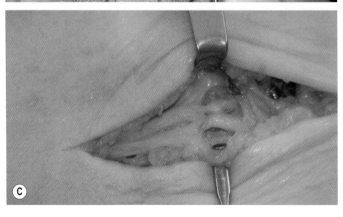

Fig. 6.16 Intraoperative views of tarsal tunnel surgery. **(A)** Left tarsal tunnel opened to demonstrate a high division of the medial and lateral plantar nerves, proximal to the tunnel, encircled with vessel loops, with the distal medial plantar nerve identified with a loop just entering the medial plantar tunnel, and from the lateral plantar nerve, a high originating calcaneal nerve, also encircled with a loop. **(B)** After release of the distal tunnels and resection of the septum, a finger can pass into the plantar aspect of the foot. **(C)** Variation in which the medial and lateral plantar nerves exchange fascicles within the tarsal tunnel. The calcaneal branch originating from the medial plantar and one from the lateral plantar are also noted.

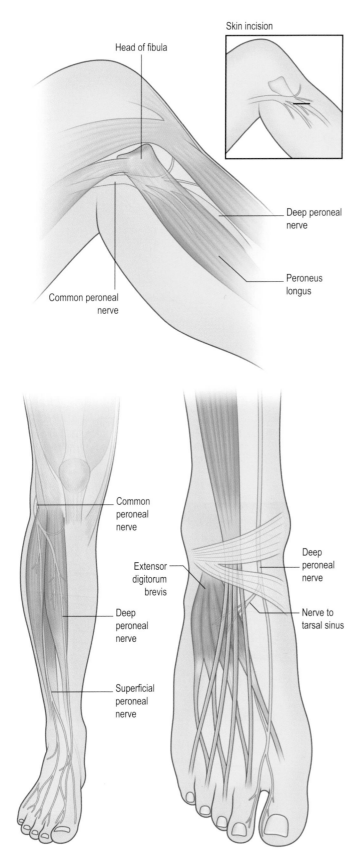

Fig. 6.17 Illustration of the sites of compression of the peroneal nerves. Common peroneal nerve entrapment at the fibular neck. Superficial peroneal nerve entrapment as it exits the fascia in the distal leg. Deep peroneal nerve entrapment beneath the tendon of the extensor hallucis brevis. (Reproduced with permission from Dellon.com.)

lipoma, so it is important not to excise it! The nerve is released into the popliteal fossa, but the entrapment site, again in the absence of trauma, is completely between the neck of the fibula and the overlying structures related to the peroneus muscles. Begin by releasing the superficial peroneus fascia transversely, proximally, and distally in a stellate fashion. There is often a septum between muscles that should be released, taking care not to extend the scissor tips too deeply and injure the nerve. Then retract the muscle. In cadavers, there is a fibrous band of fascia deep to the muscle in 20%, but this is present to some extent in 80% of those coming to surgery,[56] and this band must be carefully released to reveal the compressed, flattened, ischemic soft nerve below. Then the nerve is gently elevated. In about 15% of patients there will be a fibrous origin on the lateral head of the gastrocnemius.[56] This must be cauterized and divided. In a few patients the opening into the anterior compartment also needs to be widened by releasing some of the fibrous muscle origins. If there is intraneural fibrosis, a very gentle intraneural dissecton can be done. Intraoperative electrical stimulation that demonstrates motor function is very useful in giving the patient with a foot drop a good prognosis upon awakening from surgery. Be sure not to get any bupivacaine on to the nerve during the infiltration of the skin edges to avoid the patient awaking with poor motor function.

Neurolysis of the SPN is misleadingly simple. Despite all anatomy books illustrating the location of this nerve in the lateral compartment, the author has had the experience of resecting this nerve in this location, only to find that the patients still had sensation over the dorsum of the foot that could be relieved by a local block at the anterior ankle. The paradox is resolved by realizing that 25% of people have either the entire SPN in the anterior compartment, or, instead of this nerve dividing into its dorsomedial and dorsolateral branches at the level of the ankle, it has a high division, and will have a branch not only in the lateral compartment but also in the anterior compartment or a subcutaneous location *(Fig. 6.19)*.[52] Therefore it is critical that when you make an incision over the site of the Tinel sign, which is often where there is a slight bulge as the nerve exists the fascia accompanied by some fat, that you take care not to injure a small branch to the skin at this location, and also plan to do a fasciotomy of both the anterior and the lateral compartment. This location is on average centered 10 cm proximal to the lateral malleolus but can range from 4 to 20 cm, so be prepared to lengthen your incision if you cannot find the entrapment (exit) point. This fascia is well vascularized and can lead to postoperative bruising or hematoma, and therefore each incised side/edge should be cauterized. The SPN must be released proximally until it is surrounded by muscle, and if it is pressed up against the septum, a section of septum should be cauterized and removed. If there is no nerve identified in either compartment, it may be in the septum itself, so care should be taken when dividing this septum.

Neurolysis of the deep peroneal nerve does not require opening the anterior tarsal tunnel. The anterior tarsal tunnel is a relatively large space, and unless there has been a crush injury to the ankle, or previous surgery in this region, the usual site of compression of the deep peroneal nerve is over the dorsum of the foot, not the ankle. In this location, electrodiagnostic testing will not be helpful because the sensory nerve is small and too distal. Neurosensory testing can

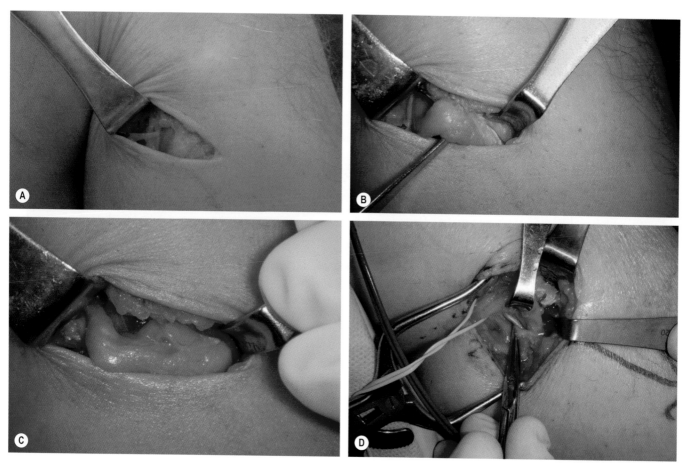

Fig. 6.18 The common peroneal nerve is **(A)** approached through an oblique incision over the fibular neck. In this location, the lateral cutaneous nerve of the calf should be protected. **(B)** The deep fascia is opened to identify the common peroneal nerve, and then the fascia of the peroneus muscles is released and these muscles are retracted. The site of compression is the fibrous band just deep to the retracted muscles. This band is carefully divided. **(C)** The swollen proximal nerve is noted. The discontinuation of the longitudinal blood supply along the nerve is noted. The flattened, compressed nerve beneath the band is noted. The deep from the superficial peroneal nerve divisions is apparent. **(D)** This view, in another patient, shown after release of the steps above, demonstrates a white fibrous band present deep to the common peroneal nerve, part of the gastrocnemius fascia, which, when present, also must be released.

document this sensory loss in the dorsal first webspace, and there will be a Tinel sign beneath the extensor hallucis brevis tendon where it compresses the nerve against the underlying prominence of the junction of the first metatarsal and the cuneiform bone. This is often the site of an exostosis, and the most common site for a ganglion. The common LisFranc fracture/dislocation can also cause this compression, as will wearing high heels or tight sports shoes, such as in ice skating. If there has been direct trauma or antecedent surgery, then it may be more appropriate to resect this nerve in the lower leg, but if not, then the neurolysis is the appropriate choice. A 2-cm oblique incision is made between the first and second metatarsals and the cuneiform bone. The SPN is protected. The deep fascia is opened overlying the visible oblique tendon or muscle belly of the extensor hallucis brevis. This tendon is resected, and the nerve is elevated from its adherence to the underlying bone.[65] There is often a clear indentation of the nerve. Proximally, the nerve is released until it is loose at the inferior extensor retinaculum. Distally, there is often a second site of compression beneath a thin fibrous band just before the nerve becomes subcutaneous in location. A small branch innervating the metatarsocuneiform joints can be observed here.

A new site of compression of the proximal tibial nerve beneath the soleal sling has been described anatomically.[62] Compression at this site is best termed "soleal sling syndrome." As the tibial nerve travels beneath the fibrous origin of the soleus muscle, it can become compressed. The sensory complaints are similar to those of tarsal tunnel syndrome except that they are not present at night. The sensory findings are the same as tarsal tunnel syndrome. The physical findings can differ in that there is weakness of toe flexion, particularly weakness in flexion of the big toe *(Fig. 6.20A)*. The innervation of the flexor hallucis longus occurs at the level of the soleal sling, causing this finding. Neurolysis at this anatomic site can recover toe flexion.[63,64] The incision is made from the medial popliteal fossa laterally and then inferiorly. The distal saphenous nerve travels in this location and is preserved. The fascia is released to bluntly dissect and posteriorly retract the medial head of the gastrocnemius muscle. The tibial nerve will be noted to be just beneath the soleal sling and just posterior (in front for the surgeon) of the popliteal vein *(Fig. 6.20B–D)*. The safest approach is to cauterize the soleus overlying the course of the tibial nerve, and then lift up on the deep posterior compartment fascia and release it. The tibial nerve can be separated from the popliteal vein, and the fascicles in this

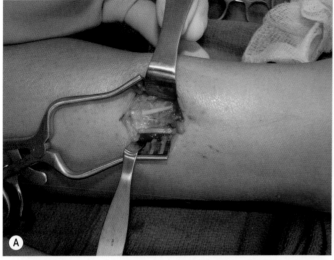

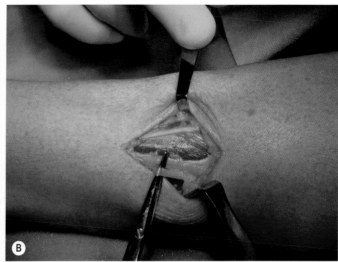

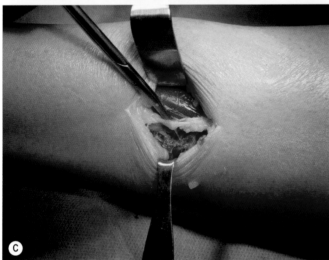

Fig. 6.19 Neurolysis of the superficial peroneal nerve must begin with the knowledge that, although this nerve is supposed to be in the lateral compartment, there is considerable variation and both the anterior and the lateral compartment must be opened. **(A)** Note a branch of this nerve in each compartment. If no nerve is found in either compartment, carefully open the septum **(B)** as the nerve can be intraseptal. **(C)** In some patients, one of the two branches may already be subcutaneously located.

location can be stimulated to demonstrate recovery of toe flexion *(Fig. 6.20E)*. Movement in the big toe can be restored.

Postoperative care/rehabilitation

The painful neuroma

The patient is allowed to ambulate immediately after surgery. The patient is instructed to change chairs, and walk around the bed every 2 hours to minimize the risk of postoperative venous thrombosis. A cane or walker can be utilized. In general, crutches are discouraged, as the patient may fall, and hurt the hands and armpits. Walking should not be for distances longer than about 50 feet (15.25 meters). For distances greater than that, a wheelchair is encouraged. Following final suture removal, the patient begins a "water walking program," beginning with 10–15 minutes a day, working up to about an hour a day, doing this 4–6 times a week *(Fig. 6.21B)*. This is a form of desensitization for the lower extremity. A therapist should not touch the leg. The patient should not touch the place where the nerve proximally has been

implanted. That site remains tender in about half of patients. The water walking will send new stimuli to the cortex to cause reorganization of the cortex, and facilitate learning about the new sensation, or lack thereof, following the denervation of that skin territory. Water therapy will help the 50% of people in whom collateral sprouting from the adjacent intact nerve, e.g., from the sural and deep peroneal and saphenous if the SPN has been resected, causes paresthesias during the third to 12th week postoperatively. Once the water walking and swimming have been accomplished, progression to the stationary bicycle and the elliptical machine can begin. Treadmill use is discouraged. By the fourth or fifth postoperative week, the patient can resume usual exercises again. At this point, if the patient had been habituated to narcotics, a withdrawal program can be initiated under the care of a certified pain management specialist.[33]

Chronic nerve compression

The same time sequence for dressing change and suture removal is used for these procedures as for the painful neuroma procedures. Since it is critical that the peripheral

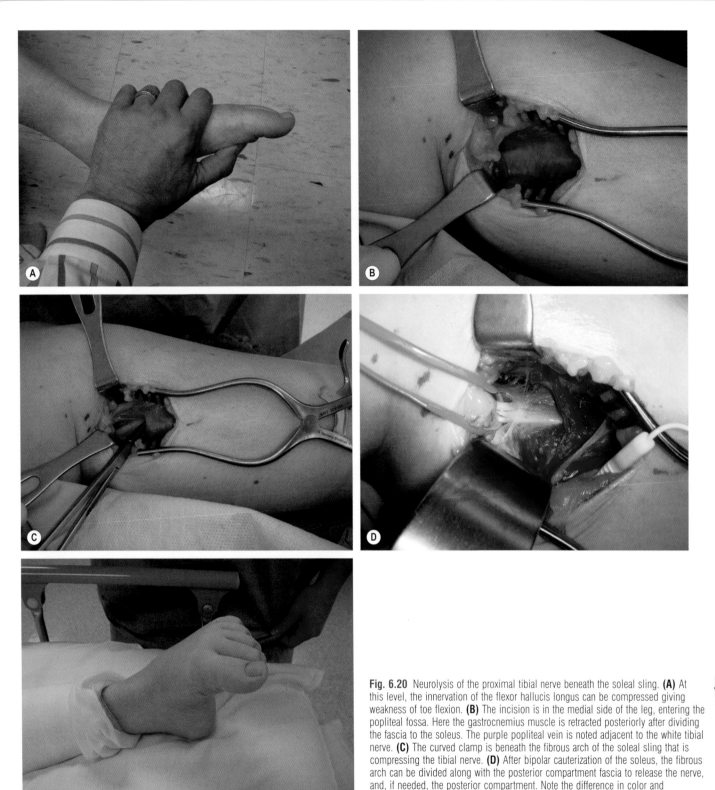

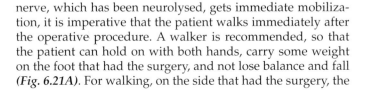

Video
1-3

Fig. 6.20 Neurolysis of the proximal tibial nerve beneath the soleal sling. **(A)** At this level, the innervation of the flexor hallucis longus can be compressed giving weakness of toe flexion. **(B)** The incision is in the medial side of the leg, entering the popliteal fossa. Here the gastrocnemius muscle is retracted posteriorly after dividing the fascia to the soleus. The purple popliteal vein is noted adjacent to the white tibial nerve. **(C)** The curved clamp is beneath the fibrous arch of the soleal sling that is compressing the tibial nerve. **(D)** After bipolar cauterization of the soleus, the fibrous arch can be divided along with the posterior compartment fascia to release the nerve, and, if needed, the posterior compartment. Note the difference in color and vascularity of the tibial nerve proximal and distal to the compression site. **(E)** Note flexion of the big toe has been achieved postoperatively.

nerve, which has been neurolysed, gets immediate mobilization, it is imperative that the patient walks immediately after the operative procedure. A walker is recommended, so that the patient can hold on with both hands, carry some weight on the foot that had the surgery, and not lose balance and fall *(Fig. 6.21A)*. For walking, on the side that had the surgery, the

operated extremity begins its step by lifting from the knee, and then leaning forward. The ankle is often prevented from moving too much, especially in those patients who have had tarsal tunnel decompression, so that ankle movement does not pull out the sutures. This is so critical in the patient with neuropathy who usually cannot tell that ankle movement is

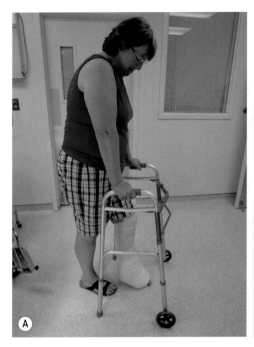
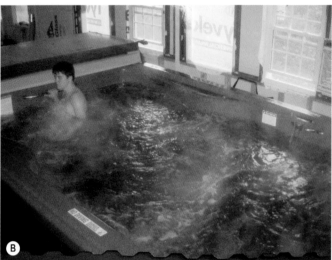

Fig. 6.21 Postoperative management following release of the four medial ankle tunnels for tarsal tunnel syndrome requires immediate mobilization of the tibial nerve and its branches, but sufficient support so that the sutures do not pull out. **(A)** The extensive soft bulky supportive dressing applied to the foot and ankle permits immediate ambulation with a walker, with the patient being reminded to lift from the knee and hip. This is continued for 3 weeks. **(B)** Following removal of the sutures at 3 weeks, a water therapy program is begun and progressed. This is helpful not only for those patients having nerve decompressions, but, and perhaps even more importantly, for those patients following neuroma resection for complex regional pain syndrome.

Table 6.5 Results of tarsal tunnel decompression

Clinical study (n)*		Excellent	Good	Poor	Failure	Worse
Tarsal tunnel syndrome						
Byank[66]	(51)	26%	53%	12%		8%
Pfeiffer and Crachhilo[67]	(32)	15%	29%	18%		32%
Mullick and Dellon[68]	(88)	82%	11%	5%		2%
*n = number of tarsal tunnel decompressions in study.						

tearing out the sutures. It is precisely for this reason that the large Robert Jones, bulky, ankle dressing is used to protect the ankle suture line in patients with insensitive feet.

The walker is used for 3 weeks. Once the sutures are out, then the same rehabilitation with water therapy is used with the same schedule as given above for the patient who has had a painful neuroma excised *(Fig. 6.21B)*.[33]

Outcomes, prognosis, and recurrence

The painful neuroma

As a general rule, if the patient responds with pain relief after a nerve block of the suspected nerve, or nerves, whether cutaneous or joint afferent, then the prognosis is 90% that the patient will achieve good to excellent relief of pain.[4,5,44,45,47–51,53] Failure to obtain the desired result is usually due to the presence of another injured nerve, whose presence was masked by the severity of the original pain. A clue to this is the original

pain level of 8–10 not being reduced to 1 or 2 after the block. Of course, not all surgery can be 100% successful, but neuroma resection with muscle implantation is highly predictable and successful. It is "ok to lose your nerve." The historic concern over "anesthesia dolorosa" is unfounded today if the nerve block is successful, and if the muscle implantation is maintained. The most common nerve to require repeat surgery is the SPN, which may pull from the extensor digitorum communis muscle during vigorous athletic jumping or repeat ankle injury. If this occurs, the nerve must be resected at a more proximal level, additional septum resected, and the nerve implanted again into the same muscle.

Chronic nerve compression

Success for neurolysis approaches 90% in the lower extremity,[46,52,59,63,65–67] as it does in the upper extremity. *Table 6.5* contains a review of the results for tarsal tunnel decompression. Prognosis is based upon the degree of axonal loss. If there is just demyelination, with primarily intermittent symptoms and some weakness, the success can be above 90%, and recovery of function can occur in the early postoperative period. Sometimes motor function recovers dramatically in the recovery room. If there is severe axonal loss, with loss of two-point discrimination, with muscle wasting or paralysis, then the success may not only be much lower, but recovery of function may extend over 1 year, and the nerve regeneration may be painful. If there are comorbidities, like diabetes or another form of neuropathy, the same general guidelines apply, but the expected recovery is 80% relief of pain, 80% recovery of sensation, plus prevention of ulceration and amputation.[38,41] Unless there has been a new trauma, recurrence of symptoms is unusual once successful recovery has occurred. For patients in whom the first neurolysis was not successful, repeat surgery can be done, but with a reduced expectation for success[69] and with an increased risk for complications.

Access the complete references list online at **http://www.expertconsult.com**

2. Dellon AL. *Pain solutions*. Lightning Source Publications; Dellon.com, 2007.

   A comprehensive review, told as patient vignettes, with historical background, anatomical illustrations, intraoperative photos of real patients with problems related to neuropathy, joint pain, Morton's neuroma, pain stimulators, and much more. Only available online.

4. Dellon AL. Partial joint denervation I: wrist, shoulder, elbow. *Plast Reconstr Surg*. 2009;123:197–207.

5. Dellon AL. Partial joint denervation II: knee, ankle. *Plastic Reconstr Surg*. 2009;123:208–217.

   Partial joint denervation is the concept of preservation of joint function and relief of joint pain by interrupting neural pathways that transmit the pain message from the joint to the brain. This review article focuses on the application of these principles to the knee and ankle and demonstrates that the results obtained for partial joint denervation of the upper extremity can be successfully applied to the knee and ankle joints.

32. Dellon AL. A numerical grading scale for peripheral nerve function. *J Hand Therapy*. 1993;4:152.

35. Weber RA, Schuchmann JA, Albers JH, et al. A prospective blinded evaluation of nerve conduction velocity versus pressure-specified sensory testing in carpal tunnel syndrome. *Ann Plast Surg*. 2000;45:252.

   A level I study comparing the classic electrodiagnostic testing by neurologists with painless, noninvasive neurosensory testing with the Pressure-Specified Sensory Device, demonstrating that the same information is obtainable without pain (P < 0.001), yet with the same sensitivity and specificity. This approach is used in the lower extremity.

38. Dellon AL. The Dellon Approach to neurolysis in the neuropathy patient with chronic nerve compression. Handchir Mikrochir. *Plast Chir.*, 2008;40:1–10.

   A systematic review of the literature demonstrating 80% relief of pain, 80% recovery of sensation, prevention of ulceration and amputation when the Dellon triple nerve decompression is done in patients with neuropathy who also have superimposed compression of the tibial nerve in the tarsal tunnels and compressions of the peroneal nerves.

42. Dellon AL. Neurosensory testing, Ch 43. In: Slutsky D, ed. *Master skills in nerve repair; tips and techniques.* Elsevier; 2008:575–586.

44. Dellon AL, Aszmann OC. Treatment of dorsal foot neuromas by translocation of nerves into anterolateral compartment. *Foot Ankle*. 1998;19:300–303.

46. Dellon AL. Treatment of Morton's neuroma as a nerve compression: the role for neurolysis. *J Am Pod Med Assn*. 1992;82:399.

48. Wolfort S, Dellon AL. Treatment of recurrent neuroma of the interdigital nerve by neuroma resection and implantation of proximal nerve into muscle in the arch. *J Foot Ankle Surg*. 2001;40:404–410.

7

Skeletal reconstruction

Stephen J. Kovach and L. Scott Levin

SYNOPSIS

- The reconstruction of defects of the appendicular and axial skeletal has been an evolving clinical endeavor that has mirrored our understanding of the basic science of bone biology.
- This chapter serves as an overview of the basic tenets of bone biology, methods of skeletal reconstruction, and a discussion of the most common skeletal defects and how the reconstructive surgeon can reasonably approach them.
- Perhaps no other clinical tool has had as much of an impact on the ability to reconstruct skeletal defects as the microsurgical transfer of bone. Thus, no chapter on skeletal reconstruction would be complete without a review of the microsurgical principles of bony reconstruction.
- The reader should understand how to approach skeletal defects and the algorithm for their reconstruction upon reading this chapter.

 Access the Historical Perspective section online at
http://www.expertconsult.com

Introduction

Skeletal reconstruction remains a challenging problem for both orthopedic and plastic surgeons. Skeletal defects result most often from trauma, but also may result from oncologic resection or infection. Additionally, traumatic injuries that have been treated with definitive fixation may subsequently develop a nonunion requiring bony debridement and a resultant skeletal defect that must be reconstructed. The majority of these skeletal defects are of the appendicular skeleton, but the reconstructive surgeon may also be called upon to reconstruct defects of the axial skeleton. This chapter will serve as an overview regarding skeletal reconstruction of and the basic tenets of reconstruction of bone.

Basic science

Inert bone grafts, including those that are xenogenic, have been shown to be successful through osteoinduction. There are no living cells in devitalized bone grafts, and growth of bone within the implant is dependent on creeping substitution of the living bone that is in contact with the implant via osteoinduction. These inert bone grafts maintain the ability to provoke a morphogenic response and maintain the potential for bone formation. Bone morphogenetic protein (BMP) is responsible for this differentiation and its potential was first demonstrated by Urist in the 1950s and confirmed by several additional authors.[6–8] It is this morphogenetic property of xenografts that allowed them to retain the potential for bone formation. Unfortunately, the immune response elucidated by xenografts limits their practical use by preventing their incorporation or revascularization. Urist's work did confirm the capacity of devitalized bone matrix to induce the formation of bone in heterotopic sites. Ultimately, the process of bone grafting involves osteoinduction, osteoconduction, and osteogenetic potential, which is in part modulated through the BMPs. Osteoinduction is the signaling of the graft to stimulate the formation of new bone, osteoconduction is the underlying framework over which new bone will grow, and osteogenesis is the ability of the bone graft itself to form new bone from its cellular elements. Autologous bone graft has the ability to perform all three and therefore remains the standard to which all others are compared.[9]

Allografts are, by definition, allogeneic to the recipient. Allografts are functionally strong, but their incorporation remains questionable over their lifespan and they have been associated with relatively high complication rates. These complications include nonunion, fracture, and infection, all of which necessitate their removal.[10–12] There are methods to combine the initial structural integrity of the allograft with a vascularized autograft to take advantage of both methods.[13] This will be discussed in a subsequent section. The ideal allograft is sterile cortical bone without loss of BMP activity while lowering the antigenicity of the implant. Current methods of preparation attempt to optimize on these principles while leaving enough of the matrix to elucidate the BMP response. Allograft does have the advantage of a potentially unlimited amount of bone for reconstruction and the avoidance of a donor site which has a morbidity associated with it.

Vascularized bone grafts display less resorption than non-vascularized grafts over time, and are able to heal secondary to their maintenance of viable cells within the graft and are capable of healing to the surrounding bone much in the manner of a fracture. These live bone grafts do not heal by the creeping substitution which is observed in inert bone grafts. Much like bone grafting, the use of vascularized bone grafts began in the craniofacial skeleton. Early conventional vascularized flaps were composed of vascularized calvarium that were included in full-thickness scalp flaps.[14]

The first vascularized bone flap for lower extremity reconstruction was performed in 1905 with the use of a pedicled vascularized fibula for tibial shaft reconstruction. The superior viability of vascularized bone flaps was evident, but with the advent of the operating microscope and microvascular surgery decades away, the routine use of vascularized bone flaps was not possible. In the 1970s there was an explosion of microsurgery techniques and vascularized free bone flaps, many of which took advantage of incorporating a soft-tissue envelope with the underlying bone to form osteocutaneous and osteomyocutaneous flaps (*Fig. 7.1*). Vascularized bone has the distinct advantage of being alive and able to grow as well as hypertrophy in response to stress, load-bearing, vascularity, and additional environmental signals. The concept of a vascularized bone graft undergoing hypertrophy by environmental stress is exemplified by a free fibula replacing an intercalary segment of a load-bearing bone (*Figs 7.2 and 7.3*).

The vascular supply to the bone dictates the nature of flap harvest and how best to achieve the most viable bone stock for transfer based on its anatomic vascular pedicle. The blood supply to long bones is derived from multiple sources which have a direct impact on the type of flap that may be transferred. The nutrient artery supplies the marrow cavity and the inner cortex, the periosteal vessels supply the outer cortex of the diaphysis, and the metaphyseal and epiphyseal vessels traverse the cortex and have an anastomotic arcade with the nutrient artery.[15] Thus, a long-bone free flap based on the periosteal vessels may have necrosis of the central portion of

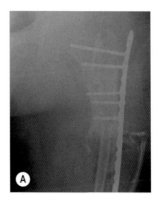
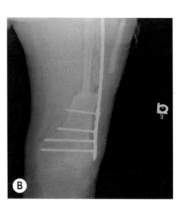

Fig. 7.2 (A, B) Immediate postoperative radiographs of reconstruction of femoral diaphyseal defect after removal of failed allograft.

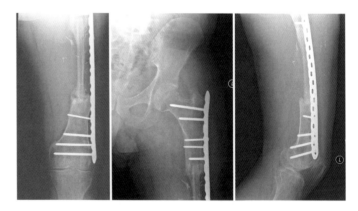

Fig. 7.3 Sequential early images of vascularized fibular graft demonstrating hypertrophy of the fibular diaphyseal shaft and bony callous formation at the proximal and distal junctions to the native femur.

the graft. Conversely, the nutrient artery supplies the majority of the vessels to the long bone. The outer cortex may become necrotic if the flap is based solely on the nutrient artery. This concept is well illustrated by a free fibular transfer based on its nutrient vessel to maintain the viability of the graft.

The blood supply to the membranous bones is distinct from the long bones. The typical pedicle to a free flap of a membranous bone is a periosteal pedicle with good filling of the nutrient vessel canals. An example of this type of flap is the free iliac crest flap which is based on a periosteal pedicle derived from the superficial circumflex iliac artery and was first described by Taylor.[16] The source of the ideal vascularized bone graft will depend upon the available donor sites, the anatomic location of the skeletal defect in need of reconstruction, and the potential of the patient to heal both the recipient and donor site. The ideal reconstruction is one in which the vascularized graft integrates well into the recipient site with rapid bony consolidation and provides structural stability to the skeletal framework.

Diagnosis/patient presentation

It is the reconstructive surgeon's responsibility to apply these basic science principles to the specific clinical situation that is

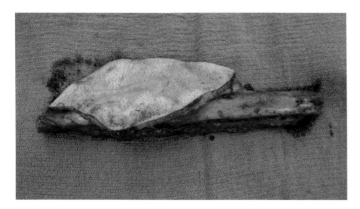

Fig. 7.1 Vascularized osteocutaneous fibular flap.

encountered in treating patients with skeletal defects. Injuries to the appendicular and axial skeleton are commonly encountered at most major medical centers. Both plastic and orthopedic surgeons are called upon to treat these challenging patients on a routine basis. These patients are best served with the "orthoplastic" approach in a multidisciplinary setting.[17,18] The evolution of the orthoplastic approach to limb salvage requires the participation of many different disciplines. The orthopedic and plastic surgeons must be supported within the multidisciplinary orthoplastic approach by prosthetists, physical therapists, vascular surgeons, infectious disease physicians, musculoskeletal radiologists, and a nursing staff well versed in patients undergoing extremity and skeletal reconstruction and convalescence.

As with any clinical problem, the approach begins with the clinical assessment of the patient. One must consider the nature of the defect, including its anatomic position, length of bony defect, other associated injuries of the ipsilateral or contralateral extremity, concomitant traumatic injuries, the potential for a functional recovery, and the cost associated with reconstruction, both financial and social. Both form and function must be considered in the reconstruction of skeletal defects, as should potentially available donor sites to obtain vascularized or nonvascularized bone grafts. While this may seem straightforward, multiply injured patients may have limited donor sites. Often, in the polytrauma patient donor sites are limited and reconstruction must be achieved with the donor sites that are available.

One of the key concerns in reconstruction of the appendicular skeleton is the blood supply to the bone graft. If a cancellous or cortical cancellous bone graft is planned, then it is the blood supply of the underlying wound bed that will be responsible for supplying the necessary blood supply to the graft. If there is poor blood supply to the wound bed, the likelihood of success of a nonvascularized bone graft is poor despite a meticulous surgical approach. There is occasionally the clinical situation of a poorly vascularized wound bed for grafting that is secondary to a reversible or treatable flow-limiting lesion. In patients with an abnormal vascular exam, angiography is indicated to discern the blood supply and to determine if there is a reversible flow-limiting lesion that can improve perfusion to the proposed site of grafting. In patients in whom a vascularized bone graft is planned there needs to be adequate inflow and outflow to achieve success. In patients with an abnormal vascular exam with weakly palpable or nonpalpable pulses, it is the authors' preference to obtain a formal arteriogram to aid in preoperative planning. It has been convention to obtain an invasive arteriogram to delineate the vascular anatomy.[19] However, invasive arteriograms are not a morbid-free procedure and computed angiography has become widely available. CT angiography has the advantage of assessing the venous system and surrounding soft tissues as well as the skeletal defect in one study.[20] Patients with known vascular disease and limited inflow with soft-tissue defects can be successfully reconstructed with free tissue transfer with acceptable flap success rates if patient selection is appropriate.[21,22]

One of the persistent questions in the treatment of patients with skeletal defects, particularly in the acute traumatic setting, is discerning who should be offered salvage versus amputation. Much of the data regarding the utility of limb salvage has been derived from the Lower Extremity Assessment Project. Functional outcomes of amputation versus limb salvage for limb-threatening injuries have been extensively studied.[23–32] Outcomes between those patients undergoing reconstruction and those receiving amputation are equivalent. Those patients who elect to undergo reconstruction for traumatic skeletal defects will require an increased number of operative interventions compared to those patients undergoing amputations, but if patients are carefully selected they have the potential to have a functional outcome. Obviously, the overwhelming majority of patients desire to keep the injured extremity if at all possible.[24,33] Ultimately, the decision to proceed with complex soft-tissue reconstruction with or without skeletal reconstruction of associated defects must be individualized to the patient and his or her potential for recovery.

Treatment and surgical technique

Methods of skeletal reconstruction

In patients with traumatic skeletal defects, osetomyelitis, or tumors requiring extirpation with subsequent bony defects, the need for skeletal reconstruction is readily apparent. More difficult clinical situations involve patients who have bone loss associated with prior treatments for oncologic disease secondary to radiation osteonecrosis, or with recalcitrant nonunions from a prior fracture. What is not always straightforward is how to achieve a stable skeletal reconstruction within the available means. To maximize the potential for skeletal stability, one must understand the methods of reconstruction and the limitations of each approach. Traditionally, there are several methods of skeletal reconstruction: conventional cancellous or corticocancellous bone grafting, nonvascularized allografts, vascularized free flap transfer of a bone or bone with associated soft tissue, and distraction osteogenesis through the use of the Ilizarov technique. These methods are not mutually exclusive and may be combined to extend the capability of one modality alone.

Bone grafting

Traditionally, corticocancellous bone grafts had been used for bony defects that are 5 cm or less in length. Conventional bone grafts require a well-vascularized bed for bone grafting that is free of underlying infection and has adequate soft-tissue coverage. These main tenets of bone grafting were put forth by Kazanjian in the 1950s[34] and still hold true today. These principles remain: the recipient site must have adequate blood supply to ensure the survival of the graft, bone-to-bone contact must be established to facilitate creeping substitution, there should be no motion at the fracture site through the use of rigid fixation, and the wound bed must be free of infection. For defects that are greater than 5–6 cm, graft resorption typically prevents complete healing.[35,36] However, Masquelet has described a technique of inducing bioactive membrane that has extended the diaphyseal defect for which cancellous bone grafting may prove to be successful.[37]

The Masquelet technique has been used with success for intercalary defects greater than 5 cm. This technique involves creating an induced membrane to reconstruct large defects with nonvascularized autograft.[37,38] The principles of reconstruction with the Masquelet technique begin with the basic tenets of wound preparation: radical debridement of devitalized tissue and delineation of the intercalary defect. If there is a concomitant soft-tissue defect, flap reconstruction to reconstitute the soft-tissue envelope is undertaken to provide for definitive soft-tissue reconstruction. A polymethyl methacrylate spacer is then placed into the defect. The second stage is then undertaken 6–8 weeks later when the spacer is removed and the membrane that is induced by the spacer is left in place. This cavity is then packed with cancellous bone graft derived from the iliac crest. The induced membrane is then closed over the autograft, resulting in a contained system. The induced membrane has been shown to have biologic properties, including a rich vascular network, a synovial-like epithelial lining, and to be biologically active, secreting growth factors such as vascular endothelial growth factor and transforming growth factor beta-1. Additionally, extracts from the membrane stimulated bone marrow cell proliferation and differentiation to osteoblastic cell lines.[39] This technique has proven to be powerful in a small series, with the authors able to achieve union of long-bone segmental defects ranging from 5 to 24 cm.[38]

Donor sites for bone grafts have evolved over time. In the early 20th century, the tibia was the preferred site for cortical as well as cancellous bone grafts. However, large grafts cannot be obtained from the tibia without a significant donor defect and the risk of chronic pain at the donor site as well as secondary pathologic fractures. Nonvascularized autografts are now harvested routinely from the iliac crest. The iliac crest contains an abundant source of cancellous bone for grafting, and may be taken as a corticocancellous graft depending on the needs of the recipient site. The bone grafts may be harvested from an anterior or posterior approach depending on the positioning needs of the patient. A cortical window is made and the underlying cancellous bone is harvested. In general, 50 cc of bone graft can be obtained from either the anterior or posterior approach, which is typically adequate for defects amenable to cancellous grafts.

Vascularized bone transfer

Intercalary defects that are larger than 5 cm typically required free vascularized bone reconstruction. Vascularized bone grafts have a significant advantage over their nonvascularized counterparts.[40] Additionally, there may be an additional soft-tissue defect associated with the underlying bone loss and an osteocutaneous free flap may be used to provide simultaneous skeletal as well as soft-tissue reconstruction. Vascularized bone grafts for use as a free flap and microsurgical reconstruction of the skeleton have become commonplace in most major medical centers and can be done with a very high patency rate of the graft. Additional factors to consider when choosing a free vascularized bone graft is the available pedicle length that is characteristic of the flap, the available bone stock of the flap in terms of its length and thickness, its osteogenic potential, and ease of harvest at the time of surgery if concomitant orthopedic procedures are to be performed.

Since it was first described in 1975,[41] the fibula has become the preferred source for vascularized bone grafts for reconstruction of defects of the axial as well as appendicular

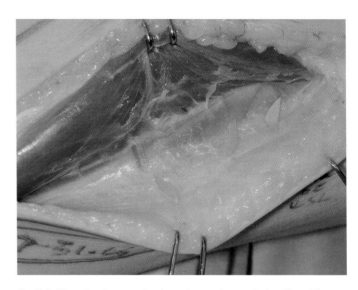

Fig. 7.4 Dissection demonstrating the perforators that supply the skin paddle through the crural septum to raise an osteocutaneous fibular flap.

skeleton. The fibula is well suited for use as a free vascularized bone graft given its potential for an abundant source of the bone, a long length of vascularized graft, and acceptable donor site morbidity.[41] Up to 26 cm of vascularized cortical bone can be harvested from the fibula in the typical adult patient. The fibula is triangular in shape and primarily a cortical bone with a small medullary component. These anatomic characteristics allow it to resist angular and rotational stress and to remodel with graduated weight-bearing in the postoperative period for intercalary defects. The blood supply to the diaphysis of the fibula is based on an endosteal and musculoperiosteal component which are both provided by the peroneal artery and vein. In a small (<1%) number of patients the peroneal artery is the dominant supply to the lower extremity.[42] Peroneus magnus may not be evident on preoperative clinical exam, but if it is encountered intraoperatively the fibular harvest should be abandoned so as not to render the foot ischemic. If the patient has an abnormal pulse exam or has a traumatized extremity that suggests possible underlying vascular injury, preoperative imaging is indicated. A skin paddle may be harvested with the fibula to reconstruct associated soft-tissue defects concomitantly. The skin paddle is supplied by perforators that exit through the posterior crural septum and are found in greatest concentration at the proximal and distal fibula (*Fig. 7.4*).

The epiphysis of the fibular head is supplied by the anterior tibial artery. If epiphyseal growth of the fibula is needed for skeletal reconstruction in the immature skeleton to allow for longitudinal growth, the epiphyseal blood supply needs to be included in the graft so that survival of the epiphysis is insured. It has been shown in studies by Taylor *et al.*[43] and Bonnel *et al.*[44] that the proximal diaphysis is supplied by small, musculoperiosteal branches and there is no need to harvest both pedicles if there is only a small, proximal diaphyseal segment needed for reconstruction. If a significant length of the fibular diaphysis is needed, then both the anterior tibial and peroneal artery must be included with the graft to ensure adequate survival of the segments (*Fig. 7.5*). Typically, a thin cuff of muscle (1 mm) is usually left attached to the graft in order to preserve the muscular

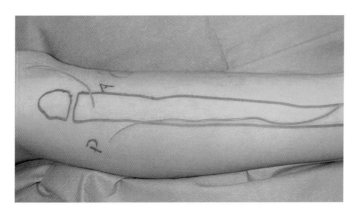

Fig. 7.5 Markings for free fibular harvest with epiphyseal segment based on the anterior tibial artery and the diaphysis based on the peroneal artery.

periosteal circulation and the distal 6 cm of the fibula should be preserved in adults in order to maintain ankle stability. If there is a question of ankle stability following harvest of the fibula, a syndesmotic screw should be placed for additional stability of the ankle joint.

Harvest of the fibula is not without its consequences. Large series have demonstrated persistent long-term deficits after free fibula harvest. Patients may have pain, ankle instability, and/or weakness after harvest of the fibula. Up to 11% of patients undergoing harvest of the free fibula may have persistent pain.[45] The incidence of motor weakness decreases over time after harvest of the fibula but persists in a subset of patients. A small number of patients will complain of subjective weakness in the follow-up period. However, when the harvested legs are compared to the nonoperated leg with isokinetic testing, strength measurements at the knee and ankle are significantly decreased.[46] These defects rarely cause a disability in the patient's postoperative functioning and should not prohibit the reconstructive surgeon from harvesting the appropriate free vascularized fibular graft for reconstruction.

There are multiple additional flaps for skeletal reconstruction. While this will not serve as an exhaustive review of vascularized bone flaps, there are additional flaps worth mentioning due to their common use in vascularized bone reconstruction. The scapular and parascapular flap remain a viable source of adequate bone stock for reconstruction. The scapular osteocutaneous flap has a reliable vascular pedicle and permits harvest of an approximately 11–13 cm length of bone from the lateral side of the scapula. This osseous segment is supplied by musculoperiosteal branches of the circumflex scapular vessels. The medial portion of the scapula can be harvested as a vascularized flap as well, although this requires detaching the serratus, teres major, and greater rhomboid muscles and theoretically has more donor morbidity. The subscapular system is a rich source of additional flaps if additional soft-tissue coverage is needed in addition to the required vascularized bone. The latissimus and serratus muscle can be included on a single subscapular vascular pedicle, depending on the needs of the reconstruction. This allows greater versatility in designing vascularized flaps from the subscapular system.

The radial forearm flap provides for a thin fasciocutaneous skin paddle and can be harvested with a length of the distal radius approximately 8–10 cm in length and 1–1.5 cm in width. The available bone stock is of reasonable length, but by virtue of its thickness does not permit it to be used for larger intercalary defects, with the exception of metacarpal or metatarsal reconstruction. Its chief advantage is a long reliable vascular pedicle and fasciocutaneous portion. Risk of fracture to the radius can occur with bone harvest and avoidance of stress risers is important when performing osteotomies for harvest of the bone segment.

The osteocutaneous lateral arm flap is a fasciocutaneous flap that is supplied by small perforators as well as the posterior radial collateral artery. The vascular pedicle length can be up to 8 cm, but is typically on the order of 4–6 cm in length. The external arterial diameter of the posterior radial collateral artery is small, with an average diameter of 1.5 mm. This flap can be harvested with an osseous segment up to 1 cm in width and 10 cm in length that is harvested from the lateral cortex of the humerus which runs parallel to the line of attachment of the lateral intermuscular septum. Much like the radial forearm, the bone stock available with this flap does not permit it for reconstruction of large intercalary defects, with the exception of metatarsal or metacarpal defects.

The iliac crest vascularized bone flap was popularized in the early 1980s. Its vascular supply is based on the deep circumflex iliac artery. It has the advantage of being able to supply a large segment of bone as well as skin. A segment of bone up to 4 × 11 cm can be harvested as a vascularized segment with a skin paddle measuring 8 × 18 cm. The curve of the native ileum limits its usefulness in intercalary defect reconstruction secondary to its curvature. In general, reconstruction of intercalary defects with the free iliac crest flap is limited to 10 cm. If the defects are more than 10 cm, then osteotomies are required to account for the curvature of the graft. Additionally, there is in inherent risk of hernia after harvest of this flap and anesthesia in the distribution of the lateral femoral cutaneous nerve of the thigh. In a large series, 9.7% of patients developed a formal hernia after harvest of the flap. These donor site hernias are challenging to repair secondary to their anatomic location. Persistent pain is a problem in approximately 8% of patients at 1 year after harvest.[47]

Periosteal and other bone flaps

Periosteum has long been known to have significant osteogenic activity.[48,49] The osteogenic properties of the periosteum can be utilized by harvesting a vascularized periosteal flap. Periosteal and osteoperiosteal grafts from the medial femoral condyle were first used as pedicled flaps[50] and subsequently as free flaps.[51] Recently, the free vascularized medial femoral condyle flap has been shown to have a plentiful and reliable blood supply based on the descending genicular artery[52] and has been used to treat recalcitrant nonunions of the appendicular skeleton. The size of the vascularized bone that is available is ideal for smaller nonunions. The vascularized medial femoral condyle flap may be harvested as an osteogenic periosteal, an osteoperiosteal, or a cutaneous osteoperiosteal flap depending on the needs of the reconstruction. Early experience in the use of this flap has been primarily with scaphoid nonunions, but has also proven useful in nonunions of long bones and mandibular defects as well.[53–57] This flap is based upon the descending genicular artery, which is a branch of the superficial femoral artery, and on the superomedial genicular artery, which is a medial branch of the popliteal artery. The pedicle is reliable and between 1.5 and 3.5 mm in diameter at its origin. The medial condyle has a rich supply of arterial perforators to facilitate harvest of a vascularized bone graft.[52] This flap lends itself well to the harvest of a smaller vascularized bone graft for the treatment of recalcitrant nonunions. Use of this flap for nonunions displayed a 75% success rate for primary union without complication over an average time period of 3.8 months.[53] Given the reliability of the pedicle and the rich vascular supply of the medial femoral condyle, this flap has great utility in both the axial and appendicular skeleton.

Distraction osteogenesis and the Ilizarov technique

The Ilizarov technique is a means of generating bony length through distraction osteogenesis as well as the capacity to generate additional soft tissue. The Ilizarov technique was developed in Siberia in the 1950s when Ilizarov observed that bone and soft tissue could be generated through the use of judiciously applied tension.[58,59] The Ilizarov technique can be used for reconstruction of defects up to 15 cm and may be combined with free vascularized bone grafts in order to achieve reconstruction.[60,61] The Ilizarov method may be used to treat fractures, nonunions, segmental loss of bone, malrotation, and congenital abnormalities. The Ilizarov technique requires the use of an external fixator that is rigid but allows axial motion. The Ilizarov device is a system of rings and thin wires that transfix the extremity at a tension of 60 and 130 kg.[62] The Ilizarov technique is incredibly powerful in its ability to adjust for deformity of the extremity and to generate bone and soft tissue as the limb is distracted (approximately 1 mm/day) over small increments. Muscle, nerves, blood vessels, and skin are generated in response to the tension applied by the frame and the components proliferate at the cellular level in response to tension.[63,64] In many patients, particularly those patients with Gustilo IIIB tibia fractures, there may be associated soft-tissue loss with an underlying bony defect. The Ilizarov method may be combined with free tissue transfer of soft tissue alone, or with a free vascularized bone flap that may subsequently be distracted *(Fig. 7.6)*. The utility of this combined technique was first elucidated by Fiebel *et al.* in 1994 and subsequently expanded upon by numerous others.[65–67]

The use of the Ilizarov frame in relation to soft-tissue reconstruction may be thought of in the framework as elucidated by Hollenbeck and colleagues.[68] In type I patients the Ilizarov frame may function as an external fixator for stabilization. In this case, there is adequate bone for fracture healing and the need for soft tissue can be managed with a pedicled or free tissue transfer. In type II patients the Ilizarov frame may be placed after free tissue transfer for ongoing correction of a potential nonunion or malunion. In type III patients the Ilizarov frame is placed in conjunction with a free flap and immediate bone shortening and corticotomy. The patient subsequently undergoes distraction in order to compensate for bone loss and limb length discrepancies. In type IV patients, the Ilizarov frame is used as a method of fixation for a free

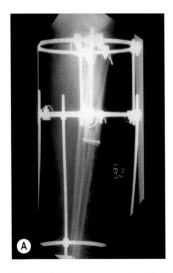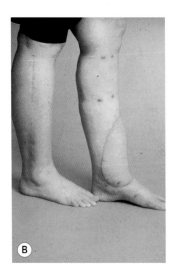

Fig. 7.6 (A) Osteocutaneous free fibular flap for reconstruction of the tibial diaphysis combined with Ilizarov frame for lower extremity reconstruction. The combination of free vascularized bone transfer and distraction with the Ilizarov frame is a very powerful tool to restore length and alignment of the affected extremity. **(B)** Postoperative result of free osteocutaneous fibular flap and Ilizarov distraction.

vascularized bone graft when the defect meets the criteria for the need of free vascularized bone transfer. This classification scheme is a useful construct to stratify the treatment of patients requiring the Ilizarov method and soft-tissue reconstruction.

The placement of the Ilizarov frame and soft-tissue reconstruction may be staged. In those patients who have a hostile or inadequate wound bed with residual infection, an antibiotic spacer may be placed in the skeletal defect at the time of debridement and soft-tissue reconstruction. Initial provisional fixation is provided by an external fixator followed by placement of an antibiotic-impregnated methylmethacrylate spacer, followed by definitive soft-tissue coverage. This allows a stable soft-tissue envelope at the time of placement of the Ilizarov frame.[69]

The combination of the Ilizarov method and modern means of vascularized soft-tissue reconstruction is a powerful methodology for limb salvage. However a subset of these patients will ultimately require amputation. In the largest series published to date the overall limb salvage rate was 84%. Within this study, the only predictor of amputation was the inability to achieve primary bony union, and increasing age was the only predictor of bony nonunion. Given these findings, it stands to reason that an aggressive approach to achieving bony union is warranted. The use of additional bone grafting, adjunctive biologic measures such as BMP, and longer periods of fixation should be considered in an attempt to achieve bony union in those patients with skeletal injuries in an Ilizarov frame.

There have been recent advances in the construct of the frame itself. The Taylor spatial frame has shown promise in the treatment of traumatic injuries with acute bone loss as well as tibial nonunions with associated bone defects.[70–73] The spatial frame differs from the standard Ilizarov construct in that it is a thin wire frame with virtual hinges and computer software support to facilitate fine corrections of bone length, angulation, and rotation. The spatial frame allows the reconstructive surgeon to have control over multiple variables through the utilization of a hexapod construct, and sophisticated computer algorithms to correct underlying deformities without frame modification, as is the case with a standard Ilizarov frame. Additionally, the spatial frame allows for potential early weight-bearing and range of motion, which may lead to improved rates of union.

Allograft reconstruction

Reconstruction of skeletal defect greater than 6 cm in length will require allograft or vascularized bone reconstruction. The reconstruction of large bony defects can be problematic and has limited surgical options. Allografts provide for reconstruction with a readily available product that can be cut to the desired size and lack the morbidity of a donor site that is required when harvesting a vascularized autograft. Allografts are typically cryopreserved grafts that are cataloged and then selected based on their specific anatomic characteristics and the reconstructive needs.[74] However, these are nonvascularized grafts and ultimately lack any osteogenic potential. The healing of these nonvascularized grafts is slow, and their incorporation is never complete.

Most studies of allografts conclude that the inner portion of the allograft remains a mechanical graft without cellularity and replacement with living tissue with the outer 2–3 mm is gradual[75–77] Allografts may be intercalary or osteoarticular. The union times of the allograft vary according to the anatomic position of the allograft, with osteoarticular grafts typically healing in less time than intercalary grafts. Union times for allograft can be as long as 23 months in the intercalary position, with union in the osteoarticular position taking as long as 12 months.[75,76,78,79] Many of the patients in need of a large allograft are patients who have an underlying bony malignancy that will require chemotherapy, which may further delay healing and union of the allograft. Despite their widespread use and availability, the avascular nature of these grafts predisposes them to complications, including infections and fracture and the need for revisions in the future *(Fig. 7.7)*.

The use and subsequent success of allografts remain dependent on the surrounding soft tissues. If there is an insufficient soft-tissue envelope, or if the surrounding soft tissue has been previously radiated, one can expect a higher complication rate which includes allograft-related infections, fractures, and nonunions.[12,80–84] When one looks at large series of long-bone reconstruction with allografts, there is a failure rate of 14% for intercalary grafts, and a wide-ranging complication rate,[85] including a nonunion rate up to 30% and failure rate of 37%.[86] The majority of these failures occur within the first 3–4 years following reconstruction, with return to function being much better for allografts in the intercalary position than when combined with a prosthesis or when used in an allograft arthrodesis.[74] In fact, when one examines the literature regarding the use of allograft reconstruction, intercalary allograft reconstruction fares much better than any other.[12,83,87–89] This fact has bearing on the current discussion as most reconstructive surgeons will be primarily involved in reconstruction of intercalary defects, with most osteoarticular or reconstructions combined with a prosthesis being performed by an orthopedic surgeon.

The Capanna technique takes advantage of both allograft and free vascularized bone reconstruction of the femoral shaft.[13,90–94] The intercalary allograft provides initial stability

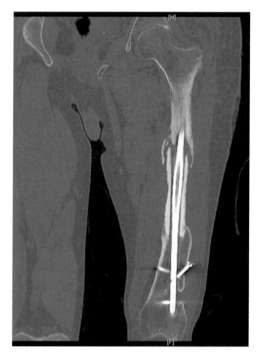

Fig. 7.7 Radiograph of failed femoral shaft reconstruction with an allograft. The patient developed a draining sinus and fractured hardware that necessitated removal of the allograft. The patient was subsequently reconstructed with a vascularized fibular flap.

and mechanical strength, while the free vascularized bone allows integration, the capacity for bony remodeling, and long-term viability of the construct and bony union. The technique involves cutting the cortical allograft to the appropriate size of the skeletal defects. The medullary portion of the allograft is then enlarged to facilitate placement of the free fibular bone graft within the medullary canal. Typically, the ends of the free fibula are left longer than the allograft so that they will have overlap with the proximal and distal ends of the bony segment. A canal or trough is cut within the allograft to provide for the vascular pedicle and to facilitate microvascular anastomoses. This method can be used to reconstruct defects of the femur, tibia, and humerus. It may be used in the immediate setting after tumor resection, or in a delayed setting for nonunion of a previously placed allograft. For patients undergoing resection for sarcoma and immediate reconstruction, the allograft will provide mechanical stability and allow for earlier ambulation without the requisite delay for hypertrophy of the free fibular graft. Additionally, patients undergoing resection for sarcoma may have delayed healing secondary to the need for adjuvant chemotherapy which would otherwise delay healing of the free fibular graft. Using the Campanna technique, recent studies have displayed a mean time for bony union of 8.6 and 9 months respectively.[13,93]

The authors have also utilized a method we have termed the "hemi-Campanna" in which the cortical allograft is bisected. This allows much easier positioning of the fibular free flap and there is no need for a slot to be cut in the allograft; it permits much easier positioning of the pedicle to facilitate microvascular anastomoses. This approach affords some of the early mechanical strength afforded by the allograft without the additional bulk and need for altering the allograft to facilitate microvascular anastomoses.

Secondary to the high complication rates associated with allograft reconstruction, some have advocated for vascularized reconstruction of skeletal defects, including the authors. Living, vascularized bone has the capacity to remodel in response to stress and hypertrophy to permit unprotected weight-bearing once union of the vascularized graft is confirmed radiographically, and the bone is of adequate caliber to withstand the anticipated forces.

Reconstruction by anatomic area

Upper extremity

Humerus

Skeletal reconstruction of any upper extremity defect must be tailored to the specific reconstructive needs. Many younger patients with bony malignancies will anticipate a functional reconstruction and have relatively high functional demands for their reconstructions. Although reconstructions of the upper extremity are not considered weight-bearing *per se*, a high degree of physiologic stress is placed on any reconstruction. Small (<6 cm) defects in well-vascularized, nonradiated, nonarticular defects may be reconstructed with conventional bone grafting. If the defect is articular, prosthetic reconstruction or a composite of prosthesis and allograft may be considered.

The treatment of segmental bone defects of the upper extremity that are greater than 6 cm has been well established with the fibular vascularized graft. Its application to large defects of the humerus, with and without the skin paddle, has become routine for reconstruction of defects after recalcitrant nonunion, tumor extirpation, hardware infection, or failure of conventional bone grafting for smaller defects.[17,68,94] The fibula is well suited to the application of humeral intercalary reconstruction given its size, length, and ease of harvest.

The operative sequence is that of a two-team approach. The humeral defect is prepared by one team, and the fibula is harvested by a second. The approach to the humerus is mandated by the previous incisions that have been used as well as the associated soft-tissue defects. The medial approach to the humerus is preferred secondary to the ease of preparation of the nearby brachial vessels to facilitate microvascular anastomoses. Any nonviable native humeral bone is resected. A standard approach to prepare cortical bone to accept the vascularized fibular graft is to maintain an intact circumferential cortex to accommodate the fibula to be placed in an intramedullary location. One can plan to excise any overlying associated scars or soft-tissue contractures that can be replaced with the supple and well-vascularized skin paddle associated with the fibula supplied by the perforators through the posterior crural septum.

The inset of the fibula involves the insertion of the fibula into the intramedullary canal of the residual ends of the native humerus. The proximal and distal ends of the humerus and the ends of the fibula may require contouring with a high-speed bur to achieve impaction of the fibular graft of 1–2 cm into the intramedullary canal. The entire construct can then be stabilized with dynamic compression plates, transcortical screws, Kirschner wires, or external fixator. This is the typical sequence that is used for placing the fibular graft for an intercalary defect.

Using this technique, primary osseous union was achieved in 11 of 15 patients (73%) in a large series. Three patients were noted to have early failure of graft fixation at the proximal or distal fixation site. These patients subsequently underwent open reduction, internal fixation with compression plates, and cancellous bone grafting for augmentation at the graft junction with the native humerus. One patient in the series required a second free fibula for graft resorption. In three patients who achieved a primary union, a secondary fracture of the fibula was noted. These patients were also subsequently treated with open reduction, internal fixation, compression plating, and an additional bone grafting and went on to achieve union within 4 months.[17]

In patients who have an existing construct with an underlying atrophic nonunion or a pathologic fracture associated with a prior allograft reconstruction, the fibular graft may be placed in an onlay fashion as a strut which spans the nonunion. There have been encouraging reports within the literature of this technique in salvage of pathologic fractures associated with allografts of the humerus and other long bones.[95–97] In the largest series in the literature of the use of the free fibular graft for salvage of a pathologic fracture, four of the 25 patients never obtained union, for a failure rate of 16% of the attempted fibular salvage of the allograft. The overall limb salvage rate was 90%; however the limbs that were salvaged after failure of the fibula were done so with an endoprosthesis.[98]

Reconstruction of the humerus with the free fibula is a well-recognized modality. Interestingly, the outcome of reconstruction of the humerus with the fibula is worse when compared to the use of the fibula for radial forearm reconstruction. The relatively high rate of fracture of the fibular graft when used for the humeral reconstruction seems to be consistent across multiple studies.[17,99] Certainly, there is an inherent rate of complications associated with complex reconstruction of the humerus. In patients who underwent oncologic resection and vascularized free fibular reconstruction in the form of glenohumeral arthrodesis, intercalary autograft, or onlay for pathologic fracture, a mean of 2.8 operations per patient was required to achieve the desired outcome. This included three of 15 patients requiring the use of their contralateral fibula for a second vascularized fibular reconstruction. Fracture and infection were the most common complications, all of which were treated successfully for limb salvage.[94]

Forearm

Reconstruction of the radius or ulna is well suited to the free osteoseptocutaneous fibular graft. The dimensions of the fibula are very similar to the dimensions of the radius and ulna, and a diaphyseal segment of bone is able to be replaced easily with the bone stock when a bed is available for use with the free fibular graft. Additionally, in many complex defects of the forearm soft tissue is required which can be replaced by the skin paddle associated with the fibula.[100] The dynamic nature of the forearm and the ability of the forearm to perform supination and pronation are crucial in the function of the upper extremity. Reconstruction of the forearm and restoration of length with an osseous union may not completely provide for the restoration of forearm rotation.[101] Any associated contracture of the interosseous space from loss of bony length can result in decreased forearm rotation and disability.

It is therefore crucial to reconstruct the radius and ulna with the kinematics of the forearm in mind.[102]

Forearm defects are typically the result of trauma, oncologic resection, or nonunion of a prior traumatic injury. However with modern methods of internal fixation the nonunion rates of diaphyseal fractures of the radius and ulna are typically less than 5%.[103-106] The reconstruction of diaphyseal defects less than 6 cm is amenable to cancellous autograft as long as there is no underlying infection or prior radiation therapy. In a large series of patients with diaphyseal atrophic nonunions, all patients were healed in 6 months after conventional cancellous bone grafting and compression plating. The diaphyseal defect averaged 2 cm and involved both bones in approximately 4% of patients.[107] This study demonstrates that excellent results can be achieved in reconstruction of diaphyseal defects with conventional, time-honored means in appropriately selected patients.

The vascularized free fibular graft remains the gold standard for reconstruction of large segmental defects of the forearm in the setting of defects longer than 6 cm or diaphyseal defects in the setting of infected nonunions and prior radiation therapy within the anticipated field of reconstruction[100,108,109] *(Fig. 7.8)*.

One should plan for excess length of the fibular graft in order to achieve the ideal final length. Having an appropriately sized fibular graft is crucial to insure that the distal radioulnar joint is in alignment.[110] During the course of reconstruction, the fibular graft is temporarily placed in its anticipated final position and a radiograph is obtained with the wrist in neutral position. This allows for verification of the appropriate anatomic position of the fibula as well as the forearm length, ulnar variance, and congruity of the distal radioulnar joint. Microvascular anastomoses are done either to the distal brachial artery in an end-to-side fashion or to the radial or ulnar arteries, ideally in an end-to-side fashion to preserve maximal flow into the distal extremity. Venous anastomoses are performed to the appropriately paired venous comitants or to a subcutaneous vein.

The outcome of the free fibular grafting for forearm reconstruction has been well documented. A survey of the literature regarding the time to union of the fibular graft to the native bone reveals a mean time to union ranging from 3.8 to 4.8 months,[100,111-117] with the majority of patients able to achieve a primary union. A small subset of patients will require a secondary procedure such as adjunctive cancellous grafting to achieve union.

An interesting application of the vascularized fibula for forearm reconstruction is the "double-barrel" technique. This allows reconstruction of both the radius and ulna with or without an associated soft-tissue defect with a single vascularized flap[118,119]; although this technique allows simultaneous reconstruction of both bones in the forearm, the limited results

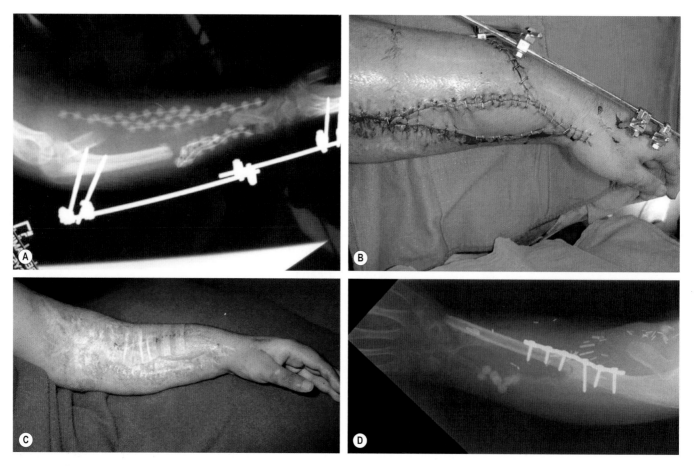

Fig. 7.8 (A) Radiograph of upper extremity with traumatic loss of radius and ulnar with provisional placement of external fixator to maintain length. **(B)** Postoperative view of upper extremity after reconstruction with vascularized osteocutaneous fibular flap to create a one-bone forearm. **(C)** Patient with healed reconstruction. **(D)** Radiograph demonstrating fibula in place after reconstruction of radius and maintenance of length of forearm.

that are available have demonstrated decreased range of motion of active pronation and supination.

Femur

Skeletal defects of the femoral shaft typically resolve from tumor resection, traumatic loss, chronic osteomyelitis, failed allografts, infected nonunions, and congenital anomalies. The femur is the longest bone in the human body and is subject to large amounts of axial loading given its position in the skeleton as well as significant rotational angular stresses. The principles of bony reconstruction as outlined above are applied to the clinical problems that are encountered. In defects that are 6 cm or less, conventional bone grafting can be applied if there is a well-suited, noninfected vascular bed. The Masquelet technique has been applied for defects over 6 cm, but in most cases for defects of 6 cm or more, vascularized fibular reconstruction of the femoral shaft is achieved as a free graft with microvascular anastomoses. Iliac crest may be used a free flap, but one must osteotimize the graft to account for the curvature of the iliac crest when using it for intercalary defects.

The maximal length of the fibula that can be harvested for reconstruction of a segmental defect remains 26 cm in a typical adult patient. The length of donor fibula available will depend on the body habitus of the individual patient. If the defect spans longer than the available fibular length, one may combine free fibular reconstruction of the femoral shaft with subsequent Ilizarov frame and distraction in order to achieve the ideal length for reconstruction and to correct for any limb length discrepancy and rotational abnormality.[68,120] Additional cross-sectional strength may be obtained with the free fibular graft by making a "double-barrel" fibular segment by performing a complete osteotomy of the fibula, taking care to protect the vascular pedicle and aligning the two fibular segments next to each other. This can only be done if the femoral segment is of a length that enables the free fibular graft to be folded in half given the available length of the donor fibula. This "double-barrel" reconstruction allows the construct to bear more force in the early postoperative period and may aid in postoperative stabilization as it is inherently a more structurally stable construct.[121,122] However, there is a requisite period of nonweight-bearing followed by reconstruction of the femur with a free fibular graft until there is adequate hypertrophy of the fibular segment as well as union of the fibula to the native femur. There is adequate evidence to demonstrate that vascularized fibular grafts have superior strength when compared with avascular bone grafts as the avascular grafts lose their strength as the graft undergoes creeping substitution after avascular necrosis.[123–125] For most patients, after demonstration of bony incorporation of the fibula into the native femur as well as a completely healed soft-tissue envelope, graduated weight-bearing may begin. This typically starts at approximately 6 months postoperatively, at which time the patient is followed through plain radiographs every several months to ensure ongoing hypertrophy of the fibula.

In order to achieve successful microvascular transfer of the fibula, one must have adequate arterial inflow and venous outflow. Depending on the approach to the femur, as well as the pedicle length and quality of the donor vessels, interposition vein grafts may be needed. The saphenous vein is the most common site for obtaining the vein grafts for additional pedicle length. The authors have previously reported a modification for the use of the ipsilateral fibula in microvascular reconstruction of the femur. The ipsilateral greater saphenous vein is transposed from its medial position and used as the venous outflow for the graft. An additional segment of vein is harvested for the interposition arterial graft. This approach obviates the need for an additional microvascular anastomosis.[126] The microvascular anastomoses are commonly performed to the superficial femoral artery and vein through a medial approach. The authors have also used the descending branch of the lateral femoral circumflex as a vascular pedicle to achieve arterial inflow and venous outflow, which obviates the need for interposition vein grafts.

When the experience of the free fibula for long bone reconstruction is reviewed, the results are favorable. Within large series of extremity reconstruction, the functional outcome is good and there is a high rate of achieving bony union.[113,127–129] The fibula should be considered the first choice for autologous vascularized reconstruction of the femur.

Tibia

Segmental defects of the tibia are commonly encountered after bone loss from trauma or after tumor resection. The use of the fibula for tibial reconstruction has been a concept that has been present within the literature for quite some time. Tibiofibular synostosis was described as early as 1941, and persisted as a means for tibial reconstruction into the 1960s. This means of reconstruction had significant limitations, including the need for large amounts of interposed cancellus bone grafts and a long time for consolidation.[130–134] Despite the advancement in microsurgical technique and the ability to harvest microvascular fibular transplants that came about in the 1970s, small series of pedicled vascularized tibial reconstructions with the ipsilateral fibula persisted in the literature with overall good results and union.[135,136] Use of the pedicled, ipsilateral fibular flap for tibial shaft reconstruction remains an alternative. However, most reconstructive surgeons prefer a free ipsilateral or contralateral vascularized fibula for tibial shaft reconstruction. Harvesting the fibula as a free flap allows an additional degree of mobility and positioning that is not afforded with a pedicled flap. Although harvesting of fibula is associated with some morbidity,[45,46,137,138] the authors' preferred approach is to harvest the ipsilateral fibula to preserve the contralateral extremity and limit the surgical undertaking to the ipsilateral extremity.

Diaphyseal tibial defects can be quite challenging problems when associated with overlying soft-tissue loss. Those gaps associated with soft-tissue loss such as seen in complex tibia fractures may require concomitant soft-tissue reconstruction as well. Segmental tibial loss is greater than 6 cm with associated soft-tissue loss of ideal candidates for reconstruction with an osteocutaneous vascularized free flap. Most patients with large tibial defects are candidates for reconstruction with a free fibular graft. The concept of reconstruction of the tibial shaft with a vascularized fibular graft was first suggested in 1981 when Chacha and colleagues[139] utilized the ipsilateral fibula as a vascularized pedicle graft for nonunion of the tibia. The use of the ipsilateral vascularized fibula for tibial reconstruction has been shown to be a reliable technique.[140] Hertel et al. used a pedicle, ipsilateral fibula for tibial shaft reconstruction in 13 patients and were able to achieve full, unprotected weight-bearing at a mean of 5.5 months. However, the majority of these patients required additional soft-tissue reconstruction in the form of a free or pedicled soft-tissue flap either pre- or postoperatively in addition to the tibial shaft reconstruction. Additionally, two of these patients required cancellous bone grafting. Since that time, microvascular reconstruction has evolved and become a reliable means for diaphyseal tibial reconstruction.

Patients undergoing segmental tibial resection for limb-sparing, oncologic surgery are candidates for the adjunctive of use of an allograft in conjunction with the free fibula via the Capanna technique. As mentioned previously, the allo-graft gives the reconstruction a mechanical strength via their strong cortical bone, but is associated with a risk of nonunion at the allograft–host junction and fracture of the allograft. The vascularized fibula contributes the potential for revasculariza-tion and remodeling through the vascularized fibula. The use of autologous bone that can grow and remodel with the patient is a particularly attractive option in younger patients requiring oncologic resection of their tibial shaft. Most authors utilize the Capanna technique with a free fibular graft, but it has also been reported with a pedicled fibular graft as well.[141,142] Utilization of the Capanna technique allows more rapid weight-bearing without the requisite time to allow fibular hypertrophy, and takes advantage of both allograft and free vascularized bony reconstruction. When one considers the anatomic location of tibial diaphyseal defects, they are more challenging than other long-bone reconstructions within the appendicular skeleton. The tibia is subject to large physical loads, relatively thin soft-tissue envelope, and a paucity of additional local soft tissue for coverage should it be needed, which makes it more prone to complication compared to reconstruction of other skeletal defects. If the tibial defect involves the articular surface, the reconstruction may be com-bined with an endoprosthesis if needed. Reconstruction of the joint in conjunction with a diaphyseal defect is beyond the scope of this chapter.

Pelvis and spine

The use of bone grafts as an adjunct in spinal surgery is indi-cated after tumor resection, traumatic defects, failed spinal fusions, and kyphoscoliosis most commonly. Historically, tho-racic spinal defects were reconstructed with pedicled rib grafts. Anterior placement of a vascularized pedicle rib graft has shown the ability to achieve bony union, but is limited in its technique to the thoracic spine.[143,144] The use of conventional cancellous bone grafting is indicated for small defects with a suitable surrounding soft-tissue envelope. Nonvascularized bone strut grafts have been described as well for defects greater than 4 cm. However, these grafts have a high fracture rate and may result in nonunions, loss of spinal height, and potentially neurologic compression.[143,145] For larger defects, free vascularized bone grafting is indicated. Both the iliac crest as well as the free fibular flap had been described as surgical options.[146] The use of the microvascular free fibular graft has been described for reconstruction of defects of the cervical spine, thoracic spine, the thoracolumbar and lumbar spine.[146–158]

Vertebrectomy defects can be reconstructed with prosthe-ses. However, if the underlying hardware is involved in infec-tion or osteomyelitis, removal of the hardware and prosthesis is mandated. Vascularized bone grafting of spinal defects after removal of hardware represents a salvage procedure. There

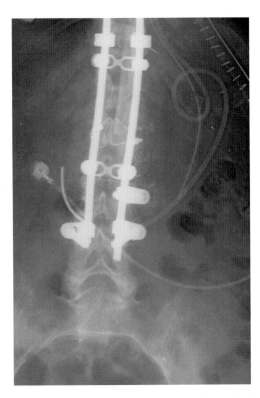

Fig. 7.9 Vertebrectomy defect reconstructed with free fibular strut graft and posterior hardware for stabilization.

are several options available for vascularized bone grafting. Vascularized rib grafts can be utilized and rotated on their vascular pedicle to facilitate vascularized reconstruction of the thoracic spine. However, one is limited by the pedicle length and proximity to the bony thoracic cage.[143,159] In most instances free vascularized bone grafting is required, and most of these cases are effectively treated with the free fibular vascularized graft (*Fig. 7.9*). The inflow and outflow vessels in the cervical region are those vessels that are typically used in microvascular head and neck reconstruction. These include the vascular branches from the external carotid artery as well as the internal jugular vein for venous outflow. For defects of the thoracic, thoracolumbar, as well as lumbar defects, seg-mental intercostal artery and veins can be used as recipient vessels. End-to-end anastomoses can be performed to the recipient vessels of the vascularized bone graft. However, if there are no suitable intercostal vessels for inflow, an end-to-side anastomosis to the aorta can be facilitated with the use of an aortic punch commonly used in cardiac surgery,[160] or end-to-side to the iliac vessels if the lumbar spine or pelvis is to be reconstructed (*Fig. 7.10*).

The use of free vascularized bone reconstruction for spinal defects is a relatively uncommon reconstructive procedure. Most reports in literature are small series or technique papers and lack long-term outcome data. The largest published series consists of 12 patients who underwent vascularized free fibular grafting after multilevel resection of their spine. Two of these patients underwent a bilateral simultaneous free fibular reconstruction following resection of one or more ver-tebral bodies or a partial or total sacrectomy. Success was measured by bony union between the fibula and the native bone. All patients required posterior fixation, and 7 of the 12

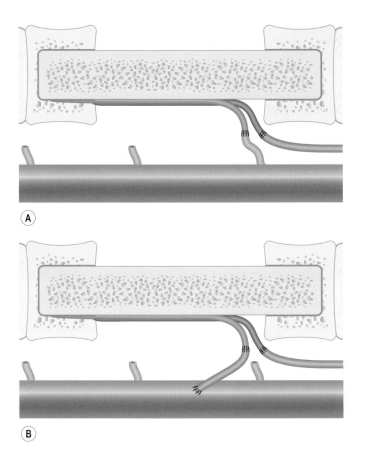

(A)

(B)

Fig. 7.10 Diagram of anastamoses of free fibular graft to aorta via an intercostal branch **(A)** and directly to the aorta in an end-to-side fashion **(B)**.

patients had additional autogenous bone graft placed at the junction of the fibula to the native bone at the time of reconstruction. All patients who underwent surgery for tumor or infection were able to achieve bony union between the free vascularized fibular graft and spine with the mean time to union of 4.5 months. While there was a relatively high complication rate associated with these reconstructions, these are difficult, complex cases without other alternatives for reconstruction.[161] The authors of this series are to be commended for their reconstructions in this very difficult patient population.

Reconstruction of the lumbosacral skeleton with vascularized bone grafts after resection results in a significant defect and discontinuity between the bony pelvis and spine. Without reconstruction, it is impossible for the patient to bear weight. This is a critical anatomic junction to allow the patient to weight-bear and be erect as well as ambulate. Any resection of the bony pelvis which involves the sacroiliac joint will need restoration of its mechanical continuity in order to distribute the weight to the lower extremities.[162] It is imperative to reconstruct this defect and give patients undergoing this complex surgical procedure their best opportunity to achieve bony union and weight distribution through their axial and appendicular skeleton and return to ambulation. In instances of large defects, there is little choice other than large vascularized bone transfers to span the significant bony gap. These large bony defects following resection have been reconstructed with vascularized fibular grafts successfully, and require a multidisciplinary approach for optimal outcomes.[161,163–167]

Clavicle

Persistent clavicular nonunion fortunately is a rare clinical occurrence. The clavicle is one of the most frequently fractured bones in the human body, and constitutes 5–10% of all fractures of the appendicular skeleton that are encountered clinically.[168,169] The clavicle typically has a rate of nonunion that is less than 1%.[169,170] Most patients with a persistent clavicular nonunion (ununited fracture after 16 weeks) will undergo a repeat open reduction and internal fixation. However, a review of the published literature reveals the failure rate of this approach was 8%, with patients suffering from persistent pain and restricted shoulder motion.[171–173] There will be a select few patients who will progress to a symptomatic nonunion and be appropriate candidates for vascularized bony reconstruction of the clavicle. The free bone flap of choice remains the fibula if there is a significant gap of 6 cm or more.

There are no large series in the literature, but the published series indicated that the fibula is a reliable source of bone and union can be achieved in complicated cases of bone loss of the clavicle, or nonunions necessitating extensive debridement and reconstruction.[174–176] However, there are several reports of success using the vascularized medial femoral condyle flap for clavicular nonunion.[55]

Vascularized epiphyseal reconstruction

Vascularized epiphyseal reconstruction has a capacity to restore the joint function as well as the growth potential of the reconstructed limb. If the epiphysis is resected secondary to tumor or lost through traumatic means in a child with skeletal immaturity, growth potential can be restored through vascularized epiphyseal transfer. The restoration of growth potential is not possible with nonvascularized autografts, allograft, a prosthesis, or vascularized bone graft without an epiphysis and maintains the potential for longitudinal growth after reconstruction.[177] The donor site for a vascularized epiphyseal reconstruction is the proximal fibular epiphysis with the diaphyseal shaft of the fibula. The proximal epiphysis of the fibula is supplied by an epiphyseal branch from the anterior tibial artery which also supplies the proximal two-thirds of the diaphysis through small, musculoperiosteal branches[43,44] *(Fig. 7.11)*. Initially, it was thought that the diaphysis was supplied through the peroneal artery and the graft must be based on both the anterior tibial as well as peroneal artery to insure survival of the epiphysis and the diaphysis respectively. Studies by Taylor *et al.*[43] and Bonnel *et al.*[44] have shown adequate perfusion of the proximal diaphysis and no need to harvest both pedicles to insure survival. The dissection can be a challenging one as the branches that supply the proximal fibular epiphysis are small and one must take care to protect the peroneal nerve during harvest. Innocenti *et al.*[178,179] have provided a beautifully illustrated technique a dissection of this difficult flap.

The proximal fibular epiphysis has several advantages over other vascularized bone grafts. The proximal head of the fibula has an articular surface and provides for a true physis and epiphysis as well as a proximal amount of diaphysis which facilitates bone fixation and diaphyseal reconstruction. The anatomic structure of the fibula and its proximal epiphysis lends itself to reconstruction of the long bones of the

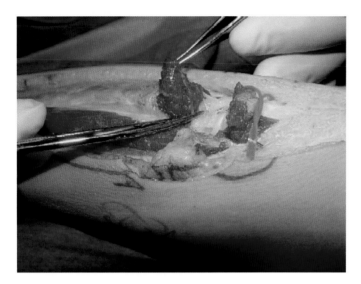

Fig. 7.11 Dissection of vascularized epiphysis of proximal fibula demonstrating the small musculoperiosteal branches.

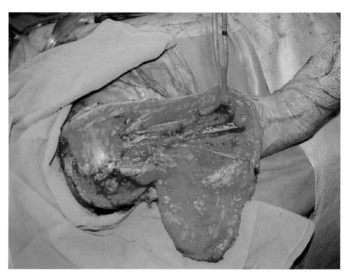

Fig. 7.12 Reconstruction of humerus with vascularized proximal fibular epiphyseal flap after resection for osteosarcoma in a child. The humeral head has been replaced with the vascularized epiphysis which will provide for longitudinal growth in the immature skeleton.

forearm as well as the humerus and the growing child. In typical vascularized bone grafts in an immature skeleton, hypertrophy of the graft is typically followed, as is growth. The addition of a true physis and epiphysis with the proximal fibular graft provides for growth but is also able to adapt to the new functional requirements as immature skeleton grows. CT studies of children who underwent reconstruction of their distal radius with vascularized proximal fibular epiphyseal graft revealed progressive remodeling of the articular surface to adapt to the proximal carpal row which translated into improvement in function of the reconstructed joint.[178] This ability to provide a vascularized articular surface, and to preserve the capacity for longitudinal growth and adaptation as to skeletal maturity, is unique to vascularized epiphyseal reconstruction. In patients with an immature skeleton who need a capacity for growth to prevent a limb length discrepancy or deformity, vascularized epiphyseal transfer from the proximal fibula should be considered (*Figs 7.12–7.14*).

Postoperative care

Postoperative monitoring

Immediate postoperative monitoring of patients who have undergone free vascularized bone transfer remains monitoring of the vascular signals of the flap. There are a multitude of options available for postoperative monitoring of free vascularized tissue transfers.[180] The authors routinely use the implantable Cook Doppler for postoperative monitoring. If the reconstruction consisted of an osetocutaneous flap, a skin perforator is marked with a 5-0 Prolene suture for additional monitoring with a surface Doppler as well as clinical examination of the skin paddle.

The other component of monitoring of patients who have undergone skeletal reconstruction typically consists of imaging the bony skeleton to assess for osseous union. This is typically done through obtaining serial conventional

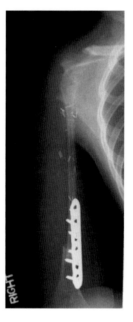

Fig. 7.13 Postoperative radiograph demonstrating flap in good position.

radiographs or cross-sectional imaging with a CT scan or MRI. The process of the ongoing osseous union is followed routinely with plain films and cross-sectional imaging is typically reserved for surveillance of those patients who underwent reconstruction after resection of malignancy, or for those patients experiencing an associated complication of their skeletal reconstruction. Technetium-99 bone scans can be performed if there is questionable viability of the skeletal construct beginning postoperatively.[181]

Adjuncts to skeletal reconstruction

Bone graft and bone substitutes used in skeletal reconstruction provide a framework for healing of the bone. They

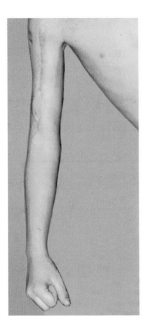

Fig. 7.14 Postoperative photograph demonstrating healed reconstruction.

provide a scaffold through which bone growth and subsequent union take place. The use of the vascularized bone graft for reconstruction of the skeleton provides living bone to bridge the bony gap but still relies on the biochemical processes of bone healing to achieve a stable skeletal union. The healing of bone is a complex biochemical pathway with multiple growth factors involved. Paramount for the healing of bone is adequate perfusion and oxygen tension of the surrounding tissues as well as stability of the bony construct to prevent motion across the reconstruction which can lead to a nonunion. There has been much research done surrounding the growth factors that are crucial in bone healing and their manipulation as an adjunctive measure to aid in achieving a stable skeletal reconstruction.

BMP has powerful osteoinductive capacity. BMP was confirmed to be osteoconductive, and the first recombinant human BMP was produced in 1988.[182,183] This ability to synthesize BMP allowed it to be used in additional basic science research and further elucidate the complex biochemical cascade that is involved in the bone-forming and osteoinductive capacity of BMP. As mentioned previously, BMP is a family of proteins with slightly different biochemical effect on bone formation. Currently, there are two commercially available recombinant BMPs available for use. RhBMP-7 has been used in a prospective randomized trial with tibial nonunions and 9 months of follow-up, which serves as the basis for its early use. The fractures had been reamed and nailed in 43% of the RhBMP-7 patients and 31% of the patients treated with allograft. At 9 months, 81% those patients treated with RhBMP-7 and 85% of allograft patients were deemed successfully treated, and radiographic evidence of fracture healing followed in a similar pattern.[184] Subsequent studies in which patients were treated with RhBMP-7 in distal tibial fractures and an external fixator were found to have more fractures healed after being treated with RhBMP-7 than those that were not treated with RhBMP-7.[185]

Despite the promising results with the use of RhBMP-7 in tibial nonunions as well as tibial fractures, there are no available clinical data to assess its usefulness when added in conjunction with vascularized bone grafting. The authors have used commercially available BMP in conjunction with the vascularized fibular flap supplemented with cancellous autograft at the proximal and distal interface with the native bone with success. However, our experience is anecdotal and small in number. This is an area of skeletal reconstruction that deserves additional research.

Other factors have been studied in their ability to aid in healing of bone, but have not reached the clinical impact that has been seen with the BMP. Vascular endothelial growth factor has been shown to enhance bone healing in a rat model of nonunion, but has not been studied in a clinical arena.[186] Platelet-rich plasma has been shown to help promote wound healing, but in experimental studies and animals was found to inhibit bone formation in a dose-dependent manner and therefore has no clinical role in the promotion of bone healing.[187]

Postoperative aesthetic considerations

Many patients who undergo skeletal reconstruction will be left with a significant scar burden, or contour deformity of the reconstructed extremity. One should not forget the aesthetic considerations in the extremity and skeletal reconstruction. Many of these patients benefit from adjunctive measures in scar reduction, improvement in appearance of other scars, or recontouring of the reconstructed extremity. There is an arsenal of reconstructive options available to aid in improving the aesthetic appearance of the extremity.

Scars may be treated through serial excision in an attempt to reduce the scar burden or completely eliminate widened or unappealing scars. If there is inadequate soft tissue to eradicate a scar completely, one may consider tissue expansion in the extremity to recruit additional soft tissue and remove unappealing, wide, or cosmetically unappealing scars. Tissue expansion has long been recognized as a valuable adjunct and soft-tissue reconstruction of the extremity.[188–191] Placement of an expander in the fascial cleft of the extremity may allow additional soft tissue for use in reconstruction and resurfacing the affected extremity. The expanders may be placed through a minimally invasive approach which shortens the time needed for reconstruction and yields a similar, more compliant flap.[192] The end result of this approach is a linear scar in the affected extremity. One must be careful not to place a linear scar over a joint, however, as this is prone to scar contracture and may limit joint mobility.

Erythematous scars may be treated with laser resurfacing to improve the erythematous nature of the scars and aid in the blending of the scars into the surrounding soft tissue. This may be performed in the office under topical or no anesthesia. The authors use the Candela V-beam laser for vascular scars with acceptable results.

Patients who have had prior soft-tissue reconstruction of their extremity with a soft-tissue free flap, or an osteocutaneous free flap with a bulky soft-tissue component, will also benefit from recontouring. This can be achieved by direct excision of the tissue bulk and thinning of the flap, or with the use of liposuction. Any plan for recontouring is delayed until a stable reconstruction is achieved and the long-term results are evident. This typically results in a minimum period of 3–6 months from the time of the initial reconstruction. If patients who have had a prior reconstruction require revision or adjunct to bone grafting, the stable soft-tissue portion of the flap may be raised and thinned at the time of the revision as well.

Conclusion

Reconstruction of the skeleton remains a challenging undertaking. There are several modalities to accomplish reconstruction of the skeleton. The optimal means of skeletal reconstruction for any existing defect is at the discretion of the reconstructive surgeon. This chapter cannot be an exhaustive review, but rather an outline of the general principles to consider when approaching these complex patients. One must be familiar with all the available techniques and the associated outcomes as well as risks and benefits of each method of skeletal reconstruction. With most reconstructive procedures there is not only the defect to be reconstructed, but potential morbidity from the donor site as well. One must not sacrifice the function of a healthy extremity in the justification of reconstruction of the contralateral one. The goal of all skeletal reconstruction is to give patients a stable bony reconstruction, and a stable and an aesthetically acceptable soft-tissue reconstruction. Additionally, it requires a multidisciplinary approach in order to achieve an optimal outcome. One needs a dedicated team to facilitate efficient and optimal care of patients undergoing skeletal reconstruction and rehabilitation.

Access the complete references list online at **http://www.expertconsult.com**

24. Bosse MJ, MacKenzie EJ, Kellam JF, et al. An analysis of outcomes of reconstruction or amputation after leg-threatening injuries. *N Engl J Med*. 2002;347: 1924–1931.

    This prospective study examined the functional outcomes of patients with severe lower extremity trauma who underwent amputation or limb salvage. Patients were rated on a self-reported health scale. This study demonstrated equivalent outcomes between amputation and limb salvage. This study lends credence to attempts at limb salvage if medically feasible.

28. MacKenzie EJ, Bosse MJ, Kellam JF, et al. Factors influencing the decision to amputate or reconstruct after high-energy lower extremity trauma. *J Trauma*. 2002;52:641–649.

38. Masquelet AC, Fitoussi F, Begue T, et al. Reconstruction of the long bones by the induced membrane and spongy autograft. *Ann Chir Plast Esthet*. 2000;45:346–353.

    This paper elucidates the Masquelet technique of inducing a bioactive membrane for the reconstruction of skeletal defects. It demonstrates that the scope of conventional bone grafting can be greatly improved by allowing the formation of a bioactive membrane to consolidate bony defects that would typically be reconstructed with vascularized bone grafting.

58. Ilizarov GA. The tension–stress effect on the genesis and growth of tissues. Part I. The influence of stability of fixation and soft-tissue preservation. *Clin Orthop Relat Res*. 1989;238:249–281.

59. Ilizarov GA. The tension–stress effect on the genesis and growth of tissues: Part II. The influence of the rate and frequency of distraction. *Clin Orthop Relat Res*. 1989;239:263–285.

    These are the seminal papers for distraction osteogenesis as initially elucidated by Ilizarov. The principles of distraction as they relate to extremity reconstruction are found in these papers. These papers demonstrated the power of distraction to generate additional soft tissue and bone length and to correct rotational deformities.

73. Feldman DS, Shin SS, Madan S, et al. Correction of tibial malunion and nonunion with six-axis analysis deformity correction using the Taylor Spatial Frame. *J Orthop Trauma*. 2003;17:549–554.

75. Bauer TW, Muschler GF. Bone graft materials. An overview of the basic science. *Clin Orthop Relat Res*. 2000;371:10–27.

90. Capanna R, Campanacci DA, Belot N, et al. A new reconstructive technique for intercalary defects of long bones: the association of massive allograft with vascularized fibular autograft. Long-term results and comparison with alternative techniques. *Orthop Clin North Am*. 2007;38:51–60, vi.

    This paper describes the use of an allograft combined with a vascularized fibula for the reconstruction of intercalary defects. It details the advantages and power of this technique which takes advantage of the strong mechanical properties of the allograft with the ability of the vascularized fibula to hypertrophy and remodel as a living graft of bone.

182. De Long Jr WG, Einhorn TA, et al. Bone grafts and bone graft substitutes in orthopaedic trauma surgery. A critical analysis. *J Bone Joint Surg Am*. 2007;89:649–658.

184. Friedlaender GE, Perry CR, Cole JD. Osteogenic protein-1 (bone morphogenetic protein-7) in the treatment of tibial nonunions. *J Bone Joint Surg Am*. 2001;83-A(Suppl 1):S151–S158.

8

Foot reconstruction

Mark W. Clemens, Lawrence B. Colen, and Christopher E. Attinger

SYNOPSIS

- Successful wound healing requires determination of wound etiology, ensuring adequate blood supply and proper identification and treatment of infection.
- This requires a team effort involving at the very least a vascular surgeon, a foot and ankle surgeon, a plastic surgeon, a diabetologist, an infectious disease specialist, a pedorthotist and a prosthetist.
- Surgical incisions and flap design relies upon a detailed knowledge of anatomy, angiosomes, and vascular status.
- Adequate debridement of the wound is critical before attempting a reconstruction. This may require a staged procedure.
- The best solution for a successful wound closure must be tailored to the patient's age and functional capacity.
- The key is to pick the optimal biomechanical result given the patient's age and functional capacity. In one patient, that may involve a free flap reconstruction while in another, it may involve a below the knee amputation,
- A successful reconstruction may ultimately fail without appropriate postoperative offloading techniques to allow healing and without addressing the biomechanical abnormalities that led to the initial breakdown.

 Access the Historical Perspective section online at
http://www.expertconsult.com

Introduction

The weight-bearing portion of the foot is subject to more repetitive trauma than any other part of the body when considering that, on average, an active individual takes over 10 000 steps a day. The foot tolerates such trauma by possessing specialized plantar tissue that can withstand the effects of such repetitive direct and shear stress forces. Blunt and/or penetrating trauma however, can cause immediate breakdown of the soft tissue and/or bone. In addition, infection, as

well as changes in blood supply, sensation, immune status, and biomechanics, render the foot and ankle susceptible to breakdown. Inability to salvage the injured foot usually leads to major amputation. This carries dramatic sequelae for the amputee because it mandates a lifetime dependence on prosthetic devices. Many never actually wear the prosthesis and are condemned to a wheelchair-bound existence. Major amputation in diabetics is associated with premature death and high likelihood of subsequent contralateral leg amputation. While foot anatomy has previously been covered in detail, this chapter will focus on the critical aspects of limb salvage, including evaluation, diagnosis, and treatment, with a focus on flap-based reconstructions.

Because the foot and ankle is such a complex body part, salvage often requires a multi-team approach. This team ideally should consist of a vascular surgeon skilled in endovascular and distal bypass techniques, a foot and ankle surgeon skilled in internal and external (Ilizarov) bone stabilization techniques, a soft tissue surgeon familiar with modern wound healing as well as soft tissue reconstructive techniques, and an infectious disease physician specializing in surgical infections. For the at-risk or biomechanically unstable foot, a podiatrist skilled in routine foot care and a pedorthotist skilled in orthotics and shoe wear are critical in preventing recurrent breakdown. Should the patient unfortunately suffer a major amputation, a skilled prosthetist is necessary to make sure that the amputee can make maximum use of his stump. To address the patient's medical co-morbidities, medical specialties are often called in to play such as endocrinology, nephrology, hematology, rheumatology, and dermatology.

Basic science

Angiosomes of the foot

In the normal patient, blood flow to the foot and ankle is redundant with three major arteries feeding the foot via multiple arterial–arterial connections. By having a thorough grasp of those arterial–arterial interconnections and by selectively Dopplering out those connections, it is possible to map out the existent vascular tree including the direction of flow. By adding the concept of angiosomes, the vascular supply becomes even clearer. G. Ian Taylor first originated the concept of angiosomes in human anatomy to describe a three-dimensional unit of tissue supplied by a single source artery. Attinger et al.[1] further developed this principle as it applies to the foot and ankle, eventually illustrating six specific foot angiosomes originating from three primary source arteries. All vascular supply to the foot and ankle enters through the popliteal fossa and the terminal branches of the popliteal artery: the anterior tibial, posterior tibial and peroneal arteries.

Above the ankle, the peroneal artery bifurcates into the anterior perforating branch and calcaneal branch. The anterior perforating branch of the peroneal artery, goes through the anterior distal intermuscular septum between the peroneal and tibial bone and sends a branch superiorly overlying the intermuscular septum (this area encompasses the area from which the supra-malleolar flap[9] can be harvested). The anterior perforating artery then connects directly with the anterior lateral malleolar artery and supplies the anterolateral ankle angiosome. The lateral calcaneal artery begins at the level of the lateral malleolus as it emerges laterally between the Achilles tendon and the peroneal tendons. It curves with peroneal tendons 2 cm distal to the lateral malleolus and gives rise to four or five small calcaneal branches. The lateral calcaneal artery terminates at the level of the fifth metatarsal tuberosity, where it connects with the lateral tarsal artery. The calcaneal branch supplies the lateral and plantar heel angiosome.

The posterior tibial artery has three terminal branches, the calcaneal branch, the medial plantar artery and the lateral plantar artery. The medial calcaneal artery branches off the posterior tibial artery inferiorly and arborizes into multiple branches that travel in a coronal direction to supply the heel. The medial calcaneal artery's angiosome boundary includes the medial and plantar heel with its most distal boundary being the glabrous junction of the lateral posterior and plantar heel.

The posterior tibial artery then enters the calcaneal canal underneath the flexor retinaculum and bifurcates into the medial and lateral plantar arteries at the level of the transverse septum between the abductor hallucis longus and the flexor digitorum brevis muscles. The medial plantar artery's angiosome boundaries encompass the instep. The lateral plantar artery's angiosome includes the lateral plantar surface as well as the plantar forefoot. The borders are: posteriorly, the distal–lateral edge of the plantar heel; medially, the central raphe of the plantar midfoot and then more distally, the glabrous juncture between the medial plantar forefoot and medial distal dorsal forefoot; laterally, the glabrous junction between the lateral dorsum of the foot and plantar surface of the foot. The distal border includes the entire plantar forefoot.

At the ankle, the anterior tibial artery gives off the lateral malleolar artery at the level of the lateral malleolus that joins with the anterior perforating branch of the peroneal artery. At the same level, it also gives off the medial malleolar artery, which anastomoses with the posteromedial artery of the posterior tibial artery. The anterior tibial artery then emerges under the extensor retinaculum of the ankle to become the dorsalis pedis artery. The dorsalis pedis artery's angiosome encompasses the entire dorsum of the foot.

The six angiosomes can be used to optimize the success of any planned treatment or procedure. The incision can be placed along the boundary of two adjoining angiosomes to ensure that the blood flow on either side of the incision is optimal. Flaps can be dissected out with a high degree of reliability. Amputations can be performed in a way that minimizes the risk of distal tissue necrosis. The revascularization can be planned to increase the chance of healing of a given wound or ulcer by 50%.[10] This detailed knowledge of vascular anatomy helps take the guesswork out of limb salvage. The surgeon is now able to determine which leg is salvageable and which has a significant chance of failure. He/she can also choose which mode of reconstruction has the most chance of success, given the existing blood supply. He/she can determine when salvage is not possible and go right to an amputation. This spares the patient needless, costly and potentially dangerous procedures, with little chance of success.

Compartment pressure measurement

Compartment syndrome of the foot, like that in the leg, must be evaluated and treated if necessary. The signs and symptoms of compartment syndrome of the foot are similar to those of compartment syndrome in general. Pain that is out of proportion to the clinical examination is often the first symptom. Weakness of the toe flexors and extensors and pain with passive dorsiflexion of the toes represents important physical signs. Pallor, paresthesia, a palpably tense compartment, and absent digital pulses on Doppler assessment eventually occur. Compartment pressure recordings should be obtained by a physician who understands the compartmental anatomy of the foot. Please refer to the section on crush injuries for a detailed discussion of the techniques to decompress the compartments of the foot.

Gait analysis

When looked for, abnormalities of gait can be detected in most patients evaluated for soft tissue repair. Working with a podiatrist and a foot an ankle surgeon is critical to determine what skeletal or muscle abnormality exists so that it can also be addressed when treating the wound. Plantar forefoot ulceration in diabetics is usually due to shortening of the Achilles tendon with resultant increases in weight-bearing pressures over the plantar foot during ambulation. Other possible causes that need to be ruled out or treated include hammer toes, long metatarsal, hallux rigidus, etc. The release of the tight Achilles tendon results in rapid healing, although at the cost of a permanent decrease in push-off forces. This however, offers long-term protection, decreasing ulcer recurrence rates by 75% at 7 months and 54% at 25 months from surgery (*Fig. 8.1*).[11,12]

Patients with prior transmetatarsal amputations and recurrent forefoot ulceration are a second group of patients with biomechanical disturbances accounting for their wounds. These problems are usually related to equinus deformity as well as varus abnormalities. Soft tissue repair should be accompanied by Achilles tendon lengthening and/or tibialis

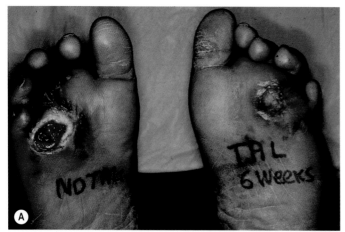

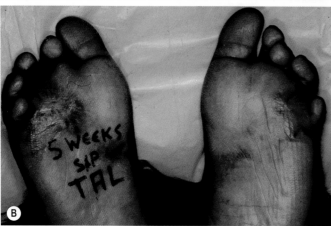

Fig. 8.1 A 39-year-old obese diabetic patient had bilateral lateral plantar metatarsal ulcers secondary to equinovarus deformity **(A)**. Both the gastrocnemius and soleus portions of the Achilles tendon were tight. The left Achilles was released percutaneously, and the left foot healed in 6 weeks with conservative wound care of the ulcer **(B)**. The right forefoot ulcer healed similarly within 5 weeks after Achilles tendon release. Correcting the biomechanical abnormality was all that was required for healing. (Reprinted with permission from Nishimoto GS, Attinger CE, Cooper PS. Lengthening the Achilles tendon for the treatment of diabetic plantar forefoot ulceration. Surg Clin North Am 2003;83(3):707–726.)

muscles at their full resting length and then with the knee flexed to assess the soleus muscle. If the ankle only dorsiflexes with knee flexion, then the gastrocnemius muscles are responsible for the tightness and can be released by performing a gastrocnemius recession. If the ankle remains tight both in extension and flexion, then both portions of the Achilles tendon have to be released, usually percutaneously. F-scan gait analysis uses multiple pressure sensing surface probes that record pressures on the sole of the foot during all phases of gait. Areas of excessive compression during weight-bearing can be displayed in graphical format and help plan the biomechanical components of the required reconstruction, as well as subsequent orthotics *(Fig. 8.2)*. The changes which occur with tendon transfer or lengthening procedures may be documented, as well, with this technique.

Patient presentation

Clinical evaluation

Principally, one has to determine a wound's etiology, previously administered wound therapies, and the patient's medical condition. The origin and age of the wound should be determined. If the wound is traumatic in origin, it should be defined in terms of high impact, low impact, repetitive, temperature related, caustic, or radiation induced. The patient's tetanus immunization status should be obtained, and the patient should be re-inoculated if indicated. In chronic wounds, the age of the wound is important because long-standing wounds can be malignant (Marjolin's ulcer). Previous topical therapy to the wound should be delineated because certain topical agents can contribute to the wound's chronicity (e.g., caustic agents such as hydrogen peroxide, 10% iodine, Dakin's solution, and so on). A careful medical history should be obtained to evaluate the most likely disease states that directly affect wound healing. Attention should be focused on diseases that may negatively affect arterial inflow into and venous outflow from the wound. Close attention should be paid to the immune system, hematological system, and to nutrition, all of which can affect wound healing. The presence of autoimmune diseases (such as rheumatoid arthritis, pyoderma gangrenosum, systemic lupus erythematosus, scleroderma, and so on) may cause inflammatory wounds that initially need medical management rather than surgical care. Compounding the care of vasculitic wounds is that they are frequently associated with coagulopathies (factor V, protein C, antithrombin III, etc.) which further complicate their management. Optimizing these vasculitic/coagulopathic wounds with medical management is critical to allow wounds to undergo the normal stages of healing. It should be noted that the medications used to treat autoimmune diseases (i.e., steroids or chemotherapy) can also contribute to poor wound healing. The nutritional status also affects wound healing and should be assessed (optimal is albumin >3.0 g/dL and/or total lymphocyte count >1500). Smoking significantly decreases local cutaneous flow and should be documented and addressed with the patient. Finally, a complete list of medications and drug allergies should be obtained. Given the complexity of various diseases affecting the healing process, multiple medical specialists may be called in to assist in the

anterior tendon transfer. Finally, patients with chronic heel ulceration will often be found to bear excessive weight on this area during gait. This may be a result of a prior Achilles tendon over lengthening procedure or a previously undetected injury to the Achilles tendon. Reconstruction should include some method of shortening and/or strengthening this important musculotendinous unit.

Other biomechanical abnormalities affecting gait can result from motor neuropathy and are most often seen in the intrinsic muscles of the foot with resultant hammer toe formation. Skeletal abnormalities can include a prominent metatarsal head, Charcot collapse, etc. Unless correction of the underlying biomechanical abnormality is part of the entire treatment plan, debriding, good wound care, and soft tissue reconstruction may prove futile.

Preoperative evaluation of gait should include a measure of ankle dorsiflexion as well as an F-scan analysis. When evaluating for equinus deformity, the leg must be held first in complete extension in an effort to keep the gastrocnemius

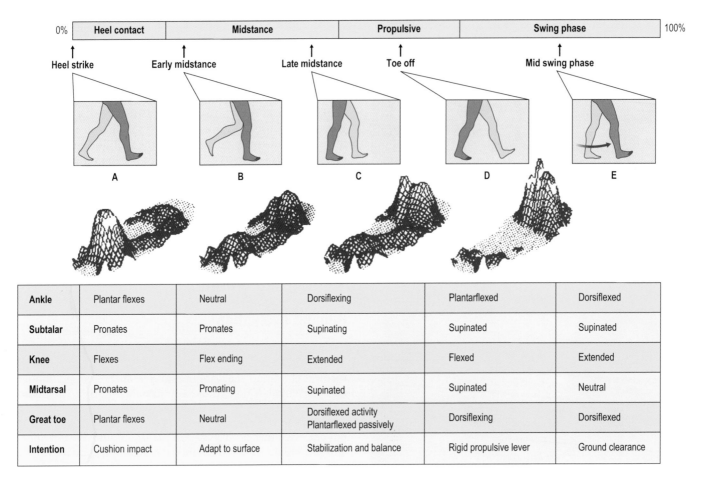

Ankle	Plantar flexes	Neutral	Dorsiflexing	Plantarflexed	Dorsiflexed
Subtalar	Pronates	Pronates	Supinating	Supinated	Supinated
Knee	Flexes	Flex ending	Extended	Flexed	Extended
Midtarsal	Pronates	Pronating	Supinated	Supinated	Neutral
Great toe	Plantar flexes	Neutral	Dorsiflexed activity Plantarflexed passively	Dorsiflexing	Dorsiflexed
Intention	Cushion impact	Adapt to surface	Stabilization and balance	Rigid propulsive lever	Ground clearance

Fig. 8.2 The normal gait cycle with representative F-Scan pressure mapping and joint function.

patient's medical management and help optimize his/her medical condition, so that the wound has a better chance of healing.

Connective tissue disorders

The connective tissue disorders (e.g., systemic lupus, rheumatoid arthritis, and scleroderma) are frequently associated with Raynaud's disease that causes distal vasospasm and cutaneous ischemia leading to lower extremity ulcers. The treatment of these connective tissue disorders frequently requires immunosuppressive drugs such as steroids or chemotherapy agents that can further inhibit healing. Although the wound retarding effects of steroids can be partially reversed with oral vitamin A (20 1000 U/day every other day while the wound is open), systemic use of vitamin A may sufficiently counter the effects of therapeutic effects steroids and this may not be desirable. Topical vitamin A at 1000U/g of ointment is usually sufficient to improve wound healing. In addition, almost half of vasculitis patients suffer from a coagulopathy leading to a hypercoagulable state. This can include any combination of Factor V Leiden deficiency, Protein C and/or S deficiency, antithrombin III deficiency, PAI 1 mutation, antiphospholipid syndrome, etc. Therefore, a coagulation blood panel should be obtained on these patients and if abnormalities exist, they should be treated with anticoagulants by the hematologist. Injectable heparin moieties, such as Lovenox, have proved to

be far more effective than warfarin in healing these ulcers.[13] The treatment of these ulcers is principally medical. Once the abnormalities have been identified and corrected, wound healing adjuncts can help in healing the wound.

Venous ulcer

Venous stasis ulcers are three to four times more prevalent than arterial ulcers and are caused by local venous hypertension. The leg has a superficial and deep venous system connected to one another by perforators. Venous blood flow is largely due to the muscle contraction that compresses the veins while directional retrograde flow is a result of the presence of unidirectional valves that prevent backflow. The valves become incompetent after thrombus formation or with old age.

Venous testing should assess for valvular competence and thrombus. A history of thrombus warrants further evaluation for coagulopathy. Surgical treatment of incompetent saphenous or lesser saphenous veins or of incompetent perforators can help relieve the local venous hypertension sufficiently to allow the wound to heal.

The mainstay of venous ulcer therapy has been compression therapy accompanied by an exercise regimen that increases venous return to the heart. Unna boots are effective in the active patient, while two, three or four-ply dressings are more effective in the sedentary patient. Chronic ulcers may benefit from aggressive wound debridement and application of cultured skin derivatives. To stay healed, the patient must wear lifetime compression therapy.

Ischemia

Atherosclerotic disease is a common cause of nonhealing foot ulcers, especially when in combination with diabetes. Hypercholesterolemia, hypertension, and tobacco use are major risk factors for atherosclerosis. Other causes of ischemia in the lower extremity include thromboangiitis obliterans (Buerger's disease, generally seen in young male smokers), vasculitis, and thromboembolic disease. The etiology of the ischemia has to be diagnosed.

If the arteries are not palpable, the Doppler signal over the posterior tibial artery, the dorsalis pedis artery and the anterior perforating branch of the peroneal artery should be evaluated. A triphasic Doppler signal indicates normal blood flow along the artery being evaluated, a biphasic signal indicates adequate blood flow, and a monophasic signal warrants further investigation. If the quality of flow is questionable, a formal noninvasive arterial Doppler evaluation has to be performed. If the flow is inadequate, the patient should then be referred to a vascular surgeon who *specializes* in endovascular techniques and in distal revascularizations. Debridement should be delayed in a stable wound with dry gangrene and inadequate blood flow, until blood flow has been corrected. Premature debridement of a de-vascularized wound may cause future loss of potentially salvageable tissue. However, immediate debridement is called for when wet gangrene, ascending cellulitis from a necrotic wound, or necrotizing fasciitis are present. Revascularization should follow as soon as possible thereafter.

Endovascular surgery has revolutionized lower extremity revascularization. This technique allows the surgeon to dilate arterial narrowing, open up an artery and keep the treated arterial segment open using drug eluting stents, or create a new subendothelial channel to reroute the blood. They are able to re-canalize occluded arteries using laser, routing, cryotherapy techniques or creating a new channel by piercing the intima. Endovascular surgery is all the more attractive because bypass surgery carries a 15–20% complication rate at the incision sites. The results of endovascular surgery are rapidly approaching those of the "gold standard", bypass surgery.[14] In bypass surgery, venous conduits remain the standard, but the availability of drug-coated grafts and the venous patch technique with or without AV fistula[15,16] are now providing an effective alternative. Combining endovascular and bypass techniques is very effective because shorter bypasses are required. It is important to remember that optimal tissue oxygenation around a wound after bypass surgery takes 4–10 days, while with endovascular surgery it can take up to 28 days. Premature wound closure attempts fail to take full advantage of the revascularization.

Brachial artery systolic pressure generally serves as a reference for determining the ankle/brachial index and gives an indication of the relative degree of ischemia. In addition, the absolute pressure measured at the ankle correlates well with the healing potential of most soft tissue wounds in the foot. A pressure cuff of 12 cm in width may be placed at the ankle level. By listening with the hand-held 10-MHz Doppler probe over the dorsalis pedis and posterior tibial vessels, the pressure at which the flow is occluded may be recorded and compared with the brachial artery occlusion pressure. In general, a normal ankle brachial index (ABI) is 1.0 or slightly greater. ABIs exceeding 0.7 have been felt to be "acceptable" for most reconstructive techniques. In diabetics, an ABI below 0.9 mandates further evaluation. Patients with indices of 0.3 or lower have rest pain, nonhealing wounds, or both. One review of vascular disease patients suggested that an ankle/brachial index of <0.5 indicates the need for a revascularization procedure before undertaking a complex reconstruction. The decision, however, is multifactorial and generally requires a complete extremity evaluation.[17] Absolute pressure measurements of <50 mmHg signify severe arterial disease with a poor prognosis for healing,[18] although neither the absolute pressure, nor the ankle/brachial index are always accurate.[19] Noncompressible arterial walls are seen in 5–30% of patients with diabetes mellitus and are caused by medial calcification, which falsely elevates the values for both tests.

Lassen et al. demonstrated that absolute toe pressures provide a highly accurate method for determining the likelihood of healing in the affected foot.[18] Barnes et al. and others[20,21] would agree that toe pressures in diabetic patients predict healing potential. A toe pressure with pressure <30 mmHg represents severe ischemia that requires vascular bypass surgery.[22]

Directional Doppler flow studies are extremely important in assessing the status of the peripheral circulation. Although many approaches to quantitative analysis of waveforms have been suggested, adequate assessment of waveforms is provided by qualitative evaluation.[23] The normal triphasic waveform becomes abnormal distal to an obstructing vascular lesion. As the obstruction becomes more significant, the waveform may deteriorate from triphasic to biphasic with a reversed flow component, to biphasic, to monophasic, to aphasic *(Fig. 8.3)*. All patients with aphasic waveforms and foot wounds should undergo vascular surgery before attempts at reconstruction. Patients with triphasic or either of the two forms of biphasic flow generally do not require vascular reconstructive procedures. Limbs with monophasic flow require further study, depending on the location of the wound and the complexity of the proposed reconstruction. If microvascular composite tissue transplantation is required for wound closure, one should attempt to obtain at least biphasic or "good" monophasic flow in the recipient vessel before the reconstruction. A narrow complex with a sharp upstroke and good amplitude characterizes "good" monophasic signals. If there is any question as to the quality of blood flow, an angiogram should be obtained. If local flap or skin-grafting techniques are employed, additional information regarding skin blood flow is needed before vascular surgical intervention can be deemed necessary.

Duplex imaging has been a component of the noninvasive vascular laboratory for more than two decades. It is most useful in the evaluation of patients with peripheral vascular disease as well as any patient who will need microvascular composite tissue transplantation (free flap) techniques in the reconstruction of their soft tissue loss. Through the use of a real time B-mode imaging system combined with a pulsed Doppler unit, it is possible to obtain a combination of anatomic, geometric, and velocity data as well as blood flow measurements from most desired locations within the vascular system.

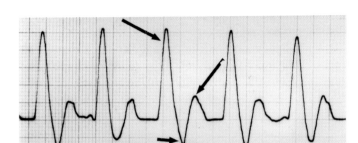

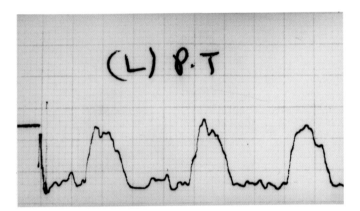

Fig. 8.3 (Top) Normal analog Doppler waveform with a forward flow component, a reverse flow component and a second forward flow component. (Bottom) With obstruction, the waveform becomes dampened and is characterized by low velocity and an attenuated or absent reverse flow component.

Diabetic foot ulcer

A total of 24 million (7.8%) of all Americans have documented diabetes mellitus and 15% of them eventually develop a foot ulcer during their lifetime.[24] Almost 15% of the healthcare budget of the US goes toward management of diabetes, with 20% of hospitalizations and 25% of diabetic hospital days for the treatment of diabetic foot ulcers.[25] Two-thirds all the major amputations performed per year in the US are performed in diabetics.[26] Diabetics battle numerous complications related to their underlying disease, but none is more devastating, both psychologically and economically, than gangrene of an extremity and its associated risk of amputation.

Diabetic peripheral polyneuropathy is the major cause of diabetic foot wounds. More than 80% of diabetic foot ulcers have some form of neuropathy present. The neuropathy is a consequence of chronically elevated blood sugars that cause vascular and metabolic abnormalities. Elevated intraneural concentrations of sorbitol, a glucose byproduct, are thought to be one of the principle mechanisms for nerve damage. Further damage can result when the damaged nerve swells within anatomically tight spaces such as the tarsal tunnel. The combination of nerve swelling and tight anatomic compartments leads to the "double crush syndrome," which can sometimes be partially reversed with nerve release surgery.[27] Unregulated glucose levels elevate advanced glycosylated end-product (AGE) levels that may induce microvascular injury by cross-linking collagen molecules. Decreased insulin levels, along with altered levels of other neurotrophic peptides, may decrease maintenance or

repair of nerve fibers. Other potential causative factors of peripheral polyneuropathy include altered fat metabolism, oxidative stress, and abnormal levels of vasoactive substances such as nitric oxide.

Hyperglycemia can also affect the body's ability to fight infection. Hyperglycemia diminishes the ability of polymorphonuclear leukocytes (PMNs), macrophages and lymphocytes to destroy bacteria. In addition, the diabetic's ability to coat bacteria with antibiotics is diminished, which further helps shield bacteria from phagocytosis. As a result of this impaired immune state, diabetics are especially prone to *Streptococcus* and *Staphylococcus* skin infections. Deeper infections tend to be polymicrobial, with Gram-positive cocci, Gram-negative rods, and anaerobes being frequently present on culture. PCR has shown that there are at least 39 species within the biofilm of such wounds, with over 60% being anaerobic. Postoperative complication rates correlate directly with the level of postoperative hyperglycemia.[28,29] Finally, diabetics have decreased stem cells in their bone marrow and decreased stem cell pluripotency when mobilized.[30] This affects the healing of wounds.

Some 80–85% of amputations are preceded by nonhealing ulcers in patients with neuropathy.[31,32] Despite attempts to decrease the number of amputations in the US by various strategies from better glucose control, to monitoring screening exams for impaired sensibility, the number of amputations has continued to increase from 54 000 in 1990 to 71 000 in 2004.[33,34] In spite of a better understanding of the pathogenesis of foot ulceration in the diabetic and the institution of a multidisciplinary approach to management, trends in amputation have not shown any tendency towards improvement in recent years and foot ulceration remains the most common reason for hospitalization of the diabetic patient in the US.[35–38]

Foot ulceration is much more common in those patients with neuropathy and vascular disease: the annual incidence rises from <1% in patients who do not have neuropathy, for example, to more than 7% in those with established neuropathy.[39,40] The average cost of an ulceration was $27 500 in 1997 and the cost of an amputation ranged from $22 702 for a toe, to $51 281 for a leg, with the annual cost for diabetic neuropathy and its complications in the US being between $4.6 and $13.7 billion.[41,42] Once an amputation has been performed, the incidence of a second amputation in the contralateral limb approaches 50% within 2 years.[43–45]

Several misconceptions have perpetuated a "fatalistic" approach towards the management of the diabetic foot resulting in excessive amputations over the years. The first is that all diabetic foot problems are due to "small vessel disease." Specifically, the presumption is that distal arteriolar occlusive disease can cause ischemic wounds even in the presence of normal pedal pulses. This misconception dates back to the work of Goldenberg more than 40 years ago.[46] More recent studies do not corroborate this retrospective analysis, including a blinded study by Strandness performed in a prospective fashion.[47] Other prospective evaluations using arterial casting techniques also failed to show diabetic-specific distal arterial occlusions.[48] Blood flow studies in diabetic patients undergoing femoral-popliteal bypass have shown no difference in the responsiveness of the runoff bed to papaverine vasodilation, when compared with the same measurements made in nondiabetic patients, indicating normal reactivity of the resistance vessels (the arterioles).[49] The second misconception is that endothelial cell proliferation occurs within the small vessels of diabetic patients and thereby, results in small vessel occlusions. Prospective studies have failed to show an increase in the incidence of intimal hyperplasia in the small vessels of these individuals.[50] Thickening of the capillary basement membrane has been well documented, but capillary narrowing or occlusion has not.

Although the infrapopliteal arterial occlusive disease present in diabetic patients often results in distal vascular insufficiency, it is now well accepted that peripheral neuropathy is the primary cause of foot wounds in the diabetic population.[51] The lack of a PO_2 gradient between arterial blood and foot skin among diabetic patients without ulceration, diabetic patients with ulceration, and nondiabetic patients with normal transcutaneous oxygen tension further implicates a nonischemic etiology.[52]

Neuropathic changes

The neuropathic changes observed in the diabetic foot are a direct result of the abnormalities in the motor, sensory and autonomic nervous systems. The loss of pseudomotor function from autonomic neuropathy leads to anhidrosis and hyperkeratosis. Fissuring of the skin results and facilitates bacterial entry with subsequent infection. The lack of sensibility over bony prominences and between the toes often delays the detection of these small breaks in the skin.

Charcot deformities (neuroarthropathy) of the small joints of the foot occur in 0.1–2.5% of the diabetic population.[53,54] When present, the tarsometatarsal joints are involved in 30%; the metatarsophalangeal joints in 30%; the intertarsal joints in 24%; and the interphalangeal joints in 4% of the time. The explanation for these degenerative changes is widely debated. One theorized etiology is "neurotraumatic," i.e., joint collapse occurring as a result of damage that has accumulated because of insensitivity to pain, although small fiber functions may be preserved.[55] The destructive changes that occur in the Charcot foot cause a collapse of the medial longitudinal arch, which alters the biomechanics of gait. The normal calcaneal pitch is distorted which in turn causes severe strain to the ligaments that bind the metatarsal, cuneiform, navicular, and other small bones that form the long arch of the foot.[56] These degenerative changes further alter the gait, resulting in abnormal weight bearing stress, causing a "collapse" of the foot. Unfortunately, ulceration, infection, gangrene, and limb loss are frequent outcomes if the process is not halted in its early stages.

The process probably begins with a ligamentous soft tissue injury accompanied by synovitis and effusion. In the absence of pain perception, continued use of the extremity exacerbates the inflammatory process. Eventually, distention of the joint capsule leads to ligament distortion, resulting in joint instability. Further activity causes articular cartilage erosion, with debris being trapped within the synovium. Heterotopic bone formation and eburnation of load-bearing surfaces frequently results.

The motor component of the neuropathy further contributes to Charcot deformities as the intrinsic foot musculature atrophies and becomes fibrotic. The resulting metatarsophalangeal joint extension and interphalangeal joint flexion produce excessive pressure on the metatarsal heads and the ends of phalanges. The loss of both the transverse and longitudinal arches of the foot exacerbates the unfavorable weight distribution across the midfoot and metatarsal heads.

Histologic similarities between chronically entrapped nerves and those seen in diabetic neuropathy provide substantial evidence that diabetic patients are unusually susceptible to peripheral nerve compression.[57,58] Several authors suggest that nerve compression (subclinical) in concert with early diabetic nerve changes (subclinical) may give rise to a clinical picture of diabetic neuropathy (the "double crush hypothesis") and therefore advocate peripheral nerve release at known anatomic sites of compression.[59]

Hemorheologic abnormalities

Although "small vessel disease" has not been anatomically confirmed in diabetic patients, recent evidence suggests that a functional alteration in capillary blood flow probably exists. This abnormal hemorheology may be responsible for much of the clinical picture now defined as "diabetic complications," i.e., retinopathy, nephropathy, microangiopathy, and neuropathy.[60] Increases in blood and serum viscosity and flow abnormalities in leukocytes, erythrocytes, platelets, and plasma proteins have been reported in diabetic patients.[61] Many investigators equate these hemorheologic impairments as the functional equivalent of diabetic microangiopathy.[62,63]

The increase in blood viscosity noted in diabetic patients appears to have its origin in a stiffened red blood cell membrane as well as an increase in erythrocyte aggregation.[64–66] Since red blood cells must deform to pass through capillary beds, stiffened cells may resist passage and even traumatize the endothelium. The nonenzymatic glycosylation of the red blood cell membrane protein spectrin is responsible for the membrane stiffening and the increased aggregation that occurs.[67] Both of these result in an increase in blood viscosity. The mechanism of this glycosylation is similar to that seen with hemoglobin and is directly proportional to serum glucose levels.[68,69]

The altered flow characteristics that result from changes in viscosity trigger a compensatory rise in perfusion pressure, causing an increase in transudation across capillary beds and further increases in viscosity. Ischemia to the peripheral tissues is further exacerbated by the increased affinity of glycosylated hemoglobin for the oxygen molecule. The detrimental effects of hyperglycemia on blood flow and tissue perfusion are significant (*Fig. 8.4*).

Fortunately, many of these effects may be reversed by establishing good metabolic control of the diabetes. Juhan et al. found that the stiff red blood cell in the uncontrolled diabetic could be reversed to normal within a 24-h controlled insulin infusion.[70] Pentoxifylline, a trisubstituted methylxanthine derivative, improves the deformability of erythrocytes and may be of considerable benefit to diabetic patients with extremity wounds. Pentoxifylline increases adenosine triphosphate (ATP) levels within red blood cells. Because erythrocyte deformability is ATP-dependent,[71] the net result is a more flexible erythrocyte. Both *in vitro* and *in vivo* studies have documented measurable improvements in blood viscosity, as well as extremity blood flow, in diabetic patients with peripheral vascular disease treated with pentoxifylline.[72–74] The salutary effects of long-term administration of pentoxifylline to type I and II diabetic patients with microvascular (retinopathy and nephropathy) and macrovascular (ischemic heart disease and

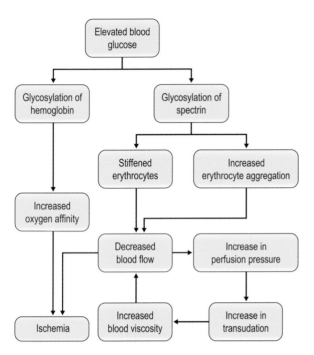

Fig. 8.4 Effects of serum glucose elevation on blood flow and tissue perfusion.

peripheral vascular disease) complications have been well documented.[75] A few studies have demonstrated the efficacy of cilostazol as an adjunct treatment of ulcers; however, the trials are small and without control groups.[76,77] Cilostazol is a selective inhibitor of 3-type phosphodiesterase (PDE3) increases cAMP and the active form of PKA, which is directly related with an inhibition in platelet aggregation.

Chronic wound evaluation

The wound is assessed carefully by measuring its size and depth and then photographed. A metallic probe is used to assist in the evaluation of the depth of the wound. If the probe touches bone, there is an 85% chance that osteomyelitis[78] is present. If tendon is involved, the infection is very likely to have tracked proximally or distally. Note the presence and extent of cellulitis and differentiate this from dependent rubor. The blood flow to the area is then evaluated by palpation and/or hand held Doppler. If the flow is inadequate, the patient should then be referred to a vascular surgeon. It is important to consider converting a "chronic wound" into an "acute wound," via surgical debridement that includes removing not only the wound base covered with excessive matrix metalloproteinases and biofilm but also the wound edges that usually consist of senescent cells. By removing the factors inhibiting the chronic wound from healing and by correcting the local and systemic factor that may also have contributed, the wound then has a chance of healing.

Bone assessment

Plain films should be obtained before any surgical intervention on the foot is planned. Bone spurs, bony prominences, malunion, nonunion, and other deformities or abnormalities

are readily identified with these simple studies. This information is extremely useful in the formation of an operative plan.

The presence of osteomyelitis in conjunction with open wound of the foot is *not* common when plain roentgenograms are normal. Whenever abnormalities on plain films suggest the presence of osteomyelitis, it is important to obtain additional studies before committing the patient to a prolonged course of parenteral antibiotics. The role of noninvasive radiologic techniques in the evaluation of the bony structures of the foot is detailed later in this chapter in the discussion of the "diabetic foot." If osteomyelitis is suspected, then a bone biopsy should be performed using a separate approach rather than obtaining tissue directly through the ulcerated wound. Most often, however, bone is sampled through the operative site because it is often present at the base of the debrided wound. In these instances, medullary tissue should be obtained with a previously unused curette and submitted for both decalcification (in formalin) and culture and sensitivity (in a few drops of normal saline solution). Based upon the results of these studies, accurate selection of antibiotics may be performed.

The precise evaluation of the extent of sequestra in patients with chronic osteomyelitis can be a formidable problem. Isosulfan blue dye may be used to help determine viable from nonviable bone. This dye has been used either via systemic administration[79] or regionally through a superficial vein.[80] The regional technique allows one to use a lower total dose of the dye and a lower concentration. An intravenous catheter is placed through a superficial vein on the dorsum of the foot. An ankle tourniquet is then inflated and 10 mL of 0.1 % isosulfidine (isosulfan) blue dye is injected followed by catheter removal. Over a period of minutes the bone and soft tissues of the foot become stained with the dye. The contrast between unstained, avascular bone and soft tissue and the stained tissue is readily apparent, thus facilitating precise debridement techniques

Infection identification and directed antibiotic therapy

Wound infection is characterized by the presence of replicating microorganisms within a wound, resulting in a subsequent host response such as erythema, warmth, swelling, pain, odor, and purulent drainage. If not recognized and treated, the infection will spread systemically leading to fever, an elevated white blood cell count, and possibly sepsis. The threshold between colonization and infection may be minute, so early identification and action are critical to healing wounds and minimizing complications. Quantitative research has shown that when the bacterial count (bioburden) reach levels more than 10^5 bacteria/g of tissue, a wound infection will result and inhibit the wound healing process.[81]

When managing the fetid foot, it is important to know the source and extent of the infection. The edge of the erythema around the wound should be delineated, timed and dated. This is then used as a reference point for effectiveness of the chosen antibiotics and/or debridement. Obtaining a radiograph of the affected area lets the physician know whether the bone is involved and whether gas is present in the soft tissue. If gas is seen within the tissue planes on the radiograph, then gas gangrene is most likely present and the wound becomes a surgical emergency. This gas is usually a byproduct of anaerobic bacteria (usually *Clostridia perfringens*); it tends to be foul smelling and to travel along the fascial planes. Compartment pressures in the affected area should be checked, because high pressures in the diabetic foot with gas gangrene are frequently missed. If there is a question of a deep abscess, ultrasound imaging or computed tomography scanning can be very useful.

If the wound is acutely infected with draining purulence, odor emanating from it and/or with proximally ascending erythema, it needs to be debrided immediately and very aggressively to prevent sepsis and possible limb loss or death. The involved compartments of the extremity should be released if there is any question that the compartment pressures are abnormally high. Wounds with foul-smelling odors should be debrided sufficiently to get rid of the odor. If the foul odor is still present at the end of the procedure, then the debridement is incomplete and more necrotic or infected tissue should be excised. It is important to remember that just because an extremity presents with gas gangrene, it should *not* be summarily amputated, as aggressive, repetitive debridement ± hyperbaric oxygen, can often salvage enough of the limb to preserve a functional extremity. Hyperbaric oxygen has been shown to be particularly helpful in the control of anaerobic infections.[82]

Aerobic and anaerobic cultures of the wound are obtained during the debridement by taking pieces deep to the surface of infected tissue and purulence. A swab or superficial tissue culture is of limited use, because it usually reflects surface flora rather than the actual underlying bacteria responsible for the infection. One should then debride the wound as specified above and start broad-spectrum antibiotics after the deep tissue cultures have been obtained. The antibiotic spectrum can be narrowed as soon as the culture results become available. It is important to remember that a deep culture may miss up to two-thirds of the bacteria species present.[83] Persisting signs of infection may be due to inappropriate antibiotics or undrained purulence or necrotic tissue.

For suspected osteomyelitis, obtain cultures of both the debrided osteomyelitic bone and the normal bone proximal to the area of debridement. It is very helpful to label the osteomyelitic bone culture as "dirty" and the normal proximal bone culture as "clean" so that the quality of the debridement can be assessed and the length of antibiotic treatment can be determined. If a wound is closed and the "clean" culture is showing no growth, then 1–2 weeks of antibiotic therapy is usually enough. On the other hand if the "clean" culture is positive for bacterial growth, then a re-resection of bone or a 6-week course of antibiotics may be necessary. A 6-week course of antibiotic therapy is no longer the accepted course of therapy if the involved infected bone has been surgically removed. When only healthy bone remains at the base of the wound, a 1-week course of appropriate antibiotics usually suffices. The exception to a 1-week course of antibiotics after closure is when the surgeon suspects that the bone left behind may still harbor osteomyelitis (e.g., calcaneus or tibia).[84] In that case, a longer course of antibiotic therapy is needed. The appropriate antibiotic course is best determined and monitored by an infectious disease physician for treatment as well as for management of untoward side-effects.

By definition, open wounds are contaminated, meaning that the bed contains planktonic bacteria and biofilm. Acute wounds have only 6% biofilm present whereas chronic wounds have greater than 90% biofilm present. Mature biofilm, older than 48 h, is resistant to topical and systemic antibiotics as well phagocytosis. It can contain over 60 different species (best identified using PCR) of which over 60% are anaerobes. Biofilm is formed when the planktonic bacteria adhere to the surface and form micro-colonies where they undergo phenotypic changes and form quorums that they protect by secreting a protective covering of extracellular polyglycolic substrates. Within the next 48 h, the protective biofilm matures and becomes resistant to both phagocytosis and antibiotics. These colonies of different species bacteria coexist at a far lower energy state and they combine their individual capacity to resist antibiotics making them less susceptible to antibiotics. The colony then spreads by breaking off fragments of biofilm (70%) or by individual seeding of undifferentiated planktonic cells (30%). Biofilm causes inflammation and while classic signs of infection may not be present, symptoms such as increased pain/tenderness, increased exudates, abnormal odor, or abnormal or friable granulation tissue signal its presence.

Patient selection

As seen in the section above, understanding and identifying the etiology of the wound is paramount before proceeding with healing of the wound. The medical conditions of the patient as well as the functional capacity of the patient are critical to determining therapeutic options. For example, microsurgical free flaps are not an option for dialysis patients. Complex reconstructions involving revascularization, microsurgery, Ilizarov and prolonged immobilization for patients with severe cardiac disease are not an option. For the noncompliant patient, the reconstruction has to assume the worse and hence a complex reconstruction may not be in the patient's best interest. Therefore, a thorough evaluation of the patient's medical capacity to undergo various reconstructive options has to be undertaken before proceeding with repair.

Identify function of the limb

The patient's current and anticipated level of activity is important to best determine if the leg should be salvaged and to what degree it should be reconstructed. If the patient is using the leg in any way, including simple transfers, then salvage, is usually indicated. However, if the limb is not going to be used, then strong consideration should be given to performing a knee disarticulation or above knee amputation to cure the problem and minimize the risk of recurrent breakdown.

The complexity of the reconstruction depends on the ultimate functional goal. For the younger patient or athlete who can tolerate microsurgery, restoration of normal function is the goal. However, a complex reconstruction for a marginally functional leg is often worse than a below the knee amputation with an athletic prosthesis. For the patient who uses the leg simply to transfer, the simplest solution that will achieve that goal should be chosen even if it means sacrificing part of the foot.

Management

Trauma and crush injuries

Crush injuries or ischemic insults to the foot can elevate pressures within the myofascial compartments. When measuring the compartment pressures of the foot, it may be difficult to determine the compartment in which the pressure is actually being recorded. If clinical indications are present, a four compartment release should be performed.[85]

The medial approach to the foot, as advocated by Henry, allows decompression of all four compartments with a single incision.[86] Mubarak and Hargens have advocated two longitudinal incisions on the dorsum of the foot through which the interosseous compartments may be decompressed (as in the hand).[87] Whitesides anecdotally described compartment syndrome of the foot secondary to burns and direct trauma and recommended decompression using the medial approach of Henry.[88]

For compartment decompression, a curvilinear incision is made on the medial side of the foot, beginning at the first metatarsal head and extending to the heel. Divide both the skin and fascia and then reflect the flap plantarly to permit visualization of the abductor hallucis muscle and its tendon, thus decompressing the medial compartment. Retract the abductor hallucis towards the plantar surface and open the medial intermuscular septum, providing for release of the central compartment. The small toe compartment may be released next using a linear incision along the lateral aspect of the foot from the level of the fifth metatarsal head to the calcaneus. This approach adequately releases the fascia enveloping the small toe compartment. Decompression of the interosseous compartment is best achieved through two linear incisions on the foot dorsum overlying the second and fourth metatarsals. The fascia overlying the four interosseous spaces may be opened *(Fig. 8.5)*.

Debridement of the chronic wound

Debriding a wound of necrotic tissue, foreign material, and bacteria/biofilm is essential as they ultimately impede the body's attempt to heal by producing or stimulating the production of proteases, collagenases and elastases that overwhelm the local wound healing process.[89] Bacteria produce their own wound inhibiting enzymes as well and consume many of the scarce local resources (oxygen, nutrition and building blocks) that are necessary for wound healing. Most of the offending bacteria reside within biofilm where they protect themselves from antibiotics and macrophages while inciting an inflammatory reaction around them.[90] The biofilm tends to penetrate the base of the wound by spreading along the blood vessels that supply the surface in a process called "perivascular cuffing". This penetration can be as deep as 4 mm suggesting that superficial scraping of the wound does little to get rid of the biofilm.

Steed reviewed the data of platelet-derived growth factor's effect on the healing of chronic diabetic wounds[91] and established level 2a evidence that wounds healed almost three fold more when the wound debridement was

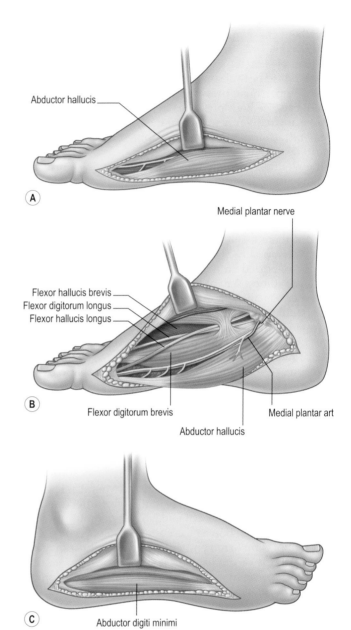

Fig. 8.5 (A) Medial instep incision and release of the great toe compartment. **(B)** Incision through the medial intermuscular septum will release the central compartment (abductor hallucis muscle retracted). **(C)** Lateral incision to release the small toe compartment.

performed weekly rather than more sporadically. Two further level 2 studies support the critical role of debridement in wound healing.[92,93]

The principal debriding technique consists of removing the grossly contaminated or necrotic tissue *en masse*, while leaving a maximal amount of viable tissue behind. It is critical not to harm the underlying tissue as they will serve as the source for future wound healing. One has to use gentle wound handling techniques such as sharp dissection instead of cautery resection, skin hooks to retract the tissue, pinpoint use of the cautery to minimize the amount of charred tissue left behind, etc. One should avoid traumatizing techniques such as crushing the skin edges with forceps or clamps, burning tissue with electrocautery, or tying off large clumps of tissue with sutures.[94] Surgical tools include a scalpel blade, mayo scissors, curettes, and rongeurs as well as power tools including a sagittal saw, a power burr, and a hydro-surgical debrider (Versa-Jet©, Smith & Nephew, Hull, UK). Debridement is performed as often as necessary until the wound is deemed clean and ready for reconstruction.

In order to be sure that the entire wound has been adequately debrided, three useful adjuncts are helpful. The first is to debride the wound until only normal tissue colors of red, white, and yellow remain at the base of the wound. The second is to first paint the wound base with blue dye using a cotton swab.[95] After adequate debridement, there should be no blue dye left in the wound base. Finally, the edges of chronic wounds contain senescent fibroblast cells[96] and an area of 3–5 mm of the tissues at the wound edge must be excised during the initial debridement to allow the healthy cells behind to help heal the wound *(Fig. 8.6)*.

In between debridements, topical antibiotics can help reduce the bacterial load: silver impregnated dressings, antibiotic beads, 0.025% acetic acid, or silver-sulfadiazine works well for all wounds. Against biofilm, silver, Iodosorb and lactoferrin have proven to effective in controlling its reaccumulation. In addition, Bactroban© is useful for MRSA, Silvadene, 0.025% acetic acid or gentamicin ointment for *Pseudomonas* infections, bacitracin for minimally infected wounds. Once the wound is *clean* and *adequately vascularized*, then it can be covered with a negative pressure wound therapy (NPWT) device. NPWT applies subatmospheric pressure to a wound via a closed suction mechanism.[97–99] NPWT increases local blood flow, reduces tissue edema, controls bacterial proliferation to 10^4–10^6 and speeds up the formation of granulation tissue. Because this dressing is changed every 48–72 h, the wound is less subject to cross contamination when compared to normal bacterial contamination that occurs when the dressing is changed every 8 h.

Wound management

Strict offloading and elevation of the extremity are essential to eliminate edema and help control infection. Adequate surgical debridement of necrotic tissue and drainage of purulent cavities are mandatory. Plantar space infection should be suspected in any patient who has cellulitis and a plantar ulcer, especially if palpation of the instep reveals tenderness or swelling. Aspiration with a 3 mL syringe and an 18 gauge needle helps confirm the presence of such a problem. If in doubt, MRI evaluation may help decide whether or not emergent surgery is indicated. Serial debridement of the ulcer and associated areas of infection are critical to controlling infection.

Although X-ray studies are not diagnostic of bone infection, they are useful for detection of bone spurs, prominences, and other osseous abnormalities.[100] While the "gold standard" for the diagnosis of osteomyelitis remains the bone biopsy of the suspected segment, the use of a metal probe to bone has been shown to be useful in increasing the index of suspicion of bone infection.[101] Of the noninvasive studies, MRI has proven to be the most reliable.[102]

Adjunctive surgical techniques alluded to earlier in this chapter are extremely important in preventing ulcer recurrence in patients with neuropathic wounds. The important role of osseous manipulation at the time of soft tissue reconstruction cannot be overemphasized. Bone spurs, joint dislocations, and other causes of improper weight dispersion on the sole of the foot must be corrected to help maintain a stable soft tissue envelope. Charcot deformities of the midfoot often are heralded by mild effusions, joint instability, crepitus, and soft tissue swelling before a fixed deformity appears. If these symptoms are identified early, casting may prevent permanent deformity.[103] When forefoot ulceration occurs over the fifth metatarsal head, resection through the metatarsal neck is recommended. This may be accomplished either through the debrided wound, if the ulcer penetrates deeply, or through a linear, tendon-splitting incision dorsally. The first metatarsal is debrided only if it is involved with the ulcer base. Complete resection is not recommended because this procedure destroys the medial column that results in excessive weight transfer to the adjacent metatarsal head. Rather, resection of the plantar flare of the metatarsal head makes the most sense. Frequently the medial or lateral sesamoid bones are the source of the ulceration. These small bones may be excised through the wound at the time of flap closure. With ulceration over the second, third, and fourth metatarsal heads, performing a "floating" metatarsal neck osteotomy at the time of wound closure offloads the ulceration site.[104] As with fifth metatarsal head resection, a linear dorsal approach may be used. This procedure allows the prominent metatarsal head to move dorsally without transferring excessive weight-bearing to the adjacent metatarsals. Address bony prominences associated with midfoot wounds with judicious resection. The medial instep wound results from deformity about the first metatarsal base, medial cuneiform, and navicular bones. The more lateral wounds seen are usually secondary to prominence of the fifth metatarsal base and cuboid bones. Limited midfoot fusions should be strongly considered when they will prevent subluxation of joints and thereby provide for more uniform weight distribution.

Many wound healing adjuncts have level-one evidence of their effectiveness in healing diabetic foot wounds.[105] The use of NPWT to prepare debrided diabetic foot wounds has been shown to hasten healing and decrease amputation rates.[106] The use of biologically active wound coverage has also been shown to speed up healing (Regranex, Apligraf and Dermagraft).[107–110] Though the use of hyperbaric oxygen therapy remains somewhat controversial, there is now level one evidence that it has been shown to decrease amputation rates and hasten healing.[111,112] These should all be considered in concert with any of the above discussed reconstructive strategies.

External fixation

A significant number of wounds will breakdown or fail to heal in the postoperative period because of repetitive shear and torque forces around a mobile joint and because of decubitus pressure or premature ambulatory pressure. This is often due to an inability of the patient able or willing to comply with postoperative offloading and immobility. The detrimental effect of motion on wound healing is well established.[113,114] External fixation has an established role for the treatment of

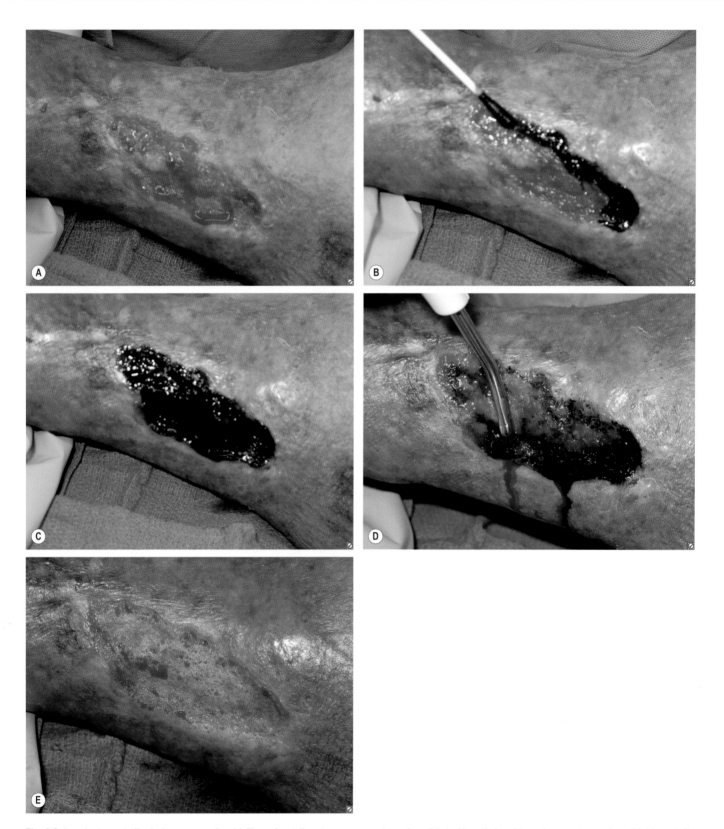

Fig. 8.6 In order to most effectively remove surface biofilm and metalloproteases, a wound may be painted with methylene blue using a cotton swab predebridement. Note after adequate debridement, there should be no blue dye left in the wound base. (Reprinted with permission from Clemens MW, Attinger CE. Functional reconstruction of the diabetic foot. Semin Plast Surg 2010;24(1):43–56.)

fracture and osteomyelitis.[115–117] The ability to immobilize the skeletal framework without utilizing internal fixation has led to the salvage of limbs that required amputation in the past.[118] The fixator maintains bone and joint alignment through rigid external fixation despite often significant bone resection for osteomyelitis and/or skeletal realignment. It does that without having to resort to internal fixation with plates and screws that are contraindicated in infected wounds. The Ilizarov fixator has been shown to shorten healing time, decrease pin track infections, and can allow early weight bearing by the addition of a protective plantar foot plate.[119]

Motion along a joint underlying a soft tissue reconstruction often leads to dehiscence or breakdown. We reviewed our experience over a 6-year period and identified 24 consecutive patients in whom external fixation was used solely to protect soft tissue reconstruction and found an overall limb salvage rate of 83% in a multiplanar external fixator group and 73% limb salvage in a monoplanar group.[120] Soft tissue reconstructions included primary closure, split thickness skin grafts, and local flaps. For larger wounds involving a free flap or Sural artery flap reconstruction, an Ilizarov frame is ideal because it not only suspends the heel and foot in good skeletal alignment, but also protects the flap from any potential trauma. Patient compliance with alternative offloading schemes has proved to be the undoing of many reconstructions and averages over 20% in our institution. Sagebien et al. have recently reported the successful use of external fixation to protect free flap soft tissue reconstruction of the lower extremity.[121] Similarly, others have previously reported the use of a fixed frame for joint immobilization to support free-flap reconstruction.[122] This is a very useful adjunct to ensuring the adequate healing of complex soft tissue reconstructions around the foot and ankle

Treatment/surgical technique

Soft tissue reconstruction

Angiosomes and clinical implications

Although the anatomy of the foot and ankle region is covered in detail above and in a previous chapter, it is worth re-emphasizing the critical significance of angiosomes and their implications in flap design and successful reconstruction.[123] The foot and ankle are composed of six distinct angiosomes; three-dimensional blocks of tissue fed by source arteries with functional vascular interconnections between muscle and fascia. The posterior tibial artery supplies the medial ankle and the plantar foot, the anterior tibial artery supplies the dorsum of the foot, and the peroneal artery supplies the anterolateral ankle and the lateral rear foot. These large angiosomes of the foot can be further broken into angiosomes of the major branches of the above arteries. The three main branches of the posterior tibial artery each supply distinct portions of the plantar foot: *the calcaneal branch* (heel); *the medial plantar artery* (instep); and *the lateral plantar artery* (lateral midfoot and forefoot). The two branches of the peroneal artery supply the anterolateral portion of the ankle and rear foot, *the anterior perforating branch* (lateral anterior upper ankle) and *the calcaneal branch* (lateral and plantar heel). The

anterior tibial artery supplies the anterior ankle and then becomes *the dorsalis pedis artery* that supplies the dorsum of the foot. Detailed descriptions of the angiosomes of the lower leg, foot, and ankle have been thoroughly illustrated elsewhere.[124–128] Because the foot and ankle comprise an end organ, their main arteries have numerous direct arterial-arterial connections that allow alternative routes of blood flow to develop if the direct route is disrupted or compromised. Understanding the boundaries of the angiosome and the vascular connections among its source arteries provides the basis for logically rather than empirically designed incisions for tissue exposure and for planned reconstructions or amputations that preserve blood flow for a surgical wound to heal.

Closure techniques

The wound is ready to close when the patient's medical condition has been addressed, the abnormal parameters surrounding the wound have been corrected, and when the signs of inflammation have disappeared. Resolution of pain, wrinkled skin edges, fresh granulation tissue, and neo-epithelialization are the necessary signs that a wound is ready for reconstruction.

The wound can then heal by secondary intention, be closed by delayed primary closure, skin grafted, or covered with a flap.

Closure techniques include: allowing the wound to heal by secondary intention or by closing it with (1) delayed primary closure, (2) skin graft (3) local flap(s) (4) pedicled flap(s) (5) free flap, or any combination thereof. If surgical closure is chosen, there should be two set-ups of instruments in the operating room. The first set of instruments is used to debride the wound. Culturing those instruments post-debridement yield a quantitative culture of up to 10^3 bacteria. Re-using those same instruments during the closure would needlessly re-contaminate the freshly debrided wound and increase the risk for postoperative infection. The freshly debrided wound should be cleansed using pulsed lavage followed by redraping with the surgeon changing his/her gown and gloves and a new set of sterile instruments being brought onto the field. These steps ensure that the wound remains as clean as possible prior to closure, thereby decreasing the risk of subsequent infection and tissue necrosis. Wounds can be allowed to heal by secondary intention by applying daily dressing changes, using wound healing adjuncts such as growth factors, cultured skin, hyperbaric oxygen and/or application of NPWT.

Delayed primary closure is easier to accomplish when the edema and induration of the wound edges has resolved. NPWT devices can be very helpful here. After primary closure, one should always check that relevant arterial pulses have not diminished because the closure was too tight. Adequate soft tissue envelope can also be created by removing bone (e.g., distal fibula in a tibial-talar fusion) or by converting a large wound to a partial foot amputation and using the resultant soft tissue envelopes for closure (*Fig. 8.7*). Technically, deep sutures should be avoided as they could potentiate re-infection. Simple vertical mattress sutures with monofilament are the least likely to facilitate reinfection. Finally, if the closure is too tight, the wound can be partially closed allowing the residual site to heal via contraction and epithelialization with the aide of NPWT.

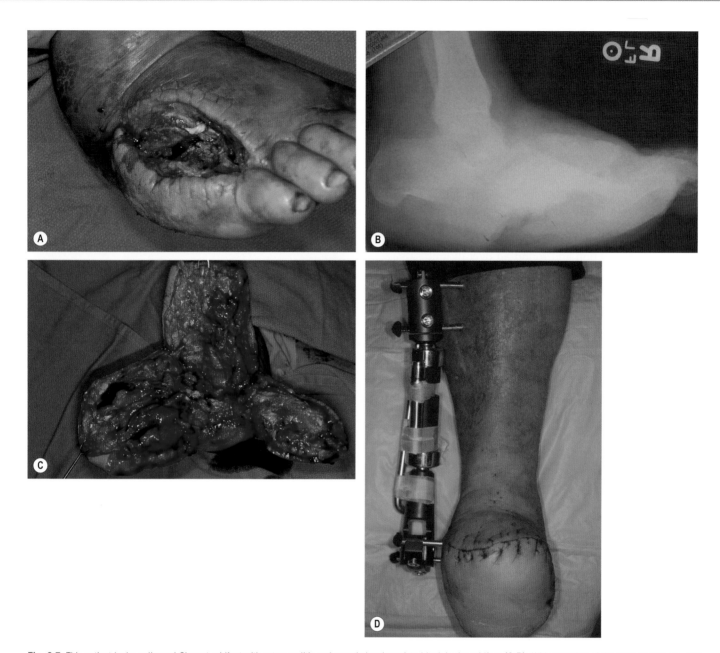

Fig. 8.7 This patient had a collapsed Charcot midfoot with osteomyelitis and a methylmethacrylate block in the midfoot **(A,B)**. With resection of the midfoot and use of the resultant soft tissue envelopes **(C)**, he underwent successful Chopart's amputation after closure, Achilles tenectomy, and immobilization with an external fixator **(D)** until he healed **(E,F)**. He has since been able walk for several years with the aid of a patellar weight-bearing brace **(G)**. (Reprinted with permission from Clemens MW, Attinger CE. Functional reconstruction of the diabetic foot. Semin Plast Surg 2010;24(1):43–56.)

Skin grafting requires a healthy granulating bed *(Fig. 8.8)* that can be achieved by using any one or combination of the following: NPWT, cultured skin derivatives, growth factor and hyperbaric oxygen. In addition, a healthy neodermis can be built up over inhospitable wounds such as bone or tendon by applying a collagen lattice framework such as Integra® (Integra Lifesciences, Plainsboro, NJ) and waiting for it to revascularize before skin grafting. Skin graft recipient bed preparation is optimized by shaving off the superficial granulation tissue prior to skin grafting to remove any residual bacteria that may still reside in the interstices of the granulation buds. Painting the wound base with the blue dye

technique and removing all stained material as described earlier is the key to limiting residual biofilm. This is often facilitated with the use of the Versajet. The wound is then pulse lavaged and new instruments are used to avoid re-contaminating the wound base. The skin graft can be meshed or pie crusted to prevent build up of seroma or hematoma that could prevent graft revascularization. The use of NPWT on low continuous suction as a temporary dressing for the first 3–5 days will ensure the highest possible skin graft take rate.[129]

On the plantar surface, however, split-thickness skin grafts are usually unstable over prolonged periods if on the

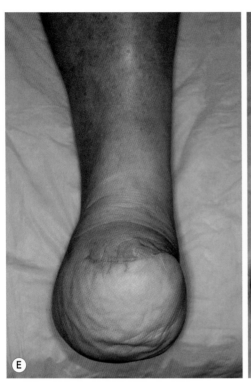 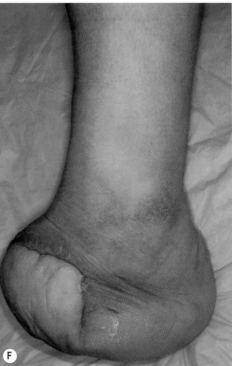 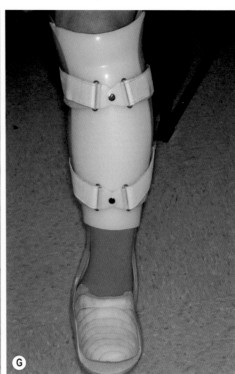

Fig. 8.7, cont'd

weight-bearing portions of the plantar foot, and about 50% of patients require additional reconstructive procedures.[130,131] Glabrous skin grafts harvested at 30/1000 inches can be an effective alternative. The instep is an ideal harvest site and should be skin grafted with a thin autograft to speed up healing.[132] Innervated full-thickness skin grafts have been employed in selective patients using a defatted skin flap in the sural nerve territory, leaving the nerve intact,[133] or by the transfer of grafts from the great toe or forearm, with nerve repair being performed between donor and recipient tissues.

Local flaps are flaps with unidentified blood supply adjacent to a given defect that are either rotated on a pivot point or advanced forward to cover the defect. They come in various shapes (square, rectangular, rhomboid, semi-circular or bi-lobed). They usually consist of skin and the underlying fat or skin, fat, and the underlying fascia. It is important to carefully pre-plan the flap by first accurately determining the size of the defect that needs to be covered after debridement. *Only exposed bone, tendon, nerve, or joint need flap coverage while the rest of the wound can be skin grafted.* This combination of limited local flap and skin graft frequently obviates the need of larger pedicled or free flaps. With good pre-planning, a local flap can also improve the surgical exposure of the underlying tissue if corrective bone surgery has to be performed. The harvesting of an appropriately designed flap allows for better exposure of joints, bone or tendons so that an extra incision can be avoided. Equally important, local flaps are a very useful mode of reconstruction when trying to close a wound within the tight confines of an external fixator.

The ratio of length to width is critical for the survival of the random patterned flap.[134] Because the capillary beds in the blood flow to the skin in the foot and ankle are not as dense as in the face, the length to width ratio should not exceed a 1:1 or 1:1.5 ratio. The length to width ratio of a flap may be increased when one can Doppler a cutaneous perforator at the base of or within the planned flap. To ensure adequate tension free coverage, the flap should be designed in the area where the tissue is the most mobile and a slightly larger pattern should be used than what would anatomically be necessary. A force of 25 mm Hg causes enough venous congestion for flap necrosis unless the tension is released within 4 h.[135] If the flap remains pale when inset, it should be rotated back into its bed and delayed for four to seven days while it develops more robust blood supply. During that time, the NPWT can be placed on the open wound to ensure that no edema develops and the tissue edges remain malleable. Finally, we have found that placement of NPWT for 3–5 days postoperatively on the local flaps as well as the skin grafted recipient site helps ensure flap viability.[136]

The *transposition flap* is the most frequently used flap to cover the malleoli or exposed tibial-talar fusion around an Ilizarov frame *(Fig. 8.9)*. The flap is designed to cover exposed bone, joint, or tendon only and not the entire defect. The flap is taken from the side that is the most mobile and that has a definable perforator at its base. That means that four possible designs exist: proximally or distally based and medial or lateral to the wound. Sometimes, the defect is large enough that a flap from both sides is necessary, with one being proximally based and the other distally based. What the flaps do not cover is then skin grafted. NPWT can be placed on the entire construct for 3–5 days to ensure good skin graft take and to optimize flap survival.

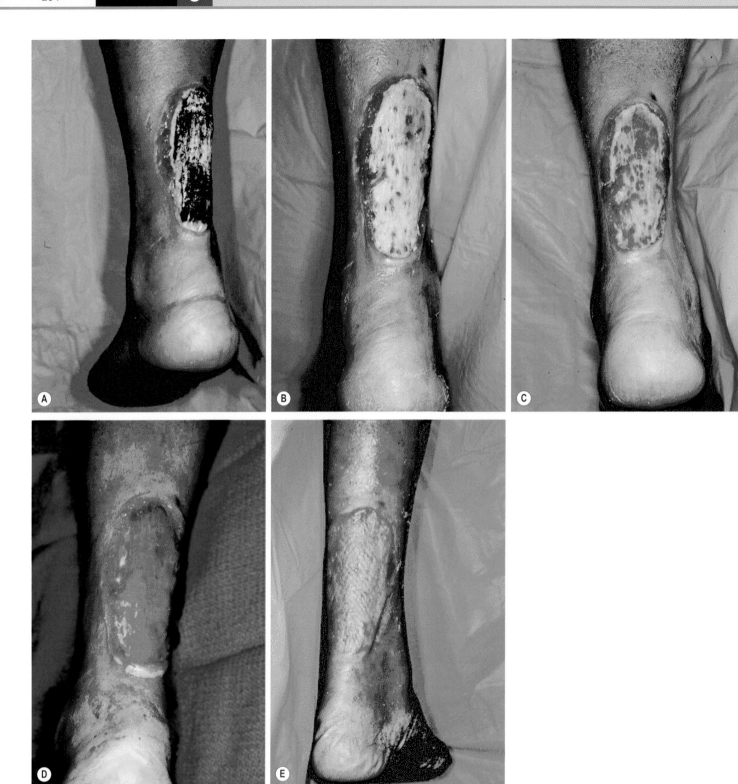

Fig. 8.8 (A) A patient presented with a gangrenous Achilles tendon. **(B)** The necrotic tendon was sharply debrided to shiny underlying tendon. Hyperbaric oxygen and topical growth factor therapies were started, and the tendon began to granulate (**B**, 1 week; **C**, 2 weeks; **D**, 3 weeks). The Achilles tendon was then successfully skin grafted and healed completely after 4 weeks **(E)**. (Reprinted with permission from Clemens MW, Attinger CE. Functional reconstruction of the diabetic foot. Semin Plast Surg 2010; 24(1):43–56.)

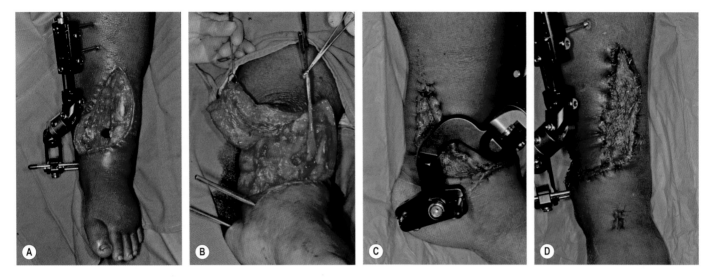

Fig. 8.9 This patient developed an infected Charcot ankle joint and was debrided and immobilized with an external fixator **(A)**. The exposed joint was a muscle flap and large transposition flap **(B)**. The donor site was skin grafted **(C)** as was the anterior portion of the wound **(D)**. The transposition flap needs to be only long and wide enough to cover exposed joint or bone and the rest can be skin grafted. (Reprinted with permission from Clemens MW, Attinger CE. Functional reconstruction of the diabetic foot. Semin Plast Surg 2010; 24(1):43–56.)

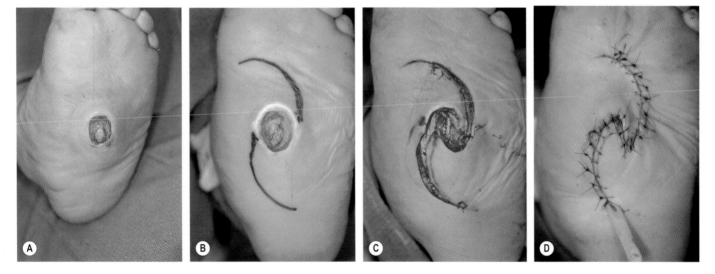

Fig. 8.10 (A–D) A double rotation flap can be used to cover a plantar defect from a collapsed Charcot midfoot. (Reprinted with permission from Clemens MW, Attinger CE. Functional reconstruction of the diabetic foot. Semin Plast Surg 2010;24(1):43–56.)

The *rotation flap* is useful on the plantar aspect of the foot where the flap is elevated off the plantar fascia and rotated into position *(Fig. 8.10)*. It can also be used over the plantar forefoot, at both malleoli and on the dorsum of the foot. If vascular anatomical considerations dictate, the flap can also include underlying fascia and or muscle.

Reconstruction by anatomic location

Large defects or "unfavorable" local tissues may require pedicled flaps from the immediate area. Pedicle flaps for soft tissue defects of the foot and ankle are invaluable and may preclude a more complex microsurgical reconstruction. Despite this, many surgeons are hesitant to attempt pedicled flaps because of the common complications of distal flap necrosis. The

following discusses critical elements of flap design to avoid these pitfalls, and postoperative management where close observation and strict offloading are essential for success. Because the reconstructive options vary according to location, it is best to differentiate between four distinct locations: (1) the Achilles' tendon area, the ankle and foot dorsum, (2) the plantar forefoot, (3) the plantar midfoot, and (4) the plantar hindfoot.

Ankle and foot dorsum

Extensor digitorum brevis muscle flap

The extensor digitorum brevis muscle may be transposed proximally to cover the anterior ankle, the proximal dorsal foot, and lateral malleolar wounds provided that the anterior tibial-dorsalis pedis artery has antegrade blood flow. The blood supply to the muscle is derived from the lateral tarsal artery, which is a branch of the dorsalis pedis artery at the level of the distal edge of the extensor retinaculum. Exposure is obtained through a curvilinear incision on the foot dorsum that communicates with the wound to be closed. The dorsalis pedis artery can be divided distal to the origin of the lateral tarsal vessels to provide for increased arc of the rotation for muscle transposition. The long extensors are then retracted off of the underlying short extensor muscle slips. The medial tarsal branches are ligated as the dissection proceeds proximally. Elevate the lateral tarsal vessels with the muscle while dividing the origin and tendinous extensions of the muscle. The four slips of the muscle are broad and thin, measuring 4.5×6 cm in the adult, making the flap useful for relatively small wounds *(Fig. 8.11)*.[137]

Lateral supramalleolar flap

The lateral supramalleolar flap has been most useful in the coverage of bony defects that accompany loss of soft tissue over the lateral malleolus and anterior ankle. The flap should be distally based as the blood supply is derived from the perforating branch of the peroneal artery as it pierces the interosseous membrane 5 cm proximal to the tip of the lateral malleolus. Cutaneous vessels then course upwards, anterior to the fibula, and anastomose with the vascular network that accompanies the superficial peroneal nerve.

The perforating branch of the peroneal artery may be located with the hand-held Doppler. The base of the flap should be centered at this point. Flap width includes the tissue between the fibula and tibia. The length should be adequate to reach the malleolus (from 6–8 cm) or more distally as dictated by wound location.[138] Most often, the tissue is developed as a fascial flap, turned over like a page of a book, and its surface skin-grafted. When performed in this manner, the donor site may be closed directly.

For the facial flap, the skin incision is made centrally over the space between the fibula and the tibia so that skin flaps may be elevated off the underlying deep fascia. The fascia is then incised along its anterior margin, and progressively reflected until the perforating branch is seen. Branches of the superficial peroneal nerve course within the fascia and must be divided to permit safe elevation and rotation. Final release of the flap will require incision through the posterior margin

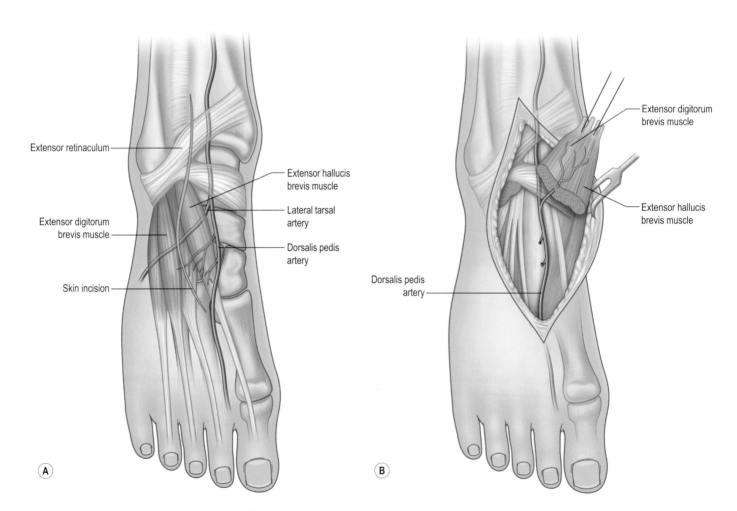

Fig. 8.11 The extensor digitorum brevis muscle flap. This type 2 muscle has a blood supply derived from the lateral tarsal artery, which is a branch of the dorsalis pedis artery. The dorsalis pedis artery can be divided distal to the origin of the lateral tarsal vessels to provide for increased arc of the rotation for muscle transposition. The four slips of the muscle are broad and thin, measuring 4.5×6 cm in the adult, making the flap useful for relatively small wounds.

and release of its attachments to the septum that separates the anterior and lateral muscular compartments.

Plantar forefoot

The area from the midshaft of the metatarsals distally is referred to as the *forefoot*. Local flaps play a major role in the reconstruction of deep wounds of the distal third of the foot. Severe injury or infection of a single toe may be managed best by toe or ray amputation. Usually plantar or dorsal flaps of the proximal toe skin may be fashioned for simple closure. If additional skin is necessary, an adjacent toe may be filleted and transposed for closure. Ray amputation (digit plus associated metatarsal) may be necessary, especially if the associated metatarsal is severely infected, devascularized or otherwise irreparable.

Transposition of local tissues may take many forms. Metatarsal head ulceration is extremely common in patients with peripheral neuropathy and associated arthropathy. Numerous techniques have been described, some of which will be discussed here. First introduced by Moberg in 1964,[139] the neurovascular island flap of a from an adjacent toe remains a useful technique today for forefoot repair.[140,141] This technique may take two forms: (1) fillet of the entire toe with transposition of the soft tissue or (2) transposition of a flap from the lateral side of the great toe without toe sacrifice.[142-144]

Toe fillet flap

This island flap is dissected most easily with the patient in the supine position under tourniquet control. The plantar wound is debrided and the flap of adjacent toe soft tissues is outlined. The flap is elevated, beginning distally, removing the entire nail complex off of the distal phalanges. An incision is then made on the dorsum of the toe to expose the underlying middle and proximal phalanx. All three bones are carefully removed while preserving the digital plantar vessels. The volar plates and flexor and extensor tendons are removed to allow for more flap pliability. A connecting incision is made between the flap and the wound to permit transposition of the flap. The tourniquet is deflated, hemostasis is obtained, and the wounds closed. If necessary, more proximal dissection of the plantar neurovascular structures may extend the flap's arc of rotation to more proximal locations. The reach of this flap is often disappointing and the flap works best with the first or fifth toe.

Neurovascular island flap

Alternatively, a neurovascular island flap from the fibular side of the great toe may be used without sacrificing the entire toe. Depending on flap size, the donor site is closed either directly or with a split-thickness skin graft.[145,146] The flap is centered over the course of the fibular neurovascular bundle of the great toe. As in the island toe flap procedure, the use of a tourniquet as well as magnifying loupes facilitates the safe performance of the procedure. The flap is outlined and then elevated from distal to proximal on the lateral plantar aspect of the great toe at the level of the phalangeal periosteum. Identifying the digital neurovascular bundle in the web space permits a more proximal dissection if necessary. A connecting

incision is made from the web space to the debrided wound in order to transpose the flap. These techniques are effective for wounds up to 2–3 cm in diameter. The preoperative workup must include assessment of the vascular status of the extremity.

V-Y plantar flap

Forefoot skin fat and fascia may be advanced in a V-Y fashion, either singly or in pairs to close wounds up to 4–5 cm^3. Anatomic studies using fresh cadavers and latex (Microfil®) injections have revealed numerous vertical perforating vessels located throughout the plantar aspect of the foot. The location of these perforators facilitates the designing of many different V-Y advancement flaps. Under tourniquet control, the wound is debrided and an adjacent V-Y flap is outlined and incised. The plantar fascia along the edge of the flap must be completely incised as well. Careful division of the septal attachments to the underlying metatarsal may further aid in flap advancement. After release of the tourniquet, hemostasis is obtained and the wound is closed. Because the advancement of a single flap is limited to 1.5 cm, wounds up to 3 cm can be closed with opposing V-Y flaps.

Forefoot amputations and associated flaps

Reconstructive surgeons managing patients with foot ulceration should be well versed in the options available for forefoot amputation as these procedures will often be the simplest way to provide stable soft tissue closure and bipedal ambulation. Transmetatarsal amputation is indicated when three or more rays have been deleted. This is usually accomplished by using a plantar flap of skin, subcutaneous tissue, and fascia to advance over the metatarsal stumps. With significant plantar ulceration, however, one may have to also use dorsal soft tissues to achieve soft tissue closure. The key is to preserve as much soft tissue as possible (both dorsal and plantar) so that length may be maintained and the suture lines remain free of tension. More proximal applications of the transmetatarsal amputation may be necessary in some patients. In these situations, care should be exercised to avoid injury to the distal perforating portion of the dorsalis pedis artery. This vessel courses between the first and second metatarsal bases to anastomoses with the lateral plantar artery and is at risk of injury when bony resection is necessary nearby. In patients with significant stenoses in their posterior tibial artery, the distal perforating portion of the dorsalis pedis artery may be the only blood supply to the plantar forefoot. By removing the first metatarsal medially and the other metatarsals laterally, the perforating dorsalis pedis can be protected.

Transmetatarsal amputation provides an excellent functional level for post-traumatic, ischemic, or neuropathic patients as long as the blood supply is adequate, the patient is nutritionally sound, and any infection or necrosis has been thoroughly eradicated.[147] No formal prosthetic or orthotic device is necessary, and the patient may wear normal shoes with a small, distal insert. Attention, however, *must* be paid to avoiding equinus deformity from loss of the extensors that will often lead to recurrent lateral plantar ulceration. Usually, the Achilles tendon is lengthened to avoid this complication. Alternatively, the flexors and extensors of the fourth and fifth toes can be tenodesed while the ankle is neutral so that distal forefoot dorsiflexion is preserved.

Plantar midfoot

The midfoot is defined as the region between the proximal tarsal row and the midshaft of the metatarsals. It comprises the medial nonweight-bearing arch as well as the more lateral weight-bearing soft tissues. Small wounds in this region may be closed using any of the options discussed previously for the forefoot. Most useful is the V-Y flap that can be advanced 1.5 cm to help close a defect or a double V-Y flap that can fill a 3 cm defect. Split-thickness skin grafts may be adequate, provided that the transverse arch of the foot has been maintained. This implies that the medial midfoot remains largely a nonweight-bearing region.

Neurovascular island flaps

The neurovascular island procedures discussed previously are useful for the repair of 2–3 cm defects. This repair necessitates a more proximal dissection of the vessels and nerves from the plantar surface of the foot. If the dominant circulation is from the first dorsal metatarsal artery, division of the deep transverse metatarsal ligament will be necessary to permit flap transfer and inset.

Suprafascial flaps

Medially or laterally based plantar flaps have been described and appear to be another reconstructive alternative.[148] Tourniquet control allows for a bloodless dissection. Medially-based flaps are raised by incising laterally and elevating the subcutaneous tissues off of the abductor digiti minimi muscle and plantar fascia from lateral to medial. The medial dissection allows for identification and preservation of the cutaneous branches of the medial plantar nerve as they emerge from the cleft between the abductor hallucis and the plantar fascia. With continued elevation of the flap off of the plantar fascia, branches of the medial plantar artery and nerve are seen coursing into the flap from the cleft between the plantar fascia and the abductor hallucis muscle. When the flap is elevated in a proximal dissection, the medial and lateral branches of the plantar nerve are separated from the main trunk for a short distance to preserve flap sensation without sacrificing flap motility. For the laterally based flap, a similar dissection may be performed; however, all perforators of the medial plantar artery are sacrificed to permit flap rotation.

Midfoot amputations

Deformities at the tarsometatarsal junctions (Lisfranc's joint) occur when a shortened gastrocsoleus complex alters normal ankle motion. The inability to fully dorsiflex at the ankle puts undue strain across Lisfranc's joint during gait. Over time, the inability to fully dorsiflex the ankle leads to increased compensatory motion at the midfoot level with breakdown of Lisfranc's joint and resultant midfoot deformity. Soft tissue ulceration is inevitable and commonly seen in diabetic patients as well as others with peripheral neuropathy.[149]

Patients who are not candidates for the reconstructive procedures previously discussed may be best served with a midfoot amputation. Midfoot amputations may be the preferred "repair," as the procedure is simple and may be performed relatively rapidly without the significant morbidity associated with more complex reconstructions. If patients are appropriately chosen, and the procedure is executed properly, one may be able to salvage a limb that provides a stable platform for ambulation with minimal increase in the energy expenditure. The two most common forms of midfoot amputation are the Lisfranc amputation and the Chopart amputation.

The Lisfranc amputation involves removal of all metatarsal remnants although the very proximal second metatarsal which serves as a keystone should be preserved if possible. Amputation at the tarsometatarsal joint (Lisfranc level) is associated with a high rate of equinovarus deformity. If blood flow is compromised, care should be taken to preserve the perforators between the dorsal and plantar circulations that occur at this level. Although some would argue that an anterior tibial tendon transfer and joint stabilization are necessary to prevent late deformity, others have found that a simple 1 cm tenotomy of the Achilles tendon, performed at the time of the midfoot amputation, effectively prevents these late changes. Patients have little need for custom footwear and generally return to their previous ambulatory level with little, if any, increase in energy expenditure.[150]

The Chopart amputation is done at the juncture between the rear foot and the midfoot separating the talus and calcaneus from the navicular and the cuboid. A modified Chopart amputation can be done by splitting the midfoot at the juncture of the navicular and cuboid from the cunieform bones. As with the Lisfranc amputation, the Chopart procedure will affect the patients' ability to dorsiflex and evert the involved foot, as the insertions of the peroneal tendons as well as the tibialis anterior tendon will be disrupted. This amputation mandates a tenectomy (1–2 cm) of the distal Achilles tendon or a combined Achilles tendon lengthening and repositioning of the tibialis anterior tendon to the lateral talus or calcaneus to help prevent recurrence. Postoperatively, the limb is cast in dorsiflexion for 4–6 weeks.[151] It is also possible to fuse the ankle in neutral with a calcaneal tibial rod to avoid any risk of equinus and subsequent breakdown.

Plantar hindfoot

Hindfoot soft tissue repair provides the greatest challenge to the reconstructive surgeon. The hindfoot is a very specialized location, with specific requirements for its repair. In addition to the thick, durable heel pad and the underlying calcaneus, the Achilles' tendon and its thin, pliable soft tissue envelope must be managed appropriately. Reconstruction should provide durable soft tissues for safe weight bearing while permitting near normal ankle motion. More than any other region in the foot, the surgeon must consider both form and function when managing wounds in this area.

Tendons from the muscles of the posterior, deep posterior and lateral compartments of the leg traverse this region as they enter the foot. One of the most important and frequently injured is the Achilles' tendon. The posterior tibial artery and tibial nerve lie between the flexor digitorum longus and the flexor hallucis longus tendons, posterior to the medial malleolus. These structures, along with the tibialis posterior tendon, travel beneath the laciniate ligament (flexor retinaculum) to enter the foot. The sural nerve and the lateral leg compartment musculature also pass posterior to the lateral malleolus to enter the foot. Loss of sufficient tissues in this location, whether through trauma or disease, can be a catastrophe that may cripple the patient permanently or mandate a below-knee amputation.

Intrinsic muscle flaps

Three intrinsic foot muscles may be used to close defects of the hindfoot. The abductor hallucis, flexor digitorum brevis, and abductor digiti minimi muscles may be used individually or together to repair small wounds in the hindfoot region.[152–155] The abductor hallucis muscle is elevated through a medial foot incision along the medial glabrous junction. The tendon is divided distally and the muscle is separated from the medial head of the flexor hallucis brevis. The blood supply enters the muscle proximally as branches from the medial plantar artery. If an increase in the arc of rotation is needed, the medial plantar artery may be ligated and divided distal to the branches of the abductor, and more proximal dissection of the medial plantar artery to its origin from the posterior tibial artery can be accomplished. The muscle will cover small defects about the heel and medial malleolus *(Fig. 8.12)*.

The flexor digitorum brevis muscle can be useful for heel pad reconstruction, especially if used to fill in an exsiting fat pad defect and then covered by residual glabrous skin. Its blood supply comes from branches of both the medial and lateral plantar arteries, with the latter usually being dominant. The lateral plantar artery courses deep to the proximal muscle belly where small arterial branches course into the muscle. A midline plantar foot incision is used to expose the muscle for elevation. The skin and plantar fascia is elevated medially and laterally off the underlying plantar fascia. The four tendons are divided distally and then the muscle may be turned on itself as it dissected off the quadratus plantae muscle. Further mobilization is possible to permit the use of this flap for posterior hindfoot reconstruction by basing the flap on the medial plantar artery and continuing the pedicle dissection to the origin of this vessel within the tarsal tunnel.

The abductor digiti minimi, the smallest of the three muscles, may be mobilized with a lateral foot incision along the lateral glabrous junction. Both motor innervation and blood supply are derived from the lateral plantar neurovascular bundle through branches entering the proximal portion of the muscle. The muscle is detached from the fifth metatarsal, and the tendinous insertion divided, allowing rotation of the flap. Use of the abductor digiti minimi muscle is useful in repairing small lateral calcaneal soft tissue defects. For larger plantar defects, it can be used in conjunction with either of the two muscles discussed above *(Fig. 8.12)*.

Medial plantar artery flap

This flap is quite useful for heel pad reconstruction, provided the instep is not a weight-bearing surface as can occur with Charcot midfoot collapse.[156] The donor site must be skin grafted; hence, when instep collapse is present, a relative contraindication to this procedure exists.

The instep of the foot may be elevated as a fasciocutaneous flap based on the medial plantar artery and transposed posteriorly to cover the heel.[157] If the lateral plantar artery is divided (not recommended), pedicle length is increased, thus allowing its use for closure of wounds more proximal to the heel. The great appeal of this procedure originates from the goal of reconstructing plantar defects with plantar soft tissue as was originally described almost 40 years ago.[158] Mir y Mir[159]

used a cross-foot flap from the instep of the opposite extremity for the repair of heel wounds. The flap is outlined over the medial instep of the foot centered on the medial plantar artery as isolated with the hand held Doppler. The extremity is exsanguinated with extremity elevation rather than with an Esmarch, and a thigh tourniquet inflated. The distal extent of the flap is incised first, through the skin and plantar fascia. The medial plantar neurovascular bundle is readily found in the cleft between the abductor hallucis and the flexor digitorum brevis muscles. The vessels are divided and elevated with the flap. An intraneural dissection of the medial plantar nerve is performed so that the cutaneous fascicles from the plantar nerve are preserved with the flap. The dissection plane is superficial to the muscles, just deep to the plantar fascia. The deep fascial septa in the clefts between the muscles must be divided. For most reconstructions, the dissection may stop where the vessels emerge from the lateral border of the abductor hallucis muscle. Further mobilization is possible by dividing this muscle and the laciniate ligament and tracing the medial plantar artery to its origin from the posterior tibial artery.

Heel pad flaps

Small wounds over the weight-bearing and posterior heel may be closed with a suprafascial flap of heel pad, based either medially or laterally.[160] After outlining the flap, an incision is made and the flap is elevated off of the underlying calcaneus and the plantar fascial attachments. If based medially, the branches of the lateral plantar vessels may need to be ligated. If based laterally, the same holds true for the perforators from the medial plantar vessels. Such flaps may be accompanied by calcanectomy, which will remove bony prominences as well as simplify the closure. Generous calcanectomy (up to one-third or more of the calcaneus) in the coronal plane may "free up" enough soft tissue to close rather large wounds without resorting to more complex reconstructive procedures. This technique is especially useful in patients who have limited ambulation and have significant comorbid factors rendering them poor candidates for free flap repair.

Sural artery flap

The retrograde sural nerve flap[161] (*retrograde sural artery*) is a versatile neurofasciocutaneous flap that is useful for ankle and posterior heel defects. Occasionally, a median superficial sural artery is seen coursing with the sural nerve however, in most cases, the arterial component is a plexus of vessels with the sural nerve and receives retrograde flow from a peroneal perforator 5 cm above the lateral malleolus. The artery first courses above the fascia and then goes deep to the fascia at midcalf while the accompanying lesser saphenous vein remains above the fascia. The venous congestion often seen with this flap can be minimized if the pedicle is harvested with 3 cm of tissue on either side of the pedicle and with the overlying skin intact.[162] Problems with the venous drainage can be further helped by delaying the flap 2–3 weeks earlier and ligating the proximal lesser saphenous vein and sural artery.[163,164] The inset of the flap is critical to avoid kinking of the pedicle. Offloading the flap and heel during the healing phase is simplified by using an Ilizarov-type frame. The major donor deficit of the flap is the loss of sensibility along the

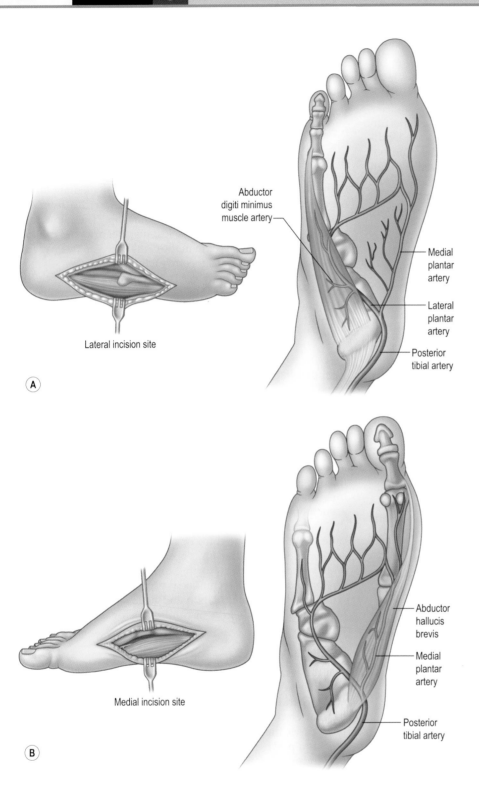

Abductor
digiti minimus
muscle artery

Medial
plantar
artery

Lateral
plantar
artery

Posterior
tibial artery

Lateral incision site

(A)

Abductor
hallucis
brevis

Medial
plantar
artery

Posterior
tibial artery

Medial incision site

(B)

Fig. 8.12 Abductor digiti minimi and abductor hallucis brevis muscle flaps. These muscles have a type 2 vascular pattern, with the dominant pedicle at the level of the distal calcaneus. They are harvested on their dominant proximal pedicles. The distal muscle bulk is often disappointingly small. However, these muscles are useful to fill small midfoot, rear foot, and distal ankle defects. **(A)** Abductor digiti minimi. **(B)** Abductor hallucis brevis. (Reprinted with permission from Attinger CE, Ducic I. Foot and Ankle Reconstruction. Grabb and Smith Plastic Surgery, 6th edn. London: Lippincott, Wilkins & Williams; 2006:Ch. 71.)

lateral aspect of the foot and a skin grafted depression at the posterior calf donor site that may pose a problem if the patient later has to undergo a below the knee amputation.

The flap is outlined over the raphe between the two heads of the gastrocnemius muscle. A line is drawn from the inferior edge of the flap to the pivot point for the pedicle approximately 5 cm above the lateral malleolus. Flap elevation is begun along its cephalic perimeter. Through this incision, the sural nerve and the lesser saphenous vein are identified just superficial to the deep fascia and ligated so that they may be elevated along with the overlying soft tissue. The deep fascia should be elevated with the flap to protect the aforementioned structures. The flap pedicle is formed by elevating a medial and lateral skin flap and then developing a 3–4 cm wide "strip" of subcutaneous fat and fascia that harbor the sural nerve and lesser saphenous vein. The flap and pedicle may then be separated from the underlying muscle and paratenon layers. The arc of rotation will provide coverage of the posterior heel/Achilles' and anterior ankle. The donor site may be closed primarily if it is small, or with the use of split thickness skin graft if larger (see Fig. 5.23). In a well vascularized extremity, the pedicle can be removed after 3–4 weeks to improve the contour of the leg.

Microvascular composite tissue transplantation (free flaps)

Large hindfoot wounds (>6 cm), defects in patients devoid of the posterior tibial vessels (from either trauma or disease), or patients who have been revascularized to the distal anterior tibial/dorsalis pedis artery via bypass grafts should be considered for reconstruction that utilize microsurgical techniques. With the exception of the sural artery flap, all of the regional flaps described for hindfoot repair require antegrade blood flow in the posterior tibial artery and its branches (medial and lateral plantar arteries).

Large dorsal foot wounds with bone and/or tendon exposure are best reconstructed with "thin" free flaps. Thin skin flaps or fascial flaps surfaced with a skin graft will provide durable, thin cover that is aesthetically pleasing and permits normal shoe wear. Some skin flaps may also be sensate if harvested with the sensory nerve that supports the flap. They can include vascularized tendon or bone for specific reconstructive tasks. Flaps that have proven to be very successful include the radial forearm flap, the lateral arm flap, the parascapular or dorsal thoracic fascia flap and the anterolateral thigh flap.

The parascapular flap (Fig. 8.13) based on the circumflex scapular artery is an excellent choice for large defects.[165,166] It is insensate, and often needs to be thinned at a later date because of its bulkiness. Colen et al. have described an adaptation of the flap where only fascia with a thin layer of overlying fat is harvested.[167] It is then skin grafted to yield an ultimately far thinner flap.

The lateral arm flap (Fig. 8.14) based on the posterior radial recurrent vascular pedicle was first described by Katseros et al.[168] It is a sensory flap (lower lateral cutaneous nerve of the arm) with a relatively long vascular pedicle (up to 14 cm). Including the skin overlying the elbow can extend the flap size.

The radial forearm flap (Fig. 8.15) is an excellent option for dorsal foot wounds.[169,170] The advantage of the radial forearm flap is that it is thin, pliable, and can be harvested with a sensory nerve (the lateral antebrachial cutaneous nerve). The palmaris longus tendon can also be used to reconstruct missing extensor tendons on the dorsum of the foot if necessary. The radial forearm flap is also very useful around the malleoli. The radial artery with the venous comitantes provides an excellent vascular pedicle up to 14 cm in length. The flap, if inset properly at the time of flap transfer, rarely needs tailoring. The donor site is skin grafted with or without Integra, and apart from the obvious resulting color disparity, is very manageable.

The anterolateral thigh (ALT) flap is a septocutaneous flap based upon perforators originating from the descending branch of the lateral circumflex femoral system.[171] Originally described by Song[172] and popularized by Koshima et al.,[173,174] the anterolateral thigh flap is well accepted and can supply a large amount of subcutaneous fat and skin on a safe and reliable pedicle with no functional donor site morbidity. The flap may be raised both sensate with the lateral femoral cutaneous nerve, and as a flow-through flap.[175] Thinning of the flap is well tolerated, even to the level of the subdermal plexus for tailoring to a particular defect.[176] The anatomy and dissection of ALT flaps has been well established for both head and neck and lower extremity defects.[177]

Pedicled instep flaps are frequently used in weight-bearing plantar reconstruction, but may not be available after severe foot injuries. Gaining popularity is the contralateral sensate free instep flap for reconstruction of a defect with "like tissue."[178] This flap yields both excellent functional and aesthetic long-term results.

Muscle flaps are preferred over exposed bone on the plantar aspects of the foot. Muscle flaps show better resistance against infection when compared with skin flaps. This holds especially true in patients with osteomyelitis. As in other locations, the use of muscle to obliterate dead space and aid in delivering both neutrophils and parenteral antibiotics to regions of chronic osteomyelitis is particularly important.[179,180] The most frequently harvested muscles include the rectus abdominus muscle, gracilis muscle, and serratus anterior muscle. A word of caution with respect to the use of the latissimus dorsi flap: while this flap is an attractive option in many other parts of the body, the functional loss of the latissimus dorsi must be taken into account in lower extremity reconstructions where many of these patients will be crutch or wheelchair-dependent for a prolonged amount of time.

There is still some debate as to whether muscle plus skin graft versus fasciocutaneous flaps on the plantar surface of the foot holds up better under the stress of ambulation. Muscle flap and a skin graft are currently favored on the plantar aspect of the foot.[181,182] Muscle flaps provide a better blood supply to the recipient site, making them the better choice for previously infected wounds.[183] If the fasciocutaneous flaps are innervated, they could potentially be more effective on the sole of the foot in nonneuropathic patients.[184] Fasciocutaneous flaps are ideal for providing skin coverage while preserving underlying tendon motion. The rectus abdominus muscle flap (Fig. 8.16)[185] is very useful because it is easy to harvest, has an excellent pedicle, and is a thin broad muscle. If the muscle is stretched over the recipient site, it may be made even thinner. The donor site morbidity is minimal. The gracilis muscle (Fig. 8.17)[186] is also an excellent choice for foot and ankle reconstruction.[187] It should be harvested from the ipsilateral

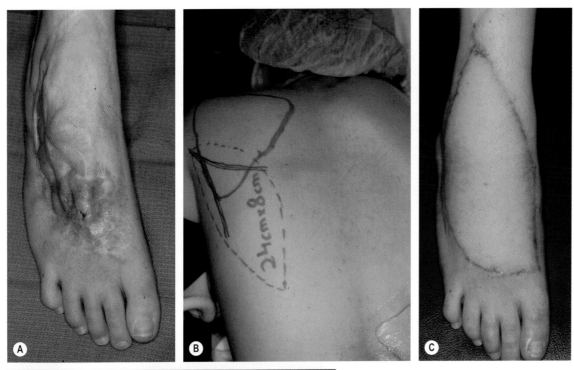

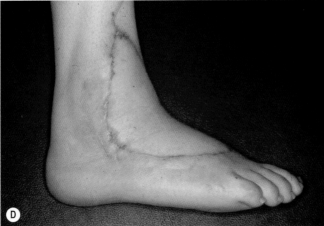

Fig. 8.13 As a child, this patient's foot was run over, leaving her with a painful, unstable foot **(A)**. Before an ankle fusion could be performed, adequate soft tissue cover was necessary. A parascapular flap was harvested from her left back **(B)**. The flap vessels were anastomosed to the anterior tibial artery and vein. The flap was subsequently debulked with liposuction **(C,D)**. (Reprinted with permission from: Attinger CE, Clemens MW, Ducic I, et al. The role of microsurgical-free flaps in foot and ankle surgery. In: Dockery GD, ed. Lower Extremity Soft Tissue & Cutaneous Plastic Surgery, 2nd edn. Oxford: Elsevier Science, Ch. 20, in press.)

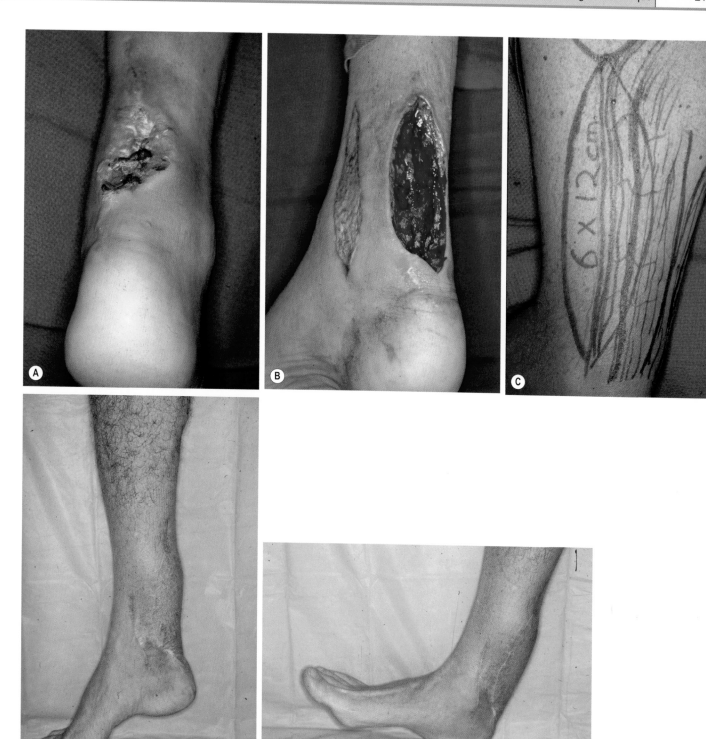

Fig. 8.14 This patient suffered a re-rupture of his Achilles' tendon and subsequent infection **(A)** that required removal of the entire lower Achilles' tendon **(B).** A lateral arm fasciocutaneous flap with a portion of the triceps tendon was harvested **(C).** The flap was connected to the posterior tibial artery and vein, and the vascularized triceps tendon was used to reconstruct the Achilles' tendon. The patient was able to flex and extend his foot and resumed playing tennis and skiing at 6 months post-procedure **(D,E).** (Reprinted with permission from: Attinger CE, Clemens MW, Ducic I, et al. The role of microsurgical-free flaps in foot and ankle surgery. In: Dockery GD, ed. Lower Extremity Soft Tissue & Cutaneous Plastic Surgery, 2nd edn. Oxford: Elsevier Science, Ch. 20, in press.)

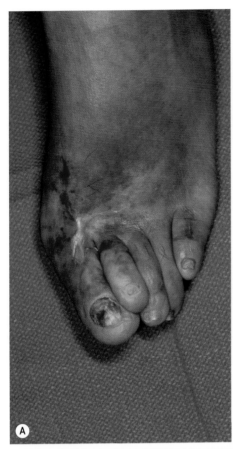
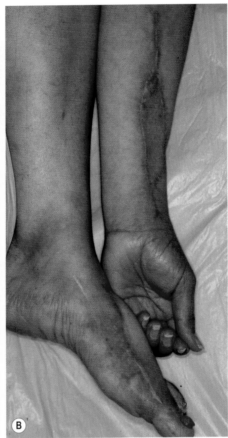
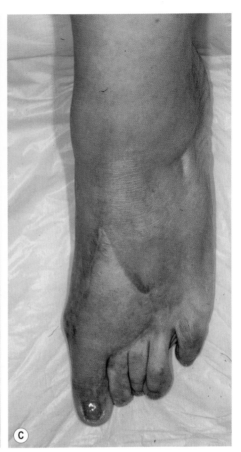
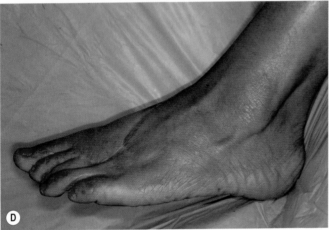

Fig. 8.15 This patient developed a severe infection and skin slough after a bunionectomy that left her with a scarred dorsal forefoot, hallux valgus, and dorsiflexed second toe **(A,B)**. The scarred tissue was excised, her first metatarsal joint fused, and the second toe straightened out. The residual defect was covered with a radial forearm flap that was anastomosed into the dorsalis pedis artery and vein **(C,D)**. (Reprinted with permission from: Attinger CE, Clemens MW, Ducic I, et al. The role of microsurgical-free flaps in foot and ankle surgery. In: Dockery GD, ed. Lower Extremity Soft Tissue & Cutaneous Plastic Surgery, 2nd edn. Oxford: Elsevier Science, Ch. 20, in press.)

leg. This limits all incisions to the same extremity. The pedicle is somewhat smaller and shorter than that of the rectus abdominus muscle. Depending on the location of the defect and the status of the recipient vessels, its use may be limited. It is most useful for heel wounds where vascular anastomoses can be performed to the nearby posterior tibial vessels. Using the bottom two or three slips of the serratus anterior muscle *(Fig. 8.18)*[188] provides an adequate amount of soft tissue with a pedicle as long as 18 cm. Wounds on the plantar surface of the foot can be reconstructed with vascular anastomoses to the foot's dorsal circulation.

Free flap muscle transfers to the foot tend to swell, which makes it more difficult to fit the foot into a shoe. To minimize

this swelling, several technical maneuvers may be helpful. First, the outflow should be optimized by performing two vein anastomoses. To minimize the profile of the flap, it should be inset under tension so that it lies flat and at the same height as that of the surrounding tissue. After the flap has survived and the skin graft has healed, compression therapy helps in improving the overall contour. Stockings with at least 30 mmHg should be worn by the patient. If that is insufficient, the muscle may need debulking. With many of the described flaps, a neurorrhaphy may be performed to improve reinnervation. Outcomes and overall benefit of this added procedure remain controversial. Some studies report no difference in flap survival or ulceration rates between innervated and

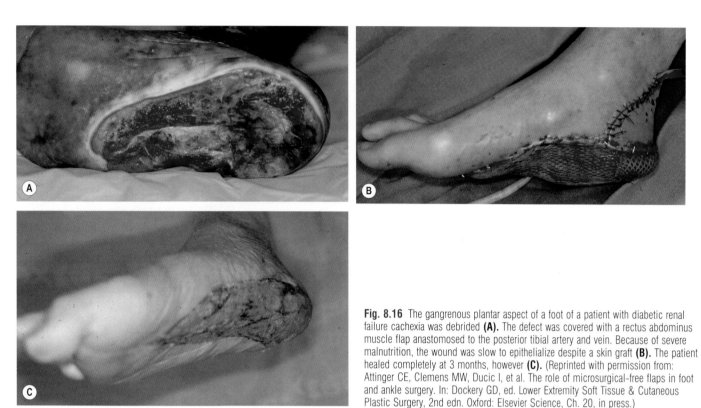

Fig. 8.16 The gangrenous plantar aspect of a foot of a patient with diabetic renal failure cachexia was debrided **(A).** The defect was covered with a rectus abdominus muscle flap anastomosed to the posterior tibial artery and vein. Because of severe malnutrition, the wound was slow to epithelialize despite a skin graft **(B).** The patient healed completely at 3 months, however **(C).** (Reprinted with permission from: Attinger CE, Clemens MW, Ducic I, et al. The role of microsurgical-free flaps in foot and ankle surgery. In: Dockery GD, ed. Lower Extremity Soft Tissue & Cutaneous Plastic Surgery, 2nd edn. Oxford: Elsevier Science, Ch. 20, in press.)

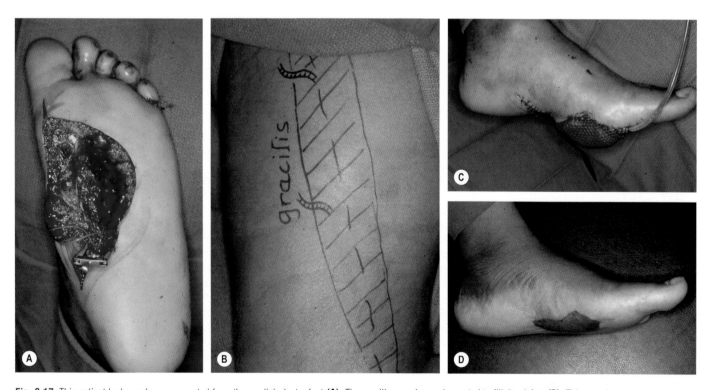

Fig. 8.17 This patient had a melanoma resected from the medial plantar foot **(A).** The gracilis muscle was harvested to fill the defect **(B).** This muscle was anastomosed to the medial plantar artery and vein **(C).** The muscle flattened as it healed and as pressure began to be applied to the foot **(D).** (Reprinted with permission from: Attinger CE, Clemens MW, Ducic I, et al. The role of microsurgical-free flaps in foot and ankle surgery. In: Dockery GD, ed. Lower Extremity Soft Tissue & Cutaneous Plastic Surgery, 2nd edn. Oxford: Elsevier Science, Ch. 20, in press.)

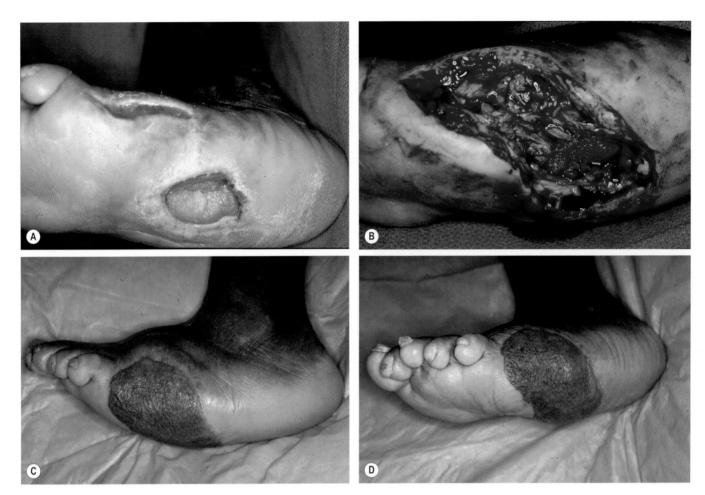

Fig. 8.18 This patient with diabetes suffered midfoot breakdown because of Charcot collapse of the midfoot **(A)**. The wound was aggressively debrided **(B)**. The bottom three slips of the serratus muscle were harvested **(C)**. The foot has remained completely healed for the last 8 years **(D)**. (Reprinted with permission from: Attinger CE, Clemens MW, Ducic I, et al. The role of microsurgical-free flaps in foot and ankle surgery. In: Dockery GD, ed. Lower Extremity Soft Tissue & Cutaneous Plastic Surgery, 2nd edn. Oxford: Elsevier Science, Ch. 20, in press.)

non-innervated flaps. Regardless of age or attempted nerve coaptation, patients with neuropathies or heavy scarring due to chronic wounds may not show improvements in flap reinnervation when compared to surrounding tissue.[189]

May and colleagues reviewed their experience with patients who underwent free muscle transplantation and split-thickness skin grafting to the weight-bearing portions of the foot and concluded that cutaneous sensibility did not appear to be necessary to maintain a functional and well-healed extremity.[190] In a similar report, Stevenson and Mathes[191] also noted successful coverage of a weight-bearing plantar defect after use of microvascular transplantation of muscle with skin-graft coverage. Levin and colleagues reviewed the Duke experience with free tissue transfer to the lower extremity and presented a subunit principle to foot and ankle reconstruction.[192] The authors noted that bulky or ill-conceived flap designs may interfere with proper shoe fitting and prevent efficient ambulation. For plantar reconstructions, flaps that developed late ulceration were more likely to include a cutaneous paddle, with the breakdown usually occurring at the flap/glabrous skin junction. Levin advocates cutting the edge of the flap and the glabrous skin obliquely to maximize the interface surface area as this may decrease the effect of shearing forces. True to all free flap reconstructions, importance

should be placed on meticulous flap inset, removal of underlying bony prominences, patient education and frequent follow-up.

Free flap repair is equally of value in the immediate or early repair of posttraumatic and postablative foot wounds. In these clinical situations the defects are commonly large and complex, and the blood supply to the available local flap alternatives is often compromised. The posterior hindfoot region presents additional challenges. Its anatomy includes a high concentration of various structures essential to normal foot function. There are five principles that must be followed in repairing wounds in this unique location: one should maintain the function of the Achilles tendon, avoid joint or tendon contractures, attempt to restore the normal anatomy, reconstruct tissue deficiencies, re-establish normal foot contour, and select donor tissues based upon the specific requirements of the wound.

Hindfoot amputations

Syme first described amputation at the ankle in 1843.[193] Then, as now, arguments continue as to its merits. The Syme's amputation has a definite role in the reconstruction of difficult hindfoot problems, especially the diabetic patient. The procedure involves using the heel pad as a soft tissue cover over the distal end of the osteotomized tibia and fibula. Amputation is preformed through the distal tibia and fibula at the level of the medial and lateral malleoli. "Fillet" of the heel pad must be performed at the level of the calcaneal and talar periosteum so that "button holing" of the thin soft tissues just distal to the ankle is avoided. It has been recommended that the approach to this amputation be modified by leaving a 1 cm thick "slice" of the plantar cortex of the calcaneus attached to the heel pad, and performing osteosynthesis between this structure and the osteotomized distal tibia. Incisional closure should always avoid tension. This usually means that medial and lateral "dog ears" can be left and revised during a second operative procedure. Significant wounds that involve the plantar heel will require the use of dorsal soft tissues as a "flap" that is turned down to provide closure over the bone ends.

For the diabetic patient with prior contralateral amputation, Syme's amputation permits weight-bearing and allows the patient to ambulate. These patients generally require no physical therapy for gait training, and energy expenditure (oxygen uptake, velocity of cadence, and stride length) is consistently better than that measured for below-knee and above-knee amputees.[194] It is this specific patient population (the diabetic with contralateral below or above knee amputation) that the Syme's amputation is the most useful. The key to the long-term success of this amputation is having a prosthetist used and skilled at creating a Syme's prosthesis.

Postoperative care

All patients who have undergone reconstructive foot surgery require a structured, well-planned, multidisciplinary recovery program to ensure success. All patients are maintained on a nonweight-bearing regimen for at least 3 weeks following procedures that place suture lines on the plantar surface of the foot. This is of paramount importance to insure uneventful healing. The use of strict bed rest and/or crutches, wheelchairs or rollabouts following reconstruction varies with the nature of the procedure performed and the physical ability and coordination of the patient. Local flaps generally require a day of elevation; skin grafts 3–5 days, and free flaps up to 2 weeks. Control of pedal edema is important and may be accomplished with bed rest and elevation followed by the careful use of elastic wraps once the patient is permitted to place the limb in a dependent position. During the bed-rest phase, the use of low molecular weight heparin significantly reduces the risk of deep venous thrombosis.

Postoperative antibiotic use should be dictated by the surgical findings. Patients who present without acute infection and the bone biopsy is negative, usually require only 5 days of broad-spectrum antimicrobials (parenteral while in hospital, enteral once discharged). Patients who present with acute infection will require a 2-week course of culture specific antibiotics. These are usually started intravenously and continued orally after discharge from the hospital. Patients that have biopsy proven osteomyelitis are a bit more complex. If the debridement procedure completely removes the offending bone, a 1-week course of culture specific antibiotics should be prescribed; otherwise a 6-week course is standard therapy.

The L'Nard splint has been a very useful tool in keeping the posterior heel off of the surface of the bed while providing the necessary immobilization of the foot and ankle. It is lightweight and therefore quite useful when the patient begins nonweight-bearing ambulation with crutches or a walker. The Cam walker boot is often used to protect foot repairs and tendon transfers/lengthenings when the patient becomes weight-bearing. Because of frequent lack of compliance (diabetics comply only 29% of the time with offloading regimens), wrapping cast material around the Cam walker to ensure compliance is very useful. A heavy device (similar to a cast), the Cam walker comfortably and effectively immobilizes the foot and ankle while allowing for adjustment of the degree of equinus required at the ankle.

Sutures are generally removed just before the patient is permitted to begin weight-bearing ambulation. Sutures will often incite callous formation on the plantar surface of the foot and trimming of the callous is extremely important. Local care may be necessary for 7–10 days after suture removal before weight-bearing is allowed.

Follow-up should be frequent and performed in a multidisciplinary manner. Plastic surgery, vascular surgery, orthopedic surgery, podiatry, and prosthetist/orthetist should all be available to participate in the patient's care. Experienced nursing personnel adept at all aspects of wound assessment and care contribute as well.

Outcomes

Only recently has there been data available regarding the outcomes from a closely supervised multidisciplinary approach to the management of diabetic foot. Several groups have reported their experience using a multidisciplinary approach within a "diabetic foot clinic." A study from the University of Louisville compared two groups of patients. One group developed ulcers while receiving prophylactic care at a multidisciplinary clinic (group I) and the other, identical group, was referred to the clinic after ulceration had already occurred (group II). The sites and sizes of the lesions were no different between the two groups. Despite similarities between the two groups, group I had significantly better prognosis than group II. The study concluded that the establishment of a dedicated diabetic foot care clinic and regular patient review can reduce the morbidity associated with diabetic foot ulceration. New ulceration, when it occurs, will be detected earlier and lead to management that is more effective in attaining limb preservation.[195]

The role of early, aggressive revascularization surgery in the long-term outcome of diabetic foot management is addressed in several recent studies. Researchers from the University of California, San Francisco, have shown that a multidisciplinary wound care program that includes vascular surgery and adjuvant HBO therapy can provide limb salvage that is both cost-effective and durable. A total of 63% of their patients healed their wounds and they remained healed during the 5 years of follow-up.[196] The vascular surgery section at the New England Deaconess Hospital similarly showed the beneficial effects of revascularization surgery in the outcome of diabetic foot management. They compared the outcomes of patients during two different time intervals. The "modern" approach included distal bypass arterial grafting and led to improved outcomes as evidenced by a decrease in major and minor amputation rates, a reduced hospital length of stay, and a reduced cost for care. In spite of this, however, they point out that reimbursement through Medicare remained insufficient, with an average loss of $7480 per admission.[197]

Studies that have specifically looked at frequent multidisciplinary wound care and its effect on the healing of diabetic foot ulceration are numerous. They repeatedly show that foot wounds will heal when pressure points are off-loaded and wound management is properly attended to at frequent intervals.[198] However, it is difficult to properly maintain off-loading with the use of orthotics alone. In one of the author's own studies, the outcomes of patients treated with plantar wound closure surgery (flap repairs) were compared to those who underwent identical surgical procedures combined with the removal of bony prominences, repair of Charcot midfoot deformities, and Achilles' tendon lengthening surgery. The former group of patients was operated upon from 1983 to 1990. The second group was treated between 1990 and 1997. All patients were followed-up for a minimum of 2 years, though the average follow-up was 5 years. All patients were fitted with footwear appropriate for the procedure performed. When wounds were closed without attention to correction of the biomechanical abnormalities, ulcer recurrence rates were 25%. With the addition of the aforementioned procedures, the recurrence rate dropped to 2%.

Internationally, the recurrence rate is closer to 60–80% at 2 years. However, the prospective randomized study on the use of Achilles tendon lengthening showed that the latter procedure decreased the chance of recurrence by half, to 40% at 27 months.

Summary

Complex lower extremity reconstructions can only be done effectively by using a team approach, which at the minimum includes a wound care team, a vascular surgeon, a foot and ankle surgeon, a plastic surgeon, an infectious disease specialist, an endocrinologist, and a prosthetist. Wounds need to be accurately assessed, debrided and cultured. The repair is then dictated by how much function of the leg and foot remain post debridement and how the wound can be closed in the most biomechanically stable construct possible. This may involve skeletal manipulation, tendon lengthening and/or partial foot and leg amputations. Soft tissue reconstruction can be as simple as allowing the wound to heal by secondary intention or as complex as coverage with a microsurgical free flap. Utilizing the techniques described in this chapter should allow for a stable functional wound closure and ultimately decrease the amputation rate.

Access the complete reference list online at **http://www.expertconsult.com**

11. Mueller MJ, Sinacore DR, Hastings MK, et al. Effect of Achilles tendon lengthening on neuropathic plantar ulcers, a randomized clinical trial. *J Bone Joint Surg Am.* 2003;85a:1436.

   Limited ankle dorsiflexion has been implicated as a contributing factor to plantar ulceration of the forefoot and chronicity of wounds in diabetes mellitus. The authors compared outcomes for 64 patients with diabetes mellitus and a neuropathic plantar ulcer treated with a total-contact cast with and without an Achilles tendon lengthening. Twenty-nine (88%) of 33 ulcers in the total-contact cast group and all 30 ulcers (100%) in the Achilles tendon lengthening group healed after a mean duration 41 (28 days and 58 (47 days, respectively (p>0.05). All ulcers healed in the Achilles tendon lengthening group, and the risk for ulcer recurrence was 75% less at 7 months and 52% less at 2 years than that in the total-contact cast group. The authors concluded that Achilles tendon lengthening should be considered an effective strategy to reduce recurrence of neuropathic ulceration of the plantar aspect of the forefoot in patients with diabetes mellitus and limited ankle dorsiflexion (5(.

13. Hairston BR, Davis MDP, Gibson LE, et al. Treatment of livedoid vasculopathy with low-molecular-weight heparin. *Arch Dermatol.* 2003;139:987–990.

27. Dellon AL, Mackinnon SE. Chronic nerve compression model for the double crush hypothesis. *Ann Plast Surg.* 1991;26:259–264.

   The authors define the concept of "Double crush hypothesis" as it pertains to the etiology of neuropathy in the diabetic foot and ankle. This study used a model of sciatic nerve minimal banding in the rat to investigate the effect on electrophysiological function of single or double band placement. This study confirmed that the existence of two sites of simultaneous compression, or a second (later) site of compression, placed either proximal or distal to the first (earlier) site of compression, will result in significantly poorer neural function than will a single site of compression. The double-crush hypothesis suggests that a particularly important cause of peripheral nerve dysfunction is an injury at more than one site, with recognition that "an underlying metabolic disease like diabetes may serve as the first crush."

36. Driver VR, Madsen J, Goodman RA. Reducing amputation rates in patients with diabetes at a military medical center: the limb preservation service model. *Diabetes Care.* 2005;28:248–253.

   The authors presented their results on initiating a multidisciplinary team approach to lower extremity wounds and reconstruction. This retrospective study on the incidence and types of lower extremity amputations was performed in patients with diabetes. The number of patients with diagnosed diabetes increased 48% from 1999 to 2003; however, the number of lower extremity amputations decreased 82% from 33 in 1999 to nine in 2003. Amputations of the foot, ankle, and toe comprise 71% of amputations among patients with diabetes. The results of this study provide evidence of the value of a focused multidisciplinary foot care program for patients with diabetes.

76. Carson SN, Overall K. Adjunctive therapy for ischemic wounds using cilostazol. *Wounds*. 2003;15(3):77–82.

77. Dean SM, Vaccaro PS. Successful pharmacologic treatment of lower extremity ulcerations in 5 patients with chronic critical limb ischemia. *J Am Board Fam Pract*. 2002;15(1):55–62.

78. Grayson ML, Gibbons GW, Balogh K, et al. Probing to bone in infected pedal ulcers: a clinical sign of osteomyelitis in diabetic patients. *JAMA*. 1995;273:721–723.

83. Cooper R, Lawrence J. The isolation and identification of bacteria from wounds. *J Wound Care*. 1996;5(7):335–340.

84. Caputo GM, Cavanagh PR, Ulbrecht JS, et al. Assessment and management of foot disease in patients with diabetes. *N Engl J Med*. 1994;331:854–860.

91. Steed DL, Donohoe D, Webster MW, et al. Effect of extensive debridement and treatment on the healing of diabetic foot ulcers. *J Am Coll Surg*. 1996;183:61–64.

    There has been a broad interest in the use of growth factors to treat patients with chronic nonischemic diabetic ulcers. The authors present a randomized, prospective, double-blind, multicenter trial comparing 118 patients treated with topically applied recombinant human platelet-derived growth factor (rhPDGF) or placebo (vehicle) and were treated until completely healed or to 20 weeks. All patients had aggressive sharp debridement of their ulcers before randomization and repeat debridement as needed. Of the patients, 48% of patients treated with rhPDGF healed compared with 25% of patients who received placebo (p = 0.01). In general, a lower rate of healing was observed in those centers that performed less frequent debridement. The improved response rate observed with more frequent debridement was independent of the treatment group. However, for any given center, the percentage of patients who healed was greater with rhPDGF than placebo. The authors concluded that wound debridement is a vital adjunct in the care of patients with chronic diabetic foot ulcers.

97. Argenta LC, Morykwas MJ. Vacuum-assisted closure: a new method for wound control and treatment: clinical experience. *Ann Plast Surg*. 1997;38:563–576.

    The authors present the new technique of subatmospheric pressure: vacuum-assisted closure (VAC) for chronic and other difficult-to-manage wounds. The technique involves placing an open-cell foam dressing into a wound cavity and applying a controlled subatmospheric pressure (125 mmHg below ambient pressure). This study reviewed their experience in 300 wounds: 175 chronic wounds, 94 subacute wounds, and 31 acute wounds. Wounds demonstrated an increased rate of granulation tissue formation, decreased chronic edema, increased localized blood flow, and the applied forces resulted in enhanced formation of granulation tissue. The authors conclude that VAC is an extremely efficacious modality for treating chronic and difficult wounds.

112. Löndahl M, Katzman P, Nilsson A, et al. Hyperbaric oxygen therapy facilitates healing of chronic foot ulcers in patients with diabetes, *Diabetes Care*. 2010;33(5):998–1003.

127. Attinger CE, Cooper P, Blume P, et al. The safest surgical incision and amputations applying the angiosomes principle and using the Doppler to assess the arterial-arterial connections of the foot and ankle. *Foot Ankle Clin North Am*. 2001;6:745.

    Understanding the angiosomes of the foot and ankle and the interaction among their source arteries is clinically useful in surgery of the foot and ankle, especially in the presence of peripheral vascular disease. The authors performed 50 cadaver dissections of the lower extremity with methyl methacrylate arterial injections to further define the angiosomes of the lower extremity. They demonstrated six angiosomes of the foot and ankle originating from the three main arteries. Blood flow to the foot and ankle is redundant, because the three major arteries feeding the foot have multiple arterial–arterial connections. By selectively performing a Doppler examination of these connections, it is possible to quickly map the existing vascular tree and the direction of flow which ultimately allows planning of vascularly sound reconstructions, safe exposures, and the ability to choose the most effective revascularization for a given wound.

132. Venturi ML, Attinger CE, Mesbahi AN. *Glabrous vs. Simple split thickness skin grafts for plantar heel reconstruction*. American Society for Reconstructive Microsurgery, Abstract Presentation, 2005.

134. Hallock GG, Distal lower leg local random fasciocutaneous flaps. *Plast Reconstr Surg*. 1990;86:304.

135. Vural E, Key JM. Complications, salvage, and enhancement of local flaps in facial reconstruction. *Otolaryngol Clin North Am*. 2001;34(4)739–751.

149. Hardcastle PH, Reschauer R, Kutscha-Lissberg E, et al. Injuries to the tarsometatarsal joint. Incidence, classification and treatment. *J Bone Joint Surg*. 1982;64(3):349–356.

162. Baumeister SP, Spierer R, Erdman D, et al. A realistic complication analysis of 70 sural artery flaps in a multimorbid patient group. *Plast Reconstr Surg*. 2003;112:129.

190. May JW, Halls MJ, Simon SR. Free microvascular muscle flaps with skin graft reconstruction of extensive defects of the foot: a clinical and gait analysis study. *Plast Reconstr Surg*. 1985;75:627.

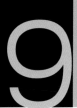

9

Comprehensive trunk anatomy

Michael A. Howard and Sara R. Dickie

SYNOPSIS

- Many workhorse flaps and reconstructive pursuits involve the trunk.
- Familiarity with the vascular relationships and tissue types within this anatomy is integral to a plastic surgeon.
- What follows is a detailed anatomy of the trunk including the chest, abdomen, back and perineum.

 Access the Historical Perspective section and Figure 9.1 online at
http://www.expertconsult.com

Basic science and disease process: embryology of the trunk

In the third week of gestation, formation of the axial skeleton begins. The bony skeleton, muscles, fascia and skin are derived from mesodermal somites bordering the central notochord. Pluripotent mesenchymal cells differentiate into fibroblasts, osteoblasts and chondroblasts and other progenitor cells that will build the tissues of the fetal body. The axial skeleton consists of skull, vertebral column, ribs and sternum. The appendicular skeleton includes the pelvic and pectoral girdles. The skeleton begins to chondrify in the 6th week of gestation. The process of ossification can last from a few months gestation until young adulthood. Progenitor skeletal muscle cells divide into dorsal (epaxial) and ventral (hypaxial) divisions along with a corresponding spinal nerve. The extensor muscles of the vertebral column, derived from the epaxial myotomes, are innervated by posterior rami of the spinal nerves. All of the other muscles of the trunk are derived from the hypaxial myotomes and are innervated by the ventral rami. Most skeletal muscles are fully developed by birth.[3]

Angiogenesis begins in the 3rd week of gestation. Primordial blood vessels begin to form in the extraembryonic mesenchyme of the yolk sac. Mesenchymal cells differentiate into angioblasts, forming aggregate blood islands. These begin to coalesce into primitive endothelium. Near the end of the 3rd week, this same process is evident within the embryo itself and by the beginning of the 4th week, the embryo has a functional circulatory system.[3] At birth, the main vessels and perforators to the skin are present. The entire body is lined by superficial fascia[4] that lies just below the dermis and is surrounded by varying amounts of adipose tissue. It serves to encase, support and protect the fatty and muscular layers of the body and to support the overlying skin in the dynamic movements of the underlying muscle. In certain areas it is adherent to the deep fascia or periosteum and at these places the body contour is defined by creases and convexities. Where there are bulges and plateaus the connections between superficial and deep systems are looser. As an individual grows, vessels stretch from their origins, usually in areas near joints or fixed fascial planes of the body. Taylor noted that areas that were mobile had cascades of arterial supply that tended to originate from the fixed areas distant from the tissue supplied by the vessel. He asserted that these perforators were present at birth and grew along the fascial planes and stretched as the individual grew and developed.[2]

Back

The back provides support for the head and shoulders while walking upright. Near the midline, the paraspinous muscles run in a vertical fashion and are mainly responsible for spinal support and protection. Moving laterally and superficially, muscles become broad and are responsible for movement of neck, shoulders, hips and extremities. The dermis of the back is thicker than any other place on the body. Dense adhesions between the superficial fascia and the skin of the back prevent shearing of the tissues. The spine has dense fascia surrounding the spinal processes and attaches to the dermis. This creates the central midline. Palpable at the base of the neck is the vertebra prominens of the C7 spinous process. The root of the scapular spine is at the level of T3 and the angle of scapula is at T7. Typically, the spinous process of T12 is palpable. The bilateral iliac crest forms the hips at the level of L4. The posterior inferior iliac spine is parallel to S2 *(Fig. 9.2)*.

The *thoracolumbar fascia* is the investing fascia of the back. It encases the paraspinous muscles as well as the quadrates lumborum. It is continuous with the nuchal fascia of the neck, attaches medially to the spinous processes of the thoracic vertebrae, laterally to the angles of the ribs and inferiorly to the posterior iliac spine. It is supplied by the lumbar and thoracic perforators, as well as the distal end arteries of the superior gluteal artery inferiorly and the thoracodorsal artery superiorly.[5]

The broad flat latissimus muscle can usually be seen on both sides of the lower midback in thin, muscular individuals. The posterior axillary fold is formed by its tendon as it crosses from the back to insert on the humerus. The *triangular space* of the posterior axilla is defined by the teres minor superiorly, teres major inferiorly and the long head of the triceps laterally *(Fig. 9.3)*. Through it courses the circumflex scapular artery and two venae comitantes.

There are two spaces referred to as the lumbar triangle. These are areas of the back that do not contain all of the muscular layers. The inferior or *petit triangle* is bound by the latissimus medially, the external oblique laterally and the iliac crest inferiorly. Its base is comprised of the internal oblique muscle *(Fig. 9.3)*. The Superior or *Grynfeltt triangle* is created

by the 12th rib superiorly, the quadrates lumborum medially and the internal oblique laterally. The floor is comprised of the transversalis muscle (not shown). No vessels or named nerves travel through these spaces. The *lumbocostoabdominal triangle* is formed by the external oblique, the serratus posterior inferior, the erector spinae, and the internal oblique.

Muscles[6]

The *trapezius* is a large flat muscle that crosses many joints and has multiple actions on the neck, back and shoulder including elevation, retraction and rotation of the scapula. Typically it is divided into superior, middle and inferior portions. Medially it is attached to the spinous processes of C7–T12 vertebrae, the superior nuchal line and ligamentum nuchae. Laterally, it attaches to the lateral third of the clavicle, the medial acromion process and the scapular spine. This is the only muscle of the back innervated by a cranial nerve. Upon exiting the skull, the spinal accessory nerve pierces the sternocleidomastoid muscle and passes through the posterior cervical triangle. It enters the trapezius muscle 5 cm above the clavicle sending a branch to the upper portion of the muscle. The remainder of the nerve runs caudally along the anterior boarder of the muscle until the fibers desiccate inferiorly. The trapezius receives sensory innervation from cervical nerves C3 and C4. Typically described, the trapezius has Mathes and Nahai type II vascular anatomy receiving blood supply from branches of the transverse cervical artery, which will be described in greater detail later.

The *levator scapulae* originates from transverse processes of C1–C4 and inserts on the superior part of medial boarder of scapula. It is innervated by dorsal scapular nerve and spinal nerves C3 and C4. Blood supply is via the dorsal scapular artery. Its main action is elevation of the scapula and depression of the glenoid.

The *Rhomboid* major and minor lay between the medial boarders of the scapula to the spinous processes of C7–T5 vertebrae. Their action is to retract the scapula, depress the glenoid and fix the scapula to the thoracic wall. They are innervated by the dorsal scapular nerve and blood supply is mainly via the dorsal scapular artery.

The *supra and infraspinatus* muscles originate in their respective scapular fossa and insert into the superior and middle facet of the greater tubercle of the humerus. They are innervated by the suprascapular nerve and receive blood supply from the suprascapular and branches of the circumflex scapular arteries. They act to help abduct the arm and stabilize the humerus in the glenoid cavity.

The *subscapularis* originates in the subscapular fossa and inserts at the lesser tubercle of the humerus. It is innervated by the subscapular nerve. It serves to medially rotate and adduct the arm. Its blood supply is via the subscapular artery.

The *teres minor* originates at the superior lateral boarder of scapula and inserts into the inferior facet of greater tubercle of humerus. It is innervated by the axillary nerve and receives blood supply via a branch of the circumflex scapular artery. It assists in lateral rotation of the arm.

The *teres major* originates at the dorsal surface of inferior angle of scapula and inserts into the intertubercular groove of humerus. It is innervated by lower subscapular nerve and receives blood supply via branches of the circumflex scapular

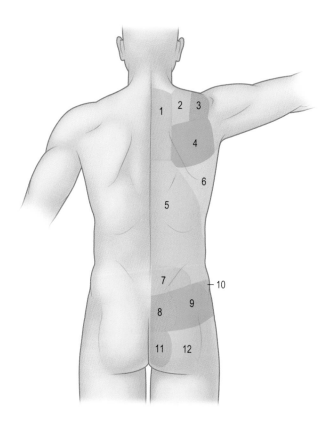

Fig. 9.2 Surface anatomy and vascular angiosomes of back and buttock. (1) Transverse cervical, (2) suprascapular, (3) acromiothoracic, (4) circumflex scapular, (5) posterior intercostals, (6) thoracodorsal, (7) lumbar perforators, (8) lateral sacral perforators, (9) superior gluteal, (10) deep circumflex iliac, (11) internal pudendal, (12) inferior gluteal.

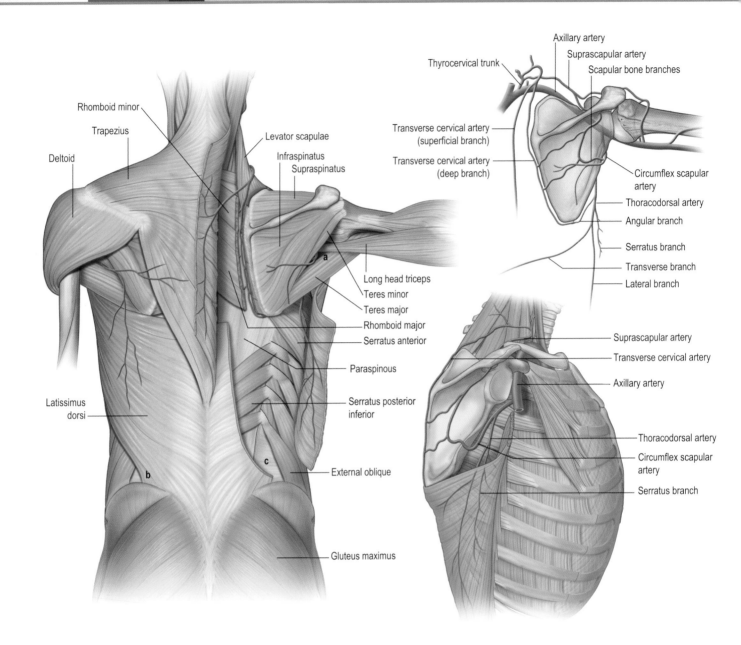

Fig. 9.3 Superficial and deep musculature of the back showing vascular relationships. (a) The triangular space is defined by the teres minor, teres major and long head of the triceps muscle; (b) lumbar triangle of petit; (c) lumbocostoabdominal triangle.

and thoracodorsal arteries. Its action is to adduct and medially rotate the arm.

The *latissimus* muscle originates at the medial attachment to spinous processes of T7–T12, thoracolumbar fascia and the iliac crest. It inserts on the intertubercular groove of the humerus. It is innervated by thoracodorsal nerve and functions to extend, adduct, and medially rotate the shoulder. The main vascular pedicle is the thoracodorsal artery, with segmental blood supply arising from intercostals and lumbar perforators medially. The latissimus dorsi is described as Mathes and Nahai type V muscle.

The *serratus posterior* (superior and inferior) are extrinsic muscles of back that lie in an intermediate layer between paraspinous and more superficial latissimus and trapezius muscles. The superior portion of serratus posterior originates

at the spinous process of C7–T3 and inserts on the superior boarder of ribs 2–5. It is innervated by intercostal nerves 2–5 and elevates the ribs during inspiration. The inferior serratus posterior originates at the spinous processes T11–L3 and the thoracolumbar fascia and inserts on the inferior boarder of ribs 9–12. It is innervated by intercostal nerves 9–11 and the subcostal nerve and serves to depress the ribs on expiration.

The *paraspinous* muscles are referred to as the intrinsic muscles of the back. These are a group of muscles that span from occiput to sacrum. They are intricate muscles that interconnect the spinous and transverse processes of the vertebral bones with the ribs and primarily support and protect the spinal column. Their movements include spinal rotation and lateral bending of neck. Innervation is via dorsal primary rami of the spinal nerves. There are three layers of the paraspinous muscles; a deep layer referred to as the transversospinal group (semispinalis, multifidus, rotators) an intermediate layer, the erector spinae group (spinalis, interspinalis, intertransverse, longissimus and iliocostalis) and a superficial layer, the spinotransverse group (splenius cervicis and capitis). The blood supply to these muscles is segmental stemming from posterior branches of intercostals, lumbar and sacral arteries, classifying these muscles as Mathes and Nahai type IV.

Vascular anatomy

The *suprascapular* artery is a branch of the thyrocervical trunk. It travels anterior to the trapezius along the shoulder and supplies the upper scapula and the scapular muscles.

The dominant blood supply to the trapezius is via branches of the *transverse cervical artery*. Originating from the thyrocervical trunk, it passes through the posterior triangle of the neck to the anterior boarder of the levator scapulae muscle.[7] Here, it divides into deep and superficial branches. Upon entering the muscle the superficial branch divides again into an ascending and descending branch. It is the descending branch, sometimes referred to as the *superficial cervical artery* (*SCA*), which supplies the middle and lateral portions of the trapezius. Once the deep branch separates from the superficial branch it courses below the levator scapulae to the undersurface of the rhomboids. A perforating branch emerges from between the rhomboid muscles and becomes the main supply to the trapezius inferior to scapular spine *(Fig. 9.3)*. The deep branch, also referred to as the *dorsal scapular artery* (*DSA*), supplies the lower middle and inferior portion of the trapezius and the skin paddle above and lateral to it overlying the latissimus. Through the years there have been many anatomical studies attempting to define the blood supply to the trapezius. Some of the confusion arises simply from nomenclature. In 2004, Hass published a large cadaver study, finding, in nearly 45% of specimens, the DSA arose from the subclavian artery or costocervical trunk. In the remaining 55%, the DSA formed a trunk with the SCA and, or the suprascapular artery. The trapezius also receives segmental blood supply medially from the intercostal arteries 3–6, leading some investigators to classify this muscle as Mathes and Nahai type V.[8]

The *subscapular artery* arises from the third portion of the axillary artery and branches into the circumflex scapular and the thoracodorsal arteries. Occasionally the circumflex scapular arises directly from the axillary artery. The *circumflex scapular artery* passes through the triangular space and gives off perforating branches to the superior lateral boarder of the scapula. There is rarely a defined medullary branch, however, a segment of bone measuring 10–14 cm along the lateral boarder, can usually be harvested reliably on these small perforators.[9] The main artery goes on to divide into a small ascending branch, which is occasionally absent, and more robust transverse and descending branches. These supply the scapular and parascapular flaps, respectively. These arteries run in the subcutaneous plane and are paralleled by two venae comitantes. The venous outflow follows the subscapular system and eventually drains into the axillary vein.[10]

After branching from the subscapular artery, the *thoracodorsal artery* passes along the deep surface of the latissimus and continues caudally 1–4 cm posterior to the lateral boarder of the muscle. As the artery descends, a branch or branches supply the lower portion of serratus anterior. After this, it divides into a lateral (or descending) branch and a transverse (or horizontal) branch. Angrigiani described three musculocutaneous perforators that reliably left the lateral branch of the thoracodorsal artery piercing the latissimus muscle and supplying the skin and subcutaneous tissue of the lateral infrascapular back. The proximal perforator exits 8 cm below the posterior axillary fold and 1–4 cm posterior to the lateral boarder of the muscle. Other smaller perforators were found along a similar trajectory inferiorly and obliquely located along the lateral boarder of the latissimus *(Fig. 9.3)*.[11]

Seneviratne et al. described the *angular artery* as a branch from the subscapular system that supplied the lower lateral segment and the angle of the scapula. It can arise from the latissimus or serratus branch of the thoracodorsal artery or at a trifurcation with both vessels. From its origin to where it penetrates the bone measures approximately 7 cm and is reliably found between the teres minor and serratus anterior on its way to the dorsal surface of the scapular angle. This artery allows a strip of bone up to 3 cm of the lateral scapular angle and 6 cm of the vertebral surface to be harvested as a composite graft with muscle, fascia or skin.[12]

The *intercostal* and *lumbar arteries* supply much of the skin and musculature of the midback. Perforators emerging from these vessels pass through the paraspinous muscles in three adjacent columns that parallel the spinous processes laterally at 3, 5 and 8 cm. These segmental perforators have longitudinal anastomotic connections to one another.[13]

The *superior gluteal artery* arises from the internal iliac artery and passes through the greater sciatic foramen. At approximately 6 cm below the PSIS and 4–5 cm lateral to the sacral midline, the artery passes between the gluteus medius and piriformis muscle to enter the gluteus maximus. It sends nutrient branches to the muscle and continues to the overlying skin and soft tissue. The *inferior gluteal artery* also arises from the internal iliac artery. It passes through the lesser sciatic foramen, inferior to the piriformis muscle to supply the lower gluteal skin and soft tissue *(Fig. 9.4)*.

Chest

The clavicle and manubrium create the cranial boarder of the chest. The midpoint of the clavicle defines a plumb line drawn down the anterior chest and is referred to as the midclavicular line. The xiphoid and the synchondrosis of ribs 7–10 create the caudal boarder of the chest. The diaphragm is attached to the posterior surfaces of the xiphoid process and the lower six ribs and costal cartilages. Laterally, the chest is bordered by the anterior axillary fold which is created by the pectoralis major tendon as it inserts on the humerus *(Fig. 9.5)*. The *deltopectoral triangle* is pierced by the cephalic vein as it joins the axillary vein. It is bound medially by the clavicle, superiorly by the deltoid and inferiorly by the pectoralis major muscle. Spanning the triangle and coursing beneath the pectoralis major is the clavipectoral fascia; a thick, dynamic fascial sling. Lateral to the triangular space discussed in the back is the *quadrangular space* of the axilla. Its boundaries include the teres major inferiorly, teres minor and subscapularis superiorly, the long head of triceps medially and the surgical neck

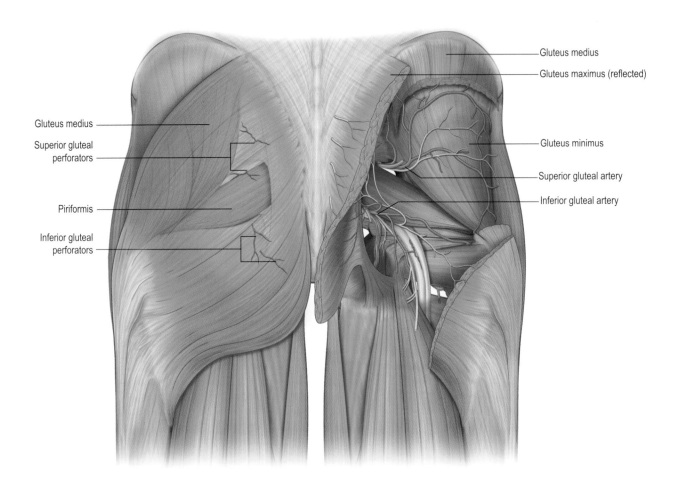

Gluteus medius

Superior gluteal
perforators

Piriformis

Inferior gluteal
perforators

Gluteus medius

Gluteus maximus (reflected)

Gluteus minimus

Superior gluteal artery

Inferior gluteal artery

Fig. 9.4 Superficial and deep musculature of the buttock showing vascular relationships of superior and inferior gluteal artery.

of the humerus laterally. Through it passes the posterior circumflex humeral artery and axillary nerve.[5]

The nipple-areolar complex is located slightly lateral to the midclavicular line and typically situated at or near the fourth rib. Innervation of the nipple is by the fourth intercostal nerve, and blood supply is via perforators from the internal mammary artery at the fourth rib as well as the intercostal arteries and the end arteries of the thoracodorsal and thoracoacromial arteries. For females, depending on the size, shape and ptosis of the breast the nipple could be any distance from the fourth rib, but the neurovascular supply remains consistent. The milk ridge refers to a primitive line of ectodermal tissue extending from the axilla to the groin. At any point along this line breast and nipple tissue can develop. During embryological development this line appears and subsequently involutes, however remnants of this tissue can give rise to supernumerary nipples or ectopic breast tissue.[14]

The superficial fascia that lies just below the skin and subcutaneous tissue is present in the chest as it is in the rest of the body. Over the area of the breast this fascia splits into a superficial and a deep layer *(Fig. 9.6)*. These layers support the breast parenchyma and glandular tissue against the chest wall. Running perpendicular between these two layers and into the deep fascia of the chest are *Cooper's ligaments*. These suspensory ligaments support the breast parenchyma yet allow breast mobility. They stretch with growth of the breast during puberty, pregnancy and weight changes. Loss of elastic fibers in Cooper's ligaments leads to breast ptosis. The superficial fascia of the chest transitions into Scarpa's fascia as it enters the abdomen below the level of the bony thorax.

There are 20–30 axillary lymph nodes draining most of the mammary gland and the anterolateral chest wall as well as the posterior thoracic and scapular regions. The parasternal nodes drain the medial mammary gland and the medial chest wall.

Muscles[6]

The *pectoralis major* is a fan-shaped muscle with a sternal and a clavicular origin. The middle and inferior portion originate at the sternum and costal cartilages of ribs 2–6. The clavicular head originates at the medial clavicle. The muscle inserts into the lateral edge of the intertubercular groove of the humerus *(Fig. 9.7)*. It is innervated by the lateral and medial pectoral nerves. Its action is to adduct and medially rotate the humerus and draw the shoulder anteriorly. The blood supply is Mathes and Nahai type V. The dominant pedicle is the pectoral branch of the thoracoacromial trunk. Secondary blood supply is via the internal mammary artery perforators along its medial

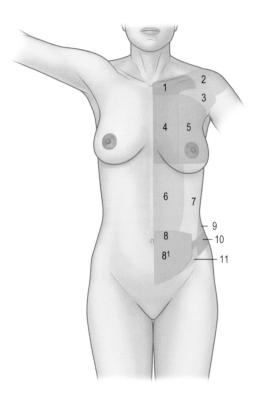

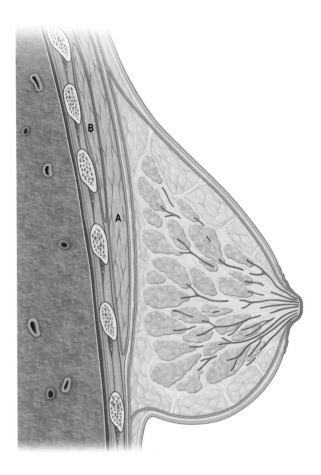

Fig. 9.5 Surface anatomy and vascular angiosomes of the chest and abdomen. (1) Clavicular branch thoracoacromial trunk, (2) acromial branch thoracoacromial trunk, (3) deltoid branch thoracoacromial trunk, (4) internal mammary perforators, (5) pectoral branch thoracoacromial trunk, (6) superior epigastric, (7) intercostal perforators, (8) deep inferior epigastric, (8′) superficial inferior epigastric (overlying angiosome of DIEP) (9), (10) deep circumflex iliac, (11) superficial circumflex iliac.

Fig. 9.6 Superficial (green) and deep (gray) fascia of the chest wall and breast. (A) Pectoralis major, (B) pectoralis minor.

boarder. Laterally, it receives perforators from the thoracic intercostal vessels and some branches from the lateral thoracic artery.

The *pectoralis minor* is a flat fan-shaped muscle which sits below the pectoralis major. It originates lateral to the costal cartilage of ribs 2–5 and inserts to the coracoid process of the scapula. The main innervation is by medial pectoral nerve. However, the lateral pectoral nerve passes directly through the muscle and a small branch of this has been reported to supply the most superior part of the muscle.[15] Along with serratus anterior and the rhomboids, the pectoralis minor stabilizes the scapula against the chest wall. The blood supply is variable, but has been reported to arise from three sources. The thoracoacromial and lateral thoracic arteries provide the main and the most consistent blood supply. The superior thoracic artery, a direct branch of the axillary artery, has also been reported to supply this muscle.[16] Mathes and Nahai originally classified this muscle as class III.

The *serratus anterior* lies below and lateral to the pectoralis major on the anterolateral aspect of the thorax. It originates on ribs 1–9 and inserts on the anterior surface of the medial boarder of the scapula. Its action is to protract and superiorly rotate the scapula, holding it against the chest wall. Innervation is via the long thoracic nerve which runs superficial to the muscle along its course.[17] The serratus has a dual blood supply to its upper and lower muscular slips from the lateral thoracic

and thoracodorsal system, classifying it as Mathes and Nahai type III.

The *intercostal muscles* include the external, internal and innermost intercostal muscles which are layered muscles between each rib. They are layered such that fibers from each pass in opposite directions aiding in expansion and compression of the ribs during respiration. The neurovascular bundles supplying these muscles run on the inferior surface of the rib between the internal and innermost intercostal muscle.

Vascular anatomy

Blood supply to the skin and soft tissues of the anterior chest is derived from a highly interconnected network of named vessels and choke anastomoses. The lateral and inferior pectoralis margins are supplied by perforators from the posterior intercostal arteries and the anterior intercostal arteries of ribs 4–6. The medial chest wall is supplied by branches of the internal mammary artery. The lateral and superior chest wall is supplied by branches of the subclavian and axillary vessels.

The *internal mammary* artery branches from the subclavian artery and runs 1–2 cm lateral to the sternum on the inner

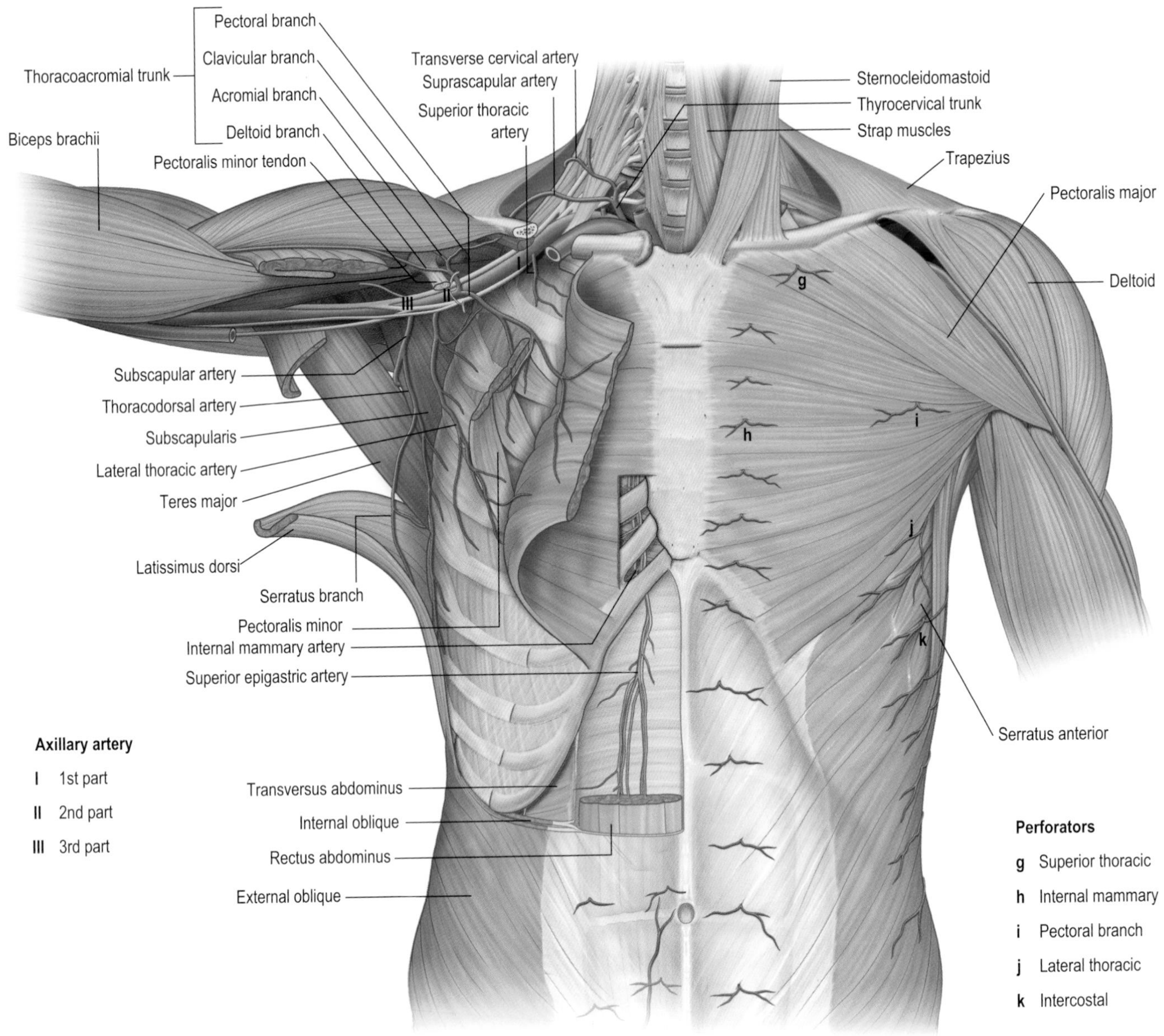

Fig. 9.7 Superficial and deep musculature of the chest and upper abdomen showing vascular relationships.

surface of the thoracic cavity. Perforating vessels arise at each intercostal space 2–6 and pass superior to the rib margin. These perforators then pass through the pectoralis major at its sternal origin and supply the anterior chest wall and the medial breast parenchyma. Typically the perforator from the 2nd or 3rd interspace is larger than the others and is referred to as the principal perforator.[18]

The *Axillary* artery begins as the subclavian artery passes out of the chest past the first rib and ends as it enters the arm passing the teres major becoming the brachial artery. It is classically divided into three parts having specific branches originating from each. The first part is medial to the pectoralis minor tendon as it inserts onto the acromion. This gives rise to the superior thoracic artery. The second part is behind the tendon and gives rise to the thoracoacromial trunk and the lateral thoracic artery. The third part is lateral to the tendon

and gives off the subscapular artery and the anterior and posterior humeral circumflex arteries *(Fig. 9.7)*.

The *superior thoracic* artery is a small vessel that courses medially to the pectoralis minor. It occasionally gives off a muscular branch along the intercostal muscles of the 1st and 2nd rib. It has anastomosis with perforators from these ribs.

The *thoracoacromial trunk* gives rise to four branches; the clavicular, acromial, deltoid and pectoral. The pectoral branch supplies the pectoralis major muscle and the superior portion of pectoralis minor. It originates below the pectoralis minor, passing medially and penetrating the clavipectoral fascia 6–10 cm lateral to the sternoclavicular joint. As it travels along the undersurface of the pectoralis major, small perforating branches pass through the muscle and supply the overlying skin of the superior and lateral chest. The pectoral artery is paralleled by two venae comitantes which coalesce near the clavicle and enter the axillary or subclavian vein as a single vessel. This is usually within 1–2 cm of where the thoracoacromial trunk arises from the second portion of the axillary artery.[19]

The *lateral thoracic* artery supplies the upper four to five slips of the serratus anterior muscle. Smaller penetrating vessels enter the underlying rib and periosteum allowing the muscle to be harvested with bone for composite flaps. Variations in blood supply to this muscle have been reported in that the lateral thoracic artery occasionally supplies the lower portion of the muscle.[20] Perforators from the lateral thoracic artery supply the skin and subcutaneous tissue of the superolateral thorax and lateral breast parenchyma.

The *subscapular* artery leaves the third portion of the axillary artery and within 1–4 cm gives rise to circumflex scapular and the thoracodorsal arteries. The prior passes through the triangular space of the back. The thoracodorsal proceeds caudally, providing a branch to the serratus anterior, then passes to the undersurface of the latissimus dorsi muscle. The serratus branch runs superficial to the muscle along with the long thoracic nerve and provides segmental branches to the lower five slips of that muscle.

The *anterior* and *posterior circumflex humeral* arteries are the last branches to arise from the axillary artery. The posterior circumflex artery passes through the quadrangular space along with the axillary nerve. It supplies the deltoid muscle and the posterior shoulder joint. It has anastomotic connections to the anterior circumflex artery on the lateral side of the humerus.

Abdomen

The abdomen is bound superiorly by the osteocartilaginous framework of the thorax, laterally, by the anterior axillary line and the iliac crest, and inferiorly at the level of the inguinal ligament and its insertion to the pubic tubercle. The umbilicus is located in the midline, approximately at the level of the iliac crest. Three tendinous inscriptions traverse the rectus muscle. Zones of adherence where the deep fascia is connected to the deep dermis by vertical fibrous septae gives rise to what is commonly known as the "six pack" abdomen *(Fig. 9.5)*.

Superficial fascial attachments to the deep fascia create contour differences between the sexes. Men tend to have a zone of adherence along the iliac crest giving rise to a square hip shape. Women tend to have a more curvilinear hip outline due to a zone of adherence several centimeters below the iliac crest.[4] The female abdomen is defined by an hourglass shape. Areas of fat accumulation tend to be inferior to the umbilicus and in the hips. The male abdomen is V-shaped with indentations at the muscular transcriptions and areas of fat accumulation tending to be circumferential in the midabdomen and flank.

Tissue layers of the abdominal wall from superficial to deep are the skin and subcutaneous fatty fascia known as Camper's fascia, deeper superficial fascial layer called Scarpa's fascia, adipose tissue, deep fascia, muscle, and peritoneum surrounding the abdominal contents.[5] The term 'Scarpa's fascia' was derived from the first description of this fascial layer in the early 19th century.[21] In modern-day vernacular, Scarpa's fascia has become synonymous with the superficial fascia of the body, however classically it is only present as the distinct membranous layer in the area of the lower abdomen. Scarpa's fascia is made-up of fibrous and adipose tissue with solitary, evenly interspersed elastic fibers. It is contiguous with the linea alba at the midline. Superiorly, it merges with the superficial fascia of the chest and laterally the external oblique fascia. The inferior lateral border includes the *fascia lata* at the thigh and medially the pubis. In males, Scarpa's is contiguous with the *fundiform ligament*, a thickening of the fascia at the pubic bone that surrounds the base of the penis.[22]

The deep fascia of the abdomen consists of the aponeurotic fascia of the paired flat muscles. The convergence of this fascia lateral to the rectus muscle bilaterally is referred to as the *linea semilunaris*. Medial to these lines, the rectus muscle is encased by the *rectus sheath* *(Fig. 9.8A)*. The anterior rectus sheath is

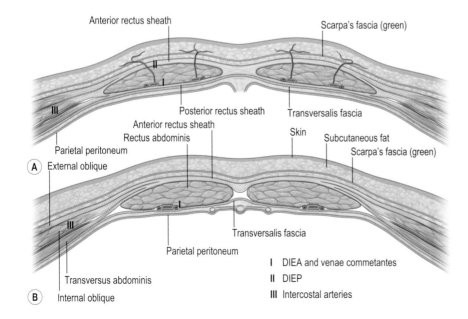

Anterior rectus sheath

Scarpa's fascia (green)

Posterior rectus sheath

Transversalis fascia

Anterior rectus sheath

Skin

Rectus abdominis

Subcutaneous fat

Scarpa's fascia (green)

Parietal peritoneum

(A) External oblique

Transversalis fascia

Parietal peritoneum

Transversus abdominis

(B) Internal oblique

I   DIEA and venae commetantes

II   DIEP

III Intercostal arteries

Fig. 9.8 (A) The rectus sheath above the arcuate line showing the layers of muscular aponeurosis **(B)** The rectus sheath below the arcuate line, showing transversalis fascia as the only posterior layer between the rectus and the peritoneum.

composed of the aponeurosis of the external oblique muscle and the anterior aponeurosis of the internal oblique muscle. The posterior rectus sheath is made-up of the posterior aponeurosis of the internal oblique and the aponeurosis of the transversus abdominis muscle. In the midline, the anterior rectus sheath fuses with the posterior rectus sheath to form the *linea alba*, which spans from the xiphoid process to the pubic symphysis. Superior to the costal margin, the posterior wall of the rectus sheath is deficient because the transversus abdominis muscle passes internal to the costal cartilages and the internal oblique muscle is attached to the costal margin. Midway between the umbilicus and the pubis is the *arcuate line*. This is the caudal most edge of the posterior rectus sheath. Caudal to this line, the aponeurosis of the transverses abdominus and the posterior aponeurosis of the internal oblique pass anteriorly to join the anterior rectus fascia and there is no longer a defined posterior rectus sheath *(Fig. 9.8B)*. Only the very thin

transversalis fascia overlying the parietal peritoneum separates the rectus muscle from the peritoneal cavity. Here, between the undersurface of the rectus muscle and transversalis fascia is a layer of adipose tissue that incases the deep inferior epigastric artery and its venae comitantes.

Muscles[6]

The *rectus abdominis* originates at the pubic symphysis and pubic crest. It inserts into the xiphoid process and costal cartilage of ribs 5–7 *(Fig. 9.9)*. It is innervated by the ventral rami of spinal nerves T7–T12. Its main action is to flex the trunk and compress the abdominal viscera. Its blood supply is via the superior epigastric artery and deep inferior epigastric artery, which classifies this muscle as Mathes and Nahai type III.

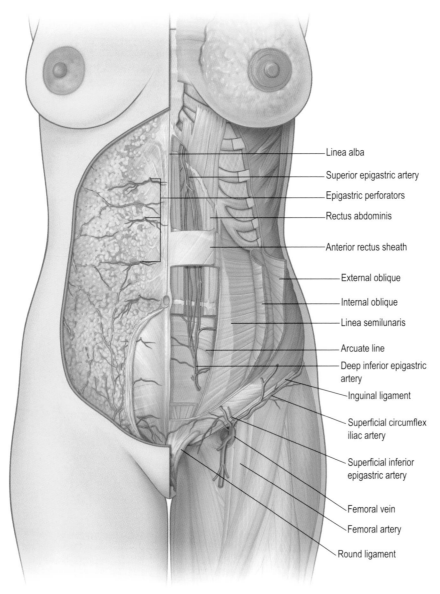

Linea alba

Superior epigastric artery

Epigastric perforators

Rectus abdominis

Anterior rectus sheath

External oblique

Internal oblique

Linea semilunaris

Arcuate line

Deep inferior epigastric artery

Inguinal ligament

Superficial circumflex iliac artery

Superficial inferior epigastric artery

Femoral vein

Femoral artery

Round ligament

Fig. 9.9 Superficial and deep anatomy of the abdomen showing muscular layers and fascial layers with vascular relationships.

The *external oblique* originates from the external surface of the lower eight ribs and inserts into the linea alba, pubic tubercle and iliac crest. The *internal oblique* muscle originates at the thoracolumbar fascia, iliac crest and lateral half of inguinal ligament. It inserts at the inferior boarder of ribs 10–12, the linea alba and the pubis. The *transversus abdominis* muscle originates from the internal surface of costal cartilage ribs 7–12, thoracolumbar fascia, iliac crest and lateral third inguinal ligament. It inserts at the linea alba, pubic crest and pectin pubis. These three layered muscles derive innervation from spinal nerves T7–T12 and L1 and act to compress and support the abdominal viscera and to flex and rotate trunk. Blood supply is segmental via the lower thoracic intercostal vessels classifying these muscles as type IV.

Vascular anatomy

In 1979, Huger described the cutaneous blood supply to the abdomen and this theory was supported by anatomical studies of Taylor. Huger's zone I is located medially and supplied by perforators from the deep epigastric system. Zone II includes the lower lateral abdomen which is supplied by the external iliac system comprising of the superficial inferior epigastric artery and the superficial and deep circumflex iliac arteries. Zone III is lateral, this is supplied by the intercostals and subcostal arteries.[23] These three zones have a rich arcade of anastomosis and choke vessels.

The *deep inferior epigastric artery* (*DIEA*) is a branch of the external iliac artery *(Fig. 9.10)*. It emerges from the medial wall of the external iliac artery and pierces the transversalis fascia to course along the posterior surface of the rectus muscle. As the DIEA approaches the arcuate line it divides into a medial and lateral branch. Occasionally, there is a third branch which will provide direct blood supply to the umbilicus. The medial and lateral branches of the DIEA give off perforating vessels to the fasciocutaneous tissue overlying the midabdomen. The dominance of one or the other branch is variable. There are between four and seven perforators in a given individual, usually clustered in the periumbilical region.[24] At the level of the umbilicus there are anastomotic

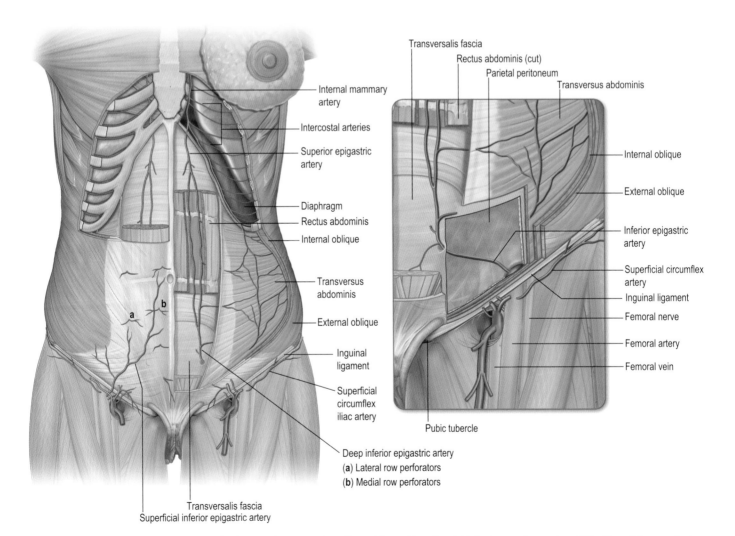

Fig. 9.10 Superficial and deep muscular layers showing vascular anatomy from iliac and femoral branches. (a) Lateral row perforators from DIEA, (b) medial row perforators from DIEA.

connections to the *superior epigastric artery* which is a continuation of the internal mammary artery in the chest.

The *deep circumflex iliac artery* (DCIA) originates from the external iliac artery near the origin of the DIEA. The DCIA travels along the iliacus muscle giving off a large ascending branch 1 cm medial to the ASIS. The artery then pierces the transversalis fascia and travels along the internal lip of the iliac crest just lateral to a line of attachment of iliacus to transversalis fascia. Along the medial surface of the iliac crest there are several periosteal branches. Approaching the flank, the transverse branch of the DCIA forms anastomotic connections with the lumbar and iliolumbar arteries. Superficial perforating branches of the DCIA supply an oval-shaped area of skin along the iliac crest *(Fig. 9.10)*. Two venae comitantes parallel the DCIA along its course and drain into the external iliac vein as a single vessel.[25,26]

The *superficial inferior epigastric artery* (SIEA) is a branch of the proximal femoral artery arising 2–3 cm below the inguinal ligament. The branching pattern is variable and reported as either an independent branch, from a common trunk with the superficial circumflex iliac artery or from another branch of the femoral artery such as the external pudendal. The SIEA was originally reported to be present in only 60% of individuals,[27] but current anatomical studies support anecdotal evidence suggesting this artery is more ubiquitous.[28] The vessel travels from its origin superolaterally and pierces Scarpa's fascia 0.5 to 4 cm above the inguinal ligament midway between the ASIS and the pubic tubercle. It travels just superficial to the fascia as it branches medially and laterally to supply the lower hemi-abdominal skin.[29] This vessel and its anastomotic connections do not reliably cross midline. Venous return of the subcutaneous tissue supplied by the SIEA is via two vessels. One vein accompanies the SIEA in its course and a larger medial vein is almost always present in a more superficial plane. The medial vein often drains into the saphenous bulb, but may at times be found to join the smaller vein and drain directly into the femoral vein.[22]

The *superficial circumflex iliac* artery is a branch of the femoral artery and usually emerges near the origin of the SIEA or shares a common trunk. This vessel passes over the inguinal ligament superiorly into the abdominal wall running in the superficial fascia along the iliac crest. It supplies the skin and subcutaneous tissue for 10–20 cm in an area of the infero-antero-lateral abdominal wall. It is paralleled by a vein which drains into the greater saphenous vein.

The *intercostal* arteries travel into the abdomen between the internal oblique and the transverses abdominis muscle.

Nerves

Sensory and motor innervation to the anterior abdominal wall is via paired spinal nerves running between the internal oblique and the transversus abdominis muscles and give rise to parallel dermatomes of the abdomen. The ventral rami of T5–T11 and subcostal (T12) provide innervation of the anterior abdominal wall from the periphery of diaphragm to the superior iliac spine. The *ilioinguinal nerve* passes between the internal oblique and transversus abdominis supplying the hypogastric region and iliac crest. The iliohypogastric nerve innervates skin of the scrotum, labia majora, mons pubis and medial thigh.

Pelvis

The pelvis consists of a bowl-shaped arrangement of bones connecting the trunk to the legs. It contains the intestines, urinary bladder, and internal sex organs. Paired ilia, ischia and pubic bones connect anteriorly at the pubic symphysis and posteriorly at the sacrum. The muscles of the pelvic floor provide the inferior most boarder of the peritoneal cavity. Below these are the perineal structures of the male and female anatomy *(Figs 9.11, 9.12)*.

Female perineum

The external genitalia are derived from ectoderm. The sex specific genital characteristics start to develop in the 7th week of gestation, appear at the 9th week and become fully differentiated by the 12th week. Estrogen produced by either the placenta or the fetal ovaries is responsible for female genital differentiation. The genital tubercle arises from mesenchyme at the superior end of the cloacal membrane and becomes the clitoris. The urogenital folds and labial scrotal folds border the cloacal membrane. These become the labia minora, fusing posteriorly to form the frenulum, and labia majora, respectively.[3] The mons pubis and labia majora are covered by stratified squamous epithelium with a thick keratinized layer containing multiple hair follicles. Below the skin of the labia majora is superficial fatty fascial tissue continuous with the Camper's fascia of the abdomen. The deep superficial fascia of the perineum is referred to as Colles fascia and is the perineal extension of Scarpa's fascia. The labia minora, clitoris, urethral and vaginal opening are covered by stratified squamous epithelium with a thin keratinized layer. There is no adipose tissue below the labia minora, only elastic and fibrous connective tissue and multiple eccrine, apocrine and sebaceous glands which serve to lubricate the surface of this delicate tissue *(Fig. 9.13)*.

The perineum is divided into two adjacent triangles *(Fig. 9.14)*. The anterior urogenital triangle is bound by the pubic symphysis, the conjoint ramus of the ischium and pubis and the deep transverse perineal muscle spanning the ischial tuberosities. The posterior anal triangle lies behind a line drawn between the ischial tuberosities and contains the anus. The urogenital triangle is divided into a deep and superficial space. Colles fascia forms the roof of the superficial perineal space. Laterally, this fascia is firmly attached to the fascia lata of the thigh at the ischiopubic ramus and defines the perineal thigh crease. Posteriorly, the fascia surrounds the superficial transverse perineal muscle and anchors to the inferior fascia of the urogenital diaphragm.[5]

The superficial perineal space contains the ischiocavernosus muscle which overlies the crus of the clitoris, the bulbospongiosus muscle which overlies the bulb of the vestibule, the superficial transverse perineal muscles, and the greater vestibular glands. The superficial perineal artery and vein travel within this space. The inferior fascia of the urogenital diaphragm, referred to in some texts as the deep perineal or Gallaudet fascia, forms the deep margin of this space. The urethral and vaginal openings pass through here. Posteriorly, the Gallaudet fascia encases the bilateral perineal muscles and fuses in the midline to form the perineal body.

Median (sagittal) section

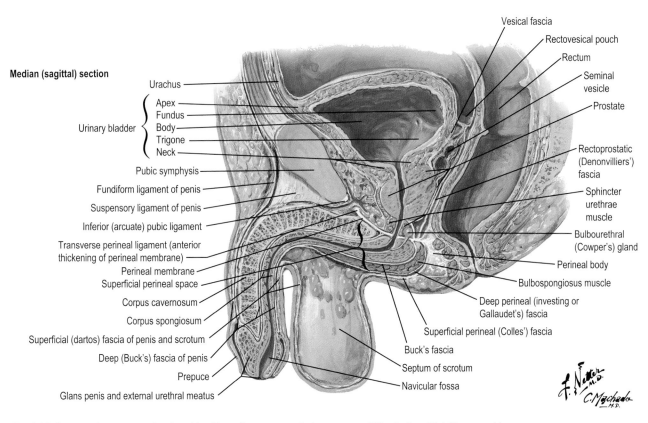

Vesical fascia

Rectovesical pouch

Rectum

Seminal vesicle

Prostate

Urachus

Apex
Fundus
Body
Trigone
Neck

Urinary bladder

Rectoprostatic (Denonvilliers') fascia

Pubic symphysis

Sphincter urethrae muscle

Fundiform ligament of penis

Suspensory ligament of penis

Inferior (arcuate) pubic ligament

Bulbourethral (Cowper's) gland

Transverse perineal ligament (anterior thickening of perineal membrane)

Perineal body

Perineal membrane

Bulbospongiosus muscle

Superficial perineal space

Corpus cavernosum

Deep perineal (investing or Gallaudet's) fascia

Corpus spongiosum

Superficial perineal (Colles') fascia

Superficial (dartos) fascia of penis and scrotum

Buck's fascia

Deep (Buck's) fascia of penis

Septum of scrotum

Prepuce

Navicular fossa

Glans penis and external urethral meatus

Fig. 9.11 Cross-section anatomy of male pelvis. (From: Netter; www.netterimages.com. ©Elsevier Inc. All rights reserved.)

Median (sagittal) section

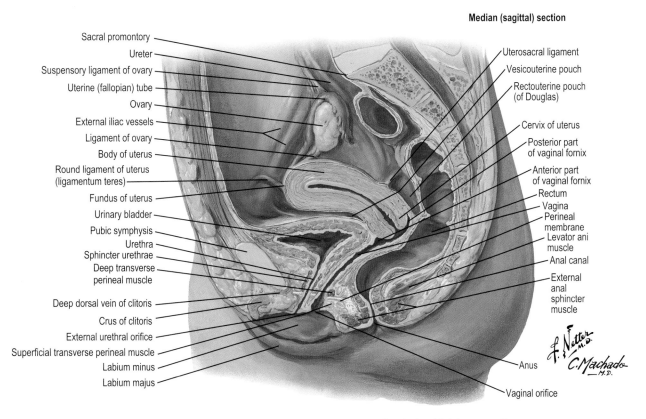

Sacral promontory

Uterosacral ligament

Ureter

Vesicouterine pouch

Suspensory ligament of ovary

Rectouterine pouch (of Douglas)

Uterine (fallopian) tube

Ovary

External iliac vessels

Cervix of uterus

Ligament of ovary

Posterior part of vaginal fornix

Body of uterus

Anterior part of vaginal fornix

Round ligament of uterus (ligamentum teres)

Rectum

Fundus of uterus

Vagina

Urinary bladder

Perineal membrane

Pubic symphysis

Levator ani muscle

Urethra

Sphincter urethrae

Anal canal

Deep transverse perineal muscle

External anal sphincter muscle

Deep dorsal vein of clitoris

Crus of clitoris

External urethral orifice

Superficial transverse perineal muscle

Labium minus

Anus

Labium majus

Vaginal orifice

Fig. 9.12 Cross-section anatomy of female pelvis. (From: Netter; www.netterimages.com. ©Elsevier Inc. All rights reserved.)

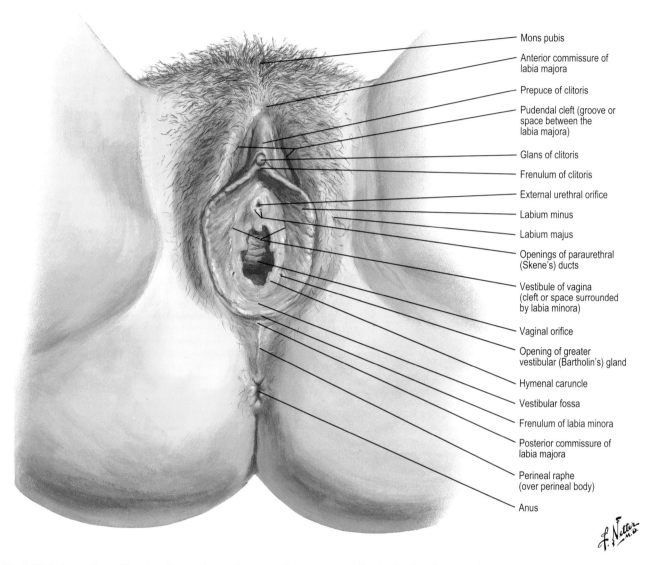

	Mons pubis
	Anterior commissure of labia majora
	Prepuce of clitoris
	Pudendal cleft (groove or space between the labia majora)
	Glans of clitoris
	Frenulum of clitoris
	External urethral orifice
	Labium minus
	Labium majus
	Openings of paraurethral (Skene's) ducts
	Vestibule of vagina (cleft or space surrounded by labia minora)
	Vaginal orifice
	Opening of greater vestibular (Bartholin's) gland
	Hymenal caruncle
	Vestibular fossa
	Frenulum of labia minora
	Posterior commissure of labia majora
	Perineal raphe (over perineal body)
	Anus

Fig. 9.13 Surface anatomy of female perineum. (From: Netter; www.netterimages.com. ©Elsevier Inc. All rights reserved.)

Deep to the Gallaudet fascia is the deep perineal space. This contains the proximal urethra, the external urethral sphincter muscle and the deep transverse perineal muscles. The terminal branches of the internal pudendal artery travel within this space as they make their way to the clitoris. As they exit the space anteriorly, between the transverse perineal ligament and the arcuate pubic ligament, they become the dorsal artery and the deep dorsal vein of the clitoris. The end branch of the pudendal nerve, the dorsal nerve of the clitoris, travels with these vessels.

Vascular anatomy

The two main vascular pedicles supplying the female perineum are the deep external pudendal artery supplying the anterior labial structures and the internal pudendal artery supplying the clitoris and posterior labial structures *(Fig. 9.15)*. The *deep external pudendal artery* is a branch of the femoral artery. It passes into the subcutaneous plane approximately 8–10 cm from the pubic symphysis and travels along the adductor longus. At 4–6 cm from the pubic symphysis the artery splits into an abdominal branch and a perineal branch. The latter is called the anterior labial artery and supplies the superior third of the labia majora. The second major pedicle arises from the internal pudendal artery supplying the posterior structures and the clitoris. The *superficial perineal artery* is a branch of the internal pudendal artery as it arises from Alcock's canal along the ischium. The superficial perineal artery has two branches, the internal posterior labial artery and the external posterior labial artery. Both supply the posterior two-thirds of the labia minora and majora.[30] The internal pudendal artery continues anteriorly within the deep perineal space to become the *dorsal artery of the clitoris*.

The venous drainage of the perineum patterns the arterial supply. Anteriorly, these vessels drain into the saphenous vein and then the femoral vein. Posteriorly, the superficial perineal veins drain into the internal pudendal vein which drains to the internal iliac vein.

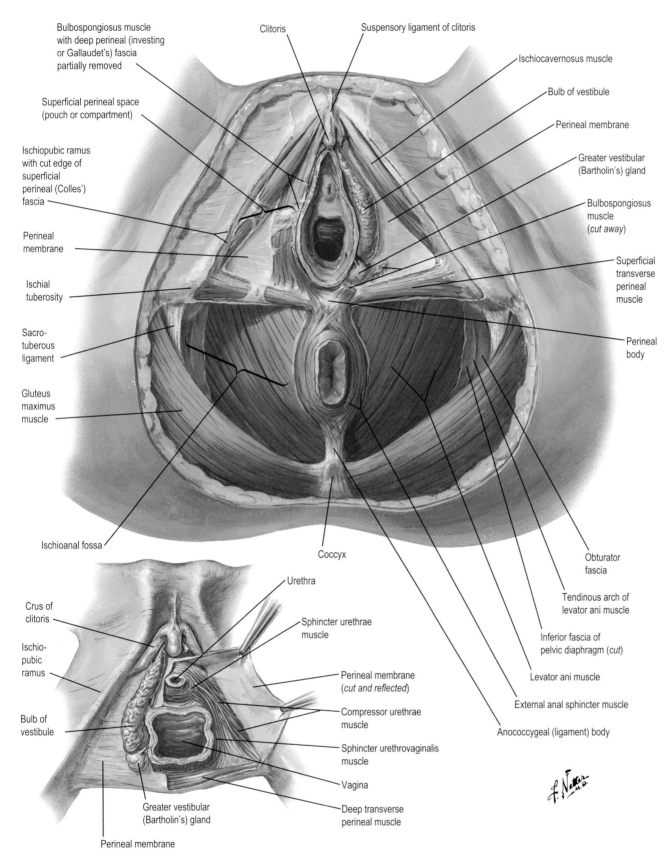

Bulbospongiosus muscle with deep perineal (investing or Gallaudet's) fascia partially removed

Superficial perineal space (pouch or compartment)

Ischiopubic ramus with cut edge of superficial perineal (Colles') fascia

Perineal membrane

Ischial tuberosity

Sacro-tuberous ligament

Gluteus maximus muscle

Ischioanal fossa

Clitoris

Suspensory ligament of clitoris

Ischiocavernosus muscle

Bulb of vestibule

Perineal membrane

Greater vestibular (Bartholin's) gland

Bulbospongiosus muscle (cut away)

Superficial transverse perineal muscle

Perineal body

Coccyx

Obturator fascia

Tendinous arch of levator ani muscle

Inferior fascia of pelvic diaphragm (cut)

Levator ani muscle

External anal sphincter muscle

Anococcygeal (ligament) body

Crus of clitoris

Ischio-pubic ramus

Bulb of vestibule

Urethra

Sphincter urethrae muscle

Perineal membrane (cut and reflected)

Compressor urethrae muscle

Sphincter urethrovaginalis muscle

Vagina

Greater vestibular (Bartholin's) gland

Deep transverse perineal muscle

Perineal membrane

Fig. 9.14 Female urogenital triangle. (From: Netter; www.netterimages.com. ©Elsevier Inc. All rights reserved.)

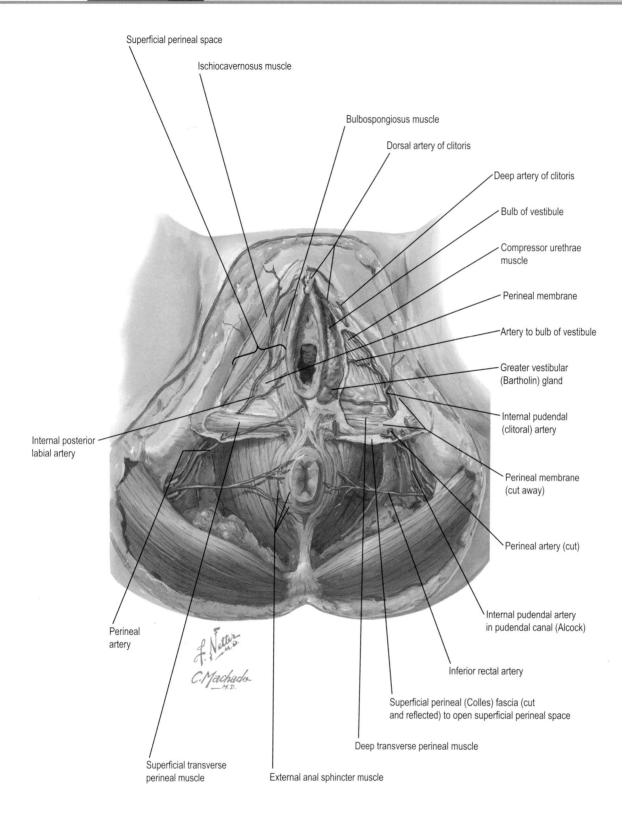

Superficial perineal space

Ischiocavernosus muscle

Bulbospongiosus muscle

Dorsal artery of clitoris

Deep artery of clitoris

Bulb of vestibule

Compressor urethrae muscle

Perineal membrane

Artery to bulb of vestibule

Greater vestibular (Bartholin) gland

Internal pudendal (clitoral) artery

Perineal membrane (cut away)

Perineal artery (cut)

Internal pudendal artery in pudendal canal (Alcock)

Inferior rectal artery

Internal posterior labial artery

Perineal artery

Superficial transverse perineal muscle

External anal sphincter muscle

Deep transverse perineal muscle

Superficial perineal (Colles) fascia (cut and reflected) to open superficial perineal space

Note: Deep perineal (investing or Gallaudet) fascia removed from muscles of superficial perineal space.

Fig. 9.15 Vascular anatomy of the female perineum. (From: Netter; www.netterimages.com. ©Elsevier Inc. All rights reserved.)

Innervation to the vulvar structures is via the ilioinguinal nerve, genitofemoral nerve, and the perineal branch of the femoral cutaneous nerve of the thigh. The superficial perineal nerve, a branch of the pudendal nerve supplies the posterior two-thirds of the labia and the terminal branch of the pudendal nerve becomes the dorsal nerve to the clitoris.

Male perineum

At the 6–7th week gestation, testosterone produced by the fetal testes induces the genital tubercle to elongate to form the phallus. An ingrowth of ectoderm along the ventral surface of the penis forms the urethral groove as surface ectoderm fuses in the midline enclosing the spongy urethra within the penile shaft. The corpora cavernosa and corpus spongiosum are developed from mesenchyme within the phallus. The labioscrotal swellings enlarge and fuse to form the scrotum. Circular ectodermal invagination at the glans forms the foreskin. The foreskin is adherent to the glans penis until birth or early infancy.[3]

Descent of the testes into the scrotum begins around the 26th week. Shortly after their descent, the inguinal canal contracts around the spermatic cord. Development of the inguinal canal involves dissention of the gubernaculum which originates at the inferior pole of the gonad. It passes through the abdominal wall and attaches to the labioscrotal swellings. The processus vaginalis develops ventral to the gubernaculum and travels along the same path carrying extensions of the layers of abdominal wall. These will become the walls of the inguinal canal. The place where the processus passes through the transversalis fascia becomes the deep inguinal ring.

Superficial structures of the male perineum include the penis and scrotum (*Fig. 9.16*). The penis consists of the root, body and glans. The paired corpora cavernosa and ventral corpus spongiosum are specialized erectile tissue surrounded by a fibrous outer layer, the tunica albuginea. At the base of the penis the corpora cavernosa split to become the crura of the penis and the corpus spongiosum thickens to become the bulb of the penis. The crura and the bulb which are surrounded by the ischiocavernosus and bulbospongiosus muscles respectively form the root of the penis and lie in the superficial perineal space (*Fig. 9.17*). Also contained in this space is the proximal spongy urethra, superficial transverse perineal muscles, superficial perineal vessels and branches of the pudendal nerve. The deep perineal space contains the transverse perineal muscles, the external urethral sphincter, the bulbourethral glands and the terminal branches of the internal pudendal vessels as they travel to become the deep artery of the penis, the dorsal artery and the deep dorsal vein of the penis.[5]

In men Colles' fascia is continuous with the spermatic cord and dartos fascia incasing the penis and scrotum. The suspensory apparatus of the penis consists of the fundiform ligament, the suspensory ligament proper and the arcuate subpubic ligament. The fundiform ligament is superficial and is an extension of Scarpa's fascia running from the level of the pubic bone around the base of the penis and attaching to the septum of the scrotum. The suspensory ligament proper is deep to the fundiform ligament and bridges between the symphysis pubis and the tunica albuginea of the corpus cavernosum. The arcuate subpubic ligament runs a similar course to the suspensory ligament proper. The suspensory ligaments maintain the base of the penis in front of the pubis and act as a major point of support for the erect penis during intercourse.[31]

The scrotum supports and encases the testicles (*Fig. 9.17*). The *dartos* fascia, which lies just under the skin is a thin musculofascial layer that regulates the temperature of the testicles by contracting and relaxing, bringing the scrotum closer or further from the ambient heat of the body. The *Cremaster* muscle originates at the inferior internal oblique muscle, inguinal ligament, pubic tubercle and pubic crest. It inserts into the investing fascia of the spermatic cord and testes. Its function is to retract the testicles. It is innervated by the genital branch of the genitofemoral nerve.[5]

Vascular anatomy

There are three main arterial pedicles to the male perineum (*Fig. 9.18*). The *deep external pudendal artery* is a branch of the femoral artery and supplies the anterior perineum. It courses from the saphenous hiatus and provides supply to anterior structures. It divides into two branches at the level of the spermatic cord to become the *internal anterior scrotal artery* supplying the base and dorsum of the penis, ventral scrotum, perineal fat and anteromedial spermatic-scrotal fascia. The *external anterior scrotal artery* supplies the lateral scrotum. The *superficial perineal artery* is a terminal branch of the internal pudendal artery. Its course takes it superficial to the superficial transverse perineal muscle and lateral to the bulbocavernosus muscle. It has three branches. The *internal posterior scrotal artery* supplies the dorsal scrotum and raphe. The *external posterior scrotal artery* supplies the posterior-lateral spermatic cord fascia. The *transperineal arteries* provide anastomotic connection to the anterior vessels. The third arterial supply is the *funicular artery*, a branch of the deep inferior epigastric artery that crosses just below the inguinal ligament and supplies the anterior perineum giving off terminal branches to the cord.[32] The deep structures of the penis are supplied by the *dorsal artery* and the *deep artery* of the penis, which are terminal branches of the pudendal artery.

Venous drainage parallels the arterial supply. Venous supply of the penile shaft is variable and can drain via the deep external pudendal system or toward the infraumbilical system of the superficial inferior epigastric or superficial external pudendal veins.[31]

Bonus images for this chapter can be found online at

http://www.expertconsult.com

Fig. 9.1 Mathes and Nehai Classification of the vascular anatomy of muscle. Type I, single vascular pedicle; type II, dominant pedicle(s) plus minor pedicles; type III, two dominant pedicles; type IV, segmental pedicles; type V, dominant pedicle plus secondary segmental pedicles. (From: Mathes SJ, Nahai F. Classification of the vascular anatomy of muscles: experimental and clinical correlation. Plast Reconstr Surg 1981; 67(2):177–187.)

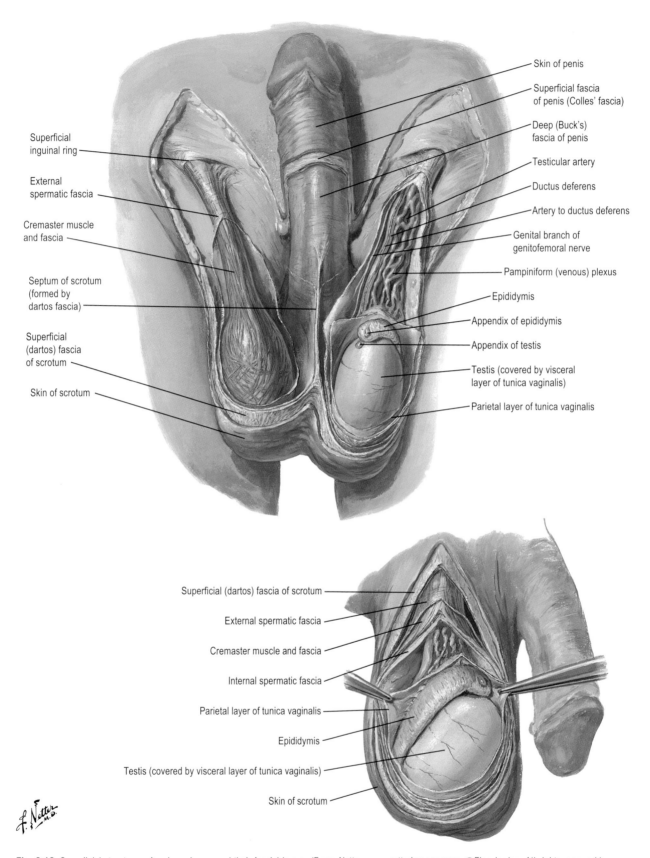

Fig. 9.16 Superficial structures of male perineum and their fascial layers. (From: Netter; www.netterimages.com. ©Elsevier Inc. All rights reserved.)

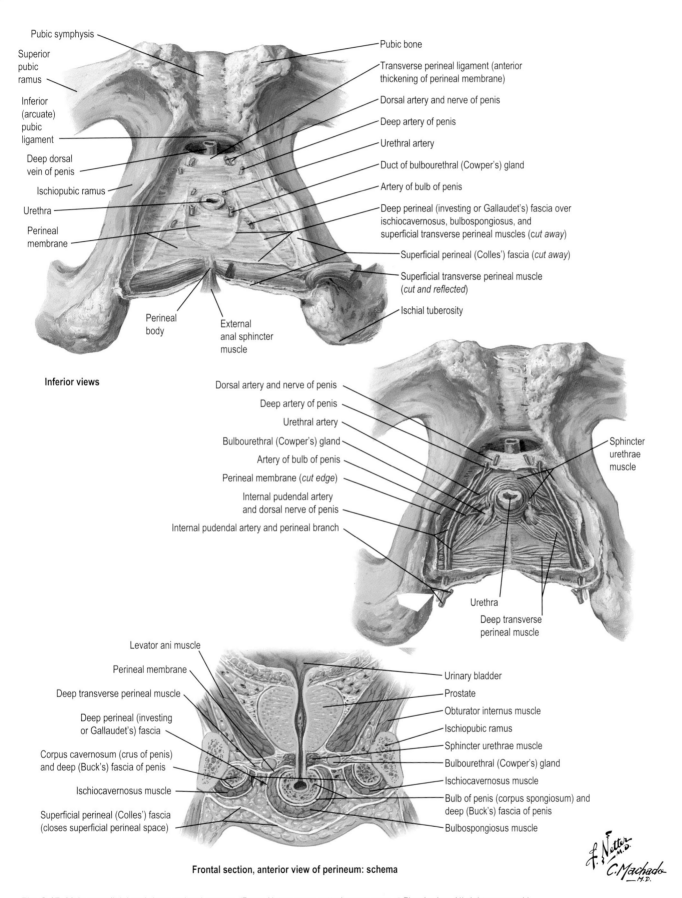

Pubic symphysis

Superior pubic ramus

Inferior (arcuate) pubic ligament

Deep dorsal vein of penis

Ischiopubic ramus

Urethra

Perineal membrane

Inferior views

Pubic bone

Transverse perineal ligament (anterior thickening of perineal membrane)

Dorsal artery and nerve of penis

Deep artery of penis

Urethral artery

Duct of bulbourethral (Cowper's) gland

Artery of bulb of penis

Deep perineal (investing or Gallaudet's) fascia over ischiocavernosus, bulbospongiosus, and superficial transverse perineal muscles (*cut away*)

Superficial perineal (Colles') fascia (*cut away*)

Superficial transverse perineal muscle (*cut and reflected*)

Ischial tuberosity

Perineal body

External anal sphincter muscle

Dorsal artery and nerve of penis

Deep artery of penis

Urethral artery

Bulbourethral (Cowper's) gland

Artery of bulb of penis

Perineal membrane (*cut edge*)

Internal pudendal artery and dorsal nerve of penis

Internal pudendal artery and perineal branch

Sphincter urethrae muscle

Urethra

Deep transverse perineal muscle

Levator ani muscle

Perineal membrane

Deep transverse perineal muscle

Deep perineal (investing or Gallaudet's) fascia

Corpus cavernosum (crus of penis) and deep (Buck's) fascia of penis

Ischiocavernosus muscle

Superficial perineal (Colles') fascia (closes superficial perineal space)

Urinary bladder

Prostate

Obturator internus muscle

Ischiopubic ramus

Sphincter urethrae muscle

Bulbourethral (Cowper's) gland

Ischiocavernosus muscle

Bulb of penis (corpus spongiosum) and deep (Buck's) fascia of penis

Bulbospongiosus muscle

Frontal section, anterior view of perineum: schema

Fig. 9.17 Male superficial and deep perineal spaces. (From: Netter; www.netterimages.com. ©Elsevier Inc. All rights reserved.)

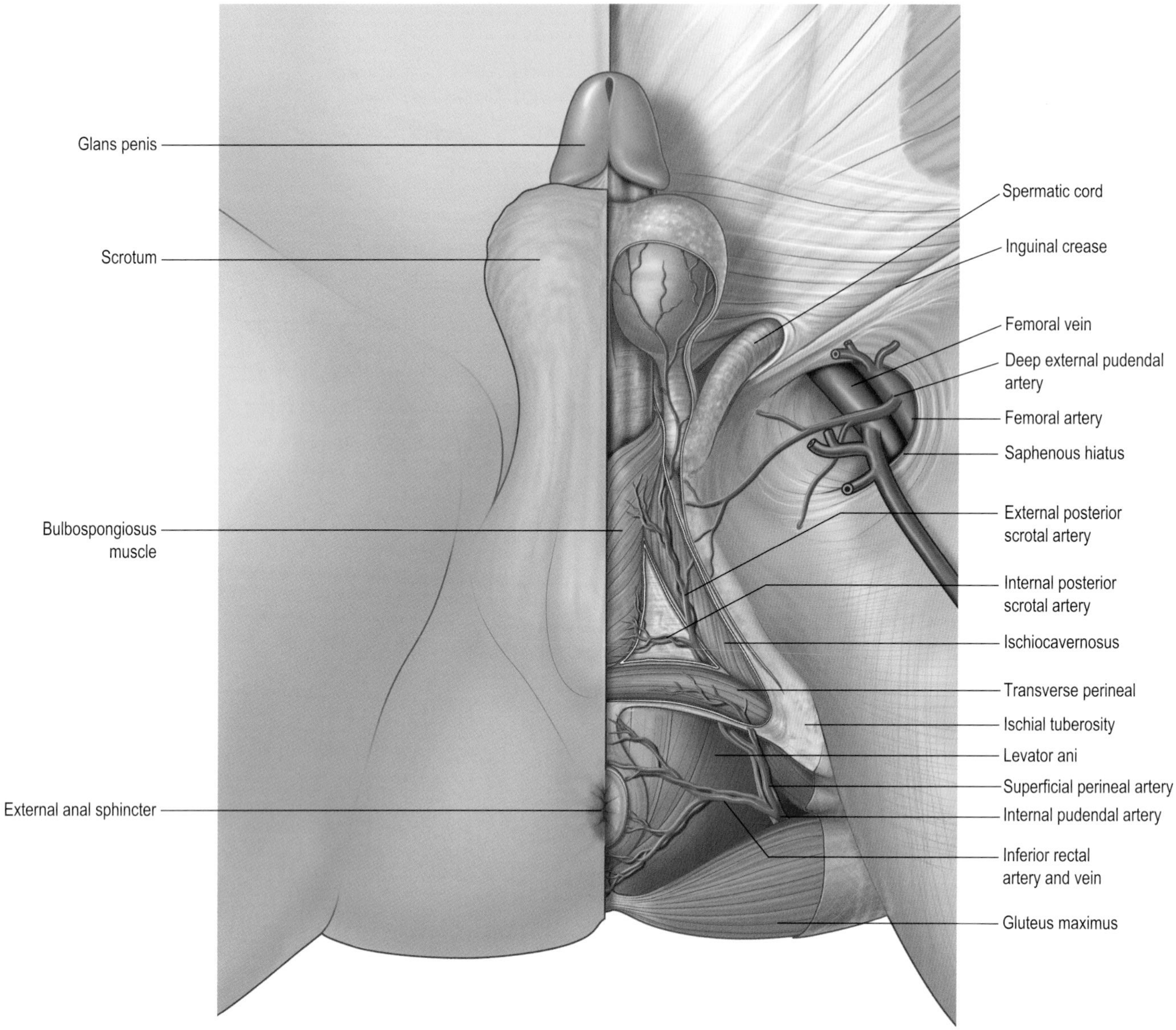

Fig. 9.18 Vascular anatomy of the male perineum.

Glans penis

Scrotum

Bulbospongiosus muscle

External anal sphincter

Spermatic cord

Inguinal crease

Femoral vein

Deep external pudendal artery

Femoral artery

Saphenous hiatus

External posterior scrotal artery

Internal posterior scrotal artery

Ischiocavernosus

Transverse perineal

Ischial tuberosity

Levator ani

Superficial perineal artery

Internal pudendal artery

Inferior rectal artery and vein

Gluteus maximus

Access the complete reference list online at http://www.expertconsult.com

1. Mathes SJ, Nahai F. Classification of the vascular anatomy of muscles: experimental and clinical correlation. *Plast Reconstr Surg*. 1981;67(2):177–187.
   Original article defining variation in muscle perfusion as it relates to reconstructive surgery.

2. Taylor GI, Palmer JH. The vascular territories (angiosomes) of the body: experimental study and clinical applications. *Br J Plast Surg*. 1987;40:113–141.
   Sentinel article laying groundwork for angiosome theory.

3. Moore KL, Persaud TVN. *Before We are Born, Essentials of Embryology and Birth Defects*, 5th edn. Philadelphia: WB Saunders; 1998.
   Used as cardinal reference for embryologic origins of trunk and perineum.

4. Lockwood TE. Superficial fascial system (SFS) of the trunk and extremities: a new concept. *Plast Reconstr Surg*. 1991;87(6):1009–1018.

5. Moore KL, Agur AM. *Essential Clinical Anatomy*, 2nd ed. Baltimore: Lippincott Williams & Wilkins; 2002.
   Textbook of anatomy for general structure and surface anatomy.

6. Olson TR, Pawlina W. *ADAM Student Atlas of Anatomy*. Baltimore: Williams & Wilkins; 1996.
   Atlas of anatomy for general structure and muscular anatomy.

10

Reconstruction of the chest

David H. Song and Michelle C. Roughton

SYNOPSIS

- Rigid chest wall support may be achieved with mesh, acellular dermal matrix, or autogenous material such as tensor fascia lata. Of these, alloplastic mesh is most prone to infection.
- Soft tissue coverage can be achieved with local muscle flaps.
- Proper treatment of mediastinitis includes debridement, rigid sternal fixation when possible, and soft tissue coverage.
- Pectoralis muscle is the workhorse for sternal and anterior chest wall defects.
- Latissimus muscle is known for its bulk and ability to reach intrathoracic defects. Caution is advised for patients with previous thoracotomy incisions as it may have been divided.
- Muscle supplies less bulk than the latissimus but will function to cover lateral chest wall defects and some intrathoracic needs.
- Rectus abdominus is an excellent choice for sternal and anterior chest wall defects, especially the lower two-thirds. Furthermore, it can be used to fill space within the mediastinum.
- The omentum can reach almost any chest wall defect. Its greatest advantage is its pedicle length, which can be extended by dividing the arcades. It does, however, require a laparotomy for harvest.

 Access the Historical Perspective section online at
http://www.expertconsult.com

Introduction

Common etiologies for chest wall defects include tumor resection, deep sternal wound infections, chronic empyemas, osteoradionecrosis and trauma. Although each mechanism carries individual nuances, they will all require adequate debridement and, when possible, replacement of like with like. Fundamentally, the chest wall must be restored for the protection of underlying viscera, maintenance of respiratory mechanics, and base for the upper limb and shoulder.

Chest wall reconstruction can be generalized to include skeletal support and soft tissue cover. Skeletal support to prevent paradoxic chest wall motion is usually required when the defect exceeds 5 cm in diameter. Generally, this corresponds to those defects exceeding a two rib resection. This rule of thumb, however, is somewhat region dependent *(Table 10.1)*. Posterior chest wall defects may tolerated up to twice the size of those in the anterior and lateral chest due to scapular coverage and support[1,2] Anecdotally, patients who have undergone radiation and have decreased chest wall compliance will tolerate larger resections without skeletal replacement due to an overall fibrosis of their viscera.

Options for skeletal support include various mesh products including PTFE (Gore-Tex®), polypropylene, Mersilene (polyethylene-terephthalate)/methylmethacrylate,[3] and acellular dermal matrix *(Fig. 10.1)*. Furthermore, use of TFL as both graft and flap reconstruction has been described. Little data exists as to outcome comparisons between these options. However, in a retrospective review of 197 patients, PTFE and polypropylene appear to be equivalent in complications and outcomes.[1] Another smaller retrospective review of 59 patients prefers Mersilene-methylmethacrylate sandwich to PTFE due of decreased paradoxic chest wall motion.[4] As alloplastic implants trend towards an increased infection rate when compared with autogenous material or acellular dermal matrix, the authors prefer to avoid mesh when possible.

Chest wall reconstruction almost always requires some form of soft tissue coverage as very few defects will close primarily. Reconstructive goals include wound closure with maintenance of intrathoracic integrity, restoration of aesthetic contours, as well as minimization of donor site deformity.

Recruitment of local muscles with or without overlying skin is often the first-line of reconstructive offense. These muscles include pectoralis major, latissimus dorsi, serratus anterior, and rectus abdominus. The omentum may also be used. Commonly the ipsilateral latissimus muscle is divided during thoracotomy incisions and the authors encourage early communication between surgeons if there are multiple teams in order to mitigate against routine division. Muscle sparing thoracotomies help to preserve both the latissimus and serratus muscles while providing adequate intrathoracic access *(Fig. 10.2)*.

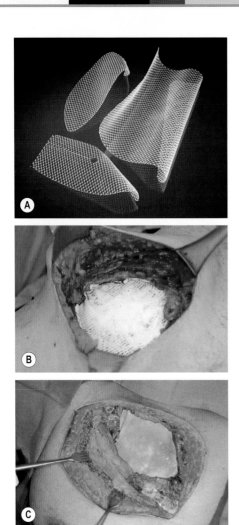

Fig. 10.1 Implantable mesh products including polypropylene, PTFE (Gore-Tex®), and acellular dermal matrix.

Table 10.1 Regions of the chest wall	
Anterior	Between anterior axillary lines
Lateral	Between anterior and posterior axillary lines
Posterior	Between posterior axillary lines and the spine

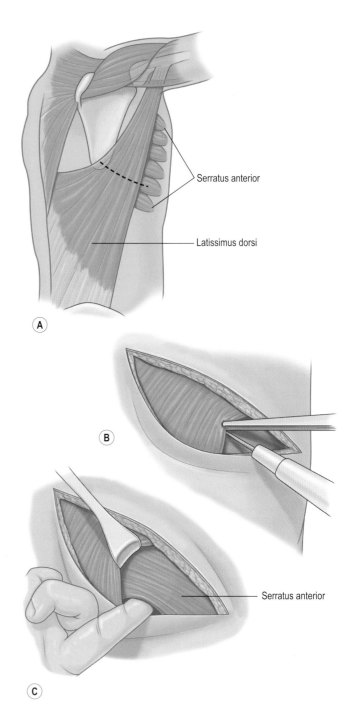

Fig. 10.2 Muscle sparing thoracotomy. (From: Ferguson MK. Thoracic Surgery Atlas. Edinburgh: Elsevier©; 2007.)

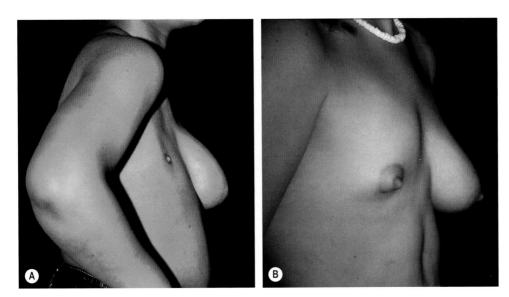

Fig. 10.3 Pectoralis major serves as the foundation for the female breast and when absent, such as in Poland syndrome, reconstruction may be indicated for aesthetic reasons.

Common flaps for reconstruction

Pectoralis major

Pectoralis major, a muscle overlying the superior portion of the anterior chest wall, is the workhorse for chest wall reconstruction, especially for defects of the sternum and anterior chest. Its main function is to internally rotate and adduct the arm. Additionally, this muscle serves as the foundation for the female breast and when absent, such as in Poland's syndrome, reconstruction may be indicated for aesthetic reasons (*Fig. 10.3*). It originates from the sternum and clavicle and inserts along the superomedial humerus in the bicipital groove. Its dominant pedicle is the thoracoacromial trunk which enters the undersurface of the muscle below the clavicle at the junction of its lateral and middle third. Segmental blood supply is derived from internal mammary artery (IMA) perforators. Based on the thoracoacromial blood supply, it will easily cover sternal and anterior chest wall defects as an island or advancement flap. Division of the pectoralis major muscle insertion can also aid in advancing the muscle flap into a properly debrided mediastinal wound. The muscle can also be turned over based on the IMA perforators and with release of its insertion, cover sternal, mediastinal, and anterior chest wall defects. Importantly, when used as a turnover flap, the internal mammary vessels and their perforators must be examined and deemed intact particularly in the setting of post-sternotomy mediastinitis. This vessel may be absent (left more commonly used than right) due to harvest for coronary artery bypass grafting or damaged during wide debridement of a post-sternotomy wound. The muscle may also be placed intrathoracically, however, this will necessitate resection of a portion of the 2nd, 3rd, or 4th rib (*Fig. 10.4*). The muscle may be harvested with or without a skin paddle. Donor site deformity including scar placement and loss of anterior axillary fold may be aesthetically displeasing.[5]

Latissimus dorsi

Latissimus dorsi, a large, flat muscle covering the mid and lower back is often recruited for chest wall reconstruction especially when significant bulk and mobility is required. It is easily placed into the chest for intrathoracic space-filling. It is known as the climbing muscle and adducts, extends, and internally rotates the arm. It originates from the thoracolumbar fascia and posterior iliac crest and inserts into the superior humerus at the intertubercular groove. Superiorly, it is attached to the scapula and care must be taken to carefully separate this muscle from the serratus at this point to avoid harvesting both muscles. Its dominant blood supply is the thoracodorsal artery which enters the undersurface of the muscle five centimeters from the posterior axillary fold.[6] Segmental blood supply is derived from the posterior intercostals arteries as well as the lumbar artery. Based upon its thoracodorsal pedicle, the muscle can easily reach the ipsilateral posterior and lateral chest wall, including those defects involving either the anterior chest wall, sternum, or mediastinum. It can also be turned over and based upon the lumbar perforators. In this fashion, it can reach across the midline back. Again, it can be moved intrathoracically with rib resection. Donor site morbidity can include shoulder dysfunction, weakness and pain, as well as unattractive scarring.[7] However, our experience suggests these concerns are minimal. Also, transposition of this muscle can blunt or obliterate the posterior axillary fold, resulting in some asymmetry (*Figs 10.5, 10.6*).[5] Care must be taken to properly drain the donor site, as seromas are common. Quilting or progressive tension sutures may mitigate against seroma formation.

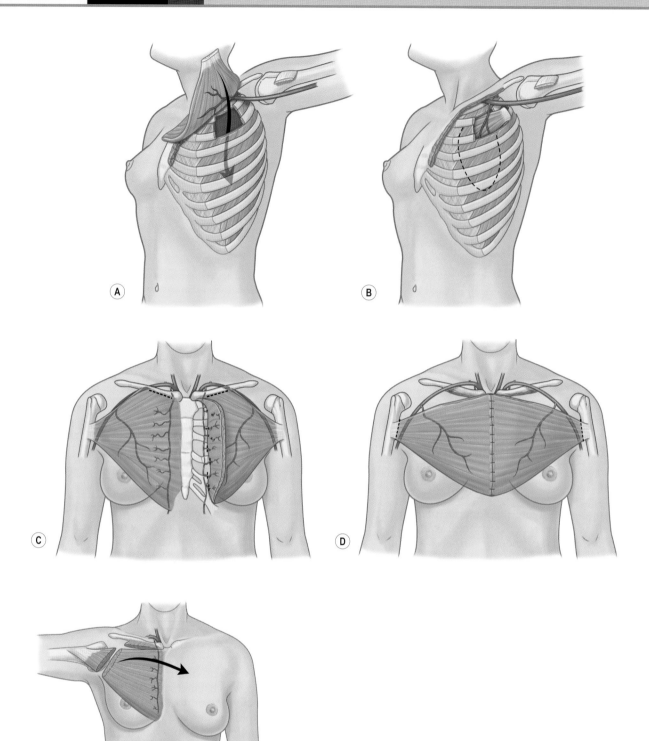

Fig. 10.4 Pectoralis anatomy and flap reach, standard and as turnover.

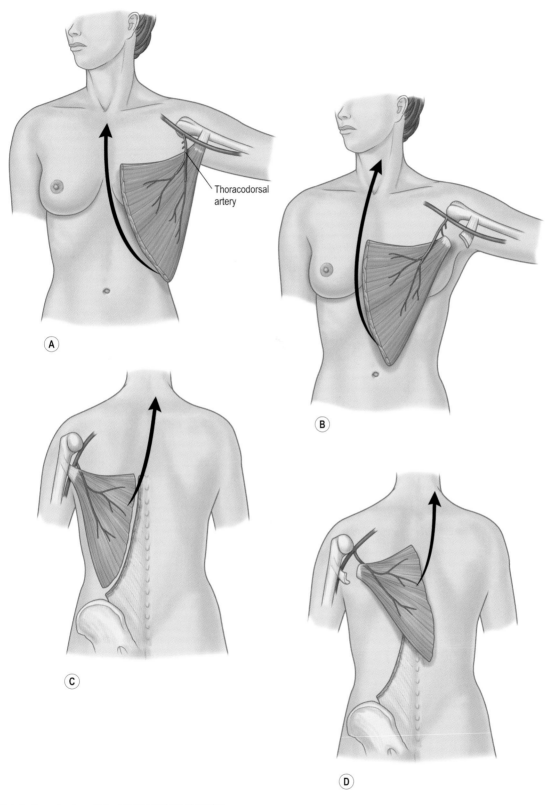

Thoracodorsal artery

Fig. 10.5 Latissimus dorsi, anatomy and standard arc of rotation.

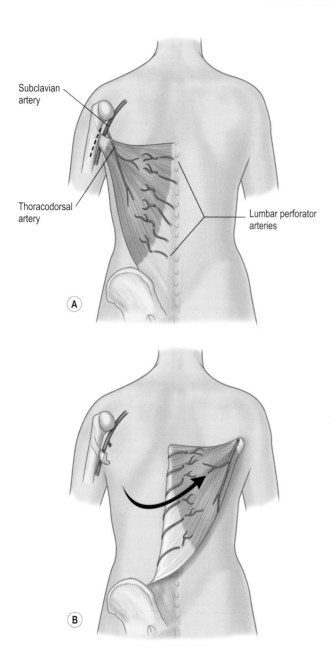

Fig. 10.6 Latissimus turnover flap. Thoracodorsal pedicle ligated, muscle turned over based upon thoracolumbar perforators. Provides coverage of contralateral posterior chest wall.

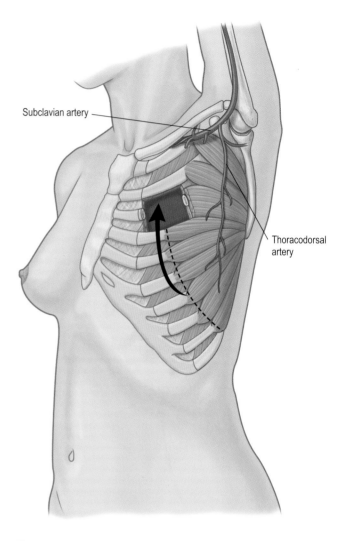

Fig. 10.7 Serratus anatomy and arc of rotation.

Serratus anterior

Serratus anterior is a thin broad multi-pennate muscle lying deep along the anterolateral chest wall. It originates from the upper 8 or 9 ribs and inserts on the ventral-medial scapula. It functions to stabilize the scapula and move it forward on the chest wall such as when throwing a punch. It has two dominant pedicles including the lateral thoracic and the thoracodorsal arteries. Division of the lateral thoracic pedicle will increase the arc posteriorly and similarly division of the thoracodorsal will increase the arc anteriorly. The muscle will

reach the midline of the anterior or posterior chest. More commonly, however, it is used for intrathoracic coverage, again requiring rib resection. An osteomyocutaneous flap may be harvested by preservation of the muscular connections with the underlying ribs. Donor site morbidity is related to winging of the scapula and can be avoided if the muscle is harvested segmentally and the superior five or six digitations are preserved *(Fig. 10.7)*.[5]

Rectus abdominus

Rectus abdominus is a long, flat muscle which constitutes the medial abdominal wall. It originates from the pubis and inserts onto the costal margin. It can easily cover sternal and anterior chest wall defects and can also fill space within the mediastinum. It has two dominant pedicles, the superior and inferior epigastric arteries and functions to flex the trunk. With division of the inferior pedicle, the muscle will cover the mediastinum and the anterior chest wall. It may be utilized

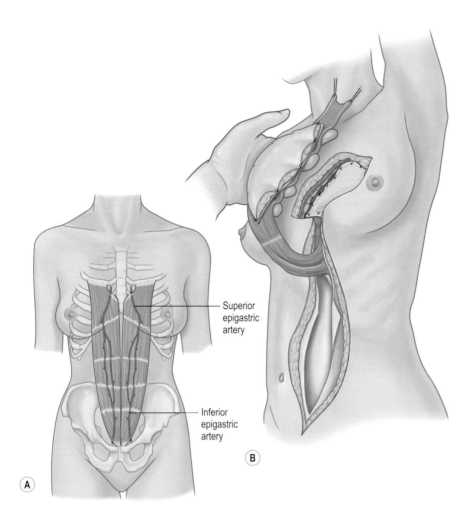

Superior
epigastric
artery

Inferior
epigastric
artery

B

A

Fig. 10.8 Rectus anatomy and arc of rotation.

despite previous IMA harvest based upon its minor pedicle, the 8th intercostals artery. It can be harvested with overlying skin paddle and usually the resulting cutaneous defect can be closed primarily. When taken with overlying fascia, there is a risk for resultant hernia, and at times, mesh reinforcement of the abdominal wall is necessary. Caution is also advised for patients with prior abdominal incisions as the skin perforators or intramuscular blood supply may have been previously violated (*Fig. 10.8*).[5]

Omentum

The omentum is comprised of visceral fat and blood vessels which arises from the greater curve of the stomach and is also attached to the transverse colon. This flap can easily cover wounds in the mediastinum, anterior, lateral and posterior chest wall. It has two dominant pedicles, the right and left gastroepiploic arteries. The greatest benefit of this flap is the pedicle length, which can be easily elongated with division of internal arcades. The flap is mobilized onto the chest or into the mediastinum through the diaphragm or over the costal margin. Ideally, the flap is mobilized through a cruciate incision in the right diaphragm as the liver helps to buttress the incision and prevent diaphragmatic hernia. Furthermore, right-sided transposition obviates the need to navigate the flap around the heart. Care must be taken when interpolating the omentum as it is often of very little substance and can easily be avulsed during passage through the diaphragm. Strategies to protect the omentum during transposition include placing the omentum into a bowel bag. The empty bag can be passed from the mediastinum into the abdomen via the diaphragm incision, past the left lobe of the liver. The omentum is then gently packed into the bowel bag with tension transferred to the bowel bag rather than the omentum during interpolation. Caution is again advised for patients with prior laparotomy incisions as the omentum may have significant intra-abdominal adhesions or have been previously resected (*Figs 10.9–10.11*).[5]

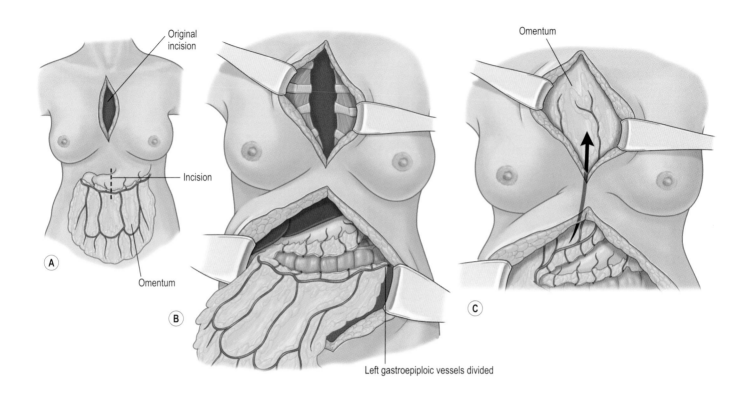

Fig. 10.9 Omentum anatomy.

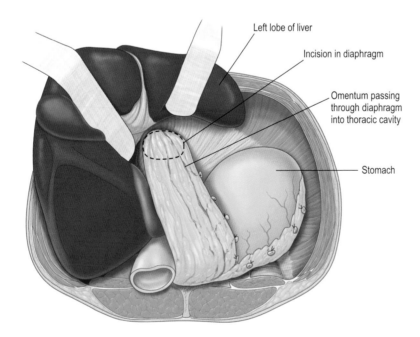

Fig. 10.10 Omentum is passed through cruciate incision in diaphragm under the left lobe of the liver.

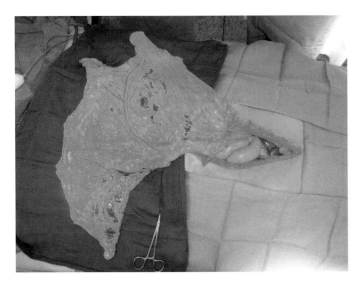

Fig. 10.11 Omentum arc of rotation.

Patient selection/approach to patient

The importance of a multidisciplinary approach to chest wall reconstruction cannot be underestimated. These patients, whether suffering from malignancy, infection, or trauma, are often also plagued with cardiac or respiratory insufficiency, diabetes, obesity, malnutrition, and generalized deconditioning. Thorough work-up including pulmonary function testing, physical therapy and nutritional assessment, and preoperative control of blood sugar may optimize outcomes. Furthermore, communication between referring surgeon and reconstructive plastic surgeon is crucial for properly defined preoperative reconstructive expectations as well as incision planning. For example, it may be advantageous to spare chest wall musculature, such as the latissimus dorsi, during thoracotomy.

Acquired chest wall deformities are commonly the result of iatrogenic injury. Usually encountered in conjunction with cardiac or thoracic surgery, wound infections, mediastinitis, osteoradionecrosis, refractory empyema and bronchopleural fistulas, can all necessitate chest wall reconstruction.

Utilizing the workhorse flaps described above combined with general principles of thorough debridement and skeletal stabilization the surgeon is generally well prepared to reconstruct any deficit. Common chest wall reconstructive problems are described below.

Chest wall tumors

Basic science/disease process

Primary tumors of the chest wall comprise only 5% of thoracic neoplasms.[21] Half of these are considered benign.[22] The most common benign tumor is osteochondroma and is resected only when symptomatic. The most common primary malignant tumors are sarcomas; chondrosarcoma from the bony structures and desmoid tumors from the soft tissue. Sarcoma resection is recommended to include a 4 cm margin of normal tissue and thus, will almost always necessitate significant

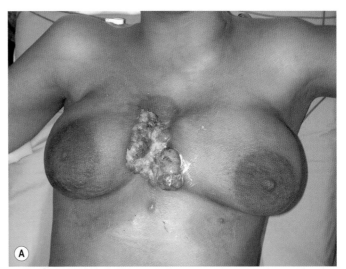

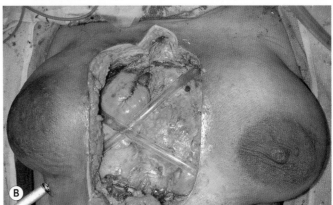

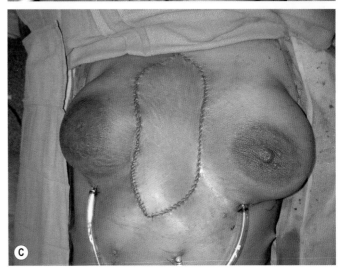

Fig. 10.12 Recurrent breast cancer, sternal metastases.

chest wall reconstruction.[23] Over half of malignant chest wall lesions represent metastatic disease with breast and lung cancers being the most common.[24]

Diagnosis/presentation/patient selection

For relief of symptoms including pain, ulceration, foul odor, and occasionally for disease-control, even metastatic lesions may necessitate resection *(Fig. 10.12)*.

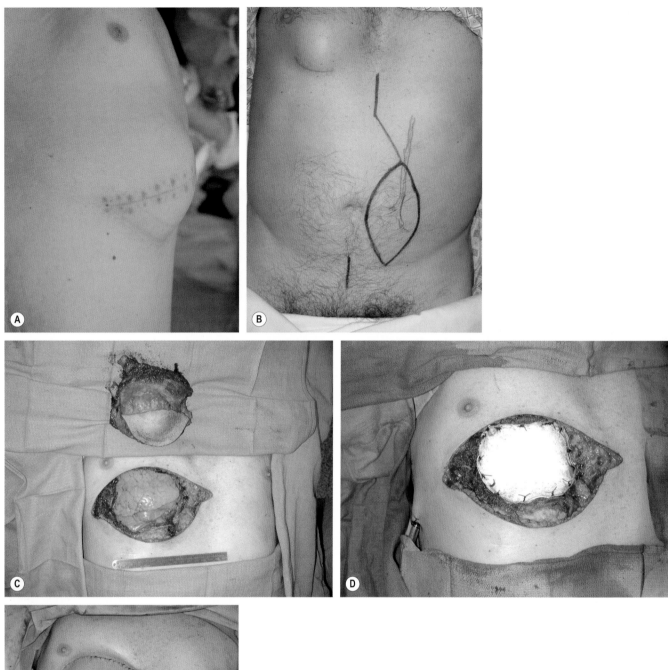

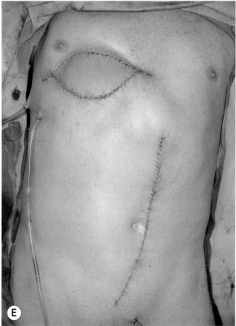

Fig. 10.13 Chondrosarcoma, resected and reconstructed with VRAM flap.

Treatment/surgical technique

Like other neoplasms, metastatic tumors are resected with a margin of normal tissue and thus, they too, will frequently require skeletal support as well as recruitment of soft tissue in the form of pedicled or free flaps *(Fig. 10.13)*.

Outcomes

Not all metastatic resections are palliative. The 5-year survival rate following resection of chest wall recurrence of breast cancer is reported to be as high as 58%.[25]

Mediastinitis and sternal nonunion

Basic science/disease process

Mediastinitis occurs in 0.25–5% of patients undergoing median sternotomy.[13,17,26] Historically, mortality approached 50% in these patients.[13] Sternal wound infections may be classified into three distinct types as described by Pairolero and Arnold[27] *(Table 10.2)*. Type 1 wounds occur in the first several postoperative days and are usually sterile. This is consistent with early bony nonunion and may represent the earliest stage of infection and perhaps even the portal of entry for skin flora. Type 2 infections, occurring in the first several weeks postoperatively are consistent with acute deep sternal wound infection, including sternal dehiscence, positive wound cultures, and cellulitis. Type 3 infections, presenting months to years later, represent chronic wound infection and uncommonly represent true mediastinitis. They are usually confined to the sternum and overlying skin and may be related to osteonecrosis or persistent foreign body.

Speculation exists that dehiscence of the sternum precedes infection of the deeper soft tissues within the mediastinum. Similar to other bones in the body such as in the lower extremity or even the mandible, sternal instability may perhaps encourage infection rather than result from it.[20] With absent bacterial contamination and resulting infection, this instability will develop into sternal nonunion as opposed to post-sternotomy mediastinitis and osteomyelitis.[28,29]

Table 10.2 Classification of infected sternotomy wounds		
Type I	**Type II**	**Type III**
Occurs within first few days	Occurs within first few weeks	Occurs months to years later
Serosanguineous drainage	Purulent drainage	Chronic draining sinus tract
Cellulitis absent	Cellulitis present	Cellulitis localized
Mediastinum soft and pliable	Mediastinal suppuration	Mediastinitis rare
Osteomyelitis and costochondritis absent	Osteomyelitis frequent, costochondritis rare	Osteomyelitis, costochondritis, or retained foreign body always present
Cultures usually negative	Cultures positive	Cultures positive

(Reprinted from Pairolero and Arnold. Chest wall tumors. Experience with 100 consecutive patients, J Thorac Cardiovasc Surg 1985;90:367-72).

Diagnosis/patient presentation

Preoperative risk factors for the development of mediastinitis include older patients, COPD, smoking, ESRD, DM, chronic steroid or immunosuppressive use, morbid obesity including large, heavy breasts, prolonged ventilator support (>24 h), concurrent infection and reoperative surgery. Other variables include off midline sternotomies, osteoporosis, use of LIMA or RIMA, long cardiopulmonary bypass runs (>2 h), and transverse sternal fractures.[30,31] A high index of suspicion is encouraged for any patient with sternal instability or 'click.' However, firm diagnosis of mediastinitis or deep sternal wound infection is made by isolation of an organism from mediastinal fluid or tissue, chest pain, or fever associated with bony instability.[32]

Sternal nonunion commonly results from failure of boney healing following median sternotomy. However, it is also seen in association with chest wall trauma. Patients with nonunion may complain of pain or clicking associated with respiration.

Treatment/surgical technique

Consistent with fundamental plastic surgery principles, treatment of infection including that of the mediastinum *(Fig. 10.14)*,[33] will require adequate drainage and debridement. Quantitative tissue culture facilitates this debridement and guides antimicrobial therapy.

If tissue culture is positive, >10^5 organisms/cm³ of tissue, indicating deep sternal wound infection rather than early sternal dehiscence, early debridement is encouraged and should be performed urgently. A thorough debridement includes the removal of sternal wires and extraneous foreign bodies including any unnecessary pacing wires and chest tubes *(Fig. 10.15)*. Sharp debridement of necrotic and/or purulent tissue is performed until remaining tissue appears healthy and bleeding.[34] Radical sternectomy is not indicated and sternal salvage should be attempted if the bone is viable. This may be determined by bleeding from the marrow and the presence of hard, crunchy cortical bone. Topical antimicrobials such as silver sulfadiazine and mafenide creams are employed to gain and maintain bacteriologic control of the wound.

Subatmospheric pressure wound therapy (e.g., V.A.C.™) may be utilized to increase wound blood flow and expedite granulation tissue, thereby decreasing dead space.[35,36] This has been shown to decrease the number of days between operative debridement and definitive closure of sternal wounds, from 8.5 to 6.2 days, as well as the number of flaps required per patient, 1.5–0.9.[19] Subatmospheric pressure wound therapy is now standard practice for the treatment of mediastinitis at many institutions.[37–40]

Fixation of the sternum or residual sternal bone is crucial for bony healing. Furthermore, this fixation prevents paradoxic motion of the anterior chest wall and may improve many complications seen with sternal nonunion such as chronic chest wall pain and abnormal rubbing or clicking sensations.[20,41] For adults, titanium plates are used *(Fig. 10.16)*.

Sternal dehiscence also occurs early in the postoperative course, consistent with type 1 sternal wound infections. This is secondary to mechanical failure of wire closure rather than

Video 1

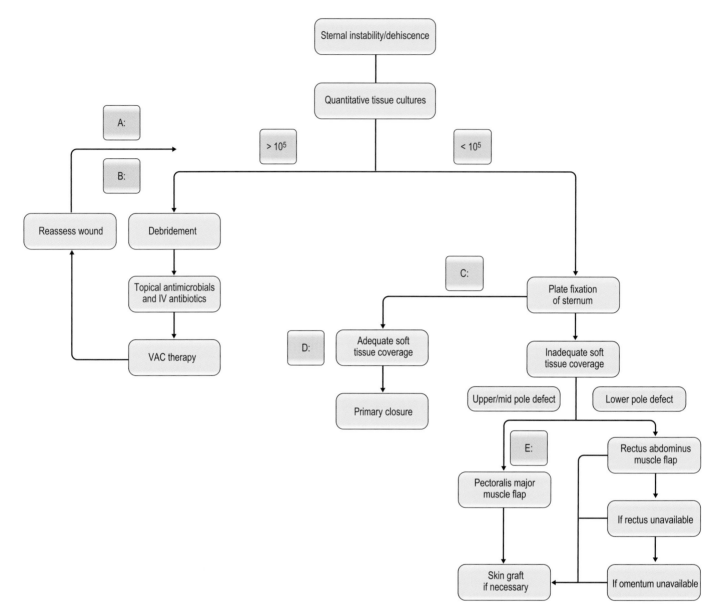

Fig. 10.14 Management of sternal wounds. (From: Roughton MC, Song DH. Sternal wounds. In: Marsh J, Perlyn C, eds. Decision Making in Plastic Surgery. St Louis, MO: Quality Medical; 2009:63.)[33]

infection. The wounds are sterile and surgeons should proceed to immediate rigid sternal fixation. More commonly, however, patients will present with sternal nonunion in a delayed fashion. In the absence of infection, the residual viable bone can be plated directly.[28] Importantly, a paradigm shift has occurred in the authors' institution such that patients who are deemed high risk for mediastinitis and sternal dehiscence are plated prophylactically.[29,42] Several plating systems exist, all designed to facilitate ease of application as well as emergent chest re-entry.

Once rigid fixation is achieved, soft tissue closure must be addressed. As very limited soft tissue exists over a normal sternum, residual local tissue following debridement of mediastinitis will often prove inadequate for plate coverage. Thus, muscle flap coverage is indicated. When the wound involves the upper two-thirds of the sternum, pectoralis major muscle

advancement or turnover flaps are easily harvested and are the first-line therapy for wound closure *(Fig. 10.17)*. Caution is advised for turnover flaps when the ipsilateral IMA has been harvested for CABG. Furthermore, emergent chest re-entry will, by definition, devascularize this turnover flap. Additionally, when the lower sternal pole lacks coverage, the pectoralis may be inadequate, based on its limited arc of rotation. For these cases, the rectus abdominus muscle flap is a better choice. It may be used despite LIMA or RIMA harvest based upon the 8th intercostal artery, its minor pedicle. If the rectus is unavailable secondary to previous surgery, a pedicled omental flap should be considered for soft-tissue sternal coverage. Finally, if the omentum has been previously resected or the patient has had multiple prior abdominal operations, the latissimus dorsi flap can be used. This may be harvested with a skin island and allow chest wound closure.[43] Skin

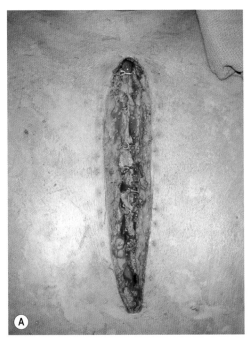

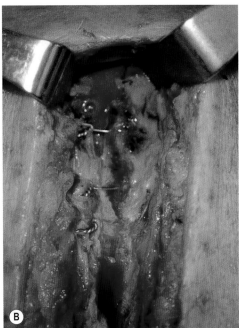

Fig. 10.15 Thorough debridement requires removal of necrotic tissue and foreign bodies.

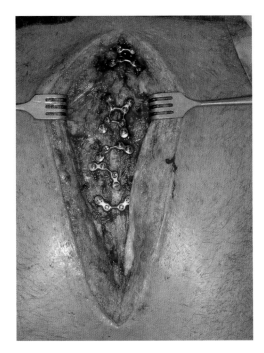

Fig. 10.16 Rigid fixation is crucial for sternal union.

grafting, if required, may be employed for closure of either the sternal wound or flap donor site.[25]

Outcomes

The importance of reconstruction is underscored when follow-up data on quality of life is assessed. When surveyed, as many as half of patients undergoing sternal debridement and muscle flap reconstruction complained of persistent chest and shoulder pain. Of the patients, 43% complained of sternal instability. This is felt to result from irritation of intercostal nerves when the residual sternal edges abut one another.[44] Although not formally addressed in the literature, however anecdotally appreciated by the authors, restoration of sternal union achieved through rigid fixation relieves the pain associated with instability.

Strength, following use of popular muscle flaps (i.e., pectoralis major, latissimus dorsi, and rectus abdominus), has been both surveyed and objectively measured and is somewhat decreased following sternectomy and muscle flap reconstruction. Interestingly, the objective decrease in pectoralis muscle function is seen on both the operated side and the contralateral side and may be more related to sternal instability than pectoralis disinsertion. Patients' ability to perform activities of daily living (ADLs) and return to preoperative activities was found to be no different when compared to their peers with uneventful healing post-sternotomy.[45]

Pulmonary function following sternectomy and reconstruction with pectoralis muscle flaps has been measured pre- and postoperatively and seems to be nearly unchanged following reconstruction. In a small group of six patients, pulmonary function testing (PFTs), specifically FVC, FEV1, retractive force, and static lung compliance were mildly diminished postoperatively, while TLC remained unchanged. This suggests maintenance of full inspiration with some decreased ability to maximally exhale. Additionally, the authors noted three patients with increased dependence on abdominal breathing.[46] Another group compared PFTs between those undergoing sternal resection and muscle flaps, $n=13$, to those with sternotomy and primary healing, $n=15$. They found no significant differences between the two groups.[47]

And perhaps most telling, when patients were surveyed regarding their general condition following sternal osteomyelitis and reconstruction, 83% of patients reported improvement in quality of life following their chest wall reconstruction.[48]

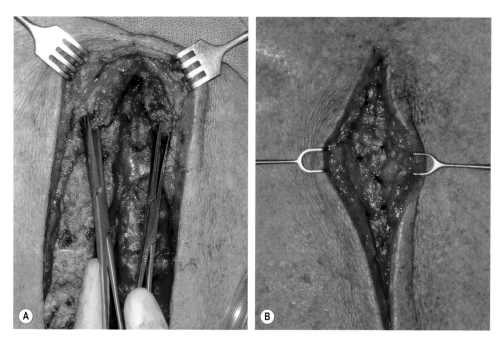

Fig. 10.17 Bilateral pectoralis advancement flaps. Allis clamps on pectoralis muscle. Muscle sutured together in midline.

Empyema, bronchopleural fistula, and chest wall osteomyelitis

Basic science/disease process

Empyema is defined as a deep space infection between the layers of visceral and parietal pleura. Empyema and bronchopleural fistulas often are found in concert and plague pneumonectomy and partial pneumonectomy defects. The chest cavity, unlike most other regions in the body, is rigid and non-collapsible. Thus, deep space infections, such as empyemas, are unlikely to heal without collapse of dead space or filling of the cavity. Older techniques, designed to decrease intrathoracic dead space, such as open chest drainage and the use of Eloesser flaps, the creation of pleural fistulas *(Fig. 10.18)*, have fallen out of favor.

The bronchial stump, created after pneumonectomy, can become a reconstructive challenge. If it dehisces, by definition, a bronchopleural fistula is created. This phenomenon, a massive airleak between the large airways and chest cavity, is unlikely to resolve without the interposition of healthy tissue in the form of flap coverage *(Fig. 10.19)*.[49]

Chest wall osteomyelitis most commonly results from contiguous spread of infection, either from pneumonia and empyema. Hematogenous spread is also possible. Infectious etiology tends to be bacterial, with mycobacterial and fungal sources less likely. Osteomyelitis produces symptoms including fever, chest pain, and localized swelling of the chest wall.[50]

Surgical technique

The omentum, latissimus dorsi, serratus anterior, pectoralis major, and rectus abdominus muscles have all been described

for space filling and reinforcement of the bronchial stump.[51,52] An often encountered problem with intrathoracic space filling is the sheer volume required to totally obliterate the thoracic cage. This can be overcome with thoracoplasty (partial rib/cage collapse) or with the use of multiple flaps.[53] As a single flap, however, the latissimus muscle is the preferred choice given its sheer size.

Similar to osteomyelitis of other areas of the body, antibiotics and surgical excision are recommended for bony infection of the chest wall. Reconstruction should proceed similarly to other areas of resection with rigid support when indicated and soft tissue coverage in the form of local muscle flaps.

Outcomes

Outcomes following muscle flap transposition are reported as quite successful, with 73% resolution or prevention of infection in Arnold and Pairolero's retrospective review of 100 patients with severe intrathoracic infections.[52] Several smaller and more recent studies report even higher rates of success.[49,54,55] In fact, prophylactic use of the latissimus muscle for reinforcement of the bronchial stump in high-risk patients is the standard of care in some centers.[56]

Osteoradionecrosis

Basic science/disease process

The use of adjuvant radiation therapy is becoming increasingly common in the treatment of both breast and lung cancer. As such, osteoradionecrosis (ORN) of the ribs is becoming an increasing problem for reconstructive surgeons. Radiation injury and tissue damage may not become clinically apparent

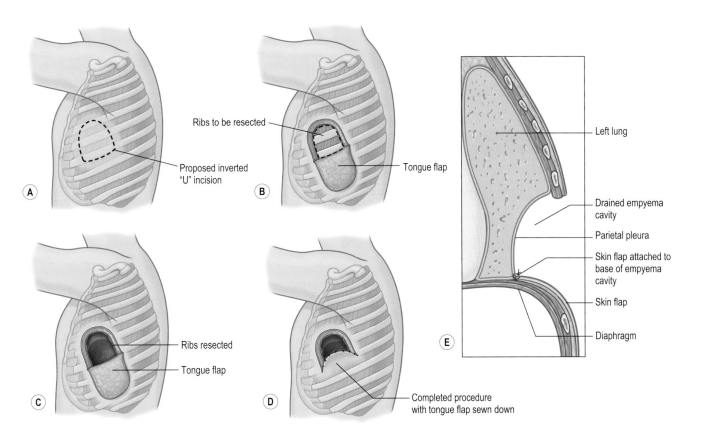

Fig. 10.18 Eloesser flap. Skin flap sewn to parietal pleura.

for months to years after exposure, especially in tissues with slow cell turnover such as bone. Although the mechanism is poorly understood, radiation leads to an increased production of cytokines, collagen deposition and scarring within affected tissues as well as vascular damage leading to relative hypoxia *(Fig. 10.20)*. The severity of radiation-induced necrosis is related to several factors including total dose, dose per fraction, frequency of administration, and whether it is combined with chemotherapy. Smaller doses per fraction appear to be better tolerated.[57]

Treatment/surgical technique

Some advocate hyperbaric oxygen (HBO) therapy for osteoradionecrosis. However, for osteoradionecrosis of the mandible, a prospective, randomized, placebo-controlled trial showed the HBO group actually fared worse than their counterparts.[58] Anecdotally, the authors have not found this therapy to be essential and do not routinely pursue it. Management of ORN of the chest wall consists of surgical excision and reconstruction. Again, should more than two ribs be resected from the anterior chest wall, skeletal support will traditionally be required. Radiation damage also affects overlying soft tissues, creating hyperpigmentation, decreased pliability, and even ulceration. Thus, recruitment of healthy tissue in the form of local myocutaneous flaps is recommended.

Traumatic chest wall deformities

Basic science/disease process

Chest trauma results from both penetrating and blunt injuries, which damage underlying bony and soft tissues. This may occur with or without further injury to vital organs or great vessels within the thoracic cage.

Diagnosis/patient presentations

Paradoxic chest wall motion, in the form of flail chest, may be seen following significant chest trauma. This results from multiple adjacent rib fractures, broken in two or more places, creating a flail segment.

Patient selection/treatment/surgical technique

Patients with traumatic chest wall deformities should initially be stabilized according to ATLS protocol. Chest tubes and positive pressure ventilation should be initiated as indicated. For patients with respiratory compromise, rigid fixation of this flail chest segment may be indicated. This is accomplished

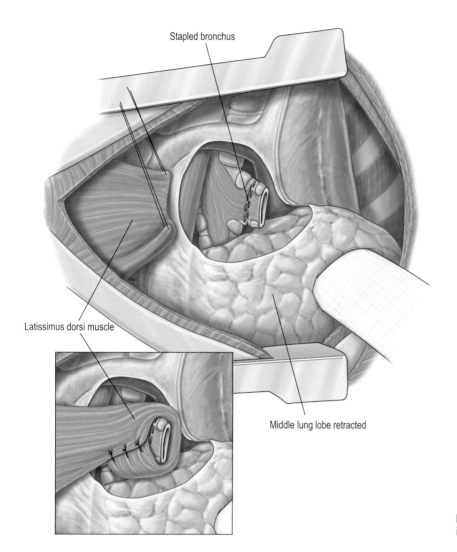

Stapled bronchus

Latissimus dorsi muscle

Middle lung lobe retracted

Fig. 10.19 Bronchopleural fistula with latissimus muscle introduced intrathoracically for reinforcement.

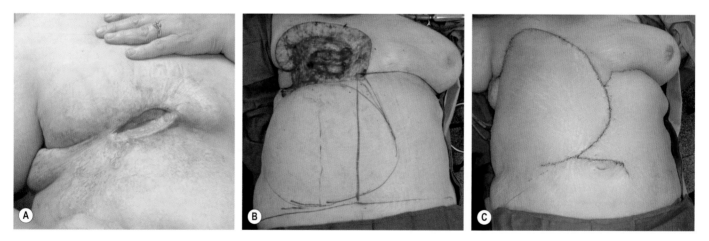

Fig. 10.20 (A) Osteoradionecrosis of ribs following chest wall radiation for breast cancer. **(B, C)** Following radical resection, serratus thoracoabdominal flap is planned and inset. Note all incisions kept supraumbilical to preserve lower abdominal donor site for future autologous breast reconstruction.

traditionally with the use of mini-plates or Judet struts *(Fig. 10.21)*. Significant chest wall loss, as can be seen in massive crush injuries, should be managed with rigid support to the remaining viable chest wall and concomitant soft tissue coverage.

Outcomes

Rib plating has been shown to reduce ventilator-dependence and ICU stay as well as incidence of pneumonia in patients with flail chest.[59]

Secondary procedures

Chest wall reconstruction has been, over the last three decades, very successful. Cases of failure commonly result from inadequate control of infection or residual tumor burden. In either case, an aggressive resection is often indicated and use of a second flap. Another unfortunate complication of skeletal chest wall reconstruction is infection of alloplastic mesh products. In these cases, removal of the infected prosthesis and use of acellular dermal matrix or autologous fascia or even contralateral ribs may be indicated.

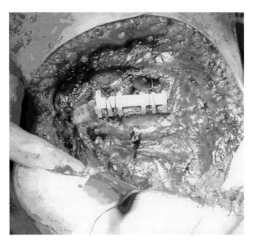

Fig. 10.21 Judet struts. (From: Surgical Stabilization of Severe Flail Chest, Fig. 7, reproduced with permission from CTSNet, Inc. ©2010. All rights reserved.)

Access the complete reference list online at **http://www.expertconsult.com**

1. Deschamps C, et al. Early and long-term results of prosthetic chest wall reconstruction. *J Thorac Cardiovasc Surg.* 1999;117(3):588–592.

   The authors review their experience with nearly 200 patients requiring chest wall reconstruction over 15 years. Mesh is utilized (polypropylene and polytetrafluoroethylene) for skeletal support and over half of the patients required muscle transposition for soft tissue coverage. Wound healing was complete for 95% of patients, although 24% experienced local cancer recurrence.

5. Mathes SJ, Nahai F. *Reconstructive surgery. Principles, Anatomy, and Technique.* Edinburgh: Churchill Livingstone; 1997.

   This textbook detailing nearly all commonly-used flaps in plastic surgery continues to be an excellent reference for relevant anatomy, flap selection, and arc of rotation.

29. Song DH, Lohman RF, Renucci JD, et al. Primary sternal plating in high-risk patients prevents mediastinitis. *Eur J Cardiothorac Surg.* 2004;26:367–372.

    This is a case-controlled study of prophylactic sternal plating in high risk patients. The group who were plated experienced no mediastinitis, while 14.8% of the control group, closed with wire, developed mediastinitis.

34. Dickie SR, Dorafshar AH, Song DH. Definitive closure of the infected median sternotomy wound: A treatment algorithm utilizing vacuum-assisted closure followed by rigid plate fixation. *Ann Plast Surg.* 2006;56(6):680–685.

    This paper contains a treatment algorithm for mediastinitis emphasizing debridement, the use of subatmospheric pressure, rigid fixation, and soft tissue coverage.

52. Arnold PG, Pairolero PC. Intrathoracic muscle flaps. An account of their use in the management of 100 consecutive patients. *Ann Surg.* 1990;211(6):656–660.

    The authors detail a 73% success rate with treatment and prevention of intrathoracic infection following muscle transposition into the chest of high risk patients.

11

Reconstruction of the soft tissues of the back

Gregory A. Dumanian

SYNOPSIS

- Reconstruction of the soft tissues of the back at first may seem to be a daunting task compounded by large wounds, unfamiliar and segmental anatomy, radiation, hardware, and difficulties with postoperative positioning.
- Many of the conditions treated require significant coordination with surgical colleagues.
- Many of the conditions are unfamiliar to the plastic surgeon and without parallel conditions elsewhere in the body, an example being pseudomeningoceles filled with cerebrospinal fluid (CSF).
- The goal of this chapter is to provide the reader with real-life solutions to difficult problems involving back wounds.

Introduction

The back is 18% of the total body surface area, yet it is an area commonly neglected in older texts of plastic surgery. From the nape of the neck, to the anterior axillary lines, to the inferior gluteal crease, the only area well known to the plastic surgeon is the buttocks for the treatment of pressure sores. In years past, the common surgical procedures that involved the back were performed in areas of good vascularity and only uncommonly required procedures to aid in coverage. Small spine procedures, thoracotomy incisions, flank incisions for access to the retroperitoneum, and removal of soft-tissue tumors of the back such as lipomas did not inspire chapters in plastic surgery textbooks. What changed the equation were the advances made in spine instrumentation.

In decades past, spinal fusions were often performed by removing discs and scraping the end plates of vertebral bodies. These procedures were not limited by the surrounding soft tissues. This changed with improvements of surgical hardware that allowed for longer and longer constructs for spinal stability. Simultaneous anterior and posterior spine exposures for rigid fixation greatly stripped and elevated the surrounding soft tissues, and correspondingly pushed the soft tissues past the point where wound healing would be automatic. For illustration, the average wound in terms of vertebral body length in a 1995 paper was three bodies long, and many wounds were due to pressure sores of the back. By 2003, the average wound length was 11 vertebral bodies long, and all of the wounds had large amounts of hardware. In response to the need created by our surgical colleagues, surgical procedures to close the back reliably were developed.

Patient presentation

Midline back wounds

When a spine surgeon calls to discuss new drainage from a midline spine wound, the thought process for treatment should be methodical and thorough. When was the last procedure performed, and did the procedure involve the placement of hardware? What type of hardware is present, and is it locally prominent or is it low-profile? Did the spine surgeons place hardware on the anterior or lateral aspect of the vertebral bodies, or rather was it only posterior? Had there been any dural tears that were repaired, and do the spine surgeons have any evidence of a CSF leak? Do the plain films demonstrate hardware immediately deep to areas of wounds or drainage? Often a computed tomography (CT) scan is obtained, but hardware artifact is substantial and prevents an adequate evaluation of fluid collections.

After obtaining an understanding of what was done, an evaluation of wound-healing issues is necessary. Is the patient markedly malnourished and catabolic? Are obesity and dead space management problems? Had the patient been radiated for a spinal cord metastasis with the associated stiff and edematous soft tissues?

Next, an examination of the patient is often telling of what needs to be done. Continued soilage of dressings with fluid and dieback of the wound edges often point to deep fluid collections that are emerging from around the spinal hardware. Is the area of wound breakdown at a pressure point due to incomplete restoration of spine architecture? Further understanding of the time course of the drainage also points to the underlying pathology. Persistent postoperative fevers ascribed to "atelectasis" are a common diagnosis made for these patients.

The time course of the presentation is critical. Early postoperative episodes of drainage less than 4–6 weeks after the spine surgery are typically successfully treated with repeat surgery and soft-tissue reconstruction with hardware preservation. However, drainage that has been only partially treated with a small debridement or treated solely with intravenous antibiotics, only to resurface months later, is more difficult to treat. In fact, a chronic hardware infection defined as bacteria in association with hardware greater than 6 months after placement is typically not a situation that plastic surgery can definitively treat without hardware removal.

Much can be learned with the simple examination of a patient's chest X-ray in terms of the existence and location of hardware. Otherwise, plain films of the spine are obtained to reveal the length of the construct when present, degenerative spine disease, and the presence or absence of fusion. CT scans and magnetic resonance imaging (MRI) are helpful to look for fluid collections, pseudomeningoceles, and inflammation of the soft tissues. A key issue is if fluid collections are above or below the standard back muscle closure. If fluid or hematoma is seen deep to the musculature, a deep hardware infection is more likely. Unfortunately, the spinal hardware causes much artifact of both CT scans and MRI, lowering their ability to demonstrate fluid collections with high accuracy.

Nonmidline back wounds

While midline wounds are either due to pressure sores or spine procedures, nonmidline wounds represent a much more heterogeneous collection of etiologies and therefore require a wide range of solutions. Much like acquired wounds elsewhere in the body, wounds of the nonmidline back are due to poor wound healing after access incisions of the chest cavity or retroperitoneum, necrotizing infections, or after tumor excision. Traumatic injuries are uncommon. A working knowledge of the conditions facing the thoracic surgeons is important in these instances. Thoracotomy incisions sometimes break down in the face of empyemas, persistent air leaks, radiation, and malnutrition. Desmoid tumors, soft-tissue sarcomas, and even neglected skin cancers can leave large defects of the back. For these patients, a more standard thought process often suffices in the absence of hardware, deep wounds, and CSF leaks. The wounds are typically flat, and often allow skin grafting. When flaps are needed to cover bone or prosthetic material, the muscles that are used to cover the midline spine are often available and even easier to mobilize to the nonmidline back due to the lateral placement of their pedicles. The lateral tissues, being more mobile than the midline tissues, are easier to transpose for adjacent tissue transfers. Free flaps are facilitated by having larger inflow vessels available, such as the subscapular arterial system, than exist for midline reconstructions.

Patient treatment

Local wound care

For superficial, relatively painless wounds without exposed hardware, local wound care with dressings is a relatively risk-free way to achieve wound closure. Draining midline incisions tend to have wide areas of undermining along the length of the closure. These tunnels can typically be opened in the office with local injection of anesthesia and finger fracturing of the incision. A long wound without tunnels with a saucer shape typically heals faster than small wounds with a fishbowl-shaped internal wound due to the improved ability to cleanse the surface of the internal wound. Therefore, tunnels should be opened along old incision lines. All necrotic tissue should be debrided. All nonabsorbable sutures such as braided polyester should be removed. Obtaining local wound control with wide exposure of the wound is a tried and true method as the first step in healing. Patients are often unaware of the real size of the wound, and must be prepared for the resulting appearance of the surgical site after opening of tunnels.

Much depends on the patient's home situation. Dressings can be simple wet-to-wet saline dressings, with twice-a-day showers to cleanse the surface of the wound. Subatmospheric-pressure dressings can be employed, but the tubing is sometimes difficult to place under back-bracing devices (*Figs 11.1–11.3*). After a wound has granulated, if it is painful, then delayed primary closure or skin grafts can be performed if the wound is sizeable. However, the risks of these secondary closure procedures often outweigh the benefits. The subcutaneous tissue stiffens during the time of obtaining local wound control, and it is difficult to re-elevate and close without a fairly sizeable procedure.

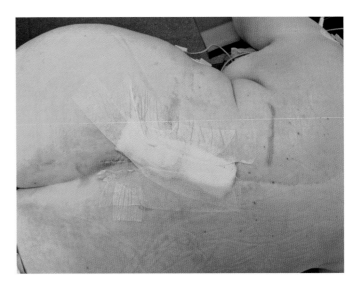

Fig. 11.1 Lumbar incision draining serous fluid 2 weeks after lumbar fusion.

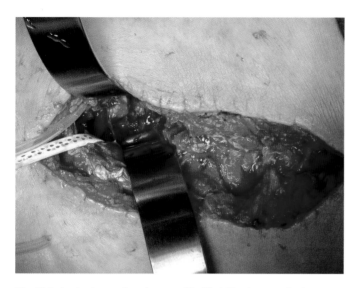

Fig. 11.2 A subcutaneous hematoma was identified. The deep muscle closure was opened and there was no purulence or fluid present. The muscles were reclosed, and a subatmospheric-pressure dressing applied.

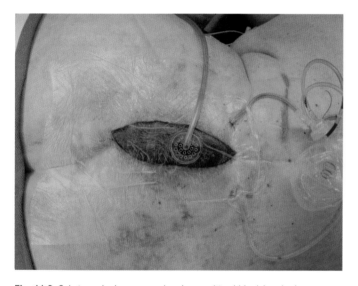

Fig. 11.3 Subatmospheric-pressure dressing used to aid in delayed primary closure of the skin flaps.

Operative debridement

Patients with persistently draining wounds after spine surgery associated with hardware should be evaluated critically for an operating room debridement. Secondary indications for a debridement include unexplained fevers and fluid collections seen on imaging scans. The patient should be readied for surgery with large intravenous lines and in a warm operating room. The large exposed surface areas can allow the patient to cool rapidly, with associated coagulopathies and increased blood loss. Blood should be available for a transfusion. Due to the segmental nature of the vascularity, surgery does not typically expose large and few blood vessels, but rather many small ones, and the blood loss is rather constant throughout the case.

The maneuvers in the operating room are a critical step in the treatment of patients with postsurgical back wounds. A thorough incision and drainage should be performed for patients with unexplained or purulent drainage through their incision. The entire length of the incision should be opened as widely as necessary to explore for purulence and drain fluid collections. The erector spinae muscle closure should be reopened for cultures and to evaluate for liquefying hematomas. The surgeon should be knowledgeable at the beginning of the debridement if a laminectomy had been performed at the original spine surgery in order to prevent injury to the spinal cord and dura during the incision and drainage.

At this point, the surgeon will need to make a decision as to the quality of the tissues. Nonpurulent benign fluid collections in the subcutaneous tissues with no purulence deep to the musculature can be reclosed over drains, or else closed secondarily with a subatmospheric-pressure dressing (see above). Purulent and deep collections require additional decisions. If the local wound is so purulent as to preclude an immediate reclosure, then all nonviable tissue should be debrided, the wound irrigated, and left open for local wound care. This can be done with dressing changes on the floor for several days until a second trip to the operating room. Alternatively, a subatmospheric-pressure dressing may be applied, but this often involves a return trip to the operating room for its next exchange.

For those deep wounds judged amenable to reclosure, a radical incision and drainage are performed. This should involve the surgical excision of scarred tissues where possible to reveal supple soft tissues with pulsatile bleeding. Scar, though it bleeds, does not bleed in pulsatile fashion due to the small size of the vessels that developed during prior wounding. Pulsatile bleeding at wound margins has been shown to correlate with wound healing in problematic incisions, such as distal foot amputations. Tissues with a pseudobursa should be excised, as this too represents scar. Tissue that is stiff is unyielding and does not conform well, and so the tissues should be removed until they are soft to palpation. Pulsatile irrigation with saline is gentle to tissues that cannot be removed and yet still is able to cleanse surface bacteria. A stronger debriding instrument has been developed (Versajet, Smith and Nephew) that can remove a thin layer of tissue at a time with pressurized streams of sterile fluid and this is effective in these large open wounds.

An interesting issue is the removal of nonviable elements such as hardware and bone graft. While plastic surgery teaching emphasizes the removal of all nonvascularized surfaces, in this case the hardware acts to stabilize the wound. An orthopedic principle is that the most effective way to fight infections is to have rigid bone fixation. Therefore, hardware that is well fixed should remain in place in early hardware infections. This is done both to stabilize the wound for improved healing as well as to avoid the surgery involved with removal and later replacement of hardware. Long-term maintenance of the hardware as well as clinical and radiographic evidence of fusion are well documented in patients who were returned to the operating room for washouts within 6–8 weeks of placement. As stated previously, hardware colonized after 6 months is defined as a chronically infected foreign body, and salvage of this hardware is much less likely long-term. Another issue is the endogenous and exogenous bone graft placed to achieve a fusion. In the absence of definitive studies, it seems reasonable to remove nonincorporated and easy-to-remove graft, but to leave in place graft that has

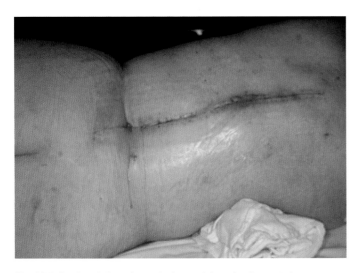

Fig. 11.4 Purulent drainage from a back wound 2 weeks after posterior spinal fusion.

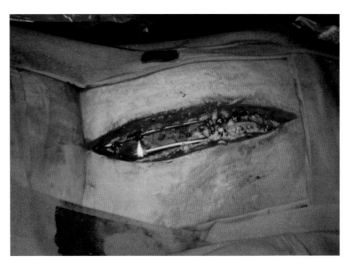

Fig. 11.5 Prominent hardware with exudate between the bars. Crosslinks create a hardware "cage" to prevent soft tissue from collapsing to the depth of the surgical dissection.

in any way begun to stick to the local tissues due to inosculation.

Wound "shape" is an important concept for reconstruction of the soft tissues of the back. The back has lordotic and kyphotic regions in the normal condition, and these contours can be dramatically changed with pathology. This serves to make postoperative positioning difficult when the surgical incision is also the most prominent portion of the back. The depth of the procedure performed by the spine surgeons is also important. A patient with a laminectomy by definition has a deeper wound than when the spinous processes are intact. Spinal hardware serves to create a local prominence in contradistinction to the depth of the surgical dissection. A prime reason for persistent fluid collections is the three-dimensional space between a laminectomy and the adjacent vertically oriented bars. Crosslinks between the bars further prevent soft tissue from collapsing into the space immediately over the midline. Finally, laterally placed hardware can be poorly covered by soft tissue and may be the originators of pressure sores. This is especially common when hardware inserts into the posterior superior iliac spines for pelvic fusions. Therefore, in the treatment of wounds of the spine, the three-dimensional shape should be evaluated and converted as much as possible to a two-dimensional wound. Prominent hardware should be exchanged for something with a lower profile *(Figs 11.4–11.7)*. Patients with incomplete corrections of the spine deformities should be revised to recreate better the natural contours. The deeper the hole, the more a flap should be "dropped into" the defect, rather than tissue simply slid towards the midline. This requires a more redundant soft-tissue flap such as an omentum to fill the defect appropriately. Teamwork between the spine and soft-tissue surgeons is often necessary to treat problems of wound shape and contour appropriately.

The status of the CSF and the dura is also critical for treatment of certain back wounds. The dura is opened and closed in a planned fashion in numerous instances, including the treatment of spinal cord malignancies, untethering of the spine for patients with a history of cord lipomas and spina

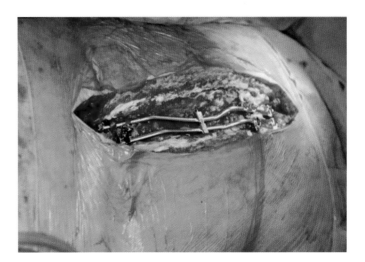

Fig. 11.6 Hardware revised to be less prominent in conjunction with erector spinae muscle flaps.

bifida, and treatment of pseudomeningoceles. Unplanned tears of the dura also occur in laminectomy procedures. The low-pressure CSF leaks and the continuing fluid buildup push the soft tissue away from the leakage site, and thereby prevent soft-tissue collapse of the space. The CSF fluid in fresh postoperative cases can also become infected, and exist in association with surgical wounds of the back. Treatment of patients with CSF leaks will be discussed later in this chapter.

Flap closure

Principles

The first step in reconstruction is a timely debridement, as has been emphasized already. The second step is local wound control with a radical debridement of all stiff and scarred

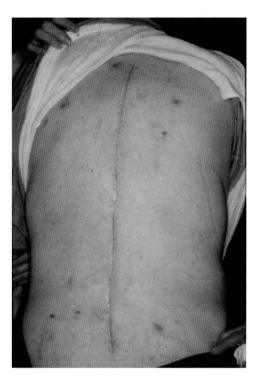

Fig. 11.7 Healed wound in this patient after optimizing both the hardware architecture and the soft tissues.

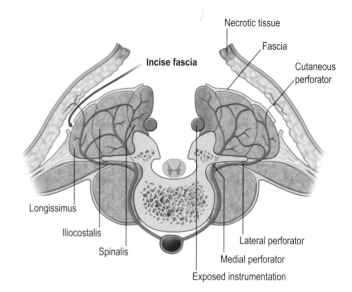

Fig. 11.8 Cross-section of lumbar spine area. Skin flaps are elevated to expose the thoracolumbar fascia and to reach the region of the lateral pedicle entering the erector spinae muscles. The thoracolumbar fascia is incised to allow a medial movement of the muscles.

tissue. For the reconstruction, the surgeon should never rely on scar to be a positive factor for wound healing. The more completely the old scar can be excised and replaced with nonscarred new soft tissues, the better the reconstruction. Finally, the reconstruction should be performed to do the "maximum for the minimum." The procedure with the highest chance for success and with the lowest morbidity should be selected for the patient.

Central questions to be answered include the presence or absence of a fusion, and the vertebral levels involved.[1] When an instrumented fusion has been performed, then the erector spinae musculature function is no longer necessary, and the muscles are completely expendable in terms of a reconstruction. The fusion rods prevent postoperative motion, and so when the erector spinae muscles are reapproximated in the midline, they tend to stay there. Spine patients without fusions still require the function of the erector spinae musculature when healing is completed for flexion and extension of the spine. These patients do better with flaps that are "dropped into the hole," rather than with erector spinae muscles that are closed side to side and that would dehisce with back flexion.

Local wound care often suffices for superficial wound problems above the erector spinae. After the deep aspect of the wound is judged to be without purulence or fluid collections, a subatmospheric dressing can be applied, often with a benign postoperative course. This does well for obese patients with thick subcutaneous tissues. Delayed closures are possible after the wound has granulated, but the failure rate in heavy patients where normal body movements pull against the suture line is substantial. Subatmospheric-pressure dressings are reported to allow soft tissues to cover over small areas of exposed hardware, but this has not been my experience.

Possible flap choices for spine closure

Erector spinae muscle flaps

The erector spinae muscles, also called the paraspinous muscles,[2] are expendable after a previous spine fusion and no longer are functional for spine extension and flexion. The dissection of the muscles proceeds in stepwise fashion in order to move the muscles towards this midline. This flap is appropriate from the high cervical area to the low lumbar area, but it will not adequately cover an occipitospinal fusion, and nor will it be sufficient for lumbosacral soft-tissue coverage. One must be careful in its use when a lateral approach to the spine has been made, because the muscle can be transected for access.

First, skin flaps are elevated superficial to the thoracolumbar fascia (*Fig. 11.8*). With a retractor putting tension on the soft tissues, with cautery the granulation tissue is entered, and with finger dissection a blunt plane is elevated. The latissimus muscle and trapezius muscle should stay attached to the skin. The dissection is easiest inferior in the lumbar area where the muscle is round and large, and most confusing superiorly where the muscle is thinnest and becomes attached to the undersurface of the trapezius. The erector spinae muscles have a convex shape, and there is a rounded aspect of the muscle that then descends laterally towards the more lateral neck, thoracic, and lumbar areas. It is in this groove that segmental blood vessels enter the lateral and deep aspects of the longissimus and iliocostalis muscles. Continuation of these blood vessels continues more superficially to the skin and to the latissimus muscle in the thoracolumbar area. While the surgeon is elevating the skin flaps, the perforators and dorsal sensory nerves going up to the skin often can be identified and preserved to maintain skin vascularity. To

Figure labels (Fig. 11.8): Necrotic tissue, Fascia, Incise fascia, Cutaneous perforator, Longissimus, Iliocostalis, Spinalis, Lateral perforator, Medial perforator, Exposed instrumentation

lessen the chance of marginal skin perfusion and to limit a future potential seroma cavity, undermining should not be overdone.

The thoracolumbar fascia is incised much like the development of any standard bipedicled flap in order to mobilize the erector spinae muscle and/or overlying skin to the midline. When the original dissection is superficial to the fascia and the fascia remains attached to the muscle, this facilitates the later closure, and the fascial release is critical to the movement of the muscle. Occasionally the fascia remains attached to the skin during the initial elevation. In this case, muscle mobilization is facile, but the skin is more difficult to close in the midline. Therefore, an incision of the fascia along its length allows the skin to move medially and to provide the excess for debridement and reclosure. The dissection up until this point is rather easy and bloodless, but only moves the muscle an estimated 30% of its potential. Complete mobilization of the muscle requires a dissection along the deep aspect of the erector spinae *(Fig. 11.9)*. Again with tension applied on to the tissue with retractors, cautery dissection of the deep and medial attachments of the erector spinae will mobilize the muscle and detach it from the lateral aspects of the transverse processes of the spine. It will by necessity divide the medial row of blood vessels entering the paraspinous muscles, but the prior dissection to identify the lateral vessels entering the muscle will suffice to preserve vascularity. One technique is to have the fingers of the nondominant hand in the lateral groove at the site of the lateral perforators while bluntly elevating the medial aspect of the muscle with the thumb and index finger. The medial muscle elevation is a powerful means to allow the paraspinous muscles to "unfold" like an accordion to be advanced toward the midline *(Figs 11.10 and 11.11)*. The muscle changes shape from being a round muscle mass to being more elliptical. Advancement of the muscle is a process much different from simply releasing the thoracolumbar fascia and "rolling" the dorsal aspect of the muscle toward the midline.

With the skin and muscle flaps so created, it is now quite easy to distinguish stiff and inflamed tissue from more normal soft tissue. The medial aspect of the skin, subcutaneous tissue, and paraspinous muscles is sharply debrided. The muscles are brought together in the midline *(Fig. 11.12)*, and any extra

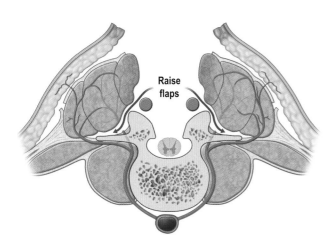

Fig. 11.9 A dissection is then performed to release the medial and deep attachments of the erector spinae muscles to the spine and transverse processes. The lateral blood supply is approached from the deep aspect of the muscle.

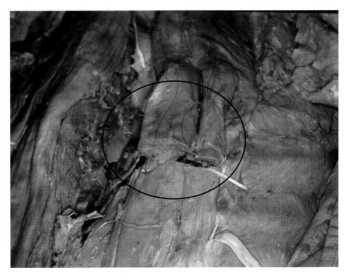

Fig. 11.10 Cadaver dissection of the erector spinae muscles at the lumbar level.

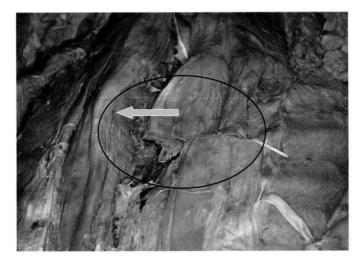

Fig. 11.11 Release and medial movement of the muscles.

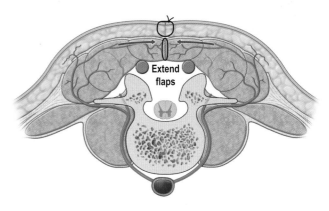

Fig. 11.12 The muscles are approximated in the midline. The erector spinae muscles unfurl, changing shape from circular to elliptical.

tissue can be imbricated to help fold the soft tissue into crevices between vertically oriented hardware bars *(Fig. 11.13)*. Drains are left both deep and superficial to the erector spinae closure, and are left in until the drainage is minimal. When the erector spinae muscle closure is of good quality, there is no need for a second overlying muscle flap using the trapezius or the latissimus muscles.

Latissimus muscle or myocutaneous flap

The latissimus muscle is a well-known and understood flap.[3] The donor site is minimal. Based on the thoracodorsal pedicle, the muscle can be moved superiorly up to the level of the top of the scapula. Based on its minor perforators that also supply the paraspinous muscles, the latissimus can reach

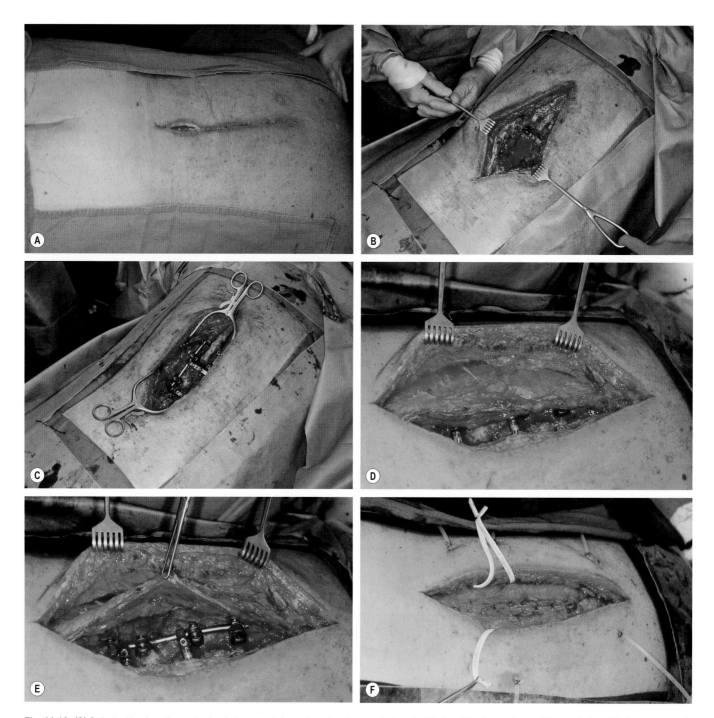

Fig. 11.13 (A) Patient with a long thoracolumbar fusion with drainage 3 weeks after a posterior spinal fusion. Note the erythema of the staple line. **(B)** Complete opening of the superficial and deep tissues reveals an infected fluid collection surrounding the hardware. A crossbar is visible. **(C)** The wound is radically debrided to reveal the entire spinal hardware construct. The hardware seems solidly fixed to the bone. **(D)** Dissection deep to the thoracolumbar fascia to the lateral border of the erector spinae muscles. A large nerve traveling through the muscle to the overlying skin is spared. **(E)** Dissection on the deep aspect of the erector spinae muscles to the level of the lateral perforators. **(F)** Erector spinae muscles closed in the midline.

the lower lumbar area. An advantage to the latissimus is being able to be "dropped in" to a hole, and so it is useful for patients who have not been fused, or for more lateral defects. The muscle can reliably carry a skin paddle, and this often helps in the inset of the flap. Caution should be taken in patients who have had thoracotomy incisions, as the muscle is often divided.

The latissimus muscle is a good but still second-line flap for the coverage of midline back wounds. In comparison to the paraspinous flaps, the latissimus flap can only cover a spine wound 10–12 cm in length, while the erector spinae flaps can cover practically the entire length of the spine. The dissection required to elevate the latissimus muscle takes more time and effort than does the erector spinae. While low, there is a donor defect from the loss of the latissimus muscle, especially in patients who may need assistive devices to ambulate. The latissimus flap is a good choice for nonfused wounds of the back *(Fig. 11.14)*, or when the erector spinae muscles have been radiated.

Patient undergoing latissimus flaps should have a thorough debridement of their wounds. The flap dissection is best begun in an area where the anatomy has not been distorted by prior incisions. For instance, flaps based on paraspinous perforators should be begun in the axilla with the identification of the muscle and division of the thoracodorsal pedicle. It is easier than one would expect to be in the wrong plane and to divide these small paraspinous perforators when the dissection is begun in the midline wound.

The orientation and design of the skin paddle should be done carefully. For flaps based on the thoracodorsal pedicle, a skin paddle oriented with its long axis perpendicular to the midline will result in the skin paddle vertically oriented. Closure of the donor site initially oriented perpendicular to the spine does not make the midline spine any more difficult to close due to added tension. Another helpful skin paddle design is a V-Y design *(Fig. 11.15)*. The donor site for the skin is in the midaxillary line. The latissimus muscle is elevated and the skin paddle moved medially, rather than turned 90°. This flap can be re-elevated and moved a second time if necessary.

Trapezius muscle flap

The trapezius flap is useful for high cervical wounds because the paraspinous musculature is of limited mobility and size at that level. The dissection begins with identification of the distal and inferior triangular aspect of the trapezius where it just overlaps the latissimus muscle, because the crossing muscle fiber directions of the two muscles are quite distinct in this area. A skin paddle overlying this inferior muscle can be taken to help with the inset. The more cephalad and larger the skin paddle, the better in terms of reliability *(Fig. 11.16)*. The inclusion of the superficial dorsal scapular artery on the lateral border of the trapezius also helps skin flap viability.[4] Further cephalad and lateral to the elevated skin paddle, the upper back skin is elevated off the trapezius. The main pedicle is the transverse cervical artery and it enters the muscle approximately 7–8 cm lateral to the midline and at the level of the spinous process of C7 on its deep aspect. Its approximate location can be ascertained with a hand-held Doppler. The deep dissection is then performed, with the muscle elevated off the paraspinous musculature and the rhomboids. The medial attachments are thickest, and then a plane between the two muscle groups is reached where dissection is easy. The main pedicle is encountered, and with this vessel under direct view, the lateral aspect of the muscle is divided. Movement of the flap is tested, and the lateral muscle division is extended if greater mobility is required for wound coverage. The higher the dissection continues, the higher the morbidity due to shoulder drop, but the greater the arc of rotation of the muscle.

Because of its sizeable donor site morbidity to the shoulder, the indication for the trapezius flap is in a nonfused patient

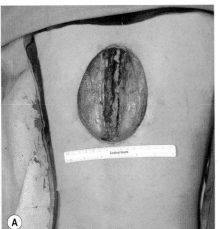
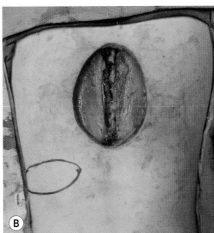
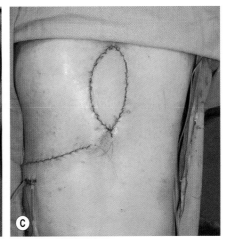

Fig. 11.14 (A) A 26-year-old man had a recurrent desmoid tumor removed from his thoracic spine area. There is exposure of the spinous processes. There is no hardware present. **(B)** A skin paddle slightly less wide than the defect and oriented at a right angle to the long axis of the wound is drawn out. **(C)** Final inset of the flap. The flap donor site is oriented perpendicular to the long axis of the defect, so that closure of the donor site will not make the recipient site more difficult to close.

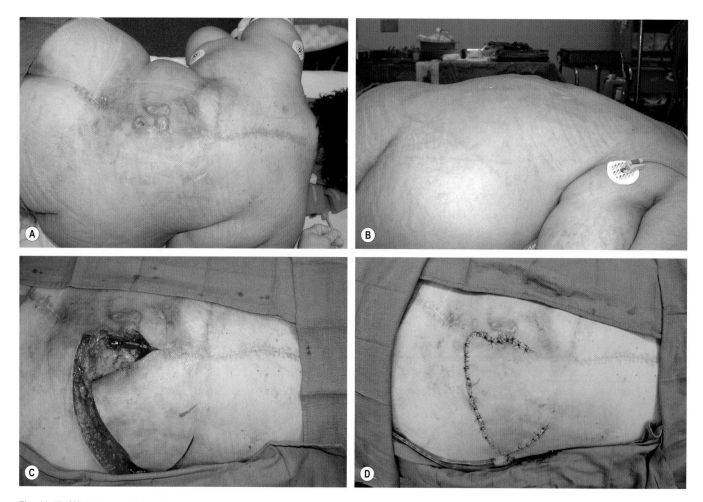

Fig. 11.15 (A) A 57-year-old female with a complex history of back surgery, revisions, and flaps. She has already had erector spinae flaps and a left latissimus flap for closure. She presents with a new area of exposed hardware due to a pressure sore. She is not fused, and removal of the hardware is not possible. **(B)** The area of the pressure sore is at a kyphotic area of the lumbosacral spine. The optimal way to treat this condition is to correct the spinal deformity at the same time as improving the soft tissues. **(C)** A myocutaneous latissimus flap with the skin paddle advanced in V-Y fashion is elevated after debridement. **(D)** Closed incisions. As might be anticipated, several months later she presented with a new pressure sore at the same spot. She subsequently underwent successful correction of the spinal deformity, and a readvancement of the V-Y flap for coverage.

with a radiated deep back wound where the erector spinae have been involved in the field of radiation. There simply do not exist other simple means for coverage. As the muscle is typically turned 90° for inset, the length of midline coverage of the trapezius is typically short, and so either a combination of two trapezius flaps, or else the trapezius flap with erector spinae flaps, should be planned for long wounds.

Superior gluteal artery

The superior gluteal artery flap technique is the most challenging of all of the reconstructive soft-tissue procedures for the spine, but it is a necessary and useful procedure.[5] The flap should not be attempted unless the surgeon has had significant experience with perforator flaps and the surgical management of sacral pressure sores. A line is drawn between the superior lateral aspect of the sacrum and the posterior superior iliac spine. From a point that bisects this line, a second line is drawn toward the greater trochanter. This second line represents the path of the superior gluteal artery, and is the long axis of the flap. A skin paddle is designed that encompasses the Doppler signal of the perforator of the superior gluteal artery and is oriented laterally towards the greater trochanter *(Fig. 11.17)*. This will be the lateralmost tissue thought to be captured by the superior gluteal artery perforator.[6] To improve the reliability of the tissue, a strip of gluteus muscle oriented underneath the skin paddle can be taken along with the perforator. This is a different orientation than the skin paddle used for closure of sacral pressure sores, where extra skin is taken medial to the Doppler signal. The superior border of the skin is incised, and the skin flap elevated until the perforator from the superior gluteal artery is seen to be entering the skin paddle. Medial to this, the gluteus muscle is split to aid in the dissection of the pedicle. These patients typically have some gluteus motor dysfunction preoperatively, and their gluteus muscles are thin and atrophic.

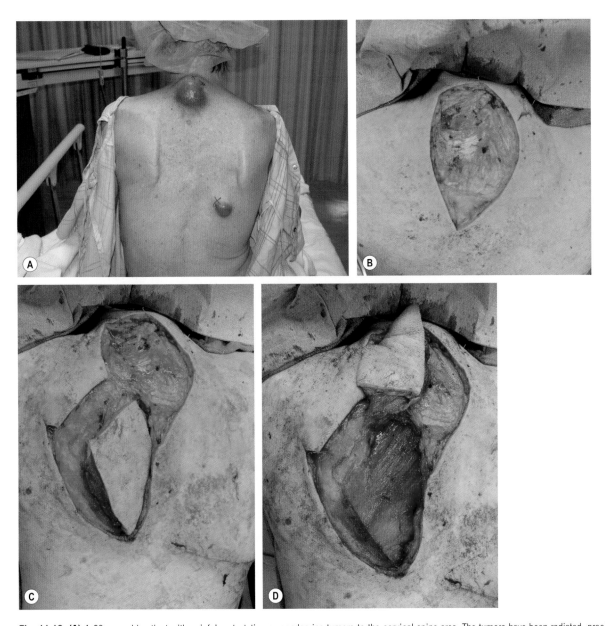

Fig. 11.16 (A) A 60-year-old patient with painful metastatic neuroendocrine tumors to the cervical spine area. The tumors have been radiated, precluding closure with skin grafts. **(B)** Wound after tumor excision. **(C)** Incised myocutaneous trapezius flap. The skin paddle was oriented at the inferior aspect of the muscle. **(D)** Trapezius flap during inset with 180° twist. The superficial dorsal scapular artery was not included with this flap, resulting in mild hypoperfusion of the skin paddle. The donor site was closed in the vertical midline.

With the pedicle under full view, the remainder of the skin paddle can be incised and the flap dissection completed. If there is difficulty with identification of the superior gluteal artery perforator, additional muscle should be elevated with the skin paddle, or a decision made to dissect the other buttock. Medially, any muscle along the pedicle will resist the 180° flip required of the pedicle for the flap to reach the midline. Muscle found around the pedicle that impedes this 180° turn should be excised so that there is no tension on the flap to reach the lumbosacral spine. The skin paddle is de-epithelialized and will be able to cover the dura. The donor and recipient sites are closed over drains. Avoidance of a three-way incision with a small skin bridge

and tunneling of the flap under this area also assists in the final closure.

The buttocks are an area not typically reached by spine surgeons. Both buttocks should be prepped into the field, in case there is an injury to the pedicle. In patients with buttock weakness preoperatively, the stronger side should be used. Caution should be taken in patients who are markedly obese, and those with prior pressure sore procedures. A complete pressure relief bed is necessary for 10–14 days after the procedure to prevent pressure on the pedicle as it runs from the lateral sacrum towards the midline. Drains are often required for several weeks in the donor site. The procedure does not cause much pain or dysfunction long-term.

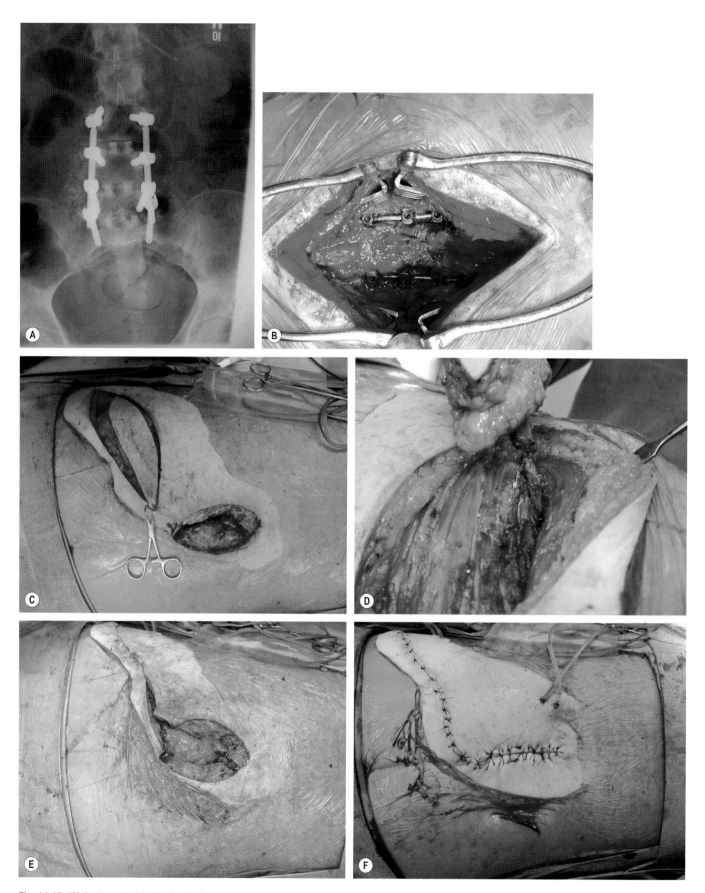

Fig. 11.17 **(A)** Radiograph of low lumbar fusion of a patient with drainage 3 weeks after spinal fusion. **(B)** Intraoperative view after debridement of fusion site. **(C)** Incised skin paddle for left superior gluteal artery perforator (SGAP) flap. The staple marks the audible Doppler signal of the SGAP perforator to the skin. **(D)** Vascular pedicle to the superior gluteal artery perforator flap. Muscle around the pedicle must be minimized to allow for a facile flip of the flap to the midline. **(E)** The skin paddle is de-epithelialized and placed to fill the lumbosacral recess. **(F)** Closed incisions.

Omentum

The primary criterion for using a pedicled omental flap includes scarred, irradiated, divided, and otherwise unusable back musculature suitable for local flap transfer in a patient in need of soft-tissue coverage of thoracolumbar spinal instrumentation *(Fig. 11.18).*[7] Secondary criteria include extremely deep wounds, such as for those patients with coverage needs of both anterior and posterior instrumentation, and for patients in whom the abdominal cavity is already entered for exposure. Absolute contraindications to the use of a pedicled omental flap include a history of intra-abdominal malignancy and a previously resected omentum. Relative contraindications include morbid obesity and the potential for intra-abdominal adhesions from previous laparotomies. The zone of coverage for an omental flap is from the lumbosacral recess inferiorly up to the level of the midscapula superiorly.

Close coordination is required between the spine and plastic surgery teams. Typically, a posterior spinal instrumentation for stabilization has been performed before the omental flap is harvested. The abdomen is entered either through an upper midline incision, a Kocher, or a right paramedian incision. After entering the peritoneal cavity and identifying the omentum, dissection begins by liberating the omentum and transverse colon such that they can be lifted out of the abdominal cavity. Traction on the tissues will aid in demonstrating the fusion plane between the omentum and transverse mesocolon. The omentum can be dissected from its attachments to the transverse colon with a minimum of sharp dissection; blunt dissection is adequate. The dissection, if performed in the correct planes, should be avascular and not require the ligation of vessels. It is critical not to confuse the transverse colon blood supply with an omental vessel. Inclusion of the middle colic vessels with the flap may potentially devascularize the colon. Performed correctly, the entire colon from the hepatic flexure to the splenic flexure can be mobilized away from the omentum and stomach. Attention to detail should be made when putting traction on the left side of the omentum. Adhesions to the spleen can cause bleeding from the splenic capsule, and in the worst case require a splenectomy.

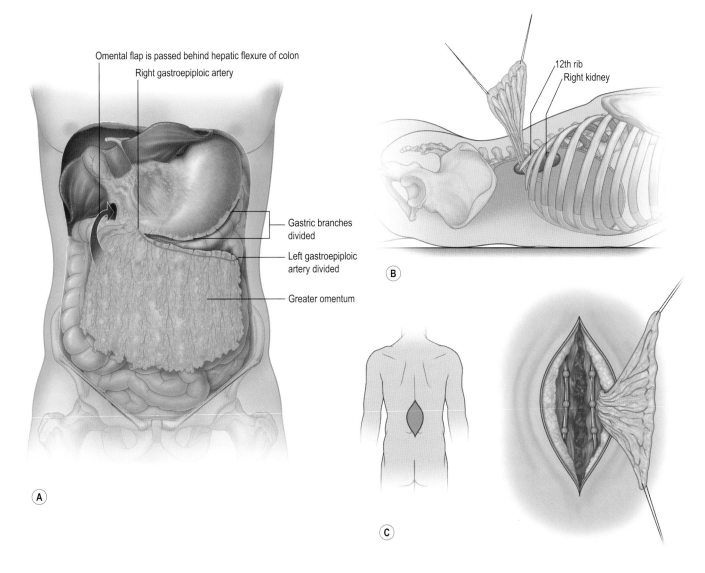

Fig. 11.18 (**A–C**) Diagram of a pedicled omental flap for coverage of the spine.

Next, a decision is made regarding whether to base the flap on the right or left gastroepiploic (gastro-omental) artery. The right-sided vessel is usually larger; the left is used when the spine exposure includes a left-flank incision. The omentum is mobilized off the stomach by taking down the short gastric vessels between snaps and ties. One should not attempt to travel great distances for each tie, as this tends to shorten the reach of the flap. The gastroepiploic vessel courses 1–2 cm from the edge of the stomach and should not be encroached by the ties. The stomach should be decompressed with a nasogastric tube, and this tube should remain in place for several days so that gastric distension will not cause any of the vessel ligatures on the greater curve to pull off. After compete mobilization of the gastroepiploic vessel off the stomach, it can be followed to the area where it emerges as the gastroduodenal artery (a branch off the hepatic artery/celiac plexus just inferior to the pylorus and still superior to the transverse colon mesentery). The artery and vein should not be skeletonized, so that the surrounding soft tissue will help to prevent unexpected tension on the vessels during the tunneling process. Sutures can also be used in this area to prevent tension and thrombosis of the pedicle.

The passage of the omentum toward the spinal column requires creativity and knowledge of anatomy of the gastroduodenal artery and its relationship to the attachments of the colon to the retroperitoneum. The most straightforward means to tunnel the omentum to the spine is to mobilize the hepatic flexure and right colon toward the midline. This is an avascular plane, and the mobilization of the colon is greatly simplified by the prior elevation of the omentum off the colon. The line of lateral peritoneal reflection (the white line of Toldt) is incised, exposing the retroperitoneum. The omental flap is then positioned behind the colon in the right paracolic gutter. The right kidney and Gerota's fascia are mobilized medially, and the omentum is "parked" on top of the 12th rib, which is confirmed by palpation. The abdomen is then closed in standard fashion and the patient reprepped in the prone position.

The 12th rib is identified by palpation after elevating the latissimus muscle and skin off the ribcage. Lateral to the paraspinous muscles, the 12th rib is excised, the periosteum opened, and the omental flap will be immediately identifiable *(Fig. 11.19)*. The only confusion would be if Gerota's fascia were entered and the perirenal fat mistaken for the omental flap. The integrity of blood flow through the pedicle is assessed with a Doppler probe. Multiple drains are used in the closure in order to avoid seroma formation and problematic fluid collections. When skin is not available for coverage of the omentum, a negative-pressure suction dressing is applied immediately on to the flap, and a delayed skin graft performed.

Adjacent tissue transfers/perforator flaps

Adjacent tissue transfers without a defined blood supply and perforator flaps are two ends of a spectrum of possible reconstructions of the soft tissues of the back. In adjacent tissue transfers such as V-Y flaps, transposition flaps, and rotation flaps, the thick soft tissues of the back will create large dog ears; donor sites will typically need to be covered with skin grafts. Perforator flaps, on the other hand, will allow transposition and insets in a more facile manner, and are especially

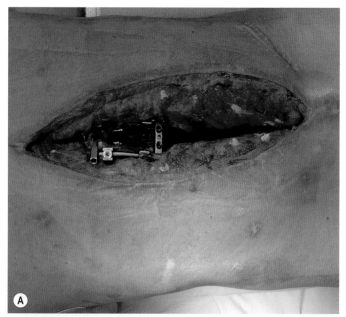

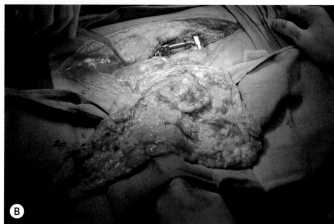

Fig. 11.19 (A) A paraplegic patient had an anterior and posterior fusion, all from the posterior approach. The spinal cord was tied off for access anteriorly. A deep infected fluid collection resulted, with the anterior and posterior hardware acting as a solid "cage." It was anticipated that flaps from the back would not be able to fill this deep hole. **(B)** The omentum has been harvested from an anterior approach, and parked under the 12th rib. From the back, the 12th rib was excised, and the omentum pulled posteriorly. The flap successfully filled the three-dimensional space created by the hardware "cage."

useful in the iliolumbar and scapular area.[8–10] However, the stresses on the soft tissues of the back with movement in and out of bed and with position changes will make the delicate nature of perforator flaps difficult to protect. In addition, these rearrangements of skin will do better with flat lateral wounds, rather than potential three-dimensional wounds of the midline spine.

External oblique flap

Patients with huge lower lateral thoracic and lumbar wounds can be closed with pedicled external oblique turnover flaps.[11]

These patients will have large radiated wounds where the remaining soft tissues would not be expected to accept a skin graft, or where there was a prosthetic material used for reconstruction of the posterior abdominal wall. These large flat flaps can be thought of as an interface to help with healing of skin grafts to the wound bed. Done either unilaterally or bilaterally, the muscle is exposed with wide elevation of the abdominal skin, done through an oblique incision paralleling the dermatomes. Then, the insertion of the muscle is divided, just as it fuses with the anterior rectus fascia. Much like a components separation procedure, the external oblique is bluntly elevated towards the posterior axillary line off the internal oblique, to the point where segmental vessels enter the muscle. The muscle is flipped on itself 180° to cover the defect and subsequently to be skin-grafted. When the flap is done unilaterally, the corresponding muscle imbalance of the anterior abdomen may cause an unusual contour of the abdominal wall.

Tissue expansion

Tissue expansion can be preferable to other solutions for reconstruction of the soft tissues of the back in certain instances. Those situations are more for pediatric cases than for adults, and include the closure of wounds for giant congenital nevi excisions. Rarely, the soft-tissue defects in children before spine surgery will be amenable to a planned prior tissue expansion. The indication for tissue expansion is scarred local tissues, laterally displaced muscles, and need for spinal instrumentation *(Fig. 11.20)*. The largest expanders possible

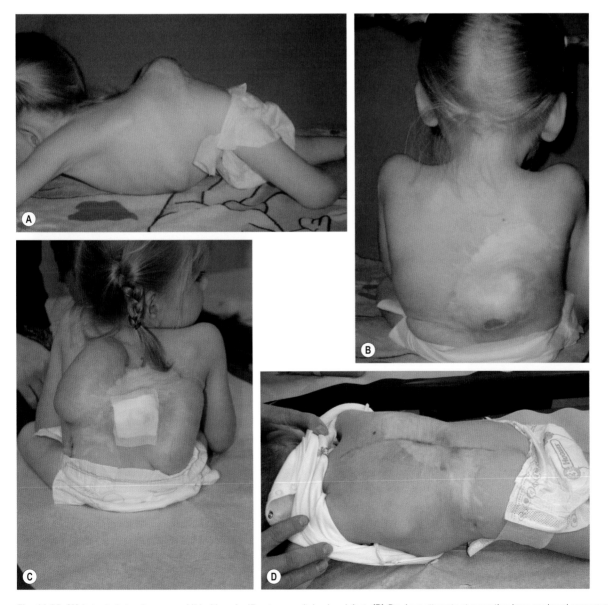

Fig. 11.20 (A) Lateral photo of a young child with a significant congenital spine defect. **(B)** Previous attempts at correction have produced numerous scars. A well-cared-for pressure sore is at the apex of the deformity. **(C)** Bilateral subcutaneous tissue expanders placed on the posterior trunk. **(D)** Healed incision after spine correction and advancement flap closure with expanded skin flaps.

should be placed immediately adjacent to the area that will require coverage, and the long axis of the expander should be oriented in a superior–inferior direction to allow for a medial sliding of the expanded tissue with a minimum of back-cuts and transposition flaps. Incisions for placement should be parallel to the axis of the expander to decrease the chance of extrusion of the implant through this newly placed scar. Ports should be placed over bony prominences to facilitate their palpability.

Free flap coverage of the back

Soft tissues

The erector spinae muscles are able to cover practically the length of the spine. However, there are patients who are not candidates for this procedure. Scarred erector spinae muscles from previous advancements or neuromuscular conditions such as polio cannot be moved to the midline. Erector spinae flaps are also not possible in patients who have received wide-field radiation. One can feel on preoperative examination of these patients a woody nonyielding feel of the soft tissues

even 6 cm from the midline. These situations are best treated with free flaps, especially when the defect is longer than 12 cm, preventing the use of a transposition of the latissimus or trapezius muscle (and when the omental flap is not possible). The difficulties with free flap coverage of the spine is finding a suitable donor vessel.[12] Possibilities include the superior gluteal artery pedicle and intercostal vessels. A long saphenous vein graft anastomosed to the common femoral artery can provide both inflow and outflow when divided for a lower trunk defect, and a long cephalic vein graft sewn to the external carotid can bring inflow for an upper trunk flap. A latissimus dorsi flap can be harvested in the prone position with proper prepping and draping *(Fig. 11.21)*.[13]

Free flaps are for defects that are both long and wide. Multiple position changes of the patient are required, and the long vein grafts, when used, are prone to twists and spasm. Some allow the vein graft loop to "mature" for a period of time to ensure that spasm will not cause a flap loss. While possible, this makes the final anastomosis to the arterial pedicle more difficult due to size mismatches, adds a separate operative procedure, and is generally not necessary.

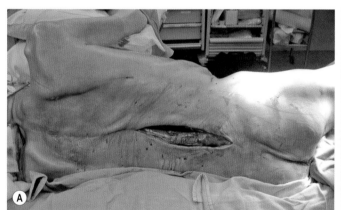

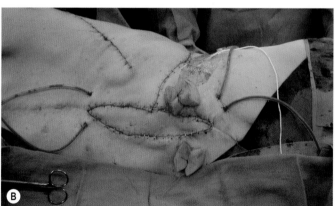

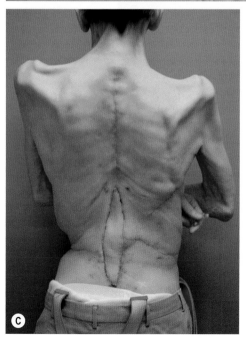

Fig. 11.21 (A) A 73-year-old man with a history of polio who has had a prophylactic closure of his spinal fusion with erector spinae flaps. Due to the fibrotic nature of his muscles, an infected fluid collection developed. He is in the lateral decubitus position at the time of his first debridement. **(B)** A myocutaneous latissimus flap is elevated and anastomosed to a long saphenous vein graft loop with inflow from the right common femoral artery and outflow through the saphenous vein to the common femoral vein. The skin paddle facilitates a solid inset of the flap. **(C)** Long-term result.

Bone

The vertebral bodies of the spine are typically reconstructed with cages and bone grafts when corpectomies are performed, and with good results. Certain patient subpopulations exist where vascularized bone is preferable. In these patients, more rapid incorporation of the bone graft due to its viable osteocytes reduces the chance of construct failure and infection. It is difficult to define exactly who should receive vascularized bone flaps, as the success rates of nonvascularized autograft and allograft are high. Fusions longer than three vertebral bodies in length, previous failed reconstructions, a history of radiation, esophagocutaneous fistula on to the fusion site, and active osteomyelitis may all be indications for a free fibula flap to the anterior spinal column.[14,15]

In the cervical esophagus, after stabilization of the posterior spine, the anterior construct is readied using a bone template of extra fibula taken from the flap. The flap is made ischemic after being preshaped on the leg according to the template, and placed into a trough created within the anterior vertebral bodies to accept the fibula flap. The trough must be slightly wider than the bone flap, so that there will be no shear or compression of the pedicle running along the side of the bone. Narrowing of the diameter of the fibula is often necessary. The bone is stabilized with kick plates superiorly and inferiorly, and the vascular anastomoses then performed to the external carotid or the transverse cervical vessels. The prior spine stabilization makes the neck by definition less mobile, and therefore the vascular repairs may best be done with loop magnification. In the thoracic area, vascular inflow is either end-to-end from a segmental lumbar vessel, or off a saphenous vein patch of the aorta fashioned by vascular surgery.

Pedicled bone flap reconstruction of the spine

A straightforward means of bringing vascularized bone to the anterior aspect of the thoracic spine is with a pedicled rib flap. For patients undergoing both anterior and posterior fusion of the spine with an associated thoracotomy for access, a pedicled rib based on its intercostal neurovascular bundle can be harvested. Unlike vascularized fibula flaps, the vascularized rib brings viable osteocytes but no structural support to the spine. The rib graft can either be placed next to or within the metal cage that is used for structural replacement of the vertebral body.[16] Rib near the costal cartilages is the actual bone that is used for the flap. Curved rib along the axillary line is excised, creating the neurovascular pedicle that is necessary for the rib flap to be positioned without tension.

Flap selection by region

Cervical region

The cervical spine area is more often instrumented from the anterior than the posterior approach. Wounds of the anterior cervical spine are uncommon, and when they occur can be in association with esophageal injuries. Wounds of the posterior cervical spine are more common. Etiologies of these wounds include pure soft-tissue defects without involvement of the spine, pressure sores, complications after laminectomy for radiated cancer excisions, and complications after placement of hardware for fusions. Soft-tissue defects without spine involvement are treated depending on the size and location of the defect either with skin grafts or adjacent tissue transfers. Pressure sores tend to be treated conservatively with pressure relief. Laminectomies are performed for spinal cord pressure from metastases, and the wound beds are typically radiated. Trapezius pedicled flaps are the preferred treatment for these patients, as the erector spinae muscles are stiff and immobile from the cancer treatment. The more laterally placed trapezius muscles are typically pliable and nonradiated, allowing them to be mobilized and "dropped in" to the defect. The erector spinae muscles also would tend to dehisce in the midline from neck flexion in the absence of spinal hardware. Complications after placement of hardware have been discussed earlier.

In most cases, the erector spinae muscles can be mobilized to the midline with both superficial and deep releases. The cervical muscles are thin, located underneath the trapezius muscle, and become smaller as they insert on the occiput. In the cervical region, the trapezius and skin should be elevated as one unit to identify the paraspinous muscles, and these planes can be confusing. Beginning inferiorly where the trapezius has a unique triangular shape and then proceeding superiorly is a means to be in the correct plane.

Thoracic region

Like the cervical region, defects of the thoracic area include pure soft-tissue defects without involvement of the spine, pressure sores, complications after laminectomy for radiated cancer excisions, and complications after placement of hardware for fusions. Soft-tissue defects without spine involvement are treated depending on the size and location of the defect either with skin grafts or adjacent tissue transfers. The scapular and parascapular flaps can be helpful in closing some of these soft-tissue defects without spine involvement, and the donor site should be oriented perpendicular to the long axis of the wound to facilitate closure.[17] Alternatively, when closure of the donor site aids in the closure of the wound, the flap can be one-half the width of the wound, and a pure 180° flip of the flap based on an underlying perforator will allow closure of both the wound and the donor site.

Pressure sores tend to be treated conservatively with pressure relief. However, in some instances, a true spine correction for deformity is what is required to treat the wound definitely. Laminectomies are performed for spinal cord pressure from metastases, and the wound beds are typically radiated. Latissimus flaps based on the paraspinous perforators are ideal to allow the muscle to be "dropped in" these defects, and thereby not manipulate the radiated and stiff erector spinae muscles. Myocutaneous latissimus flaps have easier insets with the overlying skin paddle sewn to the adjacent midline back skin.

Wounds of the thoracic back after spine surgery and placement of hardware are best treated with erector spinae flaps. There is no need for a "double muscle" closure with further mobilization of a latissimus flap if the erector spinae muscles come together normally. Rarely, the three-dimensional shape of the wound is sizeable, requiring a modification of the spinal hardware. Even more rarely, after transection of the spine or corpectomy, the wound will be extremely deep. In these circumstances, the pedicled omental flap is ideal to fill the defect and to help achieve closure. These unusual circumstances

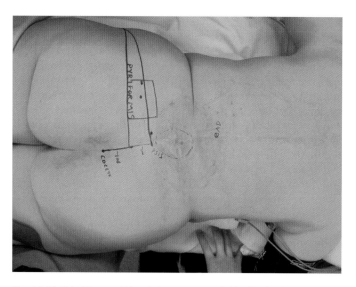

Fig. 11.22 This 50-year-old female has a recurrent fluid collection in the low lumbar spine after fusion. The initial plan is to perform a superior gluteal artery flap.

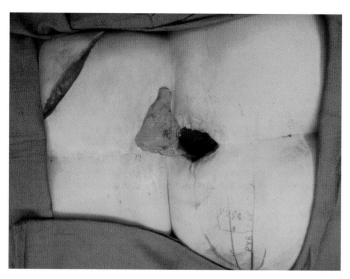

Fig. 11.23 The latissimus muscle can reach the lower lumbar spine, but only with extensive dissection, and the muscle that reaches the area is small and unable to fill the space well.

often require either erector spinae flaps or latissimus flaps to aid in the closure.

Lumbar region

The high lumbar area is the optimal area for reclosure with erector spinae flaps. The muscles are largest in this area, and exist in a lordotic area of the back that is protected from pressure. The lateral perforators are the easiest to visualize as they enter the muscle. The only difficulty in this area is management of the often-thick subcutaneous tissue. Seromas can be problematic after elevation of the skin in order to mobilize the underlying muscle. Allowing the drains to stay for a prolonged period of time, as well as quilting sutures from the subcutaneous tissue down to the muscle bed, is helpful to prevent this postoperative aggravation. Other flaps are also possible for the lumbar area. Turnover latissimus flaps can reach this area, but only with some difficulty *(Figs 11.22 and 11.23)*. Sliding of myocutaneous latissimus flaps elevated from the lower lumbar area and transposed medially provides thick coverage of the spine, but only at the expense of a skin-grafted donor site.[18] The omentum will also reach this area with some ease.

The inferior region of the lumbar spine is best covered with superior gluteal artery-based flaps as described below. Often, a gluteal flap will be combined with erector spinae flaps for coverage of a longer lumbar and lumbosacral defect. Another problem area is the posterior superior iliac spine. This area is the site where bone graft is harvested. Fluid collections, hematomas, and scar develop from procedures at this area. Lateral dissection of the erector spinae muscles can be made confusing and difficult in this area that has had a prior surgical exploration for bone graft.

Lumbosacral region

The recess between the sacrum and the inferior aspect of the spine is best filled with a superior gluteal artery-based flap. The erector spinae muscles are thin and laterally displaced in this area, precluding their use. Omental flaps require position changes in the operating room and bowel dissection.

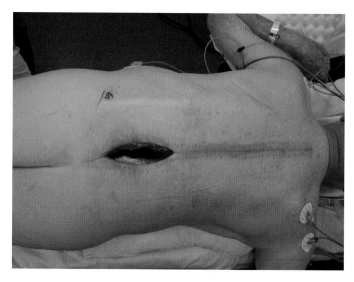

Fig. 11.24 The latissimus flap can be mobilized to reach this wound. However, the wound is large, and it would be difficult for the latissimus flap both to reach and fill this wound. This wound is better treated with a superior gluteal artery perforator flap for the lumbosacral recess, and bilateral erector spinae flaps for the lumbar area.

Random-pattern skin flaps of the lumbar tissue or perforator-based flaps are possible, but are difficult to inset and control in an area that is subjected to high shear forces with position changes. Finally, while latissimus flaps can be mobilized to reach this area, there are many wounds that are simply too big to have the latissimus muscle both reach and fill the entire cavity *(Fig. 11.24)*.

Patients undergoing a full sacrectomy for tumor can undergo bilateral gluteus myocutaneous flaps if the superior and/or inferior gluteal arteries are preserved during the sacrectomy. For these patients, the plastic surgery team can mobilize the gluteus maximus of the sacrum, exposing the pedicles to the muscle and the sacrotuberous ligaments. The spine surgeon can then perform the tumor excision. Closure of the gluteus muscles in the midline like a pressure sore can be done with V-Y advancement of the skin paddles if necessary. Finally, for low rectal tumors with invasion into the sacrum, a transabdominal flap using a flap based on the inferior epigastric artery is feasible. The oblique rectus abdominis musculocutaneous flap, using a skin paddle based in an oblique direction off the periumbilical perforators and using only the lower aspect of the rectus muscle, can easily bring nonradiated skin to the lumbosacral area.[19] The vertical rectus abdominis musculocutaneous flap is another common design to achieve wound closure, but requires the harvest of more muscle.[20] These abdominal flaps need to be parked adjacent to the sacrum and the abdomen closed. After sacrectomy, the flap can be retrieved from the posterior approach into the abdomen.

For the majority of patients with lumbosacral defects, the tissue near the trochanter can be elevated with the blood vessels in continuity with the superior gluteal artery for soft-tissue coverage *(Fig. 11.25)*. This can be done as a pure perforator flap, or else with a strip of gluteus muscle under the skin paddle (which is de-epithelialized). As the flap is typically flipped 180°, the skin paddle will rest over the dura. To re-emphasize, this is a different design than for superior gluteal artery perforator flaps done for sacral pressure sores. The proximal aspect of the pedicle must be dissected free of any muscle, as the muscle will obstruct the pedicle from being flipped towards the midline. Patients with longer wounds extending to the midlumbar area may need additional mobilization of the erector spinae muscles to the midline.

Patients undergoing this procedure do not complain of significant buttock morbidity after flap harvest. Most of these patients have chronic lower spine dysfunction and buttock weakness before surgery, and so they are not used to robust gluteus maximus muscles for ambulation. In fact, the muscle atrophy typically present facilitates dissection. If patients have any element of motor strength imbalance, then the "stronger" side should be used for the flap elevation, as that side has more to give if additional weakness develops.

Wounds of the lateral back

Soft-tissue reconstruction of the lateral back has certain special characteristics. In the thoracic area, if the ribcage is intact, then most wounds would be closeable with local wound care, latissimus flaps, parascapular/scapular flaps, serratus flaps, or posterior movement of a perforator flap from tissues in the anterior axillary line area. If the ribs are involved, then a decision about possible reconstitution of the pleural line needs to be made. Most authorities recommend that three or more ribs

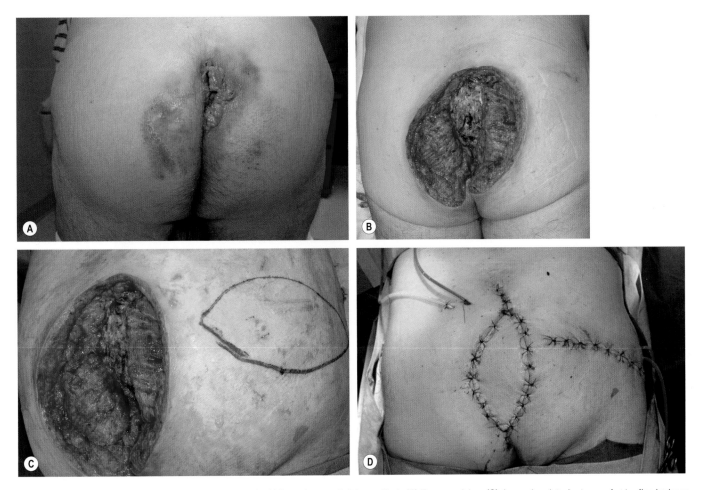

Fig. 11.25 (A) Large Marjolin's ulcer found in a chronic pilonidal cyst in an ambulatory patient. **(B)** Tumor excision. **(C)** A superior gluteal artery perforator flap is drawn out. The long axis of the skin paddle is perpendicular to the long axis of the defect to facilitate closure. The tumor excision and the final closure were staged to allow for definitive pathologic clearance of the margins. **(D)** Flap inset into defect.

be reconstructed with a prosthetic patch, and this patch would then need to be covered with soft tissues. However, when the rib defect is located under the scapula, then the scapula serves to protect and camouflage any defect, and so larger rib resections are tolerated.

The lateral lumbar area in adults typically is protected by its lordotic shape, and the only structure that needs to be reconstructed is the posterior aspect of the abdominal wall. All other wounds can be closed with local wound care, skin grafts, or transfer of the latissimus muscle. In rare instances that are radiated and require vascularized soft tissue for closure, an external oblique pedicled flap is possible.

Special clinical situations

Prophylactic closure of back incisions

Spine teams have noted the efficacy of muscle flap closure of open spine wounds, and this has led to the introduction of prophylactic use of muscle flaps at the time of spine surgery.[1,21] The same algorithms described in the chapter above are used, but now at the time of the back procedure, rather than only when there is a complication. It is difficult, if not impossible, to define exactly who should need a prophylactic soft-tissue reconstruction of the back. Patients with previous hardware infections, a woody feel to the soft tissues at the time of surgery, prior back surgery, long reconstructions greater than six vertebral bodies, CSF leaks, and a radiation history to the area all seem to be appropriate candidates to receive a soft-tissue reconstruction. However, should one prior surgery of the back require flap dissection and muscle mobilization? What about a reconstruction that is seven vertebral bodies in length in a patient who has not previously undergone a procedure? Should a remote history of a CSF leak require a prophylactic flap? Each muscle mobilization can only be performed once, and subsequently a different reconstruction would be required if there was an additional complication. At tertiary medical centers, if one includes long reconstructions in patients with prior surgeries or radiation, practically every closure would involve plastic surgery.

Studies making the case for plastic surgery closures have compared historical wound complication rates to wound rates after muscle flaps. The entire field of spine surgery has evolved over the last decade, and historical comparisons are in all likelihood not accurate. Front and back stabilizations of the spine are much more infrequent than they had been, with shorter surgeries and less stress on the patient. Better instrumentation and the use of bone morphogenic protein have improved the bone fusion rates, allowing subtle alterations in spine technique. The skill of the plastic surgeon to perform a standard soft-tissue closure is also not factored into the equation when the expected wound rate of a subpopulation of problematic patients is closed in standard fashion by spine surgeons. In an ideal world, every patient should have a closure by plastic surgery to decrease potential complication rates. In the real world, with schedules and desires for simplicity and cost containment, a more limited number of patients should receive a prophylactic closure. In our center, we limit prophylactic closures to patients with prior infections, when the muscles will not close in the midline due to

tissue loss or prior surgery, a history of radiation with a woody feel to the tissues, and CSF leaks *(Figs 11.26–11.28)*. Spine surgeons and plastic surgeons who work together frequently as teams will find a comfort zone to consult for possible closures not too early or often, and not too late.

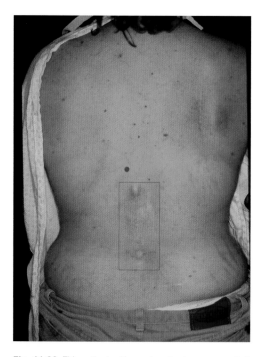

Fig. 11.26 This patient, with previous back surgery, radiation, a long planned fusion length, and a wide woody feel to the soft tissues, is a patient who should have a planned prophylactic flap closure. She underwent closure with a pedicled omental flap.

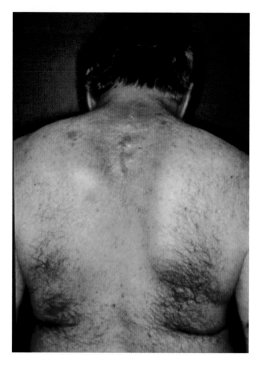

Fig. 11.27 This man has a wide radiated defect and a prior laminectomy. A long fusion is planned.

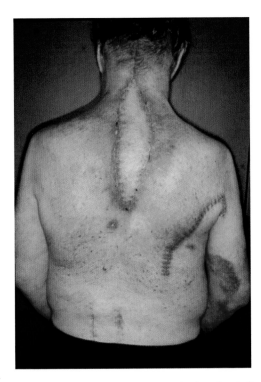

Fig. 11.28 The midline tissue was completely replaced with a free myocutaneous latissimus flap. A long cephalic vein graft loop was fashioned with inflow taken off the external carotid artery. Prophylactic flaps require a high level of coordination between spine and plastic surgery teams.

Chronic hardware exposures

Chronic hardware exposures act differently from acute exposures. Arbitrarily defined as an exposure occurring more than 6 months after placement, from experience long-term coverage of chronically exposed hardware is not successful. When patients present with small areas of drainage and by palpation a piece of hardware can be reached, this defines a hardware infection. Similarly, patients with fluid collections or "fluid cysts" in association with hardware have chronic infections. These infections can be present for months or years and yet not suppurate, nor make the patient overly ill. This is undoubtedly due to the low virulence of the organism, such as *Staphylococcus epidermidis*.

Debridement, irrigation, and soft-tissue coverage of these chronic exposures may be initially successful, but eventually fail. Perhaps these procedures can buy enough time for the spine to achieve clinical and radiographic evidence of fusion. However, for most patients the involved hardware should be removed. The question is whether all of the hardware needs to be removed, or if just a local portion (such as a large bolt) should be removed and the soft tissues closed *(Fig. 11.29)*. These are decisions made in the operating room. All hardware in association with exudative fluid should be removed. Well-incorporated hardware encased in bone can be allowed to remain. No flaps are typically required for closure when all of the hardware is removed. Patient outcomes depend more on the structural stability of the spine than on any soft-tissue work. The soft tissues are simply approximated over drains, and complete healing is the rule rather than the exception.

Antibiotics are not needed for prolonged periods in these situations.

Esophageal fistula after spine procedures

A brief mention of this spine-related soft-tissue complication will be made, despite the wound being on the anterior surface of the torso rather than the posterior surface. A small number of patients undergoing cervical spine fusion will suffer a traumatic injury to the esophagus, causing drainage and contamination of the fusion site.[22] Another group of patients will develop a pressure sore of the cervical spine hardware into the esophagus, and so the hardware can be seen during an esophagoscopy. Everything depends on the timing of the esophageal leak with the placement of the hardware. If the esophageal injury occurred at the time of hardware placement, then the spinal fusion is not solid, and the hardware is still needed. Simple repair of the esophageal defect is problematic even without the spine issues, as the standard treatment by otolaryngology is to drain fluid collections and let the wounds heal by secondary intention. Improvement of the soft tissues between the spinal hardware and the cervical esophageal repair is important. Local flaps from the neck, the pectoralis flap, and omental free flaps are all thin flaps that can be interposed into this space. The omentum is perhaps best able to deal with the contaminated drainage, and it easily conforms to the space crevices. Incisions on both sides of the neck facilitate bringing of the flap completely across the anterior body of the cervical spine. However, this would simultaneously put both recurrent laryngeal nerves at risk. Pectoralis flaps are perhaps best avoided in spinal cord patients who use their accessory chest muscles to breathe. Gastrostomy tubes obviate the need to eat in the postoperative period and are extremely helpful. Even more rarely, the esophageal leak requires removal of the previously placed construct used to fuse the anterior vertebral bodies. A short fibula-free flap "press-fit" into the defect can be used in this situation to achieve fusion, but to stay completely autogenous in the reconstruction. A longer fusion of the posterior spine is required for these cases, so that neck movement will not cause the free fibula flap to extrude anteriorly. The operative surgeon used to head and neck reconstructions for cancer will be frustrated in these cases by the lack of neck movement for positioning and the soft tissues of the neck (that did not have a lymphadenectomy) that limit exposure.

Patients who develop pressure sores of the hardware into the cervical esophagus are often found months after the cervical fusion, and the hardware can often be removed. Repair of the esophagus if possible and interposition of the soft-tissue flap are much easier in the absence of hardware and when the bone is fused. Replacement of the esophageal wall using a radial forearm flap is possible in these situations of a fused cervical spine and a persistent leak.

"Tethered cord surgery" or "lipomas of the spine"

Infants will receive procedures for closure of their spinal canal in their infancy. The spinal cord can become adherent to the spinal canal, and with growth and age, the spinal cord can be unusually stretched. Opening the dura and freeing the spinal

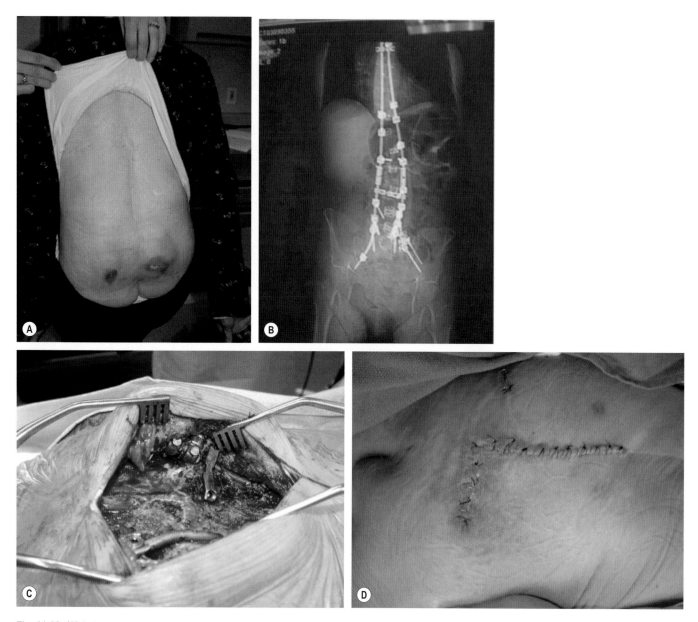

Fig. 11.29 (A) Patient over 1 year after thoracosacral fusion with bilateral lower back wounds. Large pelvic rim bolts are palpable from within the wound. The patient has not achieved clinical and radiographic evidence of fusion. **(B)** Radiograph of construct. **(C)** Large bolts from the hardware to the posterior iliac crest are visible with minimal soft-tissue cover. No purulence is noted around more superior hardware. **(D)** The bolts were excised and the superior hardware allowed to remain with a good long-term result.

cord from these attachments typically allow the cord to slide cephalad. This is an analogous procedure to what has been reported in infants.[23] The procedures have problematic postoperative healing rates. These patients tend to have a large "lipoma of the spine" overlying the area of the lumbosacral spine, and this tissue is difficult to work, with its relatively avascularity *(Fig. 11.30)*. Other patients have prior thick transverse scars from procedures performed in infancy. Preoperative debulking of the tissue can be difficult if there is an associated pseudomeningocele.

Close working between the spine and plastic surgery teams is necessary for optimal outcomes in these patients. Some patients with just thick fat over the lumbosacral recess have done well with preoperative liposuction. Patients with thick scars can be resurfaced with tissue expanders prior to the spine exploration. Others with pseudomeningoceles and need for cord re-exploration do best with superior gluteal artery-based soft-tissue reconstructions, as described below.

Pseudomeningocele repair and cerebrospinal fluid leaks

Pseudomeningoceles are contained leaks of CSF through dura into the soft tissues of the back, while CSF leaks of the spinal cord exit through drains or through the skin. The former situation typically requires treatment due to pressure of the fluid on the spinal cord with worsening motor and sensory function. The latter situation must be addressed to prevent an ascending meningitis.

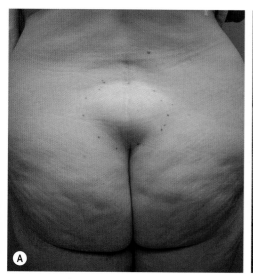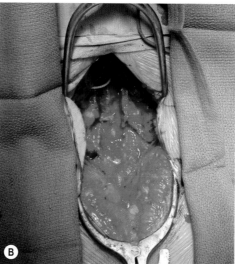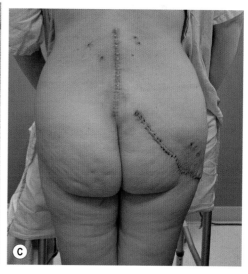

Fig. 11.30 (A) This 45-year-old female had a lipoma resected from her spinal cord in infancy. Now, she has a recurrent "lipoma" and symptoms of a tethered spinal cord. **(B)** The dura is entered and the spinal cord dissected from scar, holding it inferiorly. A dural patch is constructed. A temporary lumbar drain is visible and is used to keep cerebrospinal fluid pressure low in the immediate postoperative period. **(C)** A superior gluteal artery perforator flap is placed over the dural repair. The tissue of the flap is taken from the right buttock in this case, and near the trochanter.

The analysis of the cause of the complication is made by the spine team. Typically, the hole in the dura must be repaired or patched. It is up to the plastic surgery team to improve the soft-tissue envelope for the dural reconstruction to heal. The concepts of this chapter suffice for the management of these problems. When the patient is fused, erector spinae flaps are useful to bring new nonscarred tissue to the area. A "pants-over-vest" technique has been described to imbricate the soft tissues further on to the dural closure.[24] The lumbosacral recess is often the site of these leaks, as the dura is often opened to untether spinal cords. The superior gluteal artery-based flaps are effective to improve the soft tissues in this area with a minimum of morbidity. Important adjuncts to these procedures are a temporary or permanent decompression of the CSF pressure on the flap. This should involve flat patient positioning on a pressure relief air-fluidized sand bed for a week after the procedure. This often also involves a lumbar or head drain of CSF monitored by the neurosurgery team to keep the pressure low on the reconstruction. Drains are left in place after surgery, and the patient is carefully allowed to resume a vertical position. Postoperative CT scans and examination for chronic headaches are both means of following for recurrent CSF leaks. The CSF pressure is probably more important than the quality of the soft-tissue reconstruction long-term for pseudomeningocele recurrences.

Postoperative care

Elements of postoperative care have been introduced in this chapter, but two items deserve emphasis. Closed suction drainage between the base of the wound and the flap should be maintained until less than 30 cc/day emerges in the bulbs. The more drains the better, and for large procedures even 6–8 bulbs have been required. Second, postoperative placement on a pressure relief air-fluidized bed will allow the patient to lie directly on the flap and yet not cause a pressure injury to the tissues. It is suspected that compression of the flap directly on to the wound bed has beneficial effects in helping the wound to seal.

Access the complete references list online at **http://www.expertconsult.com**

1. Dumanian GA, Ondra SL, Liu J, et al. Muscle flap salvage of spine wounds with soft tissue defects or infection. *Spine*. 2003;28:1203–1211.

   Long-term results of successful salvage of posterior hardware with soft-tissue reconstruction of the back are presented.

2. Wilhelmi BJ, Snyder N, Colquhoun T, et al. Bipedicle paraspinous muscle flaps for spinal wound closure: An anatomic and clinical study. *Plast Reconstr Surg*. 2000;106:1305–1311.

   This is an early description of paraspinous muscle flaps for repair of soft-tissue defects after spine surgery.

6. Nojima K, Brown SA, Acikel C, et al. Defining vascular supply and territory of thinned perforator flaps: Part II. Superior gluteal artery perforator flap. *Plast Reconstr Surg*. 2006;118:1338–1348.

   This paper illustrates the performance of superior gluteal artery flaps that can then be used for spine reconstruction.

7. O'Shaughnessy BA, Dumanian GA, Liu JC, et al. Pedicled omental flaps as an adjunct in complex spine surgery. *Spine*. 2007;32:3074–3080.

   Small series illustrating the use of pedicled omental flaps in spine reconstruction surgery.

14. Lee MJ, Ondra SL, Mindea SA, et al. Indications and rationale for use of vascularized fibula bone flaps in cervical spine arthrodeses. *Plast Reconstr Surg.* 2005;116:1–7.

15. Erdmann D, Meade RA, Lins RE, et al. Use of the microvascular free fibula transfer as a salvage reconstruction for failed anterior spine surgery due to chronic osteomyelitis. *Plast Reconstr Surg.* 2006;117:2438.

16. Said HK, O'Shaughnessy BA, Ondra SL, et al. Integrated titanium and vascular bone: A new approach for high risk thoracic spine reconstruction: P34. *Plast Reconstr Surg.* 2005;116:160–162.

17. Mathes DW, Thornton JF, Rohrich RJ. Management of posterior trunk defects. *Plast Reconstr Surg.* 2006;118:73e–83e.

18. Mitra A, Mitra A, Harlin S. Treatment of massive thoracolumbar wounds and vertebral osteomyelitis

following scoliosis surgery. *Plast Reconstr Surg.* 2004;113:206–213.

20. Glass BS, Disa JJ, Mehrara BJ, et al. Reconstruction of extensive partial or total sacractomy defects with a transabdominal vertical rectus abdominis myocutaneous flap. *Ann Plast Surg.* 2006;56:526–530.

21. Garvey PB, Rhines LD, Dong Wenli, et al. Immediate soft-tissue reconstruction for complex defects of the spine following surgery for spinal neoplasms. *Plast Reconstr Surg.* 2010;125:1460–1466.

   Large series of prophylactic flaps from the MD Anderson group demonstrates improved outcomes.

23. Duffy FJ, Weprin BE, Swift DM. A new approach to closure of large lumbosacral myelomeningoceles: The superior gluteal artery perforator flap. *Plast Reconstr Surg.* 2004;114:1864–1868.

12

Abdominal wall reconstruction

Navin K. Singh, Marwan R. Khalifeh, and Jonathan Bank

SYNOPSIS

- Abdominal wall reconstruction techniques are indicated for hernia repair, reconstruction of tumor defects, congenital defects, and correction of traumatic defects (e.g., from damage control laparotomies).
- Patients may be complicated by fistulae, adhesions, infections, scarring from previous injury or surgery, and presence of dehisced prior mesh.
- Preoperative optimization of patients is requisite – smoking cessation, weight loss if indicated, and nutritional restitution.
- Autologous techniques are ideal in reconstruction, utilizing muscle and fascia – utilizing separation of components and fascia lata grafts.
- Prosthetic meshes and bioprosthetics may be utilized in addition to, or in lieu of, flaps for recalcitrant cases.
- Advanced techniques may include tissue expanders, laparoscopic methods, free flaps, and even abdominal wall transplantation.
- Postoperative management begins in the intensive care unit (ICU) and continues into postoperative rehabilitation.

 Access the Historical Perspective section online at
http://www.expertconsult.com

Introduction

The history of abdominal wall reconstruction is ensconced in the surgery-in-general literature. Abdominal wall hernias, which occur either congenitally (e.g., umbilical) or in an acquired fashion (e.g., postpartum, posttrauma, and postsurgery or iatrogenically), are routinely treated by general surgeons. Plastic surgery involvement in abdominal wall reconstruction came to the fore in complex cases where routine techniques exploiting local tissues and mesh would not suffice. Plastic surgery consultation became indicated for flap mobilization, regional tissue transfers, free flaps, and tissue

expansion techniques. A seminal paper by Ramirez et al.[1] revisited and popularized components separation as a useful technique in abdominal wall reconstruction. What has followed is an understanding of abdominal wall muscular dynamics, the role of component separation and muscle realignment as a central tenet of any reconstruction, and advances such as endoscopic or minimally invasive methods to perform component separation. Recent advances include perforator-sparing techniques, and evolution in biologic as well as synthetic meshes.

Closure of routine laparotomies itself causes many postoperative hernias. Easy to recall are the fulminant complications such as eviscerations, septic dehiscences, often despite retention sutures placed initially or at "take-back" surgery. Yet approximately 20% of laparotomies become incisional hernias in the US. Given that more than 4 million laparotomies are performed annually, this is a staggering number. Only about 90 000 are repaired annually, leaving both a huge backlog of cases that must be addressed as well as a future opportunity to deliver care to those who have limitations in activity, chronic pain, and functional issues such as chronic constipation or urinary retention from these hernias which are the sequelae of so many laparotomies.

Most surgeries are performed in the rich world – the world's wealthiest 2 billion people get 75% of all the surgery done each year while the poorest 2 billion only get 4%.[2] With increasing access to care, parts of the developing world will face similar challenges of abdominal wall reconstruction.

The ascendancy of the evidence-based medicine paradigm over the last two decades has focused attention on both the short-term failure rates of techniques as well as the long-term data. A landmark paper by Luijendijk et al.[3] showed that, if followed for 10 years, the failure rates with primary suture techniques are 2 in 3, and with synthetic meshes 1 in 3. This is unacceptably high. Consequently, there has been an escalation in interest and an introduction of novel techniques in addressing these problems, as long-term data highlight the inadequacy of previous methods. The influence of evidence-based medicine has driven a resurgence of investigations into abdominal wall reconstruction techniques, as well as multi-specialty collaboration between general surgeons, colorectal surgeons, trauma surgeons, minimally invasive surgeons, and plastic surgeons.

Patients and surgeons are seeking a decrease in herniation rates in the long term, not just a delay until reherniation. Quality measures, cost containment, and cost-effectiveness are paramount in the minds of institutions, payors, and credentialing committees, as we operate in a changing healthcare paradigm. ⊛ FIG 12.1–12.3 APPEARS ONLINE ONLY

Basic science/disease process

Hernias and abdominal wall defects may be asymptomatic or symptomatic, and range from the minor cosmetic inconvenience to major destructive processes of the abdominal wall. Congenital umbilical hernias are usually repaired in infancy or childhood. Inguinal herniorrhaphy is similarly undertaken in childhood or in adulthood when they become symptomatic. Major defects such as gastroschisis or omphalocele are not addressed in this chapter – they require multiteam approaches and staged operations.

Acquired defects resulting from straining during heavy labor, load-bearing exercises, and childbirth are defects in the fascia that tend to enlarge, if unsupported by a truss or unrepaired. Narrow-neck hernias are at greater risk for incarceration and strangulation of bowel, whereas large-neck hernias, although more dramatic, are less likely to cause bowel trauma. Success rates with smaller defects in healthy patients are high. Some recur, and may require multiple surgeries.

Analysis of the National Safety and Quality Improvement Program (NSQIP database) highlights the surgeon's intuition: comorbidities of smoking, diabetes mellitus, COPD, coronary artery disease, poor nutritional status/low serum albumin, immunosuppression, chronic corticosteroid use, obesity, and advanced age increase the risk for postoperative infection and failure. Infection, in turn, creates a higher risk of repair failure. Once the cascade is established, serial failures can turn a small, reparable defect into a challenge.

Other hernias begin as multiple small "Swiss cheese" defects, and when one defect is repaired, the other unrepaired defect(s) can enlarge. These defects may be dormant and arise as a consequence of old retention suture puncture points, prior stoma sites, or drain sites. Thus, some recurrences may not be true failures of hernia repair so much as failure of diagnosis of multiple defects. Ideally, there should be a preoperative computed tomography (CT) scan confirming the location and number of fascial defects, and at the time of repair there should be a wider dissection to identify occult hernias in proximity to the index hernia. Laparoscopic evaluation can provide a broader view of the abdominal wall and potentially identify previously occult defects as well.

Rarely, other failures may arise as a consequence of collagen vascular disorders. The patient with multiple failed attempts and signs consistent with Ehlers–Danlos syndrome, including hypermobility of skin and hyperextensibility of joints, should be referred to a rheumatologist for workup of collagen vascular disorders. This is relatively uncommon and incidence may be approximately 1 in 5000 live births worldwide.

Rectus diastases are not true abdominal wall fascial defects but are pathological stretching to the linea alba either congenitally or, most frequently, postpartum. Functionally, a diastasis is analogous to an aneurysm – wherein the adventitia (fascia) and intima (peritoneum) are intact but the muscular layer is absent *(Fig. 12.4)*. In techniques for abdominal wall reconstruction that do not centralize muscle, or cases in which the abdominal muscles have retracted beyond the possibility to be reapproximated, a functional diastasis remains, in lieu of the tendinous fusion of the paired rectus abdominis muscles. This diastasis can enlarge over time from intra-abdominal pressure, even to the point of requiring repair. Repair is achieved without intraperitoneal entry, by plicating or imbricating the defect so that the rectus abdominis muscles are returned to the midline *(Fig. 12.5)*.

Hernias are challenging problems, and a significant fraction of hernia repairs fail, occasionally further complicated by enterocutaneous fistula formation, periprosthetic mesh infection, ulceration, and tenuous skin coverage. In particular, hernias that are re-recurrent will have the highest relapse rate and also the greatest predilection for complications.

A review of the long-term data reveals that Luijendijk et al. reported 43% versus 24% for initial recurrences and 58% versus 20% for secondary recurrences at 3 years.[3] At 10-year follow-up, Burger et al. reported 63% versus 32% recurrence if primary suture techniques were used versus prosthetic mesh.[15] Despite the reduction in recurrence rates, the rates remain unacceptably high.

The development and adoption of prosthetic materials have made a tremendous impact on the treatment of hernias. Synthetic mesh was introduced in the 1950s and has become a common component of the repair process. Data from the largest prospective, randomized, multicenter study show a significant decrease in recurrence rates in relatively healthy patients with small defects (<6 cm length or width) who received synthetic mesh versus those repaired primarily with suture alone.[3]

Diagnosis/patient presentation

Hernias should be treated as a chronic disease process – a notion that is gaining ground in surgical circles – a conglomeration of collagen disorders, excess mechanical loads, comorbidities, and outdated surgical techniques, and other poorly understood factors. Success is predicated on a systematic approach from understanding the etiology of prior failure, risk factors, metabolic status, the biology and biomechanics of repair materials, employment of an appropriate surgical technique (i.e., open or laparoscopic), to postoperative vigilance.

In the elective setting, the diagnosis of an abdominal ventral defect is made on physical exam when the patient presents with a symptomatic, intermittently painful bulge. In the emergency setting, strangulated bowel is diagnosed in the presence of a firm, painful bulge in a systemically ill patient, with fever, leukocytosis, and possible bowel obstruction. Diagnosis is made on physical exam and confirmed by CT scan. An appropriate workup includes plain films of the abdomen, complete blood count, basic metabolic panel, and lactate level. After fluid resuscitation and electrolyte

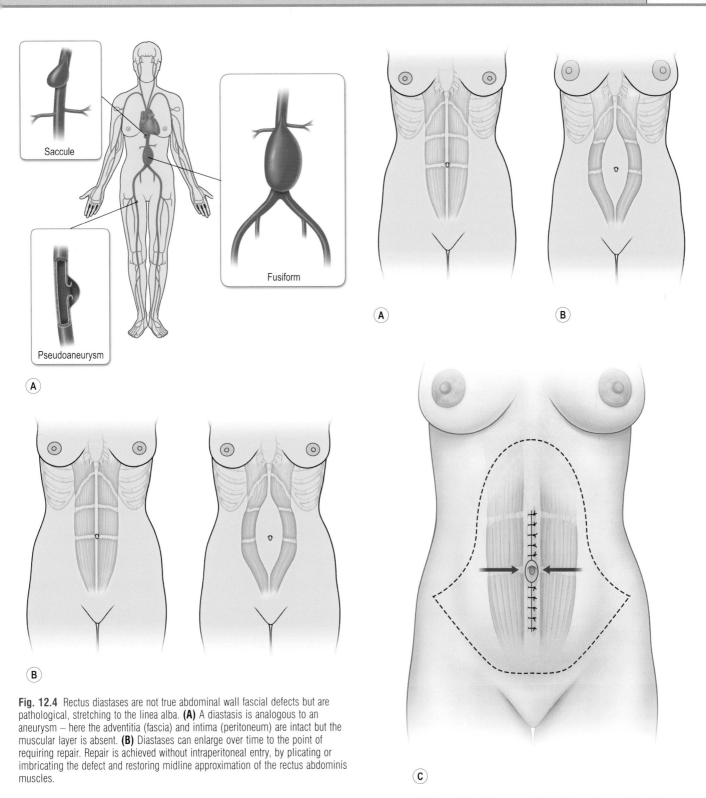

Fig. 12.4 Rectus diastases are not true abdominal wall fascial defects but are pathological, stretching to the linea alba. **(A)** A diastasis is analogous to an aneurysm – here the adventitia (fascia) and intima (peritoneum) are intact but the muscular layer is absent. **(B)** Diastases can enlarge over time to the point of requiring repair. Repair is achieved without intraperitoneal entry, by plicating or imbricating the defect and restoring midline approximation of the rectus abdominis muscles.

Fig. 12.5 (A) Normal lay of the rectus abdominis muscles on either side. **(B)** Diastasis recti. **(C)** Schematic representation of the extent of subcutaneous dissection with reapproximation at the midline and fascial plication.

correction, an urgent exploratory laparotomy must be performed. Definitive repair may or may not be performed at that time based on patient factors, comorbidities, and the contamination and condition of the wound.

Loss of domain occurs when muscle, fascia, and/or skin have necrosed or retracted and have become contracted over time and abdominal viscera extrude into the hernia sac. It is said that the bowels have "lost their domain" in the peritoneal cavity. Recreating this lost domain is the challenge and goal of the hernia surgeon.

Nonhernia abdominal defects may present from surgical oncology referral for anticipated plastic surgery closure at the time of resection of a segment of the abdominal wall.

Preoperative imaging can delineate the involved structures and thus clarify the missing anatomic components in need of reconstruction, such as skin, soft tissue, muscle, fascia, and peritoneum.

Goals of repair include both form and function. Aesthetic correction of the bulge or skin-grafted deficient contour is important, but the main impact of reconstruction is on restoration of function. Re-establishment of fascial integrity restores the function of the remaining muscular elements. Once the muscles are reconnected as part of the same aponeurosis, they have paired and gain dynamic tension and countertension. In the presence of a fascial defect, the unopposed pull of the oblique and transversus abdominis muscles on either side of the defect leads to progressive lateralization of the muscles and enlargement of the defect. In a functional repair, the muscles are restored in continuity and are balanced. This improves the ability to ventilate more effectively and efficiently, as the abdominal muscles are accessory muscles of respiration. This is particularly germane in patients with concomitant pulmonary disease. Realignment of the muscle allows patients to Valsalva, generating pressure against the rectum, assisting defecation. Similarly, patients' urinary retention improves since pressure is transmitted to the bladder to facilitate more complete emptying. Posture and back pain improve since the viscera are returned to their proper domain, and the load of the abdominal contents is replaced inside the abdomen. The moment arm of a lever is distance times force; when abdominal viscera are not contained inside the cavity, the weight of the visceral bulge causes strain on the back and postural muscles since the distance from the load axis (the spine) to the weight (viscera) is increased. With restoration of domain, the weight is returned closer to the load axis, thus decreasing the moment arm, and decreasing the strain on the supporting muscles (this is akin to why it is easier to hold a gallon of milk against the chest then to hold it at arm's length). Studies and surveys have shown that activities of daily living improve, as do patients' self-image and subjective well-being. Another functional improvement is regaining the ability to exercise, although in some recalcitrant cases it may be prudent never to allow that patient to have severe load-bearing activities again. In that setting, manual laborers may have to be trained in a different vocation.

In summary, repair and restoration of the abdominal wall provide cosmesis, postural and truncal stability, improvement in micturition, improvement in defecation, ability to perform activities of daily living, and also provide a satiety signal with restoration of physiologic intra-abdominal pressure, decreasing appetite.

Patient selection

Patient selection is less about declining the operation for certain individuals and more about eventually optimizing them for a *bona fide* chance at a durable and reliable repair. Patients who are not medically fit from a cardiopulmonary standpoint may be deferred or declined in conjunction with soliciting their wishes, risk aversion, and motivations. The only absolute contraindication is if the patient is medically unsuitable for surgical clearance.

Patients with ascites are extremely likely to have a poor outcome and should be referred to a hepatologist for management of cirrhosis or hepatic failure prior to attempt at a repair. Metastatic disease (hepatic, abdominal, or distant) is a relative contraindication, but hernia repair, as emphasized earlier in the chapter, is also about enhancing quality of life and diminishing pain. With current oncologic management, patients with metastases of certain diseases can be expected to live for years or decades, and thus cancer remains only a relative contraindication. Patients likely to need other intra-abdominal surgery may be postponed until their intra-abdominal issues are resolved, though this too remains a relative contraindication.

The largest category of denied patients is the noncompliant patient, whether this is noncompliance for weight reduction and nutritional repletion, noncompliance in nicotine avoidance, or noncompliance in seeking better glycemic control. Behavioral management, psychosocial support, and counseling can be enlisted to facilitate the goals of compliance. Those patients who lack adequate familial and social support to recover properly from surgery may also be deferred from surgery.

With weight loss in particular, patients report finding themselves in a Catch-22 situation – they cannot get their hernia fixed because they are overweight, and they remain overweight since they cannot exercise until their hernia is fixed. No easy solutions exist to this conundrum; caloric restriction, low-impact aerobic exercise, and water aerobics have been shown to be helpful. Socioeconomic barriers may prevent patients from getting these additional support modalities. For BMI > 40, a bariatric surgery referral should be considered. Patients whose BMI exceeds 40 are potential candidates for surgery if they clearly and realistically understand how their lives may change after surgery In certain circumstances, less severely obese patients (with BMIs between 35 and 40) also may be considered, since obesity-induced or exacerbated physical problems such as irreparable hernia are interfering with lifestyle or precluding or severely interfering with employment, family function, and ambulation.

Weight loss must not emperil adequate nutrition – this can be confirmed by obtaining assays of vitamin levels, albumin, prealbumin, and transferrin levels, and reticulocyte index. Even thin individuals may have diabetes or glucose intolerance. HgbA$_1$c levels can be predictive of a diabetic diathesis and serum glucose levels greater than 110 mg/dL can suggest glucose intolerance. An endocrine consult may be helpful if either of these is found to be elevated, and an additional glucose tolerance test can be administered. Better glycemic control at the time of surgery with HgbA$_1$c levels less than 7% is desirable to decrease the risk of perioperative complications.

Important vitamins and minerals include zinc for cross-linking collagen, vitamin C for collagen synthesis, vitamin A for counteracting the deleterious effects of corticosteroids in wound healing, folate, and thiamine. Other indicators of nutritional adequacy include albumin and prealbumin, transferrin, and reticulocyte index. The presence of elevated fasting blood glucose (above 110 mg/dL), recent smoking (less than 4 weeks' nicotine compliance), use of bronchodilators (presence of COPD), and absence of weight reduction attempts are all potential indicators of a patient at high risk of recurrence. At-risk subpopulations should be given thiamine, folate, and multivitamins intravenously. Massive weight loss patients from bariatric surgery should undergo a preoperative planning session with their endocrinologist, primary care physician, or surgeon. This would involve checking and restoring iron levels and fat-soluble vitamins, including vitamin A, D, and, most importantly, K. Although vitamin B_{12} is water-soluble, the altered gastric physiology of most bariatric and gastric bypass procedures can predispose to vitamin B_{12} deficiency and its level specifically will need to be assessed and restored if indicated.

Smoking has multiple deleterious mechanisms of action on healing and recovery of the abdominal wall reconstruction patient. Combustion products from tobacco include hydrogen cyanide that causes oxidative decoupling and halting of cellular respiration by inhibiting the mitochondrial enzyme cytochrome C oxidase. Another combustion product, carbon monoxide, has a 200-times greater affinity for hemoglobin than oxygen, and thus decreases oxygen-carrying capacity by left and downward shifting of the oxygen dissociation curve, thus hindering release of oxygen to cells in the healing wound.

Nicotine (whether absorbed via smoking or smoking cessation medications such as nicotine gum, lozenge, transdermal patch, inhaler, or nasal spray) is a potent vasoconstrictor, enhances platelet aggregation, and directly damages the endothelial lining of blood vessels. Thus smoking and/or nicotine directly impairs microcirculation and decreases tissue oxygenation in healing wounds.

The smoker's cough also creates mechanical pressures that are supraphysiologic in the convalescence period and can disrupt repairs in the immediate postoperative period and cause recurrence. Wound infection rates are approximately fivefold higher in smokers. Wound infection can jeopardize underlying synthetics or biologic meshes utilized in repairs, as well as increase the chance of recurrence.[18] Smoking and nicotine cessation, including exposure to second-hand smoke, is imperative for several weeks prior to surgery (preferably 4–6 weeks), and at least for several weeks postoperatively as well. In combination with behavioral therapy, it is ideal to have the patient quit smoking entirely and not just for the perioperative duration.

Smoking cessation can be enhanced via behavioral and pharmacologic methods and several psychoactive medications can enhance compliance beyond the use of nicotine replacement therapies (e.g., bupropion, clonidine, nortriptyline, varenicline, or Chantix). Compliance with nicotine abstinence may need to be independently verified via a blood, urine, or saliva test for nicotine or cotinine (a metabolite of nicotine). Urine cotinine can offer an assessment of exposure to smoking or second-hand smoking for a window of 2–3 weeks. On the morning of surgery an arterial blood gas can be sent to evaluate carboxyhemoglobin levels, which would be acutely elevated in a recent smoker. In addition to smoke and nicotine avoidance, these patients can be optimized with bronchodilators and other pulmonary medications.

Informed consent is the final cornerstone of preoperative optimization. Emphasis is placed on the risks, which include infection, bleeding, hematoma, seroma, wound dehiscence, delayed healing, poor healing, swelling, lymphedema, and scarring such as keloids, hypertrophic scar, hypo- or hyperpigmented scars. Patients may develop weakness in the abdominal wall and/or donor sites, acute and chronic pain, respiratory problems, or chronic disability. There is a reasonable expectation for further surgery (planned or unplanned) with its additional risks, financial responsibilities, and time required for surgery and recuperation, and potential rehospitalization.

A preoperative discussion of the different implant choices should be held (synthetic mesh, human and nonhuman bioprosthetics). Patients' religious and moral convictions may play a part in the choice of biologic mesh, whether the source is human, porcine, or bovine.[18] Major surgery for abdominal wall rehabilitation carries with it a risk of blood transfusion with its attendant risks of bacterial/viral infection (e.g., human immunodeficiency virus, hepatitis C virus) and transfusion reaction. The patient should be alerted that partial or total flap and tissue loss may occur or that incomplete or no relief of their pain may be a result.

The systemic risks of anesthesia, including severe nausea/vomiting, awareness, heart attack, stroke, total/partial paralysis, blindness, death, coma, or prolonged mechanical ventilator dependence, are discussed by either the surgeon or the anesthesia provider.

The risks for venous thromboembolic phenomenon are highlighted, including the role of medications such as oral contraceptive or postmenopausal estrogens which can increase the risk for deep-vein thrombosis and pulmonary embolism (DVT/PE). Even in the setting of current abstinence, past smoking or second-hand smoke exposure can increase ischemic and infective complication risks. Patients are cautioned that traveling soon after surgery and prolonged immobilization may contribute to DVT/PE. The patient with increased BMI or diabetes is educated to the elevated risks of poor healing or infection with an obese body habitus and poor glycemic control. Operating in previously distorted and scarred areas carries additional risk of injuries to surrounding structures.

Patients should acknowledge that they appreciate the best-case, worst-case, and average outcomes and scenarios and consent to following the postoperative management plan, as outlined by the surgical team, including compliance with activity limits and smoking. After a lengthy and thorough consent process, patients should feel that they are appraised of the material risks and benefits of the surgery and have participated in choosing the best option for themselves.

Treatment/surgical technique

Bioburden reduction

The first step in adherence to surgical principles is bioburden reduction. This is essential in a contaminated or infected milieu. The wound should be cleansed mechanically if needed by pulse lavage or sharp "oncologic" en bloc-type excision. Wound preparation should excise any nonvital tissues, indurated and fibrotic tissues likely to become avascular, and any retained prior foreign-body prosthetics and mesh. Debridement may necessitate removal of the umbilicus since it is often marginally attached to one of the skin flaps or may be deemed nonviable at the end of the operation. The patient should be prepared for this, and the umbilicus can always be secondarily reconstructed.

Pre-existing fistulae may be managed by controlling them with surgical drains, percutaneous drainage and diversion of collections, surgical washouts and antibiotic treatment for existing infection or colonization. In particular, patients with a history of multiple hospitalizations may be carriers of methicillin-resistant *Staphyloccocus aureus* (MRSA), and should be screened with swabs of nares, axilla, and inguinal region. They can be decontaminated prior to surgery with chlorhexidine preparations, which have antimicrobial activity against *S. aureus*, MRSA, and Gram-negatives on contact.

After nonsurgical care for a period of 24–72 hours, definitive closure can be scheduled. At the time of conclusive repair, any intra-abdominal collections and pathology such as fistulae and tumors should be addressed. Stomas may be reversed concomitantly, and diseased bowel segments may be resected. Then definitive reconstructive steps for the abdominal wall can be undertaken.

A plastic surgery adage is that "the solution is in the problem." Ventral defects of the abdominal wall create uncoupling of muscles with the lateral pull of the obliques and transversus abdominis muscles. This causes the abdominal wall musculature to become lateralized; hence the solution for lateralization is centralization of the muscles.

Negative-pressure wound therapy

If, after debridement, the wound still remains unsuitable for immediate closure, it can be temporized with topical antimicrobial creams and dressings to decrease bacterial colony counts. For frank infection or gross contamination not adequately addressable by bioburden techniques, the wound may be temporized by using negative-pressure (subatmospheric pressure) dressings. The wound may need to be temporarily managed before definitive fascial closure with an NWPT dressing such as VAC or Abthera devices, or, if fascial closure is achieved, then skin may be left open to prevent infection in the subcutaneous space and treated with a subatmospheric pressure dressing.

The proposed mechanisms by which NPWT works are: (1) compression of tissues creating shear and hypoxia which are signals for angiogenesis/granulation; (2) hypoxia which releases nitric oxide, causing vasodilatation; (3) decrease of third-space fluid; (4) compression of vessel causes, which increases velocity, leading to decrease in hydrostatic pressure by Bernoulli's law and thus less exudate; (5) increased blood velocity, which "aspirates" exudate back into the second space via Venturi effect; and (6) splinting of the wound mechanically.[19]

Primary suture technique

The primary suture technique may achieve repair for small defects by mobilizing the edges and primarily suturing them together, much like a postpartum abdomen, when a rectus diastasis is sutured by imbrication to recentralize the rectus abdominis muscles. Large sutures such as number 1 or number 2 monofilament sutures are used. They may be slowly absorbable sutures such as PDS (polydioxanone) or nonabsorbable sutures like nylon or Prolene (polypropylene). Faster-absorbing sutures such as chromic (surgical gut) or polyglactin 910 (Vicryl) are not appropriate for suture technique. There is preference for monofilament sutures, although braided sutures have been used; they are more prone to be a nidus for infection. Permanent sutures provide greater reassurance, but

may form suture granuloma or be palpable or visible in thinner patients, potentially requiring surgical removal at a later time. The matter of running suture line versus interrupted suture line remains unadjudicated by prospective peer-reviewed publications.

For small defects, such as umbilical defects or small postpartum hernias, primary suture repair can be successful and adequate. Long-term studies show that the 10-year recurrence rate for these is unacceptably high at 63% for defects larger than 6 cm.[3]

Component separation method

Component separation is the mobilization of the rectus abdominis muscles bilaterally as a musculofascial, bipedicled, neurotized flap. After the initial description by Ramirez *et al.*,[1] several authors have reported favorable outcomes with this technique and have offered improvements and variations.[16,20,21] In this technique, the skin and subcutaneous tissues are widely degloved to the anterior or midaxillary line. The transition point where the external oblique muscle becomes tendinous and attaches on to the anterior rectus sheath aponeurosis is identified as the linea semilunaris. Approximately 10–20 mm lateral to that line, a fasciotomy is made with scissors or electrocautery to separate the external oblique from the rectus abdominis. Maneuvers to identify the linea semilunaris include palpation of the rectus abdominis muscle bulk by placing four fingers intraperitoneally and pinching the abdominal wall with the thumb. Cautery stimulation can also be used to check the orientation of muscular fibers. Electrocautery stimulation starts medially, and its use will make the rectus fibers twitch vertically; once the cautery is slowly moved laterally, the fibers will twitch obliquely over the external oblique muscle (*Fig. 12.1*). Transillumination can also be used to identify the lateral extent of the rectus abdominis muscle. Its width varies by body habitus, and in the obese, it can often be splayed out wider than anticipated. In the debilitated it may be thinner and wispier than expected.

Once the fascia is incised, an avascular plane is entered, between the external oblique and the internal oblique directly below it. Orientation of the fibers can confirm that the correct plane has been entered since the fibers of the external oblique run superolateral to inferomedial, and the fibers of the internal oblique are orthogonal to the external oblique (*Fig. 12.6*). The segmental neurovascular bundles emanating from the intercostal vessels and nerves are deep to the internal oblique, and so the plane of dissection is a safe and privileged plane. Inadvertent dissection below the internal oblique might damage the innervation, resulting in a patulous and adynamic rectus abdominis muscle segment. Incision into or below the internal oblique can also create a spigelian hernia at the external oblique release site. This risk can be mitigated with an onlay or underlay technique utilizing a mesh or biologic (*Fig. 12.7*).

The intraperitoneal adhesions of the bowel to the abdominal wall should be regarded as a "component" as well, and must be separated. Wide adhesiolysis, freeing the viscera from the abdominal wall undersurface to the bilateral paracolic gutters, is an important step in mobilizing the abdominal wall.

To gain additional mobility, should it be required, a posterior release should also be done, by shelling the rectus

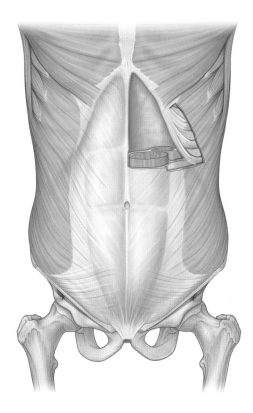

Fig. 12.6 Schematic representation of the abdominal musculature and fascial layers above the arcuate line. Note the orthogonal directionality of the oblique muscles.

abdominis out of the posterior rectus sheath by incising the posterior rectus sheath a few millimeters lateral to the free edge of the fascia where the hernia is encountered *(Fig. 12.8)*. Care should be taken to mobilize the posterior rectus sheath and attached peritoneal lining down and to reflect the rectus abdominis with its fatty areolar layer, DIEA and deep inferior epigastric vein, and nerves upward. A few centimeters of dissection usually suffice. This posterior release is not always necessary, and it offers an additional 2–3 cm of mobility on each side. It also creates a retrorectus space for placing a mesh or biologic, should that option be chosen by the surgeon.

If a stoma (colostomy, ileostomy, ureterostomy) is present, extra care should be taken in performing component separation on the involved side. If the stoma is to be preserved, wide soft-tissue attachment should be maintained around the stoma, and dissection can proceed around the stoma with a lighted retractor, and a limited external oblique release can still be performed on the involved side.

If the stoma is to be created through the rectus abdominis muscle, component separation can still be carried out as anticipated, and the stoma can be exteriorized through the skin once the fascia is closed. Otherwise there is the risk of creating a stomal obstruction by shearing the stoma between the fascial plane and skin plane.

Component separation thus performed should create musculofascial flaps, which advance 6 cm at the epigastrium, 10 cm at the waistline, and 5 cm at the suprapubic region on each side *(Figs 12.9 and 12.10)*. Superiorly, mobility becomes limited by the relatively immobile costal margin. The superior

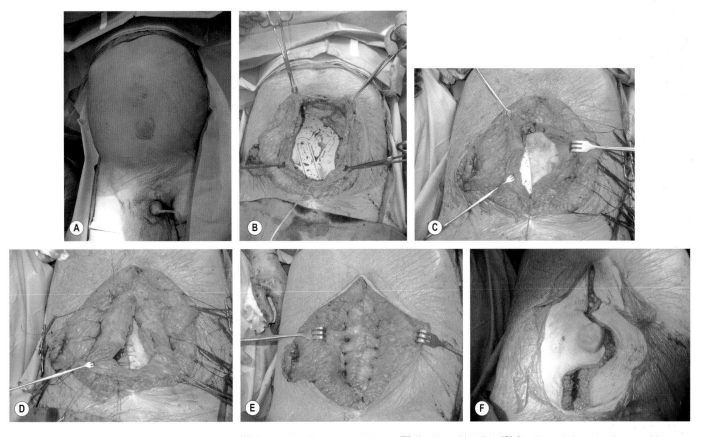

Fig. 12.7 Component separation with Strattice underlay. **(A)** Preoperative photo – ventral hernia. **(B)** Hernia sac identified. **(C)** Strattice underlay sutured to one side. **(D)** U-stitches through contralateral side. **(E)** Fascial layers closed above Strattice. **(F)** Drain placement. (Courtesy of Dr. David H. Song.)

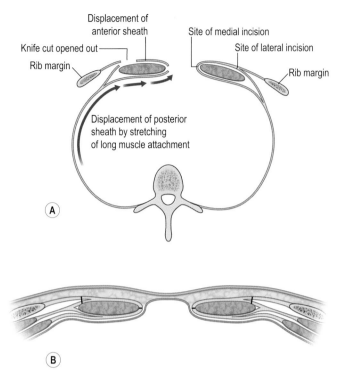

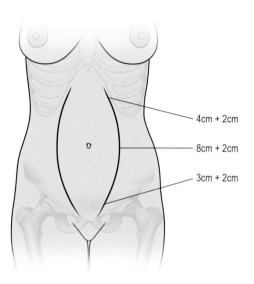

Fig. 12.9 As per Shestak *et al.*,[5] maximal unilateral rectus complex mobility in the upper, middle, and lower abdominal levels, by means of component separation of the external and internal oblique muscles to the posterior axillary line. The additional 2 cm of advancement is gained if the rectus abdominis muscle is separated off the posterior rectus fascia.

Fig. 12.8 (A) Cross-sectional diagram demonstrating medial and lateral incisions to initiate the component separation with development of the posterior rectus plane. Detachment from the lower rib margins offers additional length in the upper abdominal region. **(B)** Incision planes in the upper abdomen. Note the lateral incision traverses both components of the anterior rectus sheath.

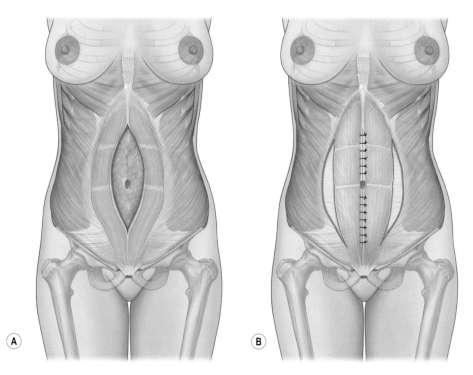

Fig. 12.10 (A) Preoperative ventral hernia schematic. **(B)** Postoperative illustration showing midline closure at the linea alba. Note the external oblique fascial release. (After Ramirez OM, Ruas E, Dellon AL. "Components separation" method for closure of abdominal-wall defects: an anatomic and clinical study. Plast Reconstr Surg. 1990;86:519–26.)

extent of the external oblique fasciotomy can be extended to above the costal margin to where the rectus abdominis widens and its fascia fuses with that of the pectoralis major. In severe cases, the rectus abdominis can also be mobilized superiosteally off the costal margin. Inferiorly, the immobile pelvis limits mobility. Surgeons have reported gaining additional mobility by subperiosteal dissection and elevation of the rectus abdominis off the symphysis pubis.

Since most hernia defects are elliptical, this technique gives the greatest advancement in the midline where it is most needed, and less advancement superiorly and inferiorly, where less is required. Some hernias however disobey this role. Notably, trauma laparotomies performed as a chevron incision, or those involving a sternotomy, leave a fascial defect in the subcostal area that is a challenge to mobilize. In these instances, closure may require suturing to ribs, suturing to heterotopic ossification, or using bone anchors.

Orthopedic-type bone anchors with attached sutures can be used to suture fascia, mesh, or a biologic matrix to the pelvis or ribs. Because the risk for osteomyelitis theoretically exists, this technique should be reserved for clean cases. It is probably preferable to use absorbable bone anchors in lieu of permanent ones. A tidy alternative to bone anchors, if unavailable or unfamiliar, is to use a 1-mm wire-passing drill to create tunnels in the bone, through which to pass the suture.

Defect size reduction via component separation is a necessary step irrespective of the method of final closure of the defect. Separation of parts allows for as much of the abdominal wall as possible to be have muscular and dynamic closure; otherwise areas without muscular coverage will tend to become lax and bulge, much like an aneurysmal dilatation. Although component separation is necessary, it is not sufficient. Prospective data have demonstrated that the rate of hernia recurrence is higher when component separation is not reinforced than when it is.[22,23] This reinforcement can be done as an onlay or an underlay, which can serve as an "internal abdominal binder," serving to offload the muscle by sharing the tensile forces across a multilayer construct.

Most surgeons prefer an underlay as opposed to an onlay reinforcement, but this has not been prospectively shown to be superior. Underlay is felt to be better because intra-abdominal distension forces apply the material into the repair as opposed to push it away and distribute the disruptive forces more uniformly, but have not been studied enough to be conclusive. It certainly is appealing based on logical principles.

The underlay material can be placed intraperitoneally, in which case it should span all the way from external oblique to the contralateral external oblique to reinforce and secure the entire operative field. U-sutures are placed full-thickness from the abdominal wall down into the peritoneum, into the mesh or biologic, and back into the abdominal wall. Devices such as a Carter–Thompson closure device (originally developed for laparoscopic methods) or a Reverdin needle can facilitate passage of the U-sutures. The biologic or mesh material used in the underlay technique should be tensioned so that the mobilized muscles passively close in the midline, if possible. There will be some instances where the muscles will not come together, and the mesh or biologic will be placed as a "bridging" material. As mentioned above, a bridged material will have greater risk for bulging and will not be a dynamic or neurotized portion of the abdominal wall. After placement of the underlay, the posterior rectus sheath and then the anterior rectus sheath can each be closed with standard technique *(Fig. 12.11)*.

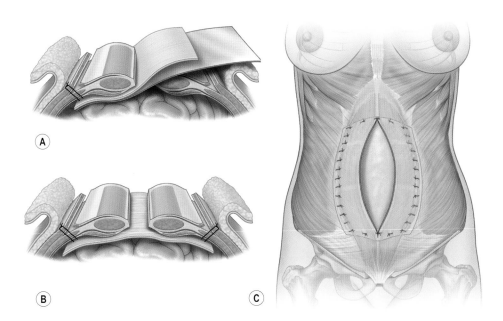

Fig. 12.11 Intraperitoneal placement of prosthetic material for ventral hernia repair. **(A)** Cross-sectional view of prosthetic placement, secured initially to one side. After initial separation of components, the underlay material is introduced and secured to the lateral musculature with a full-thickness U-suture. **(B)** If possible, the underlay is tensioned to bring both muscle complexes to the midline. If midline approximation is impossible, the mesh or biologic will be placed as a "bridging" material. This inherently poses a greater risk for bulging and will not be a dynamic or neurotized portion of the abdominal wall. After placement of the underlay, the posterior rectus sheath and then the anterior rectus sheath can each be closed with standard technique. **(C)** Anterior view of underlay suture postioning.

An underlay, alternatively, may be performed in a retrorectus position, where it is superficial to the peritoneal cavity (Rives–Stoppa method).[24] The peritoneum and posterior rectus sheath are closed, then a mesh or biologic is placed within the limits of the rectus sheath. The advantages include having the strength layer placed in proximity to the muscle sheath and muscle, and having the implant not in communication with the bowel. Disadvantages include the fact that it does not resurface the abdominal wall more broadly, and may leave the potential for herniation lateral to the rectus sheath, or through a component separation release site.

If the musculofascial edges are able to be reapproximated in such a defect, then an onlay can be performed instead. The putative advantages to an onlay include ease of use, the avoidance of a ring of U-sutures which may strangulate the fascia, and decreasing the risk of neuroma formation from injuring nerves through full-thickness sutures. Disadvantages include the possibility of contamination of the onlay material if skin edge breakdown exposes the material. Further, according to Rives–Stoppa principles, an onlay is more likely to be disrupted than an underlay, but this has not been convincingly demonstrated in the literature.

A successful onlay should also span from one external oblique to the contralateral external oblique to resurface the entire abdominal wall, and minimize the potential for a hernia in the central or lateral operative fields. Quilting sutures can be used in multiple locations to decrease seroma potential in the layer between the onlay and fascia *(Fig. 12.12)*. A drain may be placed in this layer as well.

In some instances, a "sandwich" technique involves both an underlay and an onlay for reinforcement. This has been anecdotally reported, and should be reserved for the direst of patients.

A frequent criticism of the separation of parts technique is the need for elevation of wide skin flaps. Particularly in the patient with comorbidities of obesity, diabetes, smoking history, or COPD, this predisposes the skin to edge ischemia and seroma. Saulis and Dumanian have championed a perforator-sparing technique that accounts for the fact that a single large perforator arising from the rectus abdominis in each hemiabdomen can substantially perfuse that hemiabdomen[25] *(Fig. 12.13)*. Such large-caliber perforators are found in the periumbilical region, and so if a circle of soft tissue a few centimeters wide is left attached, it will likely capture a sizeable perforator, thus minimizing ischemic soft-tissue complications. Typically, a lighted retractor is used to dissect around the stalk of tissue that is left attached. Detractors of this method raise the concern of missing a "Swiss cheese"-type hernia, yet these could be detectable from an intraperitoneal inspection. Others raise the point that, in a recurrent hernia, these perforators have likely been previously ligated, yet these do often recanalize between operations.

Perforator-sparing techniques do take slightly more time in the operating room, and may limit the degree of release to a minor extent. However, this method can be useful in those patients who are at risk for soft-tissue devitalization, such as in patients with peripheral arterial disease, obese patients, diabetics, or smokers. In the setting of a perforator-sparing technique, an underlay position for reinforcement material is preferred since the perforator and soft tissues attached to the fascia may limit the ability to place an onlay material (although slits in the mesh can be made, this may weaken the construct).

Plastic surgeons are typically not experienced with a laparoscope, and objections to laparoscopic hernia repair center around the fact that it does not realign muscles and does not

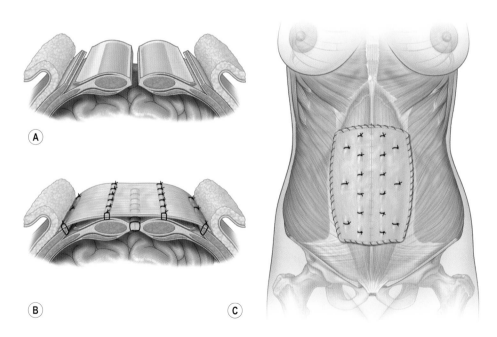

(A)

(B)

(C)

Fig. 12.12 Component separation with onlay synthetic mesh or biologic. **(A)** Cross-sectional view of separation of components, enabling midline approximation of the muscular complexes at the linea alba. **(B)** The onlay spans from one external oblique to the contralateral external oblique muscle, minimizing the potential for a hernia in the central or lateral operative fields. Full-thickness U-sutures are not necessary. Quilting sutures between the onlay and fascia can be placed to decrease seroma potential. Drains may be used above and below the onlay. **(C)** Anterior view showing a peripheral running suture and multiple quilting sutures.

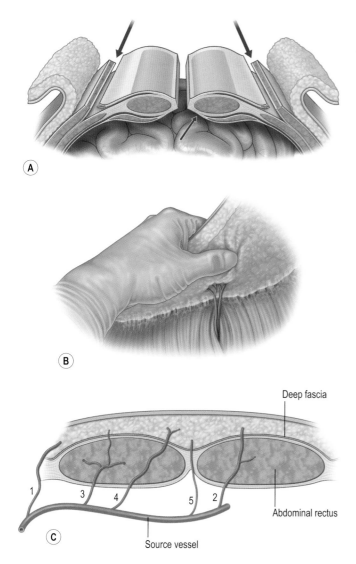

Fig. 12.13 (A) Cross-sectional illustration of the external oblique muscle release and adipocutaneous flap elevation as initial steps of component separation. **(B)** Perforator preservation during flap dissections decreases the risk of marginal skin necrosis and tissue loss. **(C)** Patterns of perforators: 1, external oblique perforator; 2, deep inferior epigastric artery perforator with large musculocutaneous branch; 3, intramuscular branching and small musculocutaneous perforator; 4, large musculocutaneous branch with no intramuscular branches; 5, septocutaneous perforator.

manage the excess skin or the hernia sac. It does not create an innervated abdominal wall with dynamic tension. Sophisticated techniques have emerged using a laparoscopic approach for component separation that is responsive to these objections.

While it is not laparoscopy of the peritoneal cavity *per se*, a laparoscope is indeed used to enter the plane between the external and internal oblique muscles via small incisions to perform essentially the same dissections as performed by open technique. The laparoscopic technique does not allow for the full advancement that an open technique does, but achieves approximately 90% of the goal, which is often sufficient. If mesh or biologic matrix is placed laparoscopically, it should be secured with absorbable tacking devices instead of permanent metallic screws to prevent future complications

of adhesions to the anchors, migration of anchors, or worse, fistulization to the anchors.[26,27]

Regional and distant autologous tissue repair

If the surgeon prefers an autologous reconstruction, and does not want to use a biologic matrix or a synthetic mesh, then the established technique of fascia lata grafting can be employed *(Fig. 12.14)*. In a 1998 report by Disa, a 32% recurrence rate was reported with this technique.[11] TFL grafting involves placing a longitudinal incision along the lateral aspect of one or both thighs. After dissecting through skin and subcutaneous tissues, the broad and dense fascia of the TFL is identified and mobilized. The tensor muscle itself (in the superior portion) is not harvested, but a broad sheet with a longitudinal "grain" of fibers is harvested. Five to 10 cm should be left above the knee to prevent lateral knee instability since the fascia lata is part of the iliotibial tract, which provides stability to the lateral knee. A graft as large as 28 × 14 cm can be harvested; if needed, two pieces can be sutured together. Drains are routinely placed in the donor site, and physical therapy for crutch or cane ambulation is recommended.

Because fascia lata is an autologous graft with low metabolic demand, it can become revascularized. It is less pliant than native rectus fascia since the lower extremity fascia is more densely developed in upright animals such as humans to decrease lymphedema and enhance venous return.

Beyond fascial grafts, a fascial flap can be utilized for closure. Rectus femoris musculocutaneous pedicled flap is one option.[28] Another option is a pedicled TFL flap based on the transverse branch of the lateral femoral circumflex vessels can reach the lower abdomen, and provide skin, subcutaneous bulk, and fascia. A more elegant solution is the free TFL musculocutaneous fascial flap. The anastomoses for the free flap can be performed to intraperitoneal vessels such as the gastroepiploic artery to create a one-step replacement for all the missing layers. Free flaps are more commonly utilized for tumor resection[12] than for hernia repair. A TFL free flap can also be taken of vascularized fascia alone, without skin.

Hershey and Butcher described the external oblique musculocutaneous flap in 1964.[29] The flap is rotational and based on the external oblique muscle and anterior rectus sheath with a small segment of skin attached. It is used to reconstruct an upper abdominal wall defect in one stage. With modification, the flap is useful in the correction of deformities in the upper two-thirds of the abdomen. Numerous other grafts and flaps have been described.[30]

Tissue expansion

The technique of fascial grafting or biologic or mesh material interposition is to provide for deficient fascia. Some patients not only have fascial deficiencies but also have skin and soft-tissue deficits. When soft-tissue coverage will be inadequate, the risk is of delayed healing, exposure, and contamination of biomaterials used in the repair, and of recurrent herniation from infection. While some biologics may be resilient in the face of exposure or contamination, it should be prevented when anticipated. Tissue expansion can meet this need.

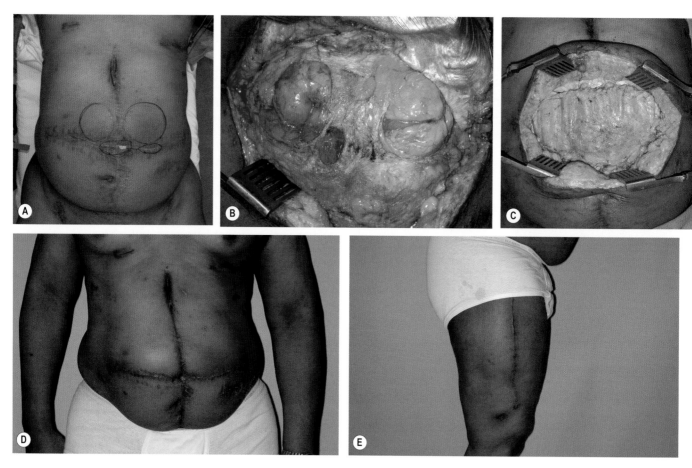

Fig. 12.14 Hernia repair with fascia lata graft. **(A)** Preoperative image with markings of multiple fascial defects. **(B)** Intraoperative image of the defects. **(C)** 20 × 15 cm fascia lata graft spanning the defects. **(D)** Postoperative image of abdomen. **(E)** Donor site. (Courtesy of Dr. David H. Song.)

Tissue expanders can be placed in the subcutaneous space, on top of the fascia and serially expanded over several weeks, recruiting additional skin. Studies have shown that the principles of tissue expansion are similar to that of the delay phenomenon.[31] After fascial reconstruction, the tissue expanders are removed, flaps elevated, and closed recruiting the viscoelastic properties of skin – creep and stress relaxation *(Fig. 12.15)*.

Not commonly done, the fascia itself can be expanded via a technique of placing tissue expanders in the plane between the internal and external oblique.[32] Both subcutaneous and interfascial tissue expander techniques are partially limited by the fact that the expander does not rest on a rigid platform (as in the scalp or on the chest wall for breast reconstruction). Because it is on mobile tissues, the expansion process expands both some tissue outward, and some tissue inward, in the path of least resistance. Hence, interfascial expansion is not commonly seen or reported.

Parastomal hernia repair

Parastomal hernias as subspecies of abdominal wall reconstruction present a notable challenge because the creation of a stoma is *de facto* the creation of a defect in the abdominal wall from which bowel emerges – the very definition of a hernia. Yet, it is a controlled defect designed only to allow the limited segment of bowel to emerge. Attenuation and enlargement of the fascial defect are sadly part of the natural history of a sizeable portion of the stoma-bearing population. Repairs may include reinforcing materials such as biologic matrices, since synthetics would be more prone to infection in the setting of stoma. Early data suggest a role for the use of a prophylactic placement of material to prevent late herniation, in combination with Sugarbaker keyhole or flap valve technique and/or resiting the ostomy.[33]

Abdominal wall transplantation

Patients undergoing intestinal or multiorgan transplantation may suffer from loss of abdominal domain, requiring reconstruction. In recent years, abdominal wall transplantation has been described and utilized in the setting of other organ transplants. Loss of volume from prior bowel surgery and loss of surface coverage of the abdominal wall from scarring, stomas, and fistulas can contribute to the problem. In addition, organ edema often prevents primary abdominal closure. The inferior epigastric vasculature is the pedicle typically used. The immunogenicity of the transplanted skin requires lifelong immunosuppression, rendering this reconstructive option to be restricted to be employed in conjunction with other transplantations.[34]

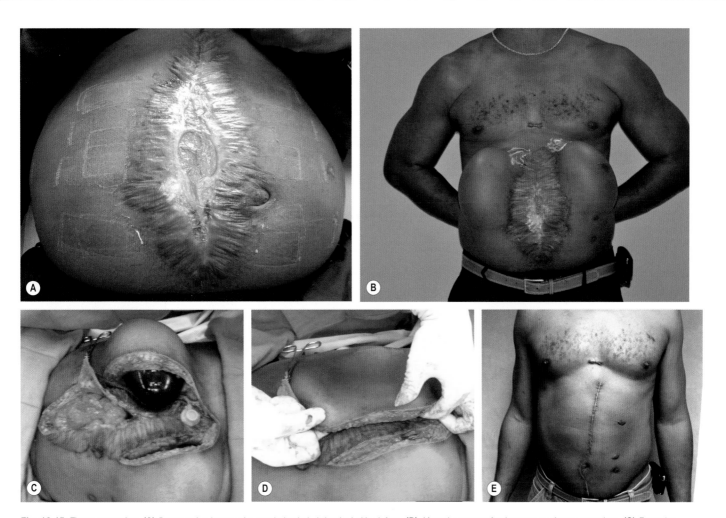

Fig. 12.15 Tissue expansion. **(A)** Preoperative image of a poorly healed abdominal skin defect. **(B)** After placement of subcutaneous tissue expanders. **(C)** Expander removal. **(D)** Transposition of expanded skin. **(E)** Postoperative result. (Courtesy of Dr. David H. Song.)

Adjuncts to repair

Adjunct techniques for optimizing outcomes include the use of drains, which may be placed in as many layers as are at risk for the formation of a collection. Drains in the paracolic gutters may be used, or placed in proximity to bowel or bladder repair sites. The potential space between an underlay and fascia can be drained, as can the layer between fascia and an overlay. At least two additional subcutaneous drains are recommended for those patients undergoing component separation, since wide degloving can cause seroma formation, especially in the obese.

In addition to drains, fibrin-based tissue glues have been reported in the subcutaneous layer to promote adherence of soft tissues to the fascia to prevent seroma formation. Alternatively, some authors note the use of quilting sutures from the skin flap down to the fascia to likewise ablate dead space and thus decrease the risk of seroma formation. A variant of quilting sutures is progressive-tension sutures (as used in abdominoplasty) whereby quilting sutures are used to advance the skin flaps on the fascia such that the final skin closure is tension-free. This technique may both facilitate closure as well as decrease seroma risk.[35]

Halsted's tenets still ring true 100 years later and are applicable to modern hernia surgery, including aseptic technique, atraumatic handling of tissues, sharp anatomic dissection, meticulous hemostasis, using nonreactive sutures, minimizing foreign body, avoiding nonphysiologic tension, and obliterating dead space. The specific steps in hernia repair are: (1) preparation of the wound by reducing bioburden; (2) realignment of muscles; (3) reinforcing attenuated areas; (4) minimizing foreign body; and (5) controlling dead space to prevent seroma which will delay revascularization *(Fig. 12.16)*.

Postoperative care

Postoperative management

Perioperative management includes DVT prophylaxis. At the very least, sequential compression devices and early ambulation are indicated. In the vast majority of cases, chemoprophylaxis is initiated, including heparin, low-molecular weight fractionated heparins, and/or coumadinization postoperatively. In many trauma centers or in those patients with an established history of venous thromboembolism, caval filters (permanent and reversible) may be utilized.

Consideration should be made to keeping the patient intubated on the night of surgery and offering a deeper extubation

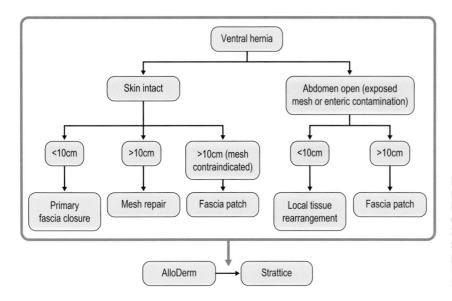

Fig. 12.16 Modified algorithm for abdominal wall reconstruction. (After Disa JJ, Goldberg NH, Carlton JM, *et al.* Restoring abdominal wall integrity in contaminated tissue-deficient wounds using autologous fascia grafts. Plast Reconstr Surg 1998;101:979–986.) The expanding usage of biologics such as AlloDerm and Strattice has replaced the use of fascial patches and augments primary fascial closure, and in many instances synthetic meshes. Other algorithms have been offered in the literature.[30]

on the first postoperative day. An agitated extubation may create nonphysiologic forces of bucking against an endotracheal tube and could disrupt the repair. Prior to considering extubation, peak airway pressures should be compared from the beginning of the operation to the end. If there is a substantial rise, the patient may benefit from ongoing ventilatory support until abdominal musculature has stretched sufficiently.

Patients with abdominal wall reconstruction may require ICU care and monitoring to support their fluid requirements since they will sequester fluids in the third space. Pulmonary optimization including ventilator support may be required since peak airway pressures may rise with embarrassment of diaphragmatic excursion. Monitoring for abdominal compartment syndrome via indwelling bladder pressure transducers may be indicated. Vasopressor support should be available if required, and a vigilant response to the systemic inflammatory response syndrome. Reported cases of abdominal wall reconstruction have a low mortality risk, depending on patient characteristics, screening out of inappropriate medical candidates, and fastidious adherences to techniques and principles.

Nutritional support

This can be provided by total parenteral nutrition (TPN) or early enteral feeds. Early feeding to the gut (via oral intake, nasogastric feeding tube, feeding gastrostomy, or jejunostomy) is contentious. Proponents suggest that returning the bowel to its normal function as early as possible will decrease the risk of bacterial translocation and septic sequelae. The further addition of immunonutrients, such as arginine, glutamine, omega-3 fatty acids, nucleotides, and others, has been shown to up-regulate host immune responses, to control inflammatory responses, and to improve nitrogen balance and protein synthesis after injury. Opponents of early enteral feeds cite the risks of abdominal pain, nausea, and vomiting, and regurgitation causing aspiration pneumonia.

TPN can incur the complications of catheter sepsis, electrolyte abnormalities, hyperglycemia, and fatty infiltration of the liver. When enteral feeding is not suitable, TPN can provide

sufficient nutrition to stave off catabolic consequences of surgical recovery.

Antibiotic therapy

Duration of antibiotics also elicits great controversy, depending on whether it is for therapeutic intent or prophylaxis. Current state-of-the art data unequivocally indicate that a dose for prophylaxis should be administered intravenously 30–60 minutes before the case starts and may require redosing depending on the duration of the case and half-life of the antibiotic. For clean cases, only the single preoperative dose may suffice, but common usage patterns are 24 hours of antibiotics for prophylaxis.

With regard to antibiotic treatment in recurrent hernias, there is emerging thought that the predisposing factors include a history of prior infection, and the potential for residual nidus of infection. A recurrent hernia repair, certainly one with retained prior synthetic mesh, should be treated not only as prophylaxis, but also as therapeutic intent for a longer course. Dirty and contaminated cases should be treated with therapeutic intent. Cases with violation of the gastrointestinal tract should be offered broader coverage for anaerobic as well as Gram-negative bacteria. Smokers may be considered at heightened risk for infection and prophylaxis may be extended in those cases for 48 hours. Additional comorbidities of COPD, diabetes mellitus, and obesity should impact on the decision of antibiotic duration. Patients who were infected in their operative interventions may retain dormant bacteria that reactivate, leading some authors to consider "once infected, always infected." Albeit an obvious overstatement, this admonition should precipitate considerations for longer duration of antibiotics than simply one preoperative dose.

The question of continuing empiric antibiotic therapy until drains are removed has not been studied in a prospective trial, and so remains unresolved. In vascular surgery, continuation of antibiotics until drains are removed has been shown to decrease the rate of infection. The indiscriminant use of antibiotics invites the emergence of multiple-antibiotic-resistant bacteria, vancomycin-resistant *Enterococcus*, and MRSA,

Clostridium difficile, as well as toxicity related to antibiotics, alteration of normal flora, and other adverse events. Topical antimicrobials such as chlorhexidine-impregnated patches at the drain site may be able to obviate the need for systemic antibiotics, by offering local protection against an ascending infection related to the drain. This is not proven with prospective data.

Drain management

Because of the risk for deep space collections near anastomoses and areas of contamination, and because of the risk for hematomas and seromas in the various dissected layers, the use of drains is essential in abdominal wall reconstruction. The range in most studies of drain use ranges from a minimum of one to as many as five, with two to three being normative. Large drains are placed in areas of potential hematoma or spillage, and smaller or thinner drains may be utilized in areas of seroma risk. Closed suction drains are used in the overwhelming majority of cases.

Drains are maintained for at least a week, and in the majority of instances for approximately 2 weeks and removed based on the criteria of amount and nature of the drainage. In porous mesh or biologic mesh use, peritoneal fluid may communicate into the subcutaneous spaces, and closed suction drains will have to be emptied frequently until the mesh is repopulated with collagen and cells. Occasionally drains may remain for several weeks until the surgeon deems them suitable for removal. Should a postoperative collection or infection develop in an area without a drain, or after drain removal, or despite a drain, interventional radiologists may be required to place additional drains as indicated.

If a seroma develops after drain removal in the subcutaneous space, it may be aspirated at frequent intervals, sclerosed with a topical sclerosant, or a percutaneous drain may have to be reintroduced. Obese patients are at particular risk for seromas since even with small movements the pannus is repeatedly avulsed off the deep layers because of its weight, preventing adhesion of the soft tissues to fascia. Because biologic meshes such as the dermal matrices and pericardial sheets are made acellular, they are porous to fluid and peritoneal fluid may drain into adjacent layers through the biologic until it is repopulated with cells over the first few weeks.

Abdominal binders

Abdominal binders can provide compression in the postoperative interval. This may help with minimizing risks for seroma and also supporting the deeper fascial repair, although this has not been scientifically proven. One must consider however that in the setting of wide subcutaneous flaps, a binder may actually compress marginally perfused tissue and lead to infarction of the tissue and suture line ischemia. A compromise is to position an abdominal binder after a period of observation of 48–96 hours once skin edges are noted to be either healing uneventfully or demarcating.

Analgesia

Pain pumps that continuously infiltrate lidocaine or bupivacaine via narrow-gauge catheters on to the muscle sheath of the rectus abdominis have gained in popularity. Literature is inconclusive since closed suction drain in proximity to the catheters may effectively aspirate out the local anesthetic. Regional anesthetic via epidurals (alone or in combination with general anesthesia) has been shown to be effective in improving pulmonary toilet, pain control, and ileus, but has limitations. Lower mean arterial pressures are reported with epidural anesthesia, and this may contribute to hypoperfusion. Timing of anticoagulation therapy for venous thromboembolism prevention is critical when placing or removing an epidural catheter to decrease the risk of hematoma formation. Heparin may have to be stopped for a few hours prior to removal of the catheter.

Muscle relaxation

Some centers have reported on use of botulinum toxin at the time of operation into the lateral musculature of the abdominal wall – the external obliques, internal obliques, and transversus muscles.[36] This temporarily attenuates the force of these muscles and decreases spasm and pain, and diminishes the lateral disruptive forces which might disrupt a healing repair. Botulinum toxin may be administered a week in advance so that maximal effect is appreciated at the time of surgery. Contraindications include neuromuscular disorders such as myasthenia gravis and Guillain–Barré syndrome.

Activity

There is broad consensus that only extremely limited activity should be undertaken for at least the first 6 weeks of convalescence. In patients felt to be at higher than average risk, prohibitions for heavy exertion may be extended for months, and for the patient undergoing reconstruction of the multiply recurrent hernia, a lifetime of limited physical activity may be indicated. Those in physically demanding vocations may need to be retrained or reassigned to different occupations.

Outcomes, prognosis, and complications

Outcomes

Current data estimate the rate of hernia recurrence in a range from 2% to 54%, depending on the type of repair (mesh 2–36% versus suture repair 12–54%). Suture repair of primary ventral has reported recurrence rates of 25–52%.[37]

Prognosis

Prognosis is a function of patient and technique factors. Patient factors for poorer outcomes are the presence of comorbidities. There are no quantitative predictive models for the relative risk associated with each independent risk factor such as obesity, diabetes, malnutrition, COPD, steroid use, and smoking status. It cannot be said if the risks are additive or multiplicative, but the greater the number of risk factors, the greater the rate of complications.

The number of prior attempts at abdominal wall herniorrhaphy is predictive of the relative risk of failure. In a population-based study of approximately 10 000 patients, the 5-year reoperative rate was 23.8% after the first reoperation, 35.3% after the second, and 38.7% after the third operation.[38]

With the addition of novel biologics and synthetic meshes, advancements in laparoscopic techniques, refinements in ICU management, and better understanding of abdominal wall mechanics, the success rate for abdominal wall reconstruction should continue to improve.

Complications

Recurrence

The chief complication would be recurrence of the hernia and this has already been discussed. Other complications include hematoma, seroma, infection, pain, bulging, and weakness of the abdominal wall, in addition to donor site considerations.

Wound breakdown

Skin breakdown leading to exposed mesh or biologic may occur. The biologic mesh should be prevented from desiccation with either moist dressings such as NPWT or topical antimicrobials such as silver sulfadiazine. Granulation is likely to form through a biologic or light-weight mesh, although the concern for infection is heightened. Alternatively, the patient may be returned to the operating room for excision of devitalized skin edges and readvancement closure over drains. Hyperbaric oxygen can be used for skin edge ischemia and hypoperfusion. Studies of hyperbaric oxygen demonstrate the increased ability to deliver oxygen locally to healing tissues by increasing the oxygen-carrying capacity of dissolved oxygen in the blood.[39]

If synthetic mesh devices are used in the operation, and a periprosthetic infection develops, it will likely necessitate its removal. Certain macroporous or light-weight meshes may be able to be treated with local wound care if exposed. Biologic meshes may be more resilient under infective or contaminative situations, but they are certainly not resistant to infection or contamination. Certain biologic meshes have been shown in case studies as well as in prospective trials to be able to withstand their use in contaminated and even dirty abdominal wall reconstruction cases. Biofilm physiology is again implicated for those cases where the wound appears to cyclically granulate-close, then ulcerate in various areas. This indicates a deep nidus, which has not been and cannot be eradicated without surgical removal of the infected nidus.

Adhesions

All surgery incites an inflammatory reaction and this reaction can cause adhesions of the intra-abdominal viscera to the abdominal wall. Any surgeon who performs a laparotomy in a nonvirgin abdomen anticipates adhesions. The reactions that cause adhesion formation can be heightened by foreign-body reaction to synthetic sutures, meshes, anchors, and contaminants. During abdominal wall reconstruction, great care should be exercised to interpose omentum between the bowel and the abdominal wall. When omentum is not available, Seprafilm (composed of hyaluronic acid and carboxymethylcellulose) may be useful as a barrier to impede adhesion formation. It is possible that biologic meshes may elicit a lower foreign-body reaction and thus have a lower rate of adhesion formation and may not require additional techniques such as Seprafilm. Autologous grafts such as fascia lata will likely have the fewest adhesions.

Minimizing adhesion formation is important to decrease the risk of bowel obstruction and internal hernia formation. Should a repeat laparotomy be needed, ideally the hernia repair and repair materials should be amenable to these purposes. It is possible to perform a routine laparotomy through native reconstructed muscle and through fascia lata graft. If a flap has been used in abdominal wall reconstruction, the plane between the flap and native tissues should be developed to prevent injury to the pedicle of the flap, which would compromise blood flow to portions of the flap which are likely still to be dependent on the original axial blood flow for perfusion. Once revascularized, biologic meshes can also be treated like fascia, entered in the midline, and sutured back, as in the case of a virgin abdomen. If synthetic meshes have not been incorporated, they cannot be simply sutured back, but must be replaced from at least one point of incorporation to the next point of incorporation into the soft tissues.

Seroma

Complications of seroma can be managed with serial aspiration with sterile technique, introduction of a sclerosant such as Betadine or tetracycline into the seroma activity, or placement of a percutaneous drain. Seromas refractory to these techniques may require operative ablation of the seroma cavity by excising the pseudobursa that has formed, and closing the new space over drains. For the seroma requiring operative intervention, additional techniques such as quilting sutures or fibrin glues should be given due consideration.

Secondary hernias

The occurrence of a hernia such as a spigelian hernia at the linea semilunaris where the external oblique tendon is released from the anterior rectus sheath aponeurosis should be considered a major complication of the components separation technique.

Pain

Most patients postoperatively will have pain. This is appropriate and is managed with either epidurals or patient-controlled analgesia pumps during the hospitalization. Thereafter the patient may be placed on long-acting opioids like continuous-release oxycodone or a fentanyl patch. If chronic pain develops, its etiology must be sought. The causes of pain may be nonneuropathic such as periosteal reaction to bone anchors or mechanical pressure. Neuropathic pain may be caused by compression from fibrosis, entanglement in suture, direct nerve injury, or transection creating an end-neuroma or neuroma-in-continuity. To minimize this occurrence in the first place, some authors advocate use of long-term absorbable sutures instead of permanent sutures during the repair. Even with absorbable sutures, if nerves have been injured, nonsurgical modalities such as massage, desensitization, ultrasound, electromagnetic pulses, and acupuncture to myofascial trigger points may be of benefit. The first line for neuropathic pain is use of neuronal stabilizing medications such as tricyclic antidepressants, anticonvulsants, corticosteroids, capsaicin, nonsteroidal anti-inflammatory drugs, and narcotic opioids. If pain can be localized to a specific trigger site such as via a positive Tinel sign, the offending neuroma can be blocked with local anesthetic to see if it alleviates the pain, and if so, it can be surgically excised. A postulated mechanism for nerve injury is when an underlay is performed; full-thickness U-stitches are placed from the fascia muscle down to the underlay mesh and back up again. These can inadvertently compress motor and/or sensory nerves of the abdominal wall. Pain may arise from segmental intercostal, ilioinguinal, iliohypogastric, or genital nerves.

Early intervention for neuropathic pain is indicated to prevent the development of intractable complications such as reflex sympathetic dystrophy or chronic regional pain syndrome. Surgical intervention may require removal of the offending sutures, staples, or mesh alongside neurolysis and/ or neurectomy of the involved nerves.

Secondary procedures

Secondary procedures for abdominal wall reconstruction include scar revision, contour improvement, correction of stretch or diastasis, reconstruction of the umbilicus, and amelioration of pain.

Scar revision techniques are employed once the patient's scars have matured over months to years. If the wound was originally closed under tension, then scar excision and closure can improve a wide, hypertrophic, or keloidal scar. A thick indurated scar can be managed with triamcinolone injections from the early postoperative period, but the scar may become wide and atrophic with too frequent injections.

Contour corrections can be afforded to those patients who have lost weight (now that they are able to exercise and have restoration of satiety signal from return of the viscera to the abdominal cavity) and have laxity of their abdominal wall. Patients may complain of a bulge and potentially even may confuse this with a recurrence of the ventral defect. This involves plication and imbrication of the fascia without necessarily entering the peritoneal cavity, and can be done on an outpatient basis.

Some laxity without true recurrence may be created when biologic or synthetic meshes are used in a bridging capacity. Where there is no muscle (if component separation has not allowed the full recentralization of the rectus abdominis muscles), there will be a bulge and stretch of the bridging material, whether it is fascia lata graft, biologic, or synthetic compounds. A bulge can be distinguished from a recurrent fascial defect by the fact that there is a continuous peritoneal border or contour, stable peritoneal volumes, no threatened visceral injury, and a normal CT scan. Intraoperative factors that may predispose to a late postoperative bulge include the presence of significant visceral edema at time of closure, significant weight gain or weight loss postoperatively, and suboptimal techniques. Plication is applicable in these situations as well.

If a concomitant panniculectomy was not performed during the hernia operation, this can be performed secondarily. It is not contraindicated to perform a panniculectomy concomitantly with the original hernia operation, but in certain scenarios with concerns for wound healing, it should be delayed to a secondary operation. Prior incisions such as a chevron incision, bucket-handle incision, or a Kocher's subcostal incision should be noted. These may preclude the ability of the surgeon to undermine flaps during a panniculectomy or abdominoplasty. Being mindful of previous incisions, which may interrupt blood supply to skin flaps, a midabdominal panniculectomy is most appropriate in a severely overweight patient. An abdominoplasty-type incision can be entertained for those patients with lower BMI and few or no comorbidities.

If the umbilicus is absent due to prior operations, it can be reconstructed via one of several techniques, which employ local flaps for a neoumbilicoplasty.

Donor site morbidity from TFL harvest is low, but physical therapy and crutch or cane ambulation are needed for a period of a few weeks until the iliotibial tract heals for knee stability. Scar revision or contour correction at donor sites is somewhat needed. Where musculocutaneous flaps are harvested, such as a TFL or rectus femoris pedicled flap or TFL free flap, donor defects are large and are frequently skin-grafted at the index operation. Revision of skin-grafted donor sites is performed via either serial scar excision or tissue expansion of the surrounding area to recruit normal skin to replace a previously skin-grafted donor area. Timing of revision should be once the skin graft is mature, without fissures or erosions, and the surrounding tissues have regained mobility and suppleness.

Donor site morbidity of component separation or rectus abdominis musculofascial advancement can include pain or bulging at the release site related to decreasing the number of muscle layers from three to two – a necessary compromise to recreate the midline. Bulging can be plicated with onlay of synthetic or biologic meshes as a secondary procedure in the subcutaneous space, using it essentially as an abdominal binder.

Secondary procedures to improve pain can be offered, such as removal of anchors or permanent sutures once the fascia has healed, or release of entrapment neuropathies if sensory nerves have become entrapped in the repair.

Conclusions

Abdominal wall reconstruction employs the full range of techniques in the plastic surgical armamentarium, including adherence to the principle of the reconstructive ladder. Simple defects may: (1) be closed primarily; (2) be closed with fascial grafts such as fascia lata; (3) be tissue-expanded to expand both skin and fascia; (4) utilize local flaps such as a "components separation"; or (5) be distant free flaps.

Utilizing the full panoply of methods, abdominal wall defects can be successfully reconstructed to minimize the recurrence of ventral fascial defects. This requires appropriate patient selection, optimization of the patient's medical status, intensive postoperative management, and ongoing psychosocial support.

Access the complete references list online at **http://www.expertconsult.com**

1. Ramirez OM, Ruas E, Dellon AL. "Components separation" method for closure of abdominal-wall defects: an anatomic and clinical study. *Plast Reconstr Surg.* 1990;86:519–526.

   This seminal paper describes 10 cadaver dissections of the abdominal wall with the purpose of determining the amount of mobilization possible by dissecting each layer of the abdominal wall versus the entire complex as a block. The mobility achieved, allowing for functional transfer of abdominal wall components, negates the need for distant muscle flaps. This set the stage for later works by multiple authors and essentially defining today's standard of care for abdominal wall reconstructions applicable in many cases.

3. Luijendijk RW, Hop WC, Van Den Tol MP, et al. A comparison of suture repair with mesh repair for incisional hernia. *N Engl J Med.* 2000;343:392–398.

   This landmark prospective multi-institutional European study evaluated 200 cases of primary hernia repair with repair reinforced with mesh. The investigators found that retrofascial preperitoneal repair with polypropylene mesh is superior to suture repair with regard to the recurrence of hernia, even in patients with small defects. However, even with this significant finding, recurrence rates remain high at 10-year follow-up (approximately 30%)

8. Gibson CL. Post-operative intestinal obstruction. *Ann Surg.* 1916;63:442–451.

9. Dixon CF. Repair of incisional hernia. *Surg Gynecol Obstet.* 1929;48:700.

11. Disa JJ, Goldberg NH, Carlton JM, et al. Restoring abdominal wall integrity in contaminated tissue-deficient wounds using autologous fascia grafts. *Plast Reconstr Surg.* 1998;101:979–986.

    After conducting animal studies, the authors present their experience with nonvascularized tensor fascia latae autografts in a series of patients in whom prosthetic mesh was contraindicated, or components separation impossible.

   Recurrence rates, local complications, and donor site morbidity were within acceptable limits. Several patients underwent subsequent laparotomy for other purposes, at which point the transferred fascia was revascularized (concordant with the authors' previous findings in animal experiments). Maximal graft dimension was 28 (14 cm. The text includes a simple algorithm quoted in this chapter (Fig. 12.16).

25. Saulis AS, Dumanian GA. Periumbilical rectus abdominis perforator preservation significantly reduces superficial wound complications in "separation of parts" hernia repairs. *Plast Reconstr Surg.* 2002;109:2275–2280; discussion 2281–2.

    Acknowledging the strengths of the "component separation" method, Saulis and Dumanian point out the weaknesses of the method, particularly regarding wound breakdown associated with the wide undermining that is part and parcel of the technique. By preserving the periumbilical rectus abdominis perforators, the authors have shown reduction in wound complications while enabling similar advancement distances and maintaining acceptable hernia recurrence rates.

29. Hershey FB, Butcher HR Jr. Repair of defects after partial resection of the abdominal wall. *Am J Surg.* 1964;107:586–590.

30. Rohrich RJ, Lowe JB, Hackney FL, et al. An algorithm for abdominal wall reconstruction. *Plast Reconstr Surg.* 2000;105:202–216; quiz 217.

    This continuing medical education article provides a good overview of abdominal wall anatomy, and provides an additional perspective to the various techniques of reconstructing abdominal wall defects and offers a reconstructive algorithm for partial and complete defects, addressing location of the defect. Autologous tissue transfer sources are discussed (cutaneous, local, and distant flaps), with critique.

13

Reconstruction of male genital defects

Stan Monstrey, Peter Ceulemans, Nathalie Roche, Philippe Houtmeyers,
Nicolas Lumen, and Piet Hoebeke

SYNOPSIS

This chapter deals with the following topics:

- Genital embryology and anatomy.
- Congenital genital defects:
  - exstrophy and epispadias
  - disorders of sex development (DSD)
  - buried penis
  - micropenis
  - reconstructive options for penile insufficiency.
- Traumatic genital defects:
  - general reconstructive options: skin grafts, pedicled flaps, microsurgery
  - specific indications: Fournier's gangrene, penile cancer.
- Reconstruction of male genitalia in the female-to-male (FTM) transsexual
  - vaginectomy, reconstruction of the fixed urethra, scrotoplasty
  - metaidoioplasty
  - complete phallic reconstruction: radial forearm phalloplasty, alternative phalloplasty
  - prostheses.

Introduction

Nowadays, reconstructive surgery of the male genitalia is increasingly performed within the context of a genitourinary reconstructive team which can include plastic surgeons, urologists, colorectal surgeons, gynecologists, and orthopedic surgeons. The essence of a reconstructive team is reflected in this chapter, which mainly is the collaborative work of plastic surgeons and urologists. Plastic surgery techniques and traditions continue to play an important role in the reconstructive armamentarium of all who aim to repair genital defects.

In this chapter, we first discuss the relevant (genital) embryology and anatomy, then provide a complete overview of congenital and acquired genital deformities and finally, present the scope of past and current surgical techniques that may be used to accomplish the reconstructive goals.

Basic science: genital embryology and anatomy

Genital embryology

Genetic sex

Genetic sex of the embryo is established at conception. The ovum, containing 22 autosomes and an X chromosome, is penetrated by one of the surrounding spermatozoa, half of which have an X chromosome and the other half of which have a Y chromosome. The sperm donates either an X or Y chromosome, thereby establishing genetic sexual assignment.

The embryos of both sexes develop identically for approximately 6 weeks' gestation, known as the indifferent stage. During this time, the embryo becomes tabularized as the primitive gut is formed to terminate in the cloacal membrane. At the 6th week, the urorectal septum begins to grow downward and inward from the sides into the cloacal cavity, thereby separating the cloaca into the bladder and rectum.

Externally, a mound of mesoderm with a midline groove develops cephalocaudal to the cloacal membrane. This is known as the indifferent genital tubercle. As the midline mesenchyme progressively fuses in a caudal direction from the umbilicus, the genital primordial fuse to form a genital eminence.

Gonadal sex

Gonadal sex (differentiated stage) begins at the 7th week of intrauterine life. Evidence suggests that a locus on the Y chromosome (H-Y antigen) induces testicular development by causing differentiation of the seminiferous tubules. Today, many genes are described that play a role in male gonadal development, such as SRY, SOX9, AMH, SF1, DHH, ATRX, and DMRT.

There are three endocrine hormones produced that explain the male differentiation. The first is müllerian-inhibiting factor produced transiently by the Sertoli cells in the seminiferous tubules, causing regression of the müllerian duct system (9–11 weeks). At the same time, Leydig cells in the seminiferous tubules begin to produce a hormone analogous to testosterone. Testosterone plays two roles: (1) completion of maturation of the seminiferous tubules, epididymis, vas deferens, and seminal vesicles and (2) extra testicular male development by irreversible reduction to dihydrotestosterone made possible by the enzyme 5a-reductase. Dihydrotestosterone is responsible for the virilization of the external genitalia and the anterior urethra.

Phenotypic sex

Phenotypic sex is 'determined' by whether the genital tubercle develops into a male or female pattern. In the male, urogenital swellings migrate ventrally and anteriorly to form the scrotum. The genital tubercle develops by elongation and cylindrical growth. At the same time, urethral folds close over the urethral groove, thereby establishing a urethra and a midline raphe. Mesenchymal tissue coalesces to surround the urethra and form the corpus spongiosum. This development is entirely under the influence (or absence) of testosterone, testosterone derivatives (i.e., dihydrotestosterone), and 5a-reductase and occurs between 6 and 13 weeks' gestation (*Fig. 13.1*). The prepuce grows to cover the penile glans but is not influenced by dihydrotestosterone.

In the female embryo, the lack of testosterone-influenced virilization holds the urogenital sinus and the genital tubercle in a fixed perineal position. The urethral groove remains unclosed (folds develop into labia minora), and the genital tubercle remains static in size but bends ventrally. The labia majora enlarge, migrate caudally, and fuse to form the posterior fourchette. It is this lack of closure of the ventral urethra (a 'nonevent') that causes the female perineum to be shorter and the introitus to be located in a more caudal position.

Genital anatomy

Male genital anatomy is unique in the human body and evolved phylogenetically as a means of protection from trauma and disease. This evolution has proved essential for the human race to continue procreation and elimination.

Genital fascia

Perhaps the most obvious protective mechanism is the testicular (and penile) withdrawal on exposure to physical stress (like hypothermia or blunt trauma), which causes the unique cremasteric muscles to contract, thereby withdrawing the testicles and shrinking the scrotum as close to the body as possible. Otherwise, the testicles hang free, ostensibly to provide the best milieu for sperm development. At the same time, the penile corporal bodies and the urethra also retract and shrink in size, although the penile skin does not have the same retraction properties of the scrotal skin. Both the penis and the

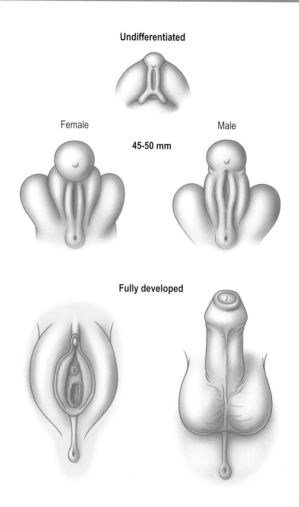

Fig. 13.1 The definitive phenotypic external genital growth that occurs *in utero* under the influence (or absence) of testosterone, dihydrotestosterone, and 5a-reductase. The influence of these virilizing hormones causes the genital tubercle to enlarge, the urethral folds to meet and close ventrally, and the scrotum to migrate medially and posteriorly. Any hormone deficit or receptor site inadequacy leads to an external female genitalia tendency ('phenotype by default').

scrotum have redundant skin coverage with their own separate blood supply and underlying supportive superficial fascial system.

The penis contains specially designed tunical tissues that surround the penile corporal bodies and have the ability to expand and hold the inflow of blood and to prevent, along with venous valve mechanisms, the egress of blood during erections. The tunica albuginea fascia envelops the corporal bodies tightly but is perforated by an intercavernosal membranous septum that allows blood flow between the corpora cavernosa. The tunical tissues are thick over the dorsal and lateral aspects of each corporal body but thin out in the ventral sulcus where the urethra and corpus spongiosum are located. The tunica also thins out beneath the glans penis cap where it has direct vascular contact with the glans.

Overlying the tunica is the deep penile fascia (Buck fascia), a strong laminar structure that tightly surrounds and binds the corpora cavernosa together and, in the case of the corpus spongiosum, envelops these tissues into a single-functioning entity. The urethra and its overlying corpus spongiosum are also protected proximally by surrounding muscles and by their location within the intercorporal groove distally. Buck

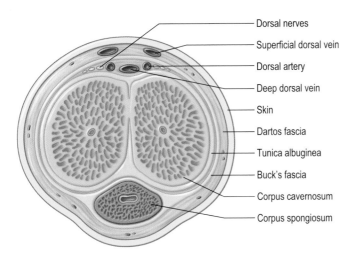

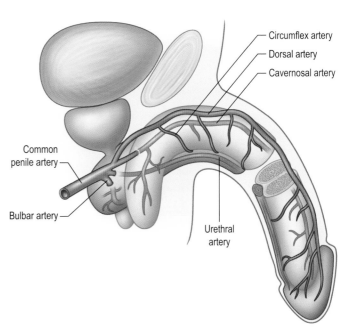

Fig. 13.2 A cross-section of the penile shaft illustrates the superficial and deep fascial layers and their relationships to the corporal bodies and neurovascular structures. (From: Quartey JK. Microcirculation of penile and scrotal skin. *Atlas Urol Clin North Am*. 1997;5:1–9.).

Fig. 13.3 The deep arterial vascularization to the penis arises from branches of the common penile arteries. (From: Quartey JK. Microcirculation of penile and scrotal skin. *Atlas Urol Clin North Am*. 1997;5:1–9.)

fascia carries important neurovascular structures to the glans penis, including the deep dorsal vein and arteries, the deep dorsal nerves of the penis, the circumflex arteries and veins, and the penile lymphatics *(Fig. 13.2)*.[1]

The penile glans itself is a vascular spongiosum containing unique sensory endings that are erogenous and tactile. The glans epithelium is a unique uroepithelium that contains sensory cells, particularly around the corona. The glans is naturally covered and protected by a prepuce that consists of inner and outer laminae. The inner lamina consists of uroepithelium that is similar to that of the glans and, in fact, developmentally separates from the glans in the last trimester and after birth. The outer lamina consists of epithelium that is consistent with the glabrous skin of the penile shaft. Superficial to Buck fascia but beneath the penile shaft skin and prepuce lays the superficial fascial system, defined by dartos fascia. This fascial layer is a continuation of the Scarpa fascia superiorly and the Colles fascia inferiorly and surrounds the penis from the penoscrotal and peno-pubic angles to the prepuce.

Dartos fascia contains its own vascular plexus that allows overlying skin islands to be elevated on its independent blood supply.

Colles fascia is a deep, tight, triangular fascial system that arises laterally from the inferior pelvic rami and posteriorly from the perineal membrane to protect the genitalia from toxins, trauma, and infections (and envelops both testicles circumferentially, as the tunica dartos). Colles fascia is analogous to the dartos fascia on the penis, and thus skin island flaps can be elevated on the vascular plexus carried on this fascia *(see Fig. 9.11)*.[2]

Overlying both testicles, the epididymis, and the cord structures is a loose, well-vascularized superficial fascial layer. The tunica vaginalis invests the testicles, and the parietal tunica vaginalis acts as the 'vaginal space,' which can be likened to the peritoneal cavity. Although the testicles are anchored within the scrotum, they move separately and independently on their cremasteric systems. The neurovascular supply to the testicles is dedicated to the viability of the

testicles, epididymis, and cord structures (vas deferens) as well as to continued sperm production.

Genital blood supply

The genitalia have two separate arterial sources. The first is the deep vascular system originating from the deep internal pudendal artery. The paired pudendal arteries originate from the internal iliac arteries, pass along the borders of the inferior pelvic rami, and then give off the perineal and scrotal branches before continuing as the common penile arteries. After exiting from the Alcock canal, a split in the obturator fascia that runs from the lesser sciatic foramen to the ischial tuberosity along the sidewall of the ischiorectal fossa, each common penile artery gives off three branches (bulbar, urethral, cavernosal), and terminates in the dorsal artery of the penis, which runs within Buck fascia distally to terminate in the balanitic arteries. Within Buck fascia, the dorsal penile arteries are coiled and tortuous compared with the deep dorsal vein, which is linear and straight. This anatomy may have something to do with erectile function *(Fig. 13.3)*.[3]

The perineal branch of the pudendal artery is just superficial to Colles fascia and has an unpredictable length, but its central location and strong collateral supply make it a mainstay of genitourinary flap reconstruction. The scrotal branch of the perineal artery passes along the fold between the lateral scrotum and medial thigh and arborizes within the tunica dartos *(Fig. 13.4)*.

The second blood supply of the penis is the superficial external pudendal system –branches of the femoral arteries. The femoral artery typically gives off a superficial external pudendal artery and a deep external pudendal artery. The superficial external pudendal artery supplies vascularity to

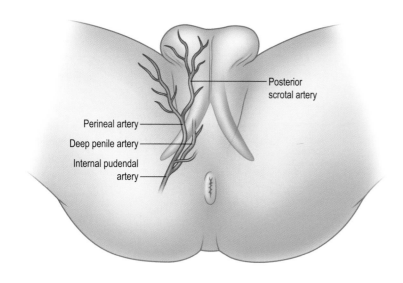

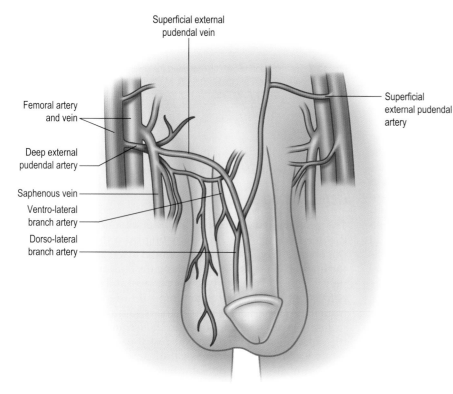

the dartos fascia and genital skin. The deep external pudendal artery arises as a separate branch and passes into the genital skin as the lateral inferior pudendal artery, which then separates into a dorsolateral branch supplying the dorsal and lateral penile shaft skin and an inferior branch supplying the ventral penile skin and the anterior plane of the scrotum (the anterior scrotal artery) *(Fig. 13.5)*. This arrangement allows surgeons to elevate long axial and transverse flaps with relative safety and still cover the shaft donor site with the adjacent skin.

The penile venous system also has an accompanying dual blood supply. The superficial system arises from the distal penile shaft and passes to the superficial dorsal vein within the dartos fascia to drain the penile shaft skin. In approximately 70% of anatomic studies, the superficial dorsal vein empties into the left saphenous vein. Other vascular patterns include connections into the right saphenous vein (10%), left femoral vein (7%), and inferior epigastric vein (3%); in 10%, the deep dorsal vein runs as a dual supply and empties into the saphenous veins bilaterally. These collateral veins are usually of different caliber and are asymmetric in their course *(Fig. 13.6)*.

The vas deferens, epididymis, and testes are vascularized from the retroperitoneal blood supply, primarily the spermatic artery, which originates from the aorta, and the deferential artery, which supplies the vas deferens. In addition,

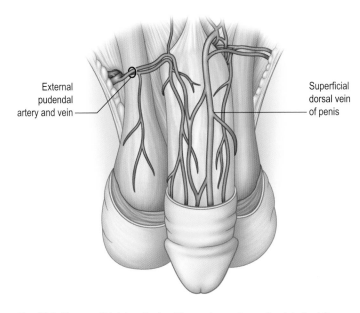

External pudendal artery and vein

Superficial dorsal vein of penis

Fig. 13.6 The superficial dorsal vein of the penis usually empties into the left saphenous system – an anatomic fact that must be taken into account in planning fasciocutaneous flaps. (From Jordan GH, Stack RS. General concepts concerning the use of genital skin islands for anterior urethral reconstruction. *Atlas Urol Clin North Am.* 1997;5:23–44.)

collateral blood supply from the retroperitoneal cremasteric artery follows the vas to become the vasal artery. As the spermatic artery and its venae comitantes approach the testis, it divides into the internal testicular artery (which supplies the testis and the adjacent epididymal head and body) and the inferior testicular artery, which passes within the testis. The epididymal tail is supplied by branches of the epididymal, vasal, and testicular arteries.[4]

The veins form in the pampiniform plexus, which coalesces around the testis and epididymis to flow into the testicular veins. The testicular veins then pass in a retroperitoneal plane to empty into the inferior vena cava on the right side and the left renal vein on the left side.

Genital nerve supply

The nerve supply of the genitalia also arises from a dual source and runs concurrently with the arterial supply. The major sensory supply to the penis arises from the pudendal nerve in the perineum. The pudendal nerve is a mixed motor, sensory, and autonomic nerve that originates from the sacral roots (S2–S4). The nerve passes through the greater sciatic foramen and then courses anteriorly across the pelvic floor to enter the pudendal canal. Within the pelvis, the nerve gives off the inferior rectal nerve, supplying the rectal sphincter and anal skin and conducting the cavernosal reflex before entering Alcock (pudendal) canal. As the nerve exits Alcock canal and passes close to the crural tips of the corporal bodies, it divides into the perineal nerve and the dorsal nerve of the penis. The perineal nerve supplies the perineal muscles, deep structures of the urogenital region, and posterior scrotal skin. The dorsal nerve of the penis gives off a proximal nerve to the urethra before arborizing into its penile branches. Branches of the nerve pass around the penile shaft within Buck fascia to innervate the distal shaft and inner lamina of the prepuce as well

as pass directly into the glans as the major tactile and erogenous source of the penis *(see Fig. 9.18)*.

The dorsal nerve of the penis does not provide sensation to the penile shaft. The shaft is innervated by ancillary erogenous nerves, including the ilioinguinal nerves, which exit through the external inguinal rings and then branch to innervate the anterior scrotum and the penile shaft skin circumferentially to the level of the prepuce, and branches of the genitofemoral nerves. The internal plate of the prepuce does contain branches of the dorsal nerve of the penis.

The scrotum has the advantage of multiple nerve supplies. In addition to the anterior scrotal branches of the ilioinguinal nerve, the anterior scrotum is also supplied by the genital branches of the genitofemoral nerve. The posterior scrotum is innervated by the posterior scrotal branch of the pudendal nerve.

Genital lymphatic supply

Lymphatics of the glans and urethra form a plexus on the ventral side before passing around to the deep vein, passing proximally to the superficial inguinal nodes. Some lymphatics also pass to the deep inguinal nodes. The distal urethral lymphatics likewise drain to the deep dorsal vein and the superficial inguinal nodes. The proximal spongy and membranous urethra drains into the external iliac nodes. The lymphatics of the testicles are contained in the spermatic cord and empty into the aortocaudal nodes.

Congenital genital defects

Exstrophy and epispadias

Exstrophy of the bladder is an uncommon condition that occurs in approximately 1 of every 30 000 live births, of which boys predominate in a 3 : 1 ratio. The defining features of epispadias and exstrophy are an open and protruding bladder, an open urethra, and a foreshortened epispadiac penis. However, the associated spectrum of anomalies may extend to involve the musculoskeletal structures and the gastrointestinal tract. Classic exstrophy –defined by bladder exstrophy, epispadias, diastasis recti, absence of fusion of the pubic symphysis, and deformed pubic escutcheon – occurs in 60% of cases; epispadias alone occurs in 30% of cases, and 10% of cases are more extensive dysmorphias including cloacal exstrophy.

The etiology of exstrophy-epispadias is controversial, but it does not represent an arrest of a normal fetal developmental stage. It occurs in early gestation between the 3rd and 9th weeks. The anomaly is associated with the formation and normal retraction of the cloacal membrane. In the normal fetus, a mesodermal layer of tissue spreads medially to replace the thin cloacal membrane by the 9th week *in utero*. According to Muecke's theory,[5] the cloacal membrane persists and resists any medial migration of mesoderm. The membrane then ruptures, thereby producing a lack of mesodermal tissue to form the anterior abdominal wall and endodermal tissue to form the anterior wall of the bladder. This lack of mesodermal migration also has a profound effect on the musculoskeletal system. The pubic rami are widely separated, and the inferior

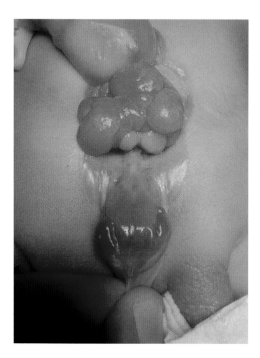

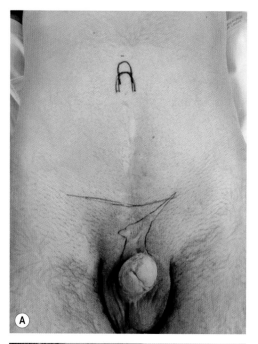

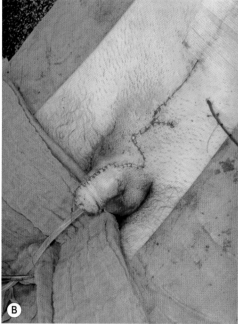

Fig. 13.7 Exstrophy in a boy.

pubic rami are consequently laterally rotated. This defect produces a widened and foreshortened urethra and bladder neck. It also produces an incompletely formed penis that remains rudimentary and, by definition, is a phallus. According to Mitchell and Bägli,[6] the anomaly is that of a fetal abdominal wall hernia and can be recreated in the laboratory in chickens because they have a persistent cloaca by induction of a localized vascular accident (J. Sumfest, pers. comm. 2002).

The defining features of exstrophy-epispadias are: an open urinary tract with protruding bladder and foreshortened epispadiac penis *(Fig. 13.7)*. The crural bodies are attached to the splayed pubic tubercles, producing a penis that is short, wide, and with dorsal chordee. Unlike in the normal anatomy, corporal bodies are independent of each other with no communication through the intercorporal septum. The neurovascular structures to the glans are laterally displaced but move medially at the distal end of the foreshortened penis; the glans is spade shaped and incompletely formed, and each side is totally dependent on the respective dorsal neurovascular supply for its viability. Little circulation passes through the corporal bodies into the glans, as opposed to a penis with normal development. The separated pelvic ring also produces a widened scrotum and lack of competent pelvic musculature. Therefore, the perineum is short and the anus can be patulous and anteriorly displaced. The rectus muscles are widely separated, and inguinal hernias are the rule.

Although the initial postnatal diagnosis and treatment of bladder exstrophy and epispadias remain in the realm of the pediatric urologist and pediatric orthopedic surgeon, it is important that the plastic surgeon be prepared, if consulted, to help reconstruct such a child. The goals of initial closure are to reconstruct a functional genitourinary system, to reduce the risk of bladder squamous metaplasia, and to close the pelvic ring. This is carried out by direct closure of the bladder and reconstitution of the pelvic ring.

Different techniques have been described for penile reconstruction[6,7] and although the results of the urethral closure

Fig. 13.8 A Z-plasty on the dorsal aspect of the penis extending into the prepubic area can be useful to obtain maximal lengthening.

have drastically improved, the ideal surgical approach is still controversial: neonatal versus delayed closure and one stage versus multi-stage repair. Phallic length mainly depends on antenatal development and the majority of these patients end-up with small and undeveloped penises, despite the best efforts of their treating surgeons. As they pass through their post-adolescent period, many of these young men will benefit from further lengthening procedures or even complete penile reconstruction. In some patients; correction of unaesthetic scars and further release of insufficiently released corpora can help to gain length *(Fig. 13.8)*.

Exstrophy patients miss an umbilicus and often they are consulting for umbilical reconstruction. Different techniques

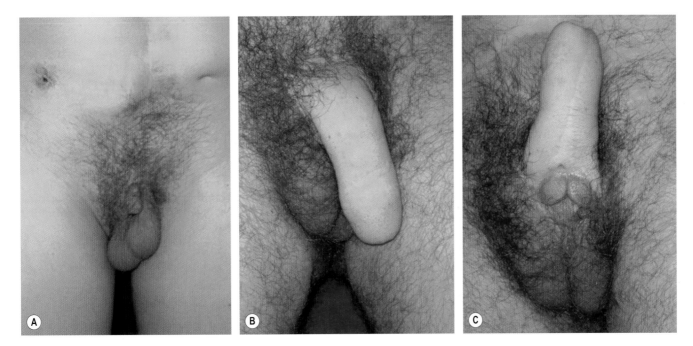

Fig. 13.9 (A) Bladder exstrophy patient with a severely underdeveloped penis who requested a complete penile reconstruction with a free radial forearm flap. **(B,C)** Postoperative result after radial forearm phalloplasty with the small glans incorporated at the base of the reconstructed penis.

have been described with good cosmetic outcomes. Neonatal preservation of the umbilicus and transposition to an abdominal position can overcome the loss of umbilicus.[8,9]

Unfortunately, in some boys there just is not enough tissue due to underdevelopment or due to partial or complete loss of penile tissue after primary closure. These patients might be a good candidate to undergo a phallic construction or further penile reconstruction with the use of microsurgical tissue transplantation techniques *(Fig. 13.9)* or local pedicled perforator flaps *(see below, Fig. 13.12A–C)*.

Most of these patients have some form of different urinary diversion and therefore a nonfunctional urethra. Although the ejaculatory ducts are mostly intact, they are often abnormally positioned as a prepubic fistula. These anatomic facts create unpredictable sperm production, and most of these patients are unable to procreate naturally. For these reasons, the urethral reconstruction may be a moot point in this group of patients thus making a phalloplasty in these 'boys without a penis,' much more easy compared to a penile reconstruction in a patient who wants to void through his new penis. The different options and peculiarities for a phalloplasty in an exstrophy patient will be addressed further in this chapter.

After neonatal closure of the exstrophy, the pubic hairline can show an asymmetry. This can easily be reconstructed by creating and mobilizing skin flaps and correcting the pubic hairline.

Disorders of sex development (formerly "intersex")

After standardization of the terminology, intersex conditions are nowadays defined as Disorders of Sexual Development (DSD).[10]

DSD is not within the scope of this text and therefore it is limited here to a short description of the conditions in which genital reconstruction is needed. Only conditions with genital ambiguity and those with the absence of Müllerian duct derived structures are mentioned.

46XX DSD: over-virilized females. The most prevalent condition here is congenital adrenal hyperplasia (CAH) where, due to a cortisol synthesis defect, androgens are overproduced in a female subject. This leads to virilization of the female genitals with urogenital sinus formation (confluence of urogenital tracts), labioscrotal fusion and clitoromegaly. Surgical correction is needed for separating the urogenital tracts bringing the urethra and the vagina separately to the perineum with a nerve sparing reduction of the clitoris size and a reconstruction of the labiae. Although the optimal timing of this surgery still is a point of controversy, most surgeons agree on early reconstruction.

46XY DSD: under-virilization in males. Testosterone synthesis defects and partial androgen receptor insensitivity are among the causes. Patients in this group present genital ambiguity with varying degrees of hypospadias, penoscrotal transposition and cryptorchidism. Surgical treatment early in life consists of hypospadias repair, correction of penoscrotal transposition and orchidopexy.

46XY/46XX DSD: consists of varying degrees of genital ambiguity and presence of both male and female or dysgenetic gonads. Reconstruction is done after gender assignment, which is not always obvious. Multidisciplinary teams with expertise in these pathologies are needed to guide the diagnosis and treatment in these children.

Genital conditions: this DSD classification includes conditions like penile agenesis, extreme penoscrotal transposition with rudimentary penis, Mayer-Rokitansky-Kuster-Hauser with absence of Müllerian duct derivates like vagina and uterus, cloacal exstrophy, micropenis and other genital mal-formations with normal chromosomes and gonads. All these conditions will eventually require genital reconstruction although due to their low prevalence these should be treated in centers of excellence with a lot of expertise in this field.

Buried penis

The buried penis deformity is present in both the pediatric and adult populations. A buried penis is defined as a penis that is of normal size for age but hidden within the peripenile fat and subcutaneous tissues *(Fig. 13.10)*.

In the pediatric population, the fat deposit is often part of the constellation of poor virilization. The abnormal mons fat pad (gynecoid mons pubis) may become associated with a generalized obesity in the adolescent patient, and the buried penis must be differentiated from a micropenis in this group. In adults, the problem is almost always associated with obesity and the development of pubic, scrotal, and peripubic ptosis, which must be addressed to correct the problem of the hidden penis. Liposuction and lipectomy are part of the treatment in adults however in children the fat resection is abandoned. With pubertal development the prepubic fat deposit often decreases in size. The focus is on the release of the penis from the fibrotic dartos tissue.[11,12] Many techniques are described but the most important steps include keeping all available skin from the start of the procedure, to resect all dartos tissue and to recover the released corpora with the skin *(Fig. 13.11)*.

Reconstructive options for severe penile insufficiency

A clear definition of severe penile inadequacy has not yet been established but can be considered as an insufficient penile length and function to obtain successful sexual intercourse. This implies that puberty must be finished and that the patient must be sexually active. Conditions with penile insufficiency include: aphallia or penile agenesis, idiopathic micropenis (stretched penile length in a full-term newborn male <2.5 cm), 46XY DSD and bladder exstrophy. Reconstructive surgery in these mostly young patients is required because of the devastating effect on psychological and sexual function.

The development of perforator flaps has given rise to some new reconstructive options in patients with such severe penile insufficiency. These perforator flaps have the advantage of reducing the donor site morbidity, increasing the range of motion of the flap and combining different tissue flaps on one single pedicle. Although, overall, the free vascularized radial forearm flap (discussed further below) is still considered as the 'standard technique' in penile reconstruction, the *pedicled anterolateral thigh (ALT) flap* has been shown to provide a valuable phalloplasty alternative specifically in patients with congenital penile insufficiency. This flap is a skin flap based on a perforator from the descending branch of the lateral circumflex femoral artery, which is a branch from the femoral artery.

There are several reasons why in the 'boys without a penis' a pedicled ALT flap can be preferred above the standard radial forearm flap *(Fig. 13.12)*:

• A pedicled flap reconstruction (the flap has a sufficiently long pedicle) avoids the technically more complex microscopic procedure and might also shorten the operation time.

• A visible donor site scar on the forearm, often considered as the signature of female-to-male transsexualism is avoided and the donor site on the leg can more easily be concealed.

• Previous reconstructive surgeries at the pelvis, groin area and lower abdomen (e.g., in case of bladder exstrophy) might have altered the local anatomy and vasculature making a microsurgical anastomosis more difficult.

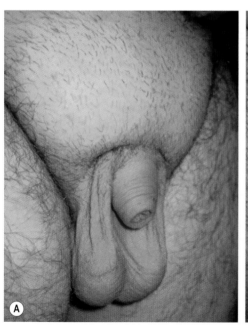
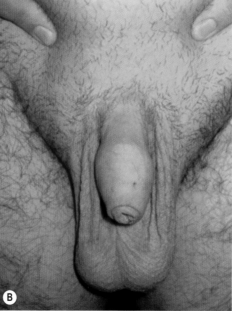

Fig. 13.10 Buried penis: retraction of the peripenile and pubic fat reveals a normal size penis.

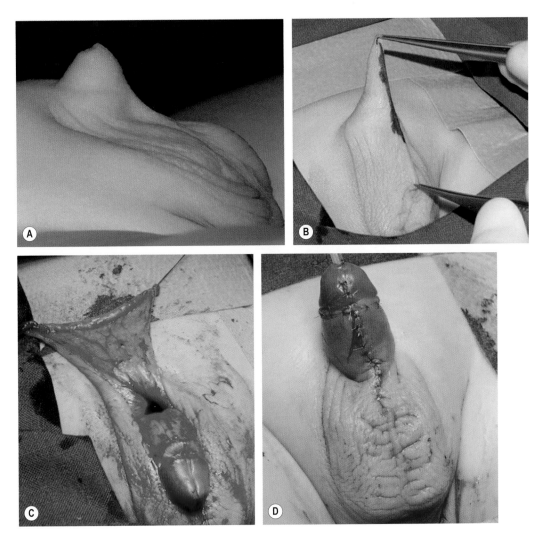

Fig. 13.11 **(A)** Typical buried penis in an infant. **(B)** Ventral incision of the skin with maximal preservation of skin at the start of the procedure. **(C)** After complete resection of the fibrotic dartos tissue the penis is released from its buried position and the skin is extendable. **(D)** Coverage of the released corpora with the extended skin creating a penis with normal length.

- The subcutaneous fat layer is much thinner than in a (biologically female) transman, facilitating the (urethral) tube-within-a-(penile)tube reconstruction of the penis; moreover, many exstrophy patients empty their bladder by catheterization through a continent diversion (e.g., appendico-vesicostomy) and don't even require a urethral reconstruction in their phalloplasty. An ejaculatory opening can be left at the ventral aspect just above the scrotum.

It is very important to preserve and incorporate any useful glandular, penile and cavernosal tissue at the basis of the newly reconstructed phallus in order to facilitate sexual stimulation and pleasure *(Fig. 13.9C)*. If available, a dorsal penile nerve is identified and connected with a cutaneous nerve of the flap; if not available, the lateral femoral cutaneous nerve is connected to the ilioinguinal nerve.

Usually, it is recommended to perform a 3D angio CT-scan preoperatively to provide detailed information on the perforator vessel(s) and the subcutaneous tissue layer.

Unfortunately, similar as to the radial forearm flap, also the ALT flap has a rather high urological complication rate with frequent strictures and/or fistula formation. Secondary procedures might be needed to treat these complications and especially the treatment of urethral strictures is challenging and difficult.

There is still a lot of controversy whether or not to perform a phalloplasty in children. Penile construction in children is similar as in adults with one added requirement – growth through puberty to adulthood. Because the phallus is constructed of somatic tissues (showing linear growth) but replaces a penis that is formed by genital tissues (demonstrating a more exponential growth), the growth rates are temporally and quantitatively different during puberty.[13] Care must be taken to accurately predict the anticipated growth rate and to design a phallic model that is larger and longer than normal genital size for that age group.[14]

Another issue that we are just now beginning to address is the 'correct' age at which to proceed with the insertion of penile prostheses. Once these boys have reached 18 years and

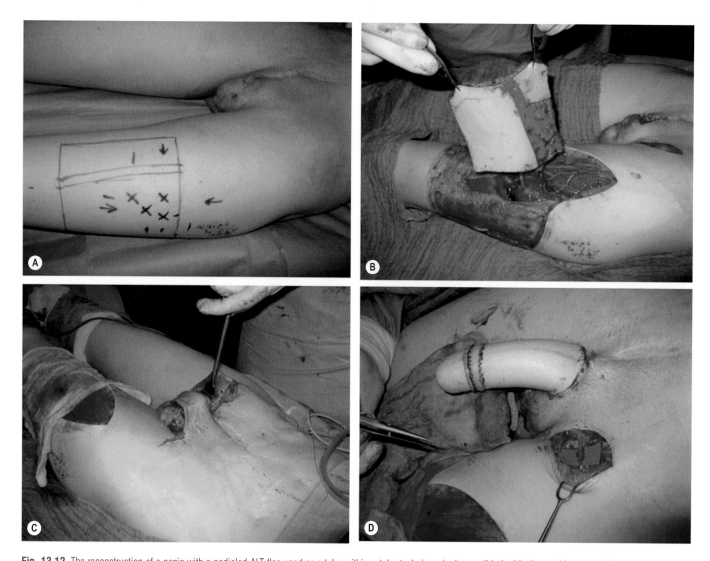

Fig. 13.12 The reconstruction of a penis with a pedicled ALT flap used as a tube-within-a-tube technique (only possible in thin 'boys without a penis' and after defatting). No real urethra was reconstructed here since the patient had a urostomy. **(A)** Preoperative view. **(B)** After flap dissection. **(C)** The flap is tunneled underneath the rectus femoris muscle. **(D)** Suturing and nerve connection (ilioinguinal nerve to lateral femoral cutaneous nerve).

the age for majority, they must be physically and psychologically prepared to manage a phallus that has previously been erectionless.

There is another nagging problem with operating on children – the lack of informed consent. Although the child's best interest and surgery's best intentions are usually served by early reconstruction, there are no long-term studies that have evaluated the results of this surgery over a lifetime or even a generation.

Finally, it comes as no surprise that the large majority of these genitally compromised boys require prolonged psychological therapy to deal with genital loss, surgical trauma, inadequacy, and scarring. These psychological issues are often closely commingled with the need for secondary surgery to complete reconstruction.

Nowhere in surgery is there a stronger need for parental and family support than with these late teenage boys who have essentially undergone years of 'surgical abuse.'

Post-traumatic genital defects

Post-traumatic genital repair is an uncommon but special chapter in surgical reconstruction. A reconstructive algorithm based on the etiology, an assessment of the extent of injury, and an anatomic inventory includes several goals and observations. First, the anatomically protected position of the genitalia implies that patients who have genital injuries often have large concomitant injuries as well and are often critically ill patients. Resuscitation and life support of the patient take precedent over any reconstruction. However, genital reconstruction is of prime relevance, and only hand, eyelid and lip reconstruction are considered more important in the reconstructive hierarchy. Second, aesthetics are foremost in genital reconstruction. Although it is not often articulated, the appearance of the genitalia is important to the self-esteem of a patient who is recovering from trauma. What is frivolous to one person may be a lifelong obsession to another, and genital aesthetics are valued as other cosmetic areas such as the face, nose, and breasts. Third, the genitalia appear to be a 'privileged site' such that the usual post reconstructive sequelae of scarring and contracture are often spared in genital reconstruction. This may be due to the fact that the average adult man has five to eight nocturnal erections every night, thereby inherently stretching scars or skin grafts on the penile shaft. This stretching may combat and overcome the tendency of myofibroblasts to contract a skin graft or scar.

General reconstructive options

Genital skin grafts

Genital skin loss occurs from burns, avulsion injuries, infections, and gangrene. As a rule, total excision of the necrotic genital tissues followed by early skin grafting produces the best results. When the wound is contaminated or infected, adequate debridement of necrotic tissues combined with wound bed preparation prior to skin grafting might be required and this can be performed with adequate (moist) wound dressings, by temporary coverage with allograft skin or with the use of topical negative pressure.

The thick split-thickness skin graft is the mainstay of penile reconstruction. The graft should be pliable, placed onto a flat bed, and secured with a tie-over bolus pressure dressing or even better with a special CaviCare cylinder type of dressing *(Fig. 13.13)* to reduce the risk of hematoma or seroma formation. Successful skin graft 'take' is directly related to a well-vascularized wound bed, meticulous hemostasis, control of erections, infection-free environment, and adequate immobilization.

The donor site should be close to the genitalia, large enough to produce a sheet skin graft and be well hidden. Ideally, the skin graft should be at least 0.018–0.02 inch in thickness and large enough to cover the whole breadth of the penile shaft or scrotum. The skin graft should be sutured circumferentially around the penile shaft with a ventral suture line. As a rule, this suture line will not contract (because of the privileged site), but a Z-plasty may often be incorporated to reduce the risk of contracture. The graft is then fixed to the surrounding skin, the underlying Buck fascia, and the tunica with dissolving sutures. Fixation with tissue-sealant has been reported to improve skin graft fixation and skin graft take in this difficult area (S. Monstrey, pers. comm. 2010).

Extended bed rest is important in the immediate postoperative period to reduce the risk of graft shearing or movement. Amyl nitrate and diazepam (Valium) can be administered to discourage erections in the early postoperative period. However, erections, massage, and stimulation are recommended for all patients after grafting as soon as there is a full take of the skin graft.

Widely meshed split-thickness skin grafts should never be used on the penile shaft. However, with the so-called 'reversed mesh graft' (= nonexpanded or 1:1 meshed skin grafts) only puncture-type perforations are made with a V1 carrier (Humeca Ltd, Enschede, the Netherlands; *Fig. 13.14*), which allow for a better fluid evacuation and thus a better skin graft take while still avoiding poor scarring and an unaesthetic mesh pattern long term. These nonexpanded meshed split-thickness grafts have also become a mainstay of complicated, staged urethral reconstruction.[15,16] McAninch[17] has described the use of (not too widely) meshed split thickness skin grafts for scrotal reconstruction. Meshed grafts in this location may produce 'good aesthetic results,' but they will never measure up to the functional capacity of sheet or 1:1 perforated grafts.

Full-thickness skin grafts also have a place in genital reconstruction, but mostly for smaller skin defects. Full-thickness grafts are particularly useful for coronal sulcus design to prevent 'coronal washout' as is usually performed in female-to-male (MTF) transsexual patients (see below; *Fig. 13.24F*).

Scrotal reconstruction adheres to the same reconstructive principles. Where possible, primary closure is the procedure of choice, particularly in partial or hemilateral injuries. However, in the case of total scrotal skin loss, split-thickness skin grafts are effective if they are placed and immobilized carefully. The testicles must be fixed in an anatomically appropriate position before proceeding with graft coverage. As already mentioned, there also is a place for meshed, non-expanded skin grafts in scrotal and perineal reconstruction because of the uneven and often biconcave contours of this region. In addition, there is an aesthetic dividend in that meshed grafts on the scrotum often emulate the scrotal rugae (see later; *Fig. 13.18*).

Buccal mucosa grafts are often used in urethral reconstruction. They can also be useful in glans reconstruction. After partial penectomy (traumatically or for cancer treatment) the residual corpora sometimes are still long enough to allow for sexual intercourse. However, the penis is completely covered with skin which leads to unnatural look. For these patients the corpora can be released by transaction of the suspensory ligament and the tip of the corpora can be covered by buccal mucosa free grafts. They create a mucosa covered glans like looking tip of the penis *(Fig. 13.15)*.

Genital flaps

Post-traumatic penile, scrotal, and perigenital anatomy dictates flap design to a great degree. Most of the serviceable flaps in genital reconstruction depend on the predictable anatomy of the superficial vascular system and, in some cases, the deep system and are designed on tissues that have recognized arterial names and vascular territories.

For small penile defects, flaps based on the superficial external pudendal system can be used for penile shaft and anterior urethral reconstruction.[18,19] Proximal penile flaps that are vascularized from the lower abdomen and pubis are recognized but are less practical for male genitalia reconstruction.

Scrotal flaps have also been employed in genital reconstruction but have limited application with the exception of hemiscrotal reconstruction. Although the scrotum has a wealth of well-vascularized skin and subcutaneous tissue that it can logically lend to its hemiscrotal twin or the adjacent penis, in fact it is ill-suited for genital reconstruction because of its rigorous and nonglabrous nature. A centrally located scrotal flap designed along the medial raphe has also been described as a reconstructive flap option for proximal urethral repair.[20] However, the unpredictable nature of scrotal hair distribution often dictates presurgical epilation of the flap.

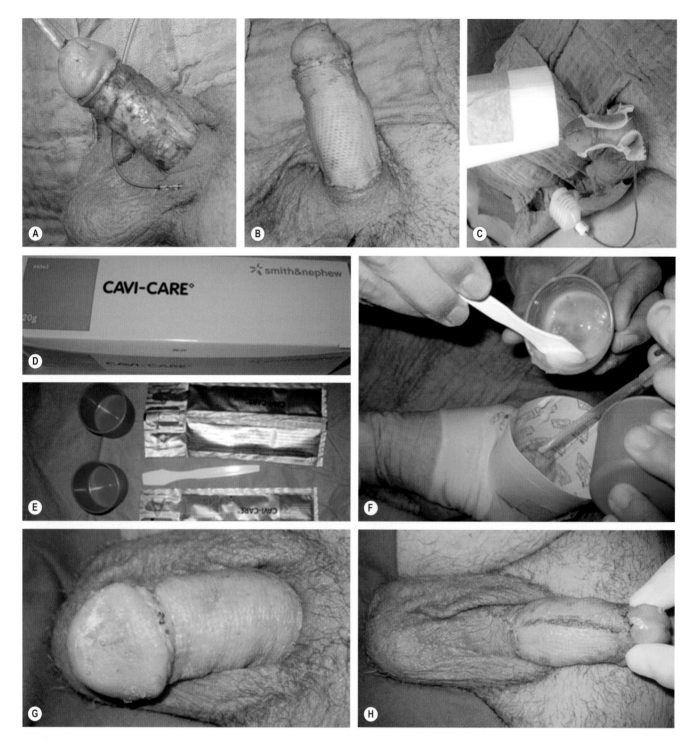

Fig. 13.13 (A) A patient with a complete defect of the skin of the penile shaft. **(B)** The 1:1 perforated split thickness skin graft is applied and sutured to the shaft. **(C–F)** A CaviCare dressing is applied around the skin graft (poured out in a cylinder form around the penis) and this dressing will stay for 1 week. **(G,H)** A complete take of the skin graft is obtained.

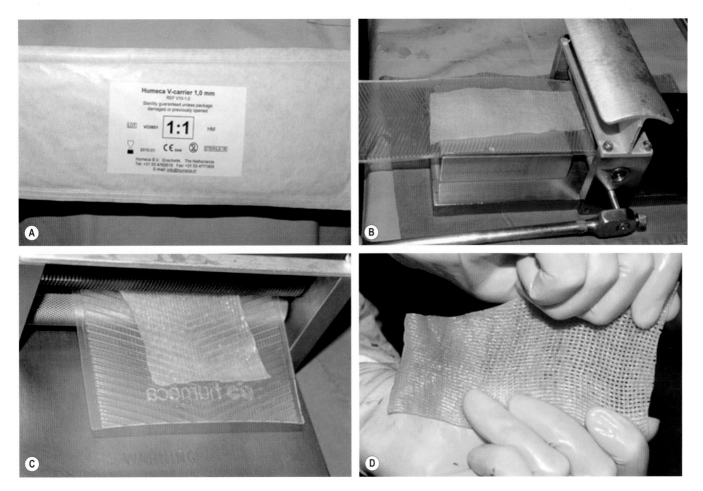

Fig. 13.14 The so-called 'reverse-meshed graft' or 1:1 perforated skin graft, obtained with a V1 mesh carrier (Humeca, the Netherlands).

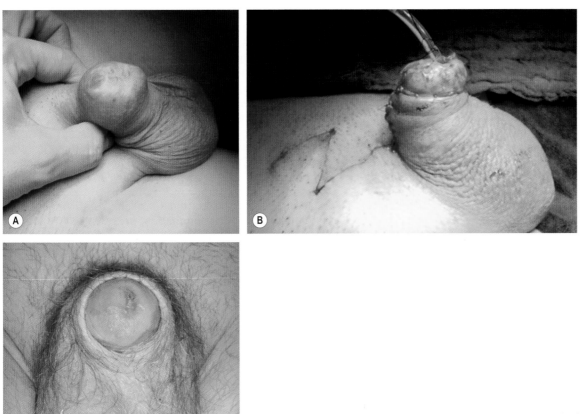

Fig. 13.15 (A) Penis after partial penectomy for spinocellular epithelioma, showing residual corpora which after release could be sufficient for sexual intercourse. **(B)** After penile elongation with release of the suspensory ligament and coverage of the distal part of the penis with buccal mucosa. **(C)** Result of glans reconstruction using buccal mucosa.

This flap is based on the posterior scrotal artery and can be difficult to mobilize extensively. In addition, when the flap has been dissected, elevated, and transferred, there can be the sequela of scrotal tethering, even after successful transfer. A free buccal mucosal graft is often a better choice for proximal urethral reconstruction.[21]

In larger defects, there often is a combined penoscrotal defect, as with Fournier's gangrene defect. Any technique of tissue expansion seems risky in this region, especially in the repair of Fournier's gangrene defect due to the bacteriological environment and the multiple stage procedure. Apart from the scrotal flap, there often is a need for the use of local muscle/myocutaneous flaps, fasciocutaneous flaps and perforator flaps in the field of male genitalia reconstruction. Nowadays, the gracilis (purely) muscle flap is no longer considered as 'the workhorse of the perineum,' but this muscle flap still is useful to cover and vascularize urethral anastomoses, to cover exposed pelvic bones, to reduce the risk of osteomyelitis, to fill the perineum after exenteration, and to vascularize the perineum in post-irradiation injuries.[22]

Fasciocutaneous paragenital flaps that have been used, often with limited application, are the superficial circumflex iliac flap,[23] the deep circumflex iliac flap (often combined with an osseous component),[24] the superficial epigastric flap,[25] the double-pedicled composite groin flap,[26] the anteromedial thigh flap,[27] the anterolateral thigh flap,[28] and the pudendal thigh flap.[29,30] The superficial groin flap is based on the superficial circumflex artery system, a branch of the femoral artery, and has an unpredictable origin, direction, and size. The flap must often be delayed, attached or 'waltzed' into a central midline position by a secondary procedure to be used as a genital flap. For these reasons, the groin flap has limited primary genital use.

Medial thigh flaps may be based inferiorly on the perineal artery system or superiorly on the external pudendal system and branches of the profunda femoris artery. The inferiorly based flap has been called by several names, including the Singapore flap[29] and the pudendal thigh flap.[31] Originally described to correct vesicovaginal fistulas, the flap is based posteriorly within the crural fold between the scrotum and the medial wall of the thigh and extends from the posterior crural fold to the medial groin area anteriorly. Although most flap descriptions have focused on vaginal reconstruction and the correction of vesicovaginal and rectovaginal fistulas, this flap has been successfully used for male genital or male urethral construction.[30]

To complete the catalogue of fasciocutaneous flaps, the gluteal-posterior thigh flap must also be included.[32,33] This flap is based on the inferior descending branch of the inferior gluteal artery. Nowadays, this flap has been replaced in most cases by perforator flaps originating from the inferior gluteal artery or IGAP flaps.[34] Additionally, various other new (pedicled) perforator flaps based (the so-called 'lotus petal flaps') on the external pudendal artery have also been described as possible options in the perineal area although more in female patients.[35]

The formerly more popular musculocutaneous flaps including the vertical and transverse rectus abdominis flap (based on the deep inferior epigastric artery),[36] the gracilis musculocutaneous flap,[37] the rectus femoris musculocutaneous flap,[38] and the tensor fasciae latae musculocutaneous flap[39] have been employed occasionally in genitourinary reconstruction

but have only limited use in the reconstruction of male genitalia.

Nevertheless, these reliable flaps still can be an important part of the surgeon's armamentarium in addressing genital injuries after trauma, infection, and cancer and for patients with co morbid health problems. These flaps are often the only tissues available for genital reconstruction. The trauma, cancer, infection, and co morbid disease that originally contributed to genital tissue loss may also preclude sophisticated microsurgical reconstruction. Thus, these flaps are the only hope for functional, albeit suboptimal, genital reconstruction.

In the last decade, the myocutaneous flaps have often been replaced by their 'perforator-type equivalent': the deep inferior epigastric artery perforator or DIEAP flap (with its skin island taken either vertically or horizontally) has been reported in a case of penile reconstruction.

However, it is mainly the pedicled anterolateral thigh or ALT flap that has become a new 'workhorse' nowadays in perineal and male genital reconstruction.[40] For the description of the use of this flap in patients with congenital penile insufficiency we refer to the beginning of this chapter.

The pedicled ALT can also be a valuable alternative for the reconstruction of a scrotum (*Fig. 13.16*).

Microsurgical genital reconstruction

Genital replantation

Microsurgical techniques and free tissue transplantation have become the state-of the-art treatment for many reconstructive problems. The first uses of the microscope in genital reconstruction for penile reattachment after amputation were reported independently by Cohen et al.[41] and Tamai et al.[42] in 1977. However, the first account of successful reattachment long predated the introduction of microsurgical techniques. In 1929, Ehrich[43] first reported a successful penile attachment by opposing and anatomizing the lacerated corporal bodies and repairing the overlying tunica only. This technique was occasionally successful but usually associated with loss of the overlying skin, glans, sensation, and erectile and voiding function.[44]

Penile replantation often mimics the algorithms of other amputated extremities that are candidates for reattachment. The penis is initially wrapped in saline-soaked gauze and placed into a plastic bag, which in turn is placed in a bag or cooler of ice with water (the so-called 'bag-in-a-bag' technique). Because genital amputations are often self-inflicted, it is important to involve the psychiatrist even before restorative surgery. After the induction of anesthesia, the proximal and distal ends of the amputated penis are examined microscopically. Minimal debridement is followed by mechanical stabilization of the urethra and reapproximation of the tunica albuginea of the corpora cavernosa.

Revascularization is completed by use of microsurgical magnification, instrumentation, and 9-0 and 10-0 nylon sutures to reanastomose the deep dorsal arteries, the deep dorsal vein, and the superficial dorsal vein. Multiple nerve coaptations are meticulously completed with 10-0 and 11-0 nylon sutures. The dartos fascia and skin are then loosely approximated to complete the reattachment. A suprapubic tube is inserted to divert the urinary flow for 2–3 weeks, and the patient is prescribed bed rest in a warm room.

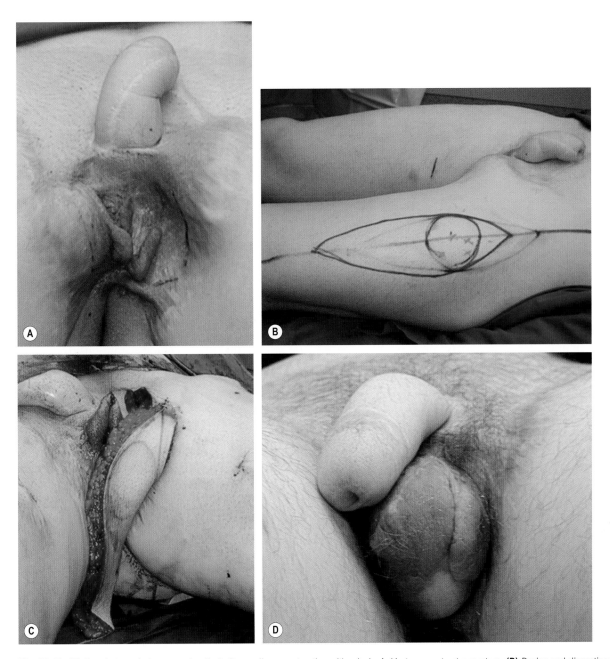

Fig. 13.16 (A) Female to male transsexual patient after penile reconstruction with a lack of skin to reconstruct a scrotum. **(B)** Design and dissection of a pedicled ALT flap. **(C)** Transfer of the ALT flap to the pubic area. **(D)** Postoperative result.

The ideal candidate for genital replantation is a patient with a clean, sharp cut in which the amputated part has been cooled *(Fig. 13.17)*.

Testicular reattachment has also been reported but requires a sharp amputation etiology for successful anastomosis of the thin-walled arteries and veins that surround and vascularize the testicle, seminiferous tubules, and vas deferens.[45,46] Unfortunately, most testicular amputations are of the avulsion or crush type and therefore are not reattachable. Clinically, the only vessel that has adequate caliber is the testicular artery with its venae comitantes.

Two other arteries are also involved in testicular vascularization: the deferens artery, which arises from the inferior vesicular artery and vascularizes the epididymis, and the

cremasteric artery, which arises from the inferior epigastric artery and vascularizes the cremasteric muscle and the other cord structures. Both of these arteries are small, filmy, and often unrecognizable in reattachment circumstances.

There are five factors to be considered before proceeding with testicular reattachment. First, it is important to understand the three different testicular blood supplies when a candidate is considered for possible reattachment. Second, the venous presence, pattern, and vascular stability may all play into the appropriateness of reattachment. Third, a devascularized testicle has only about 4–6 h of ischemia before losing its reattachment value. A reattached testicle cannot be expected to recover its sperm-producing function, and even if it does, the sperm count is often too low to be effectual. Fourth, there

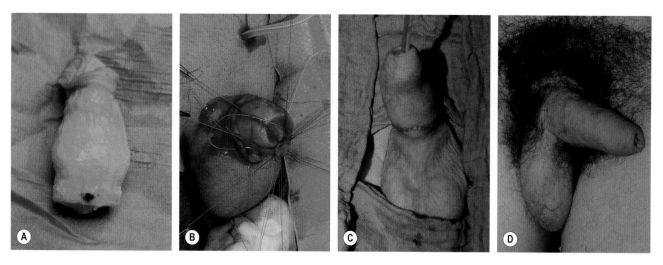

Fig. 13.17 (A) Self-inflicted penile amputation. **(B)** Preparation of microsurgical anastomoses. **(C)** Immediate postoperative result. **(D)** Late postoperative result.

is the technical issue of vas deferens anastomosis and the maintenance of patency in the face of traumatic amputation. Fifth, the post-reattachment psychological well-being of the patient (particularly in self-mutilation patients) must be considered. When all of these points are considered together, the best that can be hoped for with a reattached testicle is the maintenance of testosterone secretion. For this reason, the insertion of a testicular prosthesis combined with hormonal therapy can be a much simpler option.

Microsurgical phallic construction

Complete reconstruction of a phallus will be extensively described under the next heading: 'Reconstruction of male genitalia in the female-to-male transsexual.'

Specific reconstructive indications

Fournier disease

Fournier in 1883 was the first to describe a 'fulminant gangrene' of the penis and scrotum that: (1) developed suddenly in previously healthy young men, (2) progressed rapidly, and (3) was idiopathic. Nowadays, every necrotizing fasciitis, in the specific region of the perineum and genitalia is termed Fournier's gangrene, the etiology with or without proven infection notwithstanding.[47]

Fournier disease is rare but true genitourinary emergency when it is identified. Today, the etiology is identified in about 95% of cases. Common sources of infection include urogenital disease and trauma (renal abscess); urethral stone; urethral stricture; iatrogenic misadventure by the unrecognized rupture of the urethra when penile prostheses are inserted; colorectal (ruptured appendicitis); colon cancer; diverticulitis; perirectal, retroperitoneal, and sub diaphragmatic abscesses; and local trauma.[48]

Several systemic conditions have also been associated with Fournier gangrene and may predispose patients to its development: diabetes mellitus, alcoholism, heavy smoking (more than one pack per day), human immunodeficiency virus infection and acquired immunodeficiency syndrome,

and leukemia. Fournier disease is considered a synergistic necrotizing fasciitis that often includes Gram-positive organisms, Gram-negative organisms, and *Clostridium perfringens* anaerobes in the cultures. The disease often begins as a cellulitis adjacent to the portal of entry. The affected area is swollen, erythematous, and tender as the infection begins to include the deep fascia. There is prominent pain as well as fever and systemic toxicity. Scrotal swelling and crepitus quickly increase with the appearance of dark purple areas that become gangrenous. Specific urinary symptoms include dysuria, urethral discharge, and obstructed voiding. Gram-negative sepsis is probable if symptoms include a change in mental status, tachypnea, tachycardia, and hyperthermia or hypothermia.

A high degree of suspicion is crucial to an early diagnosis. A clinical differentiation between necrotizing fasciitis and simple cellulitis may be difficult initially because the initial signs of pain, edema, and erythema are not distinctive. However, the presence of marked systemic toxicity out of proportion to the local findings should alert the surgeon.

Once the disease is identified, intravenous fluid therapy and broad spectrum antibiotics should be deployed in preparation for surgical debridement. Once culture results are available, antibiotic coverage can be tailored to the specific organisms obtained. However, anaerobic coverage should be continued regardless of culture results because of the difficulty in culturing these organisms. The immediate surgical debridement is critical and is the definitive treatment. Initial debridement should be aggressive and continue along fascial plains until all of the devitalized tissues have been removed and viable tissue borders the wound.

Some authors also recommend hyperbaric oxygen therapy in conjunction with debridement and antibiotics to speed up wound healing and minimizing the gangrenous spread, particularly in patients with *C. perfringens* infection. In addition to hyperbaric oxygen, mechanized wound debridement tools (i.e., topical negative pressure therapy) have promoted granulation wound contracture and the reduction of bacterial colonization before reconstruction.

In most cases, reconstruction of the genitalia includes release of the penis and testicles from surrounding granulation tissue; release of scar contracture; and split-thickness sheet grafts on the penile shaft and peripenile tissues and nonexpanded meshed split-thickness grafts of the scrotum, perineum, and crural folds *(Fig. 13.18)*. Flap reconstruction is seldom required.

The mortality rate in Fournier disease averages approximately 20% but can range from 7% to 75%. Higher mortality rates are found in diabetics, alcoholics, and those with colorectal sources of infection, who often have a greater delay in diagnosis and more widespread extension. To reduce morbidity and mortality, the key is early diagnosis, aggressive treatment with antibiotics, and surgical debridement.

Penile cancer

In the past, treatment of penile cancer ranged from techniques of local excision to emasculation. Classically, penile cancer involving the redundant preputial and penile skin could be adequately treated with circumcision. Superficial penile cancer involving the glans was in recent years treated by laser excision. As penile cancer invaded the glans, the standard of care became partial penectomy; and as the deep structures were invaded, the excision amounted to subtotal or total penectomy. In recent years, it has been appreciated that penile cancer involving the spongy erectile tissue of the glans could be treated by 'glansectomy.' In other words, excision did not necessarily have to involve the underlying corpora cavernosa. Thus, reconstructive surgery after these techniques often was limited to a redefinition procedure or coverage procedure of the distal corporal bodies. Often, just grafting the tips of the corporal bodies provided an excellent functional as well as cosmetic result. Buccal mucosa grafts can be used and create a natural looking glans *(Fig. 13.15)*.

Another surgical method of treating penile cancer involves Mohs surgery. In Mohs surgery, sequential excisions are accomplished until clean margins in all quadrants are achieved. In classic Mohs surgery, the defect is then left to granulate or can be skin grafted.

In patients in whom a true partial penectomy has been performed, reconstructive efforts were directed toward an augmented reconstruction. In these patients, either local flaps or microvascular transplanted flaps were appended to lengthen the penis. The hope was then to incorporate prostheses at a later date. These techniques, however, were found to lack both in cosmetic and functional considerations. However, it is better to sacrifice some superficial penile tissue, saving the remaining corporal bodies, and to accomplish a true phallic construction. The corporal bodies are incorporated in the base of the microvascular free transfer flap. In patients requiring total penectomy, observation for 1 year confirms adequate tumor margins without recurrence. After clearance by the oncologic surgeon, a total phallic reconstruction is planned by microvascular composite tissue *(Fig. 13.19)*. In patients who have had extensive superficial lymph node dissections, there are considerations with regard to recipient vessels. In these patients, angiography is performed to define the deep inferior epigastric vessels, to define the iliofemoral system, and to use delayed films to attempt to define the venous anatomy of the groin. In addition, in cases in which reconstruction is envisioned, if possible, at the time of the extensive exenterative surgery, it is preferable to place intravenous and arterial lines in the dominant forearm, saving the vascularity of the nondominant forearm for subsequent use in phallic construction. Many surgical oncologists are consulting reconstructive surgeons before the exenterative surgery to ensure that these considerations are recognized.

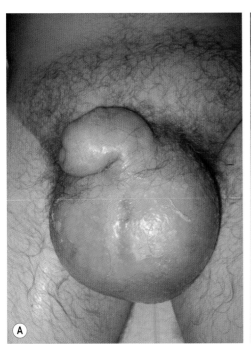 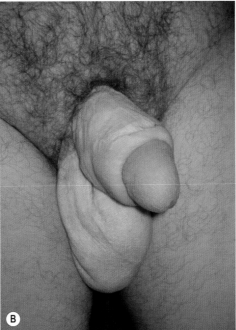

Fig. 13.18 Fournier gangrene. **(A)** Prior to debridement. **(B)** After skin grafting.

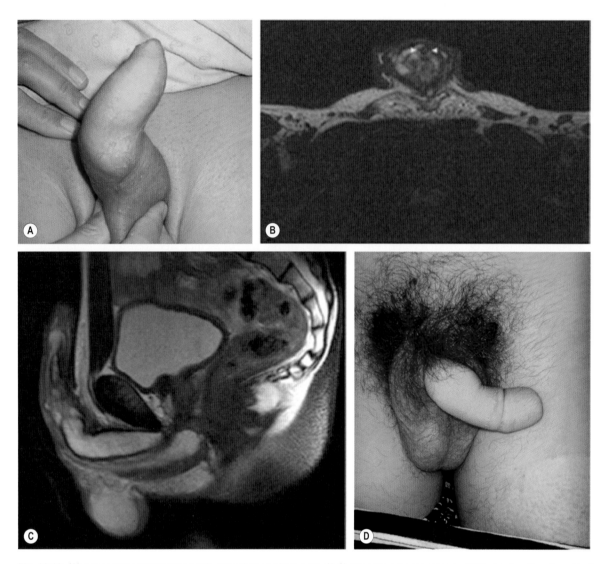

Fig. 13.19 **(A)** A hard tumor involving the whole circumference of the penis. **(B,C)** Magnetic resonance images (MRI) showing disruption of both corpora cavernosa. **(D)** Postoperative result after total penile reconstruction with a free radial forearm flap.

Reconstruction of male genitalia in the female-to-male transsexual

The reconstruction of the male genitalia in a female-to-male transsexual individual is more complex than the penile reconstruction in a biologically male patient because of the added difficulties in reconstructing the fixed part of the urethra and the combination with a vaginectomy and a scrotoplasty.

Vaginectomy, reconstruction of the pars fixa urethra and scrotoplasty

This first part of the procedure is usually done by the urological team, while the team of plastic surgeons is harvesting the flap. The patient is positioned in the lithotomy position with supportive boots to avoid compression of the *N. fibularis* and to avoid compartment syndrome. A roman-aqueduct-like incision is made at the prepubic area where the phallus will

be implanted and the vascular anastomosis will be prepared *(Fig. 13.20A)*. The prepubic space is created with division of the suspensory ligament of the clitoris.

First the vesico-vaginal space is infiltrated with a diluted solution xylocaine-adrenalin to provide a hydrodissection and hemostasis. The vaginal introitus is incised and the external urethral sphincter is gently dissected away from the submucosal vaginal tissue. Four mosquito clamps are placed at the vaginal mucosa for retraction *(Fig. 13.20B)*. The space between the posterior vaginal wall and the rectum is freed in a blunt manner. After this the space between the anterior vaginal wall and the bladder is dissected. In this area, blunt dissection is mostly not possible but must be done by electrocautery. Now the lateral dissection is started. The levator muscle is released from the lateral vaginal wall using electrocautery which ensures a better hemostasis compared to sharp dissection is this well-vascularized area. The dissection is continued until fibrotic tissue of the former hysterectomy is reached. The left and right lateral dissection is now continued to the midline following this fibrotic plane and the vagina is

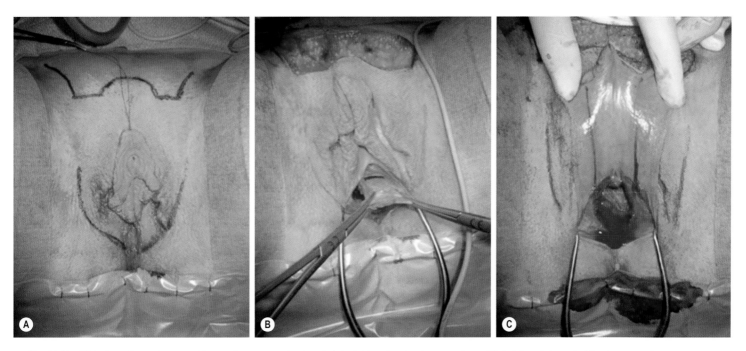

Fig. 13.20 (A) Incision lines of the prepubic area ('roman-aqueduct') and of the labia majora for the scrotoplasty. **(B)** Incision of the vaginal introitus starts the vaginectomy. **(C)** Incision lines of the urethral plate between the external urethral orifice and the tip of the clitoris.

removed in toto and the reconstruction of the urethra is started.

First an 18Fr silicone drain is inserted and attraction suture is placed through the enlarged clitoris. The mucosa between the external urethral orifice and the clitoral glans will serve as the urethral plate for the pars fixa of the urethra. *(Fig. 13.20C)*. The incision lines are marked (minimum width 2.5 cm) and the urethral plate is dissected away from the inner surface of the labia minora. Now, tabularization of the urethral plate is started at the external urethral orifice, with inclusion of the orifices of the para-urethral glands of Skène. Closure of the urethral plate is continued towards the clitoral glans with a running suture Monocryl 3.0 leaving an oblique distal end to anastomose with the phallic urethra *(Fig. 13.21A)*. The preputial skin is released from the clitoral shaft and the clitoral glans is denuded *(Fig. 13.21B)*. A dorsal clitoral nerve (1 or 11 o'clock position) is identified and prepared for later anastomosis. The clitoris with urethra is tunneled towards the prepubic area and fixed to the pubic symphysis with a suture Vicryl 2.0 *(Fig. 13.21C)*.

Now the scrotoplasty is performed: the borders of the posterior part of the labia majora are incised in a semicircular fashion *(Figs 13.20A, 13.22B)*. The subcutaneous fat is dissected in order to create two flaps *(Fig. 13.22C)*. The superficial pelvic floor muscles are now well exposed and are sutured around the pars fixa of the urethra and this closes the superficial perineal space *(Fig. 13.22A)*. The abduction and flexion of the hips are diminished in order to facilitate the closure of the subcutaneous tissue of the perineum with Vicryl 1. These labia majora flaps are now rotated 180° anteriorly towards the base of the foreskin of the clitoris *(Fig. 13.22A)*. By this maneuver, a scrotum is created which is located in front of the patient's legs. The skin of the scrotum and of the perineum is closed with Monocryl 3.0 *(Fig. 13.22)*.

The anastomosis of the pars fixa with the phallic pars of the urethra is prepared. The oblique distal end of the pars fixa is easily reached by the prepubic incision and 12–16 separate sutures Vicryl 4.0 are placed. In order to prevent fistula formation, it is advised only to include submucosa into the suture.

At the end of the perineal procedure, a suprapubic catheter is inserted.

Metaidoioplasty

A metaidoioplasty uses the (hypertrophied) clitoris to reconstruct the microphallus in a way comparable with the correction of chordee and lengthening of a urethra in cases of severe hypospadias. Eicher[49] prefers to call this intervention 'the clitoris penoid.' In metaidoioplasty, the clitoral hood is lifted and the suspensory ligament of the clitoris is detached from the pubic bone, allowing the clitoris to extend out further. An embryonic urethral plate is divided from the underside of the clitoris to permit outward extension and a visible erection.[50–53] Then the urethra is advanced to the tip of the new penis. The technique is very similar to the reconstruction of the horizontal part of the urethra in a normal phalloplasty procedure. During the same procedure, a scrotal reconstruction, with a transposition flap of the labia majora (as previously described) is performed combined with a vaginectomy.

FTM patients interested in this procedure should be informed preoperatively that voiding while standing cannot be guaranteed, and that sexual intercourse will not be possible *(Fig. 13.23)*.

The major advantage of metaidoioplasty is the absence of a donor scar and the preservation of erectile function even if only in a micropenis. Another advantage is that its cost is substantially lower than that of phalloplasty. Complications

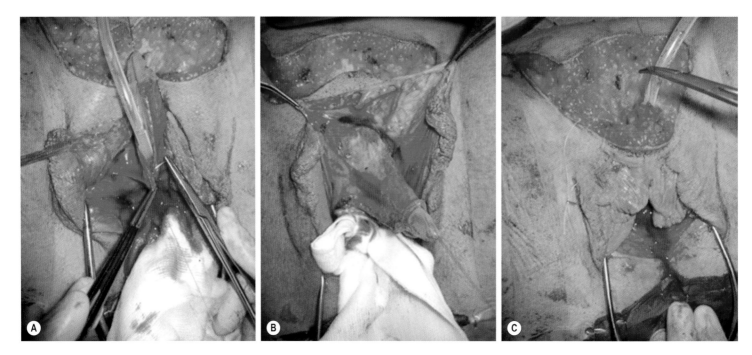

Fig. 13.21 **(A)** Creation of the pars fixa of the urethra by tabularization of the urethral plate. **(B)** Release of the foreskin of the clitoral shaft. **(C)** Tunneling of the clitoris and the distal end of the pars fixa to the prepubic area.

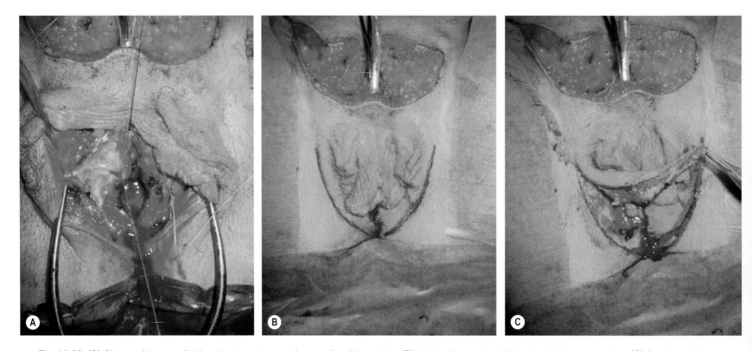

Fig. 13.22 **(A)** Closure of the superficial perineal muscles over the pars fixa of the urethra. **(B)** Incision lines at the labia majora for the scrotoplasty. **(C)** Creation of the flaps for the scrotoplasty.

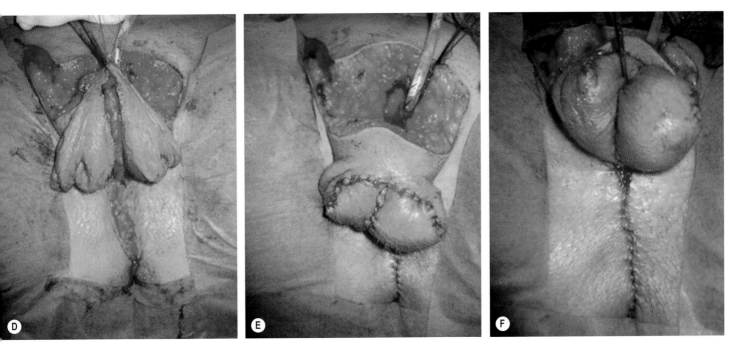

Fig. 13.22, cont'd (D) Rotation of the labial flaps 180° anteriorly. **(E,F)** Closure of the skin and final result.

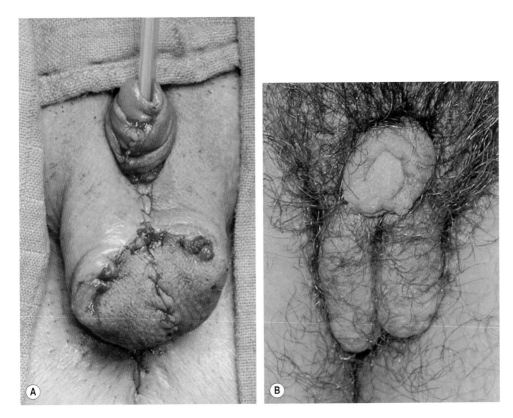

Fig. 13.23 Metaidoioplasty. **(A)** Immediate and. **(B)** Late postoperative results.

of this procedure also include urethral obstruction and/or urethral fistula.

It is always possible to perform a regular phalloplasty (e.g., with a radial forearm flap) at a later stage, and with substantially less risk of complications and operation time.

Complete phallic reconstruction

The term 'phalloplasty' was first used in 1858 by Sprengler to indicate the reconstruction of the integument after decollement (separation of the superficial tissue layers) of the penis.[54] Bogoras, the first to report on the reconstruction of the entire penis, labeled his procedure 'penis plastica totalis.'[55] He was also the first to use a single abdominal tube, a technique later applied by others. Subsequently, 'phalloplasty' was used to describe penile reconstruction.

Following the Second World War, some leading plastic surgeons showed an interest in the penile reconstructive procedure. In 1948, McIndoe[56] improved the abdominal tubed flap by constructing a neo-urethra while raising the pedicle tube employing an inlay skin graft. Maltz[57] and Gillies and Millard[58] popularized the technique when they added a costal cartilage graft as a rigidity prosthesis. Gillies was the first to report the use of this technique in a transsexual patient. The Stanford team,[53,59] refined the procedure, tubing an infraumbilical abdominal flap inside-out in order to create a skin-lined tunnel as a future urethral conduit. This method reduced the number of stages previously necessary for phalloplasty.

Snyder described a phalloplasty technique incorporating a pre-constructed superficial skin-lined conduit for intersex patients employing a single pedicled infraumbilical skin flap.[60,61] Hester performed a penile reconstruction in one stage using a vertical, superficial inferior epigastric artery flap with a subcutaneous pedicle, in a male born with ambiguous genitalia.[62] However, after McGregor introduced the groin flap in 1972,[23] Hoopes[63] commented that 'the groin flap may prove the method of choice for phallus reconstruction.' Orticochea[37] used a gracilis myocutaneous flap in a five-stage phalloplasty procedure, and claimed it produced cosmetically and functionally superior results. The Norfolk team also used a unilateral gracilis myocutaneous flap for phalloplasty.[38] Sometimes, a combination of flaps was used. Exner[64] implanted a rigidity prosthesis in a rectus abdominis muscular flap and used bilateral groin flaps to cover the neophallus.

Once microsurgery established a foothold in genital construction, plastic surgeons began to explore and map out the genital neurovascular supply and to consider expanding the applications of microsurgery to elective reconstruction of the genitalia. Chang and Hwang[65] described an ingenious adaptation of the tube-in-tube concept into a free tissue transfer with the radial forearm flap originally described by Song et al.[66]

Since these early reports, a wide variety of other free flaps have also been described for phalloplasty, including the dorsalis pedis flap,[28] the deltoid flap,[67] the lateral arm flap,[68] the fibular flap,[69] the tensor fasciae latae flap,[39] the anterolateral thigh (ALT)[70] and the deep inferior epigastric artery perforator (DIEAP) flap.[71] The fact that so many techniques for penile reconstruction exist is evidence that none is considered ideal. Still, most of these articles are only case reports or small series and even nowadays the 'old' Chinese flap or radial forearm flap is by far (>90%) the most frequently used free flap in the literature[72] and is therefore often considered as the 'gold standard' for penile reconstruction.

Radial forearm flap: technique and long-term results

Monstrey et al. recently published the only large (287 patients) and well-documented, long-term follow-up study on the use of the radial forearm phalloplasty.[71] They describe the technique they used in almost 300 consecutive cases and evaluated to what degree this supposed "gold standard" technique has been able to meet the ideal goals in phallic reconstruction.

Technique

While the urologist is operating in the perineal area, the plastic surgeon dissects the free flap of the forearm. The creation of a phallus with a tube-in-a-tube technique is performed with the flap still attached to the forearm by its vascular pedicle. A small skin flap and a skin graft are used to create a corona and simulate the glans of the penis (*Fig. 13.24A–F*).

Once the urethra is lengthened and the acceptor vessels are dissected in the groin area, the patient is put into a supine position. The free flap can be transferred to the pubic area after the urethral anastomosis (*Fig. 13.24G,H*): the radial artery is microsurgically connected to the common femoral urethra in an end-to-side fashion and the venous anastomosis is performed between the cephalic vein and the greater saphenous vein. One forearm nerve is connected to the ilioinguinal nerve for protective sensation and the other nerve of the arm is anastomosed to one of the dorsal clitoral nerves for erogenous sensation. The clitoris is usually denuded and buried underneath the penis, thus keeping the possibility to be stimulated during sexual intercourse with the neophallus.

In the first 50 patients of this series, the defect on the forearm was covered with full-thickness skin grafts taken from the groin area. In subsequent patients, the defect was covered with split-thickness skin grafts harvested from the medial and anterior thigh.

All patients receive a suprapubic urinary diversion postoperatively. The patients remain in bed during a 1-week postoperative period, after which the transurethral catheter is removed. At that time, the suprapubic catheter is clamped, and voiding is begun. Effective voiding may not be observed for several days. Before removal of the suprapubic catheter, a cystography with voiding urethrography is performed. The average hospital stay for the phalloplasty procedure is 2.5 weeks.

Tattooing of the glans can be performed after a 2–3 month period, before sensation returns to the penis. Implantation of the testicular prostheses can be performed after 6 months, but it is typically done in combination with the implantation of a penile erection prosthesis. Before these procedures are undertaken, sensation must have returned to the top of the penis. This usually does not occur for at least a year.

Ideal goals

The ideal goals or requirements of a penile reconstruction have been described by Hage and De Graaf and include the following challenges: (1) a one-stage procedure that can be predictably reproduced, (2) an aesthetically acceptable phallus, (3) that has both tactile and erogenous sensibility, (4) with a competent neourethra to allow voiding while standing, (5) involving minimal complications and (6) an acceptable donor site morbidity. Moreover (7) it must include a natural-looking scrotum and (8) provide enough phallic bulk to tolerate the insertion of a prosthetic stiffener allowing sexual intercourse.

What can be achieved with this radial forearm flap technique?

A one-stage procedure

It has been accepted that a complete penile reconstruction with erection prosthesis can never be performed in one single operation. Monstrey et al. however, early in their series and in order to reduce the number of surgeries, performed a (sort of) all-in-one procedure, which included a SCM and a complete genito-perineal transformation.[71] However, later in their series they performed the SCM first most often in combination with a total hysterectomy and oophorectomy.

The reason for this change in protocol was that lengthy operations (>8 h) resulted in considerable blood loss and increased operative risk.[73] Moreover, an aesthetic SCM is not to be considered as an easy operation and should not be performed 'quickly' before the major phalloplasty operation.

An aesthetic phallus

Phallic construction had become predictable enough to refine its aesthetic goals, which include the use of a technique that can be replicated with minimal complications. In this respect, the radial forearm flap has several advantages: the flap is thin and pliable allowing the construction of a normal sized, tube-within-a-tube penis; the flap is easy to dissect and is predictably well vascularized making it safe to perform an (aesthetic) glans-plasty at the distal end of the flap. The final cosmetic outcome of a radial forearm phalloplasty is a subjective determination, but the ability of most patients to shower with other men or to go to the sauna, is the usual cosmetic barometer *(Fig. 13.25)*.

The potential aesthetic drawbacks of the radial forearm flap are the need for a rigidity prosthesis and possibly some volume loss over time.

Tactile and erogenous sensation

Of the various flaps used for penile reconstruction, the radial forearm flap has the greatest sensivity.[74,75] Monstrey et al. always connect one antebrachial nerve to the ilioinguinal nerve for protective sensation and the other forearm nerve with one dorsal clitoral nerve. The denuded clitoris was

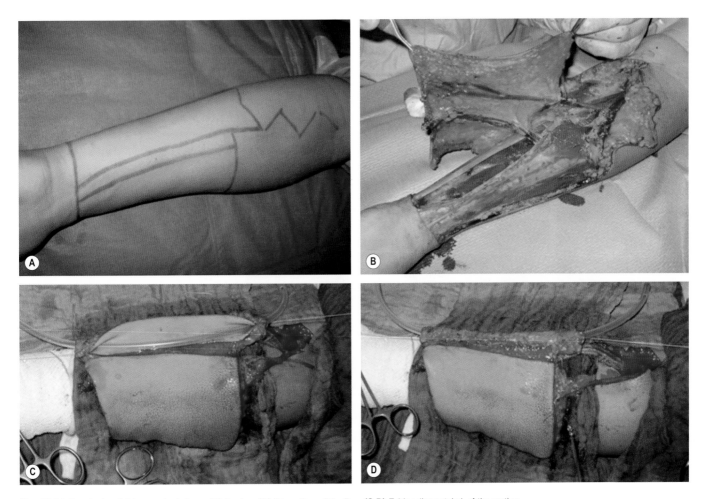

Fig. 13.24 Standard radial forearm technique. **(A)** Design. **(B)** Dissection of the flap. **(C,D)** Tubing (inner tube) of the urethra.

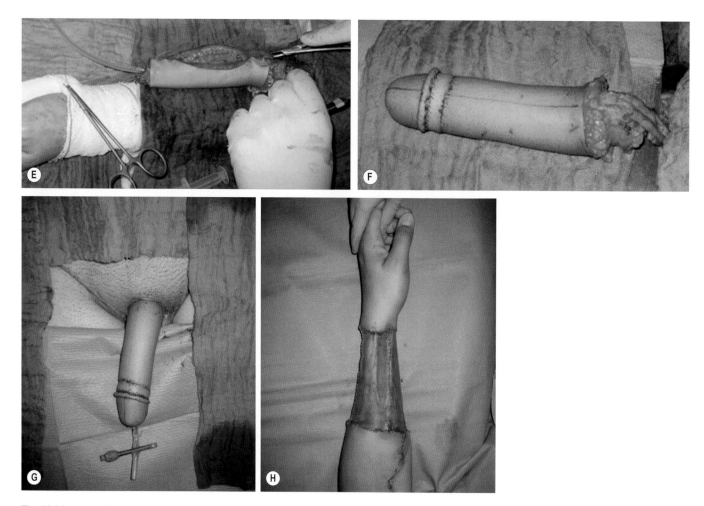

Fig. 13.24 cont'd, **(E)** Outer tube of the penis itself. **(F)** Creation of the glans of the penis (with penis still attached to the forearm, just prior to transfer to the pubic area. **(G)** Immediate postoperative result of the penis and. **(H)** The donor site on the arm.

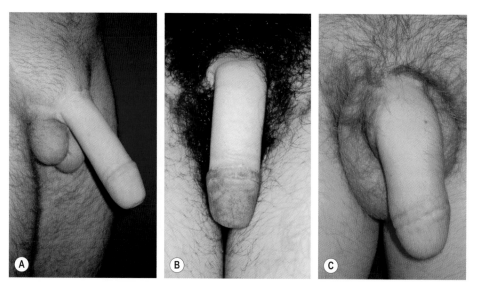

Fig. 13.25 **(A–C)** Late postoperative results of radial forearm phalloplasties.

always placed directly below the phallic shaft. Later manipulation of the neophallus allows for stimulation of the still-innervated clitoris.

After 1 year, all patients had regained tactile sensitivity in their penis, which is an absolute requirement for safe insertion of an erection prosthesis.[74]

In a long-term follow-up study on postoperative sexual and physical health, more than 80% of the patients reported improvement in sexual satisfaction and greater ease in reaching orgasm (100% in practicing postoperative FTM transsexuals).[76]

Voiding while standing

For biological males as well as for FTM transsexuals undergoing a phalloplasty, the ability to void while standing is a high priority.[77] Unfortunately, the reported incidences of urological complications, such as urethrocutaneous fistulas, stenoses, strictures, and hairy urethras are extremely high in all series of phalloplasties, even up to 80%.[33] For this reason, certain (well-intentioned) surgeons have even stopped reconstructing a complete neo-urethra.[70,78]

In their series of radial forearm phalloplasties, Monstrey et al.[71] still reported a urological complication rate of 41% (119/287) but the majority of these early fistulas closed spontaneously and ultimately *all* patients were able to void through the newly reconstructed penis.[79] Since it is unknown how the new urethra – a 16 cm skin tube – will affect bladder function in the long term, lifelong urologic follow-up was strongly recommended for all these patients.

Minimal morbidity

Complications following phalloplasty include the general complications attendant to any surgical intervention such as minor wound healing problems in the groin area or a few patients with a (minor) pulmonary embolism despite adequate prevention (interrupting hormonal therapy, fractioned heparin SC, elastic stockings). A vaginectomy is usually considered a particularly difficult operation with a high risk of postoperative bleeding but in their series no major bleedings were seen.[73] Two early patients displayed symptoms of nerve compression in the lower leg but after reducing the length of the gynecological positioning to under two hours, this complication never occurred again. Apart from the urinary fistulas and/or stenoses, most complications of the radial forearm phalloplasty are related to the free tissue transfer. The total flap failure in their series was very low (<1%, 2/287) despite a somewhat higher anastomotic revision rate (12% or 34/287). About 7.3% of the patients demonstrated some degree of skin slough or partial flap necrosis. This was more often the case in smokers, in those who insisted on a large-sized penis requiring a larger flap, and also in patients having undergone anastomotic revision.

With *smoking* being a significant risk factor, under our current policy, they no longer operate on patients who fail to quit smoking one year prior to their surgery.

No functional loss and minimal scarring in the donor area

The major drawback of the radial forearm flap has always been the unattractive donor site scar on the forearm (*Fig. 13.26*). Selvaggi et al. conducted a long-term follow-up study[80]

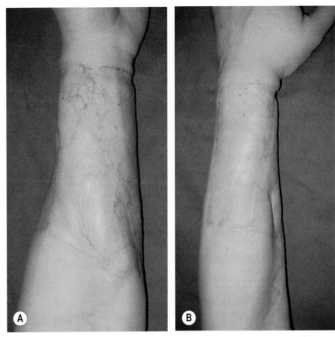

Fig. 13.26 Late result of the donor site at the forearm.

of 125 radial forearm phalloplasties to assess the degree of functional loss and aesthetic impairment after harvesting such a large forearm flap. An increased donor site morbidity was expected, but the early and late complications did not differ from the rates reported in the literature for the smaller flaps as used in head and neck reconstruction.[80] No major or long-term problems (such as functional limitation, nerve injury, chronic pain/edema or cold intolerance) were identified. Finally, with regard to the aesthetic outcome of the donor site, they found that the patients were very accepting of the donor site scar, viewing it as a worthwhile trade-off for the creation of a phallus.[80] Suprafascial flap dissection, full thickness skin grafts and the use of dermal substitutes may contribute to a better forearm scar.

Normal scrotum

For the female-to-male patient, the goal of creating natural-appearing genitals also applies to the scrotum. As the labia majora are the embryological counterpart of the scrotum, many previous scrotoplasty techniques left the hair-bearing labia majora *in situ*, with midline closure and prosthetic implant filling, or brought the scrotum in front of the legs using a V-Y plasty. These techniques were aesthetically unappealing and reminiscent of the female genitalia. Selvaggi in 2009 reported on a novel scrotoplasty technique which combines a V-Y plasty with a 90° turning of the labial flaps resulting in an anterior transposition of labial skin (*Fig. 13.27*). The excellent aesthetic outcome of this male-looking (anteriorly located) scrotum, the functional advantage of fewer urological complications and the easier implantation of testicular prostheses make this the technique of choice.[81]

Sexual intercourse

In a radial forearm phalloplasty, the insertion of an erection prosthesis is required in order to engage in sexual intercourse. In the past, attempts have been made to use bone or cartilage

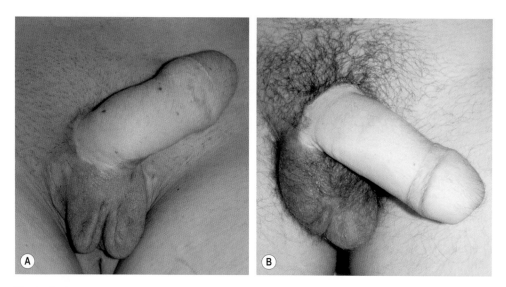

Fig. 13.27 (A,B) Reconstruction of a lateral looking scrotum with two transposition flaps before and after implantation of prostheses.

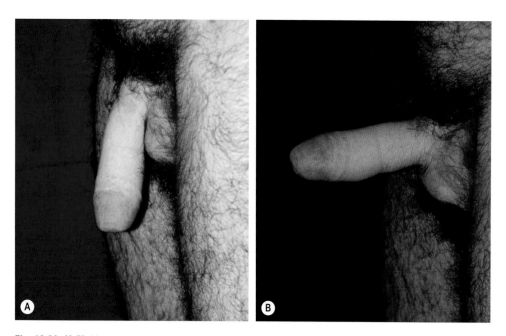

Fig. 13.28 (A,B) After implantation of an erection prosthesis.

but no good long term results are described. The rigid and semi-rigid prostheses seem to have a high perforation rate and therefore were never used in our patients. Hoebeke et al., in the largest series to date on erection prostheses after penile reconstruction, only used the hydraulic systems available for impotent men. A recent long-term follow-up study showed an explantation rate of 44% in 130 patients, mainly due to malpositioning, technical failure, or infection. Still, more than 80% of the patients were able to have normal sexual intercourse with penetration.[79] In another study, it was demonstrated that patients with an erection prosthesis were more able to attain their sexual expectations than those without prosthesis *(Fig. 13.28)*.[75]

A major concern regarding erectile prostheses is long-term follow-up. These devices were developed for impotent (older) men who have a shorter life expectancy and who are sexually less active than the mostly younger FTM patients.

Conclusion

The authors in this review article conclude that the radial forearm phalloplasty is a very reliable technique for the construction, usually in two stages, of a normal looking penis always allowing the patient to void while standing and also to experience sexual satisfaction.

The main disadvantages of this technique are the rather high number of initial fistulas, the scar on the forearm and the potential long-term urologic complications.

Alternative phalloplasty techniques

Fibula flap

There have been several reports on penile reconstruction with the fibular flap based on the peroneal artery and the peroneal vein.[69,82,83] It consists of a piece of fibula which is vascularized by its periosteal blood supply and connected through perforating (septal) vessels to an overlying skin island at the lateral site of the lower leg. The advantage of the fibular flap is that it makes sexual intercourse possible without a penile prosthesis. The disadvantages of this technique however are the poor quality of the flap sensation, a pointed deformity to the distal part of the penis when the extra skin can glide around the end of fibular bone, and that a permanently erected phallus is impractical.

Perforator flaps

Perforator flaps are considered the ultimate form of tissue transfer. Donor site morbidity is reduced to an absolute minimum, and the usually large vascular pedicles provide an additional range of motion or an easier vascular anastomosis. At present, the most promising perforator flap for penile reconstruction is the anterolateral thigh (ALT) flap, which can be used both as a free flap[84] or rather as a pedicled flap (S. Suominen, pers. comm. 1994),[40] then avoiding the problems related to microsurgical free flap transfer (see above).

The fabrication of an inner tube for urethral conduit makes the ALT flap procedure in reconstruction of a phallus more complex, especially in the biologically female transman.

Theoretically, a tube-within-a-tube technique providing a good quality inner lining of the reconstructed urethra, similar to the conventional RFAF phalloplasty procedure, can also be constructed in case of a pedicled ALT flap, especially in a thin individual. In most cases however, when folding the flap on itself, a very large and bulky phallus is obtained.

An inner urethral tube can also be provided by prefabricating the ALT flap with a split thickness skin graft. The skin grafted area should have at least a width of 5 cm to provide an adequate inner tube and prevent a future stricture. Still, the quality of the inner urethral tube when lined with skin grafts is inferior compared to normal skin, resulting in a higher rate of urological complications (strictures, fistulas) when compared to a RFAF tube-within-tube phalloplasty. The shape of a prefabricated ALT phalloplasty is comparable with or even somewhat better than the RFAF phalloplasty if the patient is not too fat and the flap is defatted.

In the search for a better inner tube, the use of well vascularized tissue is necessary. Therefore, the inner tube can be made from another flap.

A pedicled peritoneal flap, elevated together with the posterior rectus fascia pedicled on a branch of the deep inferior epigastric artery pedicle[85] has been tried in order to reconstruct an urethral conduit but this was not suitable[40,86]: the inner peritoneal lining easily causes fibrosis resulting in a permanent obliteration of the lumen.

The use of a pedicled groin flap is another alternative for the creation of an inner tube. The flap is turned 180° on his pedicle and transferred to the pubic area. The proximal part is buried subcutaneously. The donor scar can be closed primarily. Because of the thickness of the flap, the same objections can be made as mentioned with the tube within tube technique.

Finally, the inner tube can also be made from a narrow free RFAF. This flap is thin and very well vascularized *(Fig. 13.29)*. The results of this combined (pedicled ALT + freeRFAF) phalloplasty procedure, were similar to the results of the RFAF (only) phalloplasty, as to the urologic complication rate and were even more pleasing from an aesthetic point of view. The resulting scar on the arm is small and located on the inner side *(Fig. 13.29)*. This scar is easily concealed and acceptable for most female to male transsexuals willing to avoid the circumferential scar. The scar on the leg, although conspicuous, never poses a problem in these patient since it can be better hidden than the scar on the arm which is sometimes considered as 'the signature' of a phalloplasty procedure.

Summary

The importance of a multidisciplinary approach

Gender reassignment, particularly reassignment surgery, requires close cooperation between the different surgical specialties. In phalloplasty, the collaboration between the plastic surgeon, the urologist and the gynecologist is essential.[87] The actual penile reconstruction is typically performed by the plastic and reconstructive surgeon, but, in the long term, the urologist's role may be the most important for patients who have undergone penile reconstruction, especially because the complication rate is rather high, particularly with regard to the number of urinary fistulas and urinary stenoses. The urologist also reconstructs the fixed part of the urethra. He is likely the best choice for implantation and follow-up of the penile and/or testicular prostheses. He must also address later sequelae, including stone formation. Moreover, the surgical complexity of adding an elongated conduit (skin-tube urethra) to a biological female bladder, and the long-term effects of evacuating urine through this skin tube, demand lifelong urological follow-up.

Therefore, professionals who unite for the purpose of creating a gender reassignment program should be aware of the necessity of a strong alliance mainly between the plastic surgeon and the urologist, which is an absolute requisite to consistently obtain the best possible results. In turn, the surgeons must commit to the extended care of this unique population which, by definition, will protract well into the future.

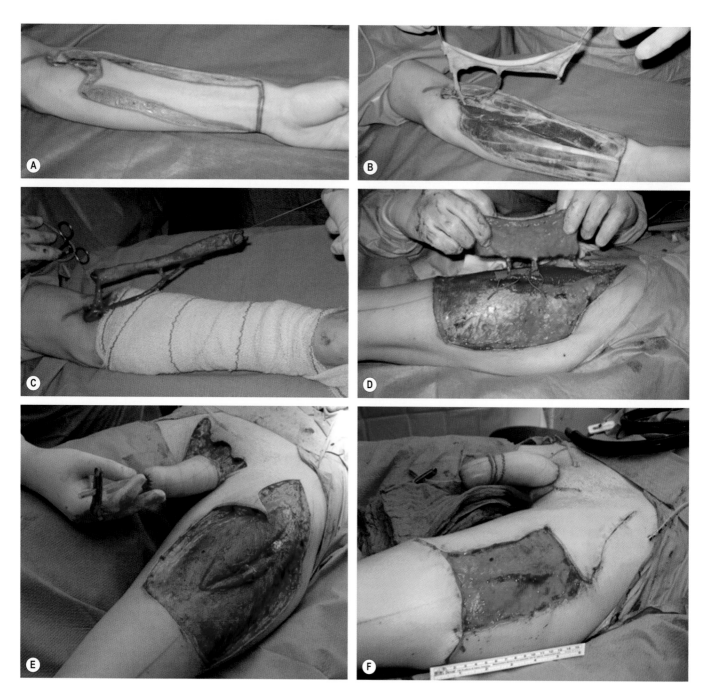

Fig. 13.29 (A,B) Dissection of a narrow free vascularized radial forearm used for the urethra. **(C)** The radial forearm flap urethra is ready to be transferred to the pubic area. **(D)** Dissection of the ALT flap will be used to wrap around the urethra. **(E)** RFAF urethra and ALT wrap-around put into position in the pubic area. **(F)** After coronoplasty and grafting of the donor area.

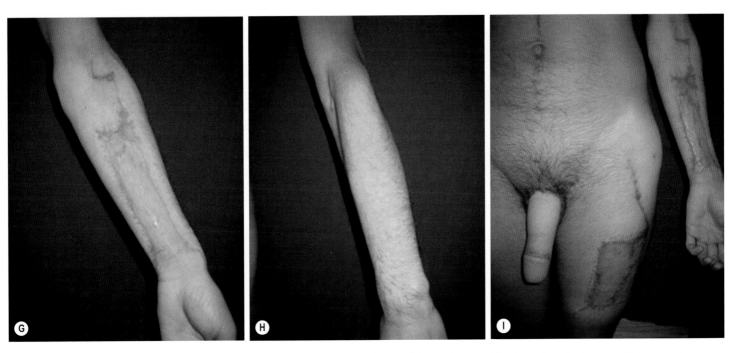

Fig. 13.29 continued (G–I) Result after 3 months: the donor site on the inner aspect of the arm is inconspicuous and the donor site on the leg can easily be covered even with shorts.

Access the complete reference list online at **http://www.expertconsult.com**

6. Mitchell ME, Bägli DJ. Complete penile disassembly for epispadias repair: the Mitchell technique. *J Urol.* 1996;155(1):300–304.

    The authors present their technique for epispadias repair in the context of a case series. Phallic disassembly into the urethral plate and bilateral hemicorporeal glandular bodies is the basis for their reconstruction.

10. Lee PA, Houk CP, Ahmed SF, et al. Consensus statement on management of intersex disorders. International Consensus Conference on Intersex. *Pediatrics.* 2006;118(2):e488–e500.

    This paper represents the responses of 50 international experts to a series of literature-based questions. Topics ranging from diagnosis to medical and surgical management, as well as the important role of psychosocial support are discussed.

23. McGregor IA, Jackson IT. The groin flap. *Br J Plast Surg.* 1972;25:3.

32. Hurwitz DJ, Swartz WM, Mathes SJ. The gluteal thigh flap: a reliable, sensate flap for the closure of buttock and perineal wounds. *Plast Reconstr Surg.* 1981;68:521.

    The authors describe the results of anatomic dissections detailing the gluteal thigh flap's neurovascular morphology. A case series demonstrating the clinical utility of the flap is also presented.

37. Orticochea M. A new method of total reconstruction of the penis. *Br J Plast Surg.* 1972;25:347–366.

47. Eke N. Fournier's gangrene: a review of 1726 cases. *Br J Surg.* 2000;87:718.

    This is a meta-analysis of Fournier's gangrene publications from 1950–1999. The authors investigate trends in diagnosis and management, and conclude that while precise definitions vary, treatment is based on clinical presentation.

41. Cohen BE, May JW, Daly JS, et al. Successful clinical replantation of an amputated penis by microneurovascular repair. *Plast Reconstr Surg.* 1977;59:276.

62. Hester Jr TR, Nahain F, Beeglen PE, et al. Blood supply of the abdomen revisited, with emphasis on the superficial inferior epigastric artery. *Plast Reconstr Surg.* 1984;74(5): 657–666.

66. Song R, Gao Y, Song Y, et al. The forearm flap. *Clin Plast Surg.* 1982;9:21.

65. Chang TS, Hwang YW. Forearm flap in one-stage reconstruction of the penis. *Plast Reconstr Surg.* 1984;74:251–258.

    Single stage free forearm-based penile reconstruction is described in this case series.

14

Reconstruction of acquired vaginal defects

Laura Snell, Peter G. Cordeiro, and Andrea L. Pusic

SYNOPSIS

- Acquired vaginal defects are most commonly the result of oncologic resections.
- Current approaches to reconstruction of these defects most commonly involves local or regional flaps if primary closure is not an option.
- Flap selection based on defect type is described *(Table 14.1)*.
- A cautious approach to postoperative management, as well as careful adjustment of patient expectations, is critical in the care of these patients.

 Access the Historical Perspective section online at
http://www.expertconsult.com

Introduction

Acquired vaginal defects most commonly result from the resection of pelvic malignant neoplasms. Advanced colorectal carcinomas frequently involve the posterior bladder wall. Carcinoma of the bladder may extend into the anterior vaginal wall. Primary tumors of the vaginal wall may result in any number of vaginal defects. Local extension or recurrence of uterine or cervical malignant neoplasms can necessitate pelvic exenteration and total vaginal resection. Trauma or burns to the vaginal area may also result in vaginal distortion; however the relatively protected position of the vagina makes these deformities much less common.

Irrespective of their etiology, vaginal defects may range from a small mucosal defect to total circumferential loss. In addition, tumor ablation may necessitate the resection of vulvar and perineal tissue, further complicating the reconstruction. Although reconstruction is usually performed at the time of the oncologic resection, delayed procedures are not uncommon. In these delayed cases, scarring and soft-tissue contracture may add to the technical difficulty of the reconstruction.

Basic science/anatomy

The close anatomic relationship between the bladder, vagina, and rectum needs to be well appreciated by the reconstructive surgeon. Ligamentous support of these organs is interrelated, and surgical dissection of any one structure may lead to prolapse and herniation of the remaining components. In addition, pelvic exenteration may disrupt or devascularize the pelvic floor musculature. The pelvic sidewalls define a fixed anatomic space that, once cleared of the pelvic organs, will either delineate a dead space or invite small-bowel prolapse and adhesions.

The vagina is essentially a distensible cylindrical pouch *(Fig. 14.1)*. Normal length is 6–7.5 cm along its anterior wall and 9 cm along the posterior wall.[7] It is constricted at the introitus, dilated in the middle, and narrowed near its uterine extremity. In its normal anatomic position, the vagina tilts posteriorly as it extends up into the pelvis, forming a 90° angle with the uterus. Careful orientation of the neovagina is important to successful reconstruction and ultimate sexual function. The introitus is a frequent site of contracture after reconstruction, and any distortion of its normal position relative to other structures such as the urethral orifice, perineal body, and anus should be addressed. If no resection of the external vulva and perineum is required, great care must be taken to avoid their distortion because this may also have an impact on sexual function and body image.

Diagnosis

The classification of acquired vaginal defects is based on their anatomic location *(Fig. 14.2)*. This classification will help to guide reconstructive efforts. There are two basic types of vaginal defect: partial (type I), and circumferential (type II). These basic types can be further subclassified. Type IA defects are partial, and involve the anterior or lateral wall. These defects may result from the resection of urinary tract malignant neoplasms or primary malignant neoplasms of the

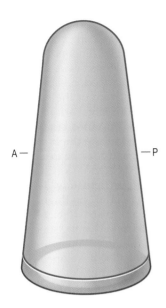

Fig. 14.1 Vaginal vault. A, anterior; P, posterior.

Table 14.1 Previously described flap options for vaginal reconstruction

Defect type	Flap option
IA	Singapore flaps (aka pudendal fasciocutaneous flap)
IB	Pedicled rectus myocutaneous flap Pedicled rectus musculoperitoneal flap Muscle-sparing rectus myocutaneous flap
IIA/B	Vertical rectus abdominis myocutaneous Gracilis Singapore flaps Pedicled jejunum Sigmoid colon

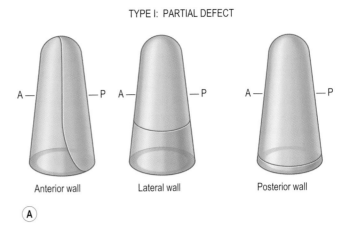

TYPE I: PARTIAL DEFECT

Anterior wall   Lateral wall   Posterior wall

(A)

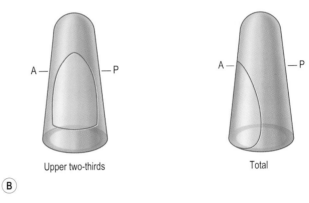

TYPE II: CIRCUMFERENTIAL DEFECT

Upper two-thirds   Total

(B)

Fig. 14.2 (A, B) Classification system of acquired vaginal defects. (A) Type I: partial defect; (B) type II: circumferential defect. A, anterior; P, posterior.

vaginal wall. Type IB defects are partial, and involve the posterior wall. These defects, which tend to be the most common type of vaginal defect requiring reconstruction, result primarily from extension of colorectal carcinomas. Type IIA defects are circumferential defects involving the upper two-thirds of the vagina. These defects are typically the result of uterine and cervical diseases. Type IIB defects are circumferential, total vaginal defects that are commonly the result of pelvic exenteration. These defects result in considerable soft-tissue loss, dead space, as well as distortion of the introitus.

Patient selection

Successful management of patients undergoing vaginal reconstruction is dependent upon a multidisciplinary approach. The oncologic and reconstructive surgeons need to communicate well in terms of both the expected defect and the reconstructive options that are available to that specific patient. The anesthesia team needs to be well advised of the nature of the procedure and the hemodynamic stress that can be expected

intraoperatively. Also, early involvement of a psychiatrist and a sex therapist may be warranted.

The radiation oncologist is an important participant in the overall treatment plan. Many patients have had previous radiotherapy, and many other patients may be receiving intraoperative radiotherapy or placement of a brachytherapy cannula. The radiotherapy plan has important implications for the choice of flap as both the recipient and donor sites can be affected by radiation injury. In addition, the medical oncologist should be involved with the decision-making as many patients may receive pre- and postoperative chemotherapy. Surgical procedures should be timed to minimize the effects of chemotherapy on wound healing, as well as to avoid unnecessary delays in starting chemotherapy protocols.

Most important to the success of the reconstruction is the full and informed involvement of the patient and her family. It is important to be specific about the goals of vaginal reconstruction with patients, which include effective wound healing and restoration of body image and sexual function[8] (Box 14.1). For those women motivated to preserve sexual function, a comprehensive program of sexual rehabilitation may be warranted. Ratliff et al. investigated sexual adjustment after vaginal reconstruction with gracilis myocutaneous flaps and found that, although 70% of patients were judged to have a physically adequate vagina, fewer than 50% resumed sexual activity.[9] Absence of pleasure (37%), problems with vaginal dryness (32%), excess secretions (27%), self-consciousness about ostomies (40%), and self-consciousness about nudity in front of their partner (30%) were the most considerable concerns. Preoperative and postoperative counseling, in addition to postoperative rehabilitation strategies (vaginal dilators, lubricants, topical estrogens), have been suggested as the best way to influence these outcomes positively and give patients the best hope of functional and psychological recovery.[8,10] The psychologist and sex therapist should be an integral part of the ablative-reconstructive team. In addition, at most tertiary care institutions, specialized nursing teams can help the patient and her family prepare for the psychological distress that they may experience.

Treatment/surgical technique

There are five basic goals in vaginal reconstruction (*Box 14.1*). Selection of the optimal reconstructive method to achieve these goals is based on the type of defect and the characteristics of the patient. Small defects that can be closed without tension will ideally be closed primarily. In the case of the irradiated wound, however, one must proceed cautiously with primary closure. Rarely is skin grafting alone an adequate alternative in oncology patients.

Proceeding along the reconstructive ladder, regional flaps continue to be the most frequently used and effective procedures. Many flaps have been described, none of which is ideal for all defect types (*Table 14.1*).[11–17] To simplify surgical decision-making, a reconstructive algorithm has been developed on the basis of defect type (*Fig. 14.3*).[18]

Box 14.1 The major goals of vaginal reconstruction

- To promote effective wound healing, facilitating postoperative radiation therapy and chemotherapy
- To decrease pelvic dead space, thus decreasing fluid loss, metabolic demands, and infection
- To restore the pelvic floor, preventing herniation and small-bowel fistula
- To re-establish body image
- To re-establish sexual function

Type IA defects, which involve only the anterior or lateral vaginal walls, usually require little tissue bulk and small to moderate surface coverage. The modified Singapore (vulvoperineal or pudendal thigh) fasciocutaneous flap is ideal in this setting.[15,16] It provides a highly vascularized, reliable, and pliable flap that conforms well to the surface of the vaginal cylinder. This flap is based on the posterior labial arteries and innervated by perineal branches of the posterior cutaneous nerve of the thigh.[19] The flaps are raised in the thigh crease, lateral to the hair-bearing labia majora, and may be designed to measure 9 × 4 cm to 15 × 6 cm.[15,16] The posterior skin margin is marked at the level of the posterior fourchette (*Fig. 14.4A*). The skin, subcutaneous tissue, deep fascia of the thigh, and epimysium of the adductor muscles are raised (*Fig. 14.4B*). Posteriorly, the base of the flap is undermined at the subcutaneous level to facilitate rotation and insetting. Depending on the defect, unilateral or bilateral flaps may be developed (*Fig. 14.4C*). The flaps may be inset by tunneling under the labia majora or by division of the labia at the level of the fourchette. The donor site is closed primarily (*Figs 14.4D and 14.5*).

Type IB defects, which encompass the posterior vaginal wall, frequently require greater soft-tissue bulk to fill the dead space made by resection of the rectum. Here, the preferred choice is the pedicled rectus myocutaneous flap. This highly reliable flap provides both a large surface area and large volume. The skin can be used to replace the entire posterior vaginal wall. The healthy muscle and subcutaneous tissue bring well-vascularized tissue to the pelvis, obliterate dead space, and separate the contents of the abdominal cavity from the zone of injury. When used for vaginal reconstruction, the flap is based on the deep inferior epigastric vessels that arise from the common femoral arteries and enter the rectus muscle along its posterolateral surface 6–7 cm above its insertion on the pubis (*Fig. 14.6*). In planning the flap, one must ensure that these vessels are not divided as part of the cancer resection. One must also ensure that the muscle itself is not violated during placement of the stoma. Stoma planning requires communication between the reconstructive surgeon and the colorectal surgeon. Usually the stoma is placed on the patient's left side, thus sparing the right rectus for reconstruction. If there is only one available rectus for both stoma placement and the reconstructive donor site, the colorectal surgeon may be able to place the stoma through an empty rectus sheath, or through the external oblique. Communication with the colorectal

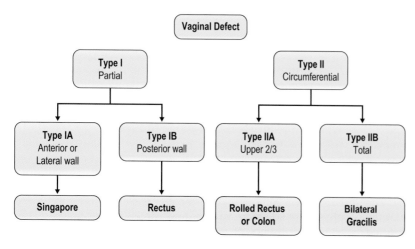

Fig. 14.3 Algorithm for reconstruction of the vagina based on defect type.

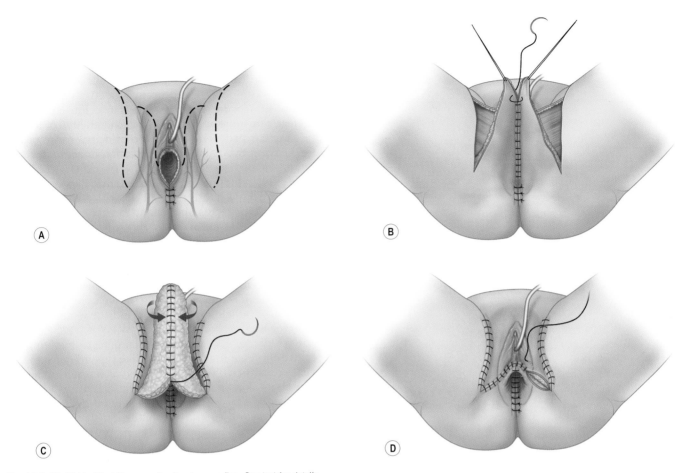

Fig. 14.4 **(A–D)** Modified Singapore fasciocutaneous flap. See text for details.

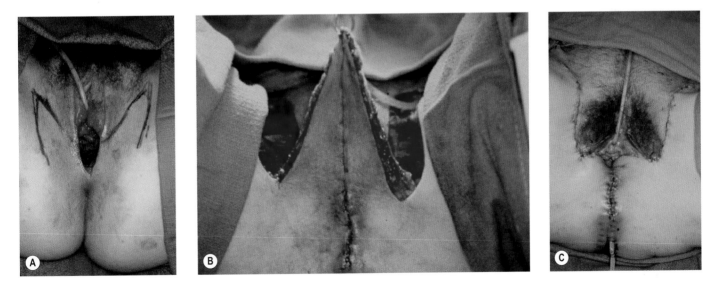

Fig. 14.5 **(A)** Marking of the modified Singapore fasciocutaneous flap. **(B)** Flap elevation. **(C)** Flap inset.

surgeon is also required for incision planning. If the right rectus is to be used for reconstruction, ask the colorectal surgeon not to plan the abdominal incision around the left side of the umbilicus, as this will lead to vascular compromise of the umbilicus when harvesting the rectus flap.

Either a vertical or transverse skin island design may be used for the rectus myocutaneous flap, depending on the size of the defect and the characteristics of the patient's abdominal wall. For posterior wall reconstruction, the vertical rectus abdominis myocutaneous (VRAM) design is usually preferable because it maximizes blood supply by centering the skin island over the medial and lateral rows of perforators, and does not interfere with the contralateral muscle and stoma placement.

Both the vertical and transverse rectus abdominis myocutaneous flaps can be designed up to 10×20 cm in size with easy donor site closure. When the flap is inset into a posterior-wall defect, care must be taken to avoid constriction or tension on the vascular pedicle as this is the principal cause of flap failure. Leaving the distal muscle insertion intact to decrease tension on the pedicle is helpful in this regard *(Fig. 14.7)*.

The rectus abdominis musculoperitoneal flap is a recent modification rectus flap for type I vaginal defects where a patch of posterior rectus sheath and peritoneum above the arcuate line is harvested with the rectus to the exact dimensions of the resected vaginal mucosa. The pedicled flap is then transposed into the vaginal canal and the peritoneal patch is sutured to the edges of the vaginal mucosa. This technique avoids the need for harvesting skin and anterior rectus sheath. The peritoneum has previously been shown to re-epithelialize to squamous epithelium, making it indistinguishable from vaginal mucosa.[17]

Type IIA defects are circumferential defects involving the upper two-thirds of the vagina and, like type IB defects, they are well reconstructed with the pedicled rectus myocutaneous flap due to its skin and soft-tissue bulk. The rectus is preferable to bilateral gracilis flaps because the intervening vulvar and pelvic floor musculature prohibits transfer of the gracili to the defect. When using the rectus myocutaneous flap for these defects, the cutaneous portion of the flap is tubed. A

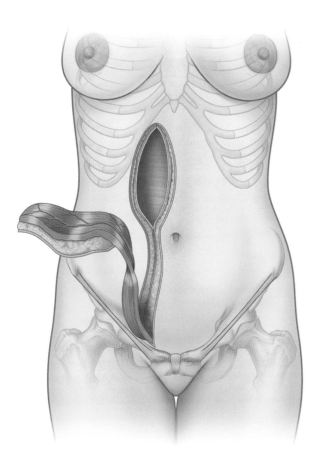

Fig. 14.6 Pedicled rectus myocutaneous flap.

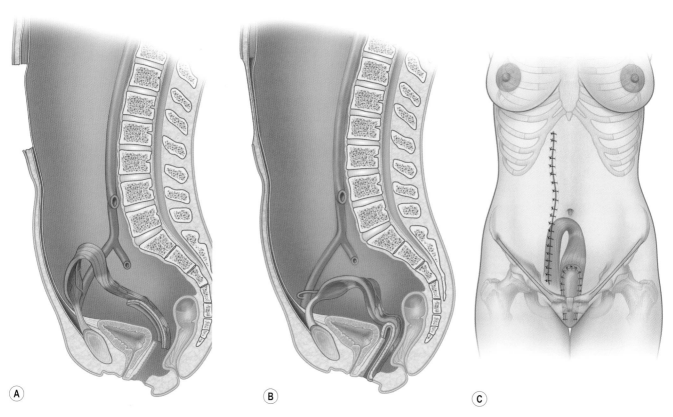

(A) (B) (C)

Fig. 14.7 (A–C) Rotation and insetting of a pedicled vertical rectus abdominis myocutaneous flap for a posterior wall defect.

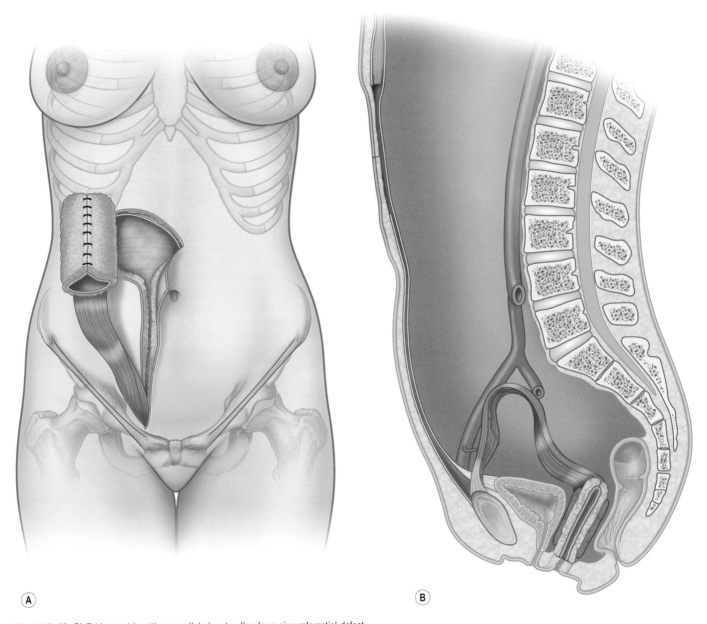

Fig. 14.8 (A, B) Tubing and insetting a pedicled rectus flap for a circumferential defect.

transverse skin island is easier to manipulate and leaves a slightly longer pedicle than the VRAM). A flap width of 12–15 cm will provide a neovagina with a 4-cm diameter.[20] Once tubed, the flap is then sutured to the remaining vaginal cuff from above *(Fig. 14.8)*.

The sigmoid colon or jejunum may also be used to reconstruct type IIA defects for patients in whom the rectus flap cannot be utilized. For the sigmoid colon flap, a segment of colon is isolated and pedicled on a branch of the inferior mesenteric artery.[11] For the jejunum flap, a 15-cm segment of jejunum is isolated and pedicled on the fourth branch of the superior mesenteric artery, approximately 30 cm distal to the ligament of Treitz.[21] For both of these flaps the bowel is stapled closed superiorly, and sutured inferiorly to the vaginal cuff. Excessive secretions and unpleasant odor, especially for the

sigmoid colon, persist as common complaints of patients, limiting the usefulness of these techniques.[22]

Type IIB defects are circumferential defects involving the entire vagina and frequently the introitus. These are usually total pelvic exenteration defects. Given the need for a large skin island, bilateral gracilis flaps are an excellent reconstructive choice for these defects. The subcutaneous tissue and muscle of the two conjoined flaps will provide a large volume of soft tissue that can obliterate the dead space within the pelvis. The vascular supply of the gracilis flap is the medial femoral circumflex artery, which enters the gracilis muscle 7–10 cm below the pubic tubercle *(Fig. 14.9A)*. An elliptical skin island approximately 6 × 20 cm can be designed centered over the proximal two-thirds of the muscle, with the anterior border of the incision lying on a line between the pubic

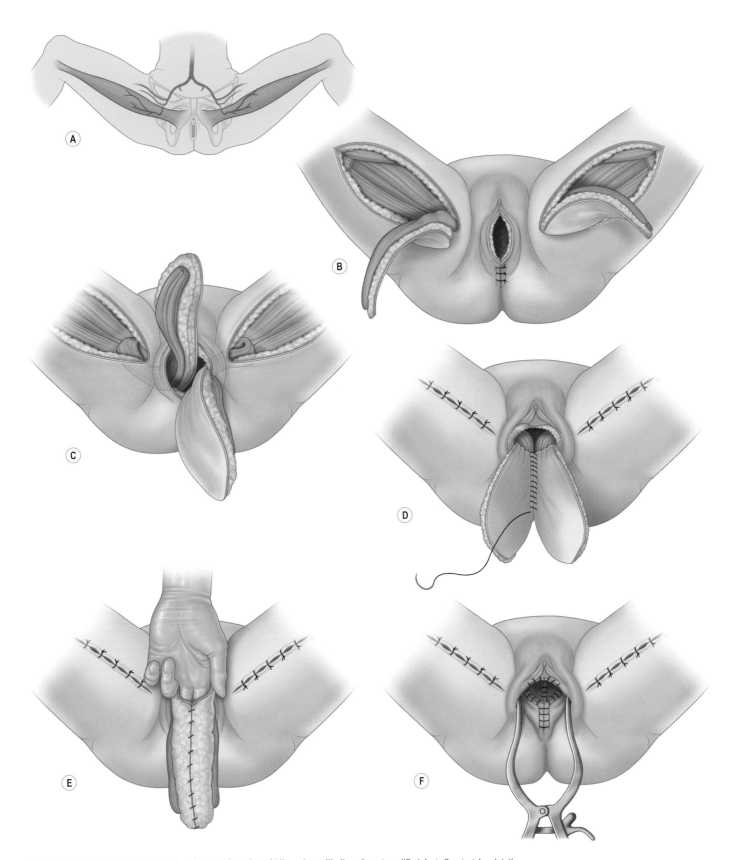

Fig. 14.9 (A–F) Anatomy, design, elevation, and insetting of bilateral gracilis flaps for a type IIB defect. See text for details.

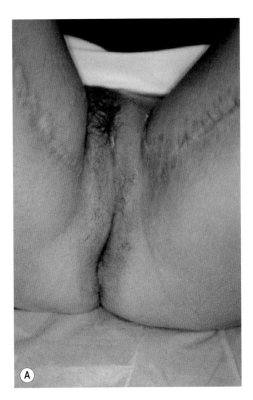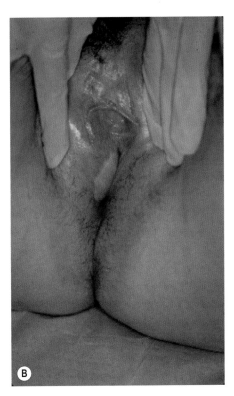

Fig. 14.10 (A, B) Postoperative results of a vaginal reconstruction using bilateral gracilis flaps.

tubercle and the semitendinosus tendon. Once elevated, the flaps are tunneled subcutaneously into the vaginal defect *(Fig. 14.9B, C)*. The flaps are then sutured in the midline, and a neovaginal pouch is formed *(Fig. 14.9D, E)*. The neovaginal pouch is then inserted into the defect, and the proximal flap edges are sutured to the introitus *(Figs 14.9F and 14.10)*. The flap can maintain some sensation for pressure through branches of the obturator nerve.[22]

Flap selection is based on both the type of defect and the individual patient's characteristics. While the majority of patients can be reconstructed by using an algorithm based on defect type, a few may require a modified approach. Obesity, for example, has been shown to be a significant risk factor for poor wound healing after rectus flap reconstruction.[6] Obese patients with type IIB defects therefore may be better reconstructed with thin, bilateral Singapore flaps. Alternatively, the rectus may be used without its cutaneous portion and a skin graft applied directly to the muscle over a vaginal stent. In heavily irradiated patients, the rectus muscle may be desirable for APR defects that appear small externally because its muscle bulk will aid pelvic revascularization, lowering the risk of perineal wound abscess and wound dehiscence.[12] In elderly patients or patients with significant comorbidities who are unlikely to resume intercourse after reconstruction, a full vaginal reconstruction may be omitted. Using a rectus muscle flap to obliterate dead space within the pelvis may still be of wound-healing benefit to these patients. In patients with previous vaginal reconstruction and recurrent disease, the choice of regional flap may be extremely limited, perhaps warranting free flap reconstruction.

Postoperative care

Immediate perioperative period

At the end of the reconstructive case, it is imperative to leave a pelvic drain in place in order to drain the fluid that will inevitably collect in any remaining dead space. While these drains typically drain a large amount, the goal should be to keep it in place until the patient is mobile and the drainage begins to decrease, rather than reaching below a certain set point.

Postoperatively, careful attention must also be paid to the patient's hemodynamic and nutritional support. All patients should receive deep-vein thrombosis prophylaxis. They should be placed on a fluidized mattress and given instructions not to sit for a minimum of 3 weeks. Positioning is difficult due to these restrictions, and patients should be encouraged to lie on either side, stand, or walk. Prophylactic perioperative antibiotics are often used.

Long-term recovery

The placement of a vaginal stent intraoperatively is not routine for all flap reconstructions. However, once the flap is healed, gradual dilatation with a lubricator may be important in order to increase the size of the orifice. If the patient wishes to use the neovagina for intercourse, she must be told that dilatation must be continued on an ongoing and regular basis for life.

Dilatation can begin at approximately 2 months postreconstruction, as long as everything is well healed. Custom dilators are usually constructed for each patient. Estrogen creams applied to reconstructed type I defects can also be helpful to maintain lubrication.

Outcomes, prognosis, and complications

Although poor tissue vascularity, dead space, and loss of pelvic support are the main causes of problems in the early postoperative period, long-term issues relating to sexual function and body image are also considerable. After pelvic exenteration, 5-year survival among patients with gynecologic cancer is 40–60%. Among APR patients, 5-year survival is 25–40%.[4] For the patients who do well with their disease, sexual function and body image are fundamental quality-of-life issues.

The principal early complications after vaginal reconstruction include infection, delayed wound healing, and flap loss. While the risk of infection and pelvic abscess is decreased when flap reconstruction is performed after vaginal resection, it still remains significant at approximately 10%.[5,12,14] Perioperative antibiotics, adequate drainage, and patient positioning, as mentioned in the previous section, are all important preventive measures. Once a pelvic infection is established, percutaneous or operative drainage is generally necessary to prevent worsening sepsis.

The incidence of delayed wound healing or wound dehiscence varies widely in the literature, ranging up to 46% of patients.[23] Radiotherapy, obesity, and smoking are all risk factors for poor wound healing that should be considered preoperatively. The most common location for wound separation is the posterior perineal closure site, which usually responds to conservative management.

Flap loss, both partial and complete, is a major postoperative problem that will delay adjuvant therapy and increase morbidity of the patient. The incidence of flap loss depends on the type of flap used, surgical technique, and patient characteristics. When used for vaginal reconstruction, the VRAM flap is highly reliable with less than 5% incidence of total or partial flap loss; gracilis myocutaneous flaps are less reliable with a 10–20% incidence of total or partial flap loss.[24,25] The success rate of both of these flaps depends on careful attention to design and surgical technique. The modified Singapore flap is susceptible to apical necrosis, but complete flap loss occurs in up to 15%.[15,19] Partial flap loss may be managed by debridement and local wound care. In the setting of irradiated tissue, full debridement and reconstruction with an alternative flap are required.

Many potential late complications are described. These include inadequate or excessive vaginal secretions, inadequate or excessive vaginal size, flap prolapse, vaginal or donor site dysesthesia, and urinary or bowel complaints. In a review of 44 patients who had undergone bilateral gracilis flap reconstruction, Ratliff et al. found that 33% of patients complained of vaginal dryness, whereas 28% complained of excess vaginal secretions. Twenty percent thought their neovagina was too small, whereas 5% found it to be too large. Eighteen percent had flap prolapse, and a further 18% had pain with intercourse.[9]

In addition to complications at the site of the vaginal reconstruction, one must also consider potential donor site complications. For all potential donor sites, hypertrophic scarring, infection, and wound-healing problems must be considered. When harvesting the rectus myocutaneous flap for vaginal reconstruction, an abdominal donor site complication rate of 16–30% has been reported, including such complications as dehiscence, delayed healing, or hernia.[12,26] However, comparing abdominal complications in similar patients without flap reconstruction shows similar abdominal complication rates, thus questioning whether harvesting the rectus muscle adds significant morbidity to these patients.[12] Thigh abscess or hematoma, infection, sensory anomalies, or hypertrophic scarring are the most common complications in patients who have had their gracilis muscles harvested, occurring in up to 40% of patients.[25,26]

Access the complete references list online at **http://www.expertconsult.com**

12. Butler CE, Gundeslioglu AO, Rodriguez-Bigas MA. Outcomes of immediate vertical rectus abdominis myocutaneous flap reconstruction for irradiated abdominoperineal resection defects. *J Am Coll Surg.* 2008;206:694–703.

   In this retrospective case series, the authors assess the impact of immediate closure of irradiated abdominal perineal resection defects with vertical rectus abdominis myocutaneous (VRAM) flaps as compared to primary closure. They conclude that VRAM flaps reduce perineal wound complications without increasing early abdominal wall complications.

13. McCraw J, Kemp G, Given F, et al. Correction of high pelvic defects with the inferiorly based rectus abdominis myocutaneous flap. *Clin Plast Surg.* 1988; 15:449–454.

14. Shibata D, Hyland W, Busse P, et al. Immediate reconstruction of the perineal wound with gracilis muscle flaps following abdominoperineal resection and intraoperative radiation therapy for recurrent carcinoma of the rectum. *Ann Surg Oncol.* 1999;6:33–37.

   This is a retrospective case review evaluating the efficacy of gracilis flaps for immediate perineal reconstructions. This modality was found to decrease the rate of major wound infections significantly in this population.

16. Woods JE, Alter G, Meland B, et al. Experience with vaginal reconstruction utilizing the modified Singapore flap. *Plast Reconstr Surg.* 1992;90:270–274.

   The authors describe a modification of the Singapore flap in which the labia majora are released, yielding good contour and no flap loss. The technique is illustrated and sample cases are described.

17. Wu LC, Song DH. The rectus abdominis musculoperitoneal flap for the immediate reconstruction of partial vaginal defects. *Plast Reconstr Surg*. 2005;115:559–562.

18. Cordeiro PG, Pusic AL, Disa JJ. A classification system and reconstructive algorithm for acquired vaginal defects. *Plast Reconstr Surg*. 2002;110:1058–1065.

    A classification system for acquired vaginal defects is presented based on a 7-year case review. From this experience, the authors derive a reconstructive algorithm and conduct an outcomes assesment.

25. Nelson RA, Butler CE. Surgical outcomes of VRAM versus thigh flaps for immediate reconstruction of pelvic and perineal cancer resection defects. *Plast Reconstr Surg*. 2009;123:175–183.

    The authors compare the efficacy of VRAM flaps to that of thigh flaps in immediate pelvic and perineal reconstruction. VRAM flaps are found to reduce major perineal wound complications without increasing early abdominal wall morbidity.

26. Soper JT, Secord AA, Havrilesky LJ, et al. Comparison of gracilis and rectus abdominis myocutaneous flap neovaginal reconstruction performed during radical pelvic surgery: flap-specific morbidity. *Int J Gynecol Cancer*. 2007;17:298–303.

15

Surgery for gender identity disorder

Loren S. Schechter

SYNOPSIS

- The goal of surgery is a successful functional and cosmetic result.
- Surgery is only one factor in the overall therapeutic process.
- Multidisciplinary care is essential for the transgendered individual.
- Surgical techniques for male-to-female transgendered individuals include penile inversion and intestinal transposition.
- Surgical techniques for female-to-male transgendered individuals include metaidoioplasty and pedicled/free flap phalloplasty.
- Secondary surgical procedures for the face and breast/chest are available for transgendered individuals.

Access the Historical Perspective section online at
http://www.expertconsult.com

Introduction

The term gender dysphoria describes a heterogenous group of individuals who express varying degrees of dissatisfaction with their anatomic gender and the desire to possess the secondary sexual characteristics of the opposite sex.[1] For these individuals, surgical therapy plays a pivotal role in relieving their psychological discomfort.[2] As noted by Dr Milton Edgerton in 1983, "transsexualism is a severe, and pathologic condition that is undesirable for both the patient and society … and nonsurgical treatment continues to be expensive, time-consuming, and enormously disappointing."[3] Recognizing that, in appropriately selected individuals, gender reassignment surgery is the best way to normalize the lives of transgendered individuals,[2] the question of how best to integrate the surgeon in the multidisciplinary team continues to undergo investigation. Although typically introduced to the patient only after diagnosis and hormonal therapy, the surgeon must actively participate in understanding the patient's diagnosis and hormonal and medical therapies. In order to do so, a collaborative effort between the surgeon, behavioral scientist, and medical physician responsible for hormonal therapy is recommended. Recognizing the limitations in access to formal multidisciplinary gender teams, the World Professional Association for Transgender Health's *Standards of Care* (Version 6) provides recommendations designed to standardize the process of surgical evaluation, treatment, and postoperative care of transgendered individuals.[4] This standardized process of surgical management will hopefully lead to uniform and consistent surgical results worldwide.

Epidemiology

While early estimates on the prevalence of gender identity disorders were focused on identification of individuals for sex reassignment surgery, it was later realized that some individuals neither desired nor were candidates for reassignment surgery.[4] Early estimates of the prevalence of transsexualism were 1 in 37000 males and 1 in 107000 females.[5] More recent data suggests that the prevalence may be as high as 1 in 11900 males and 1 in 30400 females.[4] Interestingly, approximately three times as many biological males seek genital surgery as compared to biological females. This discrepancy may exist for multiple reasons, including accessibility, cost, and surgical options available for biological females.

Distinct from gender identity disorders are disorders of sex development (DSD). DSDs represent congenital conditions in which development of chromosomal, gonadal, or anatomic sex is atypical.[6] This terminology replaces terms such as "intersex," "pseudohermaphroditism," "hermaphroditism," and "sex reversal." DSDs include a group of conditions interfering with normal sex determination and differentiation in the embryo and fetus. Although data on the prevalence and incidence of DSDs is limited, it is estimated that the incidence is 1 in 5500.[7] Congenital adrenal hyperplasia is the most common cause of ambiguous genitalia, followed in frequency by mixed gonadal dysgenesis. Gender dissatisfaction occurs more often in individuals with DSDs as compared with the general population, but it is difficult to predict, based upon karyotype, prenatal androgen exposure, degree of genital virilization, or assigned gender. A summary of DSDs is included in *Table 15.1*.[7]

The birth of a child with ambiguous genitalia is distressing to families, and management of children with DSDs benefits from a multidisciplinary approach. Clinical management includes: (1) avoidance of gender assignment prior to expert evaluation; (2) evaluation and management by a multidisciplinary team; (3) receipt of a gender assignment in all individuals; (4) communication with patients and families, as well as their participation and inclusion in decision-making; and (5) respect for patient and family concerns with strict adherence to patient confidentiality.[6] In discussions involving the

parents of newborns with DSDs, the description of the child's genitalia should include both the bipotential of the initial genital organs in addition to a discussion that the usual genetic and hormonal controls may not be fully functional. Children with DSDs may have conditions which result in excessive stimulation of female genitalia, leading to masculinization, or inadequate androgen stimulation of male genitalia resulting in incomplete formation or underdevelopment. Following appropriate testing and assessment of completeness of development of female and male structures, information should be provided to the parents so as to assist the family and physicians with the most appropriate sex assignment. Subsequent clinical discussions with the family include the need for, and benefits of, surgery, predicting future hormone production, and the projection of potential fertility.[7]

The surgical management of the genitalia of children with DSDs is made by the parents, and, when appropriate, the patient. The goal of surgery is to achieve genitalia compatible with sex, prevent urinary obstruction, urinary incontinence,

Table 15.1 Summary of the various types of disorders of sex development

Revised nomenclature	Types
Sex chromosome, DSD	45,X Turner syndrome (mosaic, isodicentric Xq, ring chromosome etc.)

46,XY DSD	Defects in testicular development
	    Complete gonadal dysgenesis (Swyer syndrome)
	    Partial gonadal dysgenesis (WT1, SOX9, SF-1 mutations)
	    Gonadal regression
	    Ovotesticular DSD
	Disorders in androgen synthesis or action
	    Androgen biosynthesis defects (e.g., 17-HSD, 5α-RD, StAR, POR, 3β-HSD, 17,20 lyase, Leydig
	      cell hypoplasia or aplasia)
	    Defects in androgen action (CAIS, PAIS)
	Others
	    Hypospadias, micropenis, cloacal exstrophy, congenital anomaly syndromes
	    Persistent Müllerian duct syndrome

46,XX DSD	Defects in ovarian development
	    Ovotesticular DSD
	    Gonadal transformation (e.g., SRY translocation)
	    Gonadal dysgenesis
	Disorders of androgen excess
	    Fetal: CAH (11 hydroxylase deficiency, 21 hydroxylase deficiency, 3β-HSD, POR)
	    Fetoplacental: aromatase deficiency, POR
	    Maternal: luteoma of pregnancy, exogenous androgen
	Others
	    Congenital anomaly syndromes, vaginal atresia, cloacal exstrophy, MURCS

Ovotesticular DSD	46,XX/ 46,XY (chimeric) 45,X/46,XY (mixed gonadal dysgenesis)
46,XX Testicular DSD	XX sex reversal (SRY translocation)
46,XY Complete gonadal dysgenesis	XY sex reversal (SF1, WT1, SOX9) Swyer syndrome

CAIS, Complete androgen insensitivity; DSD, disorder of sex development; 17-HSD, 17-hydroxysteroid dehydrogenase; 3β-HSD, 3β-hydroxysteroid dehydrogenase; MURCS, Müllerian. renal, cervicothoracic somite abnormalities; PAIS, partial androgen insensitivity, POR, P450 oxidoreductase, 5α-RD, 5α-reductase deficiency; SF1, splicing factor 1; SOX9, sex determining region box 9; StAR, steroidogenic acute regulatory protein, WT1, Wilms tumor gene. (From Nabhan ZM, Lee PA Disorders of sex development. Curr Opin Obstet Gynecol. 2007;19:440-445.)[7]

and infection, and provide good adult sexual and reproductive function.[8] Although controversy exists on the timing of genital surgery in girls with CAH, surgery is typically considered in cases of severe virilization and, when necessary, in association with repair of a common urogenital sinus. Surgery should be anatomically based so as to preserve erectile function and innervation of the clitoris. While The American Academy of Pediatric guidelines recommend genitoplasty between 2 and 6 months of age,[9] it is recognized that revision vaginoplasty will be performed at the time of puberty. For male newborns with hypospadias, standard techniques for chordee repair and urethral reconstruction apply. In patients requiring phalloplasty, the magnitude and complexity of the procedure must be discussed, especially if sex assignment depends upon it.[6] In individuals with 46,XY gonadal dysgenesis raised as females, testes, or fragments of Y-chromosome material, should be removed to prevent testicular malignancy. Gonadectomy is generally advised soon after diagnosis so as to initiate estrogen replacement when desired. In individuals with gonadal dysgenesis and scrotal testes, the current recommendation is to perform testicular biopsy at puberty to assess for malignancy. In females with ovotesticular DSD and functional ovarian tissue, early separation and removal of the testicular component is advised in an attempt to preserve fertility.[7] DSDs can be managed such that children can mature into well-adjusted individuals with a potential for sexual expression, and, in select cases, reproductive potential.[7]

Goals of therapy

The Standards of Care for Gender Identity Disorders state that the overarching treatment goal is " … lasting personal comfort with the gendered self in order to maximize overall psychological well-being and self-fulfillment."[4] While the goals of surgery include a successful cosmetic and functional result with minimal complications *(Figs 15.1, 15.2)*, surgery is only one determinant in the overall therapeutic process.[10] As such, the surgeon performing gender reassignment must assume an active and integral role in the overall care of the patient. It is the responsibility of the operating surgeon to understand the diagnosis that has led to the recommendation for genital surgery, medical co-morbidities that may impact the surgical outcome, the effects of hormonal therapy on the patient's health, and the patient's ultimate satisfaction with the surgical result.[11] Furthermore, the surgeon should assist with the coordination of the patient's postoperative care in order to assure appropriate continuity.

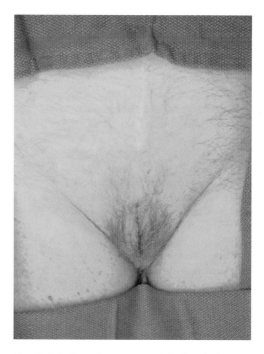

Fig. 15.1 Postoperative appearance following single-stage vaginoplasty.

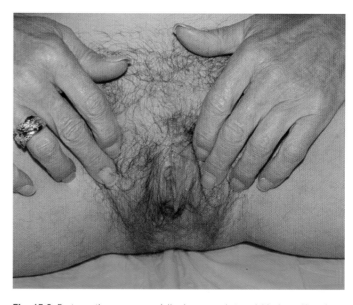

Fig. 15.2 Postoperative appearance following second stage labiaplasty. Note the neoclitoris and prepuce formed by the glans penis and urethra. Additionally, a moist appearance of the labia minora is provided by the use of a urethral flap.

Basic science/disease process

The etiology of transsexualism remains unknown[22] and has included genetic links, the hormonal milieu, family dynamics, and psychoanalytical observations.[1] Early theories were based largely in psychoanalytic contexts, followed by attempts to define transsexualism in a biological context. Psychosexual development and differentiation entails three major components: "gender identity," referring to one's sense of belonging to the male or female sex category; "gender role," sexually dimorphic behaviors and psychological characteristics within

the population, such as toy preferences and mannerisms; and "sexual orientation," one's pattern of erotic responsiveness. There are essentially three theories relating to the etiology of transsexualism: a psychological or sociological etiology, a biological etiology, or some combination thereof.

Psychoanalytic explanations have ranged from an inability to separate on the part of mother and child, psychotic disorders, and an unconscious motivation to discard bad and aggressive features.[22] As such, psychoanalysts viewed sex reassignment surgery as "psychosurgery," and argued that treatment of transsexualism could only be achieved through psychoanalysis.[22]

Proponents of a biological explanation have examined a variety of theories including anatomic differences in the brains of transsexuals as well as hormonal influences on brain development at critical gestational stages. Paralleling advances in radiographic brain imaging, early biologic theories, referred to as gender transposition, examined hormone-induced cephalic differentiation.[22] This concept relied on the "default theory;" in the absence of androgens, an embryo will feminize, and in the presence of androgens, testicles develop. However, many of these theories rested upon extrapolation from animal studies. Subsequent research later demonstrated important differences between hormone secretions in humans and animals.

Some of the most recent theories have focused attention on an attempt to identify a genetic link explaining transsexualism. However, at this time, no genetic markers have been identified which explain transsexualism. Therefore, studies have used differences in physical characteristics between transsexuals and nontranssexuals as indirect evidence of a genetic etiology. These studies include such factors as the observation of a high prevalence of left-handedness or atypical handedness in transsexuals, height differences between male-to-female transsexuals and nontransgendered males, the presence of an anomalous inframammary ligament in female-to-male transsexuals, a higher rate of polycystic ovaries in female-to-male transsexuals, and differences in bone proportion and fat distribution.[22] Still other theories have examined differences in autopsied brains of male-to-female transsexuals. These differences were noted in the region of the hypothalamus, an area of the brain involved in sexual behavior. The study noted that genetic females and male-to-female transsexuals had similar and smaller volumes of the central sulci of the stria terminalis compared to both homosexual and heterosexual males.[22]

However, in spite of continued research in this area, it must also be recognized that a spectrum of gender variance exists. Additionally, both cultural and social constructs play a significant factor in gender role. For example, while most of the studies compare transsexuals to nontranssexuals, these studies do not account for biological explanations as to cross-dressing heterosexual males or children with a history of gender identity disorder who become gender typical as adults. As Dr Randi Ettner concludes, " ... the etiology of transgenderism remains unknown. The goal of treatment, however, *is* known and is indisputable: to assist gender-variant patients who request medical interventions by providing state-of-the-art treatment."[22]

Diagnosis

Transgender is not a formal diagnosis.[4] When individuals possess concerns, uncertainties, and questions about gender identity, which persist during their development, become the most important aspect of their life, or prevents the establishment of an unconflicted gender identity, they have passed a clinical threshold. When such an individual meets the specified criteria in one of the two official nomenclatures, The International Classification of Diseases-10 or the Diagnostic and Statistical Manual of Mental Disorders-4th Edition,[23] they are diagnosed as having a Gender Identity Disorder (GID).

The International Classification of Diseases-10[24] provides five diagnoses for gender identity disorders (F64):

Transsexualism (F64.0) has three criteria:

1. The desire to live and be accepted as a member of the opposite sex, usually accompanied by the wish to make his or her body as congruent as possible with the preferred sex through surgery and hormone treatment
2. The transsexual identity has been present persistently for at least 2 years
3. The disorder is not a symptom or another mental disorder or a chromosomal abnormality
   - Dual-role Transvestism (F64.1)
   - Gender Identity Disorder of Childhood (F64.2)
   - Other Gender Identity Disorders (F64.8)
   - Gender Identity Disorder, Unspecified (F64.9).

In 1994, the DSM-IV committee replaced the diagnosis of Transsexualism with Gender Identity Disorder. According to the DSM-IV, individuals must demonstrate a strong and persistent cross-gender identification and a persistent discomfort with their sex or a sense of inappropriateness in the gender role of that sex. It is important to realize that the DSM-IV and ICD-10 are designed to guide research and treatment. The designation of gender identity disorders as mental disorders is not a license for stigmatization, or for the deprivation of gender patients' civil rights.[4]

After the diagnosis of gender identity disorder is made, the therapeutic approach commonly includes three phases (triadic therapy): a real-life experience in the desired role, hormones of the desired gender, and surgery to change the genitalia and other sex characteristics.

Patient selection

Prior to performing gender reassignment surgery, the surgeon must be satisfied that the diagnosis of gender dysphoria has been established. Although the diagnosis is typically made by the behavioral scientist the surgeon must be convinced that the diagnosis is accurate. As noted by Dr J.J. Hage (1995:18),[11] "the surgeon remains responsible for any diagnosis on the basis of which he performs surgical interventions." Direct communication between the surgeon and psychiatrist and/or psychologist is both encouraged and recommended. This serves to educate the surgeon and aid with his or her understanding of each patient's unique needs, it also helps to prevent possible falsification of letters of recommendation. The surgeon must be willing to personally communicate with other healthcare providers when questions or concerns regarding a patient's appropriateness for surgery exist. However, this communication should not be limited to the evaluation phase. It is the responsibility of the surgeon to communicate pertinent operative findings as well as postoperative instructions with the relevant members of the healthcare team.[25]

Although multiple studies conducted at a variety of international centers confirm the efficacy of surgery and low complication rates,[2,26–31] the surgeon must be familiar with preoperative psychosocial risk factors that may increase the risk of postoperative complications. It is incumbent upon the surgeon to actively investigate these potential risk factors prior to proceeding with surgery. In a study investigating the standards and policies of 19 gender clinics in Europe and North America, a high degree of consistency regarding policies and criteria for approval of reassignment surgery was identified.[32] Based upon questionnaire data, conditions that could result in delay or denial of surgery included psychosocial instability, married status, substance abuse, chronic or psychotic illness, and antisocial behavior. In addition, in a retrospective review of 136 patients who underwent sex reassignment in Sweden, several preoperative factors were identified and reported to be associated with higher rates of unsatisfactory surgical outcomes. These included personal and social instability, unsuitable body build, and age over 30 at operation. Additionally, in this study, adequate family and social support were noted to be important for adequate postoperative functioning.[10]

Though understanding potential preoperative risk factors is important, their presence is not necessarily a contraindication to surgery. In a retrospective review of 232 male-to-female transsexuals, Lawrence[28] noted that no participants regretted sexual assignment surgery outright and only 6% were occasionally regretful. In this study, dissatisfaction was associated with unsatisfactory surgical results, not other indicators of transsexual typology such as age at surgery, previous marriage or parenthood, or sexual orientation. This serves to reinforce the concept that the *Standards of Care* are intended to provide flexible direction for the treatment of transgendered individuals. It is generally recognized that individual centers may vary with regard to specific hormonal regimens and time requirements for the real life test. It must be emphasized that the *Standards of Care* are not intended as barriers to surgery, but rather as a means of identifying patients who would benefits from surgical reassignment.

Upon completion of the first or diagnostic phase, the patient is referred to a medical physician for hormonal therapy. Though specific hormonal regimens may vary between centers, the surgeon should be familiar with the possible side-effects of hormonal therapy and how they relate to the surgical care of the transgendered patient. These include issues related to liver function, risk of venous thromboembolism, electrolyte imbalance, and drug-drug interactions. It is helpful if the medical physician is a member of the multidisciplinary team. If not, the medical physician should have substantial experience in the field of transgender medicine.[11] Medical comorbidities should be investigated and treated prior to surgery. In patients with chronic medical conditions, the surgeon should work closely with medical colleagues to optimize and manage these conditions prior to surgery.

The goal of endocrine therapy is to change secondary sex characteristics in order to reduce gender dysphoria and/or facilitate a physical presentation which is consistent with one's sense of self.[33] Hormonal therapy is typically individualized to the needs and desires of the patient based upon their goals, associated medical conditions, and consideration of social and economic issues. The *Standards of Care* indicate the physician prescribing hormones should:

1. Perform an initial evaluation that includes health history, physical examination, and relevant laboratory tests

2. Explain what feminizing/masculinizing medications do and the possible side-effects/health risks

3. Confirm that the patient has the capacity to understand the risks and benefits of treatment and to make an informed decision about medical care

4. Inform the patient of the *Standards of Care* and eligibility/readiness requirements

5. Provide ongoing medical monitoring, including regular physical and laboratory examination to monitor hormone effects and side-effects.

Feminization through hormonal therapy is achieved by two mechanisms: suppression of androgen effects and induction of female physical characteristics. Androgen suppression is achieved by using medications which either suppress gonadotrophic releasing hormone (GnRH) or are GnRH antagonists (progestational agents), suppress the production of luteinizing hormone (progestational agents, cyproterone acetate), interfere with testosterone production or metabolism of testosterone to dihydrotestosterone (spironolactone, finasteride, cyproterone acetate), or interfere with the binding of androgen to its receptors in target tissues (spironolactone, cyproterone acetate, flutamide). Additionally, estrogen is used to induce female secondary sex characteristics, and its mechanism of action is through direct stimulation of receptors in target tissues (*Table 15.2*).[33]

Within the first 6 months of therapy, there is a redistribution of body fat, decreased muscle mass, softening of skin, and decreased libido. Breast growth may be expected after 3–6 months of therapy and continue for ≥2 years. Over a period of several years, body and facial hair become finer, although they are not completely eliminated by hormonal therapy alone. Progression of male pattern baldness may slow, however, hair does not typically regrow in bald areas. Many of the changes, perhaps with the exception of breast growth, are reversible with cessation of therapy.[33]

Masculinization through hormonal therapy for female-to-male individuals follows general principles of hormone replacement for treatment of male hypogonadism. Both parenteral and transdermal testosterone preparations are available and may be used to achieve testosterone values in the normal male range.[34] Testosterone therapy results in increased muscle mass and decreased fat mass, increased facial hair and acne, male pattern baldness, and increased libido. In reference to female-to-male individuals, testosterone results in clitoromegaly, temporary or permanent decreased fertility, deepened voice, vaginal atrophy, and cessation of menses. If uterine bleeding continues, a progestational agent may be added. GnRH analogs or depot medroxyprogesterone may be used to stop menses and to reduce estrogen levels to those found in biological males.[34] Individuals should be routinely monitored so as to maintain testosterone levels in the physiological normal male range and avoid adverse events such as erythrocytosis, liver dysfunction, hypertension, excessive weight gain, salt retention, lipid changes, cystic acne, and adverse psychological changes.[34]

Once the surgeon is satisfied that the diagnosis has been established, a hormonal regimen has been instituted and followed, and the patient has successfully completed the second-stage or real life test, surgical therapy is considered. A preoperative surgical consultation is obtained. During this consultation, the procedure and postoperative course are

Table 15.2 Hormone regimen

Agent	Estrogen			Androgen antagonist		
	17β-estradiol			Spironolactone		Finasteride
	Transdermal[a]	*or*	Oral	Oral	*and/or*	Oral
Pre-orchiectomy	Start at 0.1 mg/24 h. applied twice a week; gradually increase up to maximum of 0.2 mg/24 h. applied twice per week.		Start with 1–2 mg q.d.; gradually increase up to maximum 4 mg q.d.	Start with 50–100 mg q.d.; increase by 50–100 mg each month up to average 200–300 mg q.d. (maximum 500 mg q.d.). Modify if there are risks of adverse effects.[b]		Use 2.5–5.0 mg q.d. for systemic anti-androgen effect; use 2.5 mg every other day if solely for alopecia androgenetica
Post-orchiectomy	0.375–0.1 mg/24 h. applied twice per week.		1–2 mg q.d.	25–50 mg q.d.		2.5 mg q.d.

[a]Use transdermal estradiol if the patient is >40 years of age, or is at risk for DVT. Oral estradiol is an option if the patient is <40 years of age and is low risk for DVT. [b]If taking ACE-inhibitors or other potassium-sparing medication, spironolactone should not go above 25 mg q.d. and serum potassium should be closely monitored. If the patient has low blood pressure or renal insufficiency start at 50 mg and increase by up to 50 mg per week to a maximum of 300 mg q.d., with a renal function test 1–2 weeks after each increase. (From Dahl M, Feldman JL, Goldberg JM, Jaberi A. Physcial aspects of transgender endocrine therapy. Int J Transgenderism 2006;9:111-134.)[33]

described, the potential risks and benefits of surgery are reviewed, and the patient's questions are answered. Equally important is a discussion of the patient's expectations as well as limitations of surgery. In a follow-up study of 55 transsexual patients treated in Belgium, De Cuypere et al.[27] noted that the transsexual person's expectations were met at an emotional and social level, but less so at the physical and sexual level. This occurred despite an indicated improvement in sex life and sexual excitement after reassignment surgery.[27] Based upon these findings, it was recommended that discussions regarding sexual expectations be entertained prior to surgery. After deciding to proceed with surgery, written documentation of informed consent should be included in the patients chart.

Treatment of adolescents

Over the past decade, an emerging area of clinical interest involves the treatment of transgendered adolescents. Adolescents with gender identity disorder may consider the physical changes of puberty unbearable. In an effort to prevent psychological harm, some centers have initiated treatment of adolescents with puberty-suppressing medications, such as a GnRH analog, before development of irreversible secondary sex characteristics. Potential benefits of this approach to pubertal suppression may include a relief of gender dysphoria and better psychological and physical outcome.[34]

The physical changes of puberty result from maturation of the hypothalamo-pituitary-gonadal axis and development of secondary sex characteristics. In girls, the first physical sign of puberty is breast budding, while in boys, an increase in testicular volume heralds the onset of puberty. Pubertal suppression may aid with management of gender dysphoria, and the hormonal changes are fully reversible.[34] Hormone-treated adolescents may be referred for surgery when the real-life experience has resulted in a satisfactory social role change, the individual is satisfied about the hormonal effects, and the individual desires definitive surgical changes.[34] Surgery is typically considered at 18 years of age, although individual exceptions may be appropriate.

Treatment/surgical technique

Surgical options/descriptions of technique

Surgical conversion of the genitalia in male-to-female transsexuals has evolved since the use of skin grafts for creation of a neovagina in cases of vaginal agenesis.[35] The use of pedicled penile and scrotal skin flaps was described over 40 years ago, and despite technical refinements, remains the mainstay for neovaginal construction.[36,37,38] The vascular basis of these flaps is derived from one of three vascular axes: (1) the deep external pudendal artery, a branch of the femoral artery, (2) the superficial perineal artery, a branch of the internal pudendal artery, and (3) the funicular artery, a branch of the deep inferior epigastric artery[39]

A successful surgical result involves the creation of a natural-appearing vagina and mons pubis. This includes a feminine-appearing labia majora and minora with removal of the stigmatizing scrotum, a sensate neoclitoris, and adequate vaginal depth and introital width for intercourse *(Figs 15.3– 15.5)*. Although a functional vaginoplasty is performed in a single-stage, further feminization of the mons pubis is often performed at a second surgical stage. The labiaplasty, performed under local anesthesia as an outpatient three months after vaginoplasty, creates a convergent anterior commissure and provides additional clitoral hooding.

The surgical options for male-to-female genital surgery consist of one of three options: penile disassembly and inversion vaginoplasty, intestinal transplantation, or nongenital flaps. Most centers perform primary vaginoplasty using the

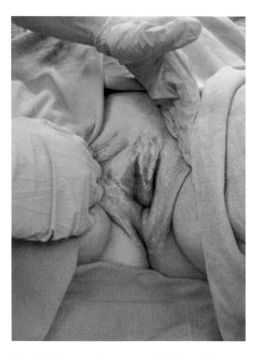

Fig. 15.3 Postoperative appearance following single-stage vaginoplasty, prior to labiaplasty. Note the width of the introitus provided by the perineal-scrotal flap and resection of the superficial muscles. Adequate introital width is essential for vaginal intercourse.

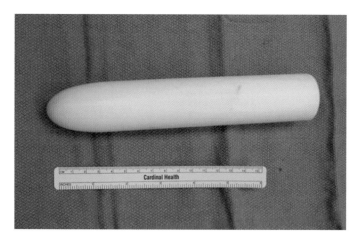

Fig. 15.4 Rigid dilator used for intraoperative blunt dissection of the neo-vaginal cavity.

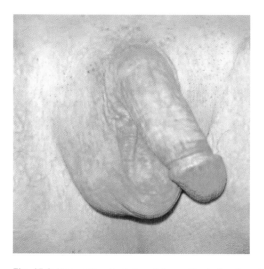

Fig. 15.6 Preoperative depilation of the penile shaft and scrotum.

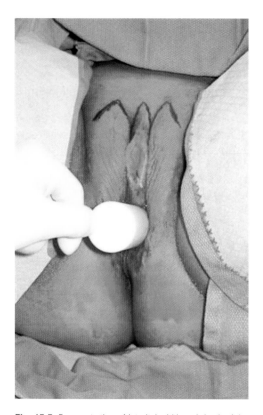

Fig. 15.5 Demonstration of introital width and depth of the neovaginal cavity. Markings on the mons pubis delineate the local tissue rearrangement for the labiaplasty. The labiaplasty will provide convergence to the labia majora as well as additional definition of the prepuce of the neoclitoris.

anterior pedicled penile skin flap. However, intestinal transposition, typically reserved for revision cases, is a first-line surgical therapy at some centers. The advantage of intestinal transposition is the creation of a vascularized 12–15 cm vagina with a moist lining. This may lessen the requirements for postoperative vaginal dilation as well as the need for lubrication during intercourse. However, the drawbacks of intestinal transposition include the need for an intra-abdominal operation with a bowel anastomosis and the potential for excess neo-vaginal secretions with a malodorous discharge. Non-genital flaps are typically considered for revision procedures in cases of vaginal stenosis. Regardless of which technique is utilized, a preoperative bowel preparation is administered. Additionally, hair removal whether by electrolysis or laser, is completed as thoroughly as possible from the penile shaft and central scrotum *(Fig. 15.6)* prior to surgery. Preoperative depilation helps to prevent intravaginal hair growth. Finally, hormones are discontinued approximately two weeks prior to surgery to reduce the risk of venous thromboembolism.

Primary surgery

Primary vaginoplasty surgery most commonly involves penile disassembly and inversion with an anteriorly based pedicled penile flap. Although a variety of technical modifications are described in the literature, the penile disassembly and inversion technique utilizes the penile skin and a second, posteriorly based, perineal-scrotal flap to construct the vaginal cavity.[40] The author's preferred technique is described herein: the labia majora are formed from the lateral aspects of the scrotum, the neoclitoris is formed from the dorsal glans penis, and the labia minora are formed with the creation of a urethral flap. The penile urethra is shortened, spatulated, and everted to create the neo-urethral meatus (*Fig. 15.7*). Depending upon the length of the penis and previous surgical history (i.e., circumcision), skin grafts may be required for additional vaginal depth. Full-thickness skin grafts may be harvested from discarded portions of the scrotum. If this is

insufficient, additional full-thickness skin grafts may be harvested with a Pfannenstiel incision.[41] Alternatively, split-thickness skin grafts may also be harvested from the lower abdomen or mons region. However, the donor site of the split-thickness skin grafts may be left with areas of hypopigmentation depending upon depth of harvest and patient's skin tone.

In the preoperative holding area, intravenous antibiotics are administered and sequential compression devices are placed. Following induction of general anesthesia, chemoprophylaxis for VTE is administered subcutaneously (either fractionated or unfractionated heparin depending upon institutional policies), the patient is positioned in lithotomy, and an indwelling urinary catheter is placed under sterile conditions after the patient is prepped and draped.

The procedure is begun with the creation of a posteriorly-based perineal-scrotal flap. This flap, which measures approximately 10 cm in greatest transverse dimension and 15 cm in length, requires sufficient width so as not to limit the neo-vaginal introitus. Additionally, the lateral aspect of the flap is designed in a "v-shaped" fashion so as not to create a circular introitus and thereby minimize the chance of introital contracture (*Fig. 15.8A*). The flap is centered cephalad to the anus and dissected to the level of the anal sphincter, with care taken not to injure the external anal sphincter (*Fig. 15.8B*).

An incision is made on the ventral penis along the midline raphe (*Fig. 15.8C*). This allows access to the testicles and performance of bilateral orchiectomies. The orchiectomy, including resection of the spermatic cords, is performed at the level of the inguinal ring. This allows the spermatic cord to retract within the inguinal canal, and prevents a palpable bulge in the groin area. The skin of the penile shaft is then circumferentially incised at the junction of the glans and penile shaft. This facilitates separation of the penile skin from the underlying corpora cavernosa and corpora spongiosum, as well as the overlying muscles, the ischiocavernosus and bulbospongiosus muscles, respectively (*Fig. 15.8D*).

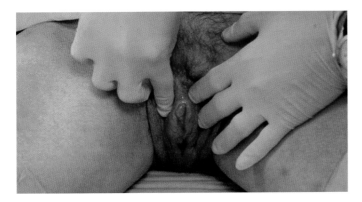

Fig. 15.7 Postoperative appearance: The labia majora are formed from the scrotum, the neoclitoris is formed from the dorsal glans penis, the labia minora are formed with a urethral flap, and the native penile urethra is shortened and spatulated to form the neourethra.

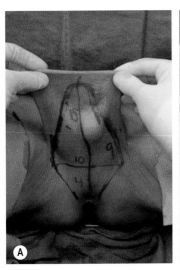 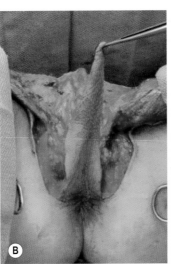 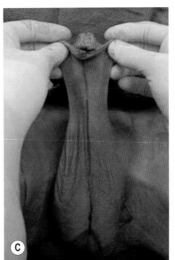 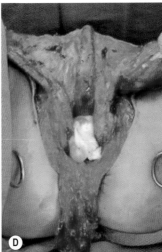

Fig. 15.8 (A) Design of the perineal-scrotal flap. Note the "v-shape" of the lateral aspect of this flap. This design assists with widening of the introitus and lessening the risks of introital scar contracture. **(B)** Elevation of the posteriorly-based perineal-scrotal flap. **(C)** Incision of the ventral penile skin along the midline raphe. **(D)** Exposure of the corpora spongiosum and ischiocavernosus muscles with underlying corpora cavernosa. A sponge is placed in the neo-vaginal cavity.

At this point, the vaginal cavity is developed by dissecting between the prostate and rectum. Care must be taken to avoid inadvertent entry into the rectum. Dissection follows Denonvillier's fascia until the peritoneal reflection is reached. Most of this dissection is performed bluntly, however, release of attachments between the prostate and rectum may require sharp division. The levator ani are then scored with electrocautery to further expand the neovaginal cavity *(Fig. 15.9)*. Adequate dissection of the neovaginal space is essential in creating and maintaining adequate vaginal depth. Once the vaginal cavity is created, the superficial perineal muscles are resected. Resection of the ischiocavernosus muscles aids with creation of the introitus and exposure of the corpora cavernosa. At this point, the corpora spongiosum is separated from the corpora cavernosa. The corpora spongiosum is resected from the bulb of the penis in order to further open the vaginal cavity. If excess erectile tissue is not removed, this tissue may become engorged during sexual arousal and restrict entry to the vaginal cavity.[42]

The neoclitoris is then fashioned from the dorsal glans penis and dissected on the dorsal neurovascular bundle *(Figs 15.10, 15.11A)*. The dissection of the dorsal vein and paired dorsal arteries and nerves is performed deep to Buck's fascia along the corpora cavernosa.[43] Dissection of the neurovascular pedicle is performed to the pubic symphysis, exposing the divergence of the underlying corpora cavernosa. The corpora cavernosa are resected at the pubis, leaving a short remnant of corpora on either side. The retained corpora will be sutured together to form a base, upon which the neoclitoris will be attached (S. Monstrey, pers. comm.).

In order to aid with advancement of the penile flap, the skin of the mons and lower abdomen is elevated to the

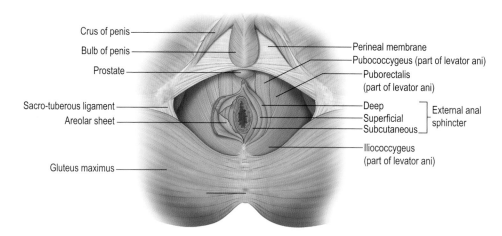

Fig. 15.9 The release of levator ani to aid with maintenance of neo-vaginal cavity.

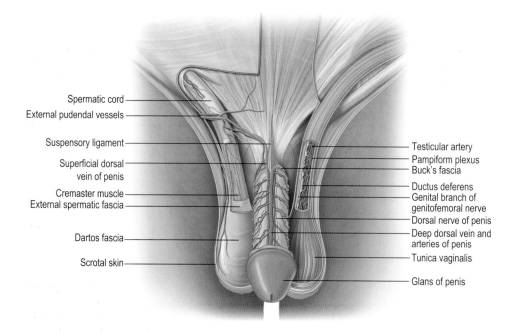

Fig. 15.10 Dissection of dorsal glans penis on dorsal neurovascular bundle.

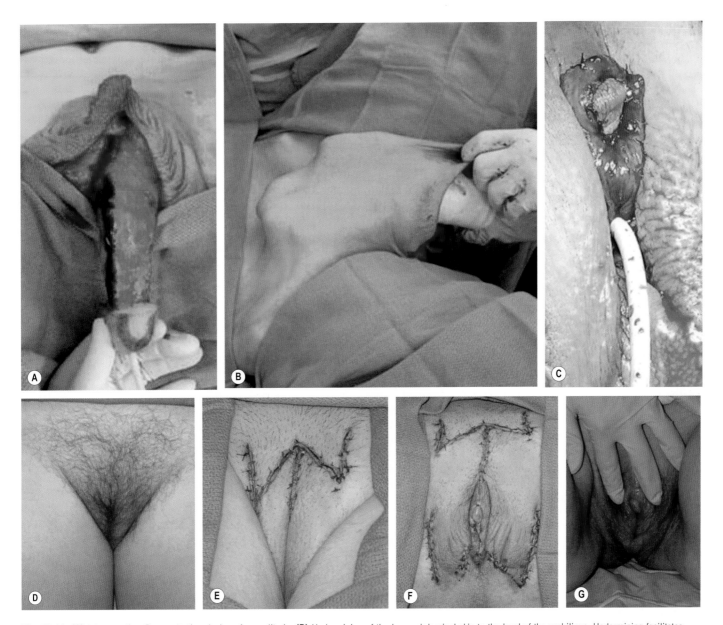

Fig. 15.11 (A) Intraoperative. Demonstrating design of neo-clitoris. **(B)** Undermining of the lower abdominal skin to the level of the umbilicus. Undermining facilitates advancement of the penile flap into the intravaginal position. **(C)** Design of the urethral flap to form the labia minora and prepuce of the neo-clitoris. **(D)** Postoperative. After single-stage vaginoplasty. **(E)** Postoperative. Following second-stage labiaplasty. Note the convergence of the labia majora in the mons pubis. **(F)** Postoperative. Following second-stage labiaplasty. Note the prepuce of the neo-clitoris. **(G)** Postoperative. Demonstrating moist appearance of labia minora and neo-clitoris with associated prepuce.

umbilicus *(Fig. 15.11B)*. This facilitates intravaginal positioning of the penile flap.[44] Depending upon the length of the penile flap, skin grafts may be required to increase vaginal depth. These may be harvested as full-thickness grafts from the nonused scrotum, groin crease, or lower abdomen. Additionally, split-thickness grafts may be harvested from the mons or lower abdominal region.[45] The scrotal-perineal flap is sutured to the penile flap over a silastic stent and advanced into the intravaginal position. A "Y"-shaped incision is made in the penile flap in order to create the urethral meatus. The penile urethra is shortened and incised ventrally. This creates a urethral flap through which the glans penis will be placed, thereby creating the labia minora and providing a prepuce to the neo-clitoris *(Fig. 15.11C)*. The scrotal skin is then tailored to form the labia majora, and the incisions are closed in a layered fashion with absorbable sutures. Drains are placed on either side of the vaginal cavity *(Fig. 15.11D)*.

Although most surgeons perform a single-stage vaginoplasty, an optional second-stage, referred to as a labiaplasty, may be performed for further feminization of the mons pubis. This procedure is usually performed under local anesthesia, approximately 3 months after the vaginoplasty. The labiaplasty involves a local tissue rearrangement, frequently in the form of multiple "z"-plasties, so as to create convergence of the labia majora, and provide for additional clitoral hooding *(Figs 15.11E–15.11G)*.

Technical variations include the use of a urethral flap inset within the penile skin designed to either lengthen or provide lubrication to the vaginal cavity.[46] Additionally, intravaginal placement of the glans penis to act as a neo-cervix has been described.[47]

Surgery for female-to-male transsexuals

The goals of genital surgery in female-to-male transsexuals may range from creation of a neourethra capable of allowing voiding while standing, to a complete penis capable of sexual penetration.[48] Metaidoioplasty, described in 1996 by Hage, has been offered as an alternative to microsurgical or pedicled flap phalloplasty in female-to-male transsexuals. The term, coined by Laub, is based upon the Greek prefix *meta-*, relating to change, and *aidoio*, relating to the genitals.[49] The procedure entails stretching the hormonally hypertrophied clitoris by resection of the ventral chordae and lengthening the female urethra with the aid of labia minora and vaginal musculomucosal flaps.[50] Additionally, buccal mucosal grafts have been utilized to aid with urethral extension. Urethral reconstruction is the major challenge associated with metaidoioplasty, and most complications involve either urethral fistulae and/or strictures.

The operative technique may involve concomitant removal of the female genitalia (hysterectomy and vaginectomy) in addition to metaidoioplasty.[51] Typically, a caudally based anterior vaginal wall flap incorporating the muscularis of the ventral vaginal wall is developed. This flap will reconstruct the fixed portion of the neourethra.[49] If a vaginectomy is not performed, the vaginal donor site is closed, thereby narrowing the retained vagina. The clitoral shaft is degloved and released by detaching the fundiform and clitoral ligaments from the pubic bone. On the ventral aspect of the clitoris, the urethral plate is dissected from the clitoral bodies. The urethral plate is divided at the level of the corona so as to release the ventral clitoral curvature allowing straightening and lengthening of the clitoris.[51] Additional lengthening of the urethra is performed with flaps developed from the labia minora. The vaginal mucosa and labial flaps are sutured to each other in a beveled fashion over a urinary catheter.

Scrotoplasty, constructed with bilateral labia majora flaps, with the addition of testicular implants may be performed as a single-stage procedure at the time of metaidoioplasty, or as an independent secondary procedure, for further masculinization of the external genitalia.

Revision surgery

In the event that vaginal depth is inadequate, revision vaginoplasty typically requires either skin grafting, local and regional nongenital flaps, or intestinal transposition. While a skin graft may alleviate the need for an intra-abdominal procedure, the dissection of the previously operated upon vaginal cavity may be difficult. Visualization and protection of the urethra anteriorly and rectum posteriorly may be limited. Additionally, donor sites for full-thickness skin grafts may be limited, and hypopigmentation from split-thickness skin graft donor sites may be undesirable. Furthermore, skin grafts require regular post-operative dilation so as to prevent contraction of the neo-vagina. Local and regional nongenital flaps include the use of various thigh or perineal-based flaps. The advantages of these nongenital flaps include less risk of post-operative contraction. However, many of these flaps are bulky, limit the size of the neovagina, and provide no intrinsic lubrication. The advantage of intestinal transposition, especially in revision cases, is the provision of a reliable length of

vascularized tissue with mucous secretion providing lubrication for vaginal intercourse. Intestinal transposition may utilize either the small or large intestine, however, the sigmoid colon is most commonly used. The advantage of the sigmoid is the larger luminal diameter and less copious secretions as compared to that of the jejunum or ileum.

Prior to performing the sigmoid vaginoplasty, a preoperative colonoscopy is performed so as to evaluate for colorectal malignancies. As with a primary procedure, a bowel preparation is prescribed preoperatively. The sigmoid vaginoplasty is also performed in the lithotomy position in conjunction with general surgery. A combined abdominal and perineal approach is utilized and allows visualization and protection of the bladder and urethra anteriorly and the rectum posteriorly. The sigmoid colon is harvested by the general surgery team, and the perineal dissection is performed concurrently by the plastic surgery team. A 12–15 cm segment of sigmoid colon is transferred in an isoperistaltic fashion *(Figs 15.12–15.14)*. The defunctionalized sigmoid colon is sutured to the introitus of

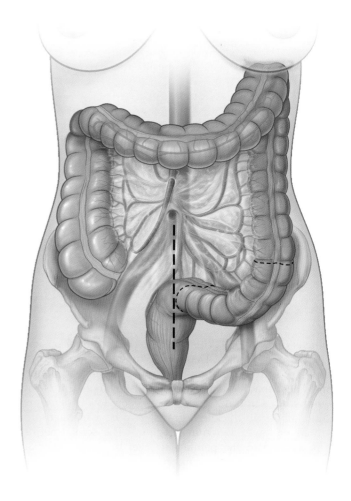

Fig. 15.12 Incision along mesentery of colon and development of the vascular pedicle.

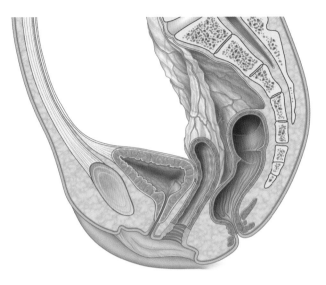

Fig. 15.14 This figure demonstrates placement of defunctionalized sigmoid colon to position of neo-vagina. The colorectal anastomosis is isolated from the sutured stump of the defunctionalized sigmoid colon.

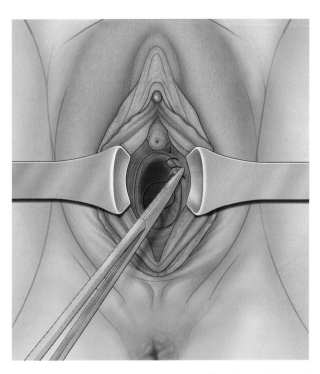

Fig. 15.15 This figure demonstrates insetting of sigmoid colon. The use of laparoscopic instruments facilitates insetting several centimeters cephalad to the introitus.

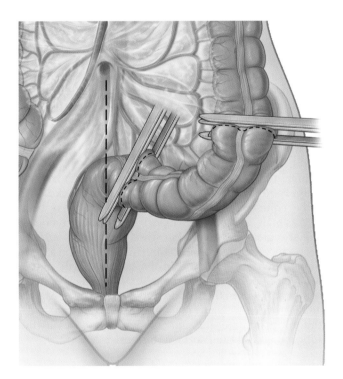

Fig. 15.13 Harvest of sigmoid colon.

the neovagina with a single layer of absorbable sutures. In order to prevent contraction of the introitus, several z-plasties are used when insetting the distal bowel segment with the perineal skin *(Fig. 15.15)*. Additionally, the mesentery of the defunctionalized sigmoid colon is gently sewn to the pelvis to prevent torsion of the vascular pedicle. A hand sewn, end-to-end colonic anastomosis is performed to restore intestinal continuity, and the distal stump of the neo- vagina is separated from the colorectal anastomosis so as to reduce the risk of fistulization. Intravenous antibiotics are maintained for 24 h postoperatively.

The neovagina is packed for 3–4 days with a soft stent, and the patient remains on bedrest with a urinary catheter. Upon return of bowel function and adequate oral intake, the patient is discharged from the hospital.

The potential drawbacks of intestinal based flaps include copious secretions, most notably with the small intestine, and possible malodorous discharge with the large intestine. Additional concerns include the possibility of diversion colitis in the defunctionalized sigmoid colon, as well as the risk of GI malignancies. Finally, the colonic mucosa may be somewhat friable, and small amounts of post-coital bleeding may occur.

Postoperative care

The postoperative care consists of a variable period of bed rest, typically 4–5 days, during which a silastic stent is used to maintain the vaginal cavity. Additionally, a urinary catheter remains in place until the vaginal packing is removed and ambulation is initiated, typically 5–6 days after surgery. Once the vaginal stent is removed, a regimen of vaginal dilation with a rigid prosthesis is begun. Initially, dilation of the neovaginal cavity is performed five to six times daily for 6 weeks. The frequency of dilation is reduced over a period of 2–3 months, ultimately requiring dilation two to three times per week. This schedule may be varied depending upon the frequency of vaginal intercourse.

Additionally, intermittent vaginal douching with a dilute povidine-iodine solution is performed to remove intravaginal debris. This is initially performed daily for 2 weeks following surgery, and reduced to two to three times per week thereafter. Vaginal intercourse may begin 6 weeks after surgery. An annual speculum and prostate exam is also recommended.

Outcome/prognosis/complications

Early postoperative complications include bleeding, infection, and delayed wound healing. Additional early or late complications include rectovaginal fistula, urinary stream abnormalities, inadequate vaginal depth or constricted introitus, partial flap loss, loss of neoclitoral sensation, and unsatisfactory cosmetic appearance.

In the event of a rectovaginal fistula recognized intraoperatively, the rectum is closed and may be left to heal. Because the patient has undergone a preoperative bowel preparation, the rectum may heal without further intervention. However, there is the potential need for a diverting colostomy, as well as the risk of neovagina stenosis. Although minor urinary stream abnormalities are not uncommon, the risk of stenosis of the neo-urethral meatus may be reduced by spatulation and eversion of the urethra. It is also imperative that the individual continue routine dilation so as to prevent the risk of vaginal stenosis. Although the frequency of dilation may be reduced with sexual intercourse, pedicled penile flaps and skin grafts still require compliance with vaginal dilation.

Routine medical care of the transgendered individual is recommended and includes clinical and laboratory monitoring. This allows assessment of the beneficial, as well as possible adverse effects, associated with cross-sex hormonal therapy. Monitoring of weight and blood pressure, directed physical examinations, complete blood counts, renal and liver function tests, lipid and glucose metabolism should be considered.

Additional monitoring considerations for male-to-female individuals on estrogen therapy include measurement of prolactin levels, evaluation for cardiac risk factors, screening guidelines for prostate disease as recommended for biological males, and screening guidelines for breast cancer as recommended for biological females.[34] For female-to-male individuals, additional monitoring considerations include evaluation of bone mineral density if risk factors for osteoporotic fracture are present, and, if mastectomy/hysterectomy/oophorectomy are not performed, mammograms and annual Pap smear, as recommended by the American Cancer Society and American College of Obstetricians and Gynecologists, respectively.[34]

A letter addressed to the relevant governmental agencies petitioning for a change of legal "sex" status may be requested by the individual following surgery. This letter may be important for the individual's legal documents (i.e., driver's license, passport, social security, etc.), and should include the nature of the treatment rendered. Individual state laws may vary in regard to the requirements for change of legal documents.

Secondary procedures

Additional procedures include both facial feminization as well as breast augmentation. The goal of these procedures is to remove the secondary sexual characteristics and stigmata associated with the biological male appearance. The timing of these surgeries in relation to genital surgery may vary between centers as well as within individual centers. It is not uncommon for feminizing procedures to be performed prior to genital surgery so as to improve the individual's sense of wellbeing and facilitate the real life test.[2]

Following hormonal therapy, there is frequently some breast growth in the male transsexual. However, the degree of breast growth is often times inadequate, and individuals continue to wear external prosthesis or padded bras. As such, augmentation mammaplasty is a frequently requested procedure. Anatomic differences between the male and female chest are relevant as to implant selection, incision choice, and pocket location.[52]

The male chest is not only wider than the female chest, but the pectoral muscle is usually more developed. Furthermore, the male areola is smaller than the female areola, the distance between the nipple and inframammary crease is less, and there is less ptosis in the natal male breast, even after hormonal therapy.[53] Based upon these characteristics, a larger implant is commonly chosen. In addition, silicone implants are usually requested. Pocket location and incision choice depend upon the individual and the degree of breast growth in response to hormone therapy. Either a prepectoral or subpectoral pocket may be used. The potential issues associated with a subpectoral pocket are implant displacement due to the activity of the overlying pectoralis muscle. However, potential concerns with the prepectoral pocket include capsular contracture and palpability due to less soft tissue coverage of the implant. In terms of incisions, transaxillary, peri-areolar, or inframammary crease approaches may be used and are tailored to the requests and anatomy of the individual *(Fig. 15.16)*.

Facial features may also be typically male or female. As such, surgery to "feminize" the face of male transsexuals is frequently requested. A variety of characteristics have been identified as male, and are often associated with the forehead, nose, malar region, and mandible. These differences include more pronounced supraorbital bossing in the male and a more continuous forehead curvature in the female. Furthermore, the chin is more pointed in the female.[54] The malar region is also more prominent in the female, and the female nose tends to be smaller, with a less acute glabellar angle than the male.[55,54] In addition, qualitative and quantitative differences in the skin, subcutaneous tissue, and hair also exist.[56]

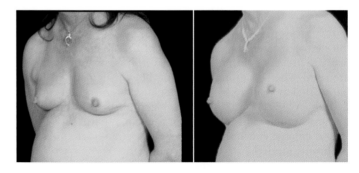

Fig. 15.16 Pre- and postoperative. Following subpectoral, silicone gel augmentation mammaplasty performed through an inframammary crease incision.

Because the female eyebrow is located above the supraorbital rim and has a more arched appearance than the male, typical procedures for facial feminization include a brow lift with advancement of the frontal hairline and frontal bone reduction. Although the brow lift may be performed with an endoscope, reduction of the frontal bone and lateral brow is facilitated with an open approach. In addition, the open approach, performed through an anterior hairline incision, allows advancement of the frontal hairline if desired (*Fig. 15.17*). Prior to proceeding with reduction of the frontal bone, lateral skull films are obtained in order to assess the thickness of the anterior table of the frontal sinus. Depending upon the thickness of the anterior table in relation to the degree of frontal bossing, craniofacial techniques may be employed for the desired correction.

A feminizing rhinoplasty typically involves dorsal hump reduction, cephalic trim, elevation of the nasal tip, and osteotomies to narrow the nasal pyramid. The chin and mandible represent additional anatomic sites which may require treatment. Based upon the individual's anatomy, either chin implants or osteoplastic genioplasty may be required. In addition, reduction of the masseter muscle or contouring of the mandibular angle may be performed through intraoral incision. Other procedures, such as facelift (*Fig. 15.18*), malar implants, and hair transplantation may also be requested.

Reduction thyroid chondroplasty is frequently requested to lessen the appearance of the "Adam's apple" or prominent thyroid cartilage (*pomus Adamus*). The procedure is typically performed as an outpatient under general anesthesia or local anesthesia with sedation. The procedure is performed through a transverse incision in a naturally occurring skin crease. Following vertical division of the middle cervical fascia, the sternothyroid and thyrohyoid muscles are retracted laterally. The perichondrium is incised and a subperichondrial dissection is performed with care taken so as not to enter the thyrohyoid membrane. On the posterior surface of the cartilage, subperichondrial dissection is performed inferiorly to the thyroepiglottic ligament. Dissection stops at this point so as not to injure the vocal cords or de-stabilize the epiglottis. Resection of the thyroid cartilage is performed between the superior thyroid notch in the midline and the superior thyroid tubercle superolaterally. The perichondrium is reapproximated and the incision is closed in a layered fashion.[57]

Voice surgery, designed to raise vocal pitch, may be requested by individuals following voice therapy. Hormonal intervention does not commonly affect vocal pitch, and this may represent a residual stigma of masculinity. As such, various techniques to shorten the vocal cords, increase vocal cord tension, or reduce the vibrating vocal cord mass may be performed.[22]

Secondary procedures for female-to-male transsexuals

Chest-wall contouring is an important early surgical step in the process of gender-confirmation for female-to-male individuals and may facilitate transition to the male role. The goals of chest surgery include the aesthetic contouring of the chest by removal of breast tissue and skin excess, reduction and re-positioning of the nipple-areola complex, release of the inframammary crease, and minimization of chest scars.[58]

Chest surgery in female-to-male transsexuals presents an aesthetic challenge due to breast volume, breast ptosis, nipple-areola size and position, degree of skin excess, and potential loss of skin elasticity. Breast binding, commonly performed by female-to-male transsexuals, may lead to a loss of skin elasticity, thereby necessitating additional skin removal. Both skin quality and elasticity are important determinants in the choice of surgical technique.[58] Technical considerations related to the subcutaneous mastectomy include preservation of subcutaneous fat on the skin flaps, preservation of the pectoralis fascia, and release of the inframammary crease.

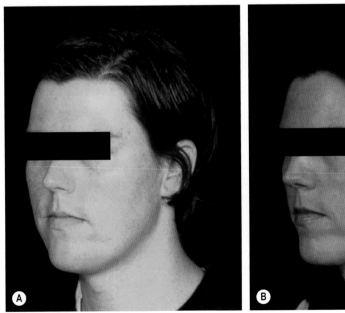
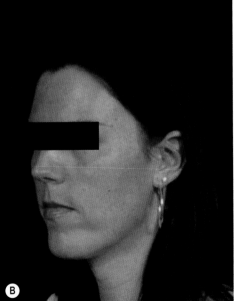

Fig. 15.17 (A) Preoperative. Prior to browlift and frontal bone reduction. **(B)** Postoperative. Following browlift and frontal bone reduction performed through an open, anterior hairline approach.

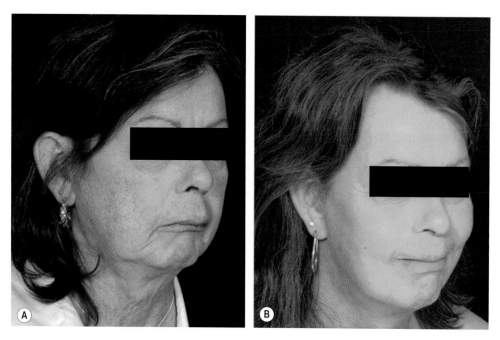

Fig. 15.18 (A) Preoperative. Prior to facelift, upper eyelid blepharoplasty, and TCA chemical peel. **(B)** Postoperative. Following facelift, upper eyelid blepharoplasty, and TCA chemical peel.

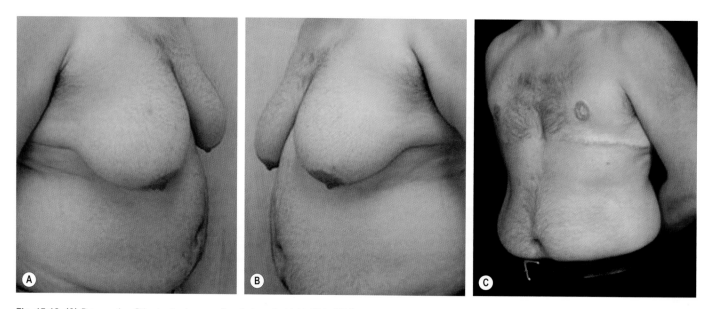

Fig. 15.19 (A) Preoperative. Prior to chest surgery female-to-male (right side). **(B)** Preoperative. Prior to chest surgery female-to-male (left side). **(C)** Postoperative. Subcutaneous mastectomy with free nipple graft.

Choice of incision is largely determined by degree of breast ptosis and skin quality/elasticity. Incisions may range from a periareolar incision in small breasts with a small areola and good skin elasticity, to circumareolar incisions, to transverse inframammary crease incisions with free nipple grafts. Liposuction may be used as an adjunct to excisional techniques. The decision as to maintenance of the nipple-areola complex on a dermoglandular pedicle versus a free nipple graft must also be considered. In positioning the nipple-areolar complex, the patient is sat upright and clinical judgment is used. In general, the nipple-areola is positioned just medial to the lateral border of the pectoralis major approximately 2–3 cm above the inferior insertion of the pectoralis major muscle

(Fig. 15.19). Post-operative management includes drains and elastic compression. Secondary revisions related to the scar and/or nipple-areolar complex are not uncommon.

Conclusion

Continued collaboration between the surgeon, behavioral scientist, and medical physician is important in providing comprehensive care to the transgendered individual. In addition, continued research focused on objective parameters and reporting of outcomes data will foster innovation and continued improvements in surgical techniques.

Access the complete reference list online at **http://www.expertconsult.com**

2. Monstrey S, Hoebeke P, Dhont M, et al. Surgical therapy in transsexual patients: a multi-disciplinary approach. *Acta Chir Belg*. 2001;101:200–209.

Excellent review article on the care of transgendered individuals.

4. WPATH. *The Standards of Care for Gender Identity Disorders*, 6th Version, World Professional Association for Transgender Health, 2001.

Flexible guidelines for the care of transgendered individuals.

6. Lee PA, Houk CP, Ahmed SF, et al. in collaboration with the participants in the International Consensus Conference on Intersex. Consensus statement on management of intersex disorders. *Pediatrics*. 2006;118:e488–e500.

Review article on disorders of sexual development.

22. Ettner R. The etiology of transsexualism. In: Ettner R, Monstrey S, Eyler E, eds. *Principles of Transgender Medicine and Surgery*. New York: Haworth Press; 2007:1–14.

25. Schechter L. The surgeon's relationship with the physician prescribing hormones and the mental health professional: review for version 7 of the World Professional Association for Transgender Health's Standards of Care. *IJT*. 2009;11:222–225.

Review of the role of the surgeon in the care of transgendered individuals.

26. Bowman C, Goldberg J. Care of the patient undergoing sex reassignment surgery. *IJT*. 2006;9(3–4):135–165.

33. Dahl M, Feldman JL, Goldberg JM, et al. Physical aspects of transgender endocrine therapy. *IJT*. 2006;9(3/4):111–134.

Guidelines for endocrine therapy for transgendered individuals.

34. Hembree WC, Cohen-Kettenis P, Delemarre-van de Waal HA, et al. Endocrine treatment of transsexual persons: an endocrine society clinical practice guideline. *J Clin Endocrinol Metab*. 2009;94:3132–3153.

37. Edgerton MT, Bull J. Surgical construction of the vagina and labia in male transsexuals. *Plast Reconstr Surg*. 1970;46:529–539.

42. Karim RB, Hage JJ, Bouman FG, et al. The importance of near total resection of the corpus spongiosum and total resection of the corpora cavernosa in the surgery of male to female transsexuals. *Ann Plast Surg*. 1991;26:554–557.

46. Perovic SV, Stanojevic DS, Djordjevic MI. Vaginoplasty in male transsexuals using penile skin and a urethral flap. *Br J Urol Int*. 2000;86:843–850.

48. Hage JJ, van Turnhout AA. Long-term outcome of metaidoioplasty in 70 female-to-male transsexuals. *Ann Plast Surg*. 2006;57(3):312–316.

50. Hage JJ, van Turnhout AVM, Dekker JJML, et al. Saving labium minus skin to treat possible urethral stenosis in female-to-male transsexuals. *Ann Plast Surg*. 2006;56(4):456–459.

16

Pressure sores

Robert Kwon and Jeffrey E. Janis

SYNOPSIS

- Pressure sores are a common problem associated with great morbidity and cost.
- They have been recognized since antiquity, though effective surgical treatment did not evolve until the 19th century.
- The pathogenesis involves not only pressure, but a multitude of additional factors including friction, shear, moisture, nutrition, and infection.
- A full evaluation of these factors, in addition to characterizing the wound in terms of stage, size, and involvement of the underlying bone, directs further treatment.
- Prevention and treatment of pressure sores should focus on correcting these risk factors, reserving operative intervention until the patient is optimized.
- Less severe pressure sores can often be treated with wound care and patient optimization.
- Thorough debridement, particularly of involved hard tissues, is critical, as with any wound.
- While flaps based on the gluteus muscles, the tensor fasciae latae, and the hamstring are workhorse flaps, a vast array of surgical options exist to treat any given wound, assuming some basic principles of flap design are respected.
- Recurrence rates are high even in the best of hands, and should be planned for preoperatively.

Access the Historical Perspective section online at
http://www.expertconsult.com

Introduction

Terminology

Though technically and semantically inaccurate, the terms "decubitus ulcer," "bedsore," and "pressure sore" are often used interchangeably. Decubitus ulcers – derived from the Latin *decumbere*, to lie down – occur over areas that have underlying bony prominences when the subject is recumbent, e.g., the sacrum, trochanter, heel, and occiput. Technically, sores resulting from pressure breakdown in areas that bear seated weight, such as the ischial tuberosities of spinal injury patients, and ulcers due to devices, such as splints, ear probes, or rectal tubes, are not decubitus ulcers.

Moreover, it has become clear that pressure is but one of many factors that contribute to the development of pressure sores. Nevertheless, it is likely the best term to use when describing these lesions which all count pressure as an important etiologic factor.

Epidemiology

There have been over 400 articles in the English-language literature alone on the incidence and prevalence of pressure sores in the last 5 years. These studies have not only examined the prevalence and incidence of pressure sores across multiple healthcare settings – specifically general acute care, long-term care, and home care – but also among specific populations and subpopulations such as the elderly, patients with hip fractures, infants and children, and terminally ill patients. Given these disparate populations and the substantial variation across individual institutions, precise determinations of incidence and prevalence are difficult.

In 1999 Amlung et al.[1] performed a 1-day pressure ulcer prevalence survey of 356 acute care facilities and 42 817 patients. The overall pressure ulcer prevalence rate was 14.8%; facility-acquired ulcers accounted for 7.1%. Ten years later, VanGilder et al.[2] reviewed the results of the International Pressure Ulcer Prevalence Survey (IPUPS) and found overall prevalence and facility-acquired ulcer rates of 12.3% and 5% respectively. Overall prevalence rates were highest in long-term acute care facilities (22%), while facility-acquired rates were highest in adult intensive care units (ICUs), ranging from 8.8% in general cardiac care units to 12.1% in medical ICUs. A total of 3.3% of ICU patients developed severe ulcers, while 10% were device-related. A broader inquiry,[3] reviewing over 400 000 records from the survey between 1989 and 2005, found overall and nosocomial pressure ulcer prevalence rates of 9.2% in 1989 and 15.5% in 2004. Rates were higher in long-term acute care facilities, at 27.3%. Overall, pressure ulcer prevalence appears relatively stable despite significant advances in treatment and prevention.

The prevalence of pressure ulcers in the nursing home population has been reported to be anywhere from 2% to 28%.[4,5] Data from the 2004 National Nursing Home Survey revealed an overall 11% prevalence rate, with elderly residents, residents with recent weight loss, and short-term residents being at even higher risk.[6] The reported prevalence of pressure ulcers in long-term acute care facilities is likewise variable, ranging from 5% to 27%,[7,8] while the IPUPS reported an overall 22% rate in this setting.

Particular populations have been identified at particularly high risk. There is a strong association between hip fractures and pressure sores, though incidences have been reported from 8.8% to 55%. A large European study[9] revealed an overall prevalence of 10% on arrival and 22% at discharge in this population, with dehydration, advanced age, moist skin, higher Braden scores, diabetes, and pulmonary disease all associated with higher rates of ulceration. The majority were stage I and none was stage IV. Baumgarten et al.[10] reported an 8.8% incidence of hospital-acquired pressure sores in a study involving multiple centers in the US. Another study by the same group,[11] with rigorous surveillance for ulcers in a slightly older population, revealed an incidence of 36.1%. Incidence was highest in the acute care setting and associated with longer wait before surgery, ICU stay, longer surgery, and general anesthetic.

Spinal cord injury (SCI) patients are at particular risk for pressure sores due to the combination of immobility and insensitivity. Rates have been reported to be 33–60%[12–14] and it is the second leading cause of rehospitalization after SCI. Gelis et al.[15] reviewed pressure ulceration in the SCI population and noted a 21–37% prevalence in the acute stage, a 2% rate leaving a rehabilitation center, and a 15–30% rate in the chronic stage. Identified risk factors included race, history of previous ulceration, and tobacco use.

Anatomic distribution

In 1964 Dansereau and Conway[16] published the results of their evaluation of 649 patients from the Bronx Veterans Administration Hospital with 1604 pressure sores among them. The authors noted that the vast majority of pressure sores developed in the lower part of the body, the ischial tuberosity being the most common site, accounting for 28% of all ulcers. In Meehan's 1994[17] review of 3487 patients with 6047 pressure sores, the most common site of occurrence was the sacrum (36%), followed by the heel (30%). More recently VanGilder et al.[2] reported that the sacrum (28.3%) and the heel (23.6%) were the most common sites for pressure ulceration, followed by the buttocks (17.2%).

Classically, in the early acute phase after SCI, the sacral area tends to be the most common site of pressure sores as patients are stabilized and treated for concomitant injuries in the supine position. In the subacute and chronic phases after SCI, the ischial area becomes the predominant site of pressure sores as the patient begins to sit up in a wheelchair during rehabilitation. However, as will be discussed later in this chapter, this division is not absolute.

Costs

Calculating the costs associated with pressure sores is complex. Monetary figures are subject to inflation and variation over time. While patients admitted with a primary diagnosis of pressure sore are simple to analyze, patients are often admitted with pressure ulcer-related problems, such as septicemia, and carry pressure sore as a secondary diagnosis. However, despite the uncertainty, it is clear pressure sores are a costly problem for the healthcare system.

The National Pressure Ulcer Advisory Panel (NPUAP) has estimated the cost to treat and heal hospital-acquired pressure sores to be up to $100 000 per patient.[18] If the additional costs, both surgical and nonsurgical, of managing pressure sores at nursing homes and home care facilities are considered, the financial burden is estimated by the Institute for Healthcare Improvement at approximately 11 billion dollars in 2006.

A review from 2006 of the Healthcare Cost and Utilization Project[19] revealed 503 300 hospital stays during which pressure sores were noted. Patients with pressure sores were inpatients nearly three times longer than patients without such a diagnosis (14.1 days versus 5.0 days). Patients with pressure sore as a primary diagnosis cost an average of $1200 a day, while patients with pressure sore as a secondary diagnosis cost an average of $1600 a day, compared with an average of $2000 a day for all other conditions. Mean cost per hospitalization was $16 800 and $20 400 for stays with a principal and secondary diagnosis of pressure sore, versus only $9900 for all other conditions. Aggregate costs were calculated to be $752 million and $10.2 billion for stays with primary and secondary diagnosis of pressure sore respectively.

Basic science

Pressure

As mentioned previously, Paget described the connection between pressure and decubitus ulcers as early as the 19th century. Though many other factors may contribute to their formation, pressure sores are thought to result from pressure applied to soft tissue at a level higher than that found in the blood vessels supplying that area for an extended time period. In 1930 Landis[30] performed a classic series of experiments and found that the average capillary closing pressure is approximately 32 mmHg. Fronek and Zweifach[31] reported similar findings in their study, noting perfusion pressures between 20 and 30 mmHg *(Fig. 16.1)*.

Lindan et al.[32] documented the human distribution of pressure points by means of a "bed of springs and nails." With the subject supine, the points of highest pressure were the sacrum, buttocks, heel, and occiput, all of which were subject to pressures of roughly 50–60 mmHg. When sitting, pressures up to 100 mmHg were recorded over the ischial tuberosities. Subjects in Lindan's study were tested on surfaces that were significantly softer than comparable wheelchair seats of beds, but even on padded surfaces with wide load distributions, all

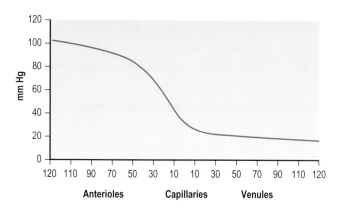

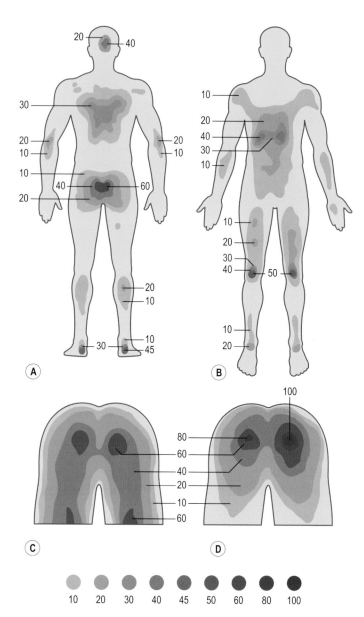

Fig. 16.1 Pressure in various components of the tissue microcirculation (diameter in μm). (Data from Fronek K, Zweifach BW. Microvascular pressure distribution in skeletal muscle and the effects of vasodilation. Am J Physiol 1975;228:791; reprinted with permission from Woolsey RM, McGarry JD: The cause, prevention, and treatment of pressure sores. Neurol Clin 1991;9:797.)

Fig. 16.2 Distribution of pressure in a healthy adult male while **(A)** supine, **(B)** prone, **(C)** sitting with feet hanging freely, and **(D)** sitting with feet supported. Values expressed in mmHg. (Adapted with permission from Lindan O, Greenway RM, Piazza JM. Pressure distribution on the surface of the human body I. Evaluation in lying and sitting positions using a "bed of springs and nails." Arch Phys Med Rehabil 1965;46:378.)

major weight-bearing areas sustained pressures in excess of end-capillary pressures *(Fig. 16.2)*.

However, simply applying pressure in excess of these levels does not necessarily result in tissue ischemia. Much of the pressure applied to tissues is carried by the connective tissues surrounding the blood vessels. Furthermore, autoregulation of local blood flow will tend to increase blood pressure in response to applied pressure within a certain range.[30,33]

Efforts have been made to quantify the degree of pressure necessary to cause tissue damage. Dinsdale[34] found that pressure roughly double capillary closing pressure, applied for 2 hours, resulted in irreversible ischemic damage to tissue. Pressures below this threshold were unlikely to cause tissue necrosis, while increased pressures were correlated with increased likelihood of ulceration. Kosiak *et al.*[35] noted similar findings in dog tissues, but noted that if the pressure was released every 5 minutes, few changes occurred. Groth[36] published a detailed study on the relationship between applied pressure and the onset of tissue damage in a rabbit model, noting an inverse relationship wherein higher pressures caused damage in less time. Husain[37] had similar results in a rat model, also noting that pressure applied over a large area was less injurious than when applied over a smaller one.

Furthermore, various tissues have different susceptibility to pressure. Nola and Vistnes[38] noted that pressure on skin over a bone is more injurious than pressure on skin over muscle. On the other hand, Daniel *et al.*[39] noted that muscle was more susceptible to injury than skin, requiring less pressure for a shorter duration likely due to its increased metabolic activity.

Friction

Friction is the force resisting relative motion between two surfaces, and is the precursor to shear. It develops between the patient's skin and any number of contact surfaces, including the patient's bedding, transfer devices such as sheets, rollers, or slide boards, various appliances and orthotics, and mobility devices such as wheelchair cushions. Excess friction may result in superficial skin injury such as abrasions, blisters, and even skin tears in patients with fragile skin.[40,41] While

relatively minor in isolation, such injuries may potentiate further damage. As the integrity of the skin is compromised, transepidermal water loss increases and allows moisture to accumulate. Moisture in turn increases the coefficient of friction and promotes adherence to sheets and other contact surfaces.[42]

Shear *(Fig. 16.3)*

Reichel[43] was one of the first authors to describe shear as a risk factor for developing decubitus ulcers, noting that patients developed more sacral pressure sores when the head of their bed was elevated. Shear develops when friction adheres skin and superficial tissues to sheets or bedding which are then

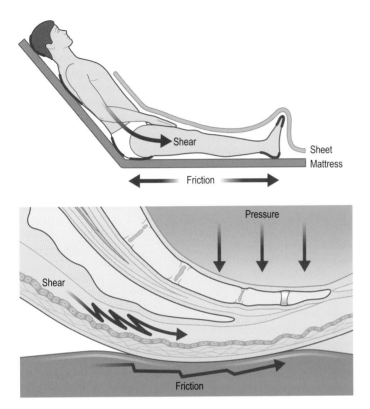

Fig. 16.3 Pressure, shear, and friction are related but distinct forces which contribute to pressure sore development.

stretched tightly over deeper structures. The underlying blood vessels are then stretched, angulated, and may be injured by this stress. Subcutaneous tissue in particular lacks tensile strength and is particularly susceptible to shear stress.[44] Dinsdale[34] noted that addition of shear forces greatly decreased the amount of pressure needed to cause ulceration in a pig model, concluding that "a shear force is more disastrous than a vertical force." Goossens *et al.*[45] noted similar results in human subjects, finding that the addition of a small shear component drastically reduces the level of pressure needed to cause critical ischemia over the sacrum.

Patient transfers, sliding or dragging the patient in bed, "boosting" patients up in bed, or allowing patients to elevate themselves in bed by pushing with elbows and heels all cause significant shear.[41] Certain positions also cause elevated levels of shear: patients in the semi-Fowler's position or sliding down in a wheelchair both experience significant shear over the lower back and buttocks.[46] This can explain why wheelchair-bound patients may still develop a sacral pressure sore if they are not sitting upright in their chair, despite the fact that theoretically the ischial tuberosities should be bearing the majority of their weight.

Moisture

Excessive moisture is not only a risk factor for pressure sores, but may also result in a separate pathology inclusive of incontinence dermatitis, perineal dermatitis, and moisture lesions.[47] Whether a separate entity resulting in skin breakdown due primarily to moisture and irritation as opposed to pressure is a legitimate or useful distinction is a matter of some debate.[48,49]

However, it is clear that moisture is an important factor to consider when evaluating pressure sores, and pressure relief should not be neglected even if lesions are thought to be primarily due to moisture. Moist skin has a higher coefficient of friction and is prone to maceration and excoriation.[44]

Though excess moisture can have many causes, urinary and fecal incontinence is of particular concern in the etiology of pressure sores. Incontinence is common in the elderly, and rates are even high in the institutionalized population, with rates from 20% to 77% for urinary incontinence[50,51] and from 17% to 50% for fecal incontinence.[52] In addition to causing excess moisture, urine also negates the acidic pH of skin through the introduction of nitrogen derivatives. Fecal contamination introduces a large bacterial load. Lowthian[48] noted a fivefold increase in pressure sores in patients who were incontinent, though he did not distinguish between urinary and fecal incontinence. While some studies have found a relationship between urinary incontinence and pressure sores,[53] others have failed to find a correlation while noting a significant correlation with fecal incontinence.[54–56]

While excess moisture is clearly deleterious, the opposite is also true. Excessively dry skin is prone to cracking, has decreased tensile strength and lipid content, and impaired barrier function, and appears to be an independent risk factor for pressure ulceration.[57,58]

Malnutrition

Patients who are chronically ill and debilitated frequently have accompanying nutritional deficiencies that manifest as low serum albumin, prealbumin, or transferrin levels. Prevalence rates range from 1% to 4% in elderly patients living at home, versus 20% in hospitalized patients and 37% in institutionalized patients.[59] The deleterious effects of poor nutrition include weight loss, negative nitrogen balance, poor wound healing, and immunosuppression.[60] Several studies have documented a clear association between protein malnutrition and wound healing,[61–63] and patients who are severely malnourished are at increased risk of sepsis, infection, in-hospital mortality, and longer hospital stays.[64,65] However, the relationship between malnutrition and pressure sore prevention, as opposed to treatment, is not entirely clear. There is certainly a strong correlation between malnutrition and pressure sores,[66–68] but a clear causal link remains elusive.

Neurological injury

Despite extensive recommendations aimed at addressing the issue, pressure sores remain the most common complication[69,70] and the second most common cause of hospital admission[71] in the SCI population. Immobility, either in bed or in a wheelchair, leads to increased pressure, friction, and shear that is a causative factor in all pressure sores. However, SCI eliminates the protective sensation that would normally stimulate them to alter their position in response to prolonged pressure, particularly during sleep. Pressure which would be innocuous with intermittent relief leads to pressure sore development.[46]

In addition to the obvious problems of immobility and decreased sensation, incontinence, spasticity, and psychosocial issues are common problems in this population. Spasticity, a common but not inevitable sequela of SCI, is a problem unique to the SCI population, affecting 65–78% patients 1 year postinjury.[72] Spasticity is characterized by hyperreflexia, clonus, and increased muscle tone. While it is not included in most pressure sore risk scales, it has effects due to direct increase in mechanical stress and altered weight distribution, as well as complicating patient positioning, skin inspection, and hygiene.[73]

Diagnosis

Classification

Multiple classification systems exist to describe pressure sores. The most commonly used system is the NPUAP staging system,[74] a modification of Shea's original classification,[74,75] most recently revised in 2007 *(Fig. 16.4)*. Though used in basic form for many years, two additional classifications, suspected deep-tissue injury and unstageable, have been added relatively recently to the NPUAP system.

"Stage" is something of a misnomer, as it implies a progression that does not reflect reality. Stage IV ulcers do not necessarily start as stage I ulcers, a fact emphasized by the addition of the suspected deep-tissue injury classification. Likewise, healing pressure sores do not progress in reverse order but instead granulate and close by secondary intention in the absence of surgical treatment. Though panel members were aware of these issues, the term "stage" was retained due to its historical use and widespread adoption.

Patient evaluation

When evaluating a new patient with a pressure sore, a wide variety of factors must be considered. Both the wound and the patient should be meticulously examined. A wound history, noting the onset, duration, prior treatments and procedures, and wound care regimen, should be noted. Wounds should be measured in three dimensions, with notes made regarding any tunneling or undermining. The tissue at the margins of the wound should be examined for any signs of occult deep-tissue injury, infection, and scarring. The base of the wound should be characterized, noting the presence of eschar, slough, or other necrotic tissue. If necrotic material obscures the base of the wound, it should be debrided until a full assessment can be performed. Granulation should be noted in terms of both character and percentage of the wound bed covered. Exposed tissues, such as bone, tendon, or joint, should be noted. If easily accessible the bone can be characterized as hard, soft, or obviously necrotic. The amount and character of the wound exudate should be documented as well. A measuring tape and camera can improve documentation and make tracking progression easier.[76]

In addition to a thorough general history and physical, some attention should be paid to the risk factors specific to pressure sores. An attempt should be made to identify the etiology of the patient's pressure sore, though it is often multifactorial. Sources of friction, shear, and pressure should be evaluated and recommendations for proper pressure relief surfaces and skin care regimens made as appropriate. If incontinence is present an effort should be made to control this, possibly involving the assistance of other specialties if needed.

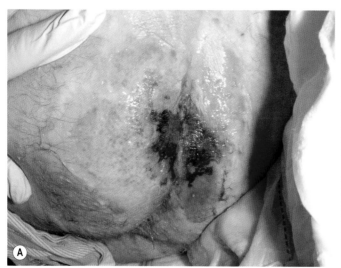 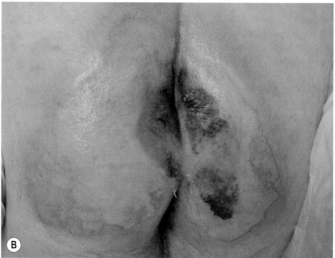

Fig. 16.4 The National Pressure Ulcer Advisory Panel staging system. **(A, E)** Stage I: Intact skin with nonblanchable redness of a localized area usually over a bony prominence. Darkly pigmented skin may not have visible blanching; its color may differ from the surrounding area. **(B, F)** Stage II: Partial-thickness loss of dermis presenting as a shallow open ulcer with a red pink wound bed, without slough. May also present as an intact or open/ruptured serum-filled blister. This should not be used to describe skin tears, tape burns, perineal dermatitis, maceration, or excoriation. **(C, G)** Stage III: Full-thickness tissue loss. Subcutaneous fat may be visible but bone, tendon, or muscle is not exposed. Slough may be present but does not obscure the depth of tissue loss. May include undermining and tunneling. **(D, H)** Stage IV: Full-thickness tissue loss with exposed bone, tendon, or muscle. Exposed bone is sufficient, but not necessary to define a stage IV pressure sore. Slough or eschar may be present on some parts of the wound bed. Often includes undermining or tunneling. May extend into muscle and/or supporting structures (e.g., fascia, tendon, or joint capsule), making osteomyelitis possible. Bone/tendon is visible or directly palpable. **(I)** Suspected deep-tissue injury: Purple or maroon localized area of discolored intact skin or blood-filled blister due to damage of underlying soft tissue from pressure and/or shear. The area may be preceded by tissue that is painful, firm, mushy, boggy, warmer, or cooler as compared to adjacent tissue. The wound may evolve and become covered by thin eschar. Evolution may be rapid, exposing additional layers of tissue even with optimal treatment. **(J)** Unstageable: Full-thickness tissue loss in which the base of the ulcer is covered by slough (yellow, tan, gray, green, or brown) and/or eschar (tan, brown, or black) in the wound bed. Until the base of the wound is exposed, the true depth, and therefore stage, cannot be determined.

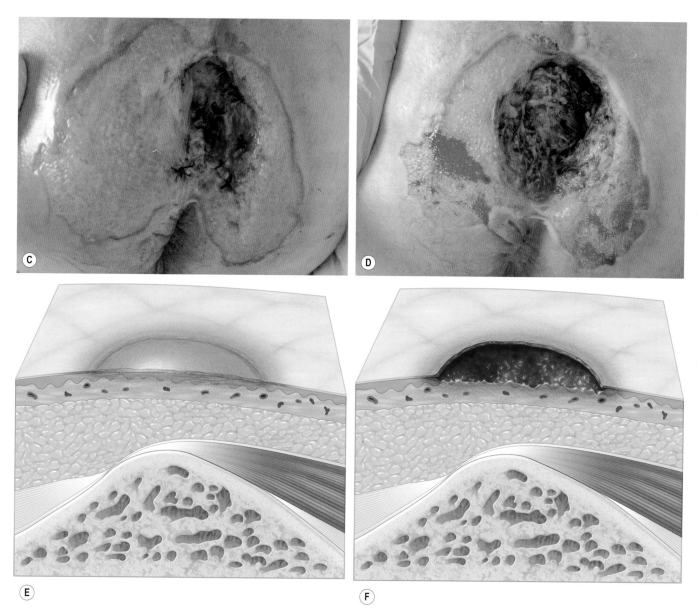

Fig. 16.4, cont'd

Likewise, spasticity should be evaluated and if needed controlled medically or surgically. Nutrition should be evaluated with serum albumin and prealbumin. If needed, nutrition should be supplemented and progress of therapy monitored with weekly serum studies. Any underlying medical problems, such as hypertension, diabetes, or history of cardiac disease, should be investigated and optimized.

A reasonable initial set of studies would include a complete blood count, basic metabolic panel, creatinine, and blood urea nitrogen. Albumin and prealbumin should be obtained at the initial consult and regularly thereafter to evaluate for malnutrition and follow the progression of therapy. C-reactive protein and erythrocyte sedimentation rate (ESR) can be obtained to evaluate for osteomyelitis, though they will almost certainly be positive in deeper ulcers. The evaluation of the pressure sore patient for osteomyelitis is discussed in the next section. Wound cultures of the open pressure sore are of little value and should not be used to direct antibiotic therapy,[77] as opposed to needle or surgical bone biopsy.

Osteomyelitis

In 1970 Waldvogel et al.[78] recognized that osteomyelitis is responsible for wound infection and breakdown after reconstruction of stage III and IV pressure sores (*Fig. 16.5*). Patients with pressure sores complicated by osteomyelitis have significantly longer hospitalizations than those who do not.[79] Establishing the diagnosis of osteomyelitis is essential before embarking on definitive surgical treatment of pressure sores. Unrecognized osteomyelitis is a major source of morbidity and increased costs.[79]

In 1988 Lewis et al.[80] tried to assess the value of some common test in diagnosing osteomyelitis by following 61 patients with pressure sores, 52 of whom eventually had confirmed histopathologic diagnosis of osteomyelitis from surgical specimens. This prospective trial examined white blood cell count, ESR, plain X-ray, technetium-99 m bone scans, computed tomography (CT) scan, and Jamshidi-needle bone biopsy. The authors felt that the most practical, revealing, and

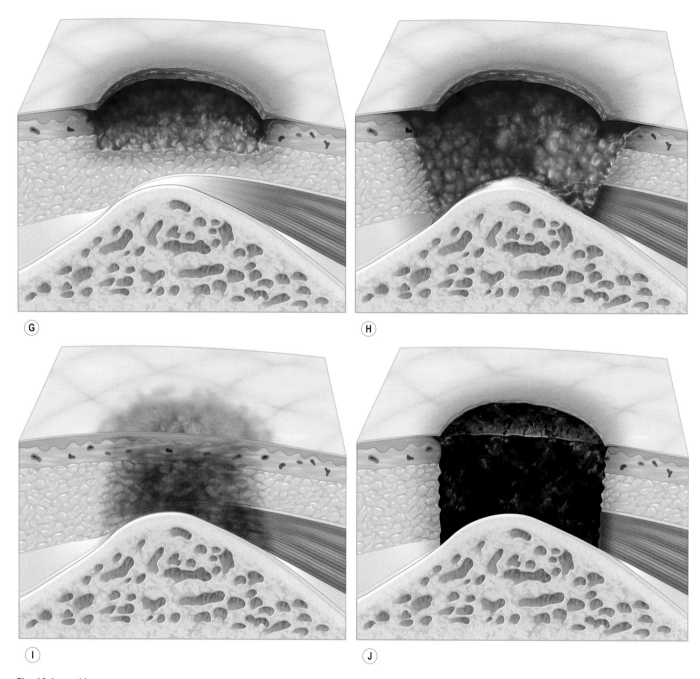

(G)   (H)

(I)   (J)

Fig. 16.4, cont'd

least invasive preoperative workup involved a combination of white blood cell count, ESR, and two-view X-ray. Only one positive test was needed to make the diagnosis. Sensitivity was 89% and specificity 88% using this protocol. Bone scans and CT scans were expensive and not very sensitive. Needle bone biopsy had a sensitivity of 73% and a specificity of 96%. Of note, magnetic resonance imaging (MRI) was not included in this analysis.

MRI has taken on a larger role in the diagnosis of osteomyelitis. Huang and colleagues[81] analyzed 59 consecutive MRIs in 44 paralyzed patients and found an overall accuracy of 97%, sensitivity of 98%, and specificity of 89%. The authors concluded that not only was MRI accurate, it helps define the extent of infection, which may help limit the surgical

resection. Ruan et al.[82] independently confirmed these findings and feel that MRI is superior to CT for the evaluation of osteomyelitis.

Han et al.[79] reviewed their series of press ulcers and noted that their high osteomyelitis-related complication rate – largely consisting of deep abscess and sinus tracts – was a result of their inability to diagnose osteomyelitis accurately preoperatively. Their group moved to a two-stage procedure, performing wound debridement and Jamshidi core needle bone biopsy at the first operation *(Fig. 16.6)*. If the biopsy results were positive, closure was delayed for 6 weeks while the osteomyelitis was treated with antibiotics; otherwise the wound was closed with a musculocutaneous flap. The authors also noted that bone cultures alone were not as useful as bone

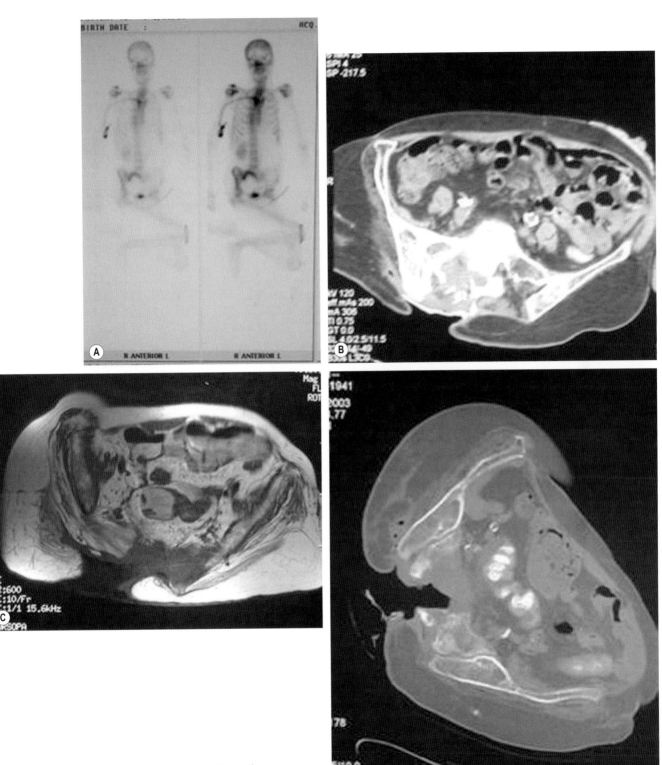

Fig. 16.5 (A–D) Bone scan, computed tomography, and magnetic resonance imaging of severe sacral osteomyelitis.

Fig. 16.5, cont'd (E) Protocol for managing patients with grade IV pressure ulcers. JNBB, Jamshidi core needle bone biopsy; IV, intravenous. (Reprinted with permission from Han H, Lewis VL, Weidrich VA, *et al.* The value of Jamshidi core needle bone biopsy in predicting postoperative osteomyelitis in grade IV pressure ulcer. Plast Reconstr Surg 2002;111:118.)

cultures and histopathology of the bone biopsy together, and found that the biopsy had a positive and negative predictive value of 93% and 100%, respectively.

These results are in keeping with several other studies that support the utility of bone biopsy in the diagnosis of osteomyelitis.[83–86] Marriott and Rubayi[87] have used the results of bone biopsy to determine the duration of antibiotic therapy, in some cases truncating treatment if pathology reveals only chronic osteomyelitis.

Ultimately, MRI appears to be accurate and noninvasive, while providing detailed anatomic information. Bone biopsy likewise has admirable accuracy, and, perhaps most importantly, is the only method that can be used to direct antibiotic therapy. Though local factors such as the availability of equipment and economic factors should be considered, used in conjunction MRI and bone biopsy allow for comprehensive evaluation of osteomyelitis in the pressure sore patient.

Psychological evaluation

Psychological problems are common in the pressure sore population. Langer[88] finds 22% of patients with SCI had diagnosable depression, considerably higher than found in the general population. Frank *et al.*[89] report 37.5% of patients with SCI had a diagnosis of major depression. Akbas *et al.*[90] report

47.4% of patients with pressure sores fulfilled the diagnostic criteria for major depression. In their prospective study, they found the depression rates to be higher in women, younger patients, and those who had undergone multiple operations for their pressure sores. The authors recommend "intensive psychological counseling" in the treatment of the pressure sore patient. Foster *et al.*[91] suggest that psychological factors play a significant role in predicting pressure sore recurrences.

Patient selection

All patients with pressure sores should be optimized with regard to the risk factors already enumerated. It is worth remembering that pressure sores are rarely life-threatening, and there is no need to rush to treatment or surgery if the patient has not been optimized. Many more superficial wounds will heal with conservative therapies if correctable risk factors are identified and addressed. On the other hand, a patient who is malnourished, bedbound on an inappropriate mattress, with undiagnosed osteomyelitis, is doomed to failure regardless of the surgical technique used.

A judgment must be made regarding whether a wound is likely to heal successfully by secondary intention or whether

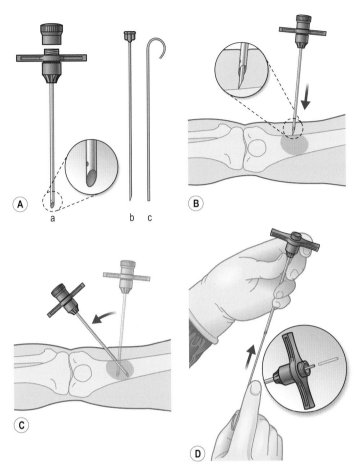

Fig. 16.6 (A) The Jamshidi bone biopsy needle, cannula, and screw-on cap (a), tapered point (b), pointed stylet to advance cannula through soft tissues (c), and probe to expel specimen from cannula (d). **(B)** With the stylet locked in place, the cannula is advanced through the soft tissue until bone is reached. The inset is a close-up view showing stylet against bone cortex. **(C)** The stylet is removed and the bone cortex is penetrated with the cannula. The cannula is withdrawn, and the procedure repeated with redirection of the instrument to obtain multiple core samples. **(D)** The probe is then inserted retrograde into the tip of the cannula to expel the specimen through the base (inset). (Reprinted with permission Powers BE, LaRue SM, Withrow SJ, *et al.* Jamshidi needle biopsy for diagnosis of bone lesions in small animals. J Am Vet Med Assoc 1988;193:206–207.)

a flap is required to resurface the wound and/or fill dead space left after debridement. In general, stage I and II pressure sores can be treated nonoperatively, while stage III and IV ulcers require flaps. Patients with suspected deep-tissue injury and unstageable ulcers should be debrided until they can be clearly staged. While surgical debridement is the gold standard, other methods can be used as appropriate.

While operative treatment is often delayed while the patient is optimized and risk factors corrected, it is a rare patient who does not qualify for any attempt at reconstruction. Obviously critically ill patients who cannot tolerate surgery should be stabilized before any sort of reconstruction is entertained. More uncommon is the patient with multiple severe comorbidities whose risk factors cannot be easily corrected, due to either medical or social factors. In such cases, chronic wound care may be preferable to attempted reconstruction that is doomed to failure and recurrence.

Treatment

Prevention

Obviously, prevention of pressure sores is preferable to treatment. As healthcare moves towards nonpayment for nosocomial pressure sores, there is ever-greater incentive to avoid these lesions. However, despite extensive study and recommendations, overall pressure sores rates have changed little in recent years.[3,92] Some pressure sores may not be preventable,[93–95] and using pressure sores as an indicator of quality is a contentious issue, particularly in light of possible negligence litigation.[96] However, though no strategy has been found which reduces pressure sore rates to zero, there are several measures, many of which now constitute standard care, which may contribute to pressure sore prevention.[58]

For the surgeon who is often consulted only after a pressure sore has developed, knowledge of prevention strategies is still critical not only to advise the consultation, but to optimize the patient before surgery, prevent additional pressure sores from developing, and perhaps most critically to prevent postoperative recurrence.

Risk assessment

The first step in pressure sore prevention is risk assessment. Multiple assessment scales have been devised, including those by Braden, Gosnell, Knoll, Norton, Waterlow, and Douglas.[97] Several are designed for specific subpopulations and each has its merits. All suffer from potential inaccuracies as their use is dependent on the competence of its assessor and the setting in which it is used.

Norton[98] developed an assessment scale for use in geriatric patients. The scale incorporates general physical condition, mental status, activity, mobility, and incontinence and ranges from 5 to 20, with lower scores associated with greater risk. Patients with a score of 11 or less had a 48% incidence of pressure sores, while those with a score of 18 or greater had a 5% incidence. Gosnell[99] added nutritional status as a variable to his method, which is often referred to as the "modified Norton scale."

The most widely used pressure sore assessment tool is the Braden scale[100] *(Table 16.1)*. The Braden scale incorporates six subscales that assess sensory perception, skin moisture, activity, mobility, friction and shear, and nutrition. Scores range from 6 to 23, with higher scores associated with an increased risk of developing pressure sores. The original study noted a score of 16 to be the threshold for pressure sore development,[100] though a different cutoff score may be more appropriate in different settings.[101,102]

Multiple studies have examined the validity, sensitivity, specificity, and predictive value of the various scales. Generally, assessment scales are superior to nurses' clinical judgment when predicting future pressure ulceration.[97] However, there is no evidence that use of risk assessment decreases pressure sore incidence.[103–105] Whether this is because interventions are not instituted or are ineffective is unclear.[104]

Skin care (Box 16.1)

Ideal skin care encompasses cleaning, hydrating, protecting, and replenishing the skin as needed. Proper skin care can be time- and labor-intensive, and is at times neglected by physicians and nurses alike.[106]

Common recommendations for skin cleansing involve the use of warm soap and water followed by drying by rubbing or patting.[107] Washing involves the use of soap and surfactants, which, while effective at removing debris, have the potential to be irritants.[108] The alkaline nature of soap also negates the protective natural acidity of the skin, which in turn alters the balance of resident flora on the skin.[109] Drying the skin by patting may cause less trauma,[110,111] though if it leaves excess moisture on the skin this can lead to maceration and increased vulnerability to friction injuries.[112] Many alternative cleansers have been marketed which address the shortcomings of soap and water, but little data exist to recommend any particular product at this time.[113]

Maintaining proper skin hydration is most often achieved through the use of emollients, which occlude the skin surface with a hydrophobic layer, and humectants, which attract and absorb water from their surroundings. Numerous formulations exist, many with additional surfactants and emulsifying agents, which vary somewhat in their effectiveness, greasiness, and potential for skin irritation. While the theoretical advantages of treating dry skin are well established,[55,57,114] as with cleansers, few data exist to recommend any one hydrating product over another.[115,116]

Box 16.1 General skin care principles

Assess the patient's skin daily
Cleanse skin when indicated using a pH-balanced cleanser
Avoid soap and hot water
Avoid friction and scrubbing
Minimize exposure to moisture (e.g., incontinence, wound leakage)
Use skin barrier product to protect vulnerable skin
Use emollients to maintain skin hydration

Table 16.1 The Braden scale for predicting pressure sore risk

Sensory perception Ability to respond meaningfully to pressure-related discomfort	1. Completely limited Unresponsive (does not moan, flinch, or grasp) to painful stimuli, due to diminished level of consciousness or sedation or Limited ability to feel pain over most of body	2. Very limited Responds only to painful stimuli. Cannot communicate discomfort except by moaning or restlessness or Has a sensory impairment which limits the ability to feel pain or discomfort over half of body	3. Slightly limited Responds to verbal commands, but cannot always communicate discomfort or the need to be turned or Has some sensory impairment which limits ability to feel pain or discomfort in one or two extremities	4. No impairment Responds to verbal commands. Has no sensory deficit which would limit ability to feel or voice discomfort
Moisture Degree to which skin is exposed to moisture	1. Constantly moist Skin is kept moist almost constantly by perspiration and urine. Dampness is detected every time patient is moved or turned	2. Very moist Skin is often, but not always, moist. Linen must be changed at least once a shift	3. Occasionally moist Skin is occasionally moist, requiring an extra linen change approximately once a day	4. Rarely moist Skin is usually dry; linen only requires changing at routine intervals
Activity Degree of physical activity	1. Bedfast Confined to bed	2. Chairfast Ability to walk severely limited or nonexistent. Cannot bear own weight and/or must be assisted into chair or wheelchair	3. Walks occasionally Walks occasionally during day, but for very short distances with or without assistance. Spends majority of shift in bed or chair	4. Walks frequently Walks outside room at least twice a day and inside room at least once every 2 hours during waking hours
Mobility Ability to change and control body position	1. Completely immobile Does not make even slight changes in body or extremity position without assistance	2. Very limited Makes occasional slight changes in body or extremity position but unable to make frequent or significant changes independently	3. Slightly limited Makes frequent though slight changes in body or extremity position independently	4. No limitation Makes major and frequent changes in position without assistance

Table 16.1 The Braden scale for predicting pressure sore risk—cont'd

Nutrition Usual food intake pattern	1. Very poor Never eats a complete meal. Rarely eats more than half of any food offered. Eats two servings or less of protein (meat or dairy products) per day. Takes fluids poorly. Does not take liquid dietary supplement or Is NOP and/or maintained on clear liquids or IVs for more than 5 days	2. Probably inadequate Rarely eats a complete meal and generally eats only about half of any food offered. Protein intake includes only three servings of meat or dairy products per day. Occasionally will take a dietary supplement or Receives less than optimum amount of liquid diet or tube feeding	3. Adequate Eats over half of most meals. Eats a total of four servings of protein (meat, dairy products) per day. Occasionally will refuse a meal, but will usually take a supplement when offered or Is on a tube-feeding or TPN regimen which probably meets most of nutritional needs	4. Excellent Eats most of every meal. Never refuses a meal. Usually eats a total of four or more servings of meat and dairy products. Occasionally eats between meals. Does not require supplementation
Friction and shear	1. Problem Requires moderate to maximum assistance in moving. Complete lifting without sliding against sheets is impossible. Frequently slides down in bed or chair, requiring frequent repositioning with maximum assistance. Spasticity, contractures, or agitation leads to almost constant friction	2. Potential problem Moves feebly or requires minimum assistance. During a move skin probably slides to some extent against sheets, chair, restraints, or other devices. Maintains relatively good position in chair or bed most of the time but occasionally slides down	3. No apparent problem Moves in bed or chair independently and has sufficient muscle strength to lift up completely during move. Maintains good position in bed or chair	
			Total score	

(Reproduced from www.bradenscale.com.)
NPO, nil per os; IV, intravenous; TPN, total parenteral nutrtion.

Barrier products protect the skin, particularly in the setting of incontinence or in the presence of stomas, fistulas, or wounds. Many preparations consist of a lipid/water emulsion that forms a protective film over the skin. Newer barrier products incorporate a polymer which forms a thin semipermeable membrane over the skin.[117] Many incorporate an antiseptic agent such as cetrimide or benzalkonium as well. Again, despite their widespread use and the proliferation of products, data on their effectiveness are scant.[118]

While data on individual agents are not very robust, there is evidence that a clear skin care protocol can benefit patients. Multiple authors have found instituting such protocols results in reduction in pressure sore incidence rates.[119] Cole and Nesbitt[120] found a reduction from 17.8% to 2% over a 3-year period, whereas Lyder et al.[121] noted an 87% reduction in a nursing home setting. Based on the available data, the American Wound Ostomy and Continence Nurses Society[122] produced a set of guidelines for skin care.

Incontinence

As noted previously, the relationship between urinary incontinence and pressure sore incidence is not clear, with limited evidence to suggest a causal relationship. Currently, the use of diapers or sanitary pads in conjunction with meticulous skin care is a reasonable option when compared to the risks associated with extended use of a urinary catheter.[123]

Fecal incontinence, on the other hand, has been shown to be a risk factor for pressure sores. At times fecal incontinence is due to factors which are not easily correctable: cognitive impairment, history of colorectal surgery, radiation proctopathy, inflammatory bowel disease, and various neurological or myogenic disorders of sphincter function are not easily correctable. The bladder and bowel dysfunction of SCI patients requires specific regimens and is generally managed by a specialist.[124]

However, many measures can be instituted to decrease the impact of fecal incontinence. Possibly the most common predisposing condition to fecal incontinence is fecal impaction, which is common in older adults and may lead to overflow incontinence.[125] Conservative measures include diet modification and a wide variety of antimotility agents, including clonidine, cholestyramine, loperamide, codeine, diphenoxylate, and atropine.[126,127] Diarrhea may be due to infection, which should be ruled out and treated prior to using antidiarrheal agents. If medical management is unsuccessful, surgery may be considered, ranging from attempts at sphincterplasty to elective colostomy when other options fail.[128] Though patients and families are often reluctant to proceed with colostomy, there is evidence overall quality of life is improved in patients with severe fecal incontinence.[129]

Spasticity

Control of spasticity may not only reduce the risk of pressure sores, but may also improve patient reports of pain and ability to perform activities of daily living (ADL).[130] However, it is worth noting that in some cases spasticity may increase stability in positioning, facilitate some transfers and ADLs, and prevent osteopenia.[131,132] Taken as a whole, the impact of spasticity on quality of life is not straightforward, and should be considered before instituting treatment.

Physical therapy is the first step in treating spasticity and an important component of care in SCI patients in general.[133] Pharmacologic treatment is the next step. Diazepam, baclofen, clonidine, tizanidine, gabapentin, and dantrolene are commonly used agents.[134–137] Each has the potential for side-effects, including sedation, nausea, diarrhea, muscle weakness, and cognitive effects, and treatment must be tailored to the individual patient.[137,138]

Patients who cannot tolerate or do not respond to oral therapy may benefit from intrathecal administration of baclofen.[136,139] As the drug directly accesses the central nervous system, systemic side-effects are minimized at the cost of the risks of surgery and possible mechanical complications with the pump. Injection with chemodenervation agents, including phenol, ethanol, and botulinum, can be effective.[140,141] Reported complications include systemic side-effects, vascular complications, skin irritation, and tissue necrosis. Though the effects are temporary, long-term use of chemodenervation agents will result in denervation atrophy.

Surgical management of spasticity is an option when medical therapy is insufficient. Baclofen pump implantation is the most common surgical procedure for spasticity in individuals with SCI and has a history of success.[137,142] In select, refractory cases, orthopedic and neurosurgical techniques may be of benefit, though such procedures are unlikely to have pressure sore prevention as their primary indication. Local tenotomy or tendon transfer has had mixed results in the treatment of spasticity.[143] Rhizotomy has been complicated by both inadequate treatment of spasticity[144] and severe atrophy,[145] depending on the technique employed. Myelotomy and T-myelotomy involving direct sectioning of the spinal cord have been reported to be effective in several case series[146,147] in patients who did not have hope of regaining motor function, though the benefits did decrease over time.[148]

Pressure relief

As befits its primary role in pressure sore pathogenesis, extensive efforts have been made in modulating the pressure through the use of various surfaces and products as well as protocols mandating patient repositioning. Though numerous support surfaces exist, most can be divided into two general categories. Constant low-pressure (CLP) devices distribute pressure over a large area and include devices such as static air, water, gel, bead, silicone, foam, and sheepskin supports *(Fig. 16.7)*. Alternating-pressure (AP) devices vary the

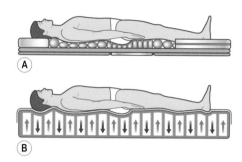

Fig. 16.7 (A) Constant low-pressure surfaces seek to distribute pressure statically, while **(B)** alternating-pressure surfaces vary applied pressure over time.

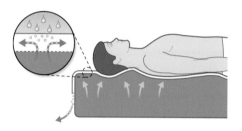

Fig. 16.8 Low air loss mattress concept.

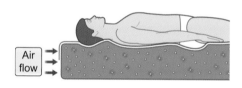

Fig. 16.9 Fluidized bed.

pressure under the patient, avoiding prolonged pressure over a single anatomic point[149] *(Fig. 16.7)*.

Two particular types of CLP device deserve special mention, as they are commonly used in the prevention and treatment of pressures sores. Low air loss (LAL) beds float the patient on air-filled cells through which warm air circulates *(Fig. 16.8)*. The circulating air both equalizes pressure exerted on the patient and keeps the skin dry. Properly utilized, LAL surfaces exert less than 25 mmHg on any part of the body.[150,151] Air-fluidized (AF) beds circulate warm air through fine ceramic beads, creating a unique support surface, while having a drying effect similar to LAL beds *(Fig. 16.9)*. With proper use these beds exert less than 20 mmHg on the patient, but are expensive, heavy, and cumbersome.[152]

Within these classifications are a multitude of beds, mattresses, overlays, pads, and cushions, each with slightly different designs by different manufacturers. There is a daunting body of literature comparing various specific products to one another and with standard hospital beds. Evaluating this literature is challenging given the often small sample sizes, poor experimental design, and lack of generalizability common in these studies. Moreover, as new products are developed and old ones are phased out, many studies refer to products no longer in production or use. Despite these limitations, some general conclusions can be drawn from the literature.[153]

Considerable evidence exists that the use of a pressure-relieving overlay is superior to a standard bed in preventing pressure sores. Multiple studies have found decreased incidence and severity of pressure sores in high-risk patients with the use of constant low-pressure devices such as overlays[154–156] or sheepskin[157,158] when compared to a standard hospital foam mattress. Pooled analysis reveals a relative risk of 0.32.[153] Data also support the use of AP devices when compared to standard mattresses. Both Andersen et al.[156] and Sanada[159] noted a significant reduction in pressure sore incidence with the use of active devices, with a pooled relative risk of 0.31.[153] Though several studies have compared CLP and AP devices,[156,160–162] no clear advantage has been identified, despite attempts at pooled analysis.[153]

LAL, like other CLP surfaces, has been shown to be effective at preventing pressure sores,[163,164] with a relative risk estimated at 0.08.[153] Comparisons with other CLP devices in regard to prevention are limited, and no clear advantage for either has been demonstrated.[165,166] Likewise, though AF beds are perhaps the most effective pressure-relieving devices in widespread use, virtually no data on its role in prevention are available, perhaps because these expensive devices are reserved for treatment. Regardless of the type of mattress used, they lose their ability to disperse interface pressure as the head is elevated to 45° or higher.[167] As such, patients should avoid prolonged periods of sitting while on these mattresses.

In addition to support surfaces, patient repositioning is often used in an attempt to prevent pressure sores, though the data are limited. Defloor et al.[168] found a significant reduction in pressure sore incidence when turning every 4 hours combined with a specialized foam mattress was compared to every 2 hours on a regular mattress. Given the study design it is difficult to determine the relative contributions of the pressure relief surface and the turning regimen. The ideal interval and posture for repositioning are not clear given the current data.[58,169] It bears mention that repositioning is not without its costs, both in terms of nursing time and effort, patient discomfort, and possible dislodgement of catheters and lines, and there is no evidence that more frequent repositioning reduces rates of pressure sores.

Cushions for wheelchairs filled with gel, foam, air, or water are available to relieve pressure. A typical wheelchair sling seat exerts a "hammocking" effect that can produce abnormal scoliotic posture and pelvic obliquity *(Fig. 16.10)*. This in turn causes asymmetrical pressure on both trochanter and ischium that requires specialized cushions for prevention.[170] Hip adduction and internal rotation of thighs, with consequent reduction in stability, are also seen in most paraplegics, who lack trunk or pelvic muscle innervation and tend to sit on their coccyx. Rigid-base cushions provide lumbar support and decrease ischial pressure by allowing wider weight distribution on the posterior thighs.[170] A direct correlation between buttock–cushion interface has been noted[171] *(Fig. 16.11)*.

Houle[172] and Souther et al.[173] studied the effects of various wheelchair seats and found decreased pressures over the ischium, although none was below the capillary pressure

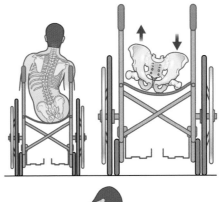

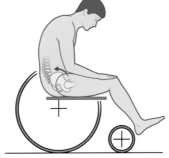

Fig. 16.10 Hammocking effect of wheelchair sling seat producing pelvic obliquity. Paraplegics lack innervation of the lower trunk muscles and sit on their coccyx, with exaggerated posterior pelvic tilt. (Reprinted with permission from Letts RM. Principles of seating the disabled. Boca Raton, FL: CRC Press, 1991.)

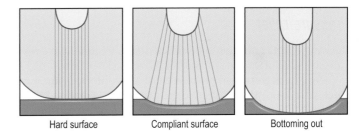

Hard surface   Compliant surface   Bottoming out

Fig. 16.11 Compressive force exerted on tissue by bone in an individual lying or sitting on (left) a hard surface; (center) an effective pressure-reducing device; and (right) an ineffective pressure-reducing device that "bottoms out." (Reprinted with permission from Woolsey RM, McGarry JD. The cause, prevention, and treatment of pressure sores. Neurol Clin 1991;9:797.)

benchmark. The authors recommend additional measures for pressure relief to prevent ulceration. Ragan et al.[174] studied seat interface pressures on wheelchair cushions of various thicknesses. They found the highest subcutaneous stress concentrated within 2 cm of the ischial tuberosity. The subcutaneous pressures decreased with thicker cushions, with the maximum effectiveness obtained with an 8-cm cushion. Increasing the thickness beyond 8 cm did not give further benefit in reducing subcutaneous stress. As with pressure relief mattresses, no data exist to recommend a particular type of cushion over another at this time.[153,160,175,176]

The development of pressure consciousness by the patient is an essential part of pressure sore prevention.[177] Pressure release maneuvers are reinforced to patients and should be performed at least every 15 minutes while the patient is seated.[178]

Nutrition

Multiple studies have examined the effect of nutritional supplementation on pressure sore prevention. Despite improvement in secondary measures such as caloric intake, body weight, and serum nutritional markers, most studies have failed to find reduction in pressure sore rates.[179–181] Bourdel-Marchasson and Rondeau[182] found a modest reduction in pressure sore rates when patients were given oral dietary supplementation. A more recent meta-analysis by Stratton et al.[183] found a modest reduction in pressure sore rates in patients treated with enteral tube feeds, estimating that 19.25 patients would need to be given enteral nutritional support to prevent one pressure sore. Overall, the evidence that pressure sores can be prevented by nutritional supplementation, much less specific formulations or micronutrient additives, is limited.[184]

Nonsurgical management

Limited wounds may heal spontaneously without surgical intervention so long as the wound is cleansed meticulously, pressure is avoided, and risk factors are corrected. The measures implemented in pressure sore prevention become doubly important once the transition is made to treating an established ulcer.

Pressure relief

Pressure relief continues to be critical in the treatment of pressure sores. While more advanced LAL and AF surfaces would in theory be preferred in the treatment of established pressure sores, the literature is mixed on this point. Ferrell et al.[185] found similar results when comparing LAL beds to foam mattresses. Ochs et al.[186] in turn found AF beds to be superior to both standard overlays and LAL beds. On the other hand Branom and Rappl[165] found LAL mattresses inferior to an advanced foam surface, while Economides et al.[187] failed to find any superiority of an AF bed over a foam overlay. Overall there is insufficient evidence to recommend any particular pressure relief surface in the treatment of pressure sores, though given the theoretical advantages of improved pressure relief and moisture control afforded by LAL and AF surfaces, their use is not unreasonable.[153,188]

Spasticity

Spasticity should be addressed not only to improve patient positioning, weight distribution, and hygiene, but also to prevent tension on the healing wound, particularly if surgical intervention is planned.[189,190] Spasticity treatment may be complicated by a reluctance to perform surgery or implant devices in a patient with an open wound, though this has been reported with favorable results.[189] If pump implantation is not an option then temporary chemodenervation should be considered, with delayed pump placement once the wound is healed.[73]

Malnutrition

Malnutrition should be corrected and nutritional markers followed and trended. While many small studies have been published examining the effect on nutritional supplementation of the healing of pressure sores, many suffer from design flaws that limit their application. In 2003 Langer et al.[184] felt the quality of the existing literature was inadequate to perform a meta-analysis and that no firm conclusions could be drawn. More recently both Heyman et al.[191] and Frias Soriano et al.[192] found improved wound healing with oral supplementation, but did not include controls in their studies. Van Anholt et al.[193] and Lee et al.[194] both found accelerated healing with the use of oral nutritional supplement in randomized control trials. There is currently little evidence to support supplementation of micronutrients such as vitamin C or zinc in the absence of a specified deficiency state.[184,195]

Infection

Osteomyelitis is a common complication of deep pressure sores and, as previously mentioned, often mandates operative therapy. Many authors rightly emphasize the importance of adequate debridement in the treatment of osteomyelitis.[196] However, biopsy-directed antibiotic therapy is still an important adjunct to surgery.[79] While traditional therapy calls for 6 weeks of intravenous antibiotic therapy, there is some evidence that shorter courses many be effective.[87]

Wound care

Debridement, regardless of the method used, should be the first step in the care of pressure sores. Only once the wound is thoroughly debrided can the full extent of the wound be examined and staged. Necrotic material impedes wound healing and acts as a nidus for infection. Traditional wet to dry dressing may debride effectively, but may remove healthy tissue and granulation in addition to necrotic tissue.[197] They may also aerosolize bacteria from the wound.[198] Allowing the wound to desiccate despite evidence that wound healing proceeds best in a moist environment is also counterproductive.[199] Enzymatic debridement can be effective, though papain preparations are no longer available in the US. Biological debridement is enjoying something of a resurgence, using maggots that consume necrotic material while sparing living tissue. Currently no evidence suggests superiority of one agent over another.[200] Ultimately, though many complementary methods of debridement are available, they are no substitute for proper sharp debridement.[76]

Selection among the many available dressings must be guided by the characteristics of the wound. Lionelli and Lawrence[200] review the multitude of dressings available. In the context of pressure sores, occlusive films and hydrocolloids are frequently used on more shallow ulcerations while alginates find use in deeper, heavily exudating wounds (**Fig. 16.12**). It is worth noting that, even within a classification, individual products may differ widely in their capacity for absorption, occlusion, permeability, and cohesion.[200] There exists little evidence to recommend a particular dressing in this context. When Bradley et al.[201] performed a meta-analysis of the various dressings and topical agents used for pressure sore treatment, no significant differences were found.

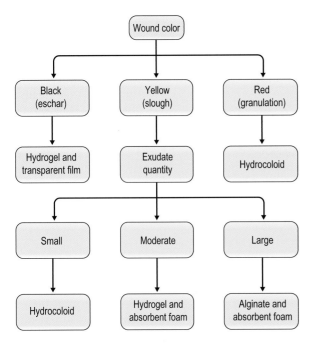

Fig. 16.12 Suggested guidelines for the use of wound products in the full-thickness, noninfected, chronic wound. (Reprinted with permission from Ladin DA. Understanding dressings. Clin Plast Surg 1998;25:433.)

As with dressings, numerous topical agents are used in the hopes of improving wound healing. Antiseptic solutions are commonly used in hopes of reducing the bacterial burden of a wound. However, while mafenide,[202] acetic acid,[203,204] Dakin's solution,[205] and iodine preparations[206] have broad-spectrum antibacterial activity, they have all been shown to kill fibroblasts and impede wound healing.[207] If they are used at all, they should be reserved for instances of active infection. Silver sulfadiazine and other silver agents may be less toxic to fibroblasts.[208,209] A review by Reddy et al.[188] failed to find any convincing data to support a particular dressing or topical agent, which correlates with the results of multiple Cochrane reviews which also failed to identify a superior dressing for arterial ulcers,[210] venous stasis ulcers,[211] or surgical wounds.[212] Ultimately the dressing selection should be guided by the characteristics of the wound and should balance moisture, bacterial control, and debridement.

Negative-pressure wound therapy

Negative-pressure wound therapy (NPWT) entails applying topical negative pressure to a wound. The most common commercially available system, the vacuum-assisted closure (VAC) system, consists of an open-cell polyurethane or polyvinyl alcohol foam sponge with a pore size ranging from 400 to 600 μm in diameter. This sponge is cut to the appropriate dimensions to fill the entire wound. Suction is then applied to the sponge after it is covered with an adhesive drape to create an airtight seal. This suction can be adjusted in intensity and frequency. The most common settings are 125 mmHg negative pressure and either continuous or intermittent frequency.

The NPWT dressing has been applied to a multitude of clinical problems,[213] and its mechanism of action[214] has been extensively studied. Given its success in multiple arenas, pressure sores seem a task to which it is well suited. Evidence for its use is somewhat limited however. Deva et al.[215] noted positive results in treated grade III ulcers but did not utilize any controls. Ford et al.[216] reported improved healing with VAC dressings when compared to standard wound care but results did not reach significance. Joseph[217] noted a greater decrease in wound depth with NPWT dressing when compared to saline dressings, but had limited follow-up and endpoints did not include wound closure. On the other hand, Wanner et al.[218] failed to find any advantage to NPWT therapy in treating pressure sores, a finding echoed in a larger review by Reddy et al.[188] It is perhaps surprising that more evidence does not support the use of NPWT in this clinical scenario, but is unclear whether this is due to inadequate data or a reflection of the altered physiology associated with pressure sores, which at times may render them resilient to closure by secondary intention.

Surgical treatment

Surgical guidelines

The basic tenets of surgical treatment of pressure sores remain essentially unchanged since they were enumerated in Conway and Griffith's report[219] over half a century ago:

- Excision of the ulcer, surrounding scar, underlying bursa, and soft-tissue calcifications, if any
- Radical removal of underlying bone and any heterotopic ossification
- Padding of bone stumps and filling dead space
- Resurfacing with large regional pedicled flaps
- Grafting the donor site of the flap, if necessary.

The authors also stressed two points of flap design that are still applicable today. First, the flap should be designed as large as possible, placing the suture line away from the area of direct pressure. Second, the flap design should not violate adjacent flap territories so as to preserve all options for coverage in the event that breakdown or recurrence dictates further reconstruction.

Debridement

Complete debridement is the crucial first step in the operative treatment of these lesions. Chronic pressure sores will generally have a relatively well-defined bursa in continuity with the base of the ulcer. Application of methylene blue can make dissecting around the margins of the bursa easier. The bursa and any surrounding scarred tissue, calcifications, or heterotopic ossification should be excised completely, leaving only healthy, pliable tissues **(Fig. 16.13)**. The bursa commonly extends much farther than the surface wound would indicate. Taking a small skin margin around the wound and following the contours of the bursa as it undermines adjacent tissues ensures it is entirely excised. After the initial excision the wound base should be palpated to identify any residual areas of woody, scarred tissues which require excision.

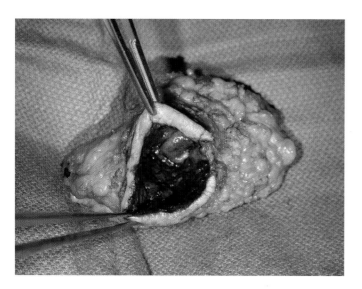

Fig. 16.13 Depiction of excision of bursa and chronic scar tissue.

Once the soft tissue has been debrided, the underlying bone must be evaluated and, if necessary, debrided. There should be a very low threshold to debride back to healthy, hard, bleeding bone using an osteotome or rongeurs. A bone biopsy can also be taken at this time if desired.

Debridement should never be compromised to facilitate wound closure, as incomplete debridement is a common cause of flap failure. The affected tissue must be debrided radically, and flap coverage designed as appropriate to fill the resulting defect, even if this may require larger, or even multiple, flaps for complete obliteration of dead space and wound closure.

Procedure selection

Once the wound has been adequately debrided, a reconstruction method must be selected. Options for surgical coverage of pressure sores include random skin flap, myoplasty plus skin graft, pedicled muscle, myocutaneous, fascial, or fasciocutaneous flap, free flaps, and tissue expansion. The choice of flap depends on many factors, including location of the ulcer, the patient's level of spinal injury, history of prior ulceration and surgery, ambulatory status and potential, daily habits, educational status, motivational level, and associated medical problems.

Muscle flaps

The indications for using muscle in pressure sore surgery remain poorly defined. As previously noted, muscle is more susceptible to ischemic necrosis than either skin or subcutaneous tissue,[35] at times resulting in necrotic muscle under intact overlying skin.[220] On the other hand, interposing muscle between skin and bone resulted in a decreased rate of skin ulceration in a rat model,[38] presumably because the increased mass of muscle can help diffuse the effects of pressure on the skin.

Compared with skin grafts and flaps, muscle flaps have the advantages of greater bulk for filling the wound cavity and obliterating dead space,[219] the ability to cover larger wounds, and a better local vascular supply.[221,222] Despite their theoretical advantages, whether the improved vascularity of muscle flaps results in clinically significant effects on infection and wound healing when compared to other options has not been determined.[223]

Anthony and associates[224] reviewed their experience with pressure sore therapy in 60 consecutive patients treated between 1979 and 1990, during which time their practice transitioned toward an increased use of muscle and musculocutaneous flaps. During this interval the number of operations per ulcer declined from 1.9 to 1.1 and the time to complete healing dropped from 12.8 to 4.8 weeks. Though they recognize that advances in supportive care certainly have played a role, the authors conclude that widespread use of muscle flaps, which allow debridement and wound closure at a single operation, is the single most important factor contributing to the improved outcome.

Musculocutaneous flaps

Bruck et al.[225] raised random skin flaps and latissimus dorsi musculocutaneous flaps in pigs, which were then transferred for coverage of iatrogenically created pelvic pressure sores. The wounds were subsequently inoculated with *Staphylococcus aureus* and *Escherichia coli*, and the flaps evaluated for their resistance to infection-induced necrosis. Only the skin flaps showed necrosis, leading the authors to conclude that the muscle acts as a barrier for vertical spread of infection and strongly recommend their use in patients with a history of osteomyelitis.

Perforator flaps

In a break from previous literature to that point, Kroll and Rosenfield[226] challenged the assumption that muscle is necessary when reconstructing pressure sores. In 1988 they reported favorable results using fasciocutaneous flaps based on parasacral perforators to cover midline and sacral wounds. Koshima et al.[227] developed the superior gluteal artery perforator flap, which they used to cover trochanteric and ischial pressure sores with good results.

Advocates of perforator flap techniques argue that such flaps not only preserve muscle, but also conserve future reconstructive options and adhere to the basic tenet of placing suture lines away from areas of direct pressure. Higgins et al.[228] state that, until further studies are performed, "muscle sparing should always be a goal in the ambulatory and sensate patient, as it may prevent some functional loss and potentially reduce postoperative pain."

Free flaps

Though not a common option, several authors have described free tissue transfer in the reconstruction of pressure sores, with and without preservation of sensation. Nahai et al.[229,230] and Hill et al.,[231,232] among others, have described transferring the tensor fasciae latae muscle–skin unit as a free flap for lower trunk reconstruction. Sensation is maintained by including the lateral femoral cutaneous nerve in the neurovascular pedicle.

Chen et al.[233] reported coverage of multiple extensive pressure sores with a single filleted lower leg musculocutaneous free flap, with satisfactory results. Yamamoto et al.[234] report successful coverage of a sacral pressure sore with a free lateral thigh fasciocutaneous flap based on the first and third direct cutaneous branches of the deep femoral vessels. A second successful reconstruction involved an ischial pressure sore covered with a free medial plantar fasciocutaneous flap based on the posterior tibial vessels.

Sekiguchi et al.[235] confirm the value of free sensory plantar flaps in the treatment of paraplegic patients who have ischial ulcers. They reason that "while the ischial region is being subject to enormous pressure, the plantar region with its more resilient skin pad is no longer functioning as a weight-bearing area. Thus [transferring] a plantar flap on to the ischial region … offers a long-term solution to the problem of chronic pressure sores."

Tissue expansion

Expanders are tolerated very well in SCI patients. According to Esposito et al.,[236] the main advantage of tissue expansion is the advancement of sensitive skin that can be used for pressure awareness and future ulcer prevention. Tissue expansion is also useful in the event of an unstable wound secondary to previous skin graft or secondary healing. Multiple reports by Braddom and Leadbetter,[237] Yuan,[238] Esposito et al.,[236] Neves et al.,[239] and Kostakoglu et al.[240] attest to the success of tissue expansion in the treatment of recalcitrant ulcers in paraplegics.

Kostakoglu et al.[240] also described pre-expansion of tensor fasciae latae and lumbosacral fasciocutaneous flaps in 6 patients. The authors felt expansion allowed the closure of large wounds while still allowing for primary closure of the donor site, while speculating that "additional benefits may include a reduction in the mechanical shear potential for these flaps and an improvement in their vascularity."

Critics question the wisdom of placing a foreign body (the expander) into a contaminated wound (all pressure sores). At this time, the primary indication for skin expansion is to cover shallow ulcers with no dead space to fill, particularly if sensate skin can be used to resurface a previously insensate area.

Single- versus multiple-stage reconstruction

Several reports in the literature describe single-stage surgical management of pressure sores.[241,242] Most of these reports involved few patients, however, until a retrospective analysis of 120 patients operated on during a 10-year period was published in 1999.[243] Although there was a large discrepancy between the number of patients treated in a single stage versus the number treated in multiple stages (120 versus 10), the hospital stay was decreased by an average of 10 weeks in the single-stage group – 9.5 weeks versus 19 weeks. This led to a considerable cost savings per admission. The authors list the disadvantages of single-stage surgical management as longer operative time and higher intraoperative blood loss. The advantages of single-stage pressure sore management include fewer anesthetic episodes, shorter hospital stays, earlier rehabilitation, and lower costs. The authors reserve multistage procedures for patients who have concurrent pressure sores on the anterior and posterior trunk that are difficult to address simultaneously.

Reconstruction by anatomic site

Many of the published descriptions of musculocutaneous flaps offer considerable flexibility in flap design to allow subsequent rerotation of the cutaneous component. In most cases this involves expanding and reshaping the skin margins towards a more rotational flap design and away from the limitations imposed by transposition and island flaps.

A number of techniques are available for closure of sacral pressure sores, including wide undermining and primary closure, random skin flaps, gluteus myoplasty, advancement flaps, pedicle island flaps, fasciocutaneous flaps, musculocutaneous flaps, and free flaps [219,226,227,244–267] (Table 16.2). Though dozens of variations have been described, musculocutaneous rotation and advancement flaps based on the gluteus maximus remain a proven option in this area.

Parry and Mathes[259] reported favorable results after sacral coverage of pressure sores with bilateral gluteus maximus musculocutaneous advancement flaps in ambulatory patients. Foster et al.[268] had high success rates with V-Y gluteus maximus flaps (36/37 or 97%) as well as with gluteal island flaps (20/22 or 91%). When the patient is ambulatory the authors recommend closure by means of bilateral V-Y gluteus maximus advancement flaps based on the superior half of the gluteus muscle to preserve muscular function.

Borman and Maral[244] describe a modification of the gluteal rotation flap, incorporating a V-Y closure, allowing closure of defects up to 12 cm with a unilateral flap. The suggested advantages include a smaller incision compared to a class V-Y advancement and the ability to convert to a musculocutaneous V-Y advancement if necessary. Though quite hardy in thinner patients, it can be unreliable in obese patients with abundant presacral subcutaneous tissue. Additional modifications include the expansive gluteus maximus flap described by Ramirez and colleagues,[260] which is advanced in a V-Y fashion either unilaterally or bilaterally to cover sacral ulcers.

Multiple authors have reported their success with gluteal artery perforator flaps, and variations abound.[269–271] Wong et al.[272] modified the classic gluteal rotation flap to spare the perforators down to the level of the piriformis. Xu et al.[273] designed a multi-island perforator propeller flap for use in large sacral defects. Cheong et al.[274] described an innervated variant of the superior gluteal artery perforator flap for sacral coverage.

Moving superiorly, both Hill et al.[252] and Vyas et al.[263] described random flaps from the thoracolumbar area to close sacral wounds. Hill et al.[252] described the transverse lumbosacral back flap, which is based on the contralateral lumbar perforators. The donor site is most commonly skin-grafted. Vyas et al.[263] described the thoracolumbar sacral flap, which is a very large rotational flap based on thoracolumbar perforators, which may or may not require back grafting.

Kroll and Rosenfield[226] and Koshima et al.[227] described perforator-based flaps from the parasacral area for coverage of low posterior midline defects. Kato et al.[256] took this concept a step further in their anatomical study on the lumbar artery perforator-based island flap, identifying the second lumbar perforator as the preferred vessel. Advantages of this flap include sparing of the muscle, a large arc of rotation, and a donor site that can be closed primarily.

Unless the skin flaps have been reinnervated at a preliminary operation or are harvested from a site that has intact sensation,[275] the reconstructed sites will not be sensible. The advantage of using sensory flaps for pressure sore coverage in patients with distal SCI is the hope that sensation will prompt behavior modifications by the patient to

Table 16.2 **Reconstructive options in sacral pressure ulcers**

Primary closure
  White and Hamm, *Ann Surg 124:1136, 1946*
	Gluteal fasciocutaneous rotation-advancement flap with V-Y closure
	  Burman and Maral, *Plast Reconstr Surg 109: 23, 2002*

Reverse dermal graft
  Wesser and Kahn, *Plast Reconstr Surg 40:252, 1967*
	Bilateral gluteus advancement flap
	  Parry and Mathes, *Ann Plast Surg 8:443, 1982*

Interiorly based random skin flap
  Conway and Griffith, *Am J Surg 91–946, 1956*
	Gluteus plication closure
	  Buchanan and Agris, *Plast Reconstr Surg 72:49, 1983*

Tranverse lumbosacral arterial and random flap
  Hill, Brown, and Jurkiewicz, *Plast Reconstr Surg 62: 177, 1978*
	Sensory island flaps
	  Synder and Edgerton, *Plast Reconstr Surg 36: 518, 1965*
	  Dibbell, *Plast Reconstr Surg 54: 220, 1974*
	  Daniel, Terzis, and Cunningham, *Plast Reconstr Surg, 58: 317, 1976*
	  Little, Fontana, and McColluch, *Plast Reconstr Surg 68: 175, 1981*

Thoracocolumbar-sacral arterial/random flap
  Vyas, Binns, and Wilson, *Plast Reconstr Surg 65:159, 1980*
	Gluteal thigh arterialized flap
	  Hurwitz, Swartz, and Mathes, *Plast Reconstr Surg, 68: 521, 1981*

Superior gluteus myoplasty
  Ger, *Surgery 69:106, 1971*
  Ger and Levine, *Plast Reconstr Surg 58: 419, 1976*
	Expansive gluteus maximus flap
	  Ramirez, Hurwitz, and Futrell, *Plast Reconstr Surg 74: 757, 1984*

Turnover gluteus myopathy
  Stallings, Delgado, and Converse, *Plast Reconstr Surg 54:52, 1974*
	Parasacral perforator-based musculocutaneous flap
	  Kroll and Rosenfield, *Plast Reconstr Surg 81:561, 1988*
	  Koshima et al., *Plast Reconstr Surg, 91:678, 1993*

Gluteus maximus musculocutaneous flap
  Minami, Mills, and Pardoe, *Plast Reconstr Surg 60: 242, 1977*
	Parasacral peforator-based fasciocutaneous flap
	  Kato et al., *Br J Plast Surg 52: 541, 1999*

Gluteus maximus musculocutaneous island flap
  Muruyama et al., *Br J Plast Surg 33:150, 1980*
  Stevenson et al., *Plast Reconstr Surg 79: 761, 1987*
  Dimberger, *Plast Reconstr Surg 81:567, 1988*
	Parasacral peforator-based fasciocutaneous flap
	  Kato et al., *Br J Plast Surg 52: 541, 1999*

Gluteus maximus fasciocutaneous flap Yamamoto et al., *Ann Plast Surg 30:116, 1993*	

(Reproduced from Janis JE, Kenkel JM. Pressure sores. In: Barton FE Jr. (ed.) Selected readings in plastic surgery, vol. 9, no. 39. Dallas, TX: Selected Readings in Plastic Surgery, 2003, p. 25.)

avoid pressure on ulcer-prone areas and prevent recurrent ulceration. Dibbell[248] and Daniel *et al.*[246] describe intercostal island flaps to bring sensation to the sacral area. Other reports by Coleman and Jurkiewicz[276] and Mackinnon *et al.*[277] discuss various techniques for reinnervation of the intercostal flap and the tensor fasciae latae flap, including nerve grafts to the intercostal muscles and to the territory of the lateral femoral cutaneous nerve.

Prado *et al.*[278] also described an innervation-sparing bilateral perforator fasciocutaneous and myocutaneous V-Y flaps for the closure of large sacral wounds. Though they demonstrated no recurrence at 1.5 years and sensation was preserved with this technique, it has the drawbacks of placing scars over the ischium as well as preventing further readvancement of the gluteal muscles.

DeWeerd and Weum[247] modified Kato's lumbar perforator island flap design to include two lumbar artery perforators as well as the intermediate nerve to preserve protective sensation. The flap is drawn as a butterfly design. At 8 weeks postoperatively, good protective sensation was documented over most of the flap by Semmes–Weinstein monofilament testing.

Selected technique: myocutaneous gluteal rotation flap (*Fig. 16.14 and Box 16.2*)

One of many options based on the gluteus maximus muscle, the myocutaneous gluteal rotation flap is technically straightforward, keeps scars off pressure-bearing surfaces, and is easily revised or re-rotated. The muscle is useful for obliterating the dead space which is often significant after the preparatory bursectomy and ostectomy.

The vascular supply is based on the superior gluteal artery perforator. This vessel can easily be identified in the plane beneath the gluteus maximus immediately superior to the piriformis muscle.

Skin incision is marked to follow the contour of the iliac crest and descends inferiorly, staying posterior to the greater trochanter and the footprint of the tensor fasciae latae flaps. Dissection is carried down through the thick subcutaneous tissues of the hip to the level of the muscle fascia.

The fascia and muscle are then divided. It can be helpful to bevel the incision so the muscle and fascia are divided more peripherally than the skin. This both accounts for some degree

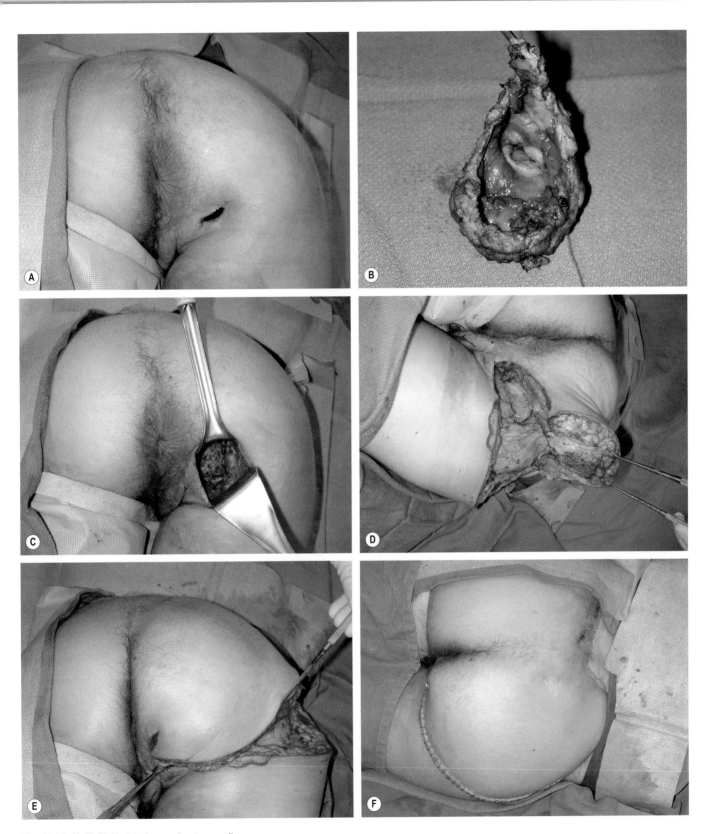

Fig. 16.14 (A–F) Right gluteal musculocutaneous flap.

of muscle retraction and provides extra soft tissue to obliterate dead space and additional fascia for added security and ease of wound closure. The flap should then be undermined in the plane beneath the gluteus maximus. The pedicle can usually be identified at this time with relative ease as it passes superior to the piriformis. It may be easier to proceed from lateral to medial, as scarring and inflammation near the ulcer can impede dissection, and the separation between the hip muscles becomes more distinct as they approach their insertion on the trochanter.

If additional length is needed or tension is excessive, the flap can be partially delaminated at either the fascial or subcutaneous level, so long as the major perforators are identified and protected. The flap is then closed in multiple layers over drains using long-lasting absorbable sutures in the muscle and superficial fascial system and either staples or nonabsorbable sutures in the skin.

Box 16.2 Myocutaneous gluteal rotation flap

As always, complete debridement is the key to any flap surgery.

This flap can survive entirely on its major vascular pedicle. The muscle can be disinserted and the skin and fascia divided circumferentially without compromising the vascularity of the flap. Creating an island design without tension is preferable to leaving a skin bridge which results in tension.

Drains remain in place until output is less than 20–30 cc/day, though some may opt to use drains for an extended period.

Ischial ulcers

Multiple techniques have been described to cover these defects, including inferior gluteal rotation flaps, island flaps, posterior V-Y advancement flaps, gluteal thigh flaps, perforator flaps, and free flaps[253,260,268,279–290] **(Table 16.3)**.

One of the most common options in ischial pressure sore coverage is the posterior V-Y advancement flap. This flap can be based on the biceps femoris muscle in ambulatory patients or on the hamstring muscle in SCI patients. This flap is able to fill the dead space with viable muscle and can be readvanced quite easily in the case of recurrence.

Some authors, however, prefer fasciocutaneous flaps over musculocutaneous flaps in this region.[291–293] Homma et al.[291] reported using a posteromedial thigh fasciocutaneous flap based on the perforators from either the gracilis or the adductor magnus muscles in the treatment of ischial pressure sores. In 11 patients with variable follow-up, they noted two flaps with distal necrosis.

The posterior thigh skin can be transferred based on perforating vessels from a cutaneous branch of the inferior gluteal artery that accompanies the posterior femoral cutaneous nerve between the semitendinosus and biceps femoris muscles.[226,281,288] The flap can be used repeatedly in the event of recurrences. When the descending branch of the infe-

---

Table 16.3 Reconstructive options in ischial pressure sores

Primary closure Arregui et al., *Plast Reconstr Surg 36: 583, 1965*	Biceps femoris musculocutaneous flap Tobias et al., *Ann Plast Surg 6: 396, 1981* Kauer and Sonsino, *Scand J Plast Reconstr Surg 20: 129, 1986*
Random posterior thigh flap ± biceps femoris myoplasty Campbell and Converse, *Plast Reconstr Surg, 14: 442, 1954* Conway and Griffith, *Am J Surg 91: 946, 1956* Baker, Barton, and Converse, *Br J Plast Surg 31: 26, 1978*	Gluteal thigh flap Hurwitz, Swartz, and Mathes, *Plast Reconstr Surg 20: 129, 1986*
Inferior gluteus maximus musculoplasty Ger and Levine, *Plast Reconstr Surg 58:419, 1976*	Sliding gluteus maximus flap Ramirez, Hurwitz, and Futrell, *Plast Reconstr Surg 74: 757, 1984*
Inferior gluteus musculocutaneous flap Minami, Mills, and Pardoe, *Plast Reconstr Surg 60: 242, 1977*	Tensor fasciae latae + vastus lateralis Krupp, Kuhn, and Zaech, *Paraplegia 21: 119, 1983*
Interior gluteus musculocutaneous island flap Rajacic et al., *Br J Plast Surg 47:431, 1994*	Lateral thigh fasciocutaneous flap Maruyama, Ohnishi, and Takeudhi, *Br J Plast Surg 37: 103, 1984* Hallock, *Ann Plast Surg 32: 367, 1994*
Gracilis musculocutaneous flap Wingate and Friedland, *Plast Reconstr Surg 62:245, 1978* Lesavoy et al., *Plast Reconstr Surg, 85: 390, 1990*	Anterolateral thigh fasciocutanous island flap Yu et al., *Plast Reconstr Surg 109: 610, 2002*
Gracilis musculocutaneous flap (with sartorius as a double muscle unit) Apfelberg and Finseth, *Br J Plast Surg 34:41, 1981*	Rectus abdominis musculocutaneous flap Bunkis and Fudem, *Ann Plast Surg 23: 447, 1989* Mixter, Wood and Dibbell, *Plast Reconstr Surg 85: 437, 1990*
Hamstring musculocutaneous flap Hurteau et al., *Plast Reconstr Surg 68: 539, 1981*	Inferior gluteal artery perforator flap Higgins et al., *Br J Plast Surg 55:83, 2002*

(Reproduced from Janis JE, Kenkel JM. Pressure sores. In: Barton FE Jr. (ed.) Selected readings in plastic surgery, vol. 9, no. 39. Dallas, TX: Selected Readings in Plastic Surgery, 2003, p. 27.)

rior gluteal artery is absent – a common vascular anomaly in this region[253] – the flap can be elevated as a superiorly based random fasciocutaneous unit supplied by multiple perforators from the cruciate anastomosis of the fascial plexus.[294]

In addition to the gluteal rotation flap, the superior and inferior gluteal arteries provide multiple options for reconstruction for ischial ulcers. The pedicle of the superior gluteal artery perforator flap is suboptimal for reaching the ischial region, and is more useful in the coverage of sacral and trochanteric ulcers. The inferior gluteal artery perforator flap, on the other hand, is well suited to ischial reconstruction, with multiple authors reporting results comparable to existing methods.[228,295,296] It has the advantage of sparing muscle for future use, is associated with minimal morbidity, and has a donor site that can often be closed directly.[290]

Alternatives for coverage of ischial pressure sores include gracilis musculocutaneous flaps,[297–300] lateral thigh fasciocutaneous flaps,[294,301] anterolateral thigh fasciocutaneous island flaps,[289,302,303] and rectus abdominis musculocutaneous flaps transferred through the space of Retzius to the perineum.[304–306] However, because the rectus initiates vertebral flexion and aids in respiration, urination, defecation, and vomiting, Bunkis and Fudem[304] speculate the muscle is more important, and thus less expendable, in paraplegics than in neuromuscularly intact patients.

Nahai et al.[229,232,307] introduced the sensate tensor fasciae latae flap for coverage of ischial and trochanteric pressure sores. The flap provides protective sensation in paraplegic patients to help avert recurrence of pressure sores, sharpens sensation of rectal filling, and enhances sitting control in a wheelchair. Dibbell et al.[308] as well as Luscher et al.[309] report successful experiences with the extended sensory tensor fasciae latae flap, which is innervated by the lateral femoral cutaneous nerve, for pressure sores in patients with meningomyelocele and paraplegia respectively. At follow-up of 1–10 years no new or recurrent sores were noted in Luscher's series.

Foster et al.[268] reviewed their experience with ischial pressure sore coverage from 1979 to 1995. During this time, 114 consecutive patients with 139 ischial pressures sores were treated. Analysis of these cases showed significant differences in healing rates and complications according to the flaps used. The inferior gluteus maximus island flap and the inferior gluteal thigh flap had the highest success rate, 94% (32/34) and 93% (25/27) respectively, while the V-Y hamstring flap and tensor fasciae latae flap had the poorest healing rates, 58% (7/12) and 50% (6/12) respectively. When Ahluwalia et al.[310] reviewed their series of 72 ischial wounds, the authors found an overall complication rate of 16% and a recurrence rate of 7%. After reviewing their results the authors felt their best results were obtained with medial thigh and biceps femoris flaps.

Selected flap: V-Y hamstring advancement *(Fig. 16.15)*

Flaps from the posterior thigh are common options for ischial reconstruction. They have the advantage of leaving the lateral hip and buttock for use in trochanteric and sacral reconstruction. The V-Y hamstring advancement is a robust flap that is relatively easy to raise and can be readvanced in necessary.

The vascular supply to the hamstring flap is based on perforators of the profunda femoris, with minor contributions from the inferior gluteal, medial circumflex, and superior geniculate arteries. These vessels are generally not specifically identified when elevating the flap, as they are well protected on the deep surface of the muscle.

Superiorly the flap is bounded by the gluteal crease or the inferior border of the ulcer. Laterally the flap extends to the posterior border of the tensor fasciae latae, while medially the dissection extends to the adductor magnus. Inferiorly the flap can be extended to the popliteal fossa, though a lesser flap can be designed as needed.

The flap is incised and dissection carried down the level of the fascia. The muscles are divided distally at the musculotendinous junction and proximally by elevating the muscles from the ischium, though this step is often partially accomplished during bony debridement of the ischium. Minimal blunt dissection may be performed at the lateral and medial margins to mobilize the flap but it is generally not necessary to perform a complete dissection on the undersurface of the muscle or to identify the major pedicle of the flap.

As with the gluteal rotation flap, it is inset in layers over drains and the donor site is closed in linear fashion.

Trochanteric ulcers

Trochanteric ulcers are generally closed with tensor fasciae latae[229,232,307–309,311–314] or vastus lateralis flaps[315–318] *(Table 16.4)*. The tensor fasciae latae can be transferred as muscle only, as skin and muscle, with the skin of the anterolateral mid and lower thigh, as an island flap, or as a free flap. For details regarding this flap's anatomy, vascularity, design, and elevation, the reader is referred to Nahai's publications on the subject.[229,232,308] Lewis et al.[312,319] described a modification of the standard tensor fasciae latae musculocutaneous flap, the tensor fasciae latae V-Y reposition: this appears to be as durable and versatile as its predecessor.

While the tensor fasciae latae is a workhorse option in this region, multiple alternative and secondary options exist. Flaps based on the gluteus maximus[320–322] or medius[323] can be used to reconstruct this region. Ramirez[320] recounts his experience with 20 distal gluteus maximus posterior thigh flaps.

A profusion of perforator flaps have found use in trochanteric reconstruction as well. The anterolateral thigh flap provides an option with considerable flexibility, allowing the option of taking chimeric flaps if necessary.[324,325] Flaps based on the gluteal,[326] ascending circumflex,[327] adductor[328] perforators all share the advantages of minimal donor morbidity and sparing of muscle for further reconstruction. The adductor perforator flap also has the advantage of being medially based and often outside the field of previous operations.

Foster et al.[268] noted a success rate of 93% (68/73) when covering trochanteric ulcers. Their most frequently used flap was the tensor fasciae latae flap, particularly in the V-Y design. Complications occurred in 15%, the most common being wound dehiscence.

If more radical treatment of the trochanter is required, e.g., a Girdlestone procedure, then the vastus lateralis becomes the flap of choice, either as a muscle or musculocutaneous flap[329–331] *(Fig. 16.16)*.

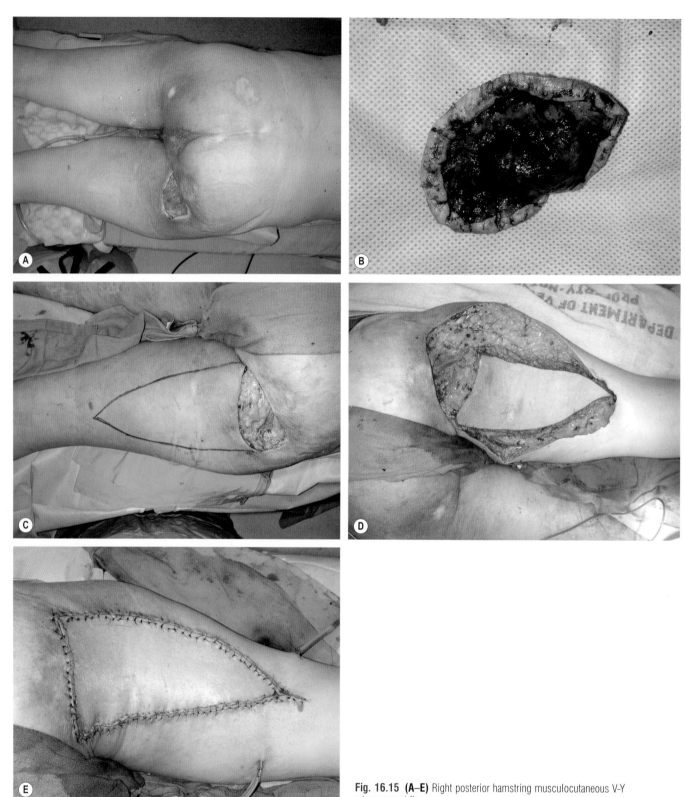

Fig. 16.15 (A–E) Right posterior hamstring musculocutaneous V-Y advancement flap.

Table 16.4 Reconstructive options in trochanteric pressure ulcers

Anteriorly based random thigh flap Vasconez, Schneider, and Jurkewicz, *Curr Probl Surg 14:1, 1977*	Tensor fasciae latae musculocutaneous flap, island Kauer and Sonsino, *Scand J Plast Reconstr Surg 20: 129, 1986*
Random bipedicle flap Conway and Griffith, *Am J Surg 91: 946, 1956*	Vastus lateralis myoplasty Minami, Hentz, and Vistnes, *Plast Reconstr Surg 60:364, 1977* Dowden and McCraw, *Ann Plast Surg 4: 396, 1980*
Tensor fasciae latae musculocutaneous flap Nahai et al., *Ann Plast Surg 1: 372, 1978* Hill, Nahai, and Vasconez, *Plast Reconstr Surg 61: 517, 1978* Withers et al., *Ann Plast Surg 4:31, 1980*	Vastus lateralis musculocutaneous flap Bovet et al., *Plast Reconstr Surg 69: 830, 1982* Hauben et al., Ann Plast Surg 10: 359, 1983 Drimmer and Krasna, Plast Reconstr Surg79:560, 1987
Tensor fasciae latae musculocutaneous flap, bipedicle Schulman, *Plast Reconstr Surg 66: 740, 1980*	Gluteus medius tensor fasciae latae musculocutaneous flap Little and Lyons, *Plast Reconstr Surg 71: 366, 1983*
Tensor fasciae latae musculocutaneous flap, V-Y advancement Lewis, Cunningham, and Hugo, *Ann Plast Surg 6:34, 1981* Siddiqui, Wiedrich, and Lewis, *Ann Plast Surg, 31: 313, 1993*	Distally based gluteus maximus flap Becker, *Plast Reconstr Surg 63: 653, 1979*
Tensor fasciae latae musculocutaneous flap, innervated Dibbell, McCraw, and Edstrom, *Plast Reconstr Surg, 64:796, 1979* Nahai, Hill, and Hester, Plast Reconstr Surg 7: 286, 1981 Nahai, Clin Plast Surg 7: 51, 1980 Cochran, Edstrom, and Dibbell, Ann Plast Surg 7: 286, 1981	Gluteal thigh flap Hurwitz, Swartz, and Mathes, *Plast Reconstr Surg 68:521, 1981*
	Expansive gluteus maximus flap Ramirez, Hurwitz, and Futrell, *Plast Reconstr Surg 74: 757, 1984* Ramirez, Ann Plast Surg 18:295, 1987

(Reproduced from Janis JE, Kenkel JM. Pressure sores. In: Barton FE Jr. (ed.) Selected readings in plastic surgery, vol. 9, no. 39. Dallas, TX: Selected Readings in Plastic Surgery, 2003, p. 29.)

Selected procedure: V-Y tensor fasciae latae flap *(Fig. 16.17)*; tensor fasciae latae rotation flap

The many variations on the tensor fasciae latae flap are common options for dealing with trochanteric ulcers. A fasciocutaneous or musculocutaneous rotation flap is technically straightforward, can reach a variety of defects, and may be readvanced if necessary.

The blood supply to the tensor fasciae latae is from branches of the lateral circumflex femoral artery, which enter the deep surface of the muscle anteriorly. The proximal, muscular portion of the tensor fasciae latae is relatively small. The distal portion of the muscle consists almost entirely of fascia, but still provides perforators to the overlying skin. If necessary, the flap can be extended just proximal to the knee and rotated to cover ischial or even sacral defects, though such extended flaps are not entirely reliable unless delayed. A much more limited dissection is possible when addressing trochanteric ulcers.

Though the blood supply to this flap is robust and relatively reliable, minor variations are common. If necessary, the flap may be based on alternate branches of the circumflex vessels. If the perforators to the muscle are not usable, dissection of the descending branch of the lateral circumflex allows relatively simple conversion to a pedicled anterolateral thigh flap.

The ulcer will generally define the posterior margin of the flap. A line from the anterior superior iliac spine to the knee marks the anterior border of the flap. Flaps up to 15–20 cm proximal to the femoral condyle are very reliable without

delay. The inferior point of the flap can be taken just short of the condyle if preferred. Though it may be excessive for single-stage ulcer coverage, a lengthier flap is easier to readvance if necessary. The pedicle is generally roughly 10 cm inferior to the anterior superior iliac spine and 10–15 cm lateral to the pubic tubercle.

After incising the skin down to fascia, dissection is easiest distally, where the tensor fasciae latae is essentially entirely fascia. Dissecting under the fascia, it is generally easy to identify the pedicle as the tensor fasciae latae transitions to muscle proximally. The fascia and muscle can then be completely divided and the flap rotated to fill the defect. As with the other flaps discussed in this section, the flap is then inset in layers over drains and the donor site closed in linear fashion.

Bone resection

Kostrubala and Greeley[26] first suggested removing the underlying bony prominences as an adjunct to the treatment of patients with pressure sores. The authors initially recommended excision of the posterior sacral promontories and greater trochanters when these areas were exposed, and subsequently expanded the resection to encompass the entire ischium. Conway and Griffith[219] noted a decrease in recurrence from 38% after partial ischiectomy to 3% after total ischiectomy.

Although total ischiectomy minimizes ipsilateral recurrence, secondary problems are frequent. Arregui et al.[332] evaluated 94 patients with pressure sores treated by total

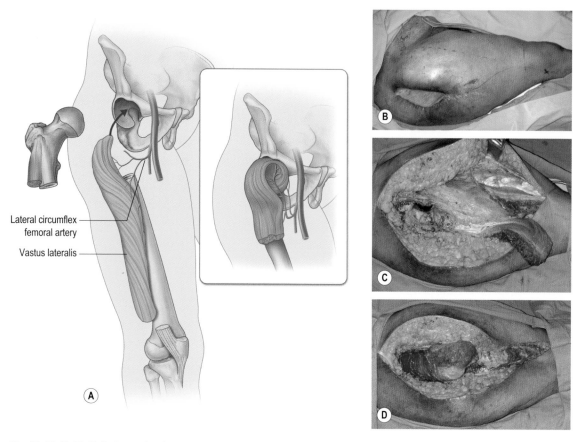

Lateral circumflex
femoral artery

Vastus lateralis

Fig. 16.16 (A–D) Girdlestone arthroplasty.

ischiectomy over a 10-year period. Despite "good" results in 81%, there was a 16% complication rate and a 28% occurrence of contralateral ischial ulcer. The authors subsequently recommended contralateral ischial resection on a prophylactic basis.

After total bilateral ischiectomy, however, weight is transferred to the pubic rami and perineum as well as the proximal femur. When sitting, pressure is borne directly by the membranous and proximal bulbous urethra.[333] Perineal ulcers, urethrocutaneous fistulas,[334] and perineourethral diverticula[28] have been reported in up to 58% of patients after complete bilateral ischiectomy. Given the high incidence of serious complications, total ischiectomy should be reserved for deep, extensive, recurrent ischial pressure sores.

Proximal femoral resection with muscle flap coverage may be indicated in instances of large and/or recalcitrant trochanteric ulcers complicated by osteomyelitis and ulcers involving the hip joint.[330] Patients who undergo proximal femoral resection may experience a piston effect that prevents

the obliteration of dead space. Klein *et al.*[331] addressed the issue through the use of an external fixator for 2–3 weeks, and reported all 10 of their patients' wounds healed, despite a 50% incidence of pin loosening. Rubayi *et al.*[335] prefer to use an abduction pillow and antispasmodic drugs to control femoral motion. A total of 24 of 26 wounds healed in the hospital, and all wounds healed eventually.

Patients with proven osteomyelitis in the bone underlying their pressure sore should be treated with at least partial ostectomy. Although in principle osteomyelitis should be treated by radical excision,[196,336] the end-point of all bony debridement should be healthy bleeding bone,[76] and osteopenia in paraplegics may cloud this goal. In these cases, preoperative imaging may be helpful in determining the extent of bony involvement. The identified areas can then be resected down to bleeding, healthy-appearing bone and cultures taken from the depths of the wound. Postoperative antibiotic therapy should be guided by the results of deep bone cultures and biopsies.[337]

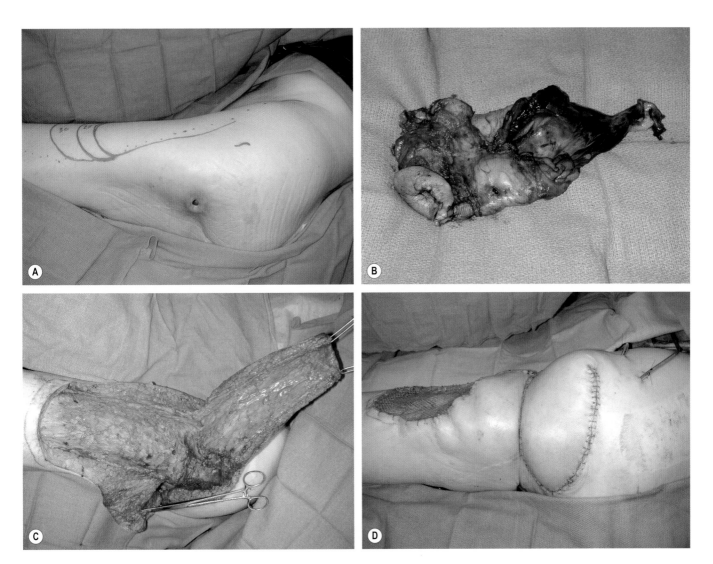

Fig. 16.17 (A–D) Left tensor fasciae latae flap with backgrafting.

Postoperative care

The care of patients after pressure sore surgery has been reviewed by multiple authors, including Vasconez et al.,[338] Conway and Griffith,[219] Stal et al.,[339] Hentz,[340] Constantian,[341] and Disa et al.[342] The measures used to address pressure relief, shear, friction, moisture, skin care, incontinence, spasticity, and nutrition should be continued aggressively through the postoperative period, in addition to standard postoperative care. Two additional issues that need to be addressed prior to discharge are length of immobilization and when to restart sitting protocols and therapy.

Traditionally pressure sore patients were kept in bed for 6–8 weeks based on experimental data indicating that wounds reached maximum tensile strength after this period.[343] More recent studies have advocated a more rapid progression to sitting. In a prospective, randomized trial Isik et al.[344] found equivalent complication rates when comparing 2 and 3 weeks of immobilization, though overall length of stay was similar and long-term follow-up was deemed inadequate to draw any firm conclusions. Likewise, Foster et al.[268] began a sitting regimen at 10–14 days and had postoperative hospital stays averaging 20 days, with short-term success rates of 89%.

Regardless of how long patients are kept in bed, they should begin active and passive range-of-motion exercises of the uninvolved extremity early in the postoperative course,[178] while the affected extremity can be ranged just prior to initiation of a sitting protocol. A typical regimen involves having the patient sit for 15-minute intervals once or twice a day, then gradually increasing the length and frequency of sitting periods until discharge.[344] Pressure release maneuvers are performed at least every 15 minutes while the patient is seated, and the surgical site is carefully monitored for signs of recurrence.[178]

Prior to discharge, patients should have their support surfaces re-evaluated *(Fig. 16.18)*. This assessment is particularly important in patients who have had bony resections or multiple procedures that may result in altered weight-bearing or pelvic and truncal instability.[345] An appropriate seat cushion should be selected, ideally with the assistance of seat mapping. Maximum recommended pressures are 35 mmHg for patients unable to relieve pressure themselves by lifting or leaning and 60 mmHg for those who can.[346]

Patient education should also be emphasized postoperatively. Though studies have demonstrated a positive effect of education on patient knowledge,[347,348] research relating education to recurrence rates is lacking at this time. However, given the evidence that recurrence rates are associated with poor patient compliance, social factors, and communication barriers,[178,349] attempts at addressing these issues through education seem reasonable.

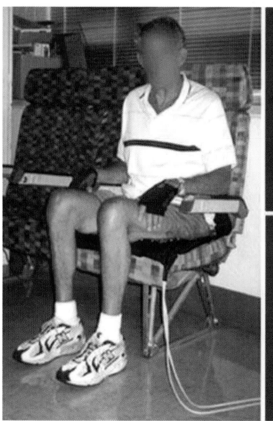
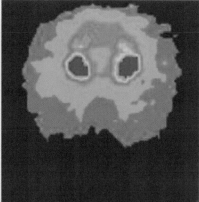
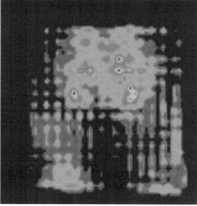

Fig. 16.18 Seat mapping. (Reproduced from the University of Washington PM&R website: http://sci.washington.edu/info/forums/reports/pressure.)

Outcomes, prognosis, and complications

Long-term outcome studies of patients with pressure sores are difficult to conduct and the existing literature reports a wide variation in recurrence rates, ranging from as low as 3–6%[279,340,350] to as high as 33–100%.[280,292,342,351]

The most extensive published experiences with pressure sore treatment are those of Conway and Griffith[219] (1000 cases) and Dansereau and Conway's[16] update of the Bronx Veterans Administration Hospital data (2000 cases). In their follow-up article from 1961, Griffith and Schultz[352] categorized the therapeutic history of the earlier series as follows:

- Sacral ulcers: Nonsurgical treatment succeeded in 29%, split-skin grafts in 30%. Excision of bone with the ulcer and closure by large rotation flap achieved healing in 84%.
- Trochanteric ulcers: 41% of patients were adequately treated without surgery; 33% needed split-thickness skin grafts. When ulcer, bursa, and trochanter were excised and the wound simply sutured, 83% healed but 20% recurred. When the trochanter was more thoroughly removed and the site reconstructed with a rotation flap, 92% healed and only 6% recurred.
- Ischial ulcers: Conservative therapy was successful in 18% of cases, skin graft in 17%, and partial ischiectomy with primary suture in 46% (but with 54% recurrence). Total ischiectomy lessened the number of recurrences to 22%, and when combined with muscle flap and regional rotation flap it further decreased the recurrence rate to 3%.

In 1994 Evans et al.[353] reviewed their experience with the surgical treatment of pressure sores in both paraplegic and non-paraplegic patients. Among paraplegics the recurrence rate was 82% with an average time to recurrence of 18.2 months. In contrast, the nonparaplegic group had no recurrence of ulceration.

Relander and Palmer[351] reviewed their experience with 66 flaps for primary coverage of pressure sores and noted a 43% recurrence rate with cutaneous flaps and a 33% recurrence rate with musculocutaneous flaps at 2–12-year follow-up, a nonsignificant difference.

Disa et al.[342] evaluated 40 consecutive patients with 66 pressure sores and, despite a cure rate of 80%, noted a 69% recurrent rate within 1 year. Two subgroups with higher recurrence rates were identified. The young, posttraumatic paraplegic subgroup demonstrated a recurrence rate of 79% at a mean of 10.9 months. The cerebrally compromised elderly subgroup had a 69% recurrence rate at a mean of 7.7 months. The authors conclude that surgical treatment of pressure sores among patients in these subgroups may not be warranted given the high recurrence rates, which they felt resulted from poor patient compliance. The ultimate causes of non-compliance were individual personalities, an unsteady social situation, and inadequate family network.

Tavakoli et al.[349] studied 27 patients with 37 ulcers who underwent musculocutaneous flap coverage of their ischial pressure sores with a mean follow-up of 62 months. Overall ulcer recurrence was 41.4% and overall patient recurrence rate was 47.8%. The recurrences were attributed by the authors to psychological and behavioral factors, such as life-style activities that led to neglect of skin care, drug and alcohol abuse, cultural barriers, and neglect of appropriate seating practices.

Kierney et al.[178] reported a lower recurrence rate in 268 pressure sores treated over a 12-year period. Mean postoperative follow-up was 3.7 years and overall recurrence rate was 19%. Unlike Evans et al.,[353] Kierney et al. did not find an association between pre-existing pressure sore risk factors and recurrence. Instead, the authors emphasize the importance of collaboration between plastic surgeons and physical medicine rehabilitation physicians as a major determinant of outcome.

In 2002 Singh et al.[354] published one of the few studies examining the outcome of surgical reconstruction of pressure sores in children. The records of 19 patients in 25 pressure sores with an average follow-up of 5.3 years were reviewed. Site-specific and patient recurrence were 5% and 20% respectively, considerably lower than generally reported in adults with similar follow-up.

Clearly, variable patient populations, risk factors, and follow-up periods make comparisons difficult. With such a wide range of outcomes, assigning a single value for recurrence is virtually impossible. Some question the wisdom of surgical intervention if the higher range of recurrence rates is legitimate.[353] It may be that select subpopulations are not good surgical candidates given their poor prognosis. However, a thorough evaluation of a patient's risk factors and a multi-disciplinary approach to treatment should be routine even for patients who initially seem like poor candidates.[178]

Complications

Common postoperative complications of pressure sore surgery include hematoma, seroma, infection, and wound dehiscence. A breakdown in the suture line should heal with local wound care within a week. If slough persists, then the wound debridement, particularly of bone, was likely inadequate.[87] The patient should be re-evaluated for risk factors and optimized, prior to return to the operating room for complete debridement, followed by flap advancement or alternative flap for coverage.[91,268]

Every chronic wound exposed to continuous trauma carries the risk of malignant degeneration.[355] Benign-appearing ulcerations are a frequent problem in our population and are usually treated conservatively, yet the suspicion of malignancy in these lesions must always be entertained, especially if the margins of the ulcer are verrucous. The term "Marjolin's ulcer" is used to describe malignant degeneration in burn scars, chronic venous ulcers, pressure sores, and sinuses from osteomyelitis. Malignant transformation is heralded by increased pain or discharge, foul odor, and bleeding. The latency period of carcinomas arising from pressure sores is approximately 20 years, compared with 30 years or more for carcinomas arising from burn scars and stasis ulcers.[356] Biopsy is indicated in all chronically draining ulcers and tracts, especially those with recent change in appearance or drainage, and should include the central area of the ulcer as well as the margins. Early recognition and proper staging offer the best chance for cure.[357]

Secondary procedures

It is critical that, before embarking on revision or repeat flap surgery, the patient be fully re-evaluated. Assuming proper surgical technique, the same risk factors that led to the patient's original ulcer are likely to be at least partially responsible for recurrence, and neglecting them will reliably result in poor outcomes.

Every pressure sore surgery should allow for the possibility of future secondary procedures. Despite favorable initial healing rates, long-term recurrence is common, even in the most favorable series. Assuming basic principles have been adhered to, multiple options should still exist, even in cases of multiple recurrences.

The simplest option may involve readvancing a previously performed flap *(Fig. 16.19)*. Flaps can often be readvanced multiple times, but, as always, excessive tension must be avoided. If tension is an issue, a change of plane, such as advancing a fasciocutaneous flap over a previous musculocutaneous flap, can provide additional length without violating another anatomic region or flap design. If a particular flap has already been readvanced or the tissue is of poor quality due to recurrent ulceration or scarring, a new, preferably virgin, anatomic area should be used to address the wound. For example, while flaps from the thigh area are commonly used to address ischial ulcers, a superiorly based gluteal flap can afford coverage if the posterior thigh is no longer a viable option.

Amputation or salvage flaps should be reserved for recalcitrant pressure sores where the ulcer is extensive to the point of precluding closure with standard flaps, or for patients who are severely ill because of uncontrollable infection, as these flaps are associated with high morbidity.[358–360] Likewise, hemicorporectomy is a highly morbid[361] last-resort measure reserved for potentially life-threatening and incurable conditions, as in patients with multiple, large, confluent ulcers in the setting of malignancy or extensive pelvic osteomyelitis[362,363] *(Fig. 16.20)*.

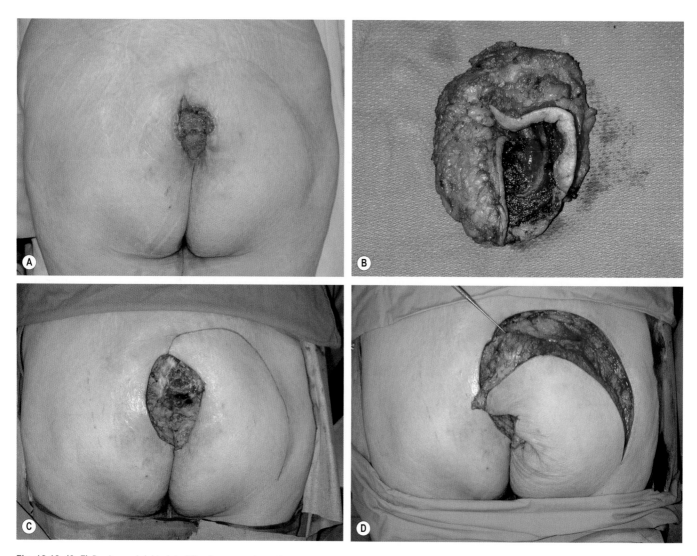

Fig. 16.19 (A–E) Readvanced right gluteal flap for recurrent sacral pressure sore.

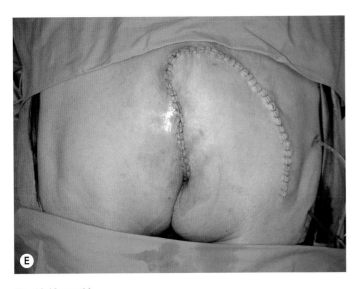

Fig. 16.19, cont'd

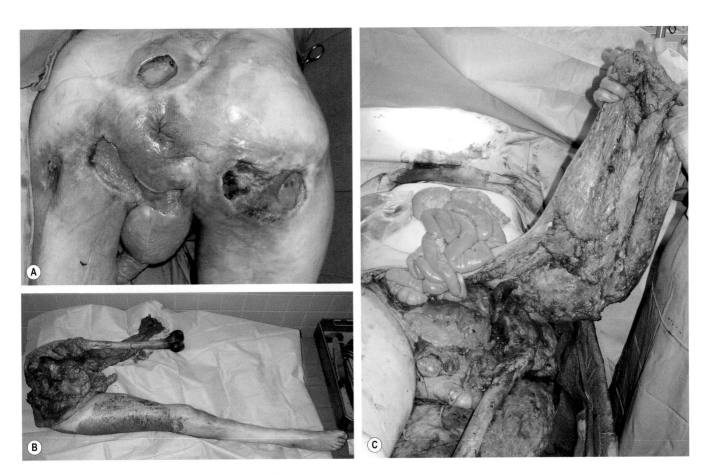

Fig. 16.20 (A–E) Hemicorporectomy with right subtotal thigh flap.

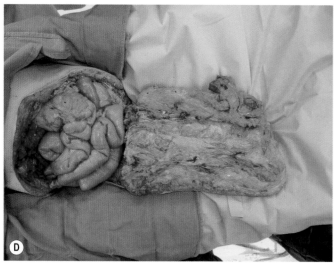

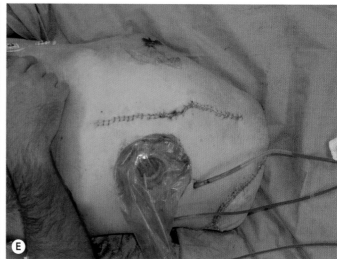

Fig. 16.20, cont'd

Access the complete references list online at **http://www.expertconsult.com**

4. Cuddigan J, Frantz RA. Pressure ulcer research: pressure ulcer treatment. A monograph from the National Pressure Ulcer Advisory Panel. *Adv Wound Care*. 1998;11:294–300; quiz 2.

   The recommendations of the National Pressure Ulcer Advisory Panel include a comprehensive set of guidelines for both operative and nonoperative treatment of pressure sores, with an emphasis on evidence-based medicine.

31. Fronek K, Zweifach BW. Microvascular pressure distribution in skeletal muscle and the effect of vasodilation. *Am J Physiol*. 1975;228:791–796.

34. Dinsdale SM. Decubitus ulcers: role of pressure and friction in causation. *Arch Phys Med Rehabil*. 1974; 55:147–152.

    This classic article describes the interplay between pressure and shear in pressure sore pathogenesis, quantifying the significant decrease in pressure required when shear is present.

58. Reddy M, Gill SS, Rochon PA. Preventing pressure ulcers: a systematic review. *JAMA*. 2006;296:974–984.

79. Han H, Lewis VL Jr, Wiedrich TA, et al. The value of Jamshidi core needle bone biopsy in predicting postoperative osteomyelitis in grade IV pressure ulcer patients. *Plast Reconstr Surg*. 2002;110:118–122.

    Han et al. not only provide a review of the various methods of evaluating pelvic osteomyelitis in the setting pressure

sores, but also provide a logical algorithm for evalaution and treatment.

188. Reddy M, Gill SS, Kalkar SR, et al. Treatment of pressure ulcers: a systematic review. *JAMA*. 2008;300: 2647–2662.

219. Conway H, Griffith BH. Plastic surgery for closure of decubitus ulcers in patients with paraplegia; based on experience with 1000 cases. *Am J Surg*. 1956;91:946–975.

     The authors report their outcomes and emphasize complete debridement and reconstruction with soft-tissue flaps. This very large series of patients is over half a century old, but the principles delineated therein have changed surprisingly little.

224. Anthony JP, Huntsman WT, Mathes SJ. Changing trends in the management of pelvic pressure ulcers: a 12-year review. *Decubitus*. 1992;5:44–47, 50–51.

226. Kroll SS, Rosenfield L. Perforator-based flaps for low posterior midline defects. *Plast Reconstr Surg*. 1988;81:561–566.

353. Evans GR, Dufresne CR, Manson PN. Surgical correction of pressure ulcers in an urban center: is it efficacious? *Adv Wound Care*. 1994;7:40–46.

     Evans et al. report their results and recurrence rate in a difficult patient population, and disuss strategies for dealing with the very high recurrence rates one can expect with flap surgery in the pressure sore population.

17

Perineal reconstruction

Hakim K. Said and Otway Louie

SYNOPSIS

- Surgical site is typically hostile after resection and/or radiation for an underlying condition.
- Healthy tissue transfer is usually necessary to mitigate wound-healing challenges.
- A proactive surgical approach can help lessen impact of complications.

Access the Historical Perspective section online at
http://www.expertconsult.com

Introduction

Perineal reconstruction poses the challenge of healing a problem area, despite a number of site-specific obstacles. Although a number of benign conditions exist which can require resurfacing perineal skin, more frequently reconstruction is needed after treatment of underlying cancer. Modern treatment of malignancies in this region has evolved to consistently use neoadjuvant radiation therapy, which can yield a high rate of complications at the time of surgical intervention. Local effects of radiation therapy and close proximity (combined in many cases with ostomies) to bowels and bladder, can all impact the perfusion to reconstructive flaps, contaminate the surgical site, and threaten surgical outcomes. Successful reconstruction takes into account these impediments and minimizes the consequences of complications in this hazardous region.

Basic science/disease process

The processes requiring reconstruction of the perineum can broadly be broken into benign and malignant processes (Table 17.1). Benign conditions primarily include hidradenitis suppurativa, infectious destructive processes such as fasciitis or

Fournier's gangrene and trauma, but can range to other rarer dermatologic conditions such as pyoderma gangrenosum and vasculitic ulcers. These entities have in common the depth of involvement, which typically leaves an external cutaneous deficit on the perineum (see Figs 9.13, 9.18). Once the primary process is addressed and resolving, the defect can begin secondary healing, although negative pressure therapy and skin grafts can often play a useful role in shortening the time to healing.

Malignant diseases include colorectal cancer, urologic and gynecologic cancers, which originate from and involve deeper structures (see Figs 9.11, 9.12). Abdominoperineal resection or exenteration has been demonstrated to provide the best cure in these cases. Typically, this extensive resection is accompanied by peri-operative radiation therapy. Treatment of these more complex defects must be individualized for the missing and exposed structures. Impediments to healing such as fistulas and radiation changes in the area generally mean these defects will not heal without the addition of a nonradiated tissue transfer. Large areas of dead space after extensive resection can allow the abdominal viscera to fall into the irradiated pelvic basin. This can lead to adhesions, obstruction, and fistulas, which can be disastrous to treat secondarily. Nearby organs such as the bladder or vagina may also be resected in part or whole as part of the treatment course.

Diagnosis/patient presentation

Patients with benign disease may present at various stages in their treatment. As a rule, reconstruction should not be initiated until the primary process is identified and resolved with repeated surgical debridements or excisions; underlying medical conditions or autoimmune disorders should be treated. Typically, areas of external perineal skin are involved and will require resurfacing in some fashion (Fig. 17.1).

Patients with malignant disease are typically treated in conjunction with a multidisciplinary oncologic team. Often the extent of the defect is not obvious until after the surgical

Table 17.1 Benign and malignant processes requiring reconstruction of the perineum

Process	Etiology	Complicating factors	Reconstructive options
Benign (simple)	Hidradenitis suppurativa Necrotizing fasciitis Fournier's gangrene Trauma Autoimmune ulcers	Usually none	Secondary healing Negative pressure therapy Skin graft
Malignant (complex)	Colorectal cancer Vulvar cancer Vaginal cancer Uterine cancer Bladder cancer	Radiation Ostomies Contamination Dead space Pelvic hernia	Rectus abdominis flap Gracilis flap Anterolateral thigh flap Singapore flap Free flap

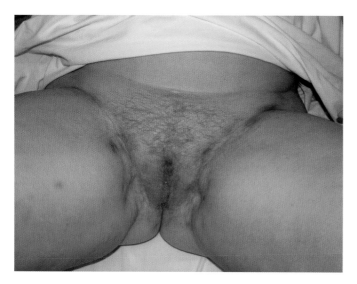

Fig. 17.1 Perineal hidradenitis.

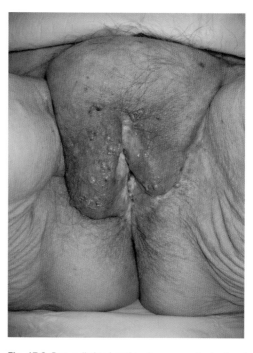

Fig. 17.2 Post-radiation lymphangiosarcoma after treatment of vulvar cancer.

resection is performed. Preoperative consultation is important to manage patient expectations, outline the possible extent of surgery and prepare for postoperative adversity. Such cases may involve more extensive external pudendal defects *(Figs 17.2, 17.3)* or deeper structures *(Fig. 17.4)*. In the event that vaginal resection is necessary, preferences regarding vaginal versus simple perineal reconstruction should be discussed, along with a thorough dialogue about sexual function. Further details and management of vaginal reconstruction is discussed in depth in Chapter 14.

Patient selection

Patients with benign disease are more straightforward in management; as their underlying process resolves, the defect begins to heal secondarily, even in response to a conventional wet to moist dressing regimen. Typically a modest, shallow perineal defect is left. A number of publications support the use of a negative pressure therapy plan to accelerate the healing process. Within a matter of weeks, a healthy wound bed can be established, confirming the suitability of these

patients for skin grafting. If the wound fails to begin the healing process despite wound healing optimization, a more complex approach and tissue transfer might be warranted.

In the case of malignancy, radiation therapy is part of the preoperative routine in most centers. This factor alone is the most significant indication for flap reconstruction at the time of resection. Large prospective series suggest that abdominal based flaps demonstrate the most favorable outcomes and mildest complication profile in this setting, even compared to thigh flap reconstruction.[16] This must be balanced with the abdominal morbidity of the harvest. Some surgeons prefer to avoid using abdominal flaps if ostomies are necessary on both sides, although these can be inset through the external oblique musculature with no additional morbidity. A vertical skin pedicle provides the most discreet scar, but an oblique paddle can provide more bulk extending off the muscle, effectively

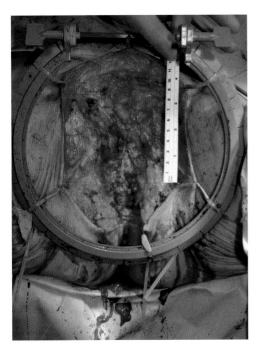

Fig. 17.3 External perineal skin and soft-tissue loss.

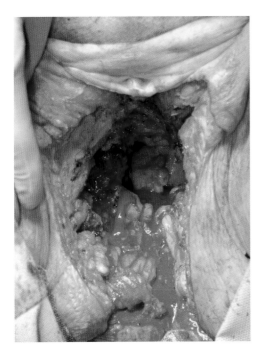

Fig. 17.4 Complex perineal defect involving external skin, soft-tissues, vagina and pelvic floor.

The complication profile of the gracilis flap is also reasonable, and represents a dramatic improvement over primary closure under these circumstances. Early studies comparing gracilis reconstruction to primary closure demonstrate a dramatic reduction in infectious complications from 46% to 12% with flap reconstruction.[18]

The anterolateral thigh flap represents an alternative option with documented excellent reliability for many applications, but with less support for its use in this setting.

Some surgeons favor a posterior thigh flap, harvested in similar fashion to the anterolateral thigh flap, but the axial nature of the perfusion off the inferior gluteal artery has been called into question. Recent series document over a 50% wound healing complication rate using this method,[19] which does not compare favorably to abdominal flaps.

For defects with less dead space or requiring less bulk, Singapore flap reconstruction can be used, although outcomes data are more mixed and overall less favorable compared with abdominal flaps. Complications are reported to range from 7% to 62%.[20–22] Recent outcome studies are not available directly comparing this method to other options in head-to-head fashion.

Massive defects in pelvic support may in fact require multiple flaps. Occasionally pelvic floor support is needed in the form of mesh reinforcement. In a hostile, radiated, often contaminated surgical site, prosthetic mesh is contraindicated. Newer bioprosthetic options provide a reinforcement alternative that is more robust in the face of complications.[23]

Finally, if the two abdominal flaps and eight thigh-based flaps are unavailable or insufficient for the defect, there are several reports of distant flaps used in conjunction with microsurgical transfer. Composite thigh tissues can be transferred en bloc, and large surface area flaps such as the latissimus dorsi have been reported in extreme cases.

Treatment/surgical technique

Skin graft reconstruction

Benign, uncomplicated wounds of the perineum that granulate in response to dressing changes or negative pressure therapy can usually be treated in staged fashion with split thickness skin grafts. However, managing these uncomplicated wounds with either negative pressure therapy or dressing changes is also a viable option. If the latter route is chosen, hydrotherapy and/or routine follow-up via a wound care center would be advised to monitor for infection, tissue necrosis or both which would require further debridement. With supportive patient counseling, particularly in cases of debridement for hidradenitis suppurativa or similar etiology of wounds, dressing changes and observant management can be an effective method of therapy *(Fig. 17.5)*.

Regional skin flaps

Processes such as Fournier's gangrene may leave more extensive but still subcutaneous defects that can be reconstructed with local flaps. Exposed subcutaneous structures such as testes can be buried under nearby intact skin if available. These adjacent areas of intact skin on the thighs or perineum

extending its reach also. Preexisting abdominal wall defects might direct some surgeons to alternative flap options. Nevertheless, Butler has shown no increased incidence of abdominal wall problems after abdominal flap harvest.[16,17] Rarely, perineal resection can be performed without laparotomy and this might predispose toward use of a nonabdominal flap option.

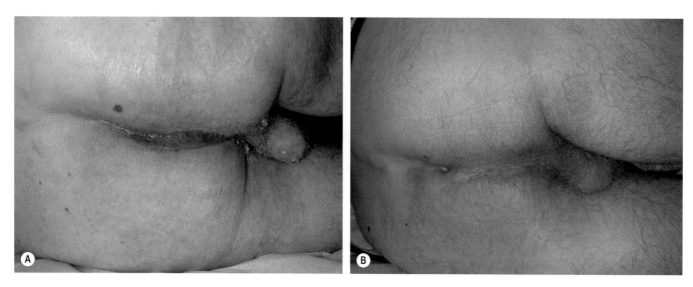

Fig. 17.5 (A) A 45-year-old male, 4 weeks after negative pressure therapy only. Initial wound was from a completion proctectomy for ulcerative colitis. **(B)** Postoperative photograph taken 12 weeks later.

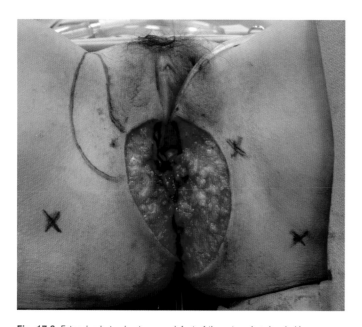

Fig. 17.6 Extensive but subcutaneous defect of the external perineal skin.

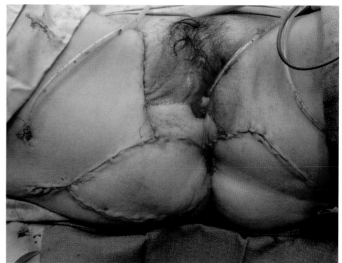

Fig. 17.7 Multiple regional flaps for reconstruction. Right Singapore flap used in conjunction with bilateral V-Y advancement flaps. (courtesy of Peter C. Neligan, MD).

can also be advanced using a V-Y pattern, rotational or keystone design to provide resurfacing *(Figs 17.6, 17.7)*. Some authors have described tissue expansion in conjunction with regional flaps to augment the amount of subcutaneous coverage available for example in the case of missing scrotal coverage.[24] Even perforator-based flaps have been described in this setting using medial circumflex femoral vessels[25] and profunda femoris perforating branches.[26]

Rectus-based reconstruction

Rectus-based flaps have emerged as workhorses for more complex perineal reconstruction. These flaps provide well-vascularized tissue with adequate bulk to fill dead-space. In addition, lining for external or vaginal wall coverage can be obtained if harvested as a musculocutaneous flap. They are

known for having a wide arc of rotation with a reliable pedicle. They have been shown to decrease the risk of perineal complications in irradiated APR defects.[27] When compared to thigh-based flaps, rectus-based flaps had lower major complications without increased abdominal morbidity.[16]

The rectus flap can be muscular or myocutaneous, depending on whether external skin or vaginal lining is needed for reconstruction. The right rectus is typically used, saving the left rectus for a colostomy if needed. After the resection is complete, the deep inferior epigastric vessels are examined to confirm they are patent, undamaged by the resection, and preferably pulsatile before proceeding with flap design. The skin paddle is based on the peri-umbilical perforators of the deep-inferior epigastric vessels, and can be oriented in vertical, transverse, or oblique directions *(Figs 17.8, 17.9; see Figs 14.6, 14.7)*. The vertical design theoretically includes more

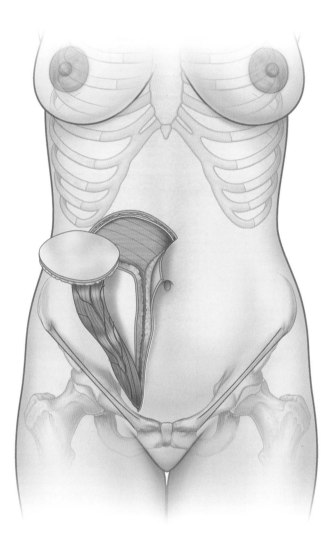

Fig. 17.8 Design of transverse rectus abdominis myocutaneous (TRAM) flap for perineal and pelvic reconstruction.

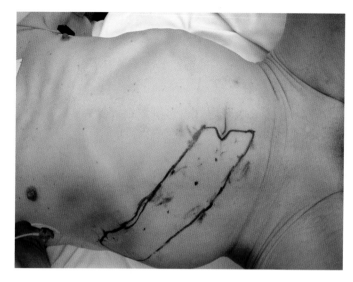

Fig. 17.9 Design of oblique rectus abdominis myocutaneous (ORAM) flap for perineal and pelvic reconstruction. Note skin paddle designed around periumbilical perforators, extending toward ipsilateral scapular tip.

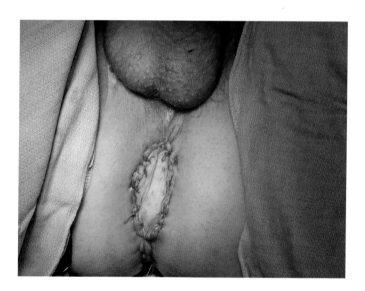

Fig. 17.10 Cutaneous paddle inset for external perineal skin reconstruction.

perforators as the skin paddle overlies the length of the rectus; however, its arc of rotation is limited by the muscle itself, and the bulk of the muscle itself can make insetting difficult, particularly in a narrow male pelvis. The transverse paddle has been well described for perineal reconstruction as well, and provides excellent cosmesis for the donor site.[28] Lee and others have had success with an oblique design for the rectus flap, noting the long, excellent arc of rotation and thin, reliable skin paddle obtained.[29,30] In addition, cadaver injection studies have shown flow in a lateral and superior oblique direction from the periumbilical perforators. After marking the periumbilical perforators with a Doppler, a skin paddle is designed with an axis towards the ipsilateral tip of the scapula, ending at the anterior axillary line. Flaps up to 12×27 cm can be obtained with this design.

Once the skin paddle has been marked in one of these orientations, the skin incisions are made and dissection carried down to the external oblique and rectus fascia. The skin paddle is dissected circumferentially, approaching the deep inferior epigastric perforators coming through the rectus muscle. The fascia immediately adjacent to these perforators is opened, and the anterior sheath elevated off the rectus muscle. The muscle is then dissected free of the rectus sheath, working down towards the deep inferior epigastric vessels. These are identified lateral to the rectus beneath the arcuate line. The superior rectus is divided, and the muscle transposed out of the rectus sheath. The vascular pedicle can be mobilized, but does not need to be skeletonized. The insertion of the rectus on the pubis typically does not need to be divided completely, and is left intact, at least in part to help prevent traction injury to the pedicle.

The flap is then delivered down through the pelvis and out to the perineum (*see Fig. 14.7*). The requisite skin for external lining or vaginal reconstruction is marked, and the remainder of the skin paddle de-epithelialized and inset under the radiated skin edges (*Fig. 17.10*). The skin paddle may be tubed if

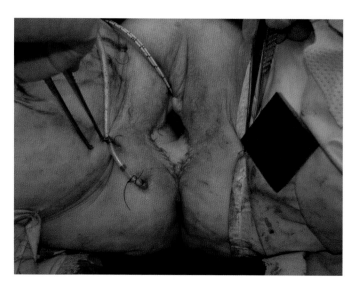

Fig. 17.11 Cutaneous paddle inset for vaginal and perineal reconstruction.

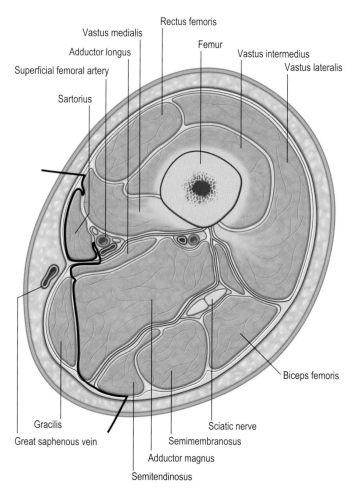

Fig. 17.12 Cross-sectional view of gracilis myocutaneous flap harvest. The fasciocutaneous vascular network around the gracilis muscle must be widely harvested to preserve perfusion to the distal tip of the skin. Adductor magnus, vastus medialis, sartorius and semitendinosus muscles are denuded by the harvest, as described by Whetzel and Lechtman (1997).[32]

needed for total vaginal reconstruction *(Fig. 17.11)*. The flap is then inset with a layered closure. The fascial donor site is closed primarily if possible, or the remaining anterior and posterior sheaths are sown together and used to span the fascial defect. Bioprosthetic mesh may be used to repair extensive anterior sheath defects. The abdominal skin is closed primarily over closed suction drainage.

Gracilis flap

The gracilis flap was first introduced in its myocutaneous form by McCraw et al. and used as a healthy tissue to augment genital reconstruction.[31] As described, it was based on the medial circumflex femoral vessels to the gracilis muscle, and to the overlying skin. Subsequent studies have shown that the perforators originating from the deep femoral system only reliably pass through the proximal gracilis directly muscle. To reliably capture the perfusion to distal portions of a longitudinal skin paddle, the fasciocutaneous vascular network around the gracilis muscle must be widely harvested as described by Whetzel and Lechtman.[32]

A line is drawn from the adductor insertion on the pubis to the semitendinosus muscle at the medial condyle of the knee. Centered on this axis at the anterior edge of the gracilis muscle, the skin flap is designed as a 6–10 cm wide ellipse, which can reach up to 30 cm in length *(see Fig. 14.9A)*. This position is slightly more anterior than the traditional design, which failed to harvest peri-gracilis fascia and was associated with a less reliable skin paddle. The skin pattern is incised distally to identify the thin, round gracilis muscle near the knee, and a bowstring technique is used to confirm its course. If necessary, the skin design is adjusted to overlie the anterior edge of the muscle. The paddle is then incised anteriorly, and beveling dissection outward ensures that the gracilis is harvested encased within its surrounding fat, vessels and fascia, essentially denuding the sartorius and adductor musculature *(Fig. 17.12; see Fig. 14.9B)*. The perforating branches off the superficial femoral vessels are divided very close to their take-off, preserving the longitudinal arcade of fasciocutaneous

vessels in communication with the primary pedicle off the deep femoral system proximally. The greater saphenous vein is divided proximally and distally and preserved within the substance of the flap as an additional venous conduit. The flap is isolated back to its pedicle off the medial circumflex femoral vessels, usually at 7–10 cm distal from the pubis *(see Fig. 14.9F)*. Upgoing adductor branches are divided to yield extra length. The muscular origin is exposed and divided off the pubis to allow rotation of the flap 180° into the perineum. To reduce the chance of flap ptosis, the flap is suspended from high within the perineal defect, or into the pelvis if possible. Layered closure over drains completes the inset *(Figs 17.13, 17.14)*.

Anterolateral thigh flap

The anterolateral thigh flap was first described by Song et al. in 1984.[33] Since that time it has become a valuable tool in the armamentarium of the reconstructive surgeon, with extensive uses in head and neck, trunk, and lower extremity reconstruction.[34] Luo et al. first described its use in perineal

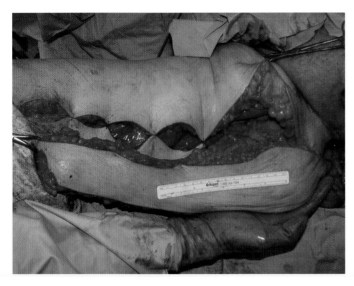

Fig. 17.13 Gracilis myocutaneous flap elevated before inset. Pedicle is visible 7–10 cm from pubis.

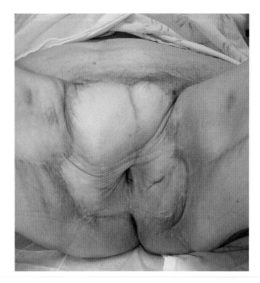

Fig. 17.14 Bilateral gracilis myocutaneous flaps for large area external perineal defect.

reconstruction after failed gracilis flaps in 2000.[35] Increasing experience with it in perineal reconstruction has confirmed its utility in complex pelvic defects.[12,13] It provides a regional flap with that can provide large, reliable skin paddles and muscle in the form of the vastus lateralis as well.

With the patient in a supine position, a line connecting the anterior superior iliac spine with the superolateral patella is marked *(Fig. 17.15)*. A circle with a 3 cm radius is marked at the center of this longitudinal axis, delineating the most common location of perforators of the descending branch of the lateral femoral circumflex vessels. Locations of perforators are confirmed by Doppler, and the skin paddle is designed as an ellipse centered on these perforators.

The anterior incision is made first, dissecting down to the fascia overlying the rectus femoris muscle *(Fig. 17.16)*. Dissection proceeds laterally, either in a subfascial or suprafascial plane, looking for septocutaneous perforators, which are then followed superomedially back to the descending branch of the lateral femoral circumflex vessels. Intramuscular perforators can be harvested with a small cuff of vastus lateralis muscle to minimize risk of injury to the perforators. The posterolateral incision is subsequently made and the harvest completed.

The flap can be delivered through either a perineal route or inguinal route, as elegantly described by Wong et al.[36] If a perineal skin defect exists, the flap is delivered under the rectus femoris and through a subcutaneous tunnel in the medial thigh to reach the perineum *(Fig. 17.10)*. If the perineal defect can be closed primarily, the inguinal ligament can be divided, and the vastus lateralis muscle delivered intraperitoneally through the abdominal wall to fill any dead space in the pelvis *(Fig. 17.17)*. The flaps are then inset with layered closure and ample drainage.

Singapore flap

First reported by Wee, Singapore flaps are fasciocutaneous flaps harvested from the groin using nonhair-bearing skin

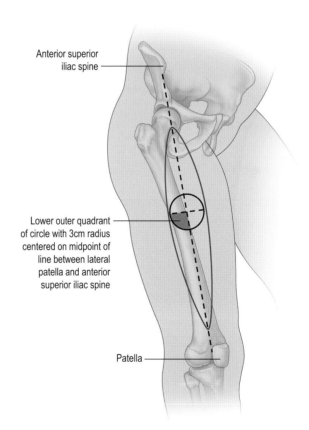

Anterior superior iliac spine

Lower outer quadrant of circle with 3cm radius centered on midpoint of line between lateral patella and anterior superior iliac spine

Patella

Fig. 17.15 Design of anterolateral thigh flap, centered midway along an axis between the anterior superior iliac spine (ASIS) and the superolateral corner of the patella.

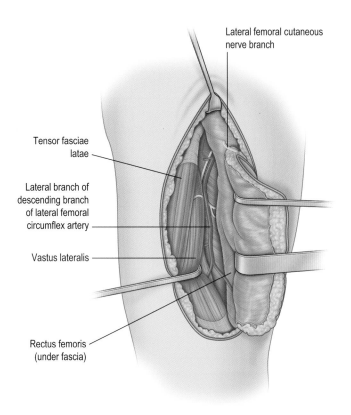

Lateral femoral cutaneous nerve branch

Tensor fasciae latae

Lateral branch of descending branch of lateral femoral circumflex artery

Vastus lateralis

Rectus femoris (under fascia)

Fig. 17.16 Elevation of anterolateral thigh flap, including skin, soft-tissue, fascia, and occasionally a small cuff of muscle. Perforators are pursued toward the septum between the vastus lateralis and rectus femoris, and then followed superomedially up to the descending branch of the lateral circumflex femoral vessels.

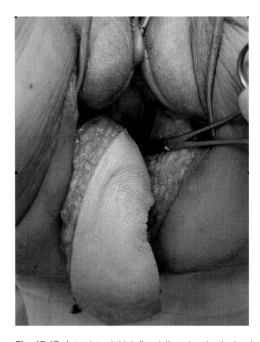

Fig. 17.17 Anterolateral thigh flap delivered under the inguinal ligament into the pelvis, then out through the pelvic defect to fill the pelvic dead space and reconstruct the perineal skin defect. The flap can be tunneled subcutaneously across the thigh if no pelvic defect is present.

just lateral to the labia majora.[11] These flaps are based on the posterior labial arteries, tracing back from the perineal arteries which in turn originate from the internal pudendal vessels. A horn-shaped flap up to 15×6 cm is designed lateral to the labia majora, and harvested to include deep fascia and adductor epimysium to preserve dermal blood supply. The original description divided the dermis at the base of the design, and tunneled the flap into the defect. In order to maximize perfusion under the most adverse circumstances, Woods subsequently described a modification to avoid dividing the skin at the base of the flap.[37] This design added an incision made at the posterior base of the labia majora in order to avoid dividing the dermal circulation to the flap entirely. The released labia are allowed to shift anteriorly and the flaps are transposed 70° through the release incision into the defect **(Fig. 17.18; see Fig. 14.4)**.

Posterior thigh flap

Although this flap has been described based on axial flow from the inferior gluteal artery, this pattern of perfusion has been called into question. A significant number of flaps in this distribution are actually based on perforators from the profunda femoris vessels,[26] which are frequently divided using the flap design as traditionally described.[38,39] This may relate to the high wound healing complication rate (53%) recently reported in a series of these flaps.[19] There are settings where this flap can be useful, especially when an abdominal approach is contraindicated and the previous flaps are not available. In such cases, using a profunda femoris perforator flap design is recommended. Not all surgeons are comfortable with this style of dissection, and the literature shows far fewer reports of its use in this manner. These various issues prevent it from being a first-line choice in comparison with the better-established and supported flaps above.

Free flap

Given the number of reliable local flap options, microsurgical tissue transfer is rarely indicated. In extenuating circumstances, however, large composite flaps of skin and muscle from the thigh can be elevated and reanastomosed using gluteal recipient vessels.[14] Alternatively, the latissimus dorsi muscle can be harvested on the thoracodorsal vascular system and anastomosed to the gluteal vessels.

Special considerations – sphincter reconstruction

For treatment of rectal cancers in patients seeking to avoid colostomy, some centers have advocated resection with sphincter reconstruction as a strategy. In such cases, functional transfer using one or two gracilis muscles wrapped around a perineal colostomy has been described with some success, although the morbidity of this approach is high. Early authors in the 1950s encountered issues generating resting sphincter tone when using a voluntary muscle to perform an autonomic smooth muscle function. This was addressed using

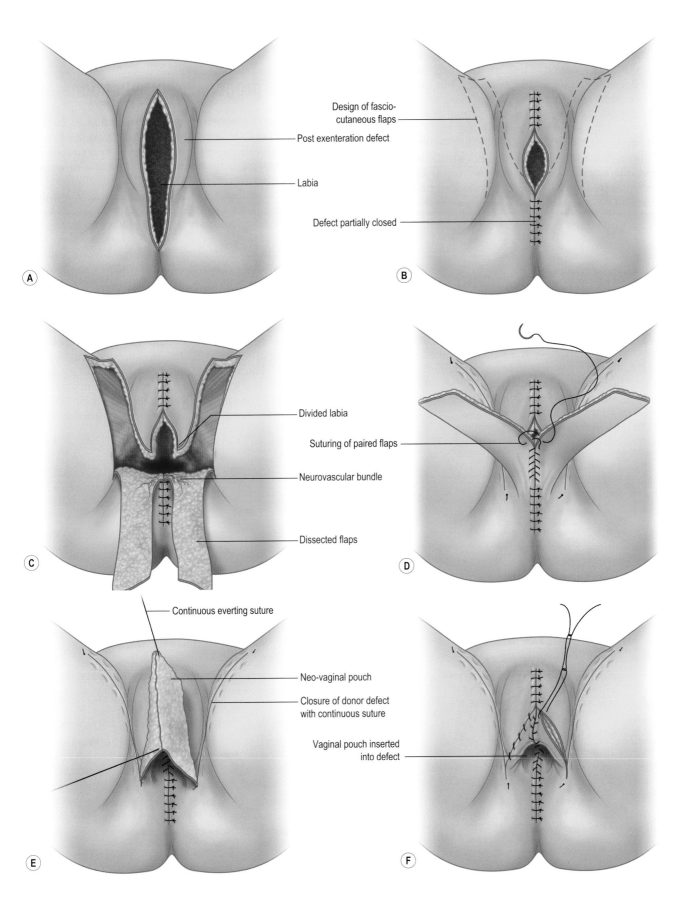

Fig. 17.18 Elevation of pudendal thigh flaps for more extensive, or vaginal defects. **(A)** Perineal defect. **(B)** Design of fasciocutaneous flaps along vascular territory of perineal arteries. **(C)** Primary closure of donor sites and suturing of flaps together. **(D)** Inset of flaps into pelvic and perineal defect.

an implantable electrical stimulator (electrically stimulated dynamic gracileplasty),[40] but a high complication rate ultimately led the manufacturer to withdraw the device from the US market in 1999.[41] Evolution of this approach has continued in Europe where the device is still available, but one meta-analysis has shown more favorable results using an artificial bowel sphincter (Acticon Neosphincter™, American Medical Systems, Minnetonka, MN).[42] All methods of sphincter preservation or reconstruction carry a significant (30–100%) risk of complications and a consensus is still not available on the best of these alternatives. Despite these newer options, in a recent review the traditional abdominal colostomy has been advocated as still having the lowest complication rate for this group of patients.[43]

Postoperative care

The management of these patients follows the basic tenets of surgical postoperative care. A key principle is to avoid excessive pressure on the flap, as this can lead to venous congestion and flap loss. The authors have the patients on bed-rest for several days, followed by progressive ambulation. However, the patients are instructed not to sit upright for several weeks. Drains are typically placed in both the donor site and the perineum. Deep venous thromboprophylaxis in the form of sequential compression devices and subcutaneous heparin is used. Nutrition must be optimized. The patient is seen regularly by all involved teams postoperatively.

Outcomes/prognosis/complications

It is important to emphasize that reconstruction of the perineum cannot eliminate complications. In fact, multiple series highlight complications even in the best of circumstances; what has improved with advances in the state of surgical treatment has been the complication profile. In earliest descriptions, extensive abdominoperineal resections and exenterations were accompanied by significant mortality, small bowel obstruction, small bowel fistulae, pelvic abscesses, perineal hernias and profound interstitial fluid losses through what frequently became a chronic draining perineal wound. In contrast, when flaps are used, the small bowels are separated from the radiated pelvic basin, which dramatically reduces or eliminates all these major sequelae in every major series.[16,17,27,44] Complications remain at a significant incidence of 5–33% overall but these manifest a shift toward minor complications. Still present are delayed wound healing at the inset incisions, seromas, or superficial dehiscence or infection, but none of these normally requires reoperation. Understanding the vulnerabilities of the surgical site and the clinical outcomes data makes it possible to employ a reconstructive plan that can limit complications and make perineal reconstruction a relatively safe, reliable process.

Access the complete reference list online at **http://www.expertconsult.com**

11. Wee JT, Joseph VT. A new technique of vaginal reconstruction using neurovascular pudendal-thigh flaps: a preliminary report. *Plast Reconstr Surg.* 1989;83(4):701–709.

16. Nelson RA, Butler CE. Surgical outcomes of VRAM versus thigh flaps for immediate reconstruction of pelvic and perineal cancer resection defects. *Plast Reconstr Surg.* 2009;123(1):175–183.

    The largest series of prospectively collected cases comparing abdominal vs thigh flap reconstruction in perineal reconstruction, demonstrating the most favorable complication profile after abdominal flap use (M.D. Anderson Cancer Center).

17. Butler CE, Gündeslioglu AO, Rodriguez-Bigas MA. Outcomes of immediate vertical rectus abdominis myocutaneous flap reconstruction for irradiated abdominoperineal resection defects. *J Am Coll Surg.* 2008;206:694–703.

    Documented improvement in outcomes using flaps in radiated perineal reconstruction.

18. Shibata D, Hyland W, Busse P, et al. Immediate reconstruction of the perineal wound with gracilis muscle flaps following abdominoperineal resection and intraoperative radiation therapy for recurrent carcinoma of the rectum. *Ann Surg Oncol.* 1999;6(1):33–37.

Early evidence that flaps can reduce complication rate from 46–12% in radiated perineal reconstruction.

27. Chessin DB, Hartley J, Cohen AM, et al. Rectus flap reconstruction decreases perineal wound complications after pelvic chemoradiation and surgery: a cohort study. *Ann Surg Oncol.* 2005;12(2):104–110.

    Documented improvement in outcomes using abdominal flaps in radiated perineal reconstruction (Memorial Sloan-Kettering Cancer Center).

29. Lee MJ, Dumanian GA. The oblique rectus abdominis musculocutaneous flap: revisited clinical applications. *Plast Reconstr Surg.* 2004;114(2):367–373.

    Variation in skin paddle design, expanding the size and the reach of the rectus abdominis myocutaneous flap.

32. Whetzel TP, Lechtman AN. The gracilis myofasciocutaneous flap: vascular anatomy and clinical application. *Plast Reconstr Surg.* 1997;99(6):1642–1655.

36. Wong S, Garvey P, Skibber J, et al. Reconstruction of pelvic exenteration defects with anterolateral thigh-vastus lateralis muscle flaps. *Plast Reconstr Surg.* 2009;124(4):1177–1185.

44. Lefevre JH, Parc Y, Kerneis S, et al. Abdomino-Perineal resection for anal cancer impact of a vertical rectus abdominis myocutaneous flap on survival, recurrence, morbidity, and wound healing. *Ann Surg.* 2009;250:707–711.

18

Acute management of burn/electrical injuries

Lars Steinstraesser and Sammy Al-Benna

SYNOPSIS

- Learn assessment and classification of burn wounds, including estimation of burn size and depth, and reduction of related morbidity and mortality.
- Gain an appreciation of stress response to acute burn injury, including hemodynamic, metabolic, nutritional and immunologic sequelae.
- Learn initial management of the acute burn patients, including fluid resuscitation, nutritional support and wound care.
- Learn wound management of burn patients including an understanding of wound healing, wound sepsis, topical antimicrobial agents, biological dressings, skin substitutes and skin grafts.
- Learn fundamental surgical principles in treatment of burn patients, including wound debridement, wound dressing and splinting, skin grafting and scar contracture release.
- Burn rehabilitation, including physical/occupational therapy, psychosocial support and reconstructive needs.
- Principles of management of special problems, including inhalation injuries, chemical burns, electrical injuries and toxic epidermal necrolysis.

 Access the Historical Perspective section online at
http://www.expertconsult.com

Aims of burn care

Restore form: Return the injured areas to as close to normality as is attainable

Restore function: Optimize patient's ability to perform activities of daily living at pre-injury level

Restore feeling: Enable psychological and emotional rehabilitation.

Acute management of burn injuries

Rescue: The aim is to get the individual away from the source of the injury and provide first aid.

Resuscitate: Immediate support must be provided for any failing organ system. This usually involves administering fluid to maintain the circulatory system but may also involve supporting the cardiac, renal, and respiratory systems.

Retrieve: After initial evacuation to an accident and emergency department, patients with serious burns may need transfer to a specialist burns unit for further care.

Resurface: The skin and tissues that have been damaged by the burn must be repaired. This can be achieved by various means, from simple dressings to aggressive surgical debridement and skin grafting.

Rehabilitate: This begins on the day a patient enters hospital and continues for years after he or she has left. The aim is to return patients, as far as is possible, to their pre-injury level of physical, emotional, and psychological wellbeing.

Reconstruct: The scarring that results from burns often leads to functional impairment that must be addressed. The operations needed to do this are often complex and may need repeating as a patient grows or the scars re-form.

Review: Burn patients, especially children, require regular review for many years so that problems can be identified early and solutions provided.

Epidemiology

The incidence of burn injuries varies from country to country, typically peaking during the country's holiday period. According to the most recent statistics compiled by the World Health Organization and the World Fire Statistics Center, fires caused 6.6 million major burn injuries and 400 000 deaths every year.[1] The burden of burn injury falls predominantly on the world's poor; 95% of fire-related burns occur in low- and middle-income countries where prevention programs are almost nonexistent and open fires for cooking, lighting or heating are commonplace. The average death rates are about three fire deaths per 100 000 inhabitants and one fire death per 100 fires. However, this average conceals a more than 100-fold variation in death rates from country to country. A better indication of typical fire risk is the median fire death rate per 100 000 inhabitants by country, which was 0.9 in 2004. In addition, the WFSC released fire-related death data by country (from lowest to highest number of deaths per 100 000 person) from 2002–2004. The countries with the lowest incidences include Singapore (0.08) and Switzerland (0.51). Those with the highest include Finland (2.08) and Hungary (2.10).The cost to society in terms of lost wages, vocational rehabilitation, and need for long-term care is staggering. Worldwide, severe burns cause disabilities that cost $80.2 billion a year in lost productivity (wages and skills) alone; medical expenses would add millions more. Lost productivity costs the world billions of dollars annually. In 2009, the WFSC noted that the cost of direct fire losses ranged from 0.06–0.26% of countries' gross domestic product (GDP) and the cost of indirect fire losses ranged from 0.002–0.95% of countries' GDP.

Males account for approximately two-thirds of the total costs of fire/burn injuries and females account for the remaining third. Fatal fire and burn injuries cost 2% of the total costs of all fatal injuries. Hospitalized fire and burn injuries are 1% of the total cost of all hospitalized injuries. Nonhospitalized fire and burn injuries cost 2% of the total cost of all nonhospitalized injuries.

Risk factors

Children under 5 years old are a vulnerable group, susceptible to injury and especially to burns. The two most common causes of burns are scalds and contact burns. The latter play a minor role since they imply injury of small extent and rarely require admission to hospital. On the other hand, scalds are often accidents of such a severity that hospitalization and resuscitation are required. In children, scald burns accounted for about two-thirds of burn injuries and in those <5 years old, scalds caused 75% of all burn injuries, most commonly occurring in the kitchen. In adults, predisposing factors to scalding include alcoholism, senility, psychiatric disorders, and neurological disease such as epilepsy.

Mechanisms of thermal injury

Types of burns

The body has very few specific protective and repair mechanisms for thermal, electrical, radiation and chemical burns. Heat changes the molecular structure of tissue and denaturation of proteins is a common effect of all types of burns. The extent of burn damage depends on the temperature of agent, concentration of heat and the duration of contact.

Thermal burns

Flash and flame burns

Flash and flame burn injuries are the most common cause of adult burn admissions. In general, flash burns reach progressive layers of the dermis in proportion to the amount and kind of fuel that explodes. In contrast to flash injuries, flame burns are invariably deep dermal if not full-thickness because of more prolonged exposure to intense heat and are often associated with inhalational injury and other concomitant trauma. Patients whose bedding or clothes have been on fire rarely escape without some full-thickness burns.

Scalds

Hot water scalds are the most common cause of pediatric burn admissions. They also often occur in elderly people. The common mechanisms are spilling hot drinks or liquids or being exposed to hot bath water *(Fig. 18.1)*. The depth of scald injury depends on the water temperature, the skin thickness and the duration of contact. Water at 60°C creates a deep dermal burn in 3 s but will cause the same injury in 1 s at 69°C. Boiling water often causes a deep dermal burn, unless the duration of contact is very short. Grease and hot oils will generally cause deep dermal or deeper burns.

Contact burns

In order to get a burn from direct contact, the object touched must either have been extremely hot or the contact abnormally long. The latter is a more common reason, and these types of burns are commonly seen in people with epilepsy or those who misuse alcohol or drugs. They are also seen in elderly people after a loss of consciousness; such a presentation requires a full investigation as to the cause of the blackout *(Fig. 18.2)*. Contact burns commonly result from hot metals, plastics, glass or hot coals. Burns from brief contact with very hot substances are usually due to industrial accidents. Although generally small in size, contact burns are

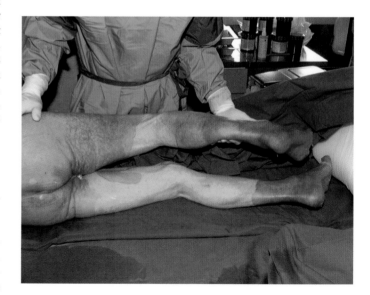

Fig. 18.1 The burn wounds may give clues to the mechanism of injury. The burn tideline associated with sitting in a bath of hot water.

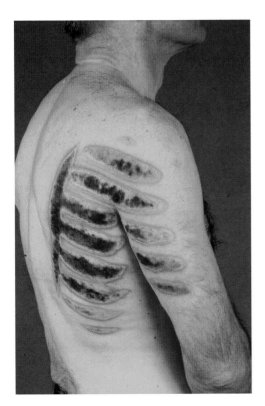

Fig. 18.2 Direct contact burn.

challenging in that the injury tends to be deep dermal or full thickness.

Tar

Tar is usually used as a protective coating in surfacing pavement and roads, roofing and other industrial applications. It is made from distillates of petroleum and is composed of long-chain hydrocarbons and waxes, which have a high boiling point. The boiling points of paving tar and roof tiling tar are 140°C and 232°C, respectively. Hence, accidents involving tar, tend to be associated with deeper burns.

When tar splatters, it cools rapidly to between 93°C and 104°C before landing. When hot tar makes contact with the skin it cools, solidifies and sticks. The tar usually retains sufficient heat to produce a significant burn by prolonged heat transfer to the skin. Once cooled, the tar quickly hardens and adheres to the skin. The aim of first aid at the scene is to reduce the effects of thermal insult. In order to expedite the cooling and solidification process one should apply cold water. Often, the tar is cool by the time the patient arrives at the medical facility. If not, the tar should be actively cooled to terminate thermal damage with room temperature water and prevent the further spread of the tar. Care must be taken not to develop hypothermia in major burns and adherent tar should not be removed in the field, but only by qualified personnel at a medical facility. The injuries are typically over the exposed skin of the face and extremities and the burn is of variable depth but is often deep second degree or third degree. Tar which has just been heated is sterile, skin is not. So, colonization of the wound from the surrounding intact skin may develop.

Burns due to hot tar are difficult to manage because of the difficulty in removing the tar without inflicting further injury to the underlying burn. As it is difficult to remove the tar rapidly and there is no pressing medical need to do so, it is best to treat the injury as a deep burn with appropriate fluid resuscitation or preparation for skin grafting as needed. Removal of the tar is not essential but it improves patient comfort and allows early assessment of the underlying tissue damage. This approach carries the risk of infection and the potential conversion of a partial thickness injury to a full thickness injury.

Numerous substances have been used in the past with variable results and selection of the appropriate agent for the removal of adherent tar is still challenging. Polyoxyethylene sorbitan, an emulsifying agent commonly used as a base in ointments, separates the tar from the skin and, as it is water soluble, easily washes off.[2]

Alternatively silver sulfadiazine, neosporin ointment (with polyoxyethylene sorbitan as a base), polysorbate or De-Solv-It (a citrus petroleum distillate with surfactant and lanolin) may be left on the burn, which is then bandaged. The tar comes away with the bandages when they are removed the next day. These may be used by themselves or in combination with an antibiotic ointment.[3] With some of these agents, it is recommended to leave it on for 12–48 h at a time until the tar has dissolved.

Organic solvents, such as alcohol, acetone, aldehydes, ether, gasoline and kerosene have had limited use. Some of these substances are relatively ineffective, have a slow solvent action, which requires continual rubbing and repeated applications and can induce further local tissue damage as well as the possibility of systemic toxicity through absorption, so these are not recommended for removing tar.

Common household agents, such as mayonnaise (15–30 min), butter (20–30 min), sunflower seed oil (20–30 min), and baby oil (1–1.5 h) placed on sterile gauze and onto the tar, have been promoted to remove tar effectively, rapidly and without further damage, over the aforementioned time periods. When large amounts of tar are present, the technique may need to be repeated. The burn depth can then be evaluated and managed by early surgical intervention if required. Organic, nonsterile agents are easy to acquire and are available in large quantities, but they carry the risk of promoting wound infection or allergic reaction. Bacterial or fungal growth can occur if the tar is not completely removed and the organic agent is not completely rinsed off.

Mechanical or manual debridement is painful, relatively ineffective, and results in the removal of underlying viable skin and hair follicles, thus extending the depth and area of the dermal injury. In addition, a degree of autodebridement will occur. Debriding is a balance between removing the tar and exposing the injured skin for evaluation and treatment. Judgment should be exercised as to how much debridement is appropriate in the emergency setting, as extensive debridement may require moderate-to-deep sedation. If the skin has a light coat of tar and the patient does not complain about the underlying skin or surrounding tissue, leaving the asymptomatic tar in place may be acceptable.[4] It has been reported that early excision and grafting may be required in some patients and this will decrease the hospitalization times. Tar that is part of an obvious burn, blister, or tissue loss should be removed and conjunctival tar, should be removed by an ophthalmologist.

Chemical burns

See 'Cold and chemical injury to the upper extremity,' Chapter 20 for details of chemical burns.

Electrical burns

Thermal injury due to electrical current is defined as tissue injury by exposure to supraphysiological electrical currents *(Table 18.1)*. Electrical burns *(Figs 18.3, 18.4)* are classified as high voltage (≥1000 V), low voltage (<1000 V), 'flash burn' (in which there is no electrical current flow through the body of the patient) and burns caused by lightning.

Low voltage injuries rarely cause significant damage beyond a small deep partial thickness burn at contact points. High-voltage injuries are more apt to cause deep tissue destruction. In fact, most electrical burns are work related (i.e., construction workers, linemen, utility and electrical workers). Typically, high-voltage injury causes extensive skin injury with necrosis at the contact point and deeper structures, resulting in a large area of necrosis. The electricity flows through the tissues and generates heat, which damages them. The resistance of tissues increases gradually from nerves to vessels, muscles, skin, tendons, fat and bone. Bones are more resistant to the flow of electricity, producing the highest amount of heat with the same current, in accordance with the Joule effect. Because of this phenomenon, multi-organ injury

can occur with significant electrical burns. This multiorgan injury (e.g., heart, kidney, nerves, eyes) must be promptly identified, controlled and treated. In addition, it is important to note that high voltage electrical injuries resemble a crush syndrome and require suitable decompression. Therefore, the degree of tissue damage is more extensive than that perceived on initial examination due to the progressive and continuing tissue necrosis. In high-voltage injuries, the victim usually does not continue to grasp the conductor. Often, these patients are thrown away from the electric circuit, which leads to traumatic injuries (e.g., multiple orthopaedic injuries, cranioencephalic trauma). As a result of these associated injuries, these patients must be considered as polytraumatized.

Despite great advances in the treatment modalities of electrical injuries in the recent decades, the magnitude of the problem remains very high both for the victim and the treating surgeon. Most of them succumb to it due to systemic effect; many of those who survive, lose one or more limbs and present with complicated defects involving different tissues at different parts of the body. These wounds are often potentially life-threatening and some are functionally disabling.

The contact wounds are usually present at the entry and exit points and the injuries are more severe at these two points. The terminology of entry and exit point, however, is an archaic term for the simple reason that they are applicable to direct current, whereas in an alternate current the exit point becomes the entry (re-entry) point also. The resultant damage is more severe.

The victims of electrical burns show certain specific features with regard to therapy and the evolution of the pathology. The very nature of electrical burns is its vascular damage leading to progressive tissue necrosis, often seen in skin and muscles. Soft tissue damage in the extremities can precipitate compartment syndrome requiring fasciotomy. This results in a gross limitation on manipulation of local tissues for reconstruction.

The damage to the tissues is three-dimensional with the current producing extensive necrosis of the tissues at different levels from skin to bone. The site and extent of tissue necrosis can be clearly identified by 99 T Cm-MDP bone scans. The optimal management of these wounds therefore has evolved

Table 18.1 Physiologic effects of different electrical currents	
	Effect current (milliamps)
Tingling sensation/perception	1–4
Let-go current	3–9
Skeletal muscle tetany	16–20
Respiratory muscle paralysis	20–50
Ventricular fibrillation	50–120

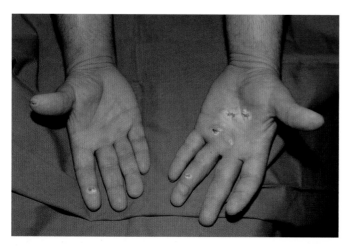

Fig. 18.3 Electrical burn wounds.

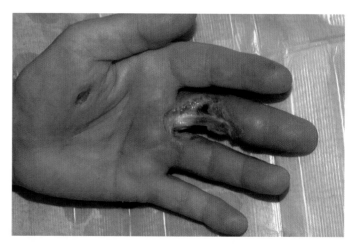

Fig. 18.4 Entry site for an electrical burn.

into a plan of early primary debridement, suitable decompression, including fasciotomy, an aggressive but cautious revision debridement and early skin cover, often composite, with an aim to preserve vital structures. Serial and multiple debridements of wounds, including superficial and deep muscles must be performed but nerves, tendons, joints and bones even if denatured can be preserved as they can partially regenerate if covered with vascularized skin.

Aggressive treatment including surgical debridement of devitalized tissues, or those with doubtful viability, frequently exposes vital structures in patients who have suffered high-voltage burns. The problem of 'high risk' wounds warranting priority in providing an early and emergency cover compounded with paucity and limitations of choice of procedures throw a great challenge to the surgeon. These require a higher necessity of flaps when compared with other burn groups, due to the characteristic compromising of deeper structures. High complication rates are reported with electrical injury including partial or complete flap failure. This fact, associated with the need to preserve the vital organs and structures like vessels, bones, tendons and nerves justifies the aforementioned cautious reconstructive approach with serial examination and debridement prior to a definitive surgery. The vascular damage and resulting thrombotic phenomenon abates during second week and tissues become healthy. This is the time when tissues around the wound withstand manipulation for a local, regional, axial or free flap. The mortality rate of patients who suffer high-voltage burns ranges from 0 to 21.7%; their main cause of death is multiorgan failure secondary to sepsis of cutaneous origin.[5,6]

Myonecrosis, with severe myoglobinemia as a result of a massive muscular destruction can lead to acute renal failure, despite aggressive volemic replacement. As the extent of injury cannot be quantified as in a cutaneous burn, fluid resuscitation must be adjusted to urine output. The treatment of myoglobinuria includes initial stabilization and resuscitation of the patient while concomitantly attempting to preserve renal function. Early aggressive fluid replacement is beneficial in minimizing the occurrence of renal failure. While osmotic diuretics (e.g., mannitol) and alkalinizing agents (e.g., bicarbonate) are considered the standard of care in preventing acute renal failure in patients with myoglobinuria, there is little clinical evidence to support the use of these agents.[7]

Cardiac dysfunction, such as atrial fibrillation or supraventricular arrhythmias, are observed in up to one-third of patients who suffered from electrical burns. Electrical function of the heart should be assessed by an initial electrocardiogram and continuous cardiac rhythm monitoring for the first 24 h after injury. According to the majority of publications, these complications are transitory and no patients were noted to have developed late cardiac complications. Chronic complications that persist after the hospitalization period, include the occurrence of peripheral nerve injuries, mainly sensory deficits such as dysesthesias and paraesthesias and cataracts.

A wide spectrum of abdominal visceral complications occur following high-voltage electrical injury. These injuries result either from direct injuries to intra-abdominal structures from the contact points over the abdomen or are a result of current passing through the abdominal viscera from more distant entrance and exit wounds. In treating high-voltage electric accidents, anticipate the entire spectrum of anatomic and pathologic alterations to the abdominal viscera. Therefore, these injuries of the abdomen warrant early exploration to determine whether there is injury of the viscera. Distribution of intravenously injected fluorescein dye may prove helpful in demarcating devascularized bowel.

Nonaccidental burns

Up to one-tenth of pediatric burns may be due to non-accidental injury. Detecting these injuries is important as up to one-third of children who are repeatedly abused die. Usually children less than 3 years old are affected. As with other nonaccidental injuries, the history and the pattern of injury may arouse suspicion. A social history is extremely important. Abuse is more common in poor households with single or young parents. Such abuse is not limited to children: elderly and other dependent adults are also at risk and a similar assessment can be made in these scenarios.

Pathophysiology

The skin is the largest organ of the body. While not very active metabolically, the skin serves multiple functions essential to our survival, functions that are compromised in the presence of a burn. These functions include: (1) Thermal regulation and prevention of fluid loss by evaporation. (2) Hermetic barrier against infection. (3) Sensory receptors that provide information about environment.

The skin is divided into three layers: (1) *Epidermis*: This is the outermost layer of skin composed of cornified epithelial cells. Outer surface cells die and are sloughed off as newer cells divide at the stratum germinativum. The outer epidermal layer provides critical barrier functions and is composed of an outer layer of dead cells and keratin, which present a barrier to bacterial and environmental toxins. The basal epidermal cells supply the source of new epidermal cells. (2) *Dermis*: This is the middle layer of skin composed of primarily connective tissue. It contains capillaries that nourish the skin, nerve endings, and hair follicles. The inner dermal layer has a number of essential functions, including continued restoration of the epidermis. The dermis is divided into the papillary dermis and the reticular dermis. The former is extremely bioactive; the latter, less bioactive. This difference in bioactivity within the dermis is the reason that superficial partial-thickness burns generally heal faster than deeper partial-thickness burns; the papillary component is lost in the deeper burns. (3) *Hypodermis*: This is a layer of adipose and connective tissue between the skin and underlying tissues.

Much of the treatment of burns is predicated on the depth and extent (percentage total body surface area, TBSA) of the initial burn injury. In this way the severity can be clarified and the treatment designed. The classification of burn depths should be referred to as:
- Epidermal burn
- Superficial partial thickness burn
- Deep partial thickness burn
- Full thickness burn.

It is critical to understand the clinical implications of accurate evaluation of the injury so that consistent and timely therapy can be instituted.

Burn injuries of the skin result in both local tissue destruction and systemic responses. Loss of the normal skin barrier function causes the common complications of burn injury. These include infection, loss of body heat, increased evaporative water loss, and change in key interactive functions such as touch and appearance.

Local response

The three mechanisms by which energy is transferred are conduction, convection and radiation. All of these mechanisms affecting heat transfer may deliver heat to, or away from, living tissues. Sustained temperatures result in cellular dysfunction and early denaturation of protein. As the temperature or the time of exposure increases, cell damage increases.

Excessively high temperatures cause graded tissue injury radiating from the point of contact and become progressively less severe at the periphery. The increased temperature kills cells in the immediate area and coagulates and denatures the surrounding extracellular matrix proteins (zone of coagulation). Circulation to this area ceases immediately. The area surrounding the injury is characterized by decreased tissue perfusion (zone of stasis). The tissue in this zone is potentially salvageable. The main aim of burn resuscitation is to increase tissue perfusion here and prevent any damage becoming irreversible. Additional insults, such as prolonged hypotension, infection, or edema, can convert this zone into an area of complete tissue loss. With proper wound care, however, these pathophysiological changes may be reversed. The zone of stasis is surrounded by a zone of hyperemia. In this outermost zone, tissue perfusion is increased. The tissue here will invariably recover unless there is severe sepsis or prolonged hypoperfusion. The three zones of a burn were described by Jackson in 1947. These three zones of a burn are three-dimensional, and loss of tissue in the zone of stasis will lead to the wound deepening as well as widening.

Primary tissue loss in burn injury occurs as a result of protein denaturation secondary to thermal, chemical, electrical, friction, or ultraviolet radiation induced insults. This process is rapidly followed by activation of toxic inflammatory mediators, especially in the perfused subsurface. Oxidants and proteases further damage skin and capillary endothelial cells, potentiating ischemic tissue necrosis Burn wound conversion is also attributed to the secondary consequences of burn injury. Sequelae such as edema, infection, and altered perfusion promote progression of injury beyond the degree of initial cell death. Burn-induced disruption of collagen cross-linking abolishes the integrity of osmotic and hydrostatic pressure gradients, resulting in local edema and larger scale fluid shifts. In addition, damage to cell membranes results in a dynamic cascade of inflammatory mediators that exacerbate already abnormal cell-to-cell permeability, worsening fluid regulation and systemic inflammatory responses. At the molecular level, both complement activation and intravascular stimulation of neutrophils result in the production of cytotoxic oxygen free radicals. Increased histamine activity, enhanced by the catalytic properties of xanthine oxidase, causes progressive local increases in vascular permeability. Toxic byproducts of xanthine oxidase, including hydrogen peroxide and hydroxyl radicals, appear to directly damage dermal structures. One major component of burn shock is the increase in total body capillary permeability. Direct thermal injury results in marked changes in the microcirculation. Most of the changes occur locally at the burn site, when maximal edema formation occurs at about 8–12 h post-injury in smaller burns and 12–24 h post-injury in major thermal injuries. The rate of progression of tissue edema is dependent upon the adequacy of resuscitation.

The temperature of the heat source and the length of exposure determine the extent of tissue destruction (time-temperature curve). Patients burned by higher temperatures (molten metal, hot grease, or flammable clothing) have deeper burns than those burned with hot water. The effect also varies over different types and parts of the body. The result of heat injury is affected by variables such as skin thickness. The thicker, glabrous skin of the palms and soles is more resistant to full-thickness injury than is the thinner skin of the eyelid or dorsum of the hand. Infant skin is also thinner than adult skin and more likely to sustain full-thickness injury from the same temperature.

The depth of any injury is not always obvious initially, and observers often disagree. Many methods have been proposed to predict the depth of the injury immediately or soon after injury (ultrasound examination, intravenous fluorescent probes), but none has been as reliable as serial examination of the wound over time. The final depth of the injury typically becomes obvious 48–72 h after injury. Very rarely does the thermal injury penetrate into the subcutaneous or deep tissue.

Systemic response

The release of cytokines and other inflammatory mediators at the site of injury has a systemic effect once the burn reaches 30% TBSA. Cutaneous thermal injury greater than one-third of the TBSA invariably results in the severe and unique derangements of cardiovascular function called burn shock. Shock is an abnormal physiologic state in which tissue perfusion is insufficient to maintain adequate delivery of oxygen and nutrients and removal of cellular waste products. Unresuscitated burn shock correlates with increased hematocrit values in burned patients, which are secondary to fluid and electrolyte loss after burn injury. Increased hematocrit values occurring shortly after severe burn injury result from fluid and protein translocation into both burned and non-burned tissues.

Burn shock is a complex process of circulatory and microcirculatory dysfunction that is not easily or fully repaired by fluid resuscitation. Severe burn injury results in significant hypovolemic shock and substantial tissue trauma, both of which cause the formation and release of many local and systemic mediators. Burn shock results from the interplay of hypovolemia and the release of multiple mediators of inflammation with effects on both the microcirculation and the function of the heart, large vessels and lungs. Subsequently, burn shock continues as a significant pathophysiologic state, even if hypovolemia is corrected. Increases in pulmonary and systemic vascular resistance (SVR) and myocardial depression occur despite adequate preload and volume support. Such cardiovascular dysfunctions can further exacerbate the whole body inflammatory response into a vicious cycle of accelerating organ dysfunction.

Hypovolemia and fluid extravasation

Burn injury causes extravasation of plasma into the burn wound and the surrounding tissues. Extensive burn injuries are hypovolemic in nature and characterized by the hemodynamic changes similar to those that occur after hemorrhage, including decreased plasma volume, cardiac output, urine output, and an increased systemic vascular resistance with resultant reduced peripheral blood flow. However, as opposed to a fall in hematocrit with hemorrhagic hypovolemia, due to transcapillary refill an increase in hematocrit and hemoglobin concentration will often appear even with adequate fluid resuscitation. As in the treatment of other forms of hypovolemic shock, the primary initial therapeutic goal is to quickly restore vascular volume and to preserve tissue perfusion to minimize tissue ischemia. The critical concept in burn shock is that massive fluid shifts can occur even though total body water remains unchanged. What actually changes is the volume of each fluid compartment, intracellular and interstitial volumes increasing at the expense of plasma volume and blood volume. In extensive burns (>25% TBSA), fluid resuscitation is complicated not only by the severe burn wound edema, but also by extravasated and sequestered fluid and protein in nonburned soft tissue. Large volumes of resuscitation solutions are required to maintain vascular volume during the first several hours after an extensive burn. Multiple formulae have been published with variations in both the volumes per weight suggested and the type or types of crystalloid or crystalloid-colloid combinations administered to approximate the fluid need of a burn patient. To date, no single recommendation has been distinguished as the most successful approach. A detailed description of various formulae appears later in this chapter. It should be emphasized that blind adherence to any formula can result in 'overresuscitation' and thereby to massive volume overload and edema. All formulae represent only a rough guideline to estimate the fluid need. Successful fluid resuscitation has to be adapted to the clinical need and to the monitoring (urinary output, sufficient mean arterial pressure). Data suggest that despite fluid resuscitation normal blood volume is not restored until 24–36 h after large burns. Edema formation often follows a biphasic pattern. An immediate and rapid increase in the water content of burn tissue is seen in the first hour after burn injury. A second and more gradual increase in fluid flux of both the burned skin and nonburned soft tissue occurs during the first 12–24 h following burn trauma.

The tissues in ischemic areas can potentially be salvaged by proper resuscitation in the initial stages and by proper burn wound excision and antimicrobial therapy in the convalescent period. Underresuscitation can convert this area into deep dermal or full-thickness burns in areas not initially injured to that extent. Reevaluation of these threatened areas over the first several days is used to determine when the first burn excision should be performed (i.e., when the depth of burn has become apparent and decisions about which areas are deep dermal or full thickness are clear).

A new area of interest with immediate resuscitation is the use of negative pressure dressings on affected areas. Animal models and early clinical work suggest that this treatment may limit the conversion of zones of hyperemia to zones of ischemia by removing edematous fluid and allowing salvage of areas that would otherwise need excision and grafting.

Mediators of burn injury

Apart from the burn shock mechanism already described, burn injury produces a veritable cornucopia of local and circulating mediators that are produced in the blood or released by cells after thermal injury. These mediators clearly play important, but complex roles in the pathogenesis of edema and the cardiovascular abnormalities of burn injury. Osteomuscular proteolysis, lipolysis, gluconeogenesis, increased metabolic rate, and a severe systemic inflammatory response are induced by local infections or surgical procedures. The increased vascular permeability post-burn is mediated by histamine and numerous vasoactive substances, including serotonin, bradykinin, prostaglandins, leukotrienes, and platelet activating factor. Hyper-metabolism is mediated by hormones such as catecholamines, glucagon, and particularly cortisol.

Hints and tips

- A burn results in three distinct zones: coagulation, stasis, and hyperemia
- The aim of burns resuscitation is to maintain perfusion of the zone of stasis
- Systemic response occurs once a burn is greater than 30% of total body surface area
- Different burn mechanisms lead to different injury patterns.

Initial evaluation and treatment

Treatment of a burned patient starts at the scene of injury with the safe removal of the patient from the cause of the burn. In all cases (especially if chemical or electrical burns), care must be taken to avoid personal injury by checking the area is safe and that appropriate protective clothing is worn if necessary. Priority should be given to assessing the person's airway, breathing, and circulation, and presence of any coexisting injuries which may require more urgent treatment than the burn. Belts, clothes, jewelry and watches that can retain heat and cause constriction should be removed and the patient kept aware. An inhalation injury should be assumed and airway should checked and oxygen given. Heat can be dissipated from the burn wound by cooling with water but cold water and ice should not be used as they can cause rapid hypothermia. A quick assessment should be made for associated trauma and the patient transported to the nearest burn unit for definitive management (Box 18.1, Fig. 18.5).

Once the patient arrives at the emergency room, an evaluation of the Airway, Breathing, and Circulation (the ABCs) should receive first priority (Box 18.2). It is also important to exclude associated trauma. The history should include the time, location and circumstances of the injury, where the patient was found, and their condition (Box 18.3). Past medical and social history, current medication usage, drug allergies, and tetanus status should be rapidly determined. It is also important to consider the possibility of nonaccidental burns or scalding (Box 18.4).

Box 18.2 **Initial assessment of a major burn**

Perform an ABCDEF primary survey:
A – Airway with cervical spine control
B – Breathing
C – Circulation
D – Neurological disability
E – Exposure with environmental control
F – Fluid resuscitation

- Assess burn size and depth
- Establish good intravenous access and give fluids (in children, the interosseous route can be used for fluid administration if intravenous access cannot be obtained)
- Give analgesia
- Catheterize patient or establish fluid balance monitoring
- Take baseline blood samples for investigation (full blood count; urea and electrolyte concentration; clotting screen; blood group; and save or cross-match serum)
- Electrical injuries
  - 12-lead electrocardiography
  - Cardiac enzymes (for high tension injuries)
- Inhalational injuries
  - Chest X-ray
  - Arterial blood gas analysis
- Dress wound
- After completion of the primary survey, a secondary survey should assess the depth and TBSA burned, reassess, and exclude or treat associated injuries
- Arrange safe transfer to specialist burns facility.

A thorough assessment of a person with a burn should then take into account:

- The type of burn (e.g., flame, scald, electrical, or chemical)
- The depth and extent of the burn, and therefore the severity
- The risk of inhalation injury (singed nasal hair, black carbon in the sputum, or carbon in the oropharynx) *(Box 18.5)*
- Any coexisting medical conditions (e.g., cardiac, respiratory, or hepatic disease; diabetes; pregnancy; or immunocompromised state)
- Any predisposing factors which may require further investigation or treatment (e.g., a burn resulting from a fit or faint)
- The possibility of nonaccidental injury
- The person's social circumstances (e.g., ability to self-care or need for admission).

The airway should be secured because upper airway obstruction can develop quickly *(Fig. 18.6)*. Smoke inhalation causes more than 50% of fire-related deaths. Patients sustaining an inhalation injury may require aggressive airway intervention *(Fig. 18.7)*. Most injuries result from the inhalation of toxic smoke; however, super-heated air may rarely cause direct thermal injury to the upper respiratory tract (see complications, below). Patients who are breathing spontaneously and at risk for inhalation injury should be placed on high-flow humidified oxygen. Patients trapped in buildings or those caught in an explosion are at higher risk for inhalation injury. These patients may have facial burns, singeing of the eyebrows and nasal hair, pharyngeal burns, carbonaceous

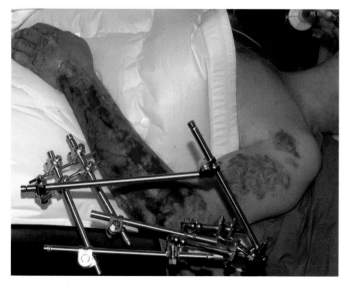

Fig. 18.5 Burns patients often have other injuries that require attention.

Box 18.3 **Key points of a burn history**

Exact mechanism
- Nature of injury (scald, flame, flash, contact, electrical, chemical)
- How did it come into contact with patient?
- What first aid was performed?
- What treatment has been started?
- Is there risk of concomitant injuries (such as fall from height, road traffic crash, explosion)?

Inhalational injuries
- Is there risk of inhalational injuries (did burn occur in an enclosed space)?
- If possible, the nature of burning materials (furniture, polyurethane foam, polyvinyl chloride, etc.)

Exact timings
- The time elapsed from burn/injury/smoke inhalation to arrival in hospital
- How long was patient exposed to energy source? *or*
- How long was the patient exposed to smoke?
- How long was cooling applied?
- When was fluid resuscitation started?

Scalds
- What was the liquid?
- Was it boiling or recently boiled?
- If tea or coffee, was milk in it?
- Was a solute in the liquid? (Raises boiling temperature and causes worse injury, such as boiling rice)
- Is there any suspicion of nonaccidental injury?

Electrocution injuries
- What was the voltage (high or low)?
- Was there a flash or arcing?
- Contact time

Chemical injuries
- What was the chemical?

Box 18.5 **Signs of inhalational injury**

- History of flame burns or burns in an enclosed space
- Full thickness or deep dermal burns to face, neck, or upper thorax
- Singed nasal hair
- Carbonaceous sputum or carbon particles in oropharynx.

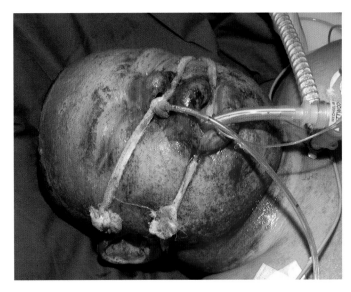

Fig. 18.6 The airway must be secured early in cases of airway involvement.

Box 18.4 **Indicators of possible nonaccidental burns or scalds**

- Delay in seeking help
- Historical accounts of injury differ over time
- History inconsistent with the injury presented or with the developmental capacity of a child
- Past abuse or family violence
- Inappropriate behavior/interaction of child or caregivers
- Glove and sock pattern scalds
- Scalds with clear-cut immersion lines
- Absence of splash marks in a scald injury. A child falling into a bath will splash; one that is placed into it may not
- Burns to palms, soles, genitalia, buttocks, perineum
- Is there sparing of flexion creases – that is, was child in fetal position (position of protection) when burnt? Does this correlate to a "tideline" of scald – that is, if child is put into a fetal position, do the burns line up?
- "Doughnut sign," an area of spared skin surrounded by scald. If a child is forcibly held down in a bath of hot water, the part in contact with the bottom of the bath will not burn, but the tissue around will
- Symmetrical burns of uniform depth
- Restraint injuries on upper limbs
- Other signs of physical abuse – bruises of varied age, poorly kempt, lack of compliance with healthcare (such as no immunizations)

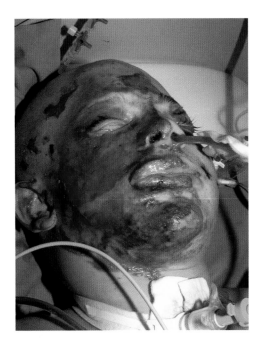

Fig. 18.7 Inhalation injury necessitates aggressive airway interventions, here nasopharyngeal suction.

sputum, or impaired mentation. A progressive change in voice quality or hoarseness, stridorous respirations, or wheezing may be noted. The upper airway may be visualized by laryngoscopy, and the tracheobronchial tree should be evaluated by bronchoscopy. Chest radiography is not sensitive for detecting inhalation injury. Patients who have suffered an inhalation injury are also at risk for carbon monoxide poisoning. The pulse oximeter is not accurate in patients with carbon monoxide poisoning because only oxyhemoglobin and deoxyhemoglobin are detected. Co-oximetry measurements are necessary to confirm the diagnosis of carbon monoxide poisoning. Other pulmonary assessments include arterial blood gas measurements and bronchoscopy. Patients exposed to carbon monoxide should receive 100% oxygen using a nonrebreather facemask.

Burn assessment

After completion of the primary survey, a secondary survey must include assessment of the depth and TBSA burned (*Figs 18.8–18.10*).

Diagnosis/patient presentation

Accurate assessment of burn depth on admission is important in making decisions about dressings and surgery (*Table 18.2*).

Age	0–1	1–4	5–9	10–14	15
A – ½ of head	9½%	8½%	6½%	5½%	4½%
B – ½ of one thigh	9½%	8½%	6½%	5½%	4½%
C – ½ of one leg	9½%	8½%	6½%	5½%	4½%

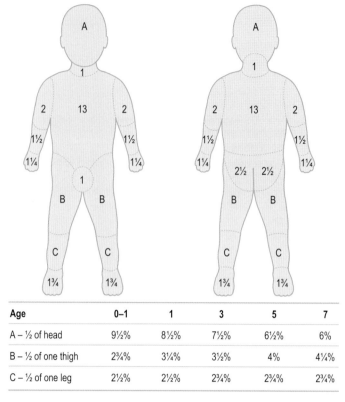

Age	0–1	1	3	5	7
A – ½ of head	9½%	8½%	7½%	6½%	6%
B – ½ of one thigh	2¾%	3¼%	3½%	4%	4¼%
C – ½ of one leg	2½%	2½%	2¾%	2¾%	2¾%

Fig. 18.9 Body surface area calculations in children must account for unique pediatric body proportions, here with the Lund and Browner method.

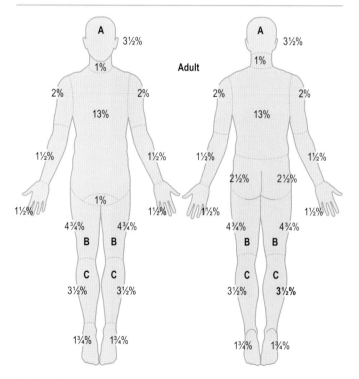

Fig. 18.8 Estimation of burn size with the Lund and Browner method. (From: Herndon DN, ed. Total Burn Care, 2nd edn. Edinburgh: Elsevier.)

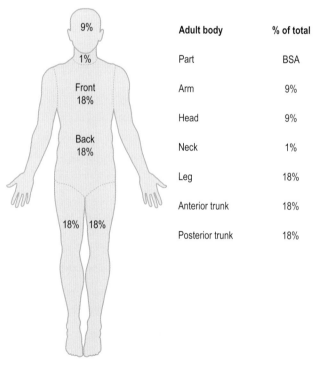

Adult body Part	% of total BSA
Arm	9%
Head	9%
Neck	1%
Leg	18%
Anterior trunk	18%
Posterior trunk	18%

Fig. 18.10 Estimation of burn size with Wallace's 'rule of nines': head and neck, 9%; each arm, 9%; anterior torso, 18%; posterior torso, 18%; each leg, 9%; genitalia/perineum, 1%. BSA, body surface area. (From: Herndon DN, ed. Total Burn Care, 2nd edn. Edinburgh: Elsevier.)

Table 18.2 Typical findings in burn injuries

Depth of burn	Skin involvement	Example	Signs	Sensation	% TBSA	Healing capacity	Healing time	Scarring
Epidermal burn	Epidermis	UV light, very short flash, sunburn	Dry and red, blanches with pressure, no blisters	May be painful	Should not be calculated in the extent of the burned surface area	Should be left to heal by itself	Within 7 days	No scarring
Superficial partial thickness burn	Epidermis and part of the papillary dermis	Scald (spill or splash), short flash	Pale pink with fine blistering, blanches with pressure	Usually extremely painful	Part of the % burned area	Should be left to heal by itself	Within 14 days	Can have color match defect. Low to moderate risk of hypertrophic scarring
Deep partial thickness burn	Epidermis, the entire papillary dermis down to reticular dermis	Scald (spill), flame, oil or grease	Dark pink to blotchy red, may be with large blisters, no capillary refill sluggish to none. In child, may be dark lobster red with mottling	May be painful or reduced/absent sensation	Part of the % burned area	Should not be left to heal by itself, but instead should probably be submitted to surgery	14–over 21 days	Moderate to high risk of hypertrophic scarring
Full thickness burn	Entire thickness of the skin and possibly deeper	Scald (immersion), flame, steam, oil, grease, chemical, high-volt electricity	White, waxy or charred, no blisters, no capillary refill. May be dark lobster red with mottling in child	No sensation	Part of the % burned area	No healing capacity and as such should always be submitted to surgery.	Does not heal spontaneously, grafting needed if >1 cm	Will scar

Box 18.6 **Burn reconstruction priorities**

Urgent and important procedures
- Deformities affecting vital function (e.g., airway, oral continence, protection of the eye, and hand function)
- Compression/entrapment or neurovascular bundles
- Severe contractures

Important procedures
- Restoration of function (e.g., joint contractures)
- Progressive deformities that prevent performing of activities of daily living not correctable by nonsurgical rehabilitation

Desirable procedures
- Aesthetics (e.g., pigmentation changes, textural irregularities)
- Contractures causing discomfort
- Resurfacing (e.g., unstable epithelium).

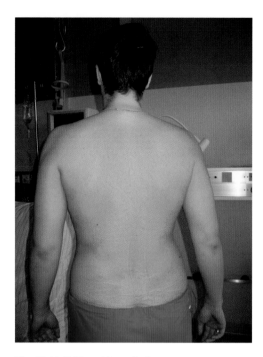

Fig. 18.11 Epidermal burn. Sunburn.

However, the burn wound is a dynamic living environment that will alter depending on both intrinsic factors (such as release of inflammatory mediators, bacterial proliferation) and extrinsic factors (such as dehydration, systemic hypotension, cooling). There is much evidence to demonstrate the beneficial effects of cooling on reducing tissue damage and wound healing time. Although immediate cooling is preferable, even a 30 min delay in application of cooling is still beneficial to the burn wound but the application of cooling 60 min after injury, does not demonstrate any benefit.[8] Tetanus prophylaxis must be considered wherever there is tissue damage, and particularly in elderly patients. It is therefore important to review the wound at regular intervals until healing.

Optimum treatment of the wound reduces morbidity and, in larger injuries, mortality. It also shortens the time for healing and return to normal function and reduces the need for secondary reconstruction *(Box 18.6)*. When epithelialization is delayed beyond 3 weeks, the incidence of hypertrophic scarring rises. Hypertrophic scars occur in 60% of burned children aged under 5 years. Optimal burn care requires early excision and grafting of all burns that will produce hypertrophic scars (typically those that will not or have not healed within 3 weeks of the injury), so an accurate estimation of burn depth is crucial. Early grafting of those burns that have not healed at three weeks has been shown to improve the result, but because of delays in the referral process, all injuries, which show no sign of healing by 10 days, should be referred for assessment. The appearance of the wound – and the apparent burn depth – changes dramatically within the first 7–10 days. A burn appearing shallow on day 1 may appear considerably deeper by day 3. This demarcation of the burn is a consequence of thrombosis of dermal blood vessels and the death of thermally injured skin cells. Superficial burns may convert to deeper burns due to infection, desiccation of the wound, or the use of vasoactive agents during resuscitation from shock.

Epidermal burns

These burns involve only the epidermis. They do not blister, but are red and quite painful *(Fig. 18.11)*. Over 2–3 days, the erythema and the pain subside. Supportive therapy is usually all that is required, with regular analgesia and intravenous fluids for extensive injuries *(Fig. 18.12)*. By about day 4, the injured epithelium peels away from the newly healed epidermis underneath, a process which is commonly seen after sunburn. By day 7, healing is complete by regeneration from undamaged keratinocytes within skin adnexae. The patient should be advised of measures to provide symptomatic relief, e.g., take a cool bath or shower; apply topical emollients; apply cold compresses; take simple analgesia (e.g., paracetamol or ibuprofen); maintain adequate hydration to prevent heat exhaustion or heat stroke.

Superficial partial thickness burns

These affect the epidermis and superficial dermis. Blistering is common. The exposed superficial nerves make these injuries painful. Healing is expected within 14 days by regeneration of epidermis from keratinocytes within sweat glands and hair follicles *(Figs 18.13, 18.14)*. First-degree burns are not considered in calculation of the TBSA burned.

They do not extend entirely through dermis and leave behind epithelial-lined dermal appendages including sweat glands, hair follicles, and sebaceous glands *(Figs 18.13, 18.14)*. When dead dermal tissue is removed, epithelial cells migrate from the surface of each dermal appendage to other epithelial cells from neighboring appendages, forming a new, fragile epidermis on top of a thin residual dermal bed. The rate of regeneration depends on the density of these skin adnexae: thin hairless skin (inner arm, eyelids, etc.) heals more slowly than thick or hairy skin (back, scalp, and face). Most superficial facial burns heal well with watchful neglect. Progression to a deeper burn is unlikely but can occur if the wound dries out or becomes infected or the patient becomes systemically unwell or hypotensive. Treatment is aimed at preventing wound progression by the use of antimicrobial creams and occlusive dressings, since epithelialization progresses faster in a moist environment. There is considerable disagreement

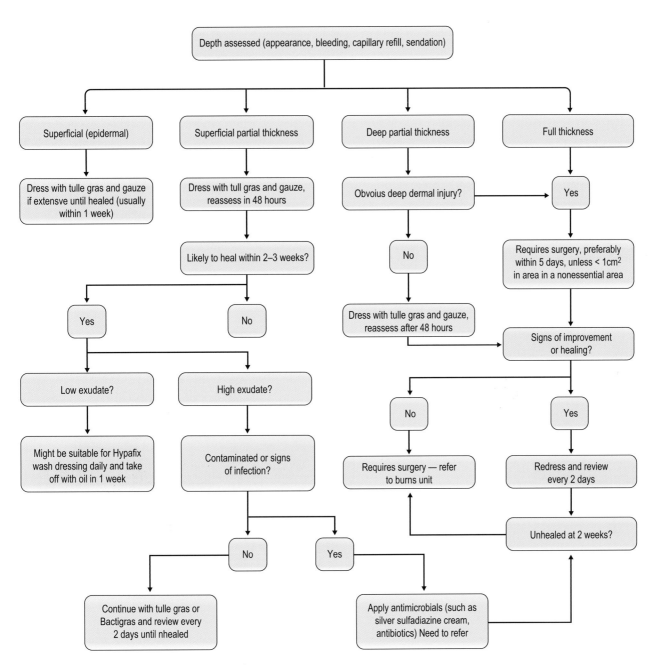

Fig. 18.12 Protocol for the management of burn wounds.

regarding the management of blisters, but there is weak evidence from one controlled study that leaving blisters intact results in fewer burns becoming colonized with bacteria at 10 days, compared with aspiration or de-roofing (15% *v* 73% *v* 78%).

All superficial partial thickness burns should heal with supervised neglect but, outcome can be improved by appropriate management. If the burn wound has not healed within 14 days of injury, the depth has probably been assessed incorrectly and referral should be made to a burns unit.

Deep partial thickness

These wounds are the most difficult to assess and treat. Nevertheless, distinguishing between deep partial thickness burns that are best treated by early excision and grafting

and superficial partial thickness burns that heal spontaneously is not always straightforward, and many burn wounds have a mixture of superficial and deep partial thickness burns, making precise classification of the entire wound difficult *(Fig. 18.12)*. They may initially seem superficial, with blanching on pressure, but have fixed capillary staining on re-examination after 48 h. With deeper burns, the density of the appendages (and hence islands of regeneration) contributing to healing is less, appendages so the burn takes longer to heal, the scarring is more severe and associated with contraction. Therefore, if these injuries are extensive or in functional or cosmetically sensitive areas, they are better excised to a viable depth and then skin grafted to reduce morbidity and to speed return to normal function. Some deep partial thickness injuries will heal if the wound environment is optimized to encourage endogenous healing. This includes keeping it

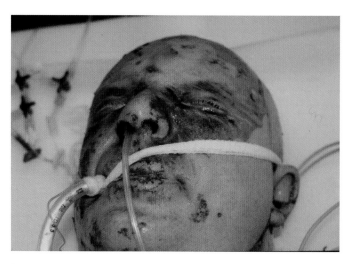

Fig. 18.13 Patient with inhalational injury must be intubated before the onset of oropharyngeal edema.

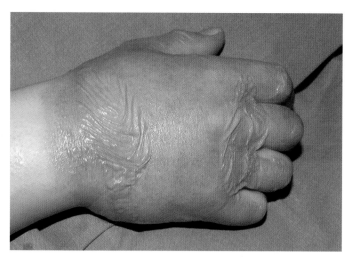

Fig. 18.15 Full thickness scald injury of the hand.

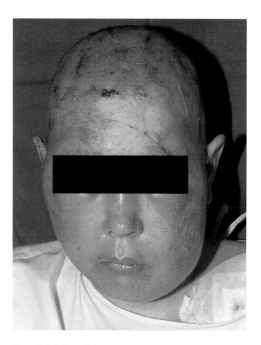

Fig. 18.14 Superficial partial thickness burns of the face.

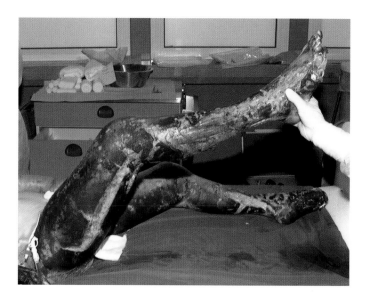

Fig. 18.16 Full thickness bilateral lower limb burns.

warm, moist, and free of infection. If infection is prevented and spontaneous healing is allowed to progress, these burns will heal in 3–9 weeks. Deep partial thickness burns that require longer than 3 weeks to heal routinely produce hypertrophic scars, frequently lead to functional impairment, even with physical therapy and provide only a thin epithelial covering that remains fragile for many weeks or months.

Full thickness injuries

Full-thickness or third-degree burns involve all layers of the epidermis and dermis and may destroy subcutaneous structures *(Fig. 18.15)*. They appear white or charred *(Fig. 18.16)*. These burns are usually insensate because of destruction of nerve endings, but the surrounding areas are extremely painful. All regenerative elements have been destroyed in

these injuries, and healing only occurs from the edges and is associated with considerable contraction. Full-thickness burns involve all layers of the dermis and often injure underlying subcutaneous adipose tissue as well. Burn eschar is structurally intact but dead and denatured dermis. Over days and weeks if left *in situ*, eschar separates from the underlying viable tissue, leaving an open, unhealed bed of granulation tissue. Without surgery, they can heal only by wound contracture with epithelialization from the wound margins. Some full-thickness burns involve not only all layers of the skin, but also deeper structures such as muscle, tendon, ligament and bone. All such injuries should therefore be excised and grafted unless they are <1 cm in diameter in an area where function would not be compromised *(Fig. 18.12)*.

Careful calculation of the burn injured TBSA is necessary to guide fluid resuscitation. For adults, Wallace's 'rule of nines' is a simple and accurate method of calculating TBSA burned *(Fig. 18.11)*. However, in children, the Lund and Browder chart is more accurate as it accounts for the different

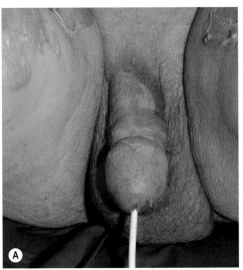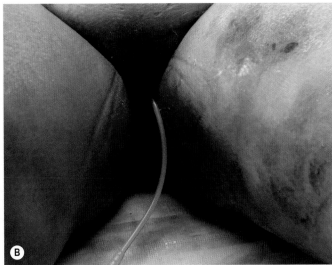

Fig. 18.17 (A,B) Burned genitalia should be catheterized in both sexes.

body proportions in infants and children *(Figs 18.9, 18.10)*. For all patients burn diagrams and photographs of the burn wounds should be placed in the medical record and updated if the burn wound extends.

Extremities should be examined for signs of circumferential burns and signs of compartment syndrome. Compartment pressures can be measured and escharotomy should be performed for pressures >40 mmHg and considered for those >25 mmHg. Fasciotomies may also be performed for electrical burns where the deep muscular compartments are effected, for diagnostic purposes such as accessing deeper tissues, evaluating the condition of the underlying muscles with direct observation and determining the extent of muscle necrosis. For patients with facial burns, fluorescent staining of the cornea and ophthalmological review are necessary. For patients with genital burns a urethral catheter should be placed *(Fig. 18.17)*. For patients with perineal burns a rectal catheter should be placed. Specific burn circumstances such as chemical and electrical burn injuries, may dictate further diagnostic studies and treatments (see later). Tetanus prophylaxis should be considered.

Inhalation injury

Smoke inhalation causes more than 50% of fire-related deaths. Smoke inhalation principally affects the respiratory system, and constitutes a major cause of mortality and morbidity in burn patients. Patients with inhalation injuries are associated with higher mortality rates than patients without inhalation injury. Inhalation injuries are likely to cause a patient's condition to weaken and to result in an increased mortality rate, but many patients with inhalation injury are also likely to sustain more severe cutaneous burns, which can also cause death.[9] Smoke inhalation has been recognized for many years but it is only relatively recently that its significance in substantially increasing the mortality in patients who also have cutaneous burns has been quantified these disasters are fortunately infrequent and contribute only a small percentage to the annual overall mortality from smoke inhalation and burns. Most smoke inhalation victims are injured in domestic fires

and therefore present sporadically. The type of respiratory injury sustained is influenced, in large part, by the magnitude of exposure, as well as the type and properties of the toxic gases and chemicals comprising the smoke to which the patient is exposed.[10]

Injury can occur to the airway during a fire or explosion and greatly complicate the cutaneous burn injury. Patients caught in an enclosed, smoke-filled space are at risk for inhalation injury. They may or may not have facial burns, erythema of the mucous membranes, and soot in the airways. Thermal injury from the flame or hot gases can damage the upper airway (supraglottic). This results in burns of the lips and oropharynx, leading to edema and airway obstruction. Heat rarely causes subglottic injury. The products of combustion, though cooled by the time they reach the lungs, act as direct irritants to the lungs, leading to bronchospasm, inflammation, and bronchorrhea. The ciliary action of pneumocytes is impaired, exacerbating the situation. The inflammatory exudate created is not cleared, and atelectasis or pneumonia follows. Acute responses to inhalation injury cause a release of inflammatory mediators, the effects of which are not limited to the lung and bronchus but also affect systemic vascular resistance. Furthermore, intravascular volume deficiency which frequency leads to reduced cardiac output and stroke volume, occurs due to increased permeability of the capillary bed and substantial interstitial fluid accumulation. This hypovolemic condition requires excessive fluid resuscitation, which could cause an overload of cardiopulmonary function during the refilling phase. The situation can be particularly severe in asthmatic patients.

Carbon monoxide binds to deoxyhemoglobin with 40 times the affinity of oxygen. It also binds to intracellular proteins, particularly the cytochrome oxidase pathway. These two effects lead to intracellular and extracellular hypoxia. In the presence of carboxyhemoglobin, conventional electrode blood gas analysers display erroneously high values for the calculated oxygen saturation and content, giving the unwary a false sense of security. In these circumstances pulse oximetry is also inaccurate as it cannot differentiate between oxyhemoglobin and carboxyhemoglobin, and may therefore give

Table 18.3 Signs of carboxyhemoglobinemia

Carboxyhemoglobin levels	Symptoms
0–10%	Minimal (normal level in heavy smokers)
10–20%	Nausea, headache
20–30%	Drowsiness, lethargy
30–40%	Confusion, agitation
40–50%	Coma, respiratory depression
>50%	Death

Box 18.7 **Indications for intubation**

- Erythema or swelling of oropharynx on direct visualization
- Change in voice, with hoarseness or harsh cough
- Stridor, tachypnea, or dyspnea
- Carbonaceous particles staining a patient's face after a burn in an enclosed space.

normal results *(Table 18.3)*. A blood oximeter, however, accurately determines oxygen saturation and content and also rapidly measures carboxyhemoglobin concentrations. However, arterial blood gas analysis will reveal metabolic acidosis and raised carboxyhemoglobin levels but may not show hypoxia. Treatment is with 100% oxygen with a non-rebreather facemask, which displaces carbon monoxide from bound proteins six times faster than does atmospheric oxygen. For instance, the amount of carbon monoxide produced in a car engine can cause fatal carbon monoxide poisoning without producing enough particulate matter to cause chemical pneumonitis. Conversely, patients can inhale significant smoke and have normal carboxyhemoglobin levels because of the rapid clearance of carbon monoxide from the blood after administration of oxygen during transport. Direct laryngoscopy and bronchoscopy more accurately assess airway injury but can still be misleading. A nuclear medicine study with technetium Tc99m uptake in the lung can also be used for diagnostic purposes. Noninvasive management can be attempted, with nebulizers and positive pressure ventilation with some positive end-expiratory pressure. However, patients may need a period of ventilation, as this allows adequate oxygenation and permits regular lung toileting. The typical adult respiratory distress syndrome picture of inhalation injury may not be manifested as altered pulmonary gas exchange and chest radiographic changes for several hours to days after injury.

Patients with carboxyhemoglobin levels greater than 25–30% indicate a significant exposure to fumes but are not always predictive of inhalation injury but should be ventilated. Hyperbaric oxygen therapy reduces the half-life of carbon monoxide to 23 min. Hyperbaric oxygen is recommended for patients with carboxyhemoglobin levels greater than 25%, myocardial ischemia, cardiac dysrhythmias, or neuropsychiatric abnormalities. Hyperbaric oxygen is also recommended for pregnant women and young children with carboxyhemoglobin levels of ≥15%.

Dicobalt edetate is standard treatment for massive cyanide poisoning in cases of ingestion or industrial accident. It may not be appropriate, however, for patients who have inhaled smoke as poisoning by inhalation is limited, with no further absorption after respiratory arrest or rescue. In the presence of low plasma concentrations of free cyanide dicobalt edetate itself can be toxic. A better approach is to use sodium nitrite, which converts hemoglobin to methemoglobin, though in a patient whose oxygen delivery is already compromised by a high carboxyhemoglobin concentration a further decrease

in the hemoglobin available for oxygen transport can be dangerous.

There is no effective treatment of inhalation injury other than supportive care, there is a real lack of motivation to develop a truly reliable test. The early accurate diagnosis of the condition has little therapeutic implication. Pulmonary injury results in sequestration of fluid in the lungs. When fluid resuscitation for the visible cutaneous thermal injury far exceeds the predicted amount, inhalation injury should be suspected. Decreasing fluid intake in these patients may decrease extravasation of fluid in the pulmonary parenchyma, but the need to maintain intravascular volume and tissue perfusion may be more important. In significant inhalation injury, fluid requirements are large, pulmonary capillary leakage is significant, and impairment of gas exchange is inevitable. Early endotracheal intubation is important in patients with upper airway or inhalation injury to safeguard patency of the airway, to deliver mechanical ventilatory support, and to provide aggressive pulmonary toilet *(Box 18.7)*. To date, we can provide only supportive care for pulmonary failure from inhalation injury because no effective therapy has been identified for prevention or treatment of the damage to the alveoli by the inhaled toxins. Hyperbaric oxygen treatment has been used for acute carbon monoxide poisoning from smoke inhalation. Hyperbaric therapy is rarely practical and has not been proved to be advantageous. It takes longer to shift the carbon monoxide from the cytochrome oxidase pathway than from hemoglobin, so oxygen therapy should be continued until the metabolic acidosis has cleared.

Management of moderate to severe burns

Initiation of fluid resuscitation should precede initial wound care. In adults, IV fluid resuscitation is usually necessary in burns involving >20% TBSA. In pediatric patients, fluid resuscitation should be initiated in all infants with burns of ≥10% TBSA and in older children with burns ≥15% TBSA. Two large-bore IV lines should be placed and fluid should be given. Intraosseous line placement may be required in children in the proximal tibia or the distal femur. Lactated Ringer's solution is the most commonly used fluid for burn resuscitation. Urine output should be used as a measure of renal perfusion and to assess fluid balance. In adults, a urine output of 0.5–1.0 mL/kg per hour should be maintained. Patients with significant burns should have a Foley catheter inserted in order to monitor urine output. The color and consistency of the initial urine in patients with severe flame or high voltage electrical burns should be noted. The urine may already be black, indicating hemoglobinuria or myoglobinuria, or both. This is of prognostic importance for subsequent renal function. In elderly patients, patients with cardiorespiratory disease, and patients who have delayed presentation consider inserting a central venous pressure line. This can play an important part in the subsequent restoration of volume in a patient with a severe burn. The risks of infection related to a central line are small in the early stages. With current methods of line management these risks are outweighed by the importance of the line for monitoring and access. A nasogastric (NG) tube should be placed in patients with burns involving ≥20% TBSA in order to prevent gastric distention and associated emesis.

Resuscitation formulae

Sufficient resuscitation to prevent burn shock is the single most important therapeutic intervention in burn treatment but due to a lack of evidence-based literature, burn resuscitation remains an area of clinical practice driven primarily by local custom of treating burn units.[11] Fluid replacement is based on the observation that fluid loss from the vascular space occurs at a constant rate during the first day after injury. The amount of replacement fluid is predicted from the extent of burn and size of the patient, and fluid replacement should proceed at the same rate as the loss *(Table 18.4)*. Fluid administered in excess of the leak is excreted by the kidney or results in increased hydrostatic pressure and extra interstitial edema. All fluid is therefore administered at a constant rate, and fluid boluses are avoided. Lactated Ringer's solution most closely resembles normal body fluids. Factors that influence fluid requirements during resuscitation besides TBSA burn include burn depth, inhalation injury, associated injuries, age, delay in resuscitation, need for escharotomies/fasciotomies, and use of alcohol or drugs. The Parkland formula has been renamed the Consensus formula because it is the most widely used resuscitation guideline. The Advanced Burn Life Support curriculum supports the use of the Consensus formula for resuscitation in burn injury. It is 4 mL/kg/% TBSA, describing the amount of lactated Ringer's solution required in the first 24 h after burn injury. Starting from the time of burn injury, half of the fluid is given in the first 8 h and the remaining half is given over the next 16 h. As an example, by the Parkland formula, a 70 kg patient with a 40% TBSA burn receives (70×40×4)=11 200 mL of lactated Ringer solution during the first 24 h after the burn (approx. 470 mL/h).

Crystalloids are the resuscitation fluids of choice given the lack of survival benefit and increased cost associated with albumin and a meta-analysis comparing albumin to crystalloid showed a more than doubled mortality rate with albumin. Albumin is contraindicated in the first 24 h post-burn, but may have a role in severe burns (>50% TBSA) after the first 24 h. Hypertonic saline has also had disappointing results, with a quadrupled increase in renal failure and twice the mortality of patients given lactated Ringer's solution. Hypertonic saline does not routinely have a place in burn resuscitation.

Table 18.4 Fluid resuscitation formulae

Formula	Electrolyte	Colloid	Glucose
Colloid formulae			
Brooke	Lactated Ringer's at 1.5 mL/kg/% TBSA burn	0.5 mL/kg/% TBSA burn	2 L 5% dextrose
Evans	0.9% NaCl at 1 mL/kg/% TBSA burn	1 mL/kg/% TBSA burn	2 L 5% dextrose
Slater	Lactated Ringer's 2 L/24 h	Fresh Frozen Plasma at 75 mL/kg/24 h	2 L 5% dextrose
Crystalloid formulae			
Modified Brooke's	Lactated Ringer's at 2 mL/kg/% TBSA burn		
Parkland	Lactated Ringer's at 4 mL/kg/% TBSA burn	20–60% estimated plasma volume	Titrated to urinary output of 30 mL/h
Hypertonic saline formulae			
Hypertonic saline solution (Monafo)	Maintain UO at 30 mL/h Fluid contains sodium 250 mmol/L		
Modified hypertonic (Warden)	Lactated Ringer's+50 mmol/L NaHCO₃ for 8 h to maintain UO at 30–50 mL/h Lactated Ringer's to maintain UO at 30–50 mL/h beginning 8 h post-burn		
Dextran formula (Demling)	Dextran 40 in saline at 2 mL/kg/h for 8 h Lactated Ringer's titrated to maintain urine output at 30 mL/h	Fresh Frozen Plasma at 0.5 mL/kg/h for 18 h beginning 8 h post-burn	

Monitoring

Heart rate and urine output are the primary modalities for monitoring fluid therapy in patients with large burns although there is a lack of evidence supporting them. Reliance on hourly urine output as the sole index of optimum resuscitation sharply contrasts with the lack of clinical studies demonstrating the ideal hourly urine output during resuscitation *(Fig. 18.17)*. A minimum of 0.5–1.0 mL/kg per hour urine output in adults and in children is recommended but 1–2 mL/kg per hour urine output is preferred. Lesser hourly urinary outputs in the first 48 h post-burn almost always represent inadequate resuscitation. Hemodynamic monitoring and treatment of deviation from normovolemia are the fundamental tasks in intensive care. A pulse rate ~110 beats/min in adults usually indicates adequate volume, with rates >120 beats/min usually indicative of hypovolemia. Narrowed pulse pressure provides an earlier indication of shock than systolic blood pressure alone.

Noninvasive blood pressure measurements by cuff are inaccurate due to the interference of tissue edema and read lower than the actual blood pressure. An arterial catheter placed in the radial artery is the first choice, followed by the femoral artery. The decision to perform invasive hemodynamic monitoring requires careful consideration. The lack of benefit associated with goal-directed supranormal therapy has resulted in waning enthusiasm for the use of pulmonary artery catheters. The most applicable cardiac output-related variable to manipulate in burn patients is preload. Pulmonary artery occlusion pressure and central venous pressure are not good indicators of preload. As long as other signs of adequate tissue perfusion are normal, the temptation to normalize filling pressures should be avoided. The use of end points demonstrating the adequacy of oxygen delivery has not yet found a place in the management of burn shock.

Management of the burn wound

Topical ointments

Many ointments serve as good temporary coverings for the wounds between dressing changes. The simplest is just a petroleum-based antibiotic ointment such as bacitracin; but for sizable burns, most clinicians use some preparation with a stronger bactericidal or bacteriostatic action.

Silver sulfadiazine is the most common ointment used. It has intermediate wound penetration and a good antibacterial spectrum. The antibacterial activity lasts 8–10 h, and the dressings are changed twice a day. Silver sulfadiazine causes transient leucopenia in some patients when it is used on large open areas. A switch to a different topical agent for a few days allows the white blood cell count to recover. Restarting silver sulfadiazine rarely causes recurrent leucopenia.

Mafenide acetate is also commonly used and looks similar. It has excellent eschar penetration and bacteriostatic action. Use of mafenide acetate on full-thickness burns prevents deeper infections. Often used on the ear, it helps against infection of the cartilage. Systemic absorption of mafenide acetate, when it is applied to large burns, produces a metabolic acidosis by inhibition of carbonic anhydrase. The effect is usually noted after 3–5 days. Use of the compound on open wounds

also causes pain on initial application. The pain subsides after several minutes, but patients usually do not like it.

Another topical dressing is Dakin solution (0.25% sodium hypochlorite). This is good for a wet-to-dry dressing for minor debridement of the wound surface. It is particularly useful if a skin graft smells or looks infected.

Silver nitrate, as a 0.5% solution, is applied as a wet dressing. It has excellent antibacterial properties but causes discoloration of the skin and all the surrounding clothing and bedding. A newer version marketed as Acticoat contains gauze material impregnated with a silver compound. This product does not discolor the skin as silver nitrate does. The dressing does not have to be removed. Instead, it is moistened occasionally to release the active ingredient into the wound.

Agents such as povidone-iodine solution and nitrofurazone are still used in some burn units but less and less often. The need to use multiple agents once one has failed is becoming less common. Burn wound infections have decreased dramatically during the last 2 decades not from better topical dressings but from a better understanding of the causes of burn wound infection. Early tangential debridement and coverage of the wound with skin have markedly decreased the opportunity for colonization of the burn eschar. Despite meticulous wound care, and even under the most sterile conditions, the patient's own microbial flora quickly colonizes and then invades the burn eschar. Only by removing the dead tissue and providing stable coverage is the risk of wound infection eliminated.

Wound dressings

The standard burn dressing consists of gauze impregnated with soft paraffin, which helps to prevent adherence to the wound. A topical antiseptic may be applied over this followed by cotton wool or Gamgee to absorb the exudate. Newer dressings have been introduced that are claimed to be less adherent and allow less water to be lost by evaporation from the wound while also protecting it from external pathogens *(Box 18.8)*. These may be classified into two groups:

1. *Biological dressings*: These can be used either fresh or after storage following preparation by freezing in liquid nitrogen or rapid dehydration (lyophilization) and later reconstitution with saline.

2. *Physiological dressings*: These consist of synthetic materials such as polyethylene or silicone, which prevent adherence to the wound, and plastic films, which reduce evaporation and contamination.

Biological wound dressings

The most widely used biologic dressing remains fresh or frozen human cadaveric split-thickness skin. Properly handled, cadaveric skin remains viable and revascularizes ('takes') when it is placed on a healthy wound bed. The dermal capillaries of the graft fill with blood and then develop nutrient flow 2–5 days after grafting by inosculation, just like autologous split-thickness grafts. The cadaveric skin functions very much like autologous grafts, decreasing fluid loss, lowering local pathogen growth, and decreasing painful stimuli during dressing changes. The need for frequent dressing changes decreases, and the overall effect on the patient's hyperdynamic state is beneficial. However, just as Medawar

Box 18.8 **Characteristics of the ideal temporary skin substitute**

- Nonantigenic
- Durable
- Flexible
- Prevents water loss
- Barrier to micro-organisms
- Drapes well
- Rapid and firm wound adherence
- Easy to secure
- Relieves pain
- Grows with a child
- Can be applied in one operation
- Hemostatic
- Stimulates wound healing
- Optimizes healing environment
- Does not cause hypertrophic tissue response
- Easy to remove when wound has re-epithelized or is ready for grafting
- Cannot transmit disease
- Inexpensive
- Long shelf-life
- Can be used off the shelf
- Does not require refrigeration.

Box 18.9 **Characteristics of the ideal permanent skin substitute**

- Bilayer structures with biologic dermal analogue and either synthetic or biologic epidermal analogue
- Rapid and excellent adherence properties
- Easily applied and secured to an excised wound
- Minimum wait period from time of burn to availability of skin substitute
- Bilayer tissue containing both epidermal and dermal eliminates to best replicate normal skin
- Rapid incorporation
- Cannot transmit disease
- Good functional and cosmetic result
- Inexpensive.

described in his Nobel Prize-winning studies in the 1940s, cadaveric skin undergoes first-set rejection 1–2 weeks after grafting. The immunosuppression found in massively burned patients may delay the rejection process some, but eventually the grafts develop an abundant inflammatory cell infiltrate and the epidermis dies and sloughs from the patient. Loss of the epidermis requires replacement with another set of cadaveric grafts, or, it is hoped, the patient is ready for coverage with permanent autologous tissue. Disease transmission from the donor to the burn patient remains a theoretical concern. Interestingly, all burn surgeons have observed over the years that the dermis of the cadaveric graft frequently remains attached to the wound bed and is eventually incorporated into the wound.

Porcine skin and freeze-dried human cadaveric skin do not have the same properties as fresh or properly preserved frozen cadaveric skin *(Table 18.5)*. These other skin substitutes do not revascularize and therefore easily detach from the wound bed during dressing changes. Whether these materials decrease fluid loss or have antimicrobial effects is debated.

The ability to grow and expand human keratinocytes in tissue culture was a major advance in wound treatment *(Table 18.6)*. No longer was an epidermal source a major limitation for restoration of the epithelial barrier. In a landmark case in 1984, twin children with burns over almost their entire bodies were treated with cultured keratinocytes taken from a small biopsy specimen of undamaged axillary skin. During the course of their treatment, the keratinocytes were successfully expanded in tissue culture and used to resurface some of their wounds. Survival of the patients was directly attributed to the use of the technique. Now several major burn centers have laboratory facilities to culture keratinocytes. Several biotechnology companies offer the service for a fee. Skin biopsy specimens sent to the company are expanded in culture and returned to the patient, usually in 2–3 weeks. The sheets of cultured epidermal autograft (CEA) are placed directly onto a cleanly debrided wound bed. The grafts survive well, and wounds close much faster than without treatment.

Despite its many advantages, CEA does not address all of the wound problems facing massively burned patients. Unlike split-thickness skin, the epithelial cultures contain no dermal matrix tissue. Typically, the CEA is placed on debrided full-thickness burns that lack any dermal elements. Because the dermis provides the elastic quality of the skin, healed wounds that lack dermis have little give and are stiff. Covered by CEA, areas around joints and over muscles, such as the face, have little motion and poor function. The dermis also provides the foundation for the formation of the basement membrane between the epidermis and dermis. CEA placed directly on muscle or subcutaneous tissue only gradually forms a basement membrane, in some cases during 6 months. The basement membrane serves an important attachment function, and epidermis lacking a well-formed basement membrane blisters and shears easily. Reopening of a healed wound is common after application of CEA.

Growth of CEA is slow and expensive. A biopsy specimen must be obtained from the patient, and growth of the CEA takes several weeks. Several centers have used cultured epidermal allograft to treat burn wounds with varying success. Because the donor keratinocytes are taken from discarded neonatal foreskins from circumcisions, cultured epidermal allografts can be available at any time and are much less expensive to produce. However, the engrafted cells undergo rejection just as cadaveric skin grafts do. The cells work best as temporary coverage in partial-thickness wounds where a supply of autologous keratinocytes is available to replace the allografts after rejection.

Dermal replacements offer better functional results once they are incorporated in the wound, but engraftment rates have been a problem *(Box 18.9)*. Replacement of lost dermis in deep second-degree or third-degree burns during the initial treatment of the wound with these materials may decrease the need for later reconstructive surgery. These dermal replacements may prevent the extensive scarring and associated poor skin elasticity often seen in burns covered with thin skin grafts. Despite the technical problems with these materials, the advantage of preventing functional and cosmetic deformities from scar contractures makes their use worthwhile in many clinical situations.

Table 18.5 Temporary skin substitutes

Product	Tissue of origin	Layers	Category	Uses	Advantages	Disadvantages
Human allograft	Human cadaver	Epidermis and dermis	Split thickness skin	Temporary dressing of partial thickness and excised burns before autografting or when there is a lack of autograft	• A bilayer skin providing epidermal and dermal properties • Re-vascularizes maintaining viability for weeks • Dermis incorporates into the wound • Antimicrobial activity	• Epidermis will reject • Difficult to obtain and store • Risk of disease transfer • Expensive • Need to cryopreserve
Human amnion	Placenta	Amniotic membrane	Epidermis Dermis	Temporary dressing of partial thickness and excised burns before autografting or when there is a lack of autograft	• Acts like biologic barrier of skin • Decreases pain • Easy to apply, remove • Transparent	• Difficult to obtain, prepare and store • Need to change every 2 days • Disintegrates easily • Risk of disease transfer • Expensive
Pig skin Xenograft	Pig dermis	Dermis	Dermis	Temporary dressing of partial thickness and excised burns before autografting or when there is a lack of autograft	• Good adherence • Decreases pain • More readily available compared to allograft • Bioactive (collagen) inner surface with fresh product • Less expensive than allograft	• Does not revascularize and will slough • Short-term use • Need to keep the fresh product frozen
Biobrane®	Synthetic with added denatured bovine collagen	Bilayer product outer silicone Inner nylon mesh with added collagen	Synthetic epidermis and dermis	Temporary coverage of superficial partial thickness burns, although it has been used for coverage of autograft and for donor	• Bilayer analog • Excellent adherence to a superficial partial thickness burn • Decreases pain • Maintains flexibility • Easy to store with long shelf-life	• Relatively expensive • Has very little direct bioactivity • Difficult to remove if left in place over 2 weeks • Not as good for deep partial and full thickness burns

	Type	Composition	Indication	Advantages	Disadvantages
Oasis®	Xenograft	Bioactive Dermal like Matrix; Extracellular wound matrix from small intestine submucosa	Temporary coverage of superficial partial thickness burns, although it has been used for coverage of autograft and for donor	• Excellent adherence • Decreased pain • Provides bioactive dermal like properties • Long shelf-life, store at room temperature • Relatively inexpensive	• Mainly a dermal analogue • Incorporates and may need to be reapplied
Transcyte®	Allogenic Dermis	Bioactive Dermal Matrix Components on Synthetic dermis and epidermis; Bilayer product Outer silicone Inner nylon seeded with neonatal fibroblasts	Temporary coverage of superficial partial thickness burns, although it has been used for coverage of autograft and for donor	• Bilayer analogue • Excellent adherence to a superficial partial thickness burn • Decreases pain • Provides bioactive dermal components • Maintains flexibility • Good outer barrier function	• Need to store frozen till use • Relatively expensive
Duoderm®	Synthetic hydrocolloid dressing	Synthetic epidermis and dermis; Monolayer	Temporary coverage of superficial partial thickness burns, although it has been used for coverage of autograft and for donor	• Long shelf-life, store at room temperature • Relatively inexpensive	• Adhesive layer barrier to diffusion of exudate from the wound so that most of the fluid never diffuses through the adhesive layer; • No transpiration of fluid to the atmosphere • The adhesive is aggressive to the intact perilesional skin so that on removal this skin may be traumatized • Loss of adhesion in a day or two due to fluid accumulation • Provides a favorable environment at the wound locus for the growth of harmful anaerobic bacteria

Table 18.5, Temporary skin substitutes—cont'd

Product	Tissue of origin	Layers	Category	Uses	Advantages	Disadvantages
Opsite®	Synthetic elastomeric polyurethane film	Monolayer	Synthetic epidermis and dermis	Temporary coverage of superficial partial thickness burns, although it has been used for coverage of autograft and for donor	• Long shelf-life, store at room temperature • Relatively inexpensive	• Not absorbent • requires fairly frequent replacement to obviate pooling of exudate and related problems • The adhesive is aggressive to the intact perilesional skin so that on removal this skin may be traumatized
Suprathel®	Synthetic copolymer of polylactide, trimethylene carbonate and ε-caprolactone	Monolayer	Synthetic epidermis and dermis	Temporary coverage of superficial partial thickness burns, although it has been used for coverage of autograft and for donor	• Long shelf-life, store at room temperature	• Relatively expensive • Not absorbent • requires fairly frequent replacement to obviate pooling of exudate and related problems
Tegaderm®	Synthetic elastomeric polyurethane film	Monolayer	Synthetic epidermis and dermis	Temporary coverage of superficial partial thickness burns, although it has been used for coverage of autograft and for donor	• Long shelf-life, store at room temperature • Relatively inexpensive	• Not absorbent • requires fairly frequent replacement to obviate pooling of exudate and related problems • The adhesive is aggressive to the intact perilesional skin so that on removal this skin may be traumatized

Table 18.6 Permanent skin substitutes

Product	Tissue of origin	Layers	Category	Uses	Advantages	Disadvantages
Apligraf®	Allogenic Composite	Collagen matrix seeded with human neonatal keratinocytes and fibroblasts	Composite: Epidermis and Dermis	Excised deep partial thickness burn	Readily available	Expensive Vascularizes slowly No epithelial barrier No antimicrobial activity
OrCel®	Allogenic Composite	Collagen sponge seeded with human neonatal keratinocytes and fibroblasts	Composite: Epidermis and Dermis	Skin graft donor site. Excised deep partial thickness burn	Readily available Live cells	Expensive Vascularizes slowly No epithelial barrier No antimicrobial activity
Epicel®	Autogenous keratinocytes	Cultured autologous keratinocytes	Epidermis only	Deep partial and full thickness burns >30% TBSA	Readily available Live cells	Expensive Vascularizes slowly No epithelial barrier No antimicrobial activity
Alloderm®	Allogenic dermis	A cellular Dermis (processed allograft)	Dermis only	Deep partial and full thickness burns	Readily available Live cells	Expensive Vascularizes slowly No epithelial barrier No antimicrobial activity
Integra®	Synthetic	Silicone outer layer on bovine collagen GAG and shark chondroitin sulfate dermal matrix	Biosynthetic dermis	Full thickness burns; definitive "closure" requires skin graft	Readily available Live cells	Expensive Vascularizes slowly No epithelial barrier No antimicrobial activity

The first product available on the market for dermal matrix was Integra. The matrix is composed of undenatured bovine collagen and shark chondroitin sulfate, a proteoglycan. A thin Silastic sheet, to serve as a barrier to the air, covers the surface. When it is placed on a wound, the material is incorporated and serves as a scaffold for infiltration and growth of fibroblasts and capillaries. Engraftment of the material takes approximately 2 weeks, and any disturbance, such as excessive movement, fluid accumulation under the material, or infection, causes loss of the material. Once the matrix is incorporated, the Silastic membrane is removed, and the material is covered by epidermis. CEA placed on Integra does not survive, and no one seems to know the explanation. After the Silastic is removed, the manufacturer recommends use of a thin split-thickness skin graft to cover the wound to establish the epidermis. An obvious disadvantage of this method is the long time from excision of the burn wound to final epithelial coverage. When multiple areas need skin grafting, this delay may be no more than waiting for donor sites to re-epithelialize. In addition, use of only thin split-thickness skin reduces donor site problems and hastens donor site healing. So far, no one has demonstrated a survival advantage with the use of Integra, but many clinicians believe that its use on extensive full-thickness wounds definitely improves the final functional results.

AlloDerm is the other commercially available dermal replacement made from freeze-dried human dermis obtained from cadaveric split-thickness skin. As with Integra, however, the engraftment process for the matrix is variable, and the matrix does not support the attachment of CEA well.

The rapidity of the engraftment process is likely to depend on the vascularity of the matrix material as much as the wound bed on which it is placed. AlloDerm placed over the wound and covered with a split-thickness skin graft acts as an extracellular dermal matrix. The matrix is incorporated into the final thickness of the skin. Studies on the long-term results of wounds treated with AlloDerm are under way.

Most burn centers, including the authors', do not use dermal replacements for extensive coverage of acute burns because of the unpredictable engraftment rate. Large clinical trials have not demonstrated a survival advantage with use of any of these products or presented data to suggest that postinjury function is improved. Therefore, most surgeons use dermal replacements for burn scar reconstruction when supplemental dermis improves functional and cosmetic outcomes of the grafting procedure and survival of the patient is not an issue.

Physiological wound dressings

Synthetic materials are often used to cover wounds but have other limitations. If they are applied correctly, they usually adhere to the wound bed. Left undisturbed, the dressing limits fluid loss and prevents stimulation of the wound. Epidermal regeneration is undisturbed beneath. The dressing falls off once the epithelial layer completely heals underneath, much like a scab falls off an open wound once it is healed. These materials work best on superficial second-degree burn wounds and skin graft donor sites that heal in 7–10 days. Placed on deeper wounds, the materials adhere poorly and as foreign material serve as a nidus for infection much like the burn eschar. These materials have no antimicrobial activity and therefore should not be placed on a contaminated wound. Most of the newly developed synthetic biologic dressings are used mainly in developed countries because most of these products are extremely expensive.

Conservative versus surgical therapy

All wounds eventually heal if they are left alone unless there is infection, lack of blood flow (tissue ischemia), or inadequate nutritional intake. Meticulous wound care helps minimize the chance of infection and maximize healing. The daily dressing changes in burn patients permit inspection of the wound to assess the need for further interventions but, more important, offer the chance to remove dead tissue that is a nidus for infection. The burn nurse dedicates a large part of the time to gently scraping off dead skin and proteinaceous debris that have gathered since the last dressing. This leaves a healthy bed for the migration of keratinocytes. Typically, the wound is covered between dressings with a moist, antibacterial covering to minimize microbial growth, fluid loss, and painful stimuli and to maximize skin regeneration. Superficial partial thickness burns heal in a short time with wound treatment only. For deep partial or full burns, the time for healing can be extensive and risks of infection greater. For these wounds, it is far better to treat by surgical debridement and coverage with skin grafts or cultured epidermis. For a deep burn over a small area or one with a patchy distribution, the time for healing by secondary intention may be no longer than the healing of a skin graft. For these wounds, surgical debridement and grafting may not be appropriate. After all, it takes a skin graft 7–10 days to stabilize on a wound and about the same amount of time for the donor site to heal. Ideally, all wounds should have epithelial cover within 3 weeks to minimize scarring, but in practice the decision whether to refer a patient must be made by day 10 to achieve this.

Surgery

Aggressive but carefully timed removal of burnt tissue and replacement with definitive wound cover is the key to survival and return to function. Early excision and grafting have been shown to reduce pain, shorten hospital stay, and accelerate return to normal function in moderate injuries. The coagulated tissue from third-degree burns does not easily separate from the wound bed until very late, and the thick layers of dead tissue retard epithelial regrowth and harbor pathogens. Removal requires sharp debridement with a knife (tangential) *(Fig. 18.18)*. Because of the intensely painful stimuli and the likelihood of a large quantity of blood loss from the debridement, these procedures are typically done in the operating room.

The main goals of surgical treatment of patients with deep burns are debridement of the burn and placement of stable permanent skin coverage. Many studies have demonstrated that early removal of the dead tissue and aggressive measures to re-establish the epithelial barrier decrease wound infections and mortality. The dead tissue continues to incite an inflammatory response, serves as a growth medium for pathogens,

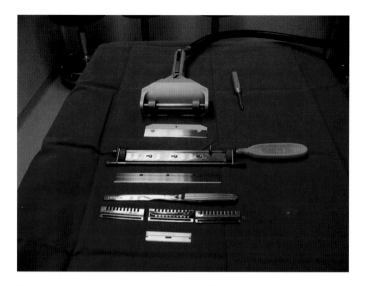

Fig. 18.18 Equipment for tangential excision. Silver knife; Watson modification of the Humby knife and air powered dermatome.

and delays wound healing. Even after removal of the dead tissue, pathogens colonize the wound and enter the patient's blood stream to seed distant sites. Open wounds leak proteins and fluids and continue to be painful. All these factors contribute to the patient's hyperdynamic and hypermetabolic state. To achieve early debridement and stable permanent coverage of the wound, the surgeon must overcome two main obstacles, the extreme physical insult of the debridement process and the limited source of replacement skin for permanent coverage of large surface area burns.

The burn eschar is shaved tangentially or excised to deep fascia. From the surgical viewpoint, the best time to graft burns is within five days of injury to minimize blood loss, and injuries that are obviously deep at presentation must be referred early. With major burns, treatment is skewed towards preservation of life or limb, and large areas of deep burn must be excised before the burnt tissue triggers multiple organ failure or becomes infected *(Fig. 18.19)*. In such cases more superficial burns may be treated with dressings until healing occurs late or fresh skin donor sites become available.

The main limitation to removal of the dead skin in large burns is severe physiologic disturbance caused by rapid and copious blood loss as a consequence of skinning patients over an extensive area. In adults, blood loss reaches 100 mL for every 1% TBSA of skin debrided. Although some units practice large (>20% TBSA) debridement in one procedure, most burn units limit each operative session to debridement of 10–20% TBSA. This keeps blood replacement, fluid administration, and anesthetic needs to levels that can be addressed by the operating room team in a timely fashion. Tangential debridement involves cutting the skin tissue at the depth of the dermal and subcutaneous capillary network. Because of the local inflammatory response in the burn, these capillaries are usually well dilated by the time of excision. After excision, blood loss can be torrential, and it is difficult to imagine such extensive hemorrhage until one participates in such a procedure. Clinical studies estimate that tangential debridement of each square centimeter of burn causes 1 mL of blood loss. Thus, in an adult, excision of each 1% TBSA of burn averages

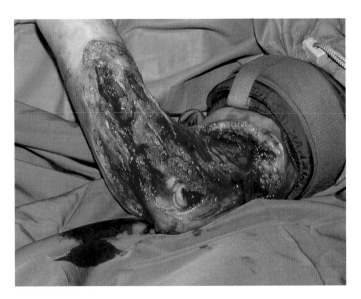

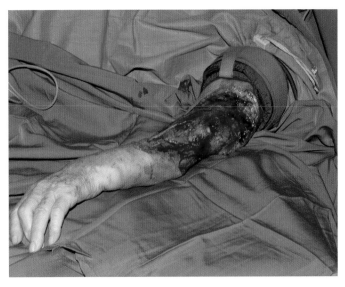

Fig. 18.19 Debridement may lead to exposed joints. Exposed elbow joint after debridement of a full thickness burn.

Fig. 18.20 Pneumatic tourniquets can minimize blood loss and improve vision during surgery.

100 mL of bleeding. Debridement of a 20% TBSA burn results in 2000 mL or 4 units of whole blood loss. Tourniquet use on extremities, pressure dressings, electrocautery, hemostatic agents, avoidance of agents that interfere with the coagulation, and subcutaneous injection of the burn with dilute epinephrine all limit blood loss but not completely *(Fig. 18.20)*. Full-thickness excision of the burn to the level of muscle fascia with electrocautery limits blood loss. The loss of such a significant amount of soft tissue requires skin grafts on muscle fascia and has poor functional and cosmetic results. The best method to control blood loss is to limit each debridement session to about 10–20% TBSA. The patient and the anesthesiologist better tolerate this amount of blood loss.

Timely coverage of the debrided wounds depends on available sources of autologous skin. Autologous split-thickness skin grafts from unburnt areas are the "gold standard" for definitive coverage of burn wounds if enough donor sites are available. When available, the extremities, minus the hands and feet, are the best areas for harvesting of skin grafts. The trunk is used next, but obtaining the grafts is technically more challenging because of contour irregularities *(Fig. 18.21)*. The scalp is a great but often underused donor site. The scalp skin is thick and re-epithelializes rapidly owing to the density of hair follicles *(Fig. 18.22)*. Tissue inflation of the scalp gives better quality of skin graft. It is even possible to harvest skin grafts from the scrotum after tissue inflation *(Fig. 18.23)*. Regrowth of the hair is rarely a problem; thus, the donor site is well camouflaged after healing.

Repeated harvesting of skin graft donor sites multiple times increases the amount of skin available, but the donor site must heal between harvest procedures, and these areas typically bleed more on the second harvest. Most important, the site has limited potential for recovery as more and more of the dermis and hair follicles are taken for the graft. Eventually, the donor site can become a full-thickness wound itself. Thickness is usually tailored to the depth of excision to obtain good cosmesis, although thinner grafts are thought to contract more. Donor sites should ideally be harvested adjacent to the injury to improve color match, and sheet graft is

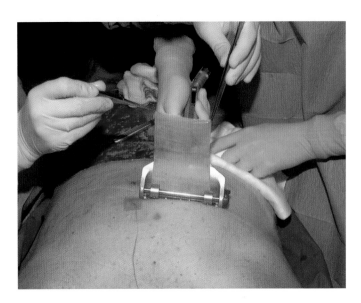

Fig. 18.21 Dermatome harvest of a split thickness skin graft.

preferred to improve the cosmetic and functional result *(Figs 18.24, 18.25)*. If donor sites are sparse, however, or the wound bed is likely to bleed profusely (because excision is carried out late, for instance) then the graft is perforated with a mesher to allow expansion *(Figs 18.26–18.28)*. Although this improves graft 'take,' where the wound bed is bleeding after tangential excision, the mesh pattern is permanent and unsightly *(Fig. 18.29)*. Unmeshed sheet graft is used on hands and faces, and over any future site for intravenous central lines and tracheostomies to obtain rapid cover. Where unburnt split skin donor sites are in very short supply, there are two possible solutions:

1. Rotation of donor sites is practised, and unexcised burn covered with antimicrobial creams

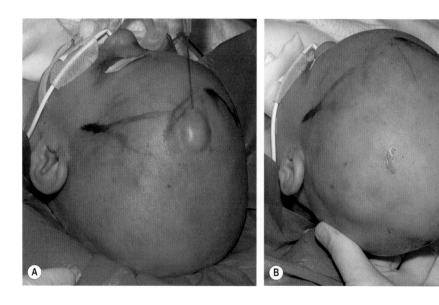

Fig. 18.22 (A) Intraoperative tissue expansion to allow harvest of split thickness skin grafts from the scalp. **(B)** Expanded scalp allows harvest of split thickness skin grafts.

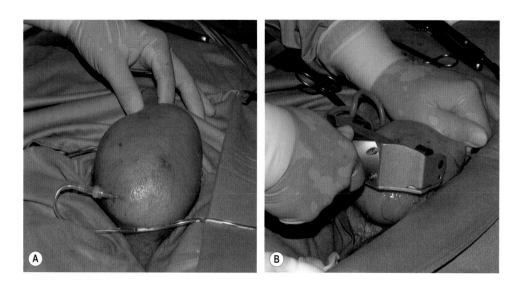

Fig. 18.23 (A) Inflation tissue expansion of the scrotum to allow skin graftings when donor sites are lacking. **(B)** Harvesting a split thickness skin graft from an inflated scrotum.

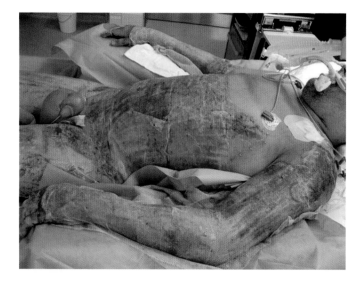

Fig. 18.24 Suprathel on superficial partial thickness burns.

2. The excised wound is resurfaced with a temporary covering until donor sites have regenerated and can be re-harvested.

Examples of a temporary covering are cadaveric allograft from an unrelated donor, xenograft, synthetic products, and cultured epithelial autograft *(Fig. 18.30)*. Development of synthetic products has allowed us to excise extremely large burns and still achieve physiological closure, with potentially lower mortality in these injuries. Cultured epithelial autografts also permits us to extend the available donor sites. The cultured cells can be applied as sheets (available after 3 weeks) or in suspension (available within 1 week). A few burns units use these cells for superficial skin loss or in combination with mesh graft to improve the cosmetic result.

Wounds are debrided and covered with skin grafts in one procedure if blood loss is acceptable. In large area burns, the patient may undergo skin grafting a few days after debridement to allow time for the debrided wounds to stop bleeding and for the patient to recover from the blood loss. Harvesting

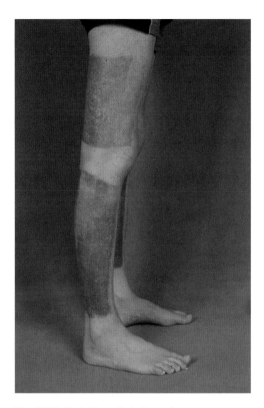

Fig. 18.25 Healed lower limb donor sites.

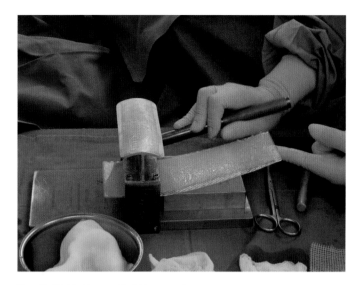

Fig. 18.26 Meshing a split thickness graft.

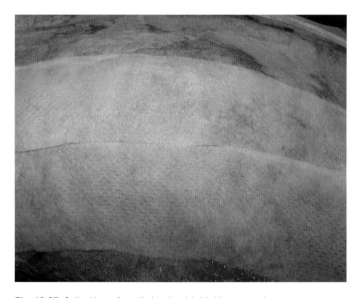

Fig. 18.27 Split skin graft applied to the debrided burn wound.

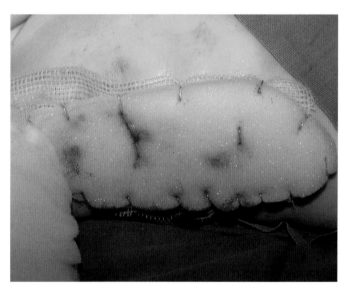

Fig. 18.28 The use of sponge and staples is a fast and easy technique to immobilize the skin graft but patients often find the removal of staples painful.

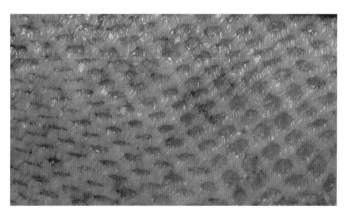

Fig. 18.29 Healing split thickness graft.

of skin grafts, although less bloody than tangential debridement of the burn, still results in significant blood loss. Between the time of excision and the skin grafting procedure, the wounds are covered with a biologic dressing (pig or cadaver skin) or a topical wound dressing. Should the patient need several debridement sessions to remove all of the burns, debridement can be alternated with grafting sessions to achieve staged coverage of each debrided area before going on to the next burned area. This strategy delays the complete removal of all burned tissue, leading to some increased risk of burn

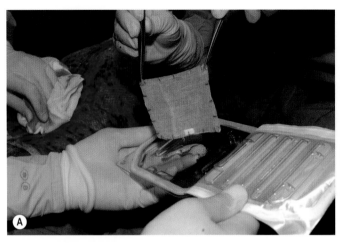

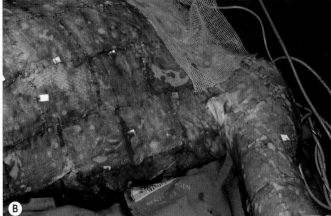

Fig. 18.30 **(A,B)** Application of a sheet of cultured epidermal autograft.

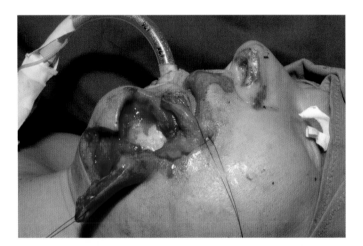

Fig. 18.31 Excised full thickness being reconstructed with local flaps.

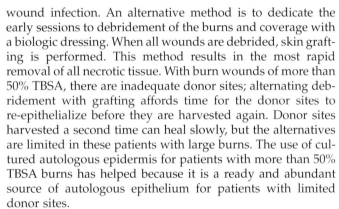

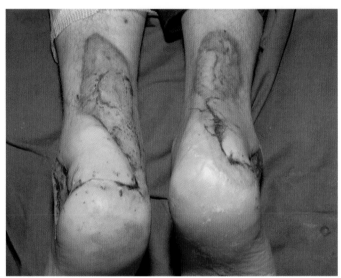

Fig. 18.32 Local pivot flaps to cover exposed tendo Achillis after a cement burn.

wound infection. An alternative method is to dedicate the early sessions to debridement of the burns and coverage with a biologic dressing. When all wounds are debrided, skin grafting is performed. This method results in the most rapid removal of all necrotic tissue. With burn wounds of more than 50% TBSA, there are inadequate donor sites; alternating debridement with grafting affords time for the donor sites to re-epithelialize before they are harvested again. Donor sites harvested a second time can heal slowly, but the alternatives are limited in these patients with large burns. The use of cultured autologous epidermis for patients with more than 50% TBSA burns has helped because it is a ready and abundant source of autologous epithelium for patients with limited donor sites.

A logical algorithm should be used in skin grafting of patients with large surface area burns. Most important for survival of the patient is to decrease the surface area of the injury, so in the absence of other restrictions, the largest area of burn should be excised and grafted first, such as the trunk, then the lower extremity, followed by the upper extremity. Burns to the hands, neck, and face warrant special consideration, however. To prevent excessive functional impairment to these areas after the burn wounds are healed, these areas

should be grafted earlier rather than later. In full-thickness burns to the hands, neck, and face, delay in grafting can result in excess scarring and functional limitations that are difficult to overcome. The scarring can make the rehabilitation of the patient very problematic. Thus, deep burns to these areas should be grafted early or closed with flaps to form healthy tissue *(Figs 18.31–18.33)* so that range of motion and hypertrophic scar management can be started early.

Summary of burn wound treatment

(Box 18.10)

Superficial wounds should heal by regeneration within 2 weeks. They should be cleaned, dressed, and reviewed on alternate days to optimize the wound healing environment. Any burn not healed within 2 weeks should be referred for assessment.

Deep partial thickness burns are unlikely to heal within 3 weeks. The incidence of unsightly hypertrophic scarring rises

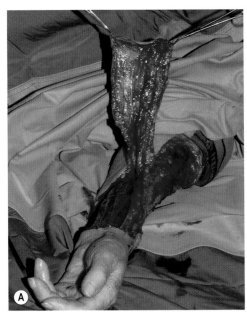
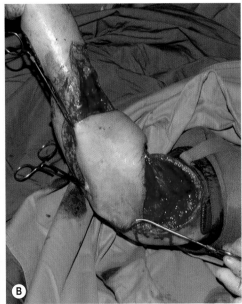

Fig. 18.33 Pedicled radial forearm flap to cover an open elbow joint.

Box 18.10 **Techniques for burn reconstruction**

Without deficiency of tissue
- Excision and primary closure
- Plasty techniques

With deficiency of tissue
- Serial excision and primary closure
- Split and full thickness skin autografts
- Dermal templates and split skin autografts
- Plasty techniques
- Local flaps
- Regional flaps
- Distant flaps
- Tissue expansion
- Free flaps.

Table 18.7 Percentage increase in metabolic rate versus burn size

% Burn (TBSA)	Metabolic rate (% increase)
20	30
30	50
40	75
50	100
60	100

Table 18.8 Catabolism-induced complications relative to loss of lean body mass

Lean body mass (% loss)	Complication	Mortality (%)
10	Impaired immunity; increased infection	10
20	Decreased healing; failure to wean	30
30	Too weak to sit; pressure sores; pneumonia	50
40	Death, usually from pneumonia	100

---

from 33% to 78% if healing is delayed from 3–6 weeks. Therefore, these injuries should also be excised and grafted within the first 5–10 days.

Full thickness injuries have no regenerative elements left. Unless they are very small they will take weeks to heal and undergo severe contraction. They should be referred for surgery as early as possible.

Clean wounds can be dressed with a nonadherant primary dressing such as tulle gras or Mepitel and an absorbent secondary dressing such as gauze or Gamgee Tissue. Antimicrobial agents are added where infection is likely (perineum, feet) or heavy colonization is evident on the dressings or invasive infection is suspected.

Metabolism/nutrition

Nutritional therapy plays a key role in the overall management of the burns patient and the aggressive dynamic approach to the nutritional management is essential for the survival of burn patients. Extensive burns elicit a pronounced metabolic response to trauma causing physiological derangements leading to the hyper-metabolic state *(Table 18.7)*.[12] The hyper-metabolic response is accompanied by severe catabolism and a loss of lean body mass and also by a progressive decline of host defenses that impairs the immunological response and leads to sepsis *(Table 18.8)*. The burn wound consumes large quantities of energy during the healing process due to the large population of inflammatory cells and the production of collagen and matrix by fibroblasts. Severe burn results in profound metabolic alterations, which include increasing nitrogen loss, malnutrition and hypermetabolism.

Catabolism as a response to thermal trauma only can be modulated, not completely reversed. Much of the morbidity and mortality after major burns may be attributed to this alteration. Nutritional therapy plays a key role in the overall strategy for burned patients.[13] Post-burn, the metabolic and catabolic responses are prolonged in severity and time course, lasting weeks to months in contrast to the days and weeks observed in other injuries. Extensive nutritional support to meet the increased energy expenditure is essential for the survival of burn patients. Effective provision of the required amount of calories can be provided with oral, enteral or parenteral route.

Controlling the 'stress response' to burn injury alters the metabolic abnormalities (*Boxes 18.11–18.13*).Optimizing nutrition to match nutrient utilization is essential. Controlling the catabolic response is the next key treatment measure. It appears that anticatabolic and anabolic agents can markedly diminish the net catabolism of burn injury during the acute and recovery phases.[12] These agents, in combination with optimum protein intake, appear to be of significant benefit in the metabolic management of the severe burn.

Therapeutic strategies should aim to prevent body weight losses of more than 10% of patient's baseline status because more profound weight losses are associated with significantly worse outcomes. Known consequences of catabolic disorders with loss of lean body mass above 10% include impaired immune function and delayed wound healing. Lean body mass reduction beyond 40% leads to imminent mortality. Therefore, complications of ongoing catabolism remain a major cause of morbidity and mortality in severely burned patients. In addition to optimizing nutrient intake, anticatabolic and anabolic agents that may counteract 'the stress response to injury or illness' may be of significant clinical

benefit. The mortality in the burns patients especially above 40% TBSA burns managed by appropriate nutrition has been found to be decreased because of decrease in negative nitrogen balance and better wound healing leading to decreased graft losses and improved immunity causing a decrease in infections.

Burn injury can increase the basal metabolic rate 50–100% of the normal resting rate. The main features include increased glucose production, insulin resistance, lipolysis, and muscle protein catabolism. Without adequate nutritional support, patients have delayed wound healing, decreased immune function, and generalized weight loss.[14] Many formulas predict the nutritional needs of these patients on the basis of lean body mass and percentage TBSA burned. Increased intake of both total calories and protein (1.5–3 g of protein/kg per day) is needed to restore the deficit. Much like fluid resuscitation, the exact nutritional requirements are debatable. The clinical response of the patient remains the best indication of nutritional repletion during recovery from the injury. The rapidity of epidermal regeneration of superficial burns and donor sites and improving serum nutritional parameters are the best indicators of adequate nutrition. Measurement of the basal metabolic rate also guides nutritional replacement therapy. Measuring weight loss and gain during treatment is

---

Box 18.11 **Body's response to injury**

Emergent Phase (Stage 1)
- Pain response
- Catecholamine release
- Tachycardia, tachypnea, mild hypertension, mild anxiety

Fluid Shift Phase (Stage 2)
- Length 18–24 h
- Begins after Emergent Phase
- Reaches peak in 6–8 h
- Damaged cells initiate inflammatory response
- Increased blood flow to cells
- Shift of fluid from intravascular to extravascular space due to leaky capillaries causing massive edema

Hypermetabolic Phase (Stage 3)
- Last for days to weeks
- Large increase in the body's need for nutrients as it repairs itself

Resolution Phase (Stage 4)
- Scar formation
- General rehabilitation and progression to normal function.

Box 18.12 **Systemic response to the release of cytokines and other inflammatory mediators at the site of injury once the burn reaches 25% of total body surface area**

- *Cardiovascular changes*: Capillary permeability is increased, leading to loss of intravascular proteins and fluids into the interstitial compartment. Peripheral and splanchnic vasoconstriction occurs. Myocardial contractility is decreased, possibly due to release of tumour necrosis factor. These changes, coupled with fluid loss from the burn wound, result in systemic hypotension and end organ hypoperfusion.
- *Respiratory changes*: Inflammatory mediators cause bronchoconstriction, and in severe burns adult respiratory distress syndrome can occur.
- *Metabolic changes*: The basal metabolic rate increases up to three times its original rate. This, coupled with splanchnic hypoperfusion, necessitates early and aggressive enteral feeding to decrease catabolism and maintain gut integrity.
- *Immunological changes*: Nonspecific down regulation of the immune response occurs, affecting both cell mediated and humoral pathways.

Box 18.13 **Major metabolic abnormalities with response to burn "stress response"**

- Increased catabolic hormones (cortisol and catechols)
- Decreased anabolic hormones (human growth hormone and testosterone)
- Marked increase in metabolic rate
- Sustained increase in body temperature
- Marked increase in glucose demands and liver gluconeogenesis
- Rapid skeletal muscle breakdown with amino acid use as an energy source (counter to normal nutrient channeling)
- Lack of ketosis, indicating that fat is not the major calorie source
- Unresponsiveness of catabolism to nutrient intake

not useful because of the large fluid shifts. Even with adequate nutritional support, most patients lose muscle mass and weight. Several studies propose the use of anabolic steroids or growth hormone to reduce muscle catabolism and weight loss during the injury and to enhance weight gain during recovery.

Nutrition

The goal of resuscitation is not only to maintain stable circulation, but also to improve the hypoxic state of the tissues and cells. Patients fed early have significantly enhanced wound healing and shorter hospital stays.[15] Meeting the extensive calorie requirement by oral route alone is practically not possible in the major burn patients. Enteral nutrition through nasogastric or nasoduodenal transpyloric tubes are the preferred supplementary route of providing calorie deficit to the acutely injured burn patient. Patients with burns 20% TBSA will be unable to meet their nutritional needs with oral intake alone and the transpyloric tube should be inserted at admission, as it is better tolerated than if inserted after the return of peristalsis. In the rare case that precludes use of the gastrointestinal tract, parenteral nutrition should be used only until the gastrointestinal tract is functioning.

Tube feedings also have an advantage over regular oral intake. Patients with large surface area burns need to consume large amounts of food to satisfy their nutritional requirements **(Fig. 18.34)**. The rigorous schedule of dressing changes, operations, and rehabilitation sessions interferes with meals. Diminished appetite from high-dose analgesics also contributes to poor feeding. Adequate nutritional support is so critical to recovery from burn injury that most clinicians will place feeding tubes in patients with inadequate oral calorie intake despite the risk of aspiration pneumonia.

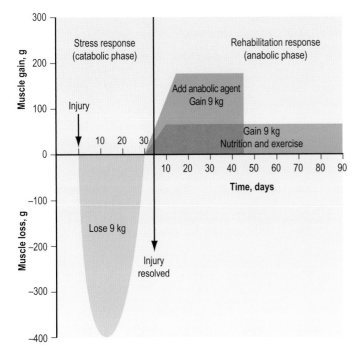

Fig. 18.34 The role of metabolic state in determining the rate of restoration of lean body mass.

Early enteral nutrition can relieve gastrointestinal damage, and maintain the integrity of intestinal mucosa after severe burn. Gastrointestinal mucosal lesions take place during ischemia and reperfusion period after severe burns. Early enteral nutrition can relieve the ischemia and reperfusion injury by means of increasing the ability of eliminating oxygen free radical. The increase of intestinal permeability is one of the early features of intestinal mucosal barrier damage. Early enteral nutrition is an effective method to keep a normal intestinal permeability through the maintenance of blood circulation and the prevention of ischemia and reperfusion injury of intestine.[13,16] Parenteral nutrition requires additional vascular access with its concomitant risks. It also lacks the beneficial effects of gut mucosal stimulation and its protective effects against bacterial translocation and stress hemorrhage. Early enteral nutrition is superior to parenteral nutrition in the early stage after burn. It might be a more effective route to preserve the secretion and motility of gastrointestinal tract, lower intestinal ischemia and reperfusion injury, reduce intestinal permeability, decrease plasma endotoxin and inflammatory mediators, and maintain mucosa barrier function.

Nutrition formulae

Burn centers continue to use a variety of formulae to estimate nutrient needs **(Table 18.9)**.[17] The number of energy estimation formulas has increased in recent years with many developed for specific patient populations.[17] Burn-specific equations have been developed both for pediatric and adult populations. A study compared 46 published energy calculations with indirect calorimetry in burn patients and found none (including, Curreri, Davies, Harris–Benedict, Muir and Wilmore formulae) precisely estimated calorie needs and most demonstrated some degree of bias.[18] In addition, formulas published before 1980 often overestimated energy needs.[18] Burn centers continue to use a variety of methods to monitor nutritional status though there appears to be less agreement regarding some methods than in years past.

Endocrine and glucose monitoring

Strict glucose control of 80–110 mg/dL can be achieved using an intensive insulin therapy protocol, leading to decreased infectious complications and mortality rates.[19,20]

Hepatic protein monitoring

Hepatic proteins (albumin, transferrin, prealbumin) have a role acute phase reactants, and are profoundly affected by fluid status and by metabolic stress, both of which are key components of the hypermetabolism present after a burn injury and therefore have limited use in the measure of nutritional status in burn injuries.

Anabolic steroids

Severe burn injuries induce a hypermetabolic response, which leads to catabolism. Oxandrolone, a synthetic derivative of testosterone, has been used in adult patients with severe

Table 18.9 Formulae for estimating calorie and protein needs

Formula	Age (years)	% TBSA Burn	Calories (kcal) per day	Protein
Adults				
Burke and Wolfe	>18	Any	$2 \times$ BMR	Not calculated
Curreri	16–59 >60	Any Any	$(25 \times$ body weight in kg$) + (40 \times \%$ TBSA burn$)$ $(20 \times$ body weight in kg$) + (65 \times \%$ TBSA burn$)$	Not calculated
Davies and Liljedahl	>18	Any	$(20$ kcal $\times$ body wt in kg$) + (70$ kcal $\times \%$ TBSA burn$)$ [>50% TBSA injuries are calculated as a 50% injury]	$(1$ g $\times$ body wt in kg$) + (3$ g $\times \%$ burn$)$
Galveston I	>18		$(2100$ kcal/m$^2 \times$ TBSA$) + (1000$ kcal/m$^2 \times \%$ TBSA burn$)$	Not calculated
Ireton-Jones	>18	Any but must be ventilator-dependent	$1784 - (11 \times$ age in years$) + (5 \times$ weight in kg$) + 244$ (sex: male$=1$; female$=0$) $+239$ (trauma: yes$=1$; no$=0$) $+804$	Not calculated
Modified Harris-Benedict	>18	<40	Male$=1.5 \times ([66 + (13.7 \times$ weight in kg$) + (5 \times$ height in cm$) - (6.8 \times$ age$))$ Female$=1.5 \times [655 + (9.6 \times$ weight in kg$) + (1.7 \times$ height in cm$) - (4.7 \times$ age$))$	1.5 g $\times$ weight in kg
		≥40	Male$=2 \times ([66 + (13.7 \times$ weight in kg$) + (5 \times$ height in cm$) - (6.8 \times$ age$))$ Female$=2 \times [655 + (9.6 \times$ weight in kg$) + (1.7 \times$ height in cm$) - (4.7 \times$ age$)$	2 g $\times$ weight in kg
Muir	>18	<20 ≥20–29.9 ≥30–39.9 ≥40–50	35 kcal/kg 40 kcal/kg 50 kcal/kg 60 kcal/kg	1.5 g/kg 2.0 g/kg 3.0 g/kg 4.0 g/kg
Wilmore	>18	Any ≥30	Use nomograms to calculate BMR, % change in BMR, energy requirements 2000–2200 kcal/m^2	Adjust nitrogen/total calorie to 1:150 15 g nitrogen/m^2
Toronto	>18	Any	$-4343 + (10.5 \times \%$ TBSA burn$) + (0.23 \times$ calorie intake$) + (0.84 \times$ Harris-Benedict energy expenditure$) + (114 \times$ mean body temperature $(^{\circ}$C$)) - (4.5 \times$ days post-burn$)$	Not calculated
Children				
Curreri Junior	0–1 1–3 4–15	Any Any Any	BMR$ + (15$ kcal $\times \%$ TBSA burn$)$ BMR$ + (25$ kcal $\times \%$ TBSA burn$)$ BMR$ + (40$ kcal $\times \%$ TBSA burn$)$	Not calculated Not calculated Not calculated
Davies Child	1–12	Any	$(60$ kcal $\times$ body weight in kg$) + (35$ kcal $\times \%$ TBSA burn$)$ [>50% surface injuries are calculated as a 50% injury]	$(3$ g $\times$ body wt in kg$) + (1$ g $\times \%$ burn$)$
Galveston Infant	0–1	Any	$(2100$ kcal/m$^2 \times$ TBSA$) + (1000$ kcal/m$^2 \times \%$ TBSA burn$)$	Not calculated
Galveston II	1–11	Any	$(1800$ kcal/m$^2 \times$ TBSA$) + (1300$ kcal/m$^2 \times \%$ TBSA burn$)$	Not calculated
Galveston Adolescent	12–18	Any	$(1500$ kcal/m$^2 \times$ TBSA$) + (1300$ kcal/m$^2 \times \%$ TBSA burn$)$	

1 g nitrogen$=6.25$ g protein; BMR, basal metabolic rate.

thermal injury to enhance lean body mass accretion, restore body weight, and accelerate wound healing. In clinical studies, oxandrolone 10 mg orally twice daily improved wound healing, restored lean body mass, and accelerated body weight gain. During the rehabilitation period, oxandrolone therapy with adequate nutrition and exercise improved lean body mass, increased muscle strength, and restored body weight.[21] Burn patients recieving oxandrolone regain weight and lean mass two to three times faster than with nutrition alone.[22]

β-blockade

β-blockers after severe burns decrease heart rate, resulting in reduced cardiac index and decreased supraphysiologic thermogenesis.[23] In children with burns, treatment with propranolol during hospitalization attenuates hypermetabolism and reverses muscle-protein catabolism. Propranolol is given to achieve a 20% decrease in heart rate of each patient compared with the 24-h average heart rate immediately before administration.[23]

Amino acids

Research into glutamine and arginine has proliferated in recent years with equivocal results. Both nutrients have been demonstrated to improve outcomes such as length of stay, infection rate, mortality in critically ill patients including burn patients. A review of randomized trials, systematic reviews and guidelines concluded that "glutamine therapy in burns is promising" but the safety and efficacy of long-term use along with the best route and dosage is debatable.[24]

Rehabilitation

Rehabilitation is the restoration to health and work capacity of a person incapacitated by burn injury. Burns rehabilitation is often challenging and has several other dimensions, entailing much more than the sole aim of preventing scarring. Burn patients have to recover full use not only of their injured part(s) but of their whole body and they have to recover confidence in their ability to work and enjoy life.

Rehabilitation starts on the day of injury. The treatment of burns is generally divided into an acute and a chronic period. Anticipation and treatment of problems resulting from the injury and edema prevent many subsequent complications. It progresses through grafting and healing to discharge from the ward, integration into society and through the sometimes endless period of reconstructive surgery to a point when, "either the patient has had enough or the surgeon suggests he can do no more, and usually it is the former."

The acute period is defined as the period from the occurrence of the burn to complete wound coverage. The chronic period has been arbitrarily defined as the period from completion of wound coverage to maturity of the scar. During the acute phase, prevention of contractures by physical therapy, traction and splinting is of paramount importance (*Box 18.14*).[25] Physiotherapy is very important in the prevention of the burn contractures and also, to show the effectiveness of the teamwork. There have been debates over whether to rest

---

Box 18.14 Physiotherapy and occupational therapy treatments

- Regular physiotherapy several times per day
- Starting physiotherapy from 1st day of patient's admission and as early as the 3rd day of grafting[25]
- Early chest physiotherapy to prevent remove secretions and prevent atelectasis
- Exercise and stretching therapy to prevent joint contracture
- Ankle pump exercise several times per day
- Prevention of muscular atrophy with passive and active (with and without load) exercises ± electrical stimulation
- Ambulation as soon as possible
- Education of the patient's family to help the patient and the burn care professionals
- Consideration and prevention of secondary complications (e.g., frozen shoulder, scoliosis, etc.)
- Use of splinting and modalities (e.g., ultrasound) based on patient's need to protecting the skin grafts and preventing the burn scar
- Encourage activities of daily living with emphasis on fine movements and joint mobilization.

---

or mobilize injuries.[26] Recently, early motion has been strongly advocated but it is important to recognize the stages of wound healing and to arrange a balance between rest and exercise. A study has demonstrated that starting good burn physiotherapy on day 1 for not grafted areas and day 3 for skin grafted areas resulted in only 6% burn contracture.[25] In addition, the results of this study indicated the following factors that could help to decrease the burn-injured complications:

1. To consider the joint position during immobilization phase after graft
2. To decrease the immobilization phase after graft
3. To increase the interval of physiotherapy treatment per day and also to organize the aim of physiotherapy based on the patient's needs
4. To pay extra attention to some areas, e.g., shoulder, neck, fingers and face.

To achieve these, everyone, including patients, must have a clear understanding of the aims of physiotherapy and the following points could be considered for decreasing the burn-injured complications:

1. To have a team activity with emphasis on psychological and nutritional supports
2. To consider the continuation of physiotherapy treatment after releasing the patient from hospital, for at least 18 months
3. To use pressure garment before starting the keloid
4. To use a suitable cream for itching.

In the acute and post-healing stages of recovery, the move out of the ward is the first defining point in a patient's post-burn life. In addition to physical considerations, wound healing and recovery after burns is promoted by good nutrition, for initial wound healing and long term scar reduction. Rehabilitation involves the whole burn team in encouraging the patient to live as normal a life as possible between dressing changes and operations; the therapists take the lead in

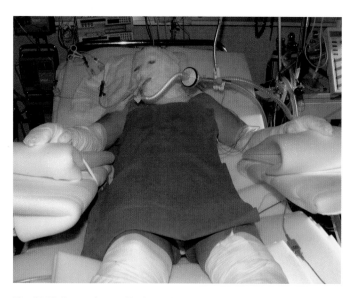

Fig. 18.35 Burn patient positioning and pressure management are important for rehabilitation.

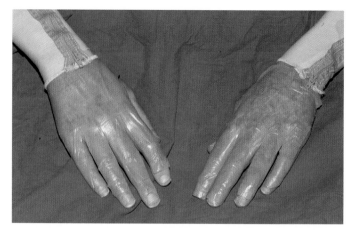

Fig. 18.36 Silicone and pressure garment therapy for burn rehabilitation.

maintaining muscle strength, joint range and activities of daily living *(Fig. 18.35)*.

In the chronic phase, the prevention of hypertrophic scarring and contractures become major concerns. Throughout treatment, the social and emotional rehabilitation of burn patients is a prime concern. Pressure garments, have pitfalls in their use and the importance of careful fitting, constant wearing of the garments and the appropriate use of pressure paddings is essential. It is obvious that close supervision is essential, particularly for children.

The rehabilitation therapist (occupational and physical) evaluates and formulates a treatment plan and begins functional range of motion, splinting, edema control, and scar modulation as needed. Hands are a primary concern, especially deep burns of the dorsal surface. They receive immediate range of motion and splinting *(Fig. 18.36)*. Although survival takes precedence in the critically ill patient, physical and occupational therapy objectives are always kept in mind. Irrespective of the patient's general condition, injured upper and lower extremities are elevated to allow adequate venous drainage and to reduce edema. Much of the functional limitations to burned areas depend on the outcome of skin grafts, the local tissue healing factors, and the baseline state of the patient. Nonetheless, the quality and availability of therapists, especially in burn injuries of the upper extremities, have been shown to influence the outcomes of surgical interventions. In some circumstances, treatment by good therapists decreases the need for surgical treatment. Early and proper splinting and stretching of flexion crease burns, such as the neck, axilla, and antecubital areas, reduce the extent of scar contractures and may prevent subsequent functional deformities and the need for reconstruction.

During the recovery phase of the burn injury, rehabilitation therapy is even more important, often occupying the majority of the patient's treatment time. Limitations to activities of daily living, strengthening and increasing of muscle mass, and even cosmetic results of burn scars are under the influence of the therapists. The therapists provide pressure garments, thermoplastic splints, serial casting, silicone inserts,

and plastic facemasks to decrease hypertrophic scars and joint contractures. There is a need for intensive post-healing rehabilitation, both for adults and for children, particularly as it will increasingly be possible to keep alive, and to heal, burns of a much greater percentage of body area. Children's burn clubs go a long way in providing confidence-building support after discharge from the ward, so the children are at present in a better position than adults, however there is still a need for intensive rehabilitation in high trauma rehabilitation centers independent of burn centers.

Many can manage well with physiotherapy and occupational therapy. Another post-healing team concept is outreach. It was introduced to try to overcome the gap recognized at this stage of recovery, to provide links with the community services and local hospitals. Rehabilitation centers start integration back into society in a protected environment with other people who had sustained physical trauma. They could receive the help in returning to work, to the home, hobbies and to society, and if necessary return for 'top up' help after reconstructive surgery.

Psychological factors such as sexuality and changed body image require careful management. Adaptation to long-term disability should be integrated into the rehabilitation treatment plan as well as the assessment of post-traumatic stress disorder as the potential to develop this disorder exists owing to the often distressing nature of many of these injuries. The input of psychological services is an invaluable aspect of burns rehabilitation.

In addition, reintroduction to society and work may provide several challenges to a burns' survivor. Issues related to a full return to the community, and their solutions such as behaviour therapy, occupational rehabilitation, and adaptive equipment may be outside the limits of this chapter. However, follow-up recommendations, including a more comprehensive checklist of potential areas of need, may be helpful.

Pain control

The adverse sequelae of inadequate pain in the burn population have been long recognized, yet control of pain remains inadequate globally. The dynamic evolution of burn pain both centrally and peripherally, and the many factors which influence pain perception illustrate the need for a therapeutic plan

Box 18.15 Pharmacological methods of burn pain management

Opioid analgesics

- Morphine: "gold standard" opioid drug
- Oxycodone: less hallucinations and histamine-induced itching than morphine
- Fentanyl: rapid onset, potent, short acting synthetic opiate. Provides good procedural analgesia but potent respiratory depressant
- Remifentanil: ultra-short acting opiate, useful only as an infusion for the management of short bursts of previous pain and to assist with weaning from mechanical ventilation
- Alfentanil: shorter acting than fentanyl and thus favored as the opiate of choice for control of procedural burn previous pain both as a sole agent and in combination with propofol
- Alfentanil: undergoes hepatic metabolism to inactive, nontoxic metabolites which are renally cleared. Safest strong opioids in severe renal impairment.
- Methadone.

Simple analgesics

- Paracetamol
- Non-steroidal anti-inflammatory drugs (NSAIDs)

Other drugs

- Gabapentin
- Ketamine
- Clonidine
- Benzodiazepines
- Amitriptyline
- Lignocaine by intravenous infusion
- Entonox

which is similarly dynamic and flexible enough to cope with the facets of background, breakthrough, procedural and post-operative pain. Regular, ongoing and documented pain assessment is key in directing this process.

Before prescribing any drug to a burn patient, the clinician must have an understanding of the altered pharmacokinetic state resulting from well-described pathophysiological changes that follow burn injury. During the first 48 h, decreased organ blood supply will reduce clearance of drugs, but the subsequent hypermetabolic phase (48 h after injury) is associated with increased clearance. Variations in levels of acute phase plasma proteins lead to changes in drug binding and free fractions available for end action. The volume of distribution of a drug may be further affected by alterations in total body water. Using regular and repeated pain assessment to quantify the effect of analgesic agents reduces the impact of these changes. Doses vary widely between individuals and over time with the same individual.

The family of opioid analgesics provides the backbone of analgesia to burn patients (Box 18.15). Together, they provide an excellent range of potencies, duration of actions and routes of administration. However, they must be used judiciously as side-effects may be clinically relevant and furthermore, recent data has implicated them as being capable of inducing pain NMDA receptor antagonist such as ketamine and gabapentin are increasingly recognized as useful adjuncts, capable of marked opiate sparing effects in this population. The simple analgesic paracetamol (acetaminophen) has both anti-pyretic and opioid-sparing properties and justly deserves its place in the pharmacological treatment of every burn patient. Nonpharmacological methods of pain control can play an important role in suitable patients but resources vary widely between units.

Severe pain with burns is a major physiologic stress that can have a negative impact on the patient's recovery. A person with burns has exposed functioning nerve endings. Dressing changes and bedside debridement often require high doses of opiates and sedatives. The availability of reversal agents for benzodiazepines has improved the safety of combining these drugs with opiates. Close monitoring of respiratory status is required when consciousness is diminished. Short-acting agents such as barbiturates and lipid-soluble agents also require careful monitoring with use. Ketamine, combined with a sedative like midazolam, provides pain control with little respiratory depression.

More emphasis on pain control not only helps the patient's psychological wellbeing but may significantly affect physical outcome as well. Some clinical evidence and common sense suggest that adequate analgesia may limit the overall hyper-metabolic and catabolic state. Painful stimuli influence the release of a number of circulatory factors that affect tissue perfusion, immune system function, and wound healing. Further research should help delineate the negative or positive effect of modulating pain.

Patients without a substance abuse problem before the injury typically do not develop opiate addiction even after receiving high doses for prolonged periods, but physical dependence often occurs after sustained treatment with opiates. Gradually reducing the doses of opiates as pain diminishes avoids opiate withdrawal.

Patients with a history of substance abuse present special problems. Heroin users require much larger doses of opiates to achieve the same analgesic effects. Methadone can be used for long-acting pain relief and to prevent opiate withdrawal. Alcoholic patients risk alcohol withdrawal and delirium tremens. Benzodiazepines prevent discomfort and the potential for progression to life-threatening delirium tremens and seizure. Skillful pain management can contribute greatly to wound healing and rehabilitation efforts and should be given a high priority in the comprehensive treatment of the burn patient.

Complications (Box 18.16)

Skin graft loss

Loss of skin graft is the most common operative complication and is caused by hematoma, infection and graft shear. Early graft examination should be encouraged with removal of any underlying hematoma. After day 3, capillary ingrowth has occurred and would be interrupted by graft movement. If examination shows that the skin grafts are grossly infected, then quantitative microbiological cultures can be performed and appropriate topical antimicrobial therapy commenced. It is very important that skin grafts are carefully immobilized with bolsters or splinting to prevent graft shear.

Infected burn

Infection should be suspected if the wound becomes increasingly uncomfortable, painful, or smelly; if cellulitis is

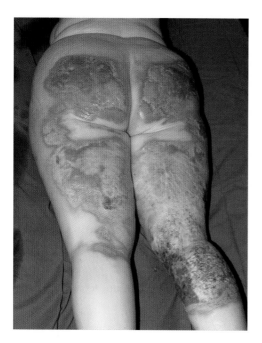

Fig. 18.37 Pseudomonas aeruginosa infection of burn wounds.

Box 18.16 **Potential complications during acute burns management**

- Respiratory distress from smoke inhalation or a severe chest burn
- Fluid loss, hypovolemia and shock
- Infection
- Increased metabolic rate
- Increased plasma viscosity and thrombosis
- Vascular insufficiency and distal ischemia from a circumferential burn of limb or digit
- Muscle damage from an electrical burn may be severe even with minimal skin injury; rhabdomyolysis may cause renal failure
- Poisoning from inhalation of noxious gases released by burning (e.g., cyanide poisoning due to smouldering plastics)
- Hemoglobinuria and renal damage
- Scarring and possible psychological consequences.

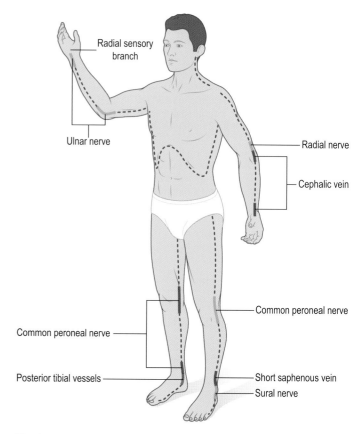

Fig. 18.38 Escharotomy lines and relevant anatomy.

---

observed; or if the person develops a fever *(Fig. 18.37)*. A swab from the burn wound should be sent for microbiology. Treatment may require wide excision of all infected tissue and administration of antibiotics. Empirical antibiotic treatment should be started after discussion with the microbiology team and the antibiotic treatment later changed according to the results from the swab. The recommended choice of antibiotic is guided by the most likely cause of infection and local patterns of antibiotic resistance should also be considered.

Adrenal insufficiency

Absolute adrenal insufficiency occurs in up to 36% of patients with major burns, but there is no association between response to corticotropin stimulation and survival. Those with >30% TBSA burns have higher cortisol levels but may be resistant to serum cortisol increases in response to stimulation. The clinical relevance of this finding has not been established.

Compartment syndrome

Pathophysiologically, any process that results in elevated pressure in a closed fascial compartment can cause a compartment syndrome *(Figs 18.38, 18.39)*. Compartment syndrome occurs when the tissue pressure within an enclosed space is elevated to the extent that there is decreased blood flow within the space, decreasing tissue oxygenation and impairing metabolic function. The final result without prompt treatment is cellular death. Extremity compartment syndromes can also result from extensive edema formation. Patients may require escharotomies, fasciotomies, or both for the release of extremity compartment syndrome. Patients with circumferential full-thickness burns (neck, thorax, abdomen, extremities) are also at risk of requiring escharotomies *(Figs 18.40–18.46)*. In extremities there is impaired capillary refill, paraesthesia, and increased pain develop earlier than decreased pulses. The orbit is a compartment limited to expansion and may require lateral canthotomy to successfully reduce intraocular pressure to normal.

Abdominal compartment syndrome is a life-threatening situation associated with fluid extravasation/edema and fluid resuscitation. It is defined as intra-abdominal pressure >20 mmHg and at least one new organ dysfunction. It is associated with renal impairment, gut ischemia, and cardiac and pulmonary malperfusion. Clinical manifestations

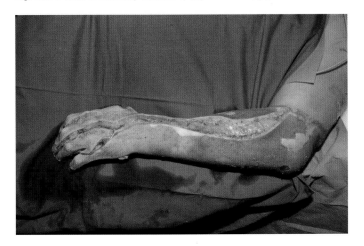
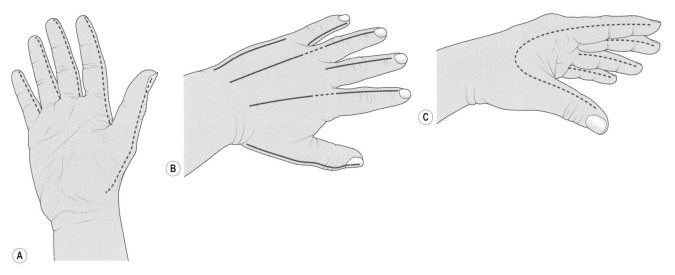

Fig. 18.39 Hand escharotomy incisions: **(A,C)** lateral view, **(B)** dorsal view.

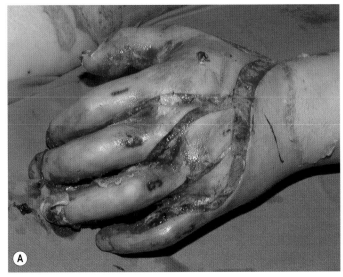

Fig. 18.40 Escharotomy for full thickness burn. It must extend into normal tissue.

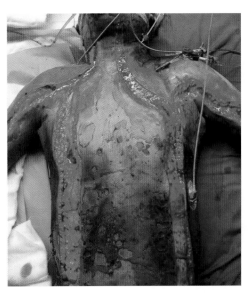

Fig. 18.41 Circumferential full thickness burns require escharotomy. It is not always possible to site intravenous access in unburnt tissue.

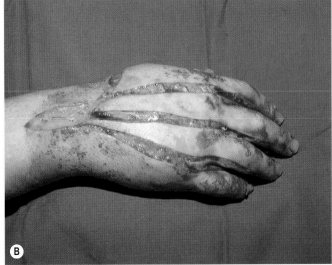

Fig. 18.42 Hand escharotomies.

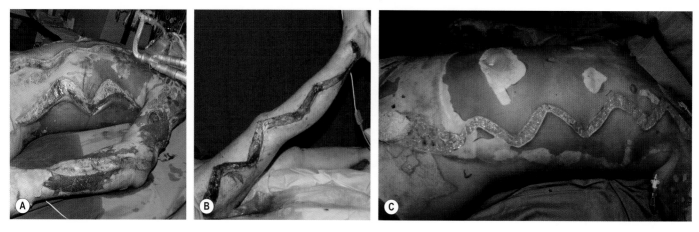

Fig. 18.43 Zigzag escharotomy incisions help prevent straight line scar contractures which may require secondary reconstruction.

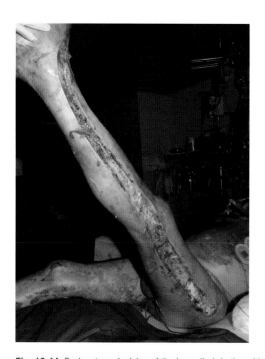

Fig. 18.44 Escharotomy incision of the lower limb in the midaxial line between the flexor and extensor surfaces.

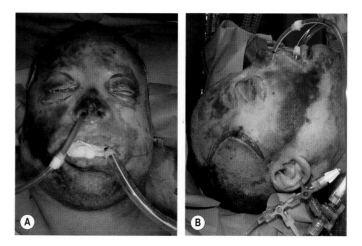

Fig. 18.45 (A) Periocular escharotomies. **(B)** Temporal and periocular escharotomies.

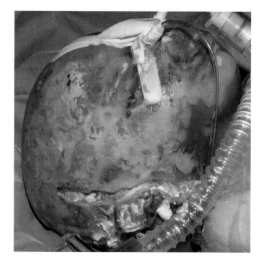

Fig. 18.46 Any circumferential burn of the face, scalp, thorax, abdomen, penis or extremity may require early escharotomy for deleterious compressional effects of the burn eschar.

include tense abdomen, decreased pulmonary compliance, hypercapnia, and oliguria. Urine output monitoring is not sensitive or specific enough to diagnose abdominal compartment syndrome. Careful monitoring and aggressive treatment should be instituted to avoid this mortal complication. Appropriate intravascular volume, appropriate body positioning, pain management, sedation, nasogastric decompression if appropriate, chemical paralysis if required, and torsoescharotomy are all interventions to increase abdominal wall compliance and decrease intra-abdominal pressures. Bladder pressure monitoring should be initiated as part of the burn fluid resuscitation protocol in every patient with 30% TBSA burn. Patients who receive >250 mL/kg of crystalloid in the first 24 h may require abdominal decompression. Percutaneous abdominal decompression is a minimally invasive procedure that should be performed before resorting to

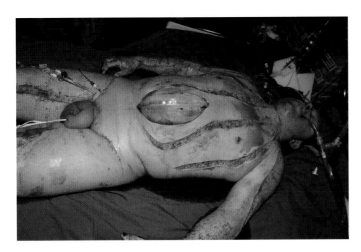

Fig. 18.47 Extensive escharotomies and decompressive laparotomy.

laparotomy. If less invasive maneuvers fail, decompressive laparotomy *(Fig. 18.47)* should be performed in patients with abdominal compartment syndrome that is refractory to other therapies and the reported mortality rates for decompressive laparotomy is as high as 100%.

Deep venous thrombosis

Deep venous thrombosis incidence ranges from 1% to 23% in burn patients and deep venous thrombosis chemoprophylaxis is recommended.

Gastrointestinal complications

Gastrointestinal (GI) complications (e.g., gastric and intestinal motor dysfunction as well as stress-related mucosal disease [SRMD]) frequently occur in burn patients and adversely affect patient outcomes. Gastrointestinal motor dysfunction may predispose patients to impaired enteral nutrition and pulmonary aspiration of gastric contents.[27] Stress-related mucosal damage – an acute erosive gastritis – occurs in many burn patients in ICUs and may develop within 24 h of admission.[28] The incidence of SRMD varies widely given the population of patients studied and the definition of bleeding used. Upper gastrointestinal tract mucosal injury detected by endoscopy is extremely common in the burns population, and stress-induced gastritis and ulceration can be shown to be endoscopically evident in up to 78% of adult burn patients. Stress induced ulcers of the stomach and duodenum in very extensively burned patients are due to a defect in the mucosal barrier to secreted acid. The cause of this defect is related partly to mucosal ischemia which is aggravated by hypotension, sepsis and hypoxia.

Occult bleeding in the adult burn population is also very common. The incidence of clinically important GI bleeding, defined as overt bleeding complicated by hemodynamic instability, decrease in hemoglobin, and/or need for blood transfusion, from SRMD in the this population is about 1–6%. In addition, the morbidity associated with this type of severe ulceration and bleeding can increase the length of stay in the ICU by up to 8 days, and mortality is as much as four-fold higher than it is in ICU patients without this complication.

The use of drugs to prevent stress-related gastric bleeding in critically ill surgical cancer patients is common. Occult bleeding in the adult burn population is also very common. However, clinically important bleeding, as defined by the need for blood transfusions or a significant alteration in the vital signs, occurs in 0.6–6% of patients. Because of marked improvements in early resuscitation and oxygenation, correction of fluid and acid–base imbalances, improvements in the care of the critically ill (including early enteral nutrition), as well as early prophylactic treatment with antacids, H2b antagonists, proton pump inhibitors or sucralfate and early enteral feedings have greatly decreased the incidence of this devastating problem. Aggressive nutritional support has probably helped with ulcer healing and also prevents acalculous cholecystitis.

Heterotopic ossification

The transformation of primitive mesenchymal cells in the surrounding soft tissue to mature lamellar bone is termed heterotopic ossification (HO). HO is a pathologic condition that adversely affects a subpopulation of burn patients. The incidence of HO in a general burn population is reported to be between 1% and 3%. HO after burns commonly occurs around major joints. Elbow, shoulder, and hip are the most commonly affected joints, in that order of frequency. HO is characterized by progressive abnormal soft tissue and periarticular bone formation that encroaches upon the joint, eventually causing decreased range of motion and functional disability, pain in the involved joint and limb, and possibly nerve entrapment. The etiology and pathogenesis of HO in burn patients is not understood. It usually occurs in patients with large (generally >20% TBSA) and/or full-thickness burns, but HO has occasionally been reported in burns under 10% TBSA. HO also usually occurs in burned extremities, but it is sometimes found in areas remote from the injured site. HO seems to be related to the extended time to wound closure and genetic predisposition. Patients who require a longer time to definitive burn excision and skin grafting tend to demonstrate a greater incidence of HO than patients who undergo successful early excision and grafting. HO also appears to be related to movement at the affected joints. However, the exact relationship is unclear. Patients who are completely immobilized and patients who receive aggressive physical/occupational therapy seem to both be at greater risk for the development of HO. A combination of immobilization, an active inflammatory state, hypermetabolism, and local trauma and hemorrhage from over-vigorous physiotherapy are thus putative causative events. Other contributing factors may include vascular stasis, tissue hypoxia, infection, deep venous thrombosis, high dietary protein intake, and abnormal calcium metabolism. Sometimes, it is difficult to differentiate HO from scar contracture by clinical symptoms and signs. Physicians should keep the diagnosis of HO in mind when burn patients complain of decreased ROM in their elbow joints. X-ray is a fast and economical tool for diagnosis of HO. Other diagnostic tools include CT, magnetic resonance imaging (MRI), bone scan and ultrasound.

The treatment of HO is largely conservative with surgery in combination with rehabilitation reserved for patients who do not respond to less invasive measures, or who have severe HO.[29,30] Adjuvants to surgical excision include perioperative radiation therapy and/or injection of corticosteroids. Attempts to prevent HO in burn patients have focused on early wound closure, early mobilization, gentle passive and active range of motion exercises, and pharmacologic therapy with salicylates, warfarin, and/or biphosphates.

Heparin-induced thrombocytopenia

Early thrombocytopenia occurs in the post-burn course in patients with extensive injury. Problems after burn injury such as pulmonary infections, multiorgan failure, sepsis, and bleeding disorders accentuate this trend. Careful observance for thrombocytopenia after the first week of hospitalization will alert the practitioner to make the diagnosis in burn patients. Although the incidence of heparin-induced thrombocytopenia is relatively low, the complications are major and include arterial and venous thromboses and increased number of surgeries.

Inflammation

There are standardized definitions for sepsis and infection-related diagnose in burn patients. Patients with large burns have a baseline temperature reset to 38.5°C, and tachycardia and tachypnea may persist for months. Continuous exposure to inflammatory mediators leads to significant changes in the white blood cell count, making leukocytosis a poor indicator of sepsis. Use other clues as signs of infection or sepsis such as increased fluid requirements, decreasing platelet counts >3 days after burn injury, altered mental status, worsening pulmonary status, and impaired renal function. The term systemic inflammatory response syndrome should not be applied to burn patients because patients with large burns are in a state of chronic systemic inflammatory stimulation.[31]

Neutropenia

Transient leucopenia is common, primarily due to a decreased neutrophil count. Maximal white blood cell depression occurs several days after admission with rebound to normal a few days later. Use of silver sulfadiazine has been associated with this transient leucopenia; resolution is independent of continued silver sulfadiazine.

Infection

Patients with large TBSA burns are immunosuppressed and at increased risk for infections, especially of the wounds, venous access sites, and lungs. Small injuries (<10% TBSA) heal rapidly, and infections are rare. Monitoring at-risk patients for infection can be a problem because many burn patients have a fever and altered white blood cell counts without infections.

In burns patients infections arise from multiple sources. Any infection in a burn patient should be considered to be from the central venous catheter until proven otherwise and the catheter should be changed.[31] Burn wounds become rapidly infected with Gram-positive bacteria, mainly staphylococci, that are normal deep inhabitants of the sweat glands and hair follicles exposed by the burn. The moist, vascular burn eschar further encourages microbial growth.

Gram-negative bacterial infections result from translocation from the colon because of reduced mesenteric blood flow at the time of burn and subsequent insults. Furthermore, there are several immune deficits in burns patients, including impaired cytotoxic T lymphocyte response, myeloid maturation arrest causing neutropenia, impaired neutrophil function, and decreased macrophage production. Finally, burns patients can incur hospital acquired infections common to other patients in intensive care units, including intravascular catheter related infections and ventilator associated pneumonia, with an overall incidence of infection higher than that of other patients in intensive care units.

Antibiotic prophylaxis reduces all cause mortality among patients in intensive care but injudicious use of antibiotics merely eliminates the patient's normal flora and allows resistant organisms to grow; therefore, prophylactic antibiotics are rarely used. Therefore, current guidelines for management do not recommend systemic antibiotic prophylaxis for burns patients, stating lack of evidence for efficacy and induction of antibiotic resistance. A recent systematic review and meta-analysis found that in burns patients, systemic antibiotic prophylaxis administered in the first 4–14 days significantly reduced all cause mortality by nearly a half and limited perioperative prophylaxis reduced wound infections but not mortality.[32] In addition, they concluded that topical antibiotic prophylaxis applied to burn wounds, commonly recommended, had no beneficial effects. Unfortunately, the methodological quality of the data was weak and they concluded that prophylaxis could not be recommended for patients with severe burns other than perioperatively and that there was a need for randomized controlled trials to assess its use.

However, these patients are often fragile, and delayed treatment of real infections risks severe episodes of sepsis leading to multisystem organ failure. Treatment is often initiated empirically before a specific organism is isolated. Patients with large enough wounds and with enough time ultimately develop life-threatening infections that must be treated. Unfortunately, treatment of one organism often leads to colonization by resistant organisms and additional infections. Bacteria, such as staphylococci and pseudomonas, resistant to many antibiotics and fungus are pathogens commonly found in burn patients late in the course of treatment. These organisms are more difficult and risky to treat. Waiting until there is good clinical evidence of an infection before initiating treatment may delay the infection by resistant organisms.

The majority of burn patients have a low-grade fever but no source of infection in the first week after injury. Contamination and then overgrowth of burn wounds by pathogens causing a systemic picture of sepsis typically occur 2–3 weeks after injury. Early debridement of the necrotic burn tissue and coverage with skin greatly reduce the incidence and morbidity of burn wound infections. Patients with large surface area burns that remain open for long periods still develop wound infections, have poor healing, and ultimately succumb to infection. Isolation of the patient in specialized unit beds along with infection precautions by the health care workers (handwashing, gloves, and gowns) reduces the transmission of pathogens from one patient to another but does not protect patients from their own pathogens (skin and gastrointestinal tract). A high level of suspicion for wound infection must be kept when the patient's condition deteriorates rapidly. Daily observation of the wounds by trained personnel is critical even after permanent skin grafts are placed. Wound cultures, particularly quantitative assessment, and biopsies for histologic examination help confirm the diagnosis and direct therapy. Prompt excision of infected and necrotic tissue, appropriate topical treatment, and systemic antimicrobial therapy are critical to survival of the patient.

Great emphasis is placed on the isolation and protection of burn patients from environmental pathogens. It is worthwhile to place these patients in protective isolation to limit contact with hospital-based pathogens, such as multidrug-resistant organisms. Despite these precautions, most severely injured patients have one or several bouts of infection through the course of their treatment. The skin and gut of the patient harbor pathogens, and no known therapy can eliminate these sources of infection for long. The best treatment is to bolster the immune system and re-establish the barrier function of the gut and skin. Suspected or proven infections warrant treatment with systemic antimicrobial medications. Treatment with an antibiotic usually controls the infections but alters the patient's microbial flora. Should the patient remain at risk for infections after the first infection is treated, a second, more drug resistant infection often occurs. Should the burn be large enough that the patient remains at risk for a month or longer, fungal infections become a serious threat. Treatment with less toxic fluconazole has greatly increased the therapeutic options, but many patients still eventually require amphotericin.

Inhalation injury and respiratory complications are still one of the major causes of mortality in severe burns. Ventilatory support and airway management in this situation is often challenging, and the need for prolonged endotracheal intubation is very common in patients affected of different degrees of respiratory distress syndrome. Despite the use of high-volume low-pressure cuffs, considerable controversy exists among burn surgeons as to whether to convert endotracheal tubes to tracheostomy in burns patients, particularly when ventilatory support is prolonged beyond two weeks or when other airway complications occur, as many studies have recorded high mortality and high tracheostomy complications.

The pathogenesis of these entities is still unclear, but the combination of the inhalation injury, infection, presence of the endotracheal tube and individual factors play an important role in the development of this complications. Tracheostomies may provide a good portal of entry for microorganisms into the respiratory tract, with a high incidence of respiratory infection and sepsis. Cross-colonization of the respiratory tract from the wound exists, but it does not show a direct relationship with cross-infection. In addition, feeding aspirations, obstructive abnormalities, increased incidence of pneumonia and trachea-innominate fistulas have been reported as high morbidity complications of tracheostomies. Long-term sequelae are no less important. Stenosis of the airway, dysphagia, alterations of speech, trachea-esophageal fistulas and tracheomalacia can compromise the favorable outcome of this selected group of patients. Every effort should be made to maintain airway pressures at the lowest range, in order to prevent tracheomalacia. Advantages of tracheostomy include minimizing dead space, ease of suctioning, presence of a more secure airway and ease of movement. Theoretically, it should prevent the appearance of subglottic stenosis.

Patients with cutaneous burns have a high incidence of pulmonary infection even without lung injury from smoke inhalation. The skin injury increases interstitial fluid in the lung, and the lung is at risk from pathogens in the blood and the respiratory tree. Chest radiographic changes, purulent sputum production, and microbiologic results help determine when and what to treat. Patients are at risk for pulmonary infection until the burn wounds are covered. Evidence of a pulmonary infection should be treated aggressively with pulmonary toilet and broad-spectrum antibiotics. A more narrow spectrum antibiotic can be selected after sputum or pulmonary lavage culture results are obtained. Mechanical ventilation support may be needed in cases of severe pulmonary compromise to augment gas exchange and to decrease the labor of respiration for the patient. On occasion, patients develop adult respiratory distress syndrome marked by worsening hypoxemia, hypercapnia, and lung compliance. Supportive treatment with supplemental oxygen, positive end-expiratory pressure, and high-frequency ventilation is effective in most patients. High-dose steroids have been used in cases of refractory pulmonary failure but have not been shown to be effective. Many patients intubated for more than a month benefit from a tracheostomy. The use of low-pressure balloons in modern endotracheal tubes has markedly decreased the incidence of tracheal erosion and life-threatening trachea-innominate artery fistulas. Tracheostomies are still useful so patients can be gradually and safely weaned from prolonged dependence on mechanical ventilation and to decrease injury to vocal cords.

Long-term vascular access plays a vital role in the management of burn patients, in which a reliable vessel to access for medications (e.g., antimicrobials and analgesics), blood draws, fluid administration and sometimes for arterial pressure monitoring is needed. Although the lines have been highly valued by patients and parents, they carry with them inherent risks *(Table 18.10)*. Most of these problems occur either at the time of insertion, such as a pneumothorax, or while the line is in place, such as a line infection. Regular monitoring following insertion or removal of a vascular access line is mandatory for the early recognition and treatment of any associated complications. Peripheral lines should be used initially whenever sites are available. These lines can become infected with blood-borne pathogens or from the skin puncture site. The diagnosis should be suspected when the patient

Table 18.10 **Complications of peripheral and central-line insertion**

Early	Late
Hematoma	Thrombophlebitis
Venous laceration	Infection
Arterial puncture	Chylothorax
Hemothorax	Horner's syndrome
Air embolism	Pseudoaneurysm
Pneumothorax	Arteriovenous fistula
Pleural effusion	Thrombosis
Dysrhythmias	Embolism

develops fever, leucocytosis, or thrombocytopenia or when organisms are grown from blood cultures. Septic thrombophlebitis should be suspected in all burn patients with unexplained infections, and all sites of prior catheter access must be carefully inspected. Many of these patients require central venous lines at some point in their treatment because peripheral access sites are usually limited. Central line-related infections can cause major morbidity, and constant attention is given to changing catheters once a line infection is suspected.

Hypertrophic scar

Hypertrophic scar formation after burn wound healing is a major problem. Hypertrophic scarring, unstable epithelium, and poor skin elasticity often occur when deep wounds are allowed to heal without grafting. Deep wounds, treated conservatively, tend to develop problems more frequently than superficial wounds because the extended period of inflammation elicits a fibrotic response. Early skin grafting of these deep wounds shortens the period of healing and inflammation and avoids some of the later problems of hypertrophic scarring. Both pressure garment and silicone therapy are associated with a reduction of hypertrophic scar formation after burn injury.

Hypothermia

The serious side-effects of hypothermia cannot be overstated. Strategies to vigorously prevent hypothermia include a warmed room, warmed inspired air, warming blankets, and countercurrent heat exchangers for infused fluids. Metabolic responses can be minimized by treating the patient in a thermoneutral environment (~30°C). During hydrotherapy, in the operating room, and in the burn unit, keep the room temperature at ~30°C to reduce heat loss and decrease metabolic rate.

Secondary sclerosing cholangitis

There are increasing reports in the literature regarding secondary sclerosing cholangitis (SSC).[11] Sepsis and shock cause endothelial and bile duct injury also through translocation of bacteria and endotoxins into the portal blood and into the bile ducts. Following cholangitis, post-inflammatory biliary strictures may develop. Moreover, burn injuries in particular can induce selective vasoconstriction of hepatic arterial blood flow. This additional hepatic ischemia and critical reduction of hepatic oxygen delivery may lead to sclerosing cholangitis. Treatment options for patients with SSC are limited. Long-term results of several trials in patients with sclerosing cholangitis suggest an improvement in clinical symptoms and liver function tests after regular endoscopic treatment (sphincterotomy, stenting, extraction of as many of the biliary casts as possible, continuous flushing of the bile ducts with saline solution through endoscopic nasobiliary drainage). Ursodeoxycholic acid treatment, in combination with repeated endoscopic interventions and opening of bile duct stenoses, may further improve both survival and the clinical outcome of patients with sclerosing cholangitis. It is recommended that biliary infection should be treated with antibiotics at doses high enough that effective concentrations of the drug are reached in the bile. The combination of endoscopic and medical treatment may result in transient clinical and biochemical improvements; however, the progressive destruction of the biliary tree cannot be prevented. If end-stage liver disease develops orthotopic liver transplantation is indicated.

Access the complete reference list online at **http://www.expertconsult.com**

8.   Nguyen N, Gun R, Sparnon A, et al P. The importance of immediate cooling – a case series of childhood burns in Vietnam. *Burns*. 2002;28:173–176.

   Early cooling will prevent a significant percentage of superficial burns from progressing to deep burns. This will not only reduce the probability that skin grafting and expensive treatment will be required, but will reduce the risk of other consequences of deep burns, which may be fatal.

14.   Cahill NE, Dhaliwal R, Day AG, et al. Nutrition therapy in the critical care setting: what is 'best achievable' practice? An international multicenter observational study. *Crit Care Med*. 2010;38:395–401.

19.   Hemmila MR, Taddonio MA, Arbabi S, et al. Intensive insulin therapy is associated with reduced infectious complications in burn patients. *Surgery*. 2008;144:629–637.

25.   Okhovatian F, Zoubine N. A comparison between two burn rehabilitation protocols. *Burns*. 2007;33:429–434.

31.   Greenhalgh JR, Saffle JH, Holmes RL, et al. American Burn Association consensus conference to define sepsis and infection in burns. *J Burn Care Res*. 2007;28:776–790.

32.   Avni T, Levcovich A, Ad-El DD, et al. Prophylactic antibiotics for burns patients: systematic review and meta-analysis. *Br Med J*. 2010;340:c241.

   In burns patients, systemic antibiotic prophylaxis administered in the first 4–14 days significantly reduces all cause mortality by nearly a half; limited perioperative prophylaxis reduces wound infections but not mortality. Topical antibiotic prophylaxis applied to burn wounds, commonly recommended, had no beneficial effects The methodological quality of the evidence is weak, however, so a large, robust randomized controlled trial is now needed.

19

Extremity burn reconstruction

Lorenzo Borghese, Alessandro Masellis, and Michele Masellis

SYNOPSIS

- In electrical burn injuries, the patient's conditions often seems less critical than it really is.
- Always consider compartment syndrome when limbs have extensive burns.
- When perform escharotomy on the limbs, pay attention to dangerous sites, such as the basilic or saphenus veins, and the radial or tibial nerves.
- The extremites are the most frequent areas affected by post-surgery scar contractures. Correct positioning of articualtions, good management of scars and post-operative care are mandatory.
- The Z-plasty technique (in its all variations) remains one of the most effectiveness procedure for post-burn scar retractions.
- Reconstructive surgery of burn sequelae often needs "imagination". Due to the presence of scars, to the damaged tissues, to the lack of good vessels, it is very hard to follow a single preoperative plan. You need many arrows in your quiver.

 Access the Historical Perspective section online at
http://www.expertconsult.com

Introduction

The upper and lower extremities are often involved in burn-related accidents. In particular, the arms and legs are the most exposed areas, as they constitute the first means of self-protection and are used to aid escape in accidents.

The majority of burn-related accidents involving the extremities, occur in the workplace and are mainly due to fire and electricity. In a domestic environment the majority of victims are babies, who suffer burns owing to contact with hot liquids.[1,2]

Extremity burns can be considered "difficult" burns, especially if they are extensive circumferential burns. Deep second- and third-degree burns, if not properly treated, can result in

severe *compartment syndromes*, which can cause the loss of the extremity involved if not treated in a well-equipped burn-specialized facility.[3,4]

Knee and elbow joints are often prone to severe damage related to electrocution. *The electric arc* that is formed in this type of accident often finds its entry or exit point in one of these joints, causing the joint to explode.

Scarring often represents real challenges for the plastic surgeon. Some 50% of Z-plasties, as well as other surgical techniques such as scar debridement, involve the axillary cavity. In developing countries, the percentage of scar retraction causing disabilities is significant. This results in almost grotesque thoracic-brachial and brachio-antebrachial clinical picture and presents leg adhesions that are incompatible with the physiology of the structures involved.

While the patient is hospitalized, physio-kinesitherapy is specifically aimed at maintaining mobility of the major joints. Even if they may be only marginally involved in the accident, these parts are in fact often subject to arthritis, dysplasia, and joint calcification, which are not easy to treat.

These preliminary observations serve to point out that reconstruction of the extremities, which are a person's main source of self-sufficiency, is not simply a matter of aesthetics but represents a real challenge for both the surgeon and the patient if functionality is to be restored. For the sake of clarity, the following analysis will consider the upper and the lower extremities separately.

Basic science/disease process

Electrical burns

In cases of electrocution, the upper extremities are almost always involved, especially as entry or exit points of what is known as the *electric arc*.[10]

The electric arc mainly involves the wrist, elbow, and ankle joints with devastating effects on the joints themselves, the nervous structures, and the muscular masses.

Often the most serious damage is to the wrist and ankle. Since the hands and feet are the most frequent entry and exit points, the wrist and ankle are the nearest points of electrical resistance. The patient's clinical condition on admission often looks less critical than it really is as the lesions may be misleading, with limited charring. In other cases, ample charred areas can be witnessed. These are the electric current's entry and exit points. However, the underlying damage is always more extensive and may well involve the muscular fasciae. This is because nerves and vessels are very good conductors of electricity, and they may suffer damage a few days after the accident. Venous thrombosis or ischemia can be caused by internal destruction of the vessels catalyzed by the electric current. Peripheral neurological damage may occur either with total *destruction of the nerve* (*neurotmesis*), if close to the electricity entry and exit points, or with partial *axonal damage* (*axonotmesis*), which is generally resolved within a few months.[11,12]

In cases of high-voltage electrical burns (over 1000 volts), muscles, bones, and nerve structures can be totally destroyed and, as has been said, complete destruction of the major joints is a common observation.[13]

In such cases, reconstruction should be early, i.e., within 3–5 days of the accident, in order to save the affected joints and to remove destroyed muscular tissue as soon as possible. This is to prevent any serious acidosis related to massive quantities of myoglobin, which is a difficult condition to manage if a resuscitation procedure proves necessary.

Myoglobinuria is closely linked to muscular damage, since the destruction of muscle cell causes the release of *myoglobin* and in turn catalyses myoglobinemia. The first sign of this pathology is the dark pink color of the urine.[14,15]

However, it is important to note that an accurate picture of myoglobinuria can be provided only by serum differentiation between hemoglobin and myoglobin.

All patients with myoglobinuria should be treated with mannitol IV, bicarbonate IV, and Ringer's lactate therapy in order to obtain alkaline osmotic diuresis. This can maximize the reduction of the precipitation of the pigment at the level of the renal tubules.

The damage caused by an electric current passing through the body, especially if of high voltage, depends not only on the characteristics of the electricity itself but also on the path it follows and on the characteristics of the tissues affected by the electricity. Even if adequate medical and surgical therapy is available, the risk of amputation of the extremity remains high.[11]

From a surgical point of view, debridement of necrotic tissue plays a fundamental role in the very first phase after the accident. As said, this can be very extensive compared to the skin lesion. Reconstruction in these cases rarely requires only skin graft coverage. It often also necessitates vascular reconstruction of the ulnar, radial, or tibial systems, nerve grafts, and the transposition of microvascular free flaps.

Vascular and neural reconstruction has to be carefully assessed, since electricity-related damage affecting the neurovascular structures can occur even some days after the surgical operation. This is due to irreversible endothelial damage, which affects small terminal vessels in particular. Hence it is preferable in such cases to postpone the more complex reconstruction procedures until secondary surgical procedures are performed.[16] During the acute phase, it is therefore advisable

to proceed by performing simple temporary skin coverage with a free skin graft and isolating and preparing the vascular and nervous structures that will be treated in a secondary surgical stage.[17]

Diagnosis/patient presentation

Deep burns in the entire upper extremities are statistically infrequent. The areas most often affected by burns are the hand and the forearm. The involvement of any part of the upper sleeve in any of its parts causes negative consequences below the burn, even though the burn itself does not affect that area.

Patients affected by upper extremity burns often suffer other associated traumas as a result of work-related accidents, which are the most frequent cause of this type of injury. An assessment of potential fractures, amputations, wounds, and blast and crush injuries is essential for planning subsequent reconstruction procedures. The functionality of the shoulder joints must be carefully examined.[18] If possible, the nervous functionality of the median, ulnar, and radial nerves should also be evaluated.[18]

After this first check, and after calculating the extent of the burn surface area, it is of fundamental importance to assess whether there is any need of escharotomy. This surgical procedure, which has to be performed as an emergency, helps to prevent the compartment syndrome.

Fluid infusion and edema

Burn shock is characterized by specific hemodynamic modifications on both a hypovolemic and a cellular basis, and it can be defined as a nonhemorrhagic hypovolemic shock with loss of water, sodium, and plasma proteins but not of corpusculate elements. In the first 24–48 h fluid losses cannot be stopped but only replaced.

The objective of the treatment is to restore and preserve tissue perfusion and avoid ischemia. One of the biggest complications of burn shock is the increase of capillary permeability throughout the organism due to the effects of heat on the microcirculation. Edema reaches its maximum expression within 8–12 h of the accident in minor burns and within 12–24 h in major ones.

These phenomena are caused by endothelial damage and by hypoperfusion, which lead to the liberation of vasoactive substances and cytotoxic free radicals, which in turn are responsible for cellular edema and the generalized inflammatory reaction.[12,14]

When burns exceed 20–30% TBSA, even unburned areas develop edema owing to the increase of vascular permeability secondary to hypoperfusion and because of the plasma protein deficit.

The "emergency solution" of first choice for infusion in the first 8 h is Ringer's lactate, in patients with extensive burns in whom it is not possible to achieve adequate tissue perfusion, even by doubling the infusion volume normally prescribed, it is possible to use hypertonic solutions (Ringer's lactate + 50 mEq of $NaHCO_3$ + 40 mEq Lactate). These solutions have to be used carefully, monitoring natremia (which must never exceed 160 mEq/dL) and plasma osmolarity. Note: hyperosmolar syndrome induces kidney failure.

The administration of proteins is not effective in the first 8 h post-burn; later on, it is possible to infuse solutions of albumin or fresh plasma. The quantity of proteins to infuse has to be defined: generally speaking, one can calculate 0.5–1 mL/kg/% TBSA in fresh plasma in the first 24 h, starting 8/10 h post-burn. Elderly patients and those with extensive burns (>50%) maintain better hemodynamic stability and develop less edema, thanks to the administration of proteins.

If no colloids have been used in the first hours after the trauma and oncotic pressure remains low because of the depletion of plasma proteins, it is necessary to reintegrate the losses: the 5% albumin demand during the second 24 h is 0.3–0.5 mL/kg/% TBSA. It is desirable to keep albumin blood levels above 2 g/dL to contrast peripherica edema.

The volume of fluids indicated in the resuscitation of burn patients depends on the gravity of the burn, the age and general condition of the patient, and the presence of associated lesions. In patients with burns in more than 15% TBSA, the quantity of fluid to infuse has to be calculated on the basis of the burned area and body dimensions (ABA Guidelines).[3]

Compartment syndrome

Deep second-degree and third-degree circumferential burns can trigger a serious *compartment syndrome* (*Figs 19.1–19.6,* *Box 19.1*), which if not adequately treated can easily result in the loss of the extremity involved.

Full circumferential burns, or burns involving at least three-quarters of the extremity's circumference, are liable to the risk of the *compartment syndrome*. The clinical reaction that occurs when edema develops during the first hours post-burn triggers a pressure increase at the muscular level of the extremities. The extremities are blocked by the burned skin, which has no elasticity. After the initial restriction of venous outflow, if proper treatment is not given, there is the risk of a deficit in arterial flow, resulting in ischemic tissue downstream. It is important to perform invasive monitoring of

---

Box 19.1 Emergency surgical procedures (with evidence of procedures involving limbs)

- Releasing incisions
- Unavoidable amputations
- Early debridement, excision and coverage
- Management compartment syndrome
- Deep burn of the face
- Tracheotomy (inhalation injury)
- Pin hanging of the limbs
- Colostomy.

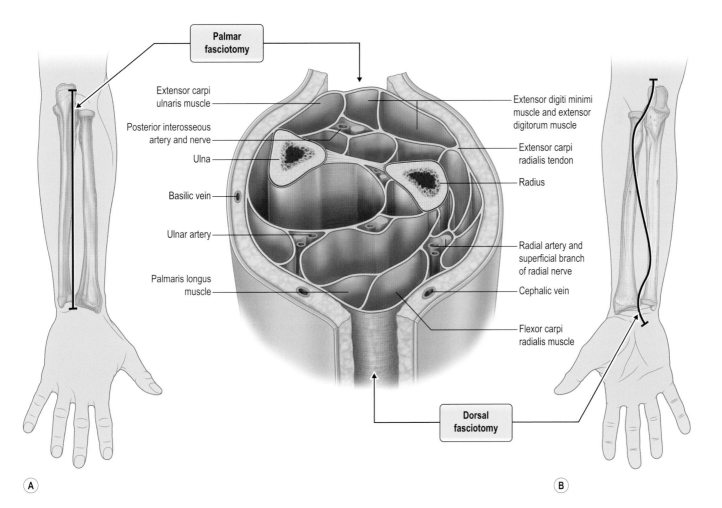

Fig. 19.1 Anatomy of forearm escharotomy incisions.

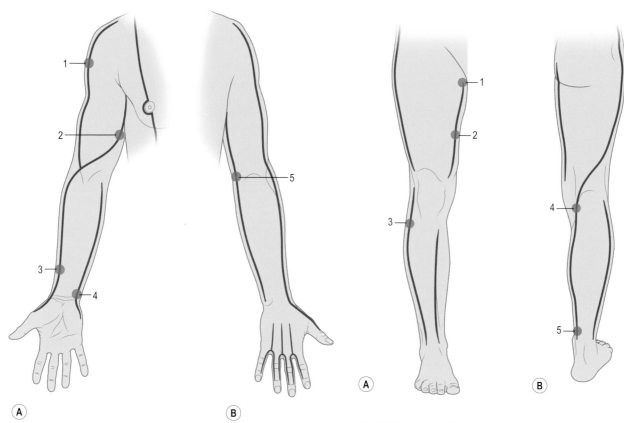

Fig. 19.2 Recommended sites for upper extremity and chest escharotomies. Numbers 1 to 5 indicate dangerous incision sites.

Fig. 19.3 Recommended sites for lower extremity escharotomies. Numbers 1 to 5 indicate dangerous incision sites.

compartment pressure. There are many external devices for measuring intramuscular pressure.

Main clinical signs of initial compartmental syndrome are failure of pulses in distal arteries, pallor and cold limb, initial intense pain which then decreases, high tension of the hand or the foot, pain at passive flexion-extension, paresthesia.

Screening with eco-color-Doppler could be useful during initial assessment, but this method cannot valuate the exact compartment pressure. If laboratory values give high levels of creatinine phosphokinase (CPK), it may indicate severe muscle damage, or ischemia.

One of the most common devices which allow a precise measurement of compartment pressure is the Stryker Set®. This Device is assembled by a monitoring unit and a syringe with 3 mL of saline solution. After an accurate identification of the muscular compartment we want to check, we proceed with a simple injection of the 0.3 mL to re-equilibrate the pressure with interstitial fluids, and then we get the compartment pressure on the monitoring unit. For measurements exceeding 35–40 mmHg, it is necessary to adopt escharotomy-fasciotomy. In all these cases, it is necessary to perform full-thickness decompressive escharotomy in the very first hours in order to restore normal blood flow.[19,20]

This procedure must involve all the burned tissues, skin, fat, and fasciae, until release of the compartment is observed. These escharotomies should follow the recommended procedures and be performed before the initial signs of either

vascular deficit (frozen hand) or neurological deficits occur. Escharotomies can be performed with an electrosurgical knife or a scalpel, ensuring complete release of the muscles (**Fig. 19.4B, 19.5).**

When treating the upper extremity, particular attention should be paid to the blood flow through the cephalic and basilic vein and superficial branch of the radial nerve at the level of the wrist. In the most serious cases, it may be necessary to perform complete decompression of the carpal tunnel (**Figs 19.1, 19.2).**

Escharotomy of the lower limb must be performed avoiding tibial anterior nerve, the medial saphenous vein and nerve, the tibial posterior nerve, the fibular nerve, and the external saphenous nerve (**Figs 19.3, 19.4, 19.6).**[21]

Medication of the extremities should be carried out after careful cleaning and debridement of the affected surface. Early mobilization of the joints is recommended unless otherwise specified. Nonadherent dressings such as Vaseline gauze are indicated for all burn-affected areas. For areas affected only superficially or at medium thickness, it is better to use medications such as Biobrane®, Mefix®, or Aquacel-Ag® to ensure good epithelialization. In areas that are deeply affected or clearly of third-degree, it is possible to proceed with occlusive dressings until the time comes for surgical procedures. Enzymatic debridement ointments or "debriders" can be useful for preparing the patient for the scheduled surgical operation. During hospitalization it is of fundamental importance to keep the upper extremities of the patient in an

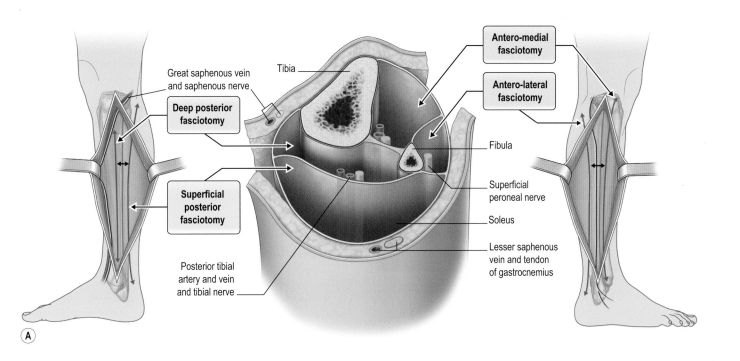

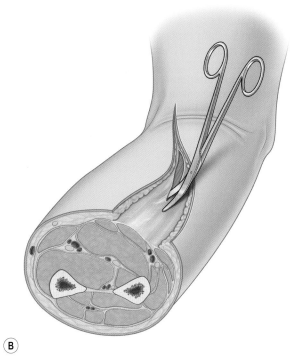

Fig. 19.4 **(A)** Anatomy of lower extremity escharotomy and fasciotomy incisions. **(B)** Schematic of fascial release after escharotomy in the lower extremity.

elevated position in order to control the formation of new edema and reduce existing edema.

Surgery of the burn areas should be performed early, since late recovery leads to a greater incidence of hypertrophic scars, weaker tissues, and delays in prompt mobilization of the extremities.[22,23]

Deep burned areas should be subjected to surgical treatment as soon as possible, while more superficial areas, if not healed within in 2 or 3 weeks, should also be considered for surgical treatment. Depending on the burn area, the extremities permit local anesthesia, but preferably only in patients with surgical indications but relatively limited burn areas. The preferred treatment remains debridement and autologous skin graft.

Related trauma

The trauma most frequently associated with burns is bone fracture. In this case, close collaboration between the plastic and the orthopedic surgeon is essential in order to choose the

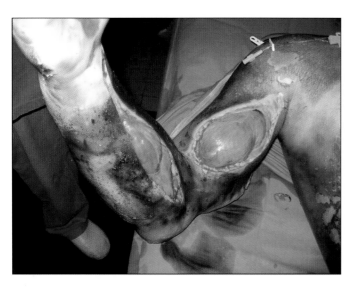

Fig. 19.5 Upper extremity escharotomy and fasciotomy.

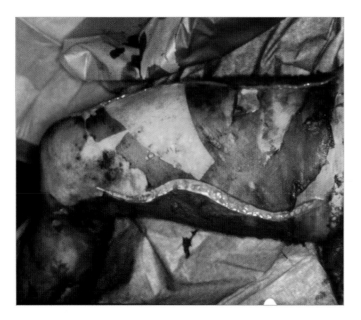

Fig. 19.6 Lower extremity escharotomy.

most appropriate surgical plan to follow. Stabilization of fractures contiguous to deeply burned areas should be performed early, preferably within the first 48 h after the accident, before bacterial colonization can hamper orthopedic action. It has frequently been reported in the literature that the early stabilization of burn patients drastically decreases the onset of complications related to the orthopedic intervention, thus reducing the risk of infective complications.

Various related trauma should be treated contextually or before their coverage with skin grafts, in order to avoid re-opening already treated burn areas.

In the deepest burn areas, especially as a result of electrocution or if accompanied by related trauma, the explosion of bones or tendons can occur, especially in the elbow, wrist, knee, and ankle areas. This condition imposes an additional priority in the planning of the surgical procedure to be performed. The exposed tendons are liable to rapid dehydration

and consequent necrosis, and prompt coverage is therefore essential. In the preparatory phase it can be useful to use cadaver skin or biological medications, while in the surgical phase it is recommended to use dermis substitutes (such as Integra, Matriderm, etc.), which permit the formation of new tissue between the tendons and the grafted skin. Grafting directly on the exposed tendons is counter-indicated in terms of graft survival and of functional results.

The same considerations apply in the case of exposed bone, which should also be covered as early as possible, even though resistance to exposure is much higher and more easily resolved than in the case of tendons. Coverage can be performed at a second stage utilizing rotation or free flaps.[24]

Patient selection

Plastic surgeons possess all the necessary tools and scientific know-how to treat burn patients. From intensive care to the surgical phase, they should be able to take the best decisions for the patient. Plastic surgeon is in fact the only professional figures that have a clear and immediate understanding of patients' overall surgical needs.

It is the plastic surgeon who decides the necessity of surgical procedures and in some cases, also decides to pursue a second-intention healing process. The preoperative care plan for scars is also crucial and should be prepared by the same medical team that treated the patient during the previous acute phase. The extremities are the most frequent sufferers from post-surgery scar contractures, often as a result of a lack of proper preventive follow-up measures (such as *massage therapy, elastic compression, physio-kinesitherapy,* and *splinting*) aimed at preventing pathological scarring. An assessment of the affected areas will suggest to the specialist whether to proceed with corrective measures or engage in additional surgical interventions.

The results of sequelae surgery can be extremely heterogeneous, ranging from scar contraction resolution at the joint level to vascular, nerve, and tendon reconstruction. The main objective of sequelae surgery in these localized areas is to re-establish the extremity's proper functionality, considering that normal walking, physical autonomy, and self-dependence at work depend on the complete rehabilitation of the areas affected.[25]

Treatment/surgical technique

Burn surgery can be subdivided into acute-phase surgery and sequelae surgery. This distinction holds also as regards localized areas only.

Acute-phase extremity surgery is not fundamentally different from surgery in any other part of the body. Procedures such as fasciotomy, debridement, and coverage with autologous skin grafts, as previously described, follow the surgical guidelines of acute-phase general burns.

With regard to sequelae surgery, the extremities have some unique characteristics, e.g., the majority of scar retractions lead to disabilities, and localized burn-related joint blockages may occur.[12]

Acute-phase surgery: skin grafting

Emergency procedures such as escharotomy and fasciotomy were largely dealt with in the foregoing section. In this section, we provide a preventative scheme concerning the incision lines to be used.

Focusing only on the extremities, the commonest surgical procedures continue to be surgical debridement and whole or meshed free-skin graft of autologous skin. These procedures should preferably be completed early, i.e., between the 5th and 7th day after the accident. As previously said, some *ad hoc* surgical variations may be necessary, depending on the type of damage affecting the extremities and the kind of structures involved. In order to limit bleeding and thus operate in a condition of controlled hemostasis, it is advisable to use a tourniquet. This procedure facilitates extremity surgery but at the same time, requires that greater attention should be paid to the assessment of vital tissue. In this way there is no microvascular bleeding.

Debridement should be performed up to the vital tissues, after careful removal of all necrotic skin, paying special attention to the flexion-extension areas and the axillary cavity areas. In these areas the necrotomy is more complex to perform. In deep or electric burns, it is advisable to reach up to the muscular fascia in order to avoid the risk of probable but undesirable liponecrosis. Unlike skin, the viable fat underneath is an unstable base for implanting free skin grafts.[26–29]

During debridement of more superficially burned areas that do however require surgical treatment, instruments like VersaJet® provide useful support as they minimize the waste of vital tissue and also permit careful debridement in nonflat surfaces, as the extremities are.[27]

Skin grafts can adhere with mesher 1:1 or 1.5:1, and it is even possible to use 2:1 if the patient does not have donor areas. The elbow joint and the axillary and popliteal cavities are preferably grafted with medium-thickness healthy skin, which provides greater elasticity and resistance in areas subject to high mobility and traumatism. All skin grafts should be positioned considering the least relaxed skin tension lines in order to obtain the aesthetically best results. In the specific case of the arms, it is recommended to position the skin grafts longitudinally for the best aesthetic outcome.

Skin grafts must be checked after 4–5 days and treated until full recovery is completed.

Skin substitutes

In the course of the last decade, the use of dermal substitutes in acute-phase burn surgery became more frequent. In particular, this technique is now used in acute-phase burn surgery in cases of extensive deep burns with exposure of bones and tendons.

The characteristics of an ideal skin substitute were defined in 1978 by Tavis, who stated that it should be adherent and impermeable to water, represent a barrier to electrolytes and proteins, be durable, and possess a bacteria barrier function. It should also show nontoxicity, nonantigenity, a hemostatic function, ease of application, and affordability. None of today's skin substitutes fulfils all these criteria.

The currently available products (Integra®, Matriderm®, Allograft®, Terudermis®, etc.) have different characteristics but they all aim at the same objective: re-establishment of a layer of dermis under a free skin graft. There is an ongoing debate as to whether these newly formed tissues can be considered dermis or not.

A fundamental prerequisite for valid results is that the application should be onto vital tissue that is free of any contamination or necrotic residue.

In acute burns of the extremities the use of skin substitutes is extremely effective in the treatment of critical areas (armpit, elbow, popliteal cavity) and exposed bones and tendons.

These products provide immediate coverage of the burned area, resulting in reduced risk of infection or necrosis of the tissue. They also facilitate the regeneration of tissues between the deep structures and the skin graft.

Applying dermal substitutes is usually easy. However, when treating the extremities, some critical aspects should be considered, such as ensuring movement, the autonomy of the various segments, and perfect adherence between the product and the wound bed, since these products are mostly indicated for the treatment of critical points such as the elbow, armpit, and popliteal cavity. It has become increasingly common to use such products together with "negative pressure systems" during the post-surgical period. It is important to recall, however, that the commonest possible complication following their use in the acute phase is infection, which can lead to complete loss of the skin grafts applied in 30–40% of cases.

In the post-surgical period it is recommended that the surgeon should be guided by the instructions of the manufacturer of the product and by personal experience.[28–30]

Negative pressure systems are often used as primary dressing for skin grafts or skin substitute sheets. The use of negative pressure devices (NPDs) improve take of the graft, perform its better adherence on the wound bed, prevent contamination, protect the graft from traumas and finally create a good environment for skin graft taking or vascularization of skin substitute. (It is the authors' opinion that it is wrong to talk about the "taking" of skin substitutes and that "vascularization" sounds more appropriate.) It is possible to use these devices on meshed and un-meshed skin grafts, on single/double layer sheets with interposition of Vaseline gauze between the graft and the NPD gauze/sponge. Many authors suggest removing the dressing directly on 6th/7th postoperative day, but it is possible to do so before. We found this kind of dressing very useful in critical areas such as hollows, axilla, popliteal region, neck, giving much more stability and a perfect adhesion of the graft on the wound bed. For the same reason, bulky gauzes, bolsters and soft collars should be used in these areas.

Joint reconstruction with dermis in acute phase *(Figs 19.7 and 19.8)*

High-voltage electricity (>1000 volts) flowing through the extremities meets the point of maximum resistance in the joints, and in such cases, severe damage involving all the anatomical joint structures affected can be observed.

Joint reconstruction and coverage of exposed joints should be managed early, in order to preserve as much functionality as possible, together with the integrity of any viable tissue that is still alive, and to prevent septic arthritis.

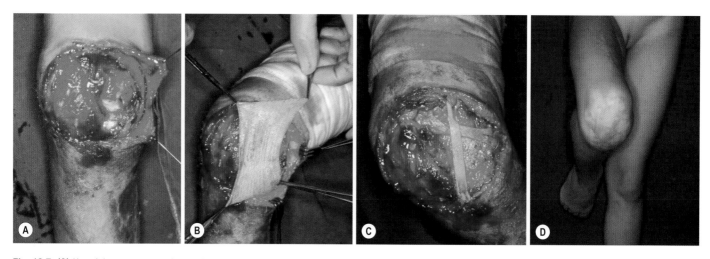

Fig. 19.7 **(A)** Knee joint space exposed secondary to high voltage electrical burn. **(B)** Dermis harvested for joint reconstruction. **(C)** Dermal grafts incorporated into joint capsule reconstruction. **(D)** Result after skin graft.

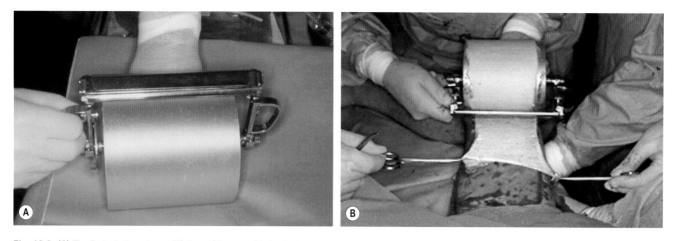

Fig. 19.8 **(A)** The Padgett dermatome. **(B)** Dermal harvest with the Padgett dermatome.

Articulation capsule and joint ligament apparatus reconstruction has priority for surgery. The dermis graft is an effective solution to this problem. Prior to using the Padgett dermatome or free blade skin graft removal, the area should be cleared, keeping the majority of the live tissue intact. The donated dermis is then carefully shaped in relation to the structures requiring reconstruction, whether an articulation capsule or a joint, and then finally grafted. Skin coverage should be ensured through flap rotation or free flap transfer.

The fibroblast-rich grafted dermis realigns its elastic fibers under the stimulation of the force applied to the joint. This contributes to the reconstruction of strong vectoral tissue, which is a characteristic feature of healthy joint structure.

The donor area can be sutured directly if the dermis has been drawn using a free blade through a small cutaneous excision. If a Padgett dermatome is used, the donor area can be covered with epidermis from the donor region. This kind of dermatome, now little used, continues to be the best instrument for performing ample dermis grafts.[31]

Postoperative care

Burn injuries cause highly scar-related disabilities characterized by major hyperplasia and marked contraction of the skin surface. The mobile segments of the extremities (armpit, elbow, wrist, knee, ankle) are among the most critical for monitoring in the post-surgical phase *(Figs 19.9, 19.10; Table 19.1)*.

Many studies have dealt with the actual effectiveness of post-surgical elastic compression and massage therapy, and in normal clinical practice these procedures are routinely performed to obtain the best results possible in terms of scarring. The use of elastic garments for the extremities, of splints for the hand and foot, and of elastic collars for the neck is widely recommended from the earliest postoperative stage in all centers specializing in burns treatment. In addition to these devices it is always advisable to perform physio-kinesitherapy daily, especially in burns involving the extremities.

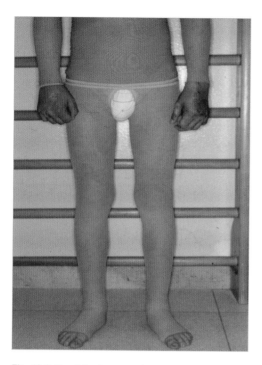

Fig. 19.9 Specialized compression garment.

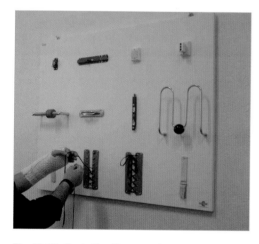

Fig. 19.10 Physio-kinesitherapy tasks to enhance post-burn mobility and minimize contracture formation.

Table 19.1 Joint position

Joint	Position
Shoulder	Abduction 65–85° Slight flexion 25°
Elbow	Extension
Wrist	Slight extension 30°
Hip	Extension Abduction 15°
Knee	Extension
Ankle	Maintain 90°

Burn patients who have to stay many hours in bed may lie in particular positions that can be defined as "antalgic." These are related to the great degree of pain suffered and to the distressing situation the patients find themselves in. The joints can easily lose their range of movement if not properly treated. It is important in these cases to apply splints to the extremities and to give daily physio-kinesiotherapy as part of burn patients' routine treatment.

Positioning the patient

The position of the patient should generally be supine with the neck slightly stretched. In nonextensive burns, lateral decubitus is also allowed.

The interposition of a thick surface (e.g., pillow, sheets) in the interscapular area ensures slight hyperextension of the neck. When necessary, it is desirable to use tutor collars. As for the extremities, these must be placed in the correct position during the postoperative period in order to prevent physiological pathologies and scar contractures.

Upper extremity

The upper extremity, excluding the hand, consists of three major joints, which must be carefully handled if crippling deficits of mobility are to be avoided.

Shoulder

The shoulder joint should usually be held in abduction and slight flexion (60–80° abduction and 15–20° flexion) through the use of special bandages, a figure of 8, and swabs. Gauze or foam should be used for the armpits. This position ensures good stability of the shoulder joint. In discharged patients in outpatient care, the use of "aeroplane" splints, with a base on the hips and 80–90° arm support, is particularly indicated.

Should greater extension prove necessary, it is desirable to use a splint, always bearing in mind that excessive abductions can create pathological tractions at the level of brachial plexus and a nerve-radial deficit.

Elbow

The elbow is another critical area that needs attention. During the period of hospitalization, the elbow joint should necessarily be maintained in a position of extension in order to avoid frequent burns sequelae. The use of splints or sticks is hence crucial, and a prone posture should be ensured to avoid having any negative effects on hand posture.[32,33]

Wrist

The wrist should be maintained in a position of slight extension (about 30°), using splints and hand braces.

Lower extremity

As said, burn patients tend to adopt an antalgic physiopathological position, which may lead them to flex major joints.

Hip

Burns that extend from the abdomen to the anterior thigh can cause troublesome retractions at the level of the hip joint.

Especially in children, scarring and retracting tissue may affect the proper alignment of the pelvis and the spinal column. In the acute phase, the hips should be kept in full extension (0°), with a physiological abduction of about 15°.

During post-surgery, babies should be monitored using braces and splints, which allow coxofemoral extension and help to prevent hyperlordosis of the lumbar region.

Knee

If not properly cared for, the knee, like the elbow, is subject to serious flexion, resulting in major mobility deficits. This kind of negative outcome should be avoided by positioning the part in extension using a splint or a cast.

Ankle

The ankle should be preserved by maintaining a position at 90° through the use of splints or special supports. Post-traumatic clubfoot is the most frequent joint complication in burn patients. The problem manifests itself a few days after hospitalization and may lead to permanent deformity that is hard to resolve. Scar contraction and shortening of the muscle tendon risk prolonging this pathological condition for some long time.[34]

All these guidelines are part of a comprehensive physio-kinesitherapy programme, which together with correct positioning of the joints should include appropriate rehabilitation exercises, which play a very important role. These exercises, which should be performed daily under the guidance of a physiotherapist, are usually performed in a passive way at the patient's bedside. The purpose is to maintain joint mobility and keep muscle tone intact. The patient must be mobilized as soon as the general and local conditions so permit.

The rehabilitation treatment using the classic principles of kinesitherapy, consist of forms of muscular activation as well as simple and complex exercises to improve the posture and the dynamics of the body. Kinesitherapy makes use of forms of active and passive mobilization.

Passive mobilization

Passive mobilization refers to the use of particular movements of the patients' joints caused by external action without any muscular contraction or nervous participation by the patients themselves. Passive kinesis employs methods of slow mobilization and methods of rapid mobilization.

Active mobilization

This indicates the overall complex of particular movements of the patients' joints with the participation of their nervous centers and active muscular contraction. Active kinesis employs assisted exercises, exercises against resistance, and free exercises. Burn patient kinesis makes use of both static and dynamic forms. Static kinesitherapy consists of forms of postural alignment and the use of rigid and mobile splints, anti-decubitus ulcer beds, and normal or elastic bandages. Dynamic kinesitherapy consists of changes of posture during mobilization of joints affected by the trauma or of undamaged joints, mobilization of the rib cage, postural drainage, and water rehabilitation therapy.[32–34]

After discharge, the patient should continue therapy for several months. The local treatment of scars, continuous elastocompression, splinting, and physical exercises during the postoperative period should all be regarded as an integral part of the management of burn patients.

Treatment usually continues on an outpatient basis until the scar tissue is well stabilized. In the assessment of outpatients with severe extremity burns, it is important to assess the degree of improvement in mobility achieved during the entire period of physio-kinesitherapy. Measuring the degree of flexure–extension of the joints and the quality of the scars will indicate whether patients may be considered to be definitively cured or whether they are capable of further improvement.

Outcomes, prognosis, complications

Unstable healing: Marjolin's ulcer

The healing of large burn areas leads to unstable scar sequelae that represent the first complication specialists have to face in the follow-up of burn patients. As soon as the first surgical operation, some areas tend to develop towards hypergranulation rather than epithelialization, while some areas that have healed spontaneously may ulcerate or develop hypertrophic scars.

The continued presence of scar tissue has a negative effect on rehabilitation procedures. Sharp pain and the lack of solid skin coverage severely limit the use of splints, massage therapy, and the use of elastic girdles. In some patients, the scarring phase is so unstable that it can go on for months, without reaching completion. In such cases, it advisable to consider performing an extensive excision followed by a skin graft because repeated ulcering for months or even years, can lead to malignant forms developing in the burn areas.

Marjolin's ulcer is an infiltrating spinocellular carcinoma, with a low level of differentiation, which forms in unstable scar areas. Statistically, its rate of incidence is 2% in burn scars, with a higher prevalence in the limbs, especially the lower limbs. As it occurs in areas with a record of instability, it is rarely diagnosed early because of confusion with other ulcerative processes. The first histological sign of this highly invasive type of carcinoma occurs at the edge of the ulcer. There is early development of lymph node metastases in 30% of cases, with a 5-year survival in <10% of cases.[35,36]

Treatment is purely surgical. First, the area is extensively excised, histological tests are performed, and – in the event of metastasis – lymph nodes can be emptied. There are no reports of preventative lymph node emptying being reliable for the purposes of prognosis.

In some cases, when bone or deep levels are affected, proximal limb amputation may be necessary.

Scar retraction

As in any other trauma, burns may also result in scarring tissue, which if not properly treated, can develop into hypertrophic scarring. The deeper the burns, the greater the risk of becoming hypertrophic scars in the future. Also, if a burn is left exposed overlong, the possibility of its becoming a pathological scar increases. Burn scars take a very long average time to become stable, i.e., 1.5–2 years.

Some factors related to burns pathophysiology are decisive for the healing of severely injured patients and the final outcome. The commonest and most evident complication is scarring of the skin. Contracting scarring tissue may cause significant functional limitation and physical deformity, which may eventually lead to permanent damage at the musculoskeletal level, deforming the joints and, in children, stimulating pathological bone growth.

Full hand motion in the burned patient is useless if significant contractures of the elbow and axilla prevent the patient from positioning the hand for optimal function. Also, severe knee contracture will interfere with correct walking. It is not easy to specify which extremity burns will or will not be disabling. As specified in other sections in this chapter, the final result is influenced by various factors such as the burn's aetiology, its precise location, surgical and post-surgical treatment, and patient compliance.

In cases of particularly deep burns in the upper extremities complicated by necrosis involving the deepest structures, it is not uncommon to witness the phenomena of osteomyelitis and necrotizing fasciitis. These severe complications often result in the amputation of the affected extremity.

The most serious burns from the point of view of complications are certainly those of electrical origin. They are frequently "subdued" burns, in a relatively small area, but with vast underlying damage below. Muscle tissue, the vascular and neural fasciae, and the joints and bones are frequent occurrences and may be associated with very severe tissue damage.

Necrosis of muscle and tendon may be extensive, with the loss of whole muscles or tendons, resulting in severe functional deficits.

Massive involvement of the extremities can result in decreased mobility and articular, vascular, and aesthetic defects that are hardly ever totally resolved.

Axillary contractures *(Fig. 19.11)*

Retraction of the main joint of the limbs is very common. Of all burn-related contractures, that of the axilla is the commonest – more frequent than elbow contractures.

Management of axilla burns is difficult, especially in pediatric patients. The favorite antalgic position of a patient with burns in this area is commonly in adduction. The problems in this unfavorable anatomical position are further aggravated by the difficulty of immobilizing the shoulder joint in the correct position.

Kurtzman and Stern's classification (1990)[37] divides axillary contractures into three main types, on the basis of their anatomical characteristics:

- *Type 1*: Contracture involving either the anterior (1A) or the posterior (1B) axillary fold alone
- *Type 2*: Contracture involving both the anterior and the posterior axillary fold but not the skin in the axillary dome
- *Type 3*: Contracture involving both axillary folds and the axillary dome.

The surgery plan has to consider the type of contracture in order to tackle the local problem in the best possible way.

In types 1 and 2, it is normally possible to use local flaps, while in type 3 it is necessary to extend the surgical area to the trunk, using large flaps from the latissimus dorsi and pectoral area.

Elbow contractures

After axilla contractures, the joint most frequently involved is the elbow. Most contractures at this level are caused by skin scars, which exert such a powerful effect that they limit the range of movement of the forearm and upper arm.

We usually distinguish between intra-articular and extra-articular contractures, depending on whether the joint structures are involved or not. The majority of elbow contractures are extra-articular, in flexion, caused only by skin scars, while extension contractures are quite rare in burn sequelae.

With regard to articular contractures, the use of local flaps or incisional release and grafting will usually suffice. In very large scar retractions, in which the excised scar tissue involves the upper arm and forearm, fasciocutaneous flaps from the chest or abdomen can be recommended. Excellent results have been reported with the use of Integra in the reconstruction of anterior and posterior elbow defects after release of the burn scar contractures.

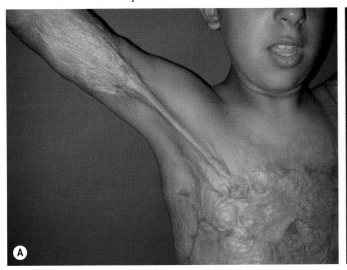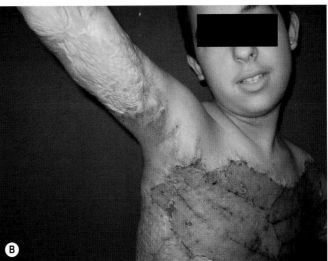

Fig. 19.11 Axillary contracture **(A)** before and **(B)** after Z-plasty release. (Courtesy of Department of Plastic Surgery and Burn Therapy, ARNAS Ospedale Civico, Palermo, Italy.)

In the postoperative period, the use of extension splints is recommended early and early physio-kinesitherapy exercises are mandatory to maintain the movement range obtained with surgery.

Heterotopic ossification

Heterotopic bone formation in burn patients is a rare occurrence but functionally speaking, it is a major complication. Only 3% of burn patients develop this complication, but if periarticular calcifications are included, which are a false form of heterotrophic ossification, about 30% of patients develop the complication.

Heterotopic bone formation is a complication that occurs when new bone develops in tissues that do not normally ossify. It is coupled with important joint movement deficit. There are many possible causes of heterotopic ossification, but the real etiology is still not well known. Usually the severity of the burn injury is considered more likely to be responsible than its extension or location. Unnecessary joint manipulation with related microtraumas has also been considered as a possible cause of the initial micro-ossification of the musculo-tendinous tissues. The elbow is the joint most frequently involved, followed by the shoulder and hip joints. The knee is not often involved.

The most serious clinical picture is bridge ossification, in which the jointed bones become linked by the new bone tissue in a condition of structural stability. The joint remains blocked even after the patient has recovered from the burns. If the new bone has not established any structural continuity, it may regress and sometimes, especially in children, even completely disappear. This ossification process usually starts a few weeks post-burn injury, the average being 10–15 weeks. The symptoms, i.e., loss of range of movement and joint pain, may be preceded by radiological evidence. We thus prescribe physio-kinesitherapy without excessive joint stress, which seems to stimulate the ossification process.

Surgical treatment is necessary only in the case of a complete osseous bridge, and it is better to treat only mature new-formed bone, in order to be able to proceed with complete removal of the defect. Particular attention must be paid to the ulnar nerve, which is sometimes trapped inside the new bone, and the nerve must be identified and carefully isolated in order to preserve it. In the postoperative period, it is necessary to apply a splint in the flexed position, if the blocking was in extension, and in extension if the ankylosis was in flexion. Early physio-kinesitherapy should start within 10 days, and continue throughout healing.[38,39]

Skeletal-muscle complications: bone exposure

In elbow and knee joint burns, the olecranon and patella bone is often exposed (*see Fig. 19.13A*). In spite of the local and general conditions, osteomyelitis is rare and after surgical toilette of the cortex, the underlying bone is vital. The cortex of these areas is thick and resists exposure-related infection and necrosis for some time, especially if properly treated. Surgically, in order to facilitate granulation, it is possible to punch the cortex in order to expose the little blood vessels under the cortex.

Additional considerations are needed for injuries involving open fractures associated with burns, where infection is perhaps inevitable. But also in this case, the infection remains localized to the fracture site for a long time, with rare involvement of the entire bone segment.

In these patients, the restraint system should be carefully chosen. Many surgeons strongly oppose plaster splints because they prevent easy inspection of the burn area and recommend instead, external fixation with Kirschner nails. This procedure – now considered the most appropriate – is not free of risk in burn patients because often the nails have to pass through the burned skin, transferring bacteria to the bone.

Surgical coverage of these exposed areas should be performed rapidly on cleared tissues. In this context, a negative pressure unit is particularly useful (VAC, Renasys, etc.), as this quickly promotes cleansing of the bed and improves promotes vascularization and granulation.

Secondary procedures

Minor surgical procedures on the extremities are usually indicated when rehabilitation therapy has been ineffective or when joint functionality is compromised. Apart from the cases just described, surgery on the joints usually occurs at this stage and not during the acute phase.

Reconstructive surgery can also be delayed whenever, following particularly deep burns, areas subject to loss of skin substance with exposure of underlying anatomical structures remain present.

Patients with secondary indication for surgery are:

- Patients with scar sequelae not resolvable by physio-kinesitherapy
- Patients with debilitating scar sequelae
- Patients with chronic skin tissue loss and exposure of nerve-vascular structures, bone, and tendons
- Patients with articulation deficit
- Patients with nervous deficit.

Before planning any surgery, the specialist should take into account certain aspects, summarized as follows:

- Scars location
- Scars thickness and quality
- Joint deficit assessment
- Extent of loss of skin substance and careful evaluation of exposed tissues
- Local conditions (presence of normal surrounding skin, surgical options).

It is appropriate to plan the surgical procedure when the scar tissue is completely stabilized and after obtaining the best possible result in terms of joint mobility.

Reduced joint mobility may depend on various factors. The commonest is obviously the contraction of scar tissue around the joint itself. Scarring masses that are so firm that they do not allow proper excision of bone segments can aggravate this condition.

The most reliable method of diagnosis is an intraoperative examination. An incision or Z-plasty of contracted scarring tissue can sometimes be the best solution for articulation contractures, as is also reconstruction of the articular capsule and debridement in periarticular scar tissue.

In joint surgery, particular attention should be paid to vascular nerve fasciae in the armpit, elbow, and wrist. Unless there are special surgical needs, it is always best to maintain the integrity of the joint capsule and the articular face.

Z-plasty

This technique is the basis of the surgical treatment of burns sequelae. Z-plasty is feasible in the presence of surrounding healthy tissue. It exploits the principle that it is possible to stretch a scarred area by the interposition of two or more triangular strips rotated from immediately adjacent areas, with maximum elongation, using strips with an angle of 60°. In scarring and contractures of the armpit and elbow, multiple Z-plasties remain one of the most effective techniques *(Fig. 19.12)*. There are many variations to the normal Z-type plastic technique, described by various authors, identifying different angles between two or more interposed flaps. It is possible, especially when treating armpits, to use two asymmetric flaps angled at 90°. This technique is also called the ¾ Z-plasty technique *(Figs 19.13, 19.14)*.

In ankle and knee injuries, Z-type fasciocutaneous flaps are used. These skin flaps are prepared including the skin, the subcutaneous tissue, and the muscular fascia, leaving in place the muscular belly. For the ankle, both frontally and at the rear, the flaps should be set up including the paratenon with its entire vascular network. Flaps thus prepared have greater strength and vitality in critical areas such as those described. This procedure, if well planned, can be performed under local or loco-regional anaesthesia.

In general, in flexion areas where the cause of the retraction is a longitudinal hypertrophic scar band with workable skin on both sides, it is possible to use a simple or multiple Z-plasty. When we observe surrounding scar tissue, with involvement of three-quarters of the circumference, we need a large transverse excision of the scar tissue, and skin grafting of the entire area.

Skin grafts

As in the previous case, this is also a preliminary technique for the treatment of burn scars. After thorough debridement of the retracted scar, it is necessary to interpose a full-thickness graft on the residual bloody area. The donor area should be intact, even if this procedure is influenced by the extent of the original burn. Donations from the groin or abdomen can be easily closed by first-stage surgery. The removed skin should be defatted with chamfers scissors up to the dermis and then applied on the wound bed. The grafting should be monitored for 4–5 days post-surgery after removal of the moulage.

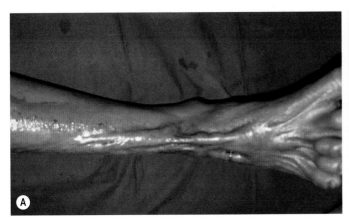
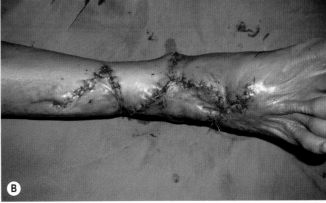

Fig. 19.12 **(A)** Severe ankle contracture. **(B)** Ankle contracture from *Fig. 19.16*, treated with multiple Z-plasties.

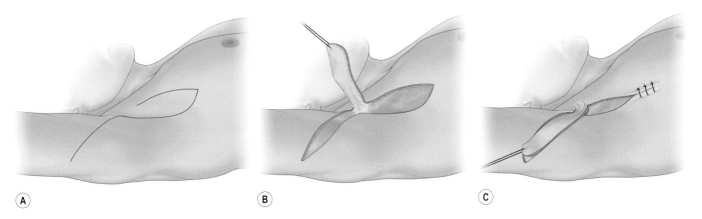

Fig. 19.13 **(A)** Designing a ¾ Z-plasty for the treatment of an axillary contracture. **(B,C)** Raising the flaps of the ¾ Z-plasty designed in *Figure 19.18*.

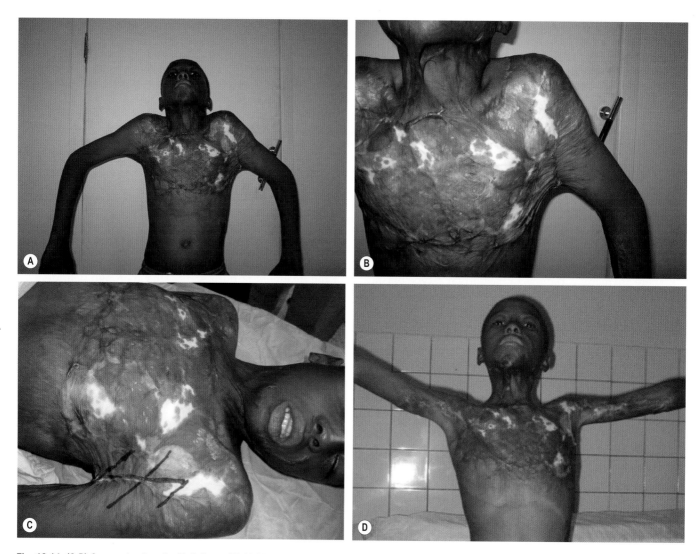

Fig. 19.14 (A,B) Severe retraction of axilla hollows. **(C)** Multiple Z-plasty plan. **(D)** Final result after 2 months. (Courtesy of the International Association of Humanitarian Medicine.)

This procedure too can be performed under local or regional anaesthesia, with minimal discomfort to the patient. Functional rehabilitation can be cautiously resumed 3 weeks after surgery.

Dermal substitutes (INTEGRA®) in the surgical treatment of sequelae

The use of dermal substitutes in today's surgical practice is increasingly widespread. It allows the adding of new tissue in scarring characterized by a basic tissue deficit with greater advantages than those offered by simple free grafts of skin.

In the surgical treatment of retractions of the armpit, elbow, and kneecap, Integra has proved to be highly effective for ensuring a good basis for epidermis tissue grafts, permitting the use of thinner samples and less morbidity in donor areas.

Integra stabilizes after about 21–28 days (it is wrong, in our view, to speak of grafting, since we are considering an acellular matrix). The newly formed tissue is therefore well vascularized and ready to receive a free skin graft (but not full-thickness).

The result is a softer and more durable grafted area than that produced by simple free grafts of skin, even compared with the full-thickness modality. The scar is also of better quality.

Integra is of great help in the surgical treatment of burns sequelae and specifically in the treatment of critical areas.[28–30]

Flaps

Numerous rotation flaps **(Fig. 19.13)** are described in all treatises on plastic surgery, representing a technical heritage through which the plastic surgeon can effectively tackle skin substance defects in an aesthetic way, always remembering that rotation flaps guarantee the same texture, thickness, and color as the adjacent skin. They also minimize the donor area.

Flaps are indicated without question when it is necessary to cover noble structures such as the vascular-nerve fasciae or areas with bone or tendon exposure.

As in all surgical procedures, rotation flaps should carefully studied, prepared and well arranged. Large rotation flaps can be sculpted in the scapular region for the resolution of major scarring of the armpit. Rotation flaps taken from the thoracic or flank region are useful in reconstructive surgery of the elbow. However, at the elbow or ankle level, it is sufficient to use small local flaps or simple Z-type plasties, which are simply rotation flaps.

The flap must be designed in such a way that its margins are never placed longitudinally over the joint.

The survival of the flap should be followed for the first 7–10 days. If there are no signs of suffering, it is possible to resume positioning of the limb and physio-kinesitherapy after 15–21 days, depending on the area involved.

Fasciocutaneous and myocutaneous flaps

Reconstructive surgery of the limbs involves extensive use of *fasciocutaneous* and *myocutaneous rotation flaps*, which successfully cover full-thickness loss of substance, especially at elbow and knee joint level and the proximal third and middle limb (*Figs 19.15, 19.16*).

Because of the unfavorable angle of rotation, large flaps are frequently required to correct small defects. It is therefore recommended that this surgical solution should be carefully considered.

Fasciocutaneous flaps from the lateral region of the arm, supplied by branches of the radial collateral artery and sometimes used as "island flaps", have good mobility and are a reliable solution for reconstruction of the lateral and posterior region of the elbow.

In reconstructive surgery of the upper extremities, *the forearm flap on the radial artery* plays an important role, thanks to its versatility. This flap, based on fasciocutaneous branches of the radial artery and used as an "island flap" with its proximal base on the radial artery, is useful for coverage of defects in the entire region of the elbow, including large defects with olecranon exposure.

Among myocutaneous flaps, *the latissimus dorsi* with and without skin are of particular importance for correction of large defects of the proximal third of the arm and armpits, while *flexor radial carpis flaps* are important for coverage of defects of the forearm and elbow.

The medial or lateral gastrocnemius flap is particularly recommended for coverage of defects of the proximal third of the leg. The same flap can be used to cover the defects in the knee. The *soleus muscle flap*, prepared preserving half the muscle, is useful in the reconstruction of defects of the medial third of the leg. Because of their segmental vasculature, the muscles

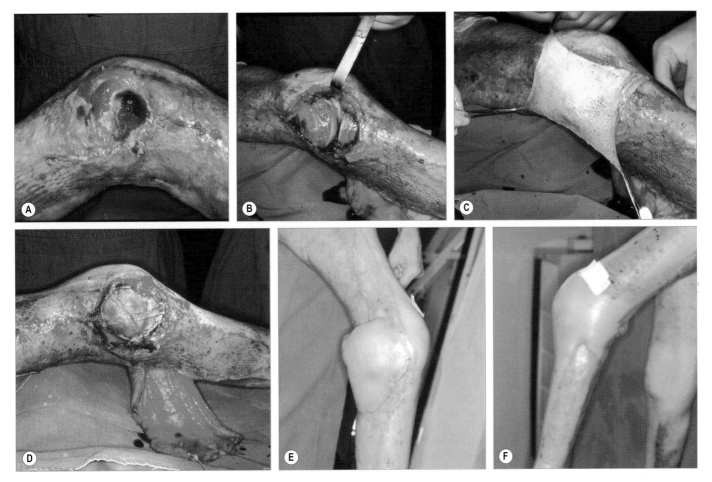

Fig. 19.15 (A) Bone exposed secondary to severe burn. **(B)** Exposed knee joint. **(C)** Dermal graft for coverage of exposed knee joint. **(D)** Dermal grafts in place reconstructing joint capsule; fasciocutaneous flap has been raised. **(E)** Fasciocutaneous flap inset to provide definitive joint coverage superficial to dermal graft. **(F)** Final result of knee reconstruction.

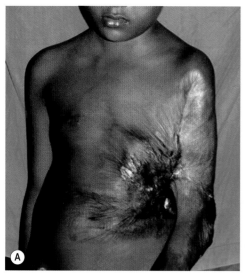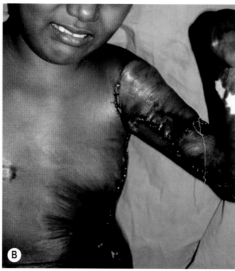

Fig. 19.16 (A) Severe axillary contracture. **(B)** Axillary release and reconstruction with locoregional flaps.

of the lower third of the leg are less suitable for rotation and can be used to cover adjacent skin deficits. The *extensor hallucis longus myocutaneous flap*, as also the *extensor digitorum longus muscle flap*, can be used to cover defects just above the medial malleolus, while short peroneal muscle flaps are useful just above the lateral malleolus.

The partial soleus muscle flap can also be for used for defects of the distal third of the leg. When properly detached from its distal pedicle, it can be rotated on its pedicle more proximally to cover large areas up to about 5–6 cm above the ankle.

The fasciocutaneous flap of greatest interest for coverage of the distal part of the leg and ankle is the *retrograde fibular flap*, the blood supply of which is based on the peroneal artery retrograde. However, it is essential that the connection between the anterior and posterior tibia artery should be intact because the retrograde blood supply will come from the terminal part. The long pedicle that can be obtained allows the flap to move easily and to be used in the entire leg and ankle.

Skin expansion

The principle for the use of skin expansion lies in the positive response of live dermal tissue when it is subjected to mechanical stimulation. The expanded tissue undergoes significant histological changes such as cell hyperplasia, an increase in the number of basal cells in the mitotic phase, an increase in vascular atrophy, and the loss of adipose tissue.[40]

In addition, the soft tissues of the extremities can also be expanded. The placement of the expander should be carefully studied in order to obtain the maximum return in terms of tissue gain, also considering scar tissue healing: theoretically, only healthy skin should be expanded but, if necessary, it is possible to expand skin areas affected by scarring. In such cases, however, the expansion will be very limited; it will also be painful for the patient.

Choice of the correct place to position the expander is crucial. It must be possible to advance or rotate the expanded skin without tension, ensuring complete covering of the area that will going to be lost.

In the upper limb, it is preferable to use radial positioning in order to avoid compression of the neurovascular structures. Expansion with medial and lateral advancement is indicated in all cases rather than unlikely advancement towards a distal position.

When skin expanders are used in the lower extremities, it is necessary to take into account local lymphatic drainage as well as venous drainage conditions because if they are compromised complications such as skin necrosis and tissue expander rejection may occur *(Fig. 19.17)*.

Free flap

The use of free flaps in the reconstruction of extremities with severe burns is infrequent in routine clinical practice. Severely burned patients do not usually have many adequate donor sites for microvascular flaps.

All patients who present a serious loss of skin substance at the level of the knee and ankle joints are potential candidates for this type of reconstructive surgery.

The free flap is commonest in reconstruction of the leg *(Fig. 19.18)*.

Nerve repair

In a step-by-step approach to reconstruction, the surgical repair of nerves comes after immediate burn coverage.

Neural deficit in burn patients is usually associated with electrical burns (and therefore to axonal damage, as described above) or related trauma.

The usual damage consists of interruptions of various length somewhere at some point of the nerve, which have to be repaired using grafts from other nerves. Statistics tell us

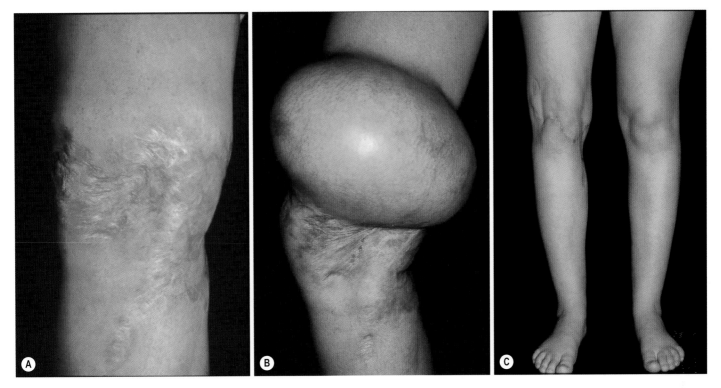

Fig. 19.17 (A) This case illustrates the painful after-burn scar strongly adherent to the joint. **(B)** The use of skin expansion of the lower medial thigh region. **(C)** The result of the use of skin expansion of lower medial thigh region, for an after-burn scar.

that the nerves most frequently damaged are the ulnar nerve and the median nerve, as result of their exposed position.

Normally, the best donor nerve is the *sural nerve*, which can be used for grafts even in excess of 10 cm. This is because it is possible to obtain the *nervus cutaneus surae medialis* connected to the communicating branch of the peroneus, providing up to 30 cm of nerve. The points of reference to be guided by are the external malleolus and the inferior saphenous.

Patients with third-degree burns in the lower limbs, who therefore have no sural nerve to be removed, can receive grafts, albeit much smaller, from the upper limb. The medial and lateral *cutaneous antebrachial nerves* are the candidates of choice because their use causes only a limited sensory deficit with little invalidating effect.

The *medial cutaneous antebrachial* nerve is located medially in the groove between the biceps and the triceps, adjacent to the vena basilica vein. Of its two branches, anterior and posterior, the anterior branch sensitizes the anterior part of the forearm, the posterior branch the elbow, and the remainder of the forearm on all the rest. Using only the anterior branch is less incapacitating for the patient.

The *lateral cutaneous antebrachial* nerve runs along the ulnar border of the musculus brachioradialis, next to the cephalic vein. Resulting insensible areas are usually well tolerated by the patient, since the areas involved overlap the sensitive branch of the radial nerve.

If the gap is small (<3 cm), it is possible to achieve nerve regeneration guided by biodegradable laboratory-produced ducts. The findings of clinical tests have been found to be comparable with the results of small nerve grafts.

Surgery of tendon retraction

The action of scar contractures on the joints causes abnormalities in the tendon structures involved in the deformity. An extreme tendency towards hyperflexion or hyperextension of a joint will ultimately modify the length of the tendons, making them shorter on the flexion side and longer on the opposite side. If the defect persists over time, it will become permanent.

It is possible to intervene with lengthening plastic reconstruction *(Fig. 19.19)*. The technique usually employed consists of a partial horizontal section of the tendon in two distant points, continuing with a median longitudinal section that unites them. This allows the use of two specular half tendons that can slip and then be sutured together in the new location. Once healed, the tendon is longer but thinner.

For this reason, it would be useful to reinforce the elongated tendon with a dermis patch, harvested from a donor site, as described for joint reconstruction. It gives more resistance and better recovery in the postoperative period, allowing a faster FKT.

Amputation

Patients who have suffered high-voltage electrical burns account for the highest proportion of limb amputations. In such cases, the damage to the muscles, blood vessels, and nerves may be such that no other therapeutic solution is viable.

The main objective is to obtain durability of the stump so that the amputated limb can serve as an excellent base for affixing prosthesis.

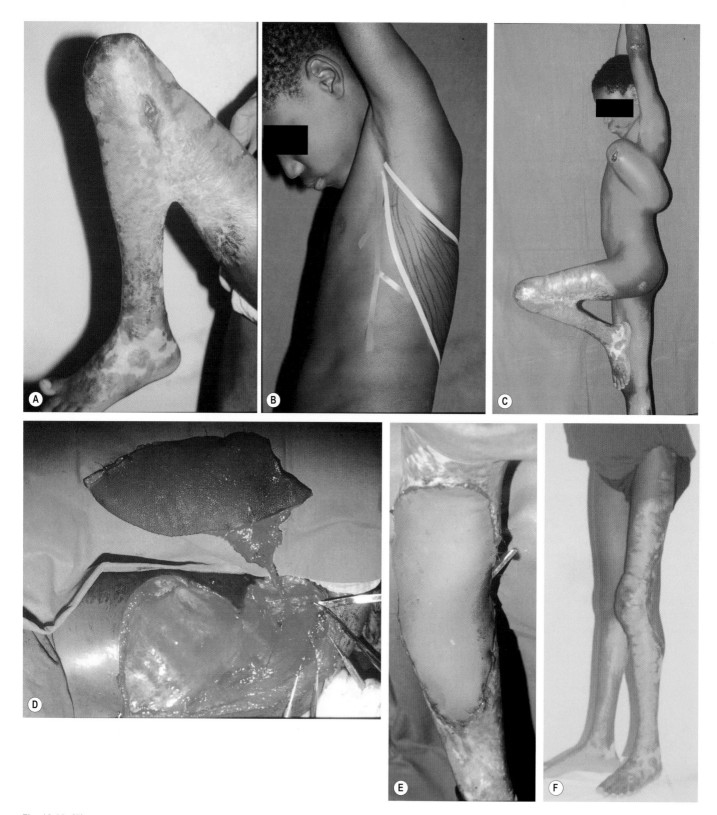

Fig. 19.18 **(A)** Knee: severe retraction. **(B)** Donor area. **(C)** Expansion of latissimus dorsi flap. **(D)** Microsurgical session. **(E)** Free pre-expanded flap. **(F)** Final result.

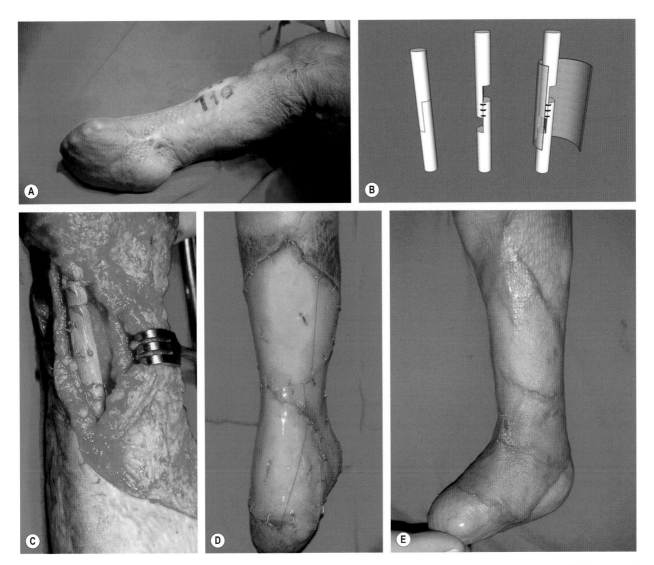

Fig. 19.19 **(A)** Scar contracture about ankle leading to imbalances in the underlying tendons. **(B)** Lengthening design and dermal patch. **(C)** Tendon lengthened and reinforced by dermal patch. **(D)** Resurfaced ankle after underlying tendons have been rebalanced. **(E)** Postoperative result after tendon rebalancing and ankle resurfacing (Courtesy of the Department of Plastic Surgery and Burn Therapy, ARNAS Ospedale Civico, Palermo, Italy.)

The point where an amputation should be performed is dictated primarily by the presence of vital tissue and by the operative technique used. The amputation stump should be covered with local skin and muscle flaps and then sutured to cover the remaining bone stump in order to obtain a soft and viable cushion. If this is not possible, it is advisable, at least initially, to proceed with full-thickness skin grafts, with possible secondary reconstructive surgery to follow.

The lower limb usually requires amputation closer to the vital tissue, while in the upper limb, it is necessary to preserve the maximum possible length in order to have better control over the future prosthesis. For the same reason, in forearm amputations it is always correct to preserve the tendon's pronosupination structures. When it is necessary to create an amputation stump that is too short for application of prosthesis, it is possible to proceed with bone distraction techniques such as the Ilizarov technique.

Lipofilling

The technique of liposculpture, originally created for aesthetic purposes, now plays a primary role in the treatment of areas of scarring. In recent years, the treatment of burn scars with this technique has yielded excellent results that are documented and histologically proven. The quality of the scar has improved in terms of texture, color, and elasticity.

The surgical technique is standard and entails the removal of adipose tissue from donor areas like the abdomen, treatment according to Coleman's technique,[41] and grafting below the areas of scarring. The action of adipose tissue, and more probably that of the stem cells inside it, histologically determines increased vascularization and remodelling of collagen fibers in the treated areas.

The use of lipofilling in the extremities is particularly recommended for reconstituting normal volume, which is

Table 19.2 Laser in scar treatment

Nd:YAG 1064	Scars immature, with vessels
IPL	Hyperpigmentation Scar with vessels
Fractional laser	
Ablative	Mature scars with heterogeneous surface
Nonablative	Mature scars, fibrotic, thick

sometimes lost during surgery, thereby restoring the extremities' conical-cylindrical characteristics.[42]

Laser

The face and neck region can be regarded as "socializing" anatomical areas which are usually exposed, enabling people to communicate and play their role in society. Not surprisingly, patients with burns in these areas often request the intervention of a plastic surgeon, with the aim of improving the quality of their scars. In recent years, we have witnessed a steady growth of laser therapy in the domain of the plastic surgeon. Even though this technique is still under scrutiny, the results have been encouraging.

The final outcome of scar tissue is variable, and many different types of lasers are available for different needs.

The *vascular laser*, such as the Nd:YAG 1064, is indicated in areas of scarring which are immature and have a particularly strong vascular component. The reduction in the blood supply induces an involution of the scar tissue treated.

The *fractional laser (ablative and nonablative)* plays an important role in the remodelling of fibrotic scar tissue, with the interruption and regeneration of collagen and elastic fibers in

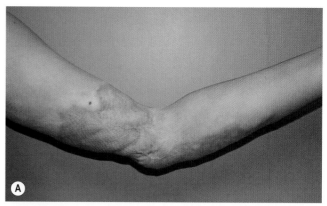

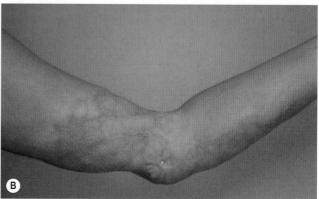

Fig. 19.20 (A) Crop to match heights. **(B)** Elbow area after 6 treatments with nonablative fractional laser. Better color matching and more quality of skin texture.

the dermis, resulting in softening and thinning of the scar itself. Their action also makes the coloring of scar areas more homogeneous, compacting their texture *(Fig. 19.20)*.[43]

IPL and *Q-switched lasers* act on hyperpigmentation and discoloring in certain areas of scarring *(Table 19.2)*.

Access the complete reference list online at **http://www.expertconsult.com**

1. Vyrostek SB, Annest JL, Ryan GW. Surveillance for fatal and non fatal injuries – United States 2001. Office of Statistics and Programming. *National Center for Injury Prevention and Control.* CDC/NCIPC/OSP; 2001.

   This comprehensive government publication reports demographic and mechanistic data for all injuries sustained in the United States during 2001. A 0.5% mortality rate is reported for injured individuals varying by age, sex, and mechanism.

3. American Burn Association. Guidelines for service standards and severity classifications in the treatment of burn injury. *Bull Am Coll Surg.* 1984;69:24–29.

9. McCauley RL, Asuku ME. Upper extremity burn reconstruction. In: Mathes SJ, Hentz VR, ed. Plastic Surgery. Vol VII. 2nd ed. Philadelphia: Saunders Elsevier; 2005:605–619.

   This encyclopaedic book chapter covers upper extremity burn care from primary excision and grafting to secondary

   procedures. An informative historical perspective is also provided.

13. Purdue GF, Arnoldo BD, Hunt JL. Electrical injuries. In: Herndon DN, ed. *Total Burn Care.* 3rd ed. Philadelphia: WB Saunders; 2008:513–520.

24. Heimbach DM, Logsetty S. Modern technique for wound coverage of the thermally injured upper extremity. *Hand Clin.* 2000;16(2):205–214.

   Advanced modalities in burn reconstruction are discussed. The authors stress, however, that the split-thickness skin graft remains the "gold standard" in burn reconstruction.

25. Borghese L, Latorre S, Montagnese A, et al. Retrospective analysis of 200 severe post-burn cases in Cambodia and Bangladesh. *Ann Burns Fire Disast.* 2005;18(1).

26. Smith MA, Munster AM, Spence RJ. Burns of the hand and upper limb – a review. *Burns.* 1998;24:493–505.

   The authors discuss the standard of care and controversial issues in hand and upper extremity burns.

28. Atiyeh BS, Hayek SN, Gunn SWA. New technologies for burn wound closure and healing – Review of the literature. *Burns*. 2005;31:944–956.

The authors of this review note the limitations of autologous skin grafting in burn reconstruction. Alternative replacement modalities are surveyed.

31. Masellis M, Conte F, Fortezza GS. Use of dermis to reconstruct hand joint capsules. *Ann Plast Surg*. 1982;9:72–80.

32. Beasley RW. Burns of the axilla and elbow. In: Converse JM, ed. Reconstructive Plastic Surgery. Vol 6. Philadelphia: WB Saunders; 1977:3391–3402.

20

Cold and chemical injury to the upper extremity

Dennis S. Kao and John Hijjawi

SYNOPSIS

Cold injury

- Frostbite should be treated with rapid rewarming in a 40–42°C hydrotherapy tank.
- Frostbite should be treated with oral ibuprofen and topical aloe vera.
- Common sequelae of frostbite, in general, include residual pain and cold intolerance.
- Less common sequelae of frostbite in children include shortened digits and angular deformity due to injury to the growth plate.

Chemical injury

- Chemical burns usually result in a deeper burn than thermal burns.
- Clothing, gloves, or other items in contact with the skin should be quickly removed to minimize contact with the chemical.
- Immediate treatment consists of copious water lavage for 2 h for most chemicals but up to 12 h for alkalis.

Extravasation injury

- Extravasation involving small to intermediate amounts of agent may be managed with elevation and observation versus liposuction or saline flushout performed within 24 h of extravasation.
- Significant extravasation carries a high risk of skin ulceration and should be addressed with early surgical intervention.
- Doxorubicin extravasation can be managed with IV administration of dexrazoxane within 6 h of extravasation.
- If compartment syndrome develops, prompt fasciotomy is indicated.

 Access the Historical Perspective sections online at
http://www.expertconsult.com

Cold injury

Frostbite is the most common local cold injury, although cold exposure does not always result in tissue freezing. Rather, there is a continuum that ranges from minimal skin chilling to tissue freezing with ice crystal formation.[1] The two key factors that determine the resultant type of cold injury are the rate of cooling and the presence or absence of ice crystal formation in the tissues.[2] Frostnip occurs due to rapid temperature drops without formation of ice crystals. It causes skin pallor and numbness but is completely reversible.[3] Flash freezing occurs due to contact with cold metal or volatile liquids that results in rapid cooling with formation of ice crystals. Frostbite occurs when the tissue is cooled slowly with formation of ice crystals when the tissue freezes at −2°C.[4] Environmental factors that predispose to the development of frostbite include windchill,[5] water immersion,[6] high altitude,[7,8] and chemical agent exposure.[9] Physiologic factors that predispose to the development of frostbite include vascular dehydration,[10,11] previous cold injury,[12] alcohol or drug consumption,[13,14] altered mental status/psychological illness, and inactivity.[15]

Basic science/disease process

Pathophysiology

The blood flow to the skin is one of the most important means of heat regulation for the human body.[19] The extremities account for approximately 50% of the total body surface area (TBSA) but are responsible for most of the protective vasoconstriction response to cold, because the skin covering the head and trunk has little capacity for vasoconstriction.[20] Peripheral vasoconstriction is a physiologic response to cold exposure in order to preserve and maintain core body temperature.[21] However, this physiologic peripheral vasoconstriction is interspersed with intermittent vasodilation, known as the hunting response. Such a response involves transient vasodilation of the vasculature of the extremities to increase blood flow through arteriovenous shunting in an effort to rewarm and perfuse the tissue. The hunting response occurs every 7–10 min until the body's core temperature falls below 28°C, at which point the hunting response is lost.[21] When the core temperature falls below 10°C, sensory nerve dysfunction occurs, leading to the loss of protective sensation. The loss of the hunting response and protective sensation in combination with subfreezing ambient temperature will lead to progressive tissue cooling and subsequent tissue freezing with ice crystal formation at $-2°C$.

Freezing phase

Tissue injury and death occur not only during the cooling/freezing process, but also during the rewarming/reperfusion process.[22] During the cooling phase, prolonged vasoconstriction leads to cell ischemia, which activates the inflammatory cascade and initiates the release of a group of cytokines, including prostaglandins,[23] bradykinins,[24] thromboxane,[23] and histamine.[25] Inflammatory cells such as leukocytes[26] and platelets[27] are also recruited. Cell death during the freezing phase is believed to result from cellular dehydration.[28] Slow cooling causes the extracellular fluid to freeze first. As the water in the extracellular space freezes and forms ice crystals, the water concentration in the extracellular space decreases and the extracellular space becomes more hypertonic than the intracellular space. As a result, water is drawn out of the cell by the osmotic gradient and leads to cellular dehydration. Cellular dehydration alters the protein and lipid composition of the cell membranes, making them less stable. The cellular pH also falls, which causes disruption of enzymatic activities. If the freezing process continues, ice crystals will form within the cell and cell membrane, causing disruption of membrane integrity and cell death. Rapid freezing (defined as a drop in tissue temperature >10°C per min) is less deleterious than slow freezing, because rapid freezing allows near simultaneous ice crystal formation in both the extracellular and intracellular space, therefore creating minimal osmotic gradient and minimal fluid shift.[29] Furthermore, different cell types have different resistance to cold injuries. Nerve, cartilage, bone, and especially endothelial cells are more susceptible to freezing injury than are skin, fat, or connective tissue.[3,4,26] This is why neuropathic pain is a common sequelae of frostbite injury, even without soft tissue loss, and also why frostbitten children can develop shortened or angular deformity in affected digits due to injury to the cartilaginous growth plates.

Rewarming phase

Although freezing and ice crystal formation may fatally injure a certain number of cells; the clinical significance of this direct injury to the soft tissue is thought to be limited. This was demonstrated when frostbitten skin transplanted to a new, vascularized recipient site survived, but developed necrosis if left *in situ* and not transplanted.[30] The indirect cell injury that occurs during the rewarming/reperfusion process is believed to be more critical. The endothelial cells are very vulnerable during the rewarming stage and become highly permeable if injured.[26] The increased permeability leads to significant interstitial edema as the blood flow is restored. In severe endothelial cell injuries, erythrocyte extravasation and perivascular hemorrhage occur and produce hemorrhagic blisters.[26,29,31] The injured endothelial cells also detach from the basement membrane, leaving a raw vessel surface that is thrombogenic. The restoration of blood flow then leads to immediate platelet aggregation in the arterioles, followed by leukocyte aggregation and activation. These events result in thrombosis and

progressive vascular obstruction. If thrombosis is limited to only some areas of the microcirculation, only partial soft tissue loss will occur. If the larger arterioles and arteries are affected, the entire limb is at risk of necrosis. The major determinant of tissue necrosis is the degree of endothelial cell injury and the extent of microvascular thrombosis during the rewarming process.

Diagnosis/patient presentation

Physical exam

A thorough history and physical exam is crucial. Host risk factors such as peripheral vascular disease, diabetes, tobacco or alcohol use, altered mental status, and sensitivity to cold from previous exposure all need to be identified. Environmental risk factors such as wet clothing, windchill factor, the exposure temperature, and the duration of exposure all need to be documented if possible.

Physical examination of the patient with frostbite injury includes measurement of the core body temperature, as well as inspection and palpation of the affected area. Superficial frostbite occurs more commonly in the face and upper extremities. It may have a waxy appearance with blanching or whitening in color. After rewarming, it is supple and painful, with reactive hyperemia and minimal to moderate edema. Deep frostbite occurs more commonly in the lower extremities. It has a bluish-gray appearance. After rewarming, it is firm and anesthetic, with significant edema due to the increased permeability of the injured endothelial cells. In addition to reactive hyperemia and edema, significant frostbite is also associated with blister formation. Blisters containing clear fluid form 6–24 h after rewarming as blood flows into the area and extravasated fluid accumulates beneath the detached epidermal sheet. Hemorrhagic blisters indicate disruption of the subdermal plexus and carry a less favorable prognosis than areas with clear blisters. If the tissue appears severely frost bitten but shows no edema or blister formation after rewarming, it may be an indication of complete absence of blood flow restoration, and signals the likelihood of subsequent complete tissue loss of that affected area.

Staging

The extent of the frostbite injury is determined by clinical examination and the final outcome of the injured sites. Frozen skin is cold, white, and firm to the touch. No descriptive or prognostic assessment can be made until the tissues have been rewarmed.[32] The older classification defines injury grades as first- to fourth-degree, much like thermal burns.[33] Currently, most clinicians classify frostbite as either superficial or deep.[34] However, early clinical assessment of tissue viability has poor accuracy, and progressive changes in clinical appearance are anticipated.[7] Definitive classification may not be possible for several weeks.

Radiographic studies

^{99m}Tc pertechnetate scintigraphy (^{99m}Tc bone scans) can be used to evaluate perfusion of bone and soft tissue and predict the final extent of tissue damage from frostbite. ^{99m}Tc bone scan images are acquired over three phases: the blood flow phase, the blood pool phase, and the delayed bone phase.

Patterns of radioactive tracer uptake in each phase may show normal uptake, decreased uptake, or nonuptake. Several studies have shown that the delayed bone phase correlates best with the true extent of tissue injury and final outcome.[35] The areas of nonuptake in the delayed bone phase will usually require amputation, while the areas of normal uptake typically heal uneventfully. The areas of decreased uptake are regions with marginal viability and may subsequently evolve into areas of normal uptake or areas of nonuptake.[36] This explains why the predictive power of ^{99m}Tc bone scans is time-dependent. The diagnostic accuracy of bone scans performed at 48 h post-injury is only 84%, but can be improved when bone scans are delayed until 7–10 days post-injury, because during this time, the areas of marginal viability (decreased uptake) would have evolved and declared themselves as either viable (normal uptake) or nonviable (nonuptake).[37] Interestingly, one study suggests that areas of nonuptake on bone scans 10 days after frostbite does not always lead to complete tissue necrosis.[38] The possible explanation is that these areas may have marginal perfusion that is adequate to support tissue viability, but below the detection level of the ^{99m}Tc bone scans. Therefore, bone scans may be used to predict the extent of worst possible outcome, but if given enough time to heal and recover, the final amount of tissue loss may not be as extensive as predicted by the bone scans.

Magnetic resonance imaging and angiography (MRI/MRA) may be superior to ^{99m}Tc bone scans in the evaluation of frostbite due to the ability to visualize occluded vessels and line of demarcation between viable and nonviable tissue.[39] However, the high cost associated with MRI/MRA, along with contraindications in patients having metallic implants, may limit their clinical application. Perfusion status of the frostbitten area can also be assessed with angiography. However, it is invasive and perhaps is better reserved only when thrombolytic therapy is also being considered.

Patient selection

Initially, all patients should receive medical management for frostbite. For patients who sustained frostbite due to psychological disorders (e.g., hallucination from schizophrenia), their psychological illness must be addressed to optimize their outcome and prevent similar injuries in the future. For patients with severe frostbite injury, thrombolytic therapy or length salvage surgery should only be considered if the patient has no major medical or psychological contraindications (e.g., schizophrenia).

Treatment/surgical technique

Nonoperative management

Field management

Initial treatment in the field should focus on protecting the affected extremity from mechanical trauma and avoiding rewarming. Cyclic thawing and cooling or inadequate rewarming can worsen a frostbite injury.[22] The patient should be transferred to centers that are familiar and equipped to perform rapid rewarming.

Rapid rewarming

The core temperature of the patient should be measured, and if hypothermia is present, it should be treated appropriately with core rewarming. The core temperature should rise above 35°C prior to attempting rapid rewarming of the frostbitten area. Any attempt of extremity rewarming prior to this may cause a paradoxical core body temperature drop, as the peripheral vessel beds reopen and the cold peripheral blood returns to the core body. The ideal temperature for rapid rewarming has been experimentally determined to be between 40° and 42°C.[40] Rewarming at this temperature results in the least amount of tissue injury. It is best achieved in a hydrotherapy tub. Rewarming should be continued for 15–30 min or until thawing is complete, which is marked by the red or purple appearance of the affected area, indicating the restoration of blood flow. This often coincides with extreme pain in 75% of the patients, and may require parenteral narcotic administration.[29] Active motion during rewarming is helpful, but massage of the affected part is not recommended, as it may traumatize the friable frostbitten skin.

Adjunctive therapy

White or clear blisters contain fluid that is high in prostaglandin $F_{2\alpha}$ and thromboxane B_2.[23] These cytokines promote vasoconstriction, leukocyte adherence, and platelet aggregation. They have been shown to mediate dermal ischemia in burns and pedicled flaps.[23,41] The fluid should be aspirated but the deflated blisters should be left in place to prevent desiccation of the underlying wound bed. Ibuprofen, a specific thromboxane inhibitor, can be used to counter the effects of these vasoconstrictive cytokines and has been associated with the best tissue salvage.[29] It is currently the standard pharmacologic treatment for frostbite. Topical aloe vera may also be applied to the affected area, as it is an effective thromboxane inhibitor and has been shown to reduce the degree of tissue loss.[42] Systemic antibiotics are generally not indicated unless clinical infection is present.[32] However, tetanus prophylaxis should be given or updated. Tetanus killed thousands of Napoleon's troops during the invasion of Russia, and clinical tetanus infection in frostbite patients has been reported as recently as 1990.[29,43]

Splinting

The affected extremity should also be splinted in a functional position. The hand should be splinted in the intrinsic plus position to prevent late deformities caused by intrinsic muscle contracture.

Operative management

Amputation

Distinguishing between viable and nonviable tissue in the early stages of frostbite injury is difficult, if not impossible. Therefore, every effort should be made to preserve as much tissue as possible while waiting for the frostbitten tissue to declare its viability, hence the classic adage of "freeze in January, amputate in July." The only absolute indication for early debridement is uncontrollable infection.[4] Mummification and black eschar occur at approximately 3–4 weeks post-injury.[29] Amputation can generally be performed at that time, once there is a clear line of demarcation occurring between viable and nonviable tissue (*Fig. 20.1*).

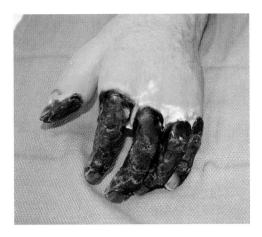

Fig. 20.1 Frostbite injury of the nondominant hand. Two months have been allowed to elapse since injury to ensure maximum length preservation.

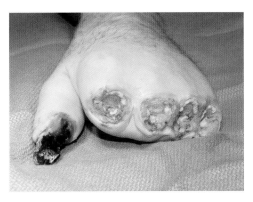

Fig. 20.2 Amputation back to viable tissue performed without tourniquet control.

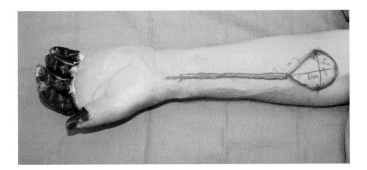

Fig. 20.3 A pedicled radial forearm flap designed for thumb coverage to maximize the preservation of bony length. This procedure was performed under regional anesthesia with sedation due to an unstable cardiac condition. Any reconstruction requiring general anesthesia was felt to be contraindicated by the cardiology service.

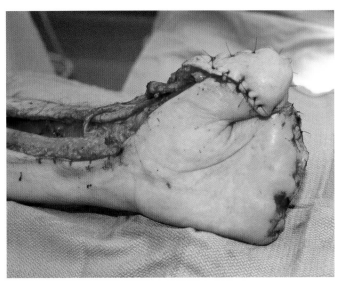

Fig. 20.4 Radial forearm flap inset on the thumb.

Amputation can be done without the use of tourniquet, which allows the surgeon to determine the level of viable tissue intraoperatively. Tissue is debrided until a bleeding wound edge is encountered *(Fig. 20.2)*. The level of amputation should be conservative in order to preserve length and function.[44] If the overlying soft tissue has sloughed but the underlying bony and tendinous structures are viable, a negative wound pressure dressing can be used to provide temporary coverage to prevent desiccation. Local or free tissue transfer can be utilized for length salvage *(Figs 20.3, 20.4)*.[45] However, function, and not length, ought to be the priority.

Length salvage

Advocates of early surgery utilize the results of ^{99m}Tc bone scan to guide surgical intervention. At 48 h post-injury, an initial bone scan is obtained. If there is any perfusion abnormality, the bone scan is repeated 72 h later. Areas with a persistent deficit in the delayed bone phase are treated with surgical excision of the nonperfused skin and soft tissues. The underlying tendon, nerve, and bone are covered with appropriate flaps to prevent desiccation. Follow-up bone scans demonstrated revascularization of structures covered by the flaps. This treatment algorithm limited the extent of required amputation with some length preservation in selected patients.[46] However, there has not been any published long-term functional outcome study to demonstrate

the efficacy of early surgical intervention when compared to initial observation followed by revision amputation at 4–6 weeks.

Postoperative care

If the patient sustained frostbite due to psychological illness, special precautions should be taken to protect the incisions to prevent self-mutilation. Elevation is important to minimize edema. Once the incisions have healed, rehabilitation should be started to prevent stiffness and improve range of motion.

Outcomes/prognosis/complications

Common early complications of frostbite are infection and gangrene. Frequent late sequelae are residual pain and cold intolerance of the affected site.[7] Less common complications include hyperhidrosis, pigmentation changes, and skin atrophy.[47] Localized osteoporosis and pronounced subchondral bone loss have been reported as early as 4 weeks post-injury and as late as several months later.[48] Physeal injury with subsequent growth disturbance has been observed in children.[49–51] The most frequently affected site is the phalangeal epiphyses, following a pattern of decreasing frequency from distal to proximal. Direct injury to the vulnerable chondrocytes in the cartilaginous growth plate results in shortened digits or asymmetric growth of the digit leading to angular deformity. Radiographic evidence of premature epiphyseal closure may not be evident until 6–12 months after cold exposure.[52] Long-term complications that involve joints and soft tissue injury may result in joint contracture and spontaneous joint fusion.

Secondary procedures

Sympathectomy

Surgical sympathectomy has been used to treat frostbite. It has been shown to be effective in decreasing the late sequelae of frostbite, including improved circulation, decreased hyperhidrosis and pallor, and reduced vasospastic symptoms and pain upon cold exposure.[53–55] It has also been shown to expedite resolution of edema and the healing of ulcers.[56,57] However, neither surgical sympathectomy nor chemical sympathectomy has been shown to decrease the amount of tissue loss after frostbite injury.[58–60]

Hyperbaric oxygen

The role of hyperbaric oxygen therapy in the treatment of frostbite remains unclear. In theory, it is attractive due to its ability to increase dissolved oxygen in the plasma, resulting in increased oxygen delivery to the tissue. It has been shown to accelerate capillary formation.[61] Several anecdotal case reports describe improvement of wound healing and salvage of frostbitten digits with hyperbaric oxygen.[62,63] However, there has not been any controlled clinical trial to demonstrate the therapeutic efficacy of hyperbaric oxygen therapy.

Thrombolytics

Since the major determinant of frostbite injury outcome is the severity of microvascular thrombosis that occurs after rewarming, thrombolytics are conceptually attractive because they potentially correct the pathology leading to tissue necrosis.[1,64] Thrombolytic therapy involving either intravenous or intra-arterial tissue plasminogen activator (tPA) administration was found to improve the tissue viability after frostbite and decrease the need for amputation.[65,66] The reported digit salvage rate for severe frostbite with perfusion deficits is approximately 75%.[2] However, this involves invasive procedure with potential hemorrhagic complications. Its use has not yet been widely accepted.

Chemical injury

Chemical injuries are similar to thermal injuries, in that they are usually associated with damage to the skin only. However, the major difference is that some chemical may remain active at the contact site and cause continual tissue damage until neutralized. The level of injury depends on the duration of contact, and the nature and concentration of the chemical agent. Chemical burns represent only a small percentage of burn unit admissions. Yet more than 60% of these are work-related and have major occupational morbidity.[67,68] Other exposures occur accidentally, in assaults, or during military conflicts.[69] Alkalis are the most common chemical involved in cutaneous burns, but the most frequent single chemical agent involved is sulfuric acid.[70] The silicon chip manufacturing industry is often associated with hydrofluoric acid burns.[71,72]

Many chemical burns involve the upper extremity and specifically the digits. Although the traditional measure of burn severity (percentage of total body surface area burned or %TBSA) is low compared with the usual burn population, chemical burns have a significant morbidity because the percentage of full-thickness burn is high and the patient's hospital stay tends to be long.[69] It is important to remember that while only about 3% of all burns are due to chemical exposure, 30% of burn deaths are due to chemical injuries.[73]

Basic science/disease process

Pathophysiology

There are similarities between thermal and chemical burns; they both involve protein denaturation and produce wounds that look alike superficially. Yet, important differences exist. First, thermal injuries typically are produced by very brief exposure to intense heat. Chemical injuries are produced by longer exposure to chemicals, which may still be continuing at the time of presentation. Second, there are fundamental differences between thermal and chemical burns at the molecular level. Proteins are composed of chains of amino acids. Different protein chains interact with each other and form complex three-dimensional structures that are held together by weak forces such as van der Waals' forces and hydrogen bonds. Application of heat or chemicals can disturb these forces and cause protein structures to fall apart. In thermal injuries, there is a rapid coagulation of protein due to cross-linking reactions followed by termination of that reaction once the heat source is removed. In chemical injuries, pH disturbance leads to ongoing hydrolysis that damages proteins until the original tissue pH has been restored. Third, chemical agents usually cause injury by direct chemical reaction rather than by the production of heat. Finally, chemical agents may act in a systemic fashion as they are absorbed and circulated throughout the body, causing metabolic toxicity and multi-system organ failure.

Classification

The chemicals can be classified into six categories based on their mechanism of action: oxidizing agents, reducing agents, corrosive agents, desiccants, vesicants, and protoplasmic poisons.[74] The pathophysiology of each category is briefly discussed below, and examples of representative agents commonly encountered from each category are described in further detail.

Oxidizing agents

Oxidizing agents introduce oxygen, sulfur, or halogen atoms into proteins and destroy the proteins' ability to function. In some cases, the oxidation product can become a competitor for active metabolic binding sites. Common examples are chromic acid and sodium hypochlorite (bleach).

Chromic acid

The active chemical in chromic acid is chromic trioxide. It is a pungent viscid yellow liquid. This hexavalent chromium, Cr(VI), is rapidly absorbed through the skin and reaches peak serum level by 5 h post-injury.[75] Once in the circulation, Cr(VI) binds to hemoglobin, followed by parenchymal uptake by kidney, liver, bone, lung, and spleen within the first 24 h.[76] Its toxic effect on the kidney may lead to renal failure.

Sodium hypochlorite

Also known as common household bleach, it is a potent oxidizing agent in a strong alkaline solution that causes protein coagulation. The active ion is hypochlorous (OCl^-), but free chlorine (Cl_2) is also present. The severity of injury is dependent more on the concentration of the solution rather than the duration of exposure.

Reducing agents

These are highly reactive chemicals that bind free electrons in tissue proteins, cause reduction of the amide link and lead to protein denaturation. Common examples are alkyl mercuric compounds used in batteries and paints, hydrochloric acid, and nitric acid.

Hydrochloric acid

It protonates skin proteins into chloride salts. While it is in contact with tissue, the wound will progress as the acid continues to denature protein.

Corrosive agents

Corrosive agents cause extensive protein denaturation. Agents commonly encountered include phenol, white phosphorus, and lyes.

Phenol

Phenol is an aromatic hydrocarbon derived from coal tar. It has antiseptic properties and is used in chemical face peels, nerve injections, and topical anesthetic for skin and mucous membranes.[77]

White phosphorus

White phosphorus is a yellow, waxy, translucent solid element that ignites spontaneously at temperature greater than 34°C unless preserved in oil. It is used in the manufacture of various insecticides, fertilizers, fireworks, and incendiary weapons. It is extremely lipid soluble and readily penetrates the dermis. White phosphorus causes tissue injury in two ways. It oxidizes adjacent tissue, causing protein denaturation, and generate considerable amount of heat in the process. Therefore, it causes both chemical and thermal injury.

Desiccants

These cause injury by extracting water from tissue, causing dehydration. The damage is often exacerbated by heat production, as these reactions are usually exothermic. A common example is sulfuric acid.

Sulfuric acid

Sulfuric acid has a high affinity for water since the hydration process of sulfuric acid is very thermodynamically favorable. Its reaction with water is highly exothermic. It has many applications and is one of the top products of the chemical industry. Principal uses include lead-acid batteries, fertilizer manufacturing, wastewater processing, and chemical synthesis. It is the most common chemical involved in chemical burns.

Vesicants

These agents are characterized by their ability to produce cutaneous blisters. They are potent chemical warfare agents and include mustards, arsenicals, and halogenated oximes. These compounds affect not only the skin, but also all epithelial tissues with which they come into contact, particularly the eyes and respiratory tract.

Mustard gas

Mustards are alkylating agents that cause damage to DNA, making them toxic to proliferating cells. Evidence suggests that alkylation of DNA may not be the critical step in producing skin manifestations. Rather, following cell death of the basal cells, proteases are released from lysosomes, causing the epidermis to separate from the dermis.[78] It is highly lipid soluble and can be readily absorbed through the skin.

Protoplasmic poisons

Some poisons produce their effects by causing the formation of esters with proteins or by acting as metabolic inhibitors when they bind inorganic ions that are necessary for normal cellular function. Ester formers include formic acid. Metabolic competitors include hydrofluoric acid (HF).

Formic acid

Formic acid is used industrially as a descaling agent and a textile tanning substance. It forms esters with cellular proteins and is cytotoxic especially to red blood cells.

Hydrofluoric acid

Hydrofluoric acid is commonly used in glass etching, rust removers, and heavy-duty cleaners. HF has a dual mechanism of injury that makes its injury amongst the most severe and lethal. HF produces dehydration and corrosion of tissue due to the free hydrogen ions. Fluoride anions bind bivalent cations such as calcium and magnesium to form insoluble salts. This process may occur at a rate exceeding the body's ability to mobilize bone calcium and magnesium into serum, thus leading to hypocalcemia and hypomagnesemia. Fluoride anions may also inhibit the Na-K ATPase in the cell membrane, leading to a massive potassium efflux.[79] The resultant ionic shifts, particularly of potassium, are thought to be responsible for the excruciating pain associated with HF burns. In addition, fluoride ions may cause direct activation of myocardial adenylate cyclase, which leads to myocardial irritability and potentially fatal arrhythmias.[80]

Diagnosis/patient presentation

The severity of a chemical burn is often under-estimated on first examination.[81] Corrosive material blackens the skin and converts it to a firmly adherent, dry eschar, making the true assessment of the depth of injury difficult.

Oxidizing agents

Chromic acid

Chromic acid burns produce protein coagulation, blister formation, and ulceration. Ingestion will lead to severe gastroenteritis, vertigo, muscle cramps, peripheral vascular collapse, and coma.

Sodium hypochlorite

Systemic symptoms include vomiting, dyspnea, hoarseness, airway edema, confusion, cardiovascular collapse, cyanosis, coma, peritonitis, and mediastinitis.

Reducing agents

Hydrochloric acid

Hydrochloric acid burns produce shallow ulcers that are covered by a coagulum of damaged skin. Pneumonitis and airway obstruction secondary to glottic edema can develop from inhalation injury due to hydrochloric acid fumes.

Corrosive agents

Phenol

Skin contact with phenol leads to erythema, swelling, and pain. It can also lead to subsequent hypopigmentation. Following ingestion or absorption, it is bound to serum albumin. Acute poisoning may occur with systemic manifestations, with severity proportional to the plasma concentration of free phenol. Systemic signs include initial bradycardia followed by tachycardia and a decrease in blood pressure. Phenol depresses CNS and may lead to respiratory arrest. It may also produce peripheral nerve demyelination and renal failure through direct damage to the glomeruli.[77]

White phosphorus

White phosphorus is difficult to remove and often becomes embedded in the skin. Injuries produce wounds that are similar in appearance to partial or full thickness thermal burns. The wounds are typically extremely painful, yellowish in color, and have a characteristic smell of garlic.

Desiccants

Sulfuric acid

Contact with sulfuric acid is painful and results in the release of large quantities of heat, which increases the amount of injury. The burn tends to involve only limited areas, but often produces deep ulceration.

Vesicants

Mustard gas

Early symptoms associated with mustard gas include ocular burning, throat burning, and a feeling of suffocation.[78] Skin erythema is seen after 4 h of exposure, and blisters associated with intense pruritus appear after 12–48 h. The blisters tend to rupture, leaving shallow but painful ulcers. Greater exposure produces coagulative necrosis of the skin.

Protoplasmic poisons

Formic acid

Formic acid burn wounds have a greenish hue and are followed by blister formation and edema. Vomiting and abdominal pain are usual. Cutaneous absorption from injured areas can cause metabolic acidosis, intravascular hemolysis (due to direct cytotoxic effect on erythrocytes), hemoglobinuria, renal failure, and pulmonary complications including ARDS.[82,83]

Hydrofluoric acid (HF)

The clinical presentation of HF burns is one of blanched tissue with surrounding erythema associated with severe pain. Edema and blistering occurs within 1–2 h, followed by grayish necrosis, deep ulceration, and possible tenosynovitis and osteolysis within 6–24 h. Even burns from dilute HF can progress to a similar level of destruction if left untreated.[80] It is important to monitor the patient's serum calcium and magnesium levels, as the patient can develop arrhythmia due to hypocalcemia and hypomagnesemia.

Patient selection

Most patients with chemical burns are victims of occupational injury. Therefore, many are in relatively good health. However, the systemic consequences of a chemical injury must not be underestimated. They must be anticipated and treated early.

Treatment/surgical technique

Primary treatment

The initial goal is to minimize the duration of contact with the offending chemical. Clothing, gloves, or other items in contact with the skin should be quickly removed. Immediate treatment consists of copious water lavage of the affected area. Speed is of the essence. Both animal studies and human experience confirm that copious and continuous lavage immediately following chemical exposure is critical in limiting the extent of injury.[84] A delay following contact with a chemical may allow the epidermis to be destroyed, thus exposing the more permeable dermis to the chemical. By starting the washing process before tissue pH levels reach an extreme, subsequent pH aberrations are minimized.[85] Lavage effectively dilutes the chemical that is already in contact with the skin, restores the normal skin pH, and minimizes the heat that may be generated by the chemical reaction. It has been shown to reduce the extent of full-thickness injury and decrease hospital stay.[86] Lavage should be done with copious quantities of fluid, because even small volumes of some strong acids and alkali can alter the pH of very large quantities of fluids.[69] For example, 10 mL of 98% sulfuric acid will reduce the pH of 12 L of water down to 5.0. The lavage site should also be kept well drained in order to remove the earlier, more concentrated washings and prevent it from causing additional injury to previously uninvolved areas. Monitoring the pH of the spent lavage fluid can provide a good indication of the lavage effectiveness and completion. Pain may also be used as a guide to help determine the effectiveness of chemical neutralization. However, it is not completely reliable, as some chemicals (e.g., phenol) demyelinate nerves, making the wound anesthetic.[74]

Most chemical burns should be irrigated for 2 h. However, alkalis may need up to 12 h of irrigation to neutralize the pH.[84] The use of neutralizing agents in the treatment of chemical burns is controversial. In theory, they inactivate the offending chemical in the wound and prevent further injury. However, due to the wide range of chemicals potentially involved, their correct use cannot be assured. Also, the neutralization reaction may generate heat adding thermal injury to the chemical injury. Therefore, the use of neutralizing agents is generally not encouraged. Furthermore, no agent has been found to be more effective than water lavage.[87] Time should not be wasted in search for specific antidotes at the expense of initiating immediate and copious water lavage. Specific antidotes can be sought during or after the lavage. Exceptions to the water lavage protocol are rare and include exposure to elemental sodium, potassium, and lithium. Applying water to these elements causes ignition and will lead to additional thermal injury. Mineral oil may be used to first coat the patient, followed by water lavage to remove the particles of chemical embedded in the skin.

Secondary treatment

After using copious water lavage as the primary treatment for the majority of chemical burns, multiple secondary treatment options exist depending on the offending chemical. In general, blisters should be debrided and irrigated, as they may harbor additional chemical underneath. If the chemical burn involves the nail, the nail should be removed and irrigated to ensure that there is no residual chemical in the subungual space. The following provides a brief description of secondary treatments for cutaneous and systemic manifestations caused by different chemical agents.

Oxidizing agents
Chromic acid

Primary treatment for chromic acid burns is water lavage. Chromium that is bound to hemoglobin may be removed from the circulation via exchange transfusion.[76] Chromium in the serum that has not bound to hemoglobin may be removed using dialysis within the first 24 h of exposure, before it is absorbed by parenchymal tissues. After that, dialysis is used mainly as a supportive measure for treatment of chromium-induced acute renal failure.[88,89] Systemic chromium poisoning can occur from cutaneous absorption of chromic acid burns that involve as little as 1% TBSA.[89] Specific treatments developed in the past focused on chelating the chromium or reducing the hexavalent chromium ion into the less toxic trivalent ion. These treatments include topical 10% calcium EDTA or a combination of ascorbic acid, sodium pyrosulphite, ammonium chloride, tartaric acid and glucose.[90,91] Unfortunately, no treatment has consistently produced favorable outcomes. Since systemic chromium poisoning can often be fatal, immediate excision has been recommended as the only effective way of reducing chromium absorption and decreasing the risk of systemic toxicity.[89,92] Local flap closure of the wound is not advised if one cannot be certain that all the tissues affected by chromium have been excised. Rather, split thickness skin grafting or delayed reconstruction are recommended in these situations.[89,93]

Sodium hypochlorite

Copious water lavage is the primary treatment. Depending on the severity of the injury, subsequent wound debridement and closure or skin grafting may be required.

Reducing agents
Hydrochloric acid

Copious water lavage is the primary treatment. Depending on the severity of the injury, subsequent wound debridement and closure or skin grafting may be required.

Corrosive agents
Phenol

Phenol burn should be treated with water lavage. Avoid gentle swabbing of the affected area with sponges soaked in water, since dilute solutions of phenol are more rapidly absorbed through skin than concentrated ones. A quick wipe of the skin with undiluted 200–400 molecular weight polyethylene glycol (PEG) solution reduces mortality and burn severity in experimental animals.[94] These solutions can be used in phenol burns of the face because they are not irritating to eyes. However, copious water irrigation remains to be the best treatment. It should be performed in a well-ventilated room to avoid exposing healthcare providers to high concentrations of phenol fumes. Treatment of systemic symptoms is supportive.

White phosphorus

Immediate treatment involves removing all of a patient's clothing and thoroughly irrigating the area with cool water, because white phosphorous becomes liquid at 44°C and can cause additional burn to surrounding area as it liquefies. Remove any easily identifiable particles. Cover burned skin with towels soaked in cool water during transport to specialist unit.

Desiccants
Sulfuric acid

Treatment of sulfuric acid burn begins with water lavage. Yet due to the tendency for formation of deep but limited ulceration, early eschar excision and grafting has been recommended.[95]

Vesicants
Mustard gas

Initial treatment requires removal of patient's clothing followed by water lavage of all the exposed areas. Healthcare providers must be protected, and the contaminated clothing must be placed in special bags. Itching can be treated with sedatives such as benzodiazepines or antihistamines. Blisters should be unroofed and dressed with topical antimicrobials. The mustard blister fluid is harmless.[96] There is no specific antidote for mustard gas poisoning, although some evidence suggests that sodium thiosulfate and cysteine may offer some protection if administered early.[97] Early excision and grafting has not been proven to have any value. Treatment for systemic mustard gas poisoning is supportive. Pancytopenia may occur 4–5 days post-exposure due to bone marrow suppression.

Protoplasmic poisons
Formic acid

Initial treatment for formic acid burn is water lavage. The main concern with formic acid burn is metabolic acidosis. Acidosis should be corrected with intravenous sodium bicarbonate. When extensive absorption has occurred, exchange transfusion or hemodialysis may be required. Folic acid may also be administered to accelerate the breakdown of formic acid.

Hydrofluoric acid

Treatment for HF consists of water lavage followed by attempts to bind free fluoride ions at the site of injury. Both topical application and subcutaneous injection of calcium gluconate have been shown to be effective in binding free fluoride ions and reducing pain, with the subcutaneous injection being more efficacious in minimizing tissue injury.[98] Patients with significant exposure need to be placed on cardiac monitors, have intravenous access, and have serial evaluation of serum calcium, magnesium, and electrolytes. Q-T prolongation on the EKG may indicate hypocalcemia. Induction of metabolic alkalosis will enhance renal excretion of fluoride ions. They can also be removed via hemodialysis.[99]

Postoperative care

Scar management should be instituted after the wound has healed. Occupational and physical therapy should include modalities for splinting, stretching, desensitization, and compression.

Outcomes/prognosis/complications

Because many chemical burns are deep, the outcome is often less than ideal. The inflammatory response set-off by the injury induces significant scarring that leads to poor wound healing and impaired mobility. A rare and unusual sequelae of chemical burn is contact dermatitis. Contact dermatitis commonly occurs following prolonged exposure to a chemical, as often seen in occupational-related exposure.[100] However, even a single exposure to high concentration of a chemical may be enough to induce an antigenic sensitization and trigger an allergic reaction upon subsequent exposure.[101]

Secondary procedures

The need for secondary procedures is uncommon in chemical injuries, since most cases involve a small area but with often full thickness loss. If the area of injury is in the proximity of a joint and severe scarring has led to joint contracture, contracture release along with Z-plasty or other soft tissue replacement procedure may be indicated. If a large area is involved and not amendable for primary closure, local, regional, or even free flap surgery may be required to provide stable wound coverage.

Extravasation injury

A special type of chemical injury is worth mentioning. It involves extravasation injury due to malpositioning of intravenous access devices, leading to subcutaneous infiltration of chemotherapy agents or medications that have the potential to cause tissue necrosis. In essence, it is a 'subcutaneous chemical burn.'

Patients with small or fragile veins, such as the pediatric and the elderly population, are more prone to extravasation injury. Up to 11% of children receiving intravenous infusion suffer from extravasation injury.[102] Also, patients receiving chemotherapy are at higher risk of developing complications if extravasation occurs, due to the cytotoxic nature of the agents.

Basic science/disease process

Extravasation of a solution into the surrounding tissue spaces may lead to severe local tissue injury depending on the amount and concentration of the extravasated solution. Extravasation of isotonic intravenous solution used for fluid resuscitation usually only leads to local edema and minor inflammation and will resolve uneventfully with elevation. However, three groups of chemicals may lead to major tissue damage, namely (a) osmotically active agents (including concentrated cation solutions such as potassium and calcium, hyperalimentation solution for parenteral nutrition, and radiographic contrast media); (b) vasoconstrictive agents that induce tissue ischemia (such as vasopressors, epinephrine, norepinephrine, dopamine, and dobutamine); and (c) cytotoxic agents (such as chemotherapy agents, and drugs whose chemical nature renders them toxic to cells or medications carried in tissue irritant vehicles).

Osmotically active agents

Extravasated osmotically active agents cause osmotic imbalance across the cell membrane, leading to disruption of cellular transport mechanisms and subsequent cellular death. Concentrated cations such as calcium and potassium may cause ischemic necrosis by prolonging depolarization and contraction of the pre- and post-capillary smooth muscle sphincters.[103] They are also capable of precipitating proteins to cause direct cell death.[104]

Vasoconstrictive agents

Extravasated vasoconstrictive agents may lead to overlying skin and soft tissue necrosis by causing tissue ischemia if the vasoconstriction is persistent and not reversed.

Cytotoxic agents

Extravasated cytotoxic agents cause direct injury to the cells and tend to result in more severe and extensive tissue damage. Of the cytotoxic agents, doxorubicin is the agent most commonly reported to cause tissue necrosis upon extravasation, and has been widely studied.[105,106] Doxorubicin-induced ulcers are typified by a necrotic, yellowish base with surrounding erythema. The ulcers slowly enlarge over time, and show a diminished rate of wound contraction with a lack of granulation tissue formation and a paucity of peripheral epithelial ingrowth that are characteristic of normal wound healing.[107] Studies conducted in the rat model showed normal myofibroblast ultrastructure, suggesting that the observed lack of wound contraction might be owing to cellular dysfunction related to doxorubicin-DNA interaction.[108] Furthermore, histological studies of doxorubicin-induced ulcers in the rabbit model showed a necrotizing lesion with a lack of inflammatory response.[109] Doxorubicin also forms stable complexes with DNA, which can be liberated upon cell death. These complexes are then taken up by surrounding viable cells via endocytosis, thereby recycling the doxorubicin and leading to subsequent cell death in the area adjacent to the original extravasation.[110] This may explain why doxorubicin-induced ulcers tend to enlarge over time.

Diagnosis/patient presentation

Common sites of injury are the dorsum of the hand and the antecubital fossa, where veins are superficial and easy to cannulate. Symptoms and signs in the area of extravasation usually occur immediately and most notably include pain, swelling, and erythema. These presentations may be confused with the so-called flare reaction, which occurs in ~3% of patients receiving chemotherapy agents.[111,112] Flare reaction is characterized by pruritus and erythematous streak along the course of the peripheral vein receiving the infusion, but is transient and usually resolve within 30–90 min. Unlike extravasation, flares are usually not associated with pain or swelling.

Pain, swelling, or local hyperemia are not reliable predictors of the degrees of tissue damage.[113] Agents that cause pain even during intravascular injection may not necessarily cause tissue injury upon extravasation. For example, Propofol may cause substantial pain upon intravascular administration, but even large volume of Propofol rarely causes tissue necrosis upon extravasation.[114,115] Depending on the extent of extravasation and associated tissue damage, the local swelling and erythema may subside within 24 h. Persistent tissue induration for more than 24 h has been found to be the most reliable predictor of eventual skin ulceration.[116] Blisters may occur within the first few days of extravasation, indicating at least a partial thickness injury to the dermis. Ulceration usually occurs 1 or 2 weeks after extravasation and presents as a dry, black eschar (*Fig. 20.5*).

Chemotherapy agents may produce an insidious injury by spreading to the surrounding tissue and produce indolent ulcers that resemble radiation necrosis. Doxorubicin-induced ulcers have a characteristic appearance, as first described by Rudolph: "The ulcer had a characteristic indolent appearance, looking grossly, in many ways, like radiation ulcers. The base of the ulcers was filled with shaggy necrotic yellowish debris and the local tissue appeared unable to produce granulation tissue. The surrounding skin had raised rolled borders, with no evidence of epithelial spread into the ulcer."[107]

Patient selection

Although there has been a general agreement that most significant extravasations require early surgical intervention due to high risk of ulceration, controversy still exists regarding the optimal management of extravasation involving small to intermediate amounts. Some authors advocate conservative observation while others recommend early intervention such as saline flushout or liposuction. Proponents for conservative observation reason that in the majority of cases, ulceration does not occur and therefore intervention is unnecessary unless ulceration occurs.[117,118] Proponents for early intervention argue that dilution or removal of the extravasated agents minimize the risk of ulcer formation in all cases without significant complications.[119] In addition, extravasation can cause significant scarring around tendons, nerves, and joints, leading to functional deficits despite preservation of skin integrity or spontaneous healing of ulcers.[111,119] Therefore, it may be prudent to dilute or remove the extravasated agents whenever possible to optimize outcome, especially if the extravasated agents are potent tissue irritants. With the recent FDA approval, intravenous dexrazoxane has now been widely recommended as the standard initial treatment for all anthracycline extravasation.[120,121] However, the controversial remains regarding the management of nonanthracycline extravasation involving small to intermediate amounts.

The timing of referral can also dictate the treatment plan. If referral is made within 24 h of extravasation, various low-risk, minimally invasive interventions such as saline flushout may be attempted to minimize the risk of skin ulceration. However, if referral is made 24 h after the extravasation, the window of opportunity for early intervention would have been missed, as tissue necrosis may begin to occur after 24 h.[122] Observation may then be the best option in those cases.

Treatment/surgical technique

Once extravasation is noted, the infusion should be stopped and the involved intravenous catheter removed. Initial management consists of elevation of the involved extremity to minimize edema. Yet the decision to proceed with conservative observation or early intervention depends on the timing of the referral as well as the nature of the extravasated agent, as discussed previously. Various antidotes have also been suggested in the literature to reduce local inflammation or neutralize or dilute various extravasated agents. Antidotes such as hydrocortisone, sodium bicarbonate, isoproterenol, propranolol, have all failed to demonstrate any clinical benefit in the treatment of extravasation injury.[123]

Liposuction and saline flushout techniques have been reported to be useful in minimizing the development of skin necrosis if performed within 24 h of extravasation involving somatically active, vasoconstrictive, and cytotoxic agents, before overlying soft tissue injury becomes irreversible.[119,124] When the infiltrated area has adequate subcutaneous fat present, liposuction is recommended to remove the infiltrated chemical. When there is little subcutaneous fat present, as in pre-term infants, the saline flushout technique is recommended. The saline flushout involves infiltrating the involved area with 1 vial of hyaluronidase (1 vial=1500 units) to breakdown the connective tissues, followed by making multiple exit stab wounds in the periphery and flushing the area with a total of 500 cc of normal saline in 20–50 cc aliquots under sterile condition.

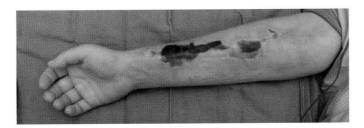

Fig. 20.5 A vancomycin extravasation injury of the volar forearm. A surgical consult was requested 1 week after injury.

If blistering occurs, it should be treated as a partial thickness burn with gentle cleaning and application of topical antimicrobial cream (e.g., Silvadene) to prevent local wound infection. Small ulcers will heal by wound contraction and re-epithelialization. Large ulcers will require excision and grafting. If after debridement and excision, tendons are exposed without intact peritenon to support skin graft, Integra may be used to provide temporary coverage until it has become vascularized, at which time, split thickness skin graft can then be applied over the vascularized Integra. Local rotational flaps may also be required to provide coverage for exposed joints, tendons, nerves, or vessels.

The following is a summary of different treatment options published in the literature according to the type of extravasation agent.

Osmotically active agents

The use of hyaluronidase has been shown to be useful in decreasing damage from extravasation of Ca^{2+} and hyperalimentation solution in the rabbit model.[125] Hyaluronidase is an enzyme that breaks down hyaluronic acid, a mucopolysaccharide that is a normal component of the interstitial fluid barrier. It has been shown to increase the rate of absorption of an injected substance by facilitating diffusion of the substance over a large area. When injected locally within 1 h of extravasation, it breaks down hyaluronic acid and decreases the viscosity of the extracellular matrix, and facilitates absorption and dispersal of the extravasated chemical.

For radiographic contrast media, small volume extravasation (<5 cc) is usually well tolerated and may be managed conservatively with limb elevation. However, with the increasing use of the automated power injector for contrast media, large volume extravasation is becoming more frequent. For large volume extravasation (>20 cc), early incision and drainage or liposuction can be efficacious in removing the infiltrated chemical, since most radiographic contrast media have a low degree of tissue binding. Based on experience from clinical case series, incision and irrigation or liposuction of large volume extravasation within 6 h is effective in preventing extensive skin necrosis.[126,127] The amount of radiographic contrast removed can be assessed by comparing preoperative and intraoperative X-rays. In addition, for large volume extravasation, if compartment syndrome is suspected, fasciotomy should be urgently performed to prevent muscle necrosis.

Vasoconstrictive agents

If discovered early, the acute ischemic effects of extravasated vasoconstrictive agents such as norepinephrine and dopamine may be reversed with local infiltration of phentolamine, which is an alpha blocking agent.[128,129]

Cytotoxic agents

Application of cold pack has been suggested to counteract the toxic effects of anthracycline drugs such as doxorubicin, while topical heat application in such cases cause increased tissue damage.[130] However, topical heat application has been recommended in vinca alkaloid extravasation such as vincristine, to promote local circulation and speed up clearance of the extravasated agent. Topical cooling in such cases has been demonstrated to increase ulcer formation in animal models.[131] Therefore, unless the identity of the extravasated chemical is known for certain, either topical cooling or heat cannot be safely recommended.

Dimethyl sulfoxide (DMSO) is a free-radical scavenger and an effective solvent. It may also have antibacterial, anti-inflammatory and vasodilatory properties. Its topical application is effective in preventing ulcerations caused by doxorubicin extravasation.[132,133] The use of hyaluronidase has also been shown to be useful in decreasing damage from extravasation of doxorubicin and vinca alkaloids when injected locally within 1 h of extravasation.[125,131]

The saline flushout technique aims to physically remove the extravasated chemical while preserving the overlying skin, and may be performed in conjunction with the use of hyaluronidase. However, with chemotherapy agents such as doxorubicin that is lipophilic and has high degree of tissue binding, the saline flushout technique may have limited benefit. Liposuction in these situations may be more efficacious.

Dexrazoxane is a specific catalytic inhibitor of DNA topoisomerase II that has been shown to antagonize the effects of several topoisomerase II poisons such as anthracycline agents, including doxorubicin.[138] It was approved by the FDA in 1995 as a treatment to reduce doxorubicin-associated cardiomyopathy. Recent clinical trials in Europe have demonstrated its efficacy in minimizing tissue damage from anthracycline extravasation if administered intravenously within 6 h of extravasation.[139] It was approved by the FDA in 2007 and now is the recommended initial treatment of anthracycline extravasation.[120,121]

In managing doxorubicin extravasation, surgical excision of all involved tissue with delay closure or skin grafting is indicated when patient has persistent pain in the extravasated area or when ulceration occurs.[111,117,118] Excision must be extensive to include all tissues containing doxorubicin. The excision may be guided by fluorescence microscopy, since doxorubicin-laden tissue glows reddish orange under ultraviolet light.[111,134–137]

Postoperative care

The involved extremity should be elevated postoperatively to minimize edema. Immobilization for at least 5–7 days is important if skin graft is applied to minimize shear force that may decrease the skin graft survival. If primary closure or flap has been performed to achieve wound closure, special precaution against wound dehiscence should be taken in patients who had recently received or currently receiving doxorubicin, as doxorubicin treated rats have demonstrated decreased wound tensile strength.[140]

Outcomes/prognosis/complications

If recognized early and the extravasation remains localized, most cases will heal spontaneously. Yet the consequences of significant extravasation are often underestimated.

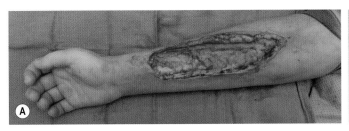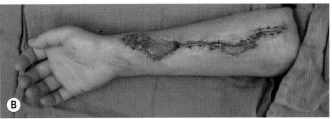

Fig. 20.6 (A) Debridement of all necrotic tissue included skin and subcutaneous fat. The necrotic subcutaneous fat extended beyond the area of obvious skin necrosis. **(B)** Primary closure was performed where possible and split-thickness skin grafts were used in areas of high tension.

Extensive extravasation may result in large wounds that require debridement and coverage with a split thickness skin graft or local flap *(Fig. 20.6)*. Severe damage to the underlying nerves and tendons can also occur. When next to a major artery in the forearm or leg, extravasation may lead to amputation.

One potential complication after doxorubicin extravasation is the 'recall phenomenon,' that is, an enhancement of the degree of existing skin necrosis from extravasation or recurrence of skin ulceration at the previous extravasation site upon additional doxorubicin administered.[141–143]

Secondary procedures

When underlying structures such as muscles and tendons have been damaged by the extravasation injury, secondary procedures may be required to improve function. When the flexor or extensor tendons or muscles have been damaged, tendon transfer using remaining functional tendons may be required to improve hand function. In severe cases when the majority of flexor or extensor muscles have also been destroyed from the extravasation, free-functional muscle transfer may be required to restore function of the wrist and hand.

Access the complete reference list online at **http://www.expertconsult.com**

1. Su CW, Lohman R, Gottlieb LJ. Frostbite of the upper extremity. *Hand Clin.* 2000;16(2):235–247.

   This article provides a comprehensive review regarding the disease process of frostbite and the rationale behind the therapeutic approaches to the management of frostbite injury.

2. Mohr WJ, Jenabzadeh K, Ahrenholz DH. Cold injury. *Hand Clin.* 2009;25(4):481–496.

   This article offers the latest review of the pathophysiology, diagnosis, and treatment of frostbite injury.

36. Cauchy E, Marsigny B, Allamel G, et al. The value of technetium 99 scintigraphy in the prognosis of amputation in severe frostbite injuries of the extremities: A retrospective study of 92 severe frostbite injuries. *J Hand Surg Am.* 2000;25(5):969–978.

    This article retrospectively evaluated the predictive power of 2-phase technetium 99 scintigraphy in determining the eventual level of amputation secondary to frostbite injury to the hand. The predictive power was found to be high when the scan was performed as early as 3 days after the frostbite.

40. Entin MA, Baxter H. Influence of rapid warming on frostbite in experimental animals. *Plast Reconstr Surg (1946).* 1952;9(6):511–524.

    This classic article used the rat model to determine the optimal rewarming temperature in the treatment of

    frostbite. It laid the foundation for the present day rapid rewarming protocol.

69. Mozingo DW, Smith AA, McManus WF, et al. Chemical burns. *J Trauma.* 1988;28(5):642–647.

84. Gruber RP, Laub DR, Vistnes LM. The effect of hydrotherapy on the clinical course and pH of experimental cutaneous chemical burns. *Plast Reconstr Surg.* 1975;55(2):200–204.

116. Heckler FR. Current thoughts on extravasation injuries. *Clin Plast Surg.* 1989;16(3):557–563.

118. Larson DL. What is the appropriate management of tissue extravasation by antitumor agents? *Plast Reconstr Surg.* 1985;75(3):397–405.

121. Kane RC, McGuinn Jr WD, Dagher R, et al. Dexrazoxane (Totect): FDA review and approval for the treatment of accidental extravasation following intravenous anthracycline chemotherapy. *Oncologist.* 2008;13(4):445–450.

    This article describes the relatively recent discovery and FDA approval of the first antidote for treating extravasation injury involving commonly used chemotherapeutic agents such as doxorubicin.

123. Loth TS, Eversmann Jr WW. Treatment methods for extravasations of chemotherapeutic agents: a comparative study. *J Hand Surg Am.* 1986;11(3): 388–396.

21

Management of facial burns

Robert J. Spence

SYNOPSIS

- Early, accurate diagnosis with early aggressive therapy of the acute burn wound is one of the keys to optimal final result, and is the beginning of restoration after facial burn injury.
- Nonoperative therapy to allow optimal natural healing and scar maturation is important to minimize the extent of reconstructive surgery and optimize the final result.
- Reconstructive surgery should be delayed until substantial burn scar maturation has occurred.
- Reconstructive surgery for the late effects of burn injury is set apart from other reconstructive surgery by the exceedingly common lack of local normal skin for donor sites.
- Specific techniques most commonly used in facial burn reconstruction practice are described in detail with emphasis on important
- An algorithm can be used to analyze facial burn scar deformities and help make decisions regarding reconstruction.
- Operatively, flaps from local donor sites should be used whenever possible.
- Technical aspects of burn reconstruction unique to specific anatomic areas are described.
- Once the reconstructive surgery operation is complete, non-operative therapy of the new surgical scars should commence.
- Secondary operations are common, and frequently follow placement of a large amount of tissue for contracture release or resurfacing to provide the optimal result.

 Access the Historical Perspective section online at
http://www.expertconsult.com

Introduction

Our face is our window to the world, and its reflection our self-image. The goal remains very straightforward and simple on paper: restore normal facial appearance, aesthetically acceptable anatomical symmetry, and the ability to express emotion through facial animation. However, the attainment of this goal presents a very significant challenge to those caring for the patient. Assessing and treating facial burns continues to be complex and controversial. Management of the acute burns is as relevant as the operations to correct deformity and dysfunction suffered from the initial injury.

Annually, there are more than 500 000 burns treated in the US. A total of 40 000 patients are hospitalized and 25 000 are hospitalized in specialized burn centers. There are 4000 fire and burn deaths per year in the US. The most common causes of burn injury are fire/flame (46%) and scald (32%), with scald burns being a particular problem in children.[1]

An estimated over 50% of burn injuries involve the head and neck region. This most likely is related to the exposed facial skin and, when one's clothes are burning, the hot gases travel upward. In the presence of fire, one instinctively protects one's face. As a result, when one sustains a severe facial burn, it frequently is associated with extensive total body burns. During the acute burn period, this means that the patient is frequently critically ill with extensive burns elsewhere on the body. During the rehabilitation and reconstruction phase, extensive burns reduce normal skin for reconstruction donor sites.

Everyone's face is exceedingly distinctive, consisting physically of shapes, contours and skin characteristics that provide an identity for each person. This is threatened and frequently destroyed by a severe burn injury. As the face provides one's identity and is the medium through which everyone interacts socially, it becomes exceedingly important to the individual. Even relatively minor deformity can have a major psychological and social impact.

Basic science

Burn injury primarily consists of damage to the skin and its immediately underlying tissues as a result of physical trauma. The most common physical trauma is thermal in nature. Essentially, the heat energy kills living cells in the tissues and denatures the proteins that make up the tissue that dies. This energy could be from fire and explosions, hot water and steam in the case of scalds, or contact with hot objects. The physical damage can be inflicted through a chemical reaction of some substances such as acids and alkalis with the skin. Electrical energy, converted to heat by the resistance imposed by the skin, and by transmission through the skin can damage the skin and the underlying tissues through which the high voltage electricity passes.

The damage to the skin is a function of the amount of heat energy transferred to the skin. An agent of very high temperature (i.e., energy) can cause the same amount of damage as a much lower temperature agent applied for a longer period of time.

The degree of tissue damage is classified by the depth of the damage to the skin and the underlying tissues *(Fig. 21.1)*. Damage to the epidermal layer alone is described as an epidermal burn scientifically, and a first-degree burn in common usage. An example of a first-degree burn is typical sunburn. An epidermal burn heals by sloughing the dead epidermal cells with immediate regrowth of new cells.

With greater energy transfer, not only are the epidermal cells lost, but the underlying dermis is damaged to varying depths. This damage consists of the denaturing of the dermal collagen, and thrombosis and destruction of the blood vessels within the dermis. The denatured collagen stays in place, and changes colors from pink to white to black depending on the number of remaining viable capillaries remaining close to the surface of the dermis. A superficial dermal injury consists of the epidermis coming off as a blister leaving a pink collagen surface due to the persistence of patent blood vessels close to the surface. A mid-dermal injury causes the remaining dermis to become increasingly pale, and a deep dermal injury causes the remaining dermis to be white in color.

Corresponding damage to the nerves within the dermis results in progressively less and less sensibility of the surface of the wound. Very superficial dermal burn wounds are very painful to contact because of the nerves at the exposed dermal wound surface. The dermal wound becomes more anesthetic as the depth of injury is greater. Although the dermal surface becomes anesthetic, the burns are still painful because the nerves are still injured at some level within the dermis.

A dermal injury heals by one of two mechanisms. Superficial injuries leave enough epidermal accessory structures such as hair follicles and sweat glands to provide epidermal cells for re-epithelialization of the dermal surface. Superficial injuries will usually re-epithelialize within 2–3 weeks if enough of the epidermal accessory structures are present. Superficial dermal injuries therefore may heal with some change in pigmentation of the new epithelium, but without burn scarring.

With deeper injuries, there are fewer epidermal accessory structures, and the wound heals by development of scar tissue and contraction mediated by fibroblasts and myofibroblasts, respectively. These cells migrate into the burn wound during the 1st week after injury, and proliferate in the granulation tissue that forms if re-epithelialization does not take place. It is, therefore, the deep dermal and deeper burn injuries that heal with burn scarring and burn scar contracture.

When the amount of energy transferred is so great that the full-thickness of the skin is destroyed, the appearance of the dermis can vary from white to cherry-red from capillary thrombosis to black from charring. Left alone, the dead dermis would separate from the underlying wound and it would go on to heal by scar formation and wound contraction.

Scientifically, 'second-degree' burns are all dermal injuries, both superficial and deep, and full-thickness burns are technically 'third-degree' burns. However, in common usage, 'second-degree' refers to the superficial burns that will heal by re-epithelialization within 2–3 weeks, and 'third-degree' refers to those deeper burns that will not. For the burn surgeon, the important diagnosis is whether the burn will heal by re-epithelialization and not require excision and grafting to prevent burn scarring and contracture. Therefore, the most useful terminology in diagnose of a burn is either "superficial" or "deep", which corresponds

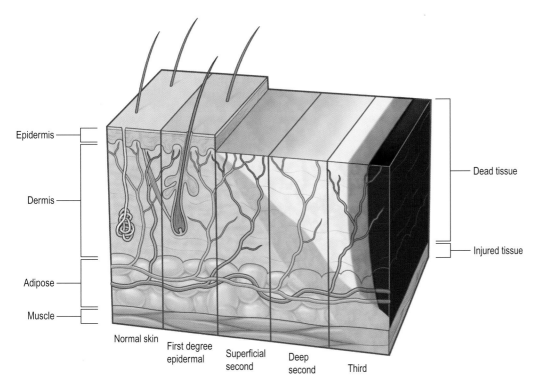

Epidermis

Dermis

Adipose

Muscle

Dead tissue

Injured tissue

Normal skin   First degree epidermal   Superficial second   Deep second   Third

Fig. 21.1 The degree of tissue damage is classified by the depth of the damage to the skin and the underlying tissues. Burns are classified by depth of burn and extent of burn in percent total body surface area (%TBSA). There is a gradation of tissue damage from necrosis to tissue injury to normal tissue seen on the surface of the skin and histologically. This diagram is an attempt to represent what is seen clinically based on the depth of burn.

most closely to the common usage of second-degree and third-degree.

Without intervention, deep facial burns heal by scarring and contraction. If the wound does not epithelialize in 2–3 weeks, fibroblasts and myofibroblasts migrate into the wound and lay down collagen and cause the wound to contract. The excess collagen becomes hypertrophic burn scar: the erythematous, thick, exuberant scar characteristic of any open wound that heals secondarily.

All scars, even primarily closed wound scars, contract. Contracted scars that limit mobility of joints or deform mobile structures, particularly of the face, are called *contractures*. Contractures of the neck are *extrinsic* to the face, but the face is affected by pulling forces from the neck transmitted to the mobile facial structures just as and frequently in conjunction with the *intrinsic* contractures represented by the scars adjacent to and deforming the mobile facial structures.

Diagnosis: determination of depth of burn

The most critical determination that the acute burn surgeon makes is whether the burn is superficial or deep because it determines whether the burn injury requires surgical intervention. A superficial burn will heal with minimal scarring, and a deep burn will heal with scarring and burn scar contracture causing significant facial distortion.

Therefore the diagnosis of burn depth is critical to determine what to do to get the best outcome for the patient's facial burn injury. Generally, this diagnosis can be made by examination of the wound for color, sensitivity to touch, and other such characteristics. The most difficult diagnosis is that of a mid-dermal injury. This injury may or may not have enough epidermal accessory structures to allow the wound to re-epithelialize within 2–3 weeks. These mid-dermal burns are often termed 'indeterminate.' The decision to excise and graft these is frequently deferred hoping that the wound will heal within 3 weeks without scarring, knowing that excision and grafting will cause a definite change in facial appearance.

Cole et al. have proposed that the decision to operate on indeterminate facial dermal burns be made at approximately 10 days, and based on the best clinical judgment, excise if indicated and graft with thick split-thickness skin graft.[8]

Recently the scanning laser Doppler has been shown to help with the diagnosis in indeterminate dermal burns.[9–11] This device determines the relative amount of blood flow in the superficial burn wound by reading the change in frequency of laser light caused by the movement of blood cells within the wound as it scans the surface of the wound. The color and numerical flux readings correspond to the likelihood of the burn wound healing within the 2–3 weeks window consistent with healing by re-epithelialization and minimal or no scarring.

Treatment of acute facial burns

Treatment of the acute facial burn injury is based on the diagnosis of the level of burn injury to both the face and the rest of the patient's body. Severe facial burn injuries frequently occur in the setting of a critically large burn injury to the rest of the patient, and critical care and saving the patient's life is often the first priority.

Because of the high degree of vascularization of the facial skin, infection of facial burn wounds is less likely than burns in other anatomic areas. This allows for some delay in making critical decisions regarding excision and grafting of facial burns. For management of the nonfacial burn, the idea of early tangential excision of deep dermal and full-thickness burns was championed by Janzekovic in the 1970s and continues to be the standard of care. Controversy still exists among surgeons regarding the early excision and grafting of facial burns. It is currently recommended to first treat a deep burn nonoperatively for 7–10 days with topical ointments, creams and local debridement.[8,12] Some deep burns are obvious and may be excised and grafted earlier, but the vast majority are initially indeterminate.

A superficial burn injury will heal by re-epithelialization within two to three weeks if the wound heals without complication. Therefore the primary task of caring for a superficial facial burn injury is to prevent infection or any other problems that might interfere with normal re-epithelialization. Generally, superficial wounds epithelialize better in a moist environment. After initial cleansing, a mild antibiotic ointment is applied. The wound is gently cleansed twice-daily and the ointment reapplied. Every effort is made to avoid disrupting the migration of epithelial cells from the epidermal accessory structures across the surface of the wound. Although stronger antibiotic preparations are available, the author usually reserves these for evidence of active infection. I believe that treating the face open is safer than covering the face with an opaque dressing that prevents observation of the wound or allows for covert infection. Also any dressing that adheres to the wound through a dry interface reduces the pace of re-epithelialization as the fibrin bond between the dressing and the wound has to be broken down before the epithelial cells can migrate.

Deep facial burn injuries that will clearly not heal by epithelialization are doomed to heal with hypertrophic scarring and contractures if there is no surgical intervention. The standard surgical intervention is early excision and grafting in facial aesthetic units. This should be done as early as possible to minimize the migration of fibroblasts into the facial burn wound. Engrav recommends that a decision be made to excise and graft by 7–10 days post-injury, and have the face entirely grafted by 21 days. Initial excision of the wound is followed by sheet split-thickness skin allograft for 1 week. After that, the patient is returned to the operating room for closure with thick split-thickness autografts in the range of 0.018–0.021 inches in adults, and 0.008–0.012 inches in children placed in facial aesthetic units *(Fig. 21.2)*.[12]

Another consideration is to use the acellular dermal matrix applied immediately after facial burn wound excision in aesthetic units, preferably after preparation with sheet allograft for up to 1 week, as above. When successful, the engrafted acellular dermal matrix is covered with split-thickness autograft which can yield facial skin that is superior to thick split-thickness autograft.

Eyes/eyelid

Generally, it is rare for a thermal injury to involve the globe. In the current literature, the reported incidence of ocular, intraocular, intraorbital foreign bodies (especially in

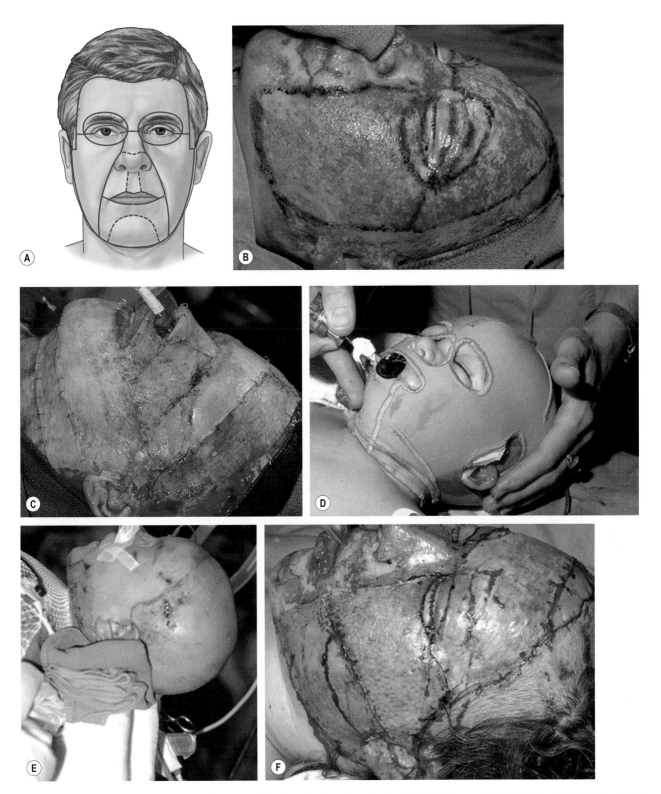

Fig. 21.2 (A) Aesthetic units. **(B)** Aesthetic unit markings. **(C)** Allograft at time of application. **(D)** Bubble facemask. **(E)** Mayfield headrest. **(F)** Allograft at 1 week.

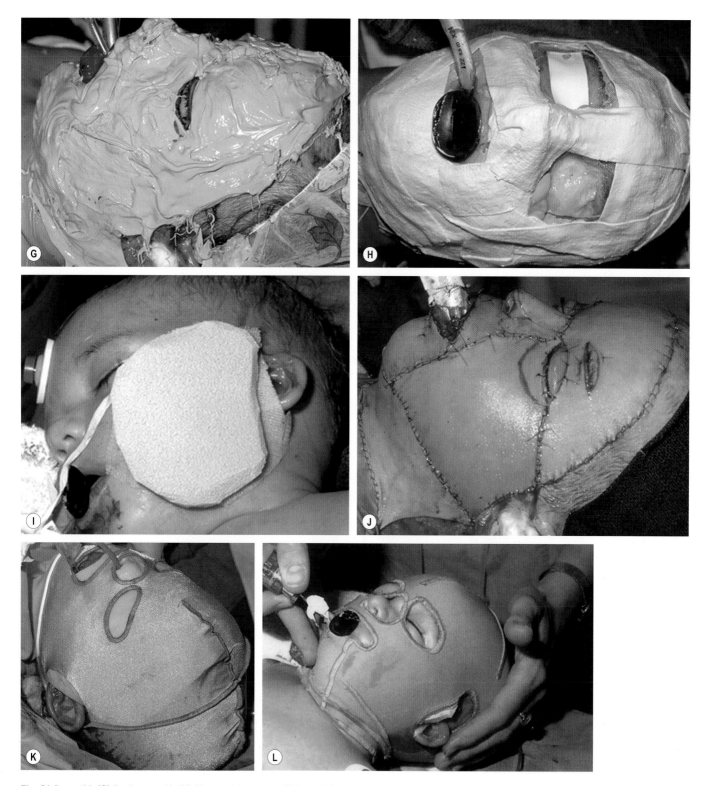

Fig. 21.2, cont'd (G) Duplicast mold. **(H)** Plaster reinforcement. **(I)** Foam. **(J)** Autograft placement. **(K)** Bubble and elastomer. **(L)** Bubble and foam. (From Cherry GW, Austad E, Pasyk K, et al. Increased survival and vascularity of random-pattern skin flaps elevated in controlled, expanded skin. Plast Reconstr Surg. 1983;72(5):680-687.)

explosions) and periorbital injury due to a burn ranges from 8% to 20% of all burn admissions.[13] This is most likely due to a significant number of protective mechanisms that include a patient's reflex protective movements of the head and arms, and more importantly, the blink reflex. It should be noted that one of the most commonly overlooked or missed foreign body is the contact lens.

All facial burns should have an ophthalmological exam on admission, preferably by an ophthalmologist.

Most commonly the problem is globe protection in burns that damage the eyelids. Various ointments, corneal shields, or protective contact lenses help shield the cornea from further injury. A temporary suture tarsorrhaphy may be useful and effective in aiding lid closure, but dehiscence and complications are common, making tarsorrhaphy use controversial.[14] Tarsorrhaphy does not prevent wound contraction, and the basic principles of early excision and grafting, and ectropion release and tissue transplantation are primary.

In the very young patient population, eyelid closure for as little as 3 days places an infant at a high risk for blindness in the affected eye. Prolonged occlusion of the eye due to scar contracture leads to decreased retinal stimulation and subsequently poor neuronal development of the corresponding optic cortex.

Ears

The vast majority of ear burns will heal without the need for excision and grafting. Aggressive debridement risks losing more tissue than natural slough of necrotic tissue and subsequent healing.

Prevention of chondritis in deeper ear burns is the main concern. Topical treatment with Sulfamylon (mafenide acetate) cream appears to be the most effective agent. The cream is applied thickly three or four times daily. Excision of the outer eschar covering the ear should not be done if there is no purulent drainage. One should minimize the use for compressive dressings and further trauma to the external ear as this may cause an increased risk of necrosis.

Nose

Treatment should be as conservative as possible. Again, aggressive debridement risks losing more tissue than natural slough of necrotic tissue and subsequent healing. Topical ointments and the avoidance of pressure, including that from feeding tubes, are of primary importance.

Mouth

Once common prior to building codes mandating local electrical outlet circuit breakers, perioral burns from children biting into electrical cords are now rarely seen. However, approximately 25% of these patients have the eschar separate and bleed from the labial artery frequently between 1–2 weeks.

Perioral and oral commissure burns may develop into microstomia which can interfere with speech, eating, oral hygiene, and cause drooling. Impairment of normal growth of the child's mandible leading to bony deformities may occur. The use of an oral splint (oral orthosis) during the period of contraction may minimize microstomia. Reconstructive surgery generally is initiated after scar maturation (6–12 months in adults and longer in children).

Wound nonoperative management of facial burn scars

Once facial burn wounds are healed, there are a number of ways that facial scars can be minimized and maturation of the scars can be encouraged. The two primary mainstays of nonoperative facial burn scar therapy are compression and contact with silicone gel. The silicone gel is thought to be effective in reducing scarring and in encouraging scar maturation.[15,16] Compression tends to keep the hypertrophy of the scars in check.

Modern facial compression masks made with clear plastic with silicone interfaces provide patients with the benefit of both, and allow the patient's face to be visible. This is an improvement over opaque elastic compression masks. Not only because they allow the patient's face to be seen, but it allows individual pressure regulation on each of the hypertrophic scars by molding the plastic to the point of blanching of the scars.

Other important modes of nonoperative therapy during the 'waiting period' before surgery and in the postoperative period include splints to maintain scars to as optimal length as possible, massage to reduce swelling and help orient new collagen fibers in as normal orientation as possible, and occasionally steroid injections into smaller hypertrophic scars.

The use of pulsed dye laser therapy has been used to reduce the erythema and pruritus, and possibly improve scar remodelling in immature hypertrophic burn scars.[17,18] Carbon dioxide fractional ablative laser therapy seems to have a positive effect on remodeling of mature burn scars sometimes many years after forming.[19,20]

Surgical management of the late effects of face, head and neck burns

Introduction

There are a myriad of techniques described to reconstruct the multiple problems of dysfunction and deformity related to the individual anatomic components located within the face, head and neck. Most of these techniques are well-described elsewhere in these volumes. This section will focus on general principles and an approach to reconstruction of the most common late effects of burn injury primarily of the face, but also the ears, scalp, and neck.

One of the primary aspects of burn reconstruction surgery that sets it apart from other reconstructive surgery is the exceedingly common lack of local normal skin for donor sites. Techniques and solutions specifically for this problem will be addressed.

Specific techniques most commonly used in a burn reconstruction practice are described in more detail with emphasis on important technical considerations that will be of particular benefit to the patients of plastic surgeons less experienced in facial burn reconstruction.

General principles

Importance of allowing total wound healing and scar maturation

Burn reconstruction should virtually never be done in the presence of residual open burn wounds. Bacteria in open wounds risk infection in the reconstructive surgery. The presence of inflammation and active scarring will compromise the result. Incomplete contraction of original wounds will affect the reconstructive outcome within that wound unless the entire burn wound is excised. Typically, one waits about 1 year to begin facial burn reconstruction. The exception to this is reconstruction to protect vital structures or restore critical functions such as eyelid closure and oral competence.

Additionally, the time waiting for reconstruction frequently results in resolution of erythema and hypertrophy of some areas of scar, and, in some cases, improving function through therapy resulting in a reduction of the extent of the scar problem requiring surgical intervention *(Fig. 21.3)*.

Reconstruction must be preceded by analysis of the problem and diagnosis of the factors causing it

Usually the most important factor is skin deficiency resulting from destruction of skin by the burn. Excisions of burn scar and contracture releases recreate the original skin deficit. The magnitude of the tissue deficit is often underestimated. Being prepared with this knowledge helps the surgeon determine whether normal donor sites will be adequate and what technique to use.

Do not assume that the entire scar must be treated similarly. Another element in diagnosis is determining whether treating only a portion of the scar will provide the desired improvement while leaving another area of the scar untreated. This is particularly true in determining the tension in a scar. By releasing tension, hypertrophy which is frequently potentiated by the tension is minimized in the rest of the scar.[21]

An overall plan for reconstruction should be developed

Once the problems are analyzed, an overall plan for surgical reconstruction and rehabilitation should be developed. Not only is this exceedingly helpful to the surgeon for planning operations and what donor sites to use, but it provides the patient with an understanding of the process required, adjusting expectations, and providing hope that there is, in fact, a positive outcome in the future.

Restoration of function usually precedes aesthetic reconstruction

This is especially important for protective functions such as the protection of the eyes by the eyelids, and oral competence. Ideally, to a degree, both goals are achieved simultaneously.

Release of contracture usually is the first priority. Extrinsic contractures, contractures of the neck in the case of facial burn scars, need to be released before the true extent of facial intrinsic contractures can be determined *(Fig. 21.4)*. Neck contracture release also allows for safer anesthetic management by allowing neck extension.

Local flaps should be used whenever possible

Local flaps tend to provide ideal color match, skin thickness and texture due to their close proximity to the skin deficit or deformity that is being replaced. Furthermore, flaps do not contract, or change color or other characteristics as skin grafts do unpredictably.

Skin grafts are used because of their thinness when a thicker flap would hide underlying anatomic contours or interfere with function

Skin grafts are less stable in their characteristics. They change color and other characteristics unpredictably, but starting with the best well-matched local skin available gives the best chance of success.[22]

All skin grafts contract to a degree and can lead to tightness that restricts facial expression or leads to recurrent contractures. Therefore, when using skin grafts, overcorrection is a general rule.

Skin replacement should generally be performed in "aesthetic units" when subtotal or total unit defects are present

This avoids the aesthetically[23] unfavorable appearance of a 'patch.' Complete excision of the entire aesthetic unit including residual normal skin should, at least, be considered if more than half the aesthetic unit is scar *(Fig. 21.5)*.

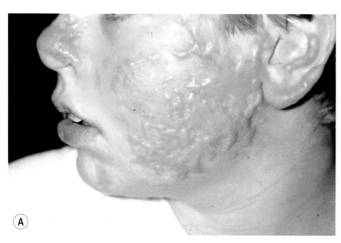
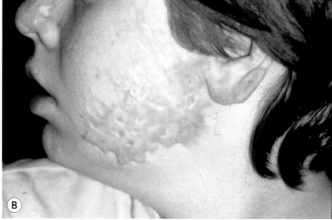

(A)   (B)

Fig. 21.3 The importance of allowing scar maturation. **(A)** Facial hypertrophic burn scar 4 months after injury. **(B)** Same scar 16 months after injury.

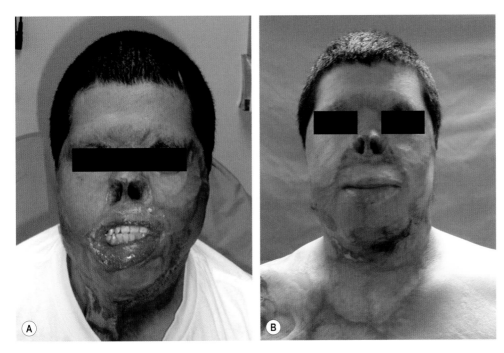

Fig. 21.4 Importance of releasing extrinsic contractures before addressing intrinsic contractures. **(A)** Posture of lower lip with severe neck burn scar contracture. **(B)** Posture of lower lip after release of severe neck contracture.

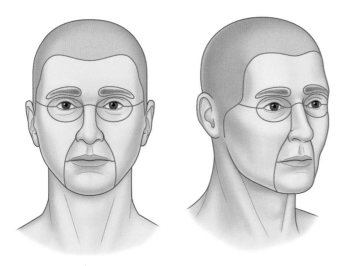

Fig. 21.5 Aesthetic units of the face.

Skin replacement should be performed with as well-matched skin as possible to the recipient site

The best donor sites matching facial skin come from the upper chest, shoulders, and scalp, commonly called the 'blush areas.'[22]

As many goals as possible should be accomplished during each operative procedure

This minimizes the number of anesthetic sessions, and the overall length of time and cost for reconstruction.

Box 21.1 Ancillary techniques in facial burn reconstruction

- Corrective cosmetics
- Laser therapy
- Steroid injection
- Prosthetics
  - Anatomic parts, e.g., ear, nose
  - Hair; hairpieces
- Hair transplantation
- Fat transplantation
- Tattooing.

Ancillary techniques should be employed to maximum advantage

The ancillary techniques are numerous and include cosmetics, tattooing, hair transplantation, prosthetics *(Fig. 21.6)*, laser therapy and others *(Box 21.1)*.

Follow-up must be diligent

The reconstructive procedure is not an endpoint. A caring doctor–patient relationship must be continued, and the surgeon must remain available, particularly in case of complications. Nonoperative modalities typically used for burn scar management such as silicone gel sheeting, compression therapy, and pulsed dye laser therapy, are frequently reinstituted to treat the new surgical scars.

An algorithmic approach to facial burn in reconstruction

Based on some of the above general principles, a framework *(Fig. 21.7)* evolved in the author's practice allows for analyzing burn-related facial deformity and dysfunction,

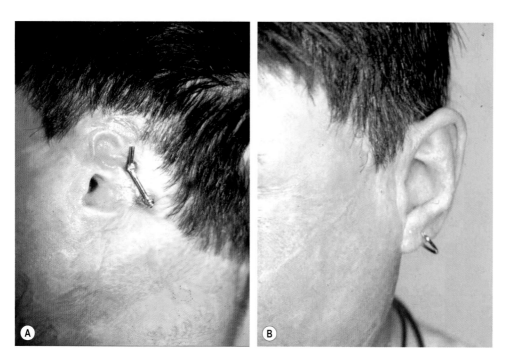

Fig. 21.6 Prosthetic total ear. **(A)** Residual ear with osseointegrated implant in place. **(B)** Prosthetic ear in place.

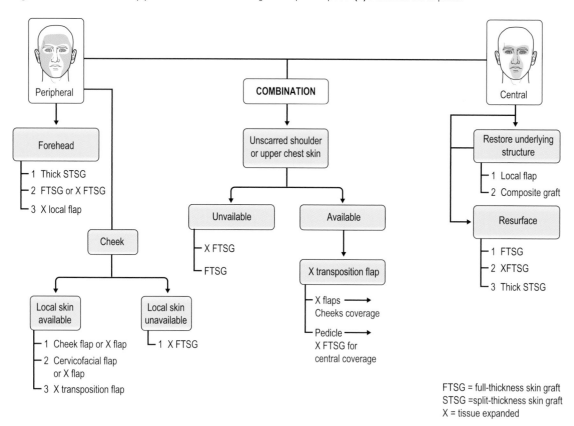

Fig. 21.7 Algorithm for the reconstruction of large facial deformities. (From Spence RJ. An agorithm for total and subtotal facial reconstruction us an expanded transposition flap: a 20-year experience. *Plast Reconstr Surg*. 2008;121(3):795–805.)

simplifying often complex problems, and guiding reconstructive surgical decisions.[24,25]

This algorithm first divides the facial aesthetic units into two broad categories: the peripheral aesthetic units of the forehead and bilateral cheeks, and the central aesthetic units of the eyelids, nose, upper lip, and the lower lip and chin aesthetic units. The peripheral facial aesthetic units are large units with minimal contour definition or structure and with relatively uniform skin characteristics. The central facial aesthetic units are smaller and have a higher degree of contour definition with intricate infrastructure and variations of skin characteristics.

Second, the algorithm analyzes the donor skin available for addition to or replacement of scarred or contracted facial skin. Specifically it asks the question whether there is donor site available locally in the 'blush' areas, the skin that is the most well-matched to replace facial skin. If this is not available, another path is taken in the decision tree.

This algorithm also incorporates all available techniques ranging from the simplest scar revision or excision and closure to complete replacement of the skin of the face. When scarred skin replacement is indicated, the algorithm recommends flap replacement of the peripheral aesthetic units as these areas are best reconstructed with broad, relatively featureless normal skin. However, when the replacement of the central facial aesthetic units is indicated, the infrastructure of the various contours needs to be reconstructed first, if necessary, and covered with a thin skin replacement usually in the form of full-thickness skin graft. As described in the literature, the expanded transposition flap[26] is central in the algorithm when major facial deformities are addressed, as it provides both relatively thin flaps for the peripheral aesthetic units and full-thickness skin grafts for the central aesthetic units (Fig. 21.8).

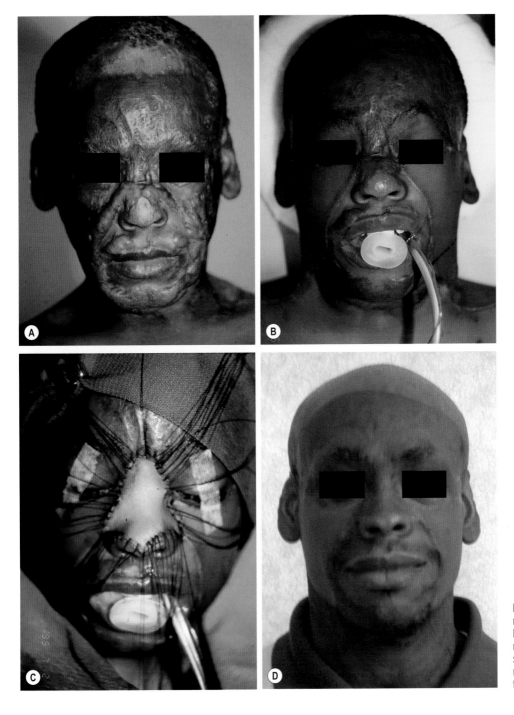

Fig. 21.8 An example of total facial reconstruction using the algorithmic approach. Bilateral expanded transposition flaps for cheek reconstruction (peripheral), and full-thickness skin graft from expanded flap pedicle for central reconstruction. Forehead was resurfaced with thick split-thickness skin graft.

Specific techniques

Scar replacement with local skin

The simplest example of scar replacement with local skin is simple scar excision with primary closure. This excises the burn scar and replaces it with a surgical scar that is designed to be better and, optimally, much less noticeable. Basic plastic surgery principles critical to obtaining the best results include: (1) performing the excision within relative adjacent tissue excess where possible; and (2) respecting resting skin tension lines (RSTL) in the planning of the new scar *(Fig. 21.9)*.[27] This repositions the new scar in a pre-existent anatomic line or contour such as the nasolabial crease, a hairline, or forehead wrinkles. It also imparts the least tension across the new scar minimizing the negative effects of tension on the scar.

Generally, there should be careful perpendicular incision through the skin to allow the most accurate re-approximation on closure of the new surgical wound. The optimal quality of the new scar is based on very careful anatomic re-approximation of the dermis and epidermis individually. The dermis is carefully re-approximated with absorbable sutures minimizing tension on surface sutures if they are used. It may make the accurate epidermal closure with surgical adhesive possible. Long-term it reduces the spreading of the new surgical scar.

The epidermis is carefully re-approximated with either surgical adhesive if the dermal sutures have brought the epidermal edges into anatomic alignment, or carefully placed sutures, with just enough tension to bring epidermal edges into anatomic alignment. If the epidermal edges overlap or are inverted, less favorable healing and suboptimal scars will form. The failure to close the epidermis results in a small open wound that will lead to increased scar formation and possible scar hypertrophy.

Serial excision

An extension of simple scar replacement by excision and primary closure is the technique of serial excision. When a scar is too large for excision and primary closure, only that portion of the scar that can be excised is, and the wound closed. The tension resulting from the first wound closure results in stretching of the surrounding skin (mechanical creep) and subsequent growth of the skin in response to the additional tension (biologic creep).[28] The increase in the amount of surrounding skin that takes place over at least 3 or 4 months allows reoperation to excise the residual scar and close the resulting wound with the expanded normal surrounding skin. With the advent of tissue expansion to develop new skin adjacent to scars, serial excision is used much less, but should be considered if the serial excision is likely to take only two or, at most, three operations.

W-plasty

A W-plasty is the closure of a wound with multiple sawtooth lines that better approximate the resting skin tension lines (RSTL) of the facial skin *(Fig. 21.10)*.[29] The resulting lines more in-line with the RSTL become less noticeable. They also break up the linear nature of the unfavorable scar. A similar effect can occur if multiple small Z-plasties are placed in the linear skin closure. Technically, this technique can be exceedingly tedious. For W-plasty closure to be safe and effective, it needs

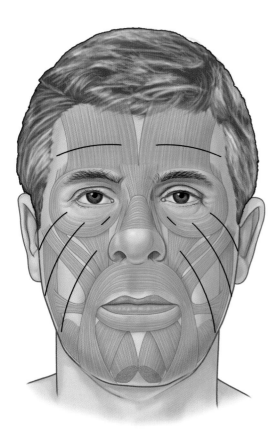

Fig. 21.9 Resting skin tension lines lie perpendicular to the action of the underlying facial muscles. Scars placed parallel to these lines are least noticeable.

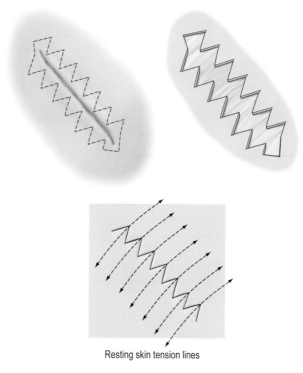

Resting skin tension lines

Fig. 21.10 W-plasty can be used to reorient scars with unfavorable position more into the resting skin tension lines.

to have limbs that are millimeters in length not to exceed 1 centimeter.

Skin grafts

Introduction

When the amount of normal skin adjacent to burn scars is inadequate to replace the scars with the adjacent skin, additional skin is required to move into the affected area to replace scar or to release contracture.

Grafts provide a technique to transplant skin without having to maintain a blood supply. As skin grafts have to be relatively thin to survive on the imbibition of nutrients and oxygen from a vascularized wound bed, they are advantageous when thin tissue is desired. Also the ability to easily transplant tissue from a distance is also advantageous. However, graft tissue tends to be less predictable in terms of maintaining the characteristics of the skin transplanted. All skin grafts contract, and change color and texture to some, unfortunately unpredictable, degree.

Generally, the more dermis within the graft, the more the skin characteristics remain stable. The use of thin split-thickness skin grafts for contracture release almost universally results in almost complete re-contracture. In the face, contraction of transplanted skin grafts is particularly troublesome as it causes a mask-like face unable to express emotion. Furthermore, recurrent contraction leads to recurrent deformity of the mobile structures of the face, and functional tightness around the mouth and eyelids.

Therefore full-thickness skin grafts, or, at least thick (0.015–0.028 inch) split-thickness skin grafts, are used much more commonly in burn reconstruction than thin split-thickness skin grafts. Furthermore, when full-thickness skin grafts are used, a general rule is to overcorrect by placing a larger graft than anatomically indicated.

Split-thickness skin grafts in facial burn reconstruction

The advantages of split-thickness skin grafts include that large grafts are possible, the donor site regenerates without losing significant additional full-thickness skin, and the take of the skin graft is relatively easy. Although split-thickness skin grafts have unpredictable pigmentation, in cases of starkly light burn scar (hypopigmentation) adjacent to dark normal skin, overgrafting with thin split-thickness skin grafts can provide improved and more uniform pigmentation. The disadvantages are that it provides the least predictable result and the most extreme negative changes in skin characteristics. The donor site wound is painful and also provides further potential for hypertrophic scar.

Split-thickness skin grafts have limited indications in facial burn reconstruction. The best indication is resurfacing of the forehead (see below). Other indications include the use of thick split-thickness graft for eyelid reconstruction, overgrafting of unfavorable burn scars, providing the epidermal component over dermal substitutes, and occasionally to close flap or full-thickness skin graft donor sites.

Because virtually any other donor site other than eyelid skin is thicker than normal eyelid skin, the author prefers using thick split-thickness skin graft in eyelid reconstruction. This is particularly true in the upper eyelid which is dynamic compared with the generally static lower eyelid.

Overgrafting of unfavorable burn scars can add pigment to hypopigmented or variegated scar color. Particularly objectionable meshed graft pattern and hypertrophic scar can be overgrafted after planing down of the irregular contours.[30]

The application of full-thickness skin grafts in facial burn reconstruction

Full-thickness skin grafts in facial burn reconstruction are most useful in releasing contractures and replacing burn scars in the central portion of the face. The thinness of the skin allows underlying contours to be seen. Although its characteristics change more than flap skin, and the changes are still unpredictable, full-thickness grafts skin can often have almost normal characteristics. Frequently, placing oversized grafts anatomically will usually contract down to normal anatomic size.

Ideally, full-thickness grafts are performed in aesthetic units, and the grafts are taken from the 'blush area.' When local skin is not available for flap reconstruction of the large peripheral aesthetic units, full-thickness grafts can be used. Expanded full-thickness grafts have been shown to behave similarly to unexpanded grafts, particularly in terms of their ability to take successfully.[5]

There are several very important technical points in the performance of full-thickness skin grafts. They are virtually always done in a clean surgical wound. They should not be attempted in or near an open wound as bacteria will lead to graft failure.

Once the surgical wound is made by either release of contracture or excision of burn scar, the wound is held out to its greatest size and a pattern is made of the defect. This pattern is transferred to the donor site and marked on the skin without stretching the donor site skin. With the possible exception of the upper lip aesthetic unit, the goal is to place the largest graft possible within the defect that is compatible with graft take. The graft will usually contract down to anatomical size, and, if it does not, excision of excess is far better than adding an additional patch of skin.

The author's preference is to defat the full-thickness graft using a scalpel blade. At the graft is stretched, epidermal side down, over an inverted bowl. Horizontal mattress, dermal sutures are placed at the periphery, the end clamped, and the curved clamp tips tucked under the edge of the bowl. This provides a more precise determination of the graft thickness, and it divides the dermal interface blood vessels more cleanly than the crushing action of scissors against the dermis. When a thick split-thickness skin graft is desired, the scalpel cut is slightly into the dermis.

Meticulous hemostasis in the recipient site is critical for full-thickness skin graft revascularization. Epinephrine is injected along the lines of the incisions before the skin incision with scalpel. Release of contracture or excision of burn scars is performed using gentle electrocautery deep to the skin to achieve the best hemostasis. In cases in which larger defects and particularly full aesthetic units are being resurfaced, delay of full-thickness skin graft placement by covering the surgical wound with sheet skin allograft for up to 3

Video 1

days allows time for hemostasis. Furthermore, the literature shows that the growth factors from the dermal surface of the allograft stimulates neovascularization and essentially begins skin graft take.[31,32] When the allograft is removed after the delay, the full-thickness skin graft vascularizes more quickly with much less risk of hematoma and graft loss.

A meticulous pressure dressing is critical to prevent hematoma and reduce graft swelling optimizing graft take. It also holds the graft out to maximal size. The traditional tie-over bolus dressing is applied by placing multiple 'pop-off' silk sutures around the graft with ample purchase of the surrounding skin margin. A bolus of mineral oil moistened cotton is wrapped in an antibacterial nonadherent dressing on the wound, and the silk sutures are tied over the bolus with moderate pressure. The softer the wound bed, the more pressure can be used. Pressure application on skin grafts overlying bony structures such as the forehead must be applied very judiciously not to exceed capillary closing pressure. Bolus dressings are usually left in place for 7–8 days during which time prophylactic antibiotics are given.

In those cases in which a large full-thickness skin graft is indicated, and there is no normal skin donor site large enough, one can pre-expand donor sites before using the skin as full-thickness skin grafts. Full-thickness skin grafts from tissue expanded skin have been shown to behave similarly to unexpanded, normal skin full-thickness skin grafts. Another option is to use composite grafts of an acellular dermal substitute and the patient's split-thickness skin graft (details below).

If the size of the defect created by a scar excision or contracture release is so large that the pattern indicates that the donor site cannot be closed primarily, the donor site can be skin grafted with a split-thickness skin graft.

Composite and nonskin grafts

Composite grafts contain more than one tissue type. The most common composite graft is skin and cartilage grafts from either the ear or the nose. They are used for replacement of specialized anatomic areas for permanent restoration of contour. The cartilage resists the normal forces of contraction in healing (e.g., philtrum reconstruction, see below).

Nonskin grafts used in facial burn reconstruction include cartilage alone from either the ear, nose, or rib, occasionally bone, fat, and hair transplants.

Acellular dermal substitute used as a dermal component covered with the patient's split-thickness skin graft as the epidermis is also a form of composite graft. This type of composite graft is used when there are inadequate full-thickness skin graft donor sites or one wishes to improve the quality of the outcome compared to using split-thickness skin graft alone (see later).

Flaps

Introduction

A flap is tissue that is transplanted while maintaining its blood supply. When unscarred skin is near burn scar, consider using it for release or replacement of the scar. Facial scar itself can be used judiciously as a flap, and this should always be considered before excising the scar. Similarly, mature, skin grafted skin can be used as flaps if adequate well vascularized underlying normal tissue is transposed with it.

With the possible exception of free flaps, flaps generally never have a significant length of time without blood supply as grafts do. This seems to correspond to the accepted fact that flap tissue characteristics generally remain unchanged after uneventful transplantation, and they sometimes do change when the flap blood supply is compromised. Change in color and contraction are generally not problems. This allows the outcome to be much more predictable than with grafts.

Furthermore, because the tissue has its own blood supply, it does not have to rely on vascularity of the recipient site, and thicker tissue can be transplanted if required. Flaps also resist infection better than grafts.

A flap's greater bulk can be a great asset, but the bulk of tissue required to maintain vascularity can be its primary disadvantage. The additional bulk frequently causes a deformity of its own when the surrounding tissue is thin. Flap thickness can hide underlying structures and contours, and mask normal facial movement and expression.

General indications for flaps are listed in *Box 21.2*.

The various types are best described elsewhere in this book and their descriptions are referred to there. The following are specific points regarding the various types of flaps that have particular importance when used in facial reconstruction.

Random flaps are the most common flap type used in facial burn reconstruction. Z-plasties, burn scar flaps, and oral mucosa flaps are all random flaps, and the rules for gentle handling and attention to blood supply need to be carefully heeded. The flaps should never be undermined more than is necessary to transpose them. Although some very small flaps of scar can live on their own blood supply, generally flaps of scar or skin grafted skin should be transposed with underlying vascularized tissue if possible.

Advancement flaps are very tempting to use in burn reconstruction, but very commonly have poor outcomes related to their predisposition to retract from normal contraction and gravity. Limited advancement flaps within the face can do well, but advancement flaps across aesthetic unit boundaries should generally be avoided. Most importantly, inferiorly based advancement flaps, particularly from the neck into the face, almost always fail, as normal contraction and gravity cause an inferior extrinsic contracture of the face and neck. Additionally frequent 'bowstringing' of the flap can obliterate the normal hyoid concavity causing further deformity.

Rotation and transposition flaps do well in the face, as the movement of these flaps and the closure of the resultant donor site tend to eliminate deforming forces on the recipient site.

Box 21.2 **General indications for flaps**

- Optimal and controllable skin appearance is important
- No contraction or undesirable skin change is desired
- Closing a wound with an avascular component
- Tissue needed for three-dimensional reconstruction and can "stand on its own."
- Need for reoperation
- Protect easily traumatized areas
- Additional function (e.g., muscle flap motor).

Other types of flaps designated by the type of blood supply have varying utility based on the requirements for the specific anatomic area. Axial, perforator, fasciocutaneous, musculocutaneous, and free flaps have all been reported for facial reconstruction, but large bulky flaps have little aesthetic usefulness.

However, when local platysma muscle is included in local flaps in the neck and face, they clearly have superior blood supply. Another good example of a musculocutaneous flap with excellent vascularity is the eyelid transposition flap. The most useful and versatile flap for extensive facial reconstruction are expanded flaps. Prefabricated flaps popularized by Khouri et al. provide an increasingly versatile tool for facial reconstruction.[33,34] Recent descriptions of 'ultra-thin' flaps suggest that random flaps in facial reconstruction can be both large and thin, and more experience will elucidate their reliability and the quality of their outcomes.[35–37]

Z-plasty

A Z-plasty is a form of local tissue rearrangement in which, in its most basic form, two V-shaped flaps are elevated and transposed to accomplish one or more functions that can benefit burn scars.

Z-plasties can reorient scars into a more favorable position relative to resting skin tension lines. They can reposition anatomic structures into more normal position, and reduce tension in scars frequently resulting in a reduction of scar hypertrophy.[21] Linear burn scar contractures that manifest themselves in lines of depressions or ridges can be lengthened and the contour normalized.

However, Z-plasties are innately limited to the area in which the flaps are raised and by the availability of excess tissue adjacent to the area being treated. They are best used in linear scar contractures, as opposed to broad scar contractures. In broad contractures, the area of the Z-plasty itself will be released, but the remainder of the tight tissues adjacent to the Z-plasty will remain tight. Furthermore, despite a Z-plasty's ability to provide more length with greater flap angles, the amount of release is also limited. In both broad scar contractures and in particularly tight contractures, transverse release with transplantation of additional skin via graft or flap, is a better choice.

Various types of Z-plasties include: the single Z-plasty, serial Z-plasties, asymmetrical Z-plasties, and double opposing Z-plasties. Other forms of a local tissue rearrangement such as V–M plasties are similar to Z-plasties and have similar reasons for use *(Fig. 21.11)*.

Technically, it is very important to protect the vascularity of each of the flaps. The flap should be undermined only to the point where the flaps can be transposed successfully. Further undermining is unnecessary and may compromise the blood supply to the flaps. Z-plasties can be performed in scarred skin, but it is particularly important to protect the vascularity of these flaps. If one of the flaps is scarred, that flap should be based proximally to optimize arterial blood flow. Gentle handling of the flaps retracting them with hook retractors rather than forceps is optimal. When suturing the flaps into position, placing the sutures somewhat diagonally across the wound closure to pull the flap tip into position relieves tension on the tip. Half buried horizontal mattress sutures placing the horizontal component on each side of the

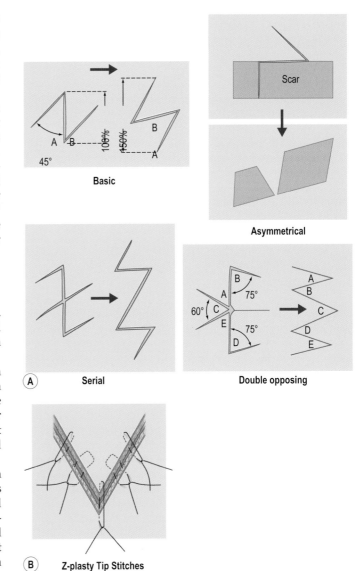

(A) Basic

Asymmetrical

Serial

Double opposing

(B) Z-plasty Tip Stitches

Fig. 21.11 (A) Various types of Z-plasties and local tissue rearrangements used to reorient facial burn scars and distorted anatomy, as well as relieve tension that potentiates hypertrophy. **(B)** Details of suture technique to protect the blood supply of small flap tips.

Z-plasty flap tip and parallel to the dermal blood supply is optimal. The suture at the very tip of the flap can be a single simple vertical suture as it does not cut off flap vascularity. An asymmetrical Z-plasty is particularly indicated for a contracture ridge that runs along the interface between normal skin and a burn scar.

Trapeze-plasty

Trapeze-plasties are very similar to Z-plasties, but designed with incisions perpendicular to the scar with small terminal 'Y' extensions, so that the flaps can be interposed with minimal transposition of the flaps, trapeze-plasties are also very effective in releasing linear scar contractures, particularly in the neck.[38]

Reconstructive options when normal skin for donor site is inadequate

When caught in a conflagration, there is an innate reflex to protect the face. When someone does sustain a serious facial burn it is often accompanied by extensive burn injuries to the entire body. With advances in wound care and critical care, more patients are surviving very large burn injuries. Frequently, the survivors of these burns are left with minimal normal skin which can be used for facial reconstruction donor sites.

Well-matched skin in terms of color and texture is particularly important in facial reconstruction, so inadequate or complete loss of the normal skin of the neck, shoulder, and upper chest can be a significant problem. Tissue expansion and the use of dermal substitutes find their best utility when normal skin donor sites are inadequate.

Tissue expansion

Historically, in order to follow the principle of using well-matched normal skin from the blush area for reconstruction of the face, large areas of full-thickness skin were removed from the shoulder and upper chest for grafting of large areas of the face. These donor sites were then closed using split-thickness skin graft from elsewhere in the body leaving very large donor site deformities.

The advent of tissue expansion has provided a mechanism to provide additional normal, well-matched skin for flaps or full-thickness skin grafts in the face.[5] More normal skin grows via the process termed 'biological creep.'[28] Although the dermis thins, the epidermis increases as the skin surface area increases. The increased metabolic demands of the growing skin causes the skin to be more highly vascularized than normal skin which may well lead to increased survival of the skin as it is transplanted as a graft or flap.[6,7]

Other advantages include the ability to grow enough extra skin to allow primary closure of the donor site. Placement of tissue expanders results in a *de facto* delay phenomenon which, along with the increased vascularity, allows even random flaps to have a greater length-to-width ratio than random flaps of normal skin.[6,7,39] Furthermore, increasing the amount of donor skin reduces tension resulting in optimal surgical scars.

Expanded full-thickness skin grafts have been used since the early 1980s.[5] They have been shown to behave similarly to unexpanded full-thickness grafts. Although very large full-thickness grafts can be 'grown' at distant donor sites and the donor site can be closed, the grafts still have the disadvantages of full-thickness skin grafts which include unpredictable change in characteristics, particularly pigmentation, and the tendency to contract to the point of masking facial expression. Change in pigmentation is particularly prominent in children with Fitzpatrick type IV–VI skin pigmentation.

Expanded advancement flaps are used commonly in scalp reconstruction where the cranium tends to splint the additional, elongated skin to prevent further contraction (*Fig. 21.12*). Expanded neck advancement flaps can be used occasionally in neck reconstruction. However, expanded advancement facial flaps and, particularly expanded neck advancement flaps into the face, are contraindicated. Unlike the scalp, expanded advancement flaps into the face have little to prevent them from contracting causing deformity of the mobile facial features. Expanded neck flaps into the face have both gravity and natural contraction causing a downward pull on the mobile facial structures.

The expanded rotation and transposition flaps tend to have much better outcomes, particularly when an ample flap is used to accommodate for a mild degree of natural contraction (*Fig. 21.13*).[24,35]

Following expanded flaps and the increased time to prepare suitable flaps for reconstruction, prefabricated, prelaminated, and super-thin flaps have evolved.[34,40–44] Increasingly impressive results are being obtained, and they currently seem to indicate the direction of local and even free flap reconstruction. Without expansion or other previous preparation, free flaps have the disadvantages of excess bulk, of being transported from a distance and not matching skin color and texture as well as local flaps, along with the increased risk of the microanastomoses.

Technical points in tissue expansion

The choice of shape of the tissue expander should be based on the proposed use of the expanded tissue. Round tissue expanders have very little utility in burn reconstruction. Crescent tissue expanders were designed specifically to develop an advancement flap used to close round defects adjacent to it. Rectangular or oval tissue expanders tend to be most commonly used and are used best for transposition flaps, rotation flaps, and advancement flaps.

Skin expanded over rectangular tissue expanders cannot be used fully as advancement flaps without making some type of incision onto the skin over the tissue expander. Zide and Karp's description of techniques to optimize the expanded skin over rectangular tissue expanders is exceedingly useful.[45]

Make the pocket of ample size and try to avoid sharp fold protrusions of foot plates or tubing that might cause pressure necrosis and exposure of the expander or tubing. At the time of insertion, assemble tissue expanders with remote ports carefully and test the system for leaks or obstruction from kinking before closing the wound. Remote ports have the advantage of placing the port at a distance from the tissue expander to prevent puncture of the tissue expander. Remember that the tissue expander will grow, and place the port far enough away so that the two will not meet. Generally the port, and tissue expanders with integrated ports, should be sutured or otherwise anchored to the surrounding tissues at three points so that it cannot migrate or flip over making the port inaccessible.

Allow plenty of time for the growth of tissue between expansions. Not only is the expanded skin better quality, but too rapid expansion will frequently lead to the skin thinning and exposure of the expander. Generally, tissue expansion is stopped 2 weeks preoperatively to allow for full tissue growth to help prevent contraction after transplantation.

Dermal substitutes

When sufficient native, normal full-thickness skin is not available for either direct transplantation or expansion with transplantation, one is left with the alternative of using a composite graft of a dermal substitutes and split-thickness skin autograft epidermis. The dermal substitute augments the dermal component of this composite graft. When

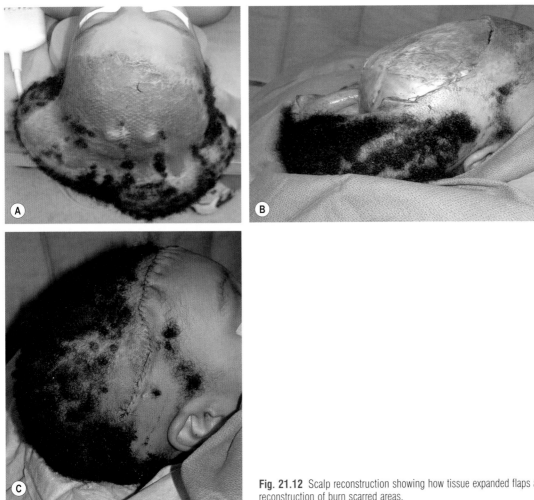

Fig. 21.12 Scalp reconstruction showing how tissue expanded flaps are typically used for advancement flap reconstruction of burn scarred areas.

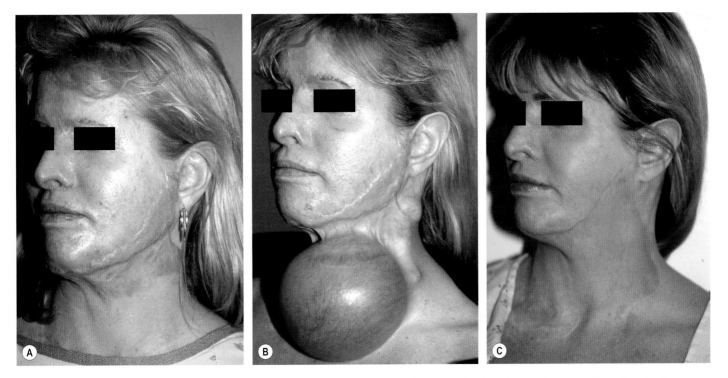

Fig. 21.13 Expanded rotation and transposition flaps tend to have better outcomes compared to advancement flaps from the neck where contraction and gravity often compromises the result.

successful, it provides a skin substitute that behaves like a full-thickness skin graft in terms of reduction of contraction and improved quality of skin compared to split-thickness skin graft alone. However, it is exceedingly rare to have a result that can simulate native full-thickness skin graft characteristics in terms of color and texture otherwise. For this reason, composite grafts using dermal substitutes find their best utility in reconstruction for function. They are most commonly used in the face, head, and neck region for release of neck contractures.

These composite grafts are still relatively new and we are still learning the best ways to achieve engraftment in a reliable way and to optimize their results.[46] When successful, composite grafts still need to be treated similarly to successful full-thickness skin grafts as they will contract usually to the extent that the anatomic area will allow.

Nonoperative facial reconstructive adjunct techniques

There are a number of techniques that, when used instead of or in conjunction with surgical reconstruction can be very helpful in facial burn reconstruction.

These techniques include: laser therapy, steroid injections, corrective cosmetics, hair and fat transplantation, and facial prostheses.

Laser therapy

Currently, the most accepted form of laser therapy for facial burn scars is pulsed dye laser therapy. 'Pulsed dye' is simply the term that is used to describe a particular laser that delivers a single beam of light with a wavelength of 585 nm. It is most effective for red, immature scars because this frequency is absorbed well by the red hemoglobin in red blood cells. It is thought that the energy from the pulsed dye laser light is absorbed by the hemoglobin, and the resulting heat damages the numerous blood vessels in immature scars. It tends to make immature, red scars become less red and also causes them to mature quickly in terms of reduction of size, firmness, and making them less pruritic. It has become well-accepted as therapy for both immature hypertrophic burn scars and as an adjunct to prevent or rapidly reduce erythema in new surgical scars (*Fig. 21.14*).[14]

Recently, CO_2 fractional ablative laser therapy has been introduced as a treatment for mature burn scars.[19,20] CO_2 laser has a wavelength of 10 600 nm, and is specifically absorbed by water. The fractional aspect of this type of therapy can best be understood as a beam of light that is broken into a number of tiny laser columns of CO_2 laser. Each column creates a tiny hole into the tissue. The tissue is totally ablated resulting in what one can picture as multiple micro-tunnels into the tissues. This results in an immediate reduction in scar tissue volume. Surrounding each one of these tunnels there is injured tissue from the heat that caused the vaporization of the tissue formerly in each tunnel. Surrounding the injured tissue, normal tissue remains intact.

The surrounding normal tissue causes rapid healing of the tunnels, but each represents a new injury to the scar tissue. Some of the scar has been totally removed, and some injured. Within these micro-injuries, all of the previous mechanisms of wound healing and scar maturation begin again with subsequent new remodelling of a burn scar. This process may stimulate new remodelling deep in scars which, in some cases, may have been dormant for years.

When this deep fractional ablative laser treatment is combined with the widely used superficial fractional ablative laser resurfacing, not only is the deep portion of the burn scars improved by new remodeling, but the superficial appearance of the scars can be improved as well.

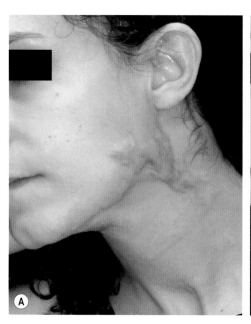 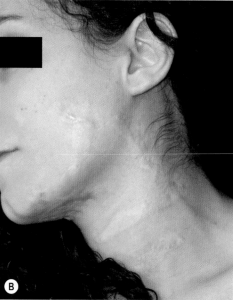

Fig. 21.14 Pulsed dye laser therapy to minimize erythema of reconstruction scars after simple excision of hypertrophic scar and advancement flap.

Steroid injections

Steroid injections have long been found to reduce inflammation and scar volume related to its biochemical action within scar tissue. They can be very helpful in smaller hypertrophic facial burn scars. It can be particularly helpful when reduction of a scar is desirable or more acceptable than the new scar caused by excision and closure primarily or with a graft. However, excessive steroid injections can result in atrophy of the scar locally or systemic effects.

Corrective cosmetics

The use of cosmetics to conceal or camouflage facial burn scars is a common practice. The plastic surgeon must understand that although irregularity of dermal color is relatively easy to hide with cosmetics, contour irregularity is much more difficult to hide due to the shadows cast by the contours from overhead lighting. For corrective cosmetics to be successful, reduction in height of hypertrophic burn scar is important. Special cosmetics that not only conceal the deformity, but are durable and do not rub off on clothing and others are available.

Hair transplantation

A large number of techniques have been described historically for reconstruction of hair bearing areas of the face and scalp.[47] The dramatic improvements in hair transplant technology in recent years have made many of these techniques obsolete. Moustaches, beards, eyebrows, and even eyelashes can be transplanted successfully using micro-transplantation of hair follicles. There has even been a recent report of hair follicle transplantation resulting in, not only hair growth in a bilayer acellular dermal substitute, but re-epithelialization of the acellular dermal substitute without epidermal autograft transplantation.[48,49]

Fat transplantation

Fat transplantation has been used for some time to fill out contour deformities, particularly under depressions formed by thin skin graft being placed over areas of relatively thick tissue loss. Recently the suggestion that stem cells originating from fat transplants may enhance the quality of the overlying skin is intriguing.[50,51]

Prosthetics

Similar to cosmetics, hairpieces have been commonplace to treat extensive burn scar alopecia, particularly while the patient is awaiting scalp reconstruction, or if scalp reconstruction is not possible because of total or subtotal hair loss.

Prosthetic ears are particularly effective as they are not dynamic structures compared to the nose. Nose prostheses should be considered when other options are not available or would provide a poorer outcome in terms of appearance, function or length of time and risks involved to achieve. Osseointegrated implants make attachment quite stable. Modern anaplastological techniques make the prosthetics exceedingly real appearing. The one disadvantage is the color change the prosthetics usually undergo over time requiring the patient to replace the prosthetic as often as annually.

Reconstruction of specific anatomic areas

Forehead

Forehead resurfacing using a moderately thick split-thickness skin graft is desirable because a single large split-thickness skin graft is relatively easily obtained and has a more reliable take over the very large surface of the forehead. The forehead has such a large surface area, a piece of full-thickness skin graft that large would be prohibitive from an unexpanded donor site, and a predictably perfect take of a full-thickness skin graft over the broad area is unlikely. Because the forehead skin overlies of the unyielding frontal bone of the cranium, a reasonably thick split-thickness skin graft is splinted against significant contraction. The disadvantage of the unpredictability of final color and texture is usually offset by the advantage of having a uniform surface over the entire expanse of the forehead. It is very important to graft up to and sometimes into the hairlines of the scalp and eyebrows to avoid the visibility of marginal scars.

Onsite tissue expansion may be used in cases where normal forehead skin is adequate to expand to replace the scarred forehead or to release a contracture causing superior displacement of the eyebrows.[52]

Eyebrows

Although historically many techniques had been described for the reconstruction of eyebrows in burn survivors, the advances in hair transplantation have been so great that it is rare in the author's practice to use any technique other than hair transplantation. Hair transplantation, particularly follicular transplants, gives by far the best chance for relatively normal appearing eyebrows when compared to techniques that have been used in the past.

Eyelids

Late reconstruction of the burn scarred eyelid is usually performed for functional correction of burn scar ectropion (*Fig. 21.15*). These releases are often required early in the recovery of the patient to protect the patient's eyes, and, because of this, it is one of the reconstructive procedures that is sometimes necessary before full maturation of the burn scars of the face. Much less frequently, residual minor deformity of the eyelid will be distressing to the burn survivor and minor eyelid ectropion releases are performed with much more emphasis on the final appearance.

Occasionally, a small linear contracture can be corrected using a Z-plasty. Most commonly, the eyelid is more broadly scarred and a formal release by incising the scarred lid transversely from medial canthus to lateral orbital rim (and sometimes beyond) is required.

The best donor site for eyelid skin is skin from another eyelid. Unfortunately, with the exception of the occasional unilateral facial burn, eyelid ectropion in one eyelid is usually associated with burn injuries to the other eyelids making the best donor site unavailable. Second choice is thick split-thickness skin from the blush area. Postauricular skin,

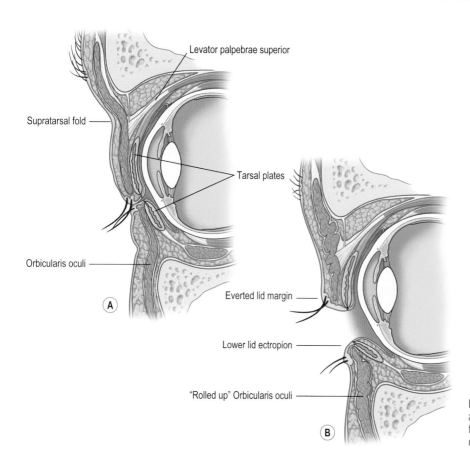

Fig. 21.15 (A) Normal eyelid anatomy. **(B)** Eyelid anatomy after burn contracture. There is shortening and eversion of the lids with flattening of contours and bunching of the orbicularis oculi muscle.

Labels in figure:
Levator palpebrae superior
Supratarsal fold
Tarsal plates
Orbicularis oculi
Everted lid margin
Lower lid ectropion
"Rolled up" Orbicularis oculi

frequently quoted as the second best donor site for eyelids, is usually too pink in color to match the facial skin and frequently is not available in major facial/head and neck burns.

Upper eyelids

The upper eyelid *(Fig. 21.16)*, in contrast to the lower eyelid, is a dynamic eyelid, which moves and folds with opening and closing of the lid. For this reason, the author believes that full-thickness skin graft from other than another eyelid skin donor site should be a thick split-thickness graft rather than a full-thickness graft.

A Frost stitch is placed for traction before marking the line of the incision. An epinephrine-containing local anesthetic is then injected. The release is performed by incising transversely several millimeters above the cilial margin depending on the severity of the ectropion and keeping the tarsal plate of the upper eyelid in mind. The incision is made from medial to the medial canthus to as much as 1 cm lateral to the lateral canthus, very commonly overlying the lateral orbital rim. Placing Y-extensions at the ends of the incisions is optional depending on the amount of eyelid skin excess in these areas. The principle of making a very large release to place an oversized skin graft is very important here.

When only a small-to-moderate sized release of the ectropion is required, incision onto the orbicularis oculi muscle while putting traction on the scarred eyelid skin with double hook retractors will often provide enough release to place a thick split-thickness skin graft to maintain the release. When moderate to severe contractures are present, the orbicularis

oculi muscle must be divided down to the orbital septum. Dividing the orbicularis oculi muscle when only a mild to moderate release is required will frequently results in an abnormal transverse groove in the eyelid. However, when a larger release is necessary, the resulting engraftment of the larger skin graft frequently provides a very normal appearance. Once the skin graft is prepared from a pattern of the release wound, it is sutured into position with multiple 4–0 silk sutures and tied over a bolus dressing. The bolus dressing is removed in as early as 5 days, but 1 week is preferable if possible.

Lower eyelids

The principles of lower eyelid release are very similar to those of the upper eyelids (see above). Placing a Frost stitch and retracting it superiorly is particularly important in lower eyelids *(Fig. 21.17)*. Again the incision should be from medial to the medial canthus and as far as 1 cm lateral to the lateral canthus, and Y-extensions of the incisions are optional. Because the lower eyelid is not dynamic and has to defy gravity, a thicker skin graft can be placed in the eyelid if deemed necessary. However, making the release wound and graft oversized is probably more important. Again, the blush area thick split-thickness skin graft is used if other eyelid skin is not available.

The lower eyelid is where a musculocutaneous transposition flap from the upper eyelid skin to release ectropion is most commonly used. This flap was described by Kostakoglu and Ozcan,[53] and has the added advantage of some lateral and superior sling action to the lower eyelid as well as adding

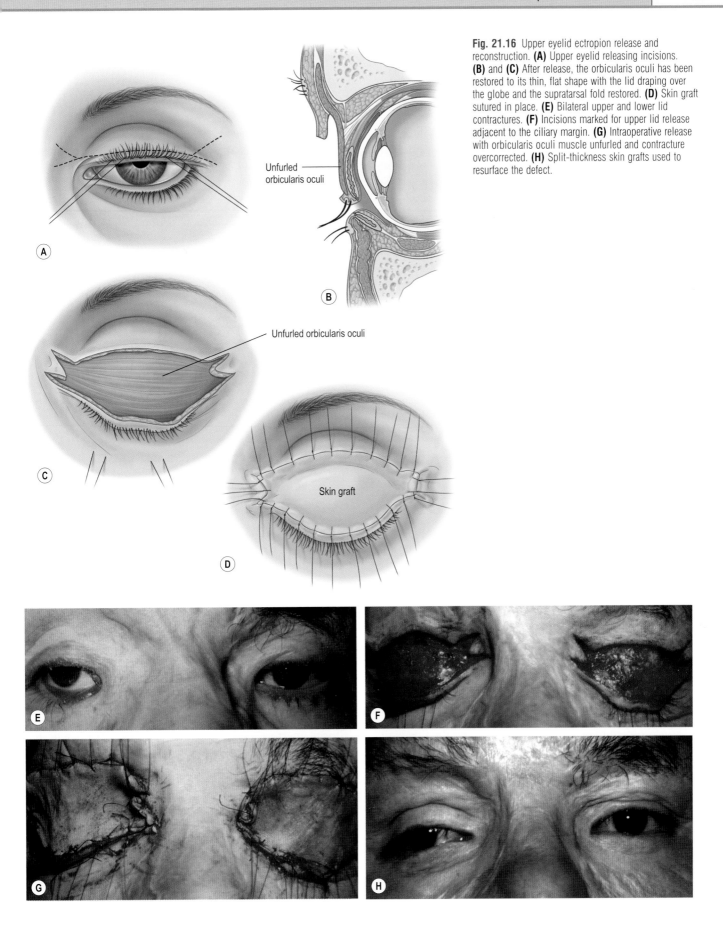

Fig. 21.16 Upper eyelid ectropion release and reconstruction. **(A)** Upper eyelid releasing incisions. **(B)** and **(C)** After release, the orbicularis oculi has been restored to its thin, flat shape with the lid draping over the globe and the supratarsal fold restored. **(D)** Skin graft sutured in place. **(E)** Bilateral upper and lower lid contractures. **(F)** Incisions marked for upper lid release adjacent to the ciliary margin. **(G)** Intraoperative release with orbicularis oculi muscle unfurled and contracture overcorrected. **(H)** Split-thickness skin grafts used to resurface the defect.

Unfurled orbicularis oculi

Unfurled orbicularis oculi

Skin graft

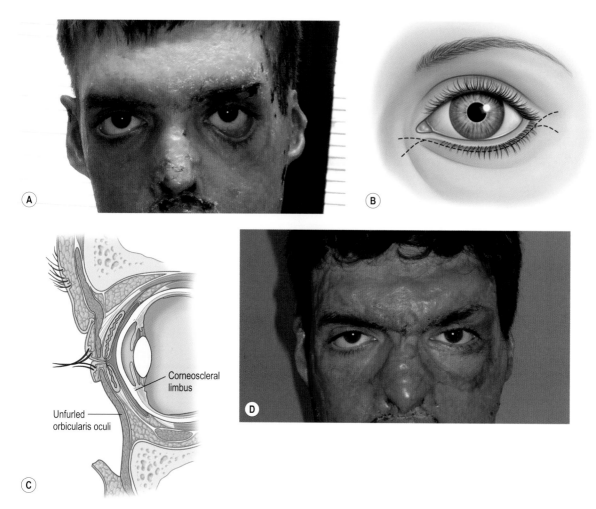

Fig. 21.17 Lower eyelid ectropion release and reconstruction. **(A)** Eyelid ectropion. **(B)** Lower eyelid releasing incision. **(C)** Lower eyelid after complete release of superficial scarring. The orbicularis oculi muscle is flat and retains its integrity. **(D)** Healed mature grafts.

skin. The flap including a strip of orbicularis oculi muscle from the upper eyelid is exceedingly hardy, and can be transposed as a flap only 8 mm in width across the entire width of the lower eyelid. Transposition from lower eyelid to the upper eyelid is also possible. A similar bipedicle flap from the upper eyelid is also described.[54]

Medial canthus scars

Burn scar contracture of the medial canthus and the side wall of the nose will often result in an epicanthal fold, sometimes with epiphora from pulling one or both of the puncta away from the globe. Careful diagnosis of the degree of tissue deficit is necessary to select the reconstructive technique. Relatively large skin deficits will require transection or excision of the scar tissue freeing-up and repositioning the medial canthus, and skin grafting the deficit. Return of the contracture is common in this situation. An attempt should be made to use a large, thick graft and apply it directly to the nasal bone periosteum after undermining the margins of the skin deficit.

Fortunately, the more frequent situation is that of a smaller tissue deficit in which very gratifying results can be obtained by using the double opposing Z-plasty technique, V–M plasty or the four-flap technique of Mustarde.[55]

Nose

The nose is a very complex structure. It is composed of the outer skin, the inner epithelial lining including both skin and mucosa, and the internal cartilages that give the nose its complex three-dimensional infrastructure. Burn injuries can result in minor external skin loss with resulting minor scarring and contractures to extensive loss of all the structures of the distal two thirds of the nose leaving only a scarred piriform aperture and a residual septum. Fortunately, the mild to moderate injuries are more common than the latter. Further complicating the situation is that extensive injury to the nose is usually accompanied by extensive injury to the surrounding tissues and particularly the forehead. Therefore, with the more extensive burn injuries to the nose, the typical median forehead flap, so commonly used for major nasal reconstruction for other reasons, is generally not available with unscarred skin or easily closable donor site.

Manson and others described an algorithm for nasal reconstruction, which stresses the characteristics of the skin of the nose divided into the upper, middle, and lower thirds.[56] Burget's concepts of nasal aesthetic subunits, the importance of the three-dimensional structure and concepts on how to maintain the infrastructure of the nose, and the multiple techniques used for minor revision of noses are exceedingly useful when approaching the burn scarred nose.[57]

A most useful technique used commonly for nasal reconstruction, both for relatively minor deformities and for major deformities is the nasal turndown flap.[58] The most common nasal burn deformity is asymmetry of the alar margins of the nose as a result of burn scar contracture of one or both alar margins. When one side of the nose is normal, one is forced to do a unilateral release of the contracted ala. Ideally the best symmetry is obtained when both alae are released. A curvilinear incision which ideally approximates the superior line of the alar subunit is marked and infiltrated with epinephrine containing local anesthetic. The incision is then made down onto the plane of the perichondrium of the nasal cartilages. The turndown flap is then undermined towards the caudal margin of the scarred ala which becomes the hinge for the turndown flap. This is done until the flap can be turned down to expose its underside . The underside of the flap and its donor site are then grafted with a single full-thickness skin graft. The reconstructed ala is usually longer than normal, but the combination of contraction and some necrosis of the new, inferior skin margin results in normalization of the ala that is surprisingly similar in length and contour to a normal ala.

Upper lip

The late effects of burn injuries to the upper lip also have a spectrum from mild to severe. Any deep burn will cause a combination of upper lip shortening and scarring. There also can be an associated injury to the base of the nose and columella.

The upper lip has a number of fine aesthetic contours and dimensions that, although subtle, are very important to its normal appearance. It is made up of the two lateral subunits, the philtral subunit, and the vermillion with the Cupid's bow. The lateral subunits have a subtle triangle superiorly on each side of the nasal alar bases, and meet the philtrum at the philtral ridges.

Minor hypertrophic scarring of the upper lip is often best left for full maturation with the addition of steroid injections or pulsed dye laser therapy as these will frequently resolve satisfactorily. Excision of any significant amount of hypertrophic scarring will require replacement with either full-thickness graft or local flap. Occasionally small nasolabial flaps can be used to advantage here. However, one must be careful not to cause a patched appearance to the lip by replacing less than the full aesthetic subunit. Small Z-plasties can be used to release tension of small contractures to the nose or to the vermillion border. Occasionally small scars can be excised and closed directly using vertical excisions including vermillion commonly used in skin cancer excisions.

Minor irregularities or loss of contour of the Cupid's bow can sometimes be corrected by transverse scar excision and advancement of the vermillion. One must be careful not to over-shorten an already shortened lip.

More major injuries to the upper lip usually result in both scarring and significant shortening that demands release and resurfacing of the upper lip. Total resurfacing of the upper lip is usually performed using a full-thickness skin graft. Ideally the patient is nasally intubated, and the upper and lower lips are sutured together. Once the upper lip is released, the scarred skin of the full aesthetic unit is excised to re-establish the shape and length of the lip. Initially the philtrum and its columns are not reconstructed. The lip is resurfaced with only a very mild overcorrection. The upper lip tends to contract less than the lower lip, where significant overcorrection is required (*Fig. 21.18*).

Once the entire lip has been replaced with full-thickness skin graft, secondary procedures can be performed to reconstruct the philtrum, and, if necessary, re-contour the Cupid's bow (*Fig. 21.19*).

Lower lip and chin

The lower lip and chin is considered a single aesthetic unit broken into the prominence of the chin subunit, the more delicate lower lip itself with the sulcus between it and the chin subunit, and the vermillion. Shortening of the lower lip results in significant ectropion commonly with loss of function as oral competence is compromised and the lower teeth exposed. Drooling and tooth damage are serious problems in severe cases. Early on, when this problem is severe, early release before the burn scar contracture is fully mature may be indicated.

The lower lip and chin aesthetic unit is quite large making a decision to do a complete aesthetic unit resurfacing a difficult one when lower lip ectropion is the primary problem. This decision is made on an individual basis. However, the rule of thumb is to overcorrect, as a combination of contraction and gravity will frequently lead to recurrence of the ectropion. Frequently the oversized full-thickness graft will contract to amazingly normal dimensions.

When total resurfacing of the entire aesthetic unit is performed, reconstruction of the chin prominence and lower lip sulcus is of particular importance. When hypertrophic scarring is present over the chin prominence, de-epithelializing the hypertrophic scar only, leaving the bulk of underlying scar will help preserve is prominence. This, combined with excising the lip scar down to the orbicularis oris muscle elsewhere, and particularly in the lower lip sulcus, provides the accentuation of the contour needed to be visible through a full-thickness skin graft (*Fig. 21.20*).

Oral commissure

Burns of the corners of the mouth create scars that result both in deformity and dysfunction. Oral commissure contractures cause microstomia and the frustrating feeling of not being able to open one's mouth adequately while eating. There often is a real problem for dentists and anesthesiologists being able to access the oral cavity well. Additionally, the deformity of microstomia is obvious particularly when the mouth is in motion while speaking and expressing emotion.

Many specific procedures are described for release and reconstruction of the oral commissure.[61,62] Almost all of them use excision of burn scar and release of the underlying tissue including the orbicularis oris muscle if necessary, before reconstructing with local flaps. The most commonly used techniques are variations of the technique described by Converse that describes a Y-shaped incision in the oral mucosal providing a mucosal flap that goes into the angle of the oral commissure.[61] Others make it even more simple by simply pulling out the entire local mucosal flap and suturing

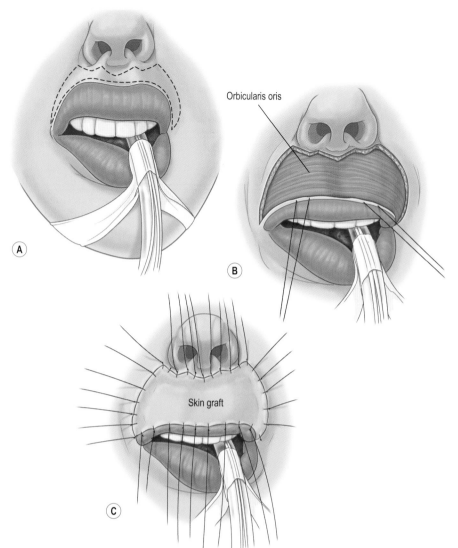

Orbicularis oris

Skin graft

Ⓐ Ⓑ Ⓒ

Fig. 21.18 Reconstruction of upper lip with full thickness skin graft. **(A)** Upper lip releasing incision. Scar is excised when indicated. **(B)** Release is carried beyond the oral commissures. The orbicularis oris muscle is unfurled, creating a concave upper lip. **(C)** Skin graft sutured in place.

it into position, but large reconstructions require at least some lateral incision of the mucosa to allow movement in the three directions necessary and to provide a lateral flap in the lateral wall to help prevent recurrence *(Fig. 21.21)*. A ventral tongue flap has been described for release and resurfacing in the case of severe oral commissure contracture.[63]

Further restriction of oral opening can result from scarring outside of the oral commissures in the area of the nasolabial folds and the cheeks. These should be look for and addressed.

Cheeks

Contrary to the aesthetic units in the central portion of the face, the cheeks represent large areas of the face that have minimal contour. They are, however, dynamic, and supple, ample cheek tissue is critical to allow movement and facial expression. Skin grafts, due to their innate contraction and change in skin characteristics, frequently limit these functions. Also skin grafts within the large aesthetic unit almost always look like a patch. For this reason, flaps are usually indicated.

Because of the cheek aesthetic unit's large size, relatively small scars have to be addressed within the aesthetic unit

using techniques that will minimize the resulting surgical scar. These techniques are myriad, and best described elsewhere.

Basic principles are important particular regarding resting skin tension lines. Both burn and incisional scars running against resting skin tension lines on the cheek will frequently be hypertrophic. Furthermore, if the burn scarring is relatively small, frequently there is ample local skin to use as flaps to replace the scar.

Larger cheek scars representing one third to one half of the cheek aesthetic unit can often be replaced using cervicofacial flaps based either anteriorly or posteriorly depending on the location of the cheek scar.[64]

When scars are more than half of the aesthetic unit, one must consider whether replacement of the entire aesthetic unit is indicated. When indicated, a large, thin flap with favorable skin characteristics from local tissue is ideal. A flap large enough is best achieved by using tissue expansion.

Expanded rotation flaps from the neck are options for subtotal replacement. The expanded transposition flap from the shoulder has yielded gratifying results for total aesthetic unit replacement, and enough skin can be left in the donor site to allow primary closure of the donor site.[26]

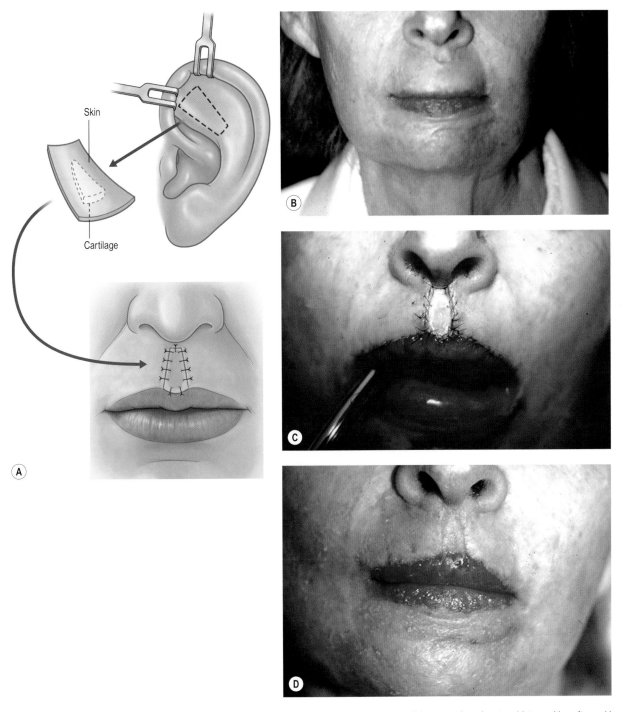

Fig. 21.19 Reconstruction of the upper lip philtrum. **(A)** Composite graft from the triangular fossa of the external ear is sutured into position after making a releasing incision in the central lip at the base of the columella. Only enough cartilage to maintain the philtral concavity is kept while maximizing the touchdown of the surrounding full-thickness skin graft. **(B)** Upper lip reconstructed with full thickness skin graft requiring philtrum. **(C)** Composite graft from ear triangular fossa in place, and upper lip vermilion advanced and re-contoured. **(D)** Final appearance.

When local skin is unavailable to cover the entire cheek, large enough full-thickness skin grafts or thin, free flaps from a distant site are further options. Tissue expansion can be helpful by developing the amount of normal skin required for a full cheek aesthetic unit from a distant location. In the case of free flaps, tissue expansion thins the flap making the donor tissue more appropriate for cheek skin replacement. In both situations, developing ample skin for the aesthetic unit to allow for some contraction is critical to provide optimal skin qualities and the ability to allow facial expression.

Ears

As with facial structures, there is a spectrum of the late effects of burn injury to ears, ranging from the very mild to total loss. At the lower end of the spectrum, the more minor deformities

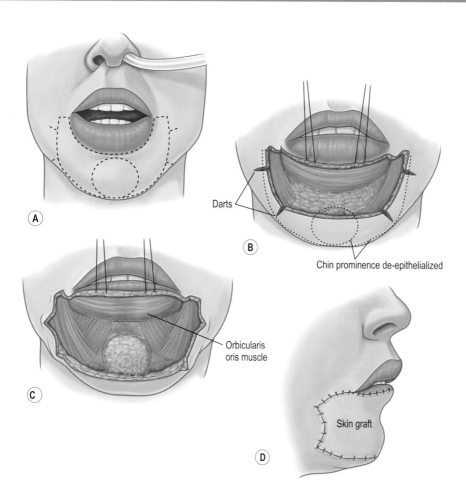

Darts

Chin prominence de-epithelialized

Orbicularis
oris muscle

Skin graft

Fig. 21.20 (A) Lower lip releasing incision. Note extension lateral to oral commissures. **(B)** Lateral darts expand the release. **(C)** After complete release, the lower lip can be elevated above the upper incisors, and the defect has expanded to include the entire lower lip–chin aesthetic unit. **(D)** The skin graft sutured in place with a concave lip-chin sulcus.

and relatively small partial losses of the ear can frequently be reconstructed using common techniques developed for reconstruction of ears after cancer excision. These techniques are discussed elsewhere. However, again, burn reconstruction of the ear is frequently made particularly difficult because of the presence of surrounding burn scar and thus the absence of normal local donor skin.

There are three common problems of burned scarred ears that are unlike the losses sustained with cancer excisions and must be addressed despite the lack of local normal skin. These problems are size reduction of the external ear particularly in the upper third, burn scar contracture of the ear lobe to the side of the neck, and total loss of the external ear.

Correction of the reduction of size of the external ear is very nicely managed with a conchal transposition flap described by Davis and popularized more recently by Donelan *(Fig. 21.22)*.[65]

Very minor releases of the ear lobe from the side of the neck can be accomplished using Z-plasty techniques. However, it is frequently much safer to simply release the ear lobe from the side of the neck and skin graft both the medial surface of the ear lobe and close or graft to the neck wound. Again, contraction of the skin graft makes overcorrection desirable to prevent recurrence of the ear lobe contracture. Alternatively, using scarred local skin as a flap for reconstruction and skin grafting the donor site can be attempted, but has the

disadvantage of often being bulky due to the inability to reduce the scar enough to make a delicate ear lobe.

Total ear loss is exceedingly difficult to reconstruct using either local or distant tissues in severe burn injury. Total loss is always associated with severe scarring of the skin in the locality of the ear canal. Although there is a great temptation to use cartilage grafts or synthetic implants with fascial turn-down flaps and skin grafts to reconstruct a total ear, very good to excellent total ear reconstruction outcomes are exceedingly difficult in the best hands.[66] Honest assessment of the usual outcomes suggests that the effort is rarely warranted. Therefore, total ear loss is one of the best indications for a prosthetic in head and neck reconstruction. Prosthetic ears can be made to look exceedingly normal in appearance and, given the adynamic nature of the ear, appearance is its primary function. Permanent osseointegrated implants can now be used to secure the prosthesis making the burn survivor confident the prosthesis will not fall off *(Fig. 21.5)*.

Scalp

Burn injuries to the scalp result in scarring and burn scar alopecia. Both are distressing to the burn survivor. Again there are a number of techniques for scalp reconstruction that are too innumerable to catalogue here.[67]

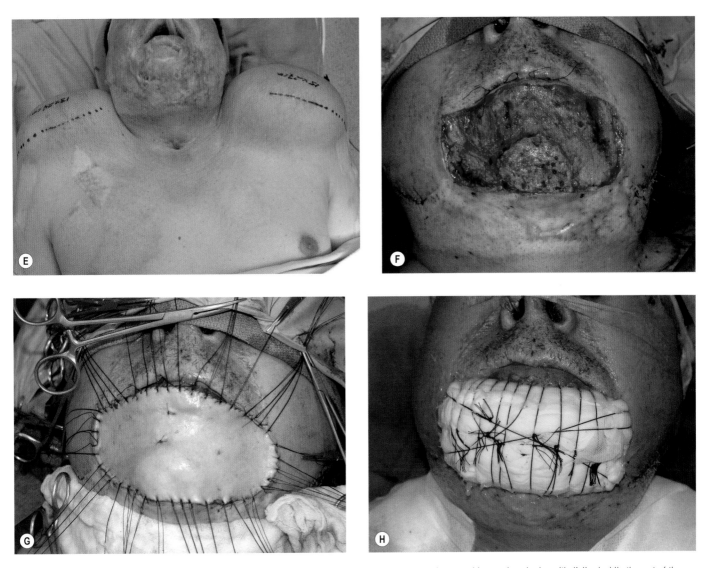

Fig. 21.20, cont'd (E) Bilateral expanded transposition flaps marked for elevation. **(F)** Chin prominence hypertrophic scar is only de-epithelialized while the rest of the lower lip is excised onto muscle. **(G)** Full thickness skin graft sutured into position. **(H)** Tie-over bolus dressing in place.

In practice, the most common problems include relatively small areas of burn scarring and burn scar alopecia that frequently can be excised and closed primarily. However, the patient must be warned that the new surgical scar will be hairless, and may tend to spread, particularly when tension is present. The unique anatomy of the scalp with the galea immediately deep to the skin makes the skin much less elastic than other areas of the body. Therefore even small excisions of the scalp tend to have tension in their closures. At the time of scalp reconstruction with flaps, any hair bearing scalp excess from the final trimming can be cut into small follicle containing grafts and inserted into the scalp incision closures. Alternatively, the patient should be advised that a secondary procedure to reduce the somewhat widened and hairless surgical scar may be required.

With larger scars, tissue expansion has become the primary technique for expanding the amount of hair bearing scalp. It provides an expanded flap to advance, rotate or transpose into a defect left by excision of burn scar alopecia **(Fig. 21.14)**. Advancement and rotation flaps usually are superior to transposition flaps as transposition flaps result in more hairless scars and frequently result in hair growing in a direction contrary to the surrounding scalp **(Fig. 21.12)**.

Neck

Severe neck contractures that cause fixed flexion deformities of the neck pose a danger to patients during anesthetic induction and emergence because of the difficulty intubating patients from restriction of neck extension. This is a primary reason early release of severe neck burn scar contractures should be considered as the first operation at the beginning of the reconstructive phase of treatment. Additionally a severe neck contracture is a major extrinsic contracture deforming

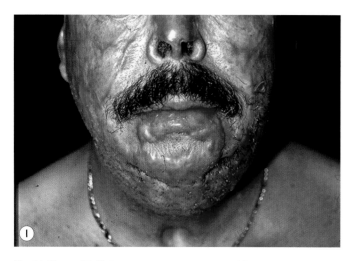
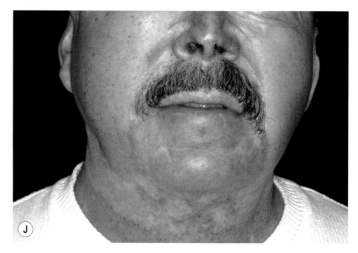

Fig. 21.20, cont'd (I) Preoperative lower lip and chin. **(J)** Postoperative lower lip and chin.

the face from tension inferiorly and should be released before addressing the intrinsic facial contractures.

Cervical burn deformities addressed during the reconstruction phase vary from relatively little scars to severely deforming and functionally limiting contractures. The smaller scars are addressed using scar revision techniques with careful attention to the resting skin tension lines of the neck.

Particularly important are the vertical, linear scars of the neck which are frequently hypertrophic because of the persistent tension caused by neck extension. These vertical scars alone may represent linear contractures that limit the extension of the neck. When excising cervical scars or transplanting skin into the neck, one should make every attempt to avoid new vertical surgical scars. When linear contractures are present, gratifying results are obtained by using Z-plasty or trapeze-plasty[38] principles to reorient these scars into the resting skin tension lines. Even broad anterior cervical burn scar contractures can be excised and occasionally there is enough normal skin in the lateral neck to advance and close anteriorly avoiding straight-line vertical scars. Sometimes, this can be done in conjunction with grafting some of the remaining open areas to get closure and leave the patient with scars oriented in lines where contracture will not recur.[68]

Severe cervical burn scars and contractures

Broad cervical contractures must be addressed by releasing the contracture and/or excising the cervical scar, and transplanting new skin in the form of skin graft or flap. Although flaps are better than grafts, no matter what type of tissue is transplanted into the neck release, the tissue will tend to contract to conform to the neck in its normal anatomic position at the midpoint between full extension and full flexion. The patient must be warned that releasing a neck contracture to the point where the neck is completely without tension when the neck is extended fully is probably not

possible. However, even with this limitation, release of neck contractures is one of the most important operations in burn reconstruction.

The patient's neck is extended as much as possible by placing a roll transversely behind the shoulders. The release is performed through a transverse incision from one midlateral line to the other. Note that as the neck contracture is released, the point marked at the midlateral line of the neck migrates anteriorly as the wound margins are widened. It is therefore important to continue to extend the incisions latterly until full release of the contracture is apparent. Placement of Y-extensions at the terminal ends of the incision is helpful to provide more release there room and avoid a linear vertical scar at the ends.

An incision above the level of the hyoid risks exposure and possible herniation of the contents of the submandibular triangle making grafting more difficult. Incision directly over the thyroid cartilage risks loss of the central portion of the graft particularly in men due to the constant movement of the cartilage during glutition. Therefore, a transverse incision in the lower third of the neck is usually the most favorable. With the exception of the rare minor broad contracture, the platysma muscle, when present, is also divided and can be undermined slightly to provide a better release.

A simple transverse release in this manner will result in loss of tension of the cervical scars with progressive improvement of the scars over time. However, if the remaining hypertrophic scars are objectionable, these can be excised, but with full knowledge that a greater amount of tissue will have to be transplanted into the neck to obtain optimal release.

My most common donor site for neck contracture releases is the thin skin of the lower abdominal and groin area. Very large grafts can be obtained from this area, and the large donor site still closed. If closure is difficult, the hip can be flexed to allow skin approximation. With a tight closure, an active suction drain should be used in the donor site to eliminate dead space.

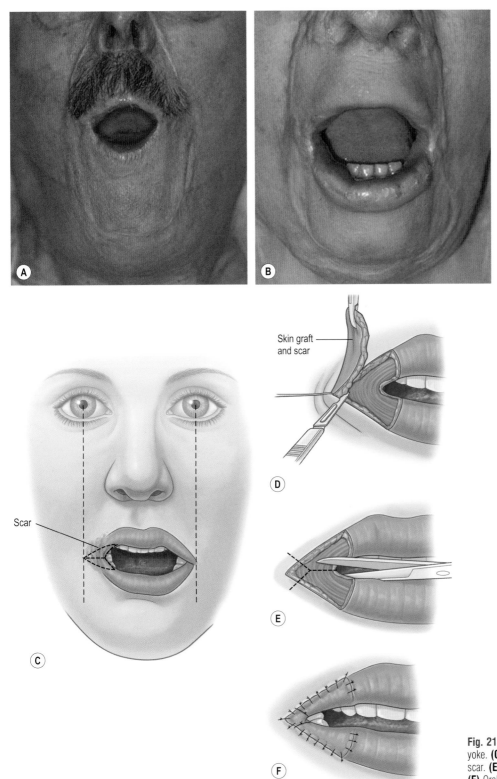

Fig. 21.21 (A) Microstomia. **(B)** Cheek, neck, cheek yoke. **(C)** The scarred commissure. **(D)** Removing the scar. **(E)** Oral mucosa advanced into the defect. **(F)** Oral mucosa sutured in place.

Skin graft and scar

Scar

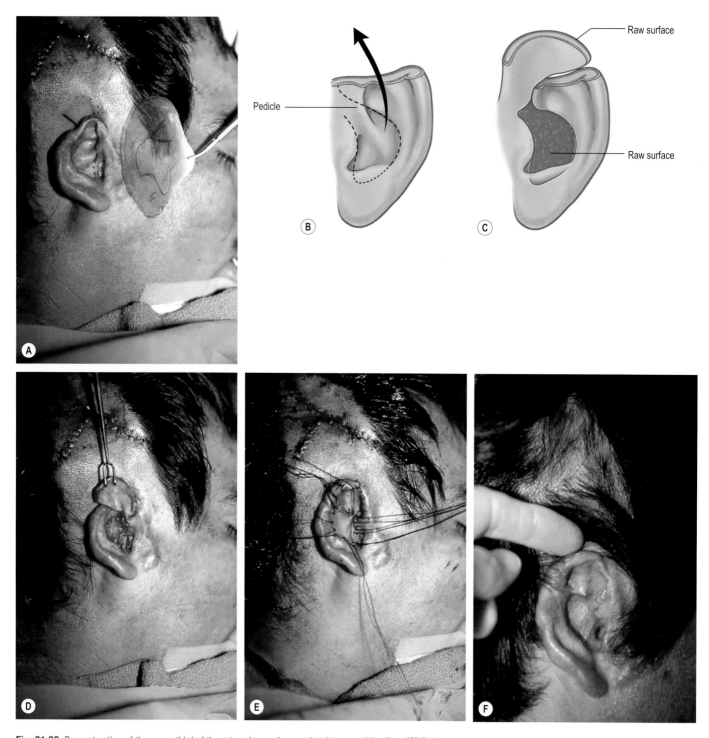

Fig. 21.22 Reconstruction of the upper third of the external ear using a cultural transposition flap. **(A)** Deformed right ear demonstrating absence of upper third compared to pattern from normal left ear. **(B)** Design of conchal flap. **(C)** Elevation and transposition of conchal flap. **(D)** Transposed conchal flap. **(E)** Conchal flap inset. **(F)** Reconstructed ear after a second operation to elevate and skin graft medial to the reconstructed ear upper third.

Postoperative care

Because of the large number of techniques that are represented in the treatment of both acute facial burns and the late effects of facial burns, it is difficult to be too specific in delineating the postoperative care of the various techniques. Most of these techniques are common to other plastic surgery problems, and the discussion of the postoperative care with these techniques is generally better discussed elsewhere. An attempt will be made here to discuss those aspects of postoperative care particularly unique to facial burns.

New split-thickness grafts for acute facial burns, and for the occasional reconstructive resurfacing with sheet split-thickness grafts, are frequently best treated open. The graft vascularizes well, and pressure is generally not necessary for split-thickness grafts. Furthermore, any accumulation of blood or pus can be seen and evacuated through small incisions in the graft preserving graft take in the area. Any conventional dressing wrapped around the face and head is somewhat tenuous, and may disrupt the graft either with the initial placement or when the dressing shifts with patient movement.

Prefabricated compression masks are another option in dressing new split-thickness grafts of the face, particularly when come compression is required as in thick split-thickness grafts *(Fig. 21.2)*. Clear plastic masks have the added advantage of direct examination of the grafted wound.

Sutured facial incisions should be kept fastidiously clean to optimize the final scar and to allow easier suture removal. Generally, facial incisions can be cleaned with soap and water. Application of an antibiotic ointment after cleansing keeps suture line drainage moist to be more easily removed at the next cleaning. Only ophthalmologic antibiotic ointment should be used around the eyes.

Drains, especially negative pressure drains, should be used in flap donor sites to prevent any accumulation of fluid, and to eliminate any dead space that would prevent wound healing. The drains are often left in for a week or more despite the absence of significant drainage simply to hold the tissues together while they heal.

Once new grafts have taken and new reconstructive incisions healed, nonoperative treatment of the new scars described above should be resumed. Use of silicone gel sheeting, compression, and pulsed dye laser are effective in optimizing the new surgical scars. Splints should be used after contracture releases of the neck with full-thickness skin grafts.

Complications

When complications occur the surgeon should be available, concerned, and proactive: available and concerned to minimize the psychological and emotional impact on the patient; and proactive to minimize the physical impact of the complication on the patient's wound and ultimate outcome.

In the management of acute burns, the most common surgical complication is loss of split-thickness skin graft due to infection or inadequate excision. When the areas of skin graft loss are large enough to require re-grafting, it should be done expeditiously with the same goals of shortening total surgical treatment time and minimize scarring. If appropriate donor sites are not available immediately, it is better to cover the recurrent facial wounds with skin allograft than to leave it open or under dressings. Skin allograft placement prevents the development of granulations tissue and minimizes subsequent recurrent scarring.

Since most of burn reconstruction surgery involves the transplantation of tissue as grafts or flaps, the most common problem is loss of that tissue from infection, bleeding, or inadequate blood supply. Again the goal is to minimize the development of hypertrophic scarring and recurrent contracture. Therefore being very proactive to excise the necrotic tissue and provide replacement usually in the form of full-thickness or thick split-thickness skin grafts is the usual rule of thumb.

When recurrent hypertrophic scarring and contracture does occur in reconstructed areas, repeat excision and replacement of tissue, or planing down the scar and split-thickness skin grafting is usually indicated. However, with recurrent scarring, just as in the original burn injury, allowing time for scar maturation to optimize the final result becomes an important consideration.

Problems related to tissue expanders represent other common complications in burn reconstruction. Infection of the tissue expander usually requires removal of the tissue expander with a several month delay before replacing it to avoid recurrent infection. If the infection occurs at the end of expansion, the expanded skin can be used as a flap with control of the infection with systemic antibiotics. The expanded skin cannot be used as a full-thickness skin graft as the skin and underlying wound bed acts as a culture medium during the period of graft avascularity.

Exposure of the tissue expander with opening of the original incision or thinning of the skin over the expander is frequently associated with infection of the expander. First, a judgment has to be made whether the expander is infected. If it is, management as above is indicated. Occasionally, in the absence of infection and if more expansion is necessary to achieve the outcome desired, suspending inflation for one or two weeks may allow skin recovery. If the skin continues to thin during this period, most likely infection is present. In any case, being proactive, available, and concerned continues to be the primary rule of thumb.

Outcomes and prognosis

Unfortunately, good evidence-based support is lacking for most of the techniques used in the treatment of acute facial burns and their late effects. Results in plastic surgery generally are so commonly visual, and almost always subjective, that precise measurements are difficult to obtain. Randomized controlled trials between reconstructive techniques discussed here, for all intents and purposes, do not exist, and other higher order evidence is distinctly rare.

In the facial burn arena, the true outcome of treatment is patient happiness, reintegration into society, and return to pre-injury level of activity and function. This and the prognosis for it usually depends more on psychological and emotional factors, the patient's support system, and the success of psychological, social, and vocational rehabilitation, in addition to the physical rehabilitation through nonoperative and operative means. This emphasizes the importance of optimizing these throughout the treatment of the facial burn injury. Always making sure that the patient has realistic expectations and showing true concern for the patient as an individual with individual needs is exceedingly important.

Secondary procedures

Just as the techniques for the treatment of acute burn injuries should be considered the first operations toward the ultimate reconstruction of the face, all of the surgical techniques for the late effects of burn injuries, or at least those used to correct problems related to the initial skin grafting and other acute procedures, could be considered secondary. However, certain techniques in facial burn reconstruction are clearly necessary only after a primary reconstructive procedure is done.

To a large extent, initial facial reconstructive operations for release of contractures and resurfacing are designed to transplant ample tissue into areas of tissue deficit. Then secondary procedures are performed to refine the tissue into more normal function and appearance. The most common example of this is 'debulking' of flaps secondarily after transplantation. Similarly, tissue transplantation can lead to linear scars that can act as their own contractures, and secondary operations to break up the straight-line scar, such as Z-plasties, are required.

Besides these general techniques, there are specific examples of common secondary procedures in facial reconstruction

In *scalp reconstruction*, even the most well done flaps result in suture lines that are hairless and frequently difficult to conceal. One valuable secondary procedure for this problem is the hair follicle or micrograft transplantation into the hairless scalp scars.

Typically *reconstruction of eyebrows* and other facial hair-bearing areas using hair transplantation is a secondary procedure that is done once the facial skin in the anatomic area is optimally reconstructed.

Residual tightness in the *eyelid reconstructions* frequently requires additional skin graft transplantation. Here, local transposition flaps can be used to achieve optimal eyelid position.[53] Occasionally, release of severe lower eyelid ectropion requiring release of the orbicularis oculi muscle results in an abnormal the transverse sulcus in the lower eyelid. This can be softened and refined using multiple serial Z-plasties.

There are multiple examples of secondary procedures in *nasal reconstruction* particularly with regard to attaining symmetry of the nose after initial reconstruction has been performed. The placement of the nasal alar base, varying the caliber of the nostril openings, release of asymmetrical contractures can be modified by the use of local flaps. (The chapter on secondary revision of the nose in Burget and Menick can be exceedingly helpful.[69])

In median *forehead flap nasal reconstructions*, when possible, not only are secondary procedures to divide the pedicle necessary, but reshaping and debulking the flaps are standard procedures. When turned-down flaps used for alar reconstruction fail to provide adequate length, the operation can be repeated.[58] When excess bulk of the reconstructed nose is present, incisions along the alar margin allow access to the excess scar and soft tissue to allow its direct excision. A wide alar caudal margin can even be thinned by direct excision or using the skin as a banner flap based either at the alar base to be transposed into the nostril or along the nostril sill, or toward the tip where it can be used to augment the columella or release a contracture in the nostril apex.

Reconstruction of the philtrum is clearly a secondary procedure. Reconstruction of the upper lip as a full aesthetic unit results in a broad, flat, contourless upper lip that clearly has an abnormal appearance until it is broken up by, at least, a simulated philtrum. The philtrum is best reconstructed using a composite graft from the triangular fossa of the ear if available *(Fig. 21.20)*.[59]

Frequently, the *reconstructed upper lip* is either tight or too long. The tightness can be improved by reconstruction of the philtrum as the lip is released centrally to reconstruct the philtrum. The length of the reconstructed upper lip can be shortened by transverse advancement of the vermillion after excising the upper lip excess. Occasionally, the upper lip excess can provide banner flaps at the nasal base to correct a nasal or perinasal deformity. The upper lip can be made even more normal appearing by creating the contour of a Cupid's bow as this transverse excision and advancement is performed.[60] In men, hair transplantation is a powerful tool. Not only does it provide normal hair, but it camouflages underlying scars.

Chin implants are commonly placed under burn scarred chins in an effort to correct the perceived flattening of the chin. Careful diagnosis is critical, as a normal chin prominence is usually compressed by tight burn scar. This should only be done secondarily once the lip contracture is completely released, ample skin has been provided, and the option of sculpting a new chin prominence from the burn scar and lower lip has been used (see above).

Once both the *upper lip and lower lip reconstruction* has been performed, bilateral oral commissure release frequently has to be done secondarily, even in the case of having a primary oral commissure release performed previously.

Secondary procedures related to *ear reconstruction* are, for the most part, releases of contractures that provide better appearance and function. The two most common secondary procedures are release of the superior helix to provide a structure on which eyeglasses may rest, and ear lobe reconstructions.

Secondary procedures in *neck reconstruction* generally consist of releases of secondary contractures caused by the reconstructive surgical scars. Any vertically oriented scar on the neck will tend to cause a secondary contracture and remain hypertrophic from persistent tension. Usually properly planned and executed local flap procedures such as Z-plasties will largely correct these problems. Surgeons inexperienced in burn reconstruction will be vexed by the recurrent tightness in extension in adequately released necks. As noted above, this is due to the almost universal contraction to normal anatomic length that happens with all types of the neck reconstructions. Even the most adequately performed release and resurfacing will tend to contract to the normal anatomic position of the neck. This position is midline and between flexion and extension, so that the extremes in extension will always feel tight to the patient. The surgeon should resist the temptation to add additional skin when the patient is comfortable in anatomic position and reasonably comfortable in extension.

The performance of secondary procedures should bring the final outcome of *facial reconstruction* closer to the ultimate, but unobtainable goal of normal appearance and function. One's zeal to reach this goal must be tempered with constant judgment of benefit versus risk. Operate when a result can clearly be improved surgically without substantial risk of unfavorable outcome. Just as in aesthetic surgery, one must learn to say 'no' to those burn survivors who seek unrealistic perfection and feel that further surgery offers it.

Access the complete reference list online at http://www.expertconsult.com

2. McIndoe AH. Total reconstruction of the burned face. The Bradshaw Lecture 1958. *Br J Plast Surg.* 1983;36(4):410–420.

8. Cole JK, Engrav LH, Heimbach DM, et al. Early excision and grafting of face and neck burns in patients over 20 years. *Plast Reconstr Surg.* 2002;109(4):1266–1273.

   This is the definitive description of what is considered the current standard for excisional therapy of acute facial burns.

12. Engrav LH, Donelan MB. Acute care and reconstruction of facial burns. In: Mathes SJ, ed. *Plastic Surgery.* Philadelphia: Saunders Elsevier; 2006:45–76.

25. Spence RJ. An algorithm for total and subtotal facial reconstruction using an expanded transposition flap: a 20-year experience. *Plast Reconstr Surg.* 2008;121(3):795–805.

40. Hyakusoku H, Ogawa R, Mizuno H. Super-thin flap. In: Hyakusoku H, Orgill DP, Teot L, et al, eds. *Color Atlas of Burn Reconstructive Surgery.* Heidelberg: Springer; 2010:356–367.

   This book is the most up-to-date reference for the specifics of facial burn wound management and facial burn reconstructive surgery.

45. Zide BM, Karp NS. Maximizing gain from rectangular tissue expanders. *Plast Reconstr Surg.* 1992;90(3):500–506.

57. Burget G, Menick FJ. *Aesthetic Reconstruction of the Nose.* St Louis, MO: Mosby; 1994.

   The entire book is excellent for the aesthetic reconstruction of the nose, and has a particularly interesting chapter with a wealth of information and innovations for small revisions in and around the nose.

58. Taylor HO, Carty M, Driscoll D, et al. Nasal reconstruction after severe facial burns using a local turndown flap. *Ann Plast Surg.* 2009;62(2):175–179.

63. Donelan MB. Conchal transposition flap for postburn ear deformities. *Plast Reconstr Surg.* 1989;83(4):641–654.

   A very good description of the most common procedure done for one of the most common problems in burn damaged ears.

66. Feldman J. Facial burns. In: McCarthy J, ed. *Plastic Surgery.* Philadelphia: WB Saunders; 1990:2196–2197.

   This chapter is encyclopedic in its overview of concepts and techniques in facial burn treatment, and remains a wealth of useful information despite being two decades old.

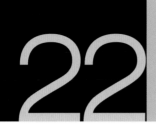

Reconstructive burn surgery

Matthew B. Klein

SYNOPSIS

- Improvements in burn survival have shifted the focus of burn care and research towards long-term outcomes. Accordingly, reconstructive burn surgery has become an increasingly relevant topic in the care of the burn patient.
- Burn reconstructive surgery seeks to restore both form and function lost to burn injury and relies on many of the basic principles of plastic surgery.
- Timing of reconstructive procedures is contingent not only on the readiness and impact of a particular scar or wound but also on the psychological preparedness of the patient.
- The majority of secondary burn defects are due to scarring and contracture. To correct deformities, scar release is necessary and then appropriate coverage is obtained from skin grafts or flaps – either local or distant.
- A postoperative plan that incorporates critical aspects of splinting and range of motion is needed to optimize outcome.

 Access the Historical Perspective sections online at
http://www.expertconsult.com

Introduction

Advances in critical care and surgical management have significantly improved survival following burn injury. In fact, survival following even severe burn injury has become the rule rather than the exception. Accordingly, there is increasing emphasis being placed on long-term outcomes following burn injury and reconstructive surgery for burn survivors has become an increasingly relevant topic in burn care.[1] Burn reconstruction refers to the numerous and varied procedures performed on healed wounds or skin grafts. The overall goal of burn reconstruction is to improve both the appearance and function of the person who sustained a burn injury. These procedures should never be considered "cosmetic" – they are

reconstructive as they seek to restore that which has been lost to injury.

Burn reconstructive surgery, as much as anything else in plastic surgery, requires a principled approach. The surgeon must accurately diagnose the problem including which types of tissue are deficient; identify which tissue is available for reconstruction, and then formulate a rational plan based on these findings. Limited availability of healthy tissue poses one of the greatest challenges in burn reconstructive surgery, as many burn patients, particularly those with extensive burn injuries, will have limited donor site availability for skin, subcutaneous tissue and, on occasion, muscle.

Timing of reconstructive procedures

The timing of reconstructive procedures vary; they could occur relatively early in the post-injury period (i.e., weeks), years or even decades, following injury. By and large, surgery on burn scars should typically occur once the scar has matured. The scar maturation process can take up to 1 year or longer. Allowing scars to fully mature could reduce or, in some cases, eliminate the need for burn reconstructive procedures altogether. As a general rule, the body should be given every chance to try and improve on its own without surgery. There are certain exceptions to waiting for scar maturation to occur including severe debilitating early contractures, severe eyelid contractures, unstable wounds and exposed vital structures.

There are several critical prerequisites that need to be met prior to embarking on any reconstructive endeavor. First and foremost, the patient must want the procedure performed and be psychologically prepared for the procedure. Unlike acute surgeries which may be life-saving, reconstructive procedures are usually elective and many patients may not be readily prepared to undergo more surgeries and to comply with postoperative splinting, garment wearing and the rigorous exercise regimens needed to achieve optimal results. In addition, many patients may not be psychologically ready to come back into the hospital for an inpatient stay. Children must also be included in the surgery decision-making process. Favorable outcome will require children to cooperate with postoperative plans and, therefore, in the cases of school-age children and adolescents, we make an effort to ensure that the patients themselves want a procedure and it is not just the desire of the parents. The cooperation of the child in terms of wearing splints, garments and performing physical therapy is critical to the success of reconstructive procedures and if the child does not want to have surgery performed, there is a high risk of poor postoperative compliance.

It is also critical that patients have realistic expectations regarding what can be achieved with reconstructive surgery. Many patients come to the burn clinic wanting their scars removed as soon as possible and many may have the unrealistic expectation that defects can be easily and rapidly fixed – that scars can simply be "erased". Expectation-reality matching must be achieved and the concept that scars cannot simply be erased must be clearly articulated. It is also crucial to explain to patients that several procedures are often needed in order to address all reconstructive needs. When possible, procedures should be grouped, yet this needs to be done cautiously. For example, a procedure that requires early mobilization of a joint, such as a capsulotomy or capsulectomy, should not be performed at the same time as a procedure that might require immobilization of an adjacent joint. Similarly, performing procedures on either both upper or lower limbs simultaneously should be avoided, so the patient will still be able to provide self-care following surgery. Unfortunately, there are deformities for which there may be no good reconstructive options or that the risks involved in a procedure may exceed the potential benefit. This too must be explained clearly to the patient but an effort should also be made to provide some hope that new techniques or technologies may one day provide a solution.

Hypertrophic scars and contractures

Hypertrophic scarring remains the most significant source of pain, discomfort, and misery for burn survivors and constitutes the chief complaint of the majority of patients seeking burn reconstruction *(Fig. 22.1)*. Despite the frequent occurrence of these scars – estimated to be as high as over 50% – still little is known about the causative factors and, therefore, a cure or effective prevention strategy remains elusive. Risk factors for hypertrophic scarring include delay in wound closure, infection and race (i.e., patients with pigmented skin are believed to be at higher risk of forming hypertrophic scar).[2] There have been several proposed prevention and treatment strategies for hypertrophic scars, including steroids, oral anti-inflammatory agents, pressure garments and silicon, and all have been reported to have varying levels of effectiveness. Steroid injection into scars and topical silicon sheeting can be used during the period of scar maturation to alleviate symptoms of pain and itch and potentially improve scar appearance. However, scar injection may be difficult to perform in children and is seldom useful for broad areas of hypertrophic scar.

Wound contraction is a natural process that occurs in all healing tissues and in all skin grafts. The amount of contraction may vary based on thickness of tissue (i.e., full thickness

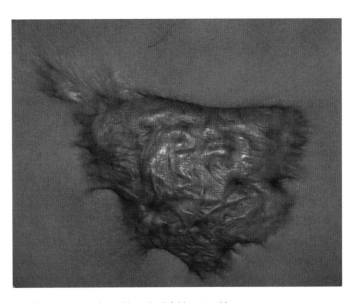

Fig. 22.1 Raised, red, pruritic and painful hypertrophic scar.

skin grafts contract less than split thickness grafts due to the presence of more dermis). Contractures result when contraction occurs over a mobile joint and leads to functional compromise; they are negative sequelae of the natural process of contraction and often require surgical correction. Contractures can involve the skin as well as underlying tissues such as muscle and tendons. Limited contractures may be overcome with aggressive range of motion and splint immobilization. However, more significant contractures will require release and subsequent grafting or flap coverage. Even after contracture releases, patients must be aware that prolonged periods of intense range of motion exercises is required as is the use of splints in order to prevent the recurrence of contractures.

Other burn injury complications can be due to mismatch in color (hypopigmentation or hyperpigmentation), texture and hair loss as well as problems of chronic pain, itch and temperature regulation.

Overview of techniques for reconstructive surgery

Scar release

Contracture release is usually achieved by incising the scar band at its point of maximal tension. Given that contracture bands typically exist in a sea of surrounding scar, full release requires incision beyond the scar band itself. In addition, in the axilla and eyelids, we typically include a superior and inferior dart at either end of the scar incision line in order disrupt the scar pull. The incision should be carried down through the scar to healthy appearing tissue. In some cases, release of the subcutaneous tissue and muscle fascia may also be required to achieve full release. This is often the case in the neck and axilla. Long-standing deformities of the digits may also require tenolysis or, in some cases, tendon lengthening or transection, as well as joint capsule release. The surgeon must be aware of the potential need to divide these underlying structures and challenges in covering the subsequent defect, since skin grafting is not possible on exposed tendon, bone and joint.

In some cases, total scar excision is necessary and practical. This is particularly true for smaller or discrete areas of scar. There are two general approaches to scar excision: intralesional and extralesional. When performing intralesional excision, a rim of scar is left in the wound and subsequently closed. The purported benefit of intralesional excision is that there will be no new tissue injury – the incision is made through previously scarred tissue only and therefore the process of scar formation has already occurred in this tissue and is unlikely to recur (*Fig. 22.2*). This is in contradistinction to extralesional excision, in which the incision is made in the healthy tissue surrounding the scar so the entire scar can be removed. The relative risks and benefits of each approach should be discussed with the patient prior to surgery. Many scars are too large to be removed in one setting and often require several "serial" excisions. We typically wait 8–12 months between serial excisions in order that the tissue can sufficiently heal and soften so that it can be optimally mobilized again to achieve closure.

Wound closure

Plastic surgeons often utilize the reconstructive ladder as a way to approach reconstructive procedures. The ladder represents a list of procedures from simple to more complex for surgical management and forms an appropriate framework for approaching burn reconstructive procedures. Below is a discussion of the most common approaches to wound closure.

Skin grafts

Skin grafts remain the workhorse coverage for burn deformities – particularly because the defect in most cases resulted from the loss of skin. Ideally, thicker grafts are utilized following contracture release because the more dermis present in a graft the less contraction that occurs during the healing process. Full thickness grafts are generally reserved for small areas on the hand and face, so the full thickness skin graft donor site can be closed primarily. The use of tissue expansion of unburned areas of skin to generate larger full thickness skin grafts is also possible for larger areas such as the face and neck. It is important to take full inventory of available donor sites in the outpatient clinic prior to operation, so one is aware what tissues are available and the patient is aware of from where the skin graft will be harvested. I will often ask the patient's input on donor site selection if there are multiple options. It is also necessary to ration donor sites appropriately based on the need for other potential procedures. For example, we will reserve the scalp if we anticipate needing to graft large areas on the face.

Skin substitutes

Skin substitutes – particularly dermal substitutes – have been used in the management of both acute burn wounds and burn reconstruction. The use of dermal substitutes is particularly useful when there are limited donor sites available. Given the general preference to use thicker skin grafts with more dermis to minimize contraction and recurrent contracture, dermal substitutes offer the potential advantage of augmenting native graft dermis. However, there are drawbacks to the use of skin substitutes including infection risk and usually the need for more than one surgical procedure – one for application of the material and the second for skin grafting following a period of time to allow for adequate vascularization.

Local flaps

There exists a veritable alphabet soup of local tissue rearrangement flap options that have been described, including Z-plasty, Y-V-plasty, V-Y-plasty and W-plasty. Each has its distinctive geometric properties, as well as relative benefits. We most commonly use Z-plasties (*Fig. 22.3*) and Y-V-plasties to address scar bands (*Fig. 22.4*). It is critical to understand that these procedures are most appropriate for scar lengthening and are not the solution to all reconstructive problems. Areas with even moderate degrees of missing tissue will be inadequately addressed by a Z-plasty and require the addition of soft tissue either in the form of a skin graft or a flap. The principal drawback to Z-plasty use is that transposition and advancement of the Z-limbs requires extensive undermining and this often means undermining scar that can result in partial flap ischemia. For this reason, in many cases we prefer

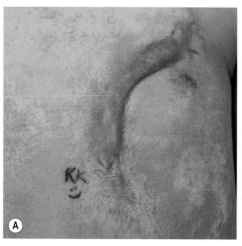
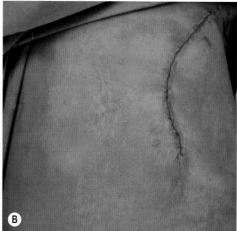

Fig. 22.2 (A) Hypertrophic scar of the chest **(B)** treated by extra-lesional incision.

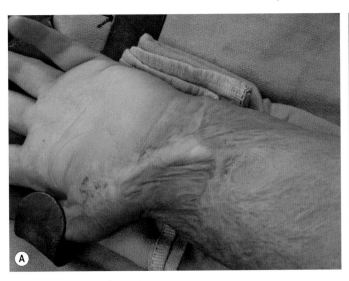
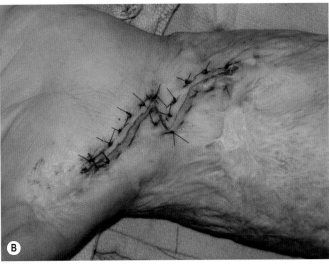

Fig. 22.3 (A,B) A Z-plasty used following excision of a scar band on the hand and wrist. Following scar excision, the Z-plasty is used to disrupt the linear band.

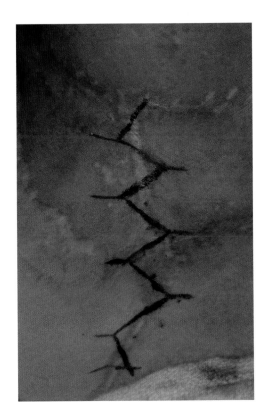

Fig. 22.4 Design of a Y-V plasty for release and reorientation of vertical neck scar band.

coverage following contracture release or for lining of facial structures such as the nose. Muscle flaps are particularly useful for areas with significant contour deformity that require bulky soft tissue. Muscle flaps are also useful for breast reconstruction (as described below) and to cover chronically exposed joints.

Tissue expansion

Tissue expansion is a useful technique for wound closure in areas where primary closure is difficult to achieve and there is insufficient tissue for local flaps. Tissue expansion is particularly useful for reconstruction of the head and neck, where the use of 'like' tissue can significantly enhance the surgical outcome. Tissue expansion is also the most effective method for treating large areas of burn alopecia, as explained below in the discussion of scalp reconstruction. There are several important caveats to tissue expansion. First, there must be adequate healthy tissue available to undergo expansion. Scarred wounds and grafts are not good candidates for expansion. In addition, expansion of distal extremities has been reported to be associated with significant high rates of expander extrusion and other complications. Patients must also be prepared to come to the clinic on a weekly basis of the course of several weeks or months to undergo expansion and children must be able to be still enough to cooperate with the filling of the expanders.

to use Y-V plasties because they require minimal flap undermining in order to achieve the desired advancement.

Other flaps

Axial flaps, fascial flaps and muscle flaps (both pedicled and free) can be used for wound closure. Fascial flaps such as the radial forearm flap are very useful for providing thin pliable

Specific reconstructive problems and procedures

The principles presented above provide a useful foundation for the evaluation and treatment of burn patients. Below we provide a description of the most common deformities and their treatments by anatomic area.

Head and neck

Scalp

Burn alopecia results from deep burns of the scalp. Clearly, acute burns that are excised and grafted are incapable of hair growth and wounds that are deep and heal spontaneously may also become areas of alopecia. There are two general options for addressing burn alopecia: serial excision and tissue expansion. Serial excision of is effective for smaller areas of alopecia that may be eliminated in two or three procedures. Larger areas typically require tissue expansion of remaining hair-bearing scalp *(Fig. 22.5)*. Significant alopecia (more than half of the scalp) may require more than one tissue expander treatment. It is important to note that tissue expansion requires a significant commitment on the part of the patient and his or her family. Expansion usually occurs over the period of several weeks to months. In addition, expanders placed under areas of scar may also be subject to infection or exposure. We typically do not perform expansion in infants and toddlers due to the potential difficulties children have with cooperation both with the installation of fluid and with avoiding activity that may lead to injury to the head and expander rupture. Often for children with extensive alopecia not yet candidates for expanders, we will begin by performing serial excisions in order to begin to reduce the burden of alopecia. As a general rule, if alopecia can be removed in its entirety (or enough that hair can cover small areas of alopecia) in two operations, it makes sense to perform serial excision and not tissue expansion since the expander process will in and of itself require two procedures (one for placement of the expanders and one for removal of the expanders).

Facial defects

Acute and reconstructive burn surgery of the face is probably the most challenging aspect of burn care. The results of facial burns are integral to appearance and feelings of self-esteem and simultaneously may be the most difficult to completely correct. The most common facial burn deformities are described below along with the most common and effective approaches for their management.

Eyelids and eyebrows

Eyelid deformities following facial burns occur quite commonly. Eyelid position can be impacted not only by eyelid burns themselves – with loss of skin or other lid structures – but also from scarring of the cheeks and forehead. Cicatricial ectropion can result from the downward pull on the lid from a scarred cheek or the upward pull of the upper lid from a contracting forehead wound. When evaluating the patient with lid deformity, one must assess the ability of the patient to close the lids completely in order to adequately protect the underlying conjunctiva and globe. Inability to adequately protect the globe is one of the few indications for early reconstructive surgery. It is important to note that minimal lid deformities may indeed improve over time with massage and scar maturation.

Surgical correction of ectropion requires scar release and subsequent skin grafting. In order to place the lids on maximal stretch and account for the invariable contraction that occurs with all grafts regardless of their thickness, silk traction sutures are placed in the lid margin. With gentle traction on the sutures a subciliary incision is made and lid release is then achieved *(Fig. 22.6)*. A template of the resulting defect is then made and skin grafts – typically full thickness – are used to fill the defect. Ideally, skin from the supraclavicular region is used to optimize graft color match with the remainder of the face but these donor sites may not be available in the case of extensive head and neck burns. Alternatively, full thickness grafts can be harvested from other locations in the body such as the inguinal region, flank or inner upper arm. The traction sutures are generally left in place for 5 days postoperatively and the graft is immobilized using a tie-over bolster. More recently, we have begun performing a lateral

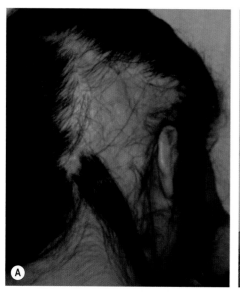
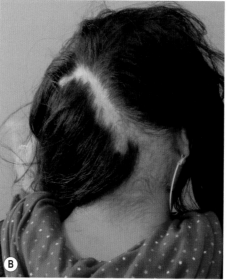
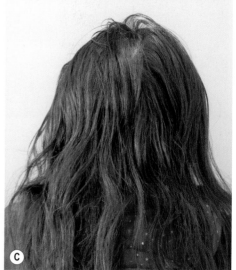

Fig. 22.5 (A) Young woman with burn alopecia, **(B)** treated with two tissue expanders. Following removal of expanders the hair-baring scalp was advanced posteriorly and laterally to reduce the area of alopecia **(C)**, so that hair could completely cover the scar.

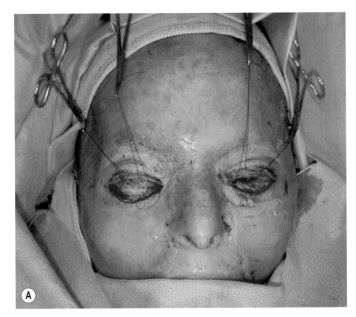

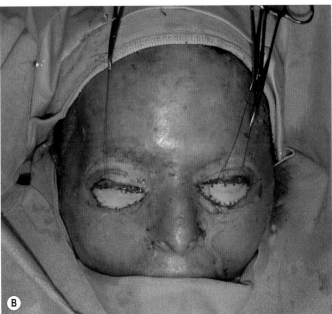

Fig. 22.6 (A) Ectropion release of the lower eyelid with silk traction sutures in place. **(B)** Following placement of full thickness skin graft.

scalp hair follicles. When reconstructing the brow care must be taken to ensure that the hairs are placed in the correct orientation for the eyebrow. Patients need to be advised that transplanted hair may grow and require intermittent trimming. Other patients will elect to have eyebrows permanently tattooed in lieu of surgery.

Nose and lips

Defects of the nose can be quite challenging. The most common deformity is alar retraction – essentially a scar contracture of the alar rim. The most effective way to deal with this deformity is to perform composite grafting of skin and cartilage. The external nasal scar can be incised and used as nasal lining and then a composite graft (typically from the ear) can be placed. More complex nasal deformities include a shortened tip and wide appearing nasal dorsum. In fact, severe facial scar contracture nasal in children can deform the nasal bones require nasal osteotomies to reposition the bones and narrow the dorsum once young adulthood is reached. Taylor et al. recently described a scar revision technique utilizing an inferior based nasal turndown flap to address the common nasal deformities including the widened dorsum.[4]

Subtotal or total destruction of the nose may require total nasal reconstruction including replacement of lining, support and skin cover. Basic principles for total nasal reconstruction need to be followed, however, it is rare that the remainder of the face has sufficient healthy tissue available to use for reconstruction. In these cases distant tissue, including microvascular free flaps, can be used to provide both lining and skin cover. One must also consider nasal prostheses either as a temporary measure until the patient is physically and psychologically prepared for a series of extensive reconstructive procedures or even as a permanent treatment.

There are several common lip deformities following burn injury including upper and lower lip ectropion, microstomia, loss of the philtral columns and dimple and loss of the mental crease. Ectropion of the lips is generally treated by release of the scar and full thickness skin grafts. However, in the case of lower lip ectropion, if there is also a severe neck contracture this may need to be addressed prior to the lip as described below. When performing lip release, we again use silk traction sutures (as with the eyelids) in order to get the lips on full stretch. These sutures remain in place for 5 days following surgery.

Commissuroplasty is used to address burn microstomia. The appropriate location of the commissure is identified by drawing a line from the medial limbus down to the lip. A triangle of scar can then be removed with the apex at the point of the medial limbus and then a flap of oral mucosa is advanced outward to close the defect and recreate the commissure. The philtrum itself can be recreated by using a skin graft the shape of the philtrum, or using a philtral-shaped cartilage graft. Philtral reconstruction can be performed simultaneously with the remainder of the upper lip or (more preferably) at a second operation once adequate lip length is established.

Ears

Ear deformities can vary from relatively small problems with simple solutions such as adherence of the ear to the mastoid, to complex problems such as severe cartilage deficiency with significant deformity. In cases of adherence of the ear to the

canthopexy in cases of severe ectropion in order to provide additional support for the lid and prevent the occurrence of recontracture.

Another common lid deformity is the medial canthal web. In fact when both the lids and nose require grafting some webbing invariably develops. We treat these webs by either Y-V plasty along the length of the web or a double-opposing Z-plasty. Both procedures disrupt and reorient the scar band in this area and tend to be highly effective.

A portion or the entirety of the eyebrow may be missing following a deep face burn. There have been several techniques described for addressing missing eyebrows including the use of strip grafts of the scalp (as described by Brent[3]), island flaps from the temporal scalp and micrografting of

mastoid area or lack of ear projection, the adherence can be divided and a full thickness skin graft placed to elevate the ear and achieve optimal angle with the scalp. A bolster is needed to secure the graft and we typically have patients keep a custom silicon block over the graft for several months to prevent the ear from losing the projection created at surgery. Cases of extensive ear deformity can be more challenging. The use of cartilage grafts to recreate the helix can be performed but typically there is a lack of adequate soft tissue coverage since the adjacent skin, including the temporoparietal region, may also be scarred. Use of autologous cartilage or Medpor implants to recreate the entire ear scaffold may be similarly difficult and impractical for the same reason, i.e., lack of adequate soft tissue coverage. Therefore, in cases of extensive ear deformity a prosthesis, either partial or complete, should be considered.

Other facial areas

Defects on the cheeks may vary from small patches of hypertrophic scar to large areas of scar that may engulf the entire cheek subunit. It is rare that a successfully grafted area on the cheek develops hypertrophic scar, however there may be small areas of scar where graft loss occurred or at the juncture of another graft or an ungrafted area. These small areas can be treated with excision and primary closure, however larger patches of hypertrophic scar will require excision and grafting or tissue expansion of local uninjured skin. Prior to excision of large areas of scar, the patient should be counseled that a prolonged period of pressure garments/facial mask may be needed in order to minimize the recurrence of hypertrophic scar. Spence provides a useful approach to reconstruction of the entire face, including the cheek regions.[5] He has had a great deal of success by utilizing tissue expanders in the shoulder/scapula region and using this tissue to resurface large areas of the face.

Neck

Neck contractures are one of the most common complications of burn injury and can significantly compromise function – both neck range of motion and oral competence – and be highly disfiguring. Neck reconstructive surgery has two distinct components: scar release and wound closure. Adequate scar release is essential to preventing recurrent contracture. In order to facilitate complete release, patients are placed in the operating room in a position of neck hyperextension, usually by placing either a towel roll or foam under the back. We create a foam wedge that places the position in the optimal position of hyperextension and then place this wedge on the patient's bed postoperatively so we are sure to maintain the desired position of hyperextension in the first week following surgery. Complete release requires division of the scar which may extend through the layer of the platysma. In cases where the platysma is not involved we will divide anyway in order to disrupt the connections between the neck and the face (the platysma continues in the face as the SMAS). Once full release is achieved, selection of appropriate tissue for wound closure is needed. A number of different approaches to neck contracture management have been described including use of grafts, skin substitutes and free tissue transfer. Our preference is to utilize Integra (Integra LifeSciences, Plainsboro, NJ) skin substitute along with a thick split thickness graft (if a donor site

is available). This requires a two-stage operation: first, for placement of the Integra, and then return to the operating room 2–3 weeks later for autografting once the Integra has adequately vascularized. There have been a number of papers in the literature advocating the use of free tissue transfers to minimize contracture recurrence. However, these are often bulky and rather than restore the natural contour of the neck, obscure the cervical mental angle. In patients who have severe neck contractures along with lower lip contractures we will address the neck contracture first, and once healed then proceed with lip reconstruction. Given the fact that the neck scar is frequently in continuity with the lip scar, treating the neck will often alter (even reduce) what needs to be done for the lip.

Breast reconstruction

Breast deformities can vary from the presence of small areas of hypertrophic scar to missing nipple-areola complex to complete amastia. Burned breast reconstruction can be quite challenging and require multiple procedures staged over several years. Breast development can be impacted by both injury to the breast bud in young girls and to surrounding scar that may restrict breast growth. As soon as bulging on the chest occurs suggestive of breast development, scar release and grafting of the chest should be performed to try and provide adequate compliance to allow breast growth. In the cases of unilateral amastia, one should wait to perform breast reconstruction until the contralateral breast growth is complete so that symmetry can be established. Prior to reconstruction with expanders and implants, an initial scar release and grafting procedure may be necessary to allow for tissue expansion to occur. Given the lack of soft tissue, submuscular expander, and subsequent implant, placement is required. Autologous tissue breast reconstruction options can be utilized depending on the availability of healthy tissue including latissimus dorsi and rectus-muscle based flap reconstructions. Nipple-areola reconstruction should be deferred until breast mound reconstruction is complete and the scars matured so that long-term positioning can be more predictable. Reconstruction of the areola can be achieved as has been described for other cases of acquired amastia including utilizing tattooing or skin graft from another area in the body. However, nipple reconstruction with local tissue flaps such as the skate flap may be challenging given the fragility of scar or grafted tissue. Therefore alternative approaches are need such as composite grafts that include cartilage (such as from the ear) or use of fat or other fillers. Split nipple grafts from the contralateral breast, if unburned, is another potential option.

Perineum

Webbing of the perineum can create difficulties for ambulation as well as hygiene. Early release is often necessary in cases of severe perianal webs or bands. These can be treated with release and grafting or in less severe cases with Z-plasty or other form of local tissue rearrangement. Contracture of the labia and the scrotum typically occur from webbing in the inguinal region and is treated by release and skin grafting. Contractures of the penile shaft can be managed as contractures elsewhere in the body, by release and skin grafting. Total phallus or scrotal reconstruction can be performed using any number of the techniques that have been described for other indications with the caveat that there may be limited suitable local tissue.

Upper extremity

The upper extremity, and the hand in particular, is commonly involved in burn injury and therefore frequently requires reconstructive procedures.

Axilla

Axillary contractures occur quite commonly and often require full release with skin grafting to be treated adequately. It is very important that prior to performing any reconstructive procedures that the patient has plateaued on range of motion progress. Often, the more range of motion a patient has pre-operatively, the better the results from surgery. In addition, the patient must be prepared to continue maximal range of motion exercises following release. While it may be attractive to perform Z-plasties or Y-V plasties on axillary bands, it is more likely that there is a deficiency of tissue that requires skin grafting. Rarely is adequate improvement possible with only a Z-plasty. Many patients have multiple bands – including one along the anterior as well as the posterior axillary folds. It is our practice to incise across all of these bands to achieve a full release. This typically leaves a large defect that is skin grafted with an intermediate to thick split thickness skin graft. The graft typically needs to be dressed with a bolster dressing given the significant concavity that results following release. We typically immobilize the patient for 5 days postoperatively and then begin a range of motion therapy at that point. Splinting then continues at night for the next several months.

If there is healthy tissue (i.e., not scarred) posterior or anterior to the axilla, a transposition flap can be used to fill the defect (*Fig. 22.7*). This flap can be a random skin and fascia flap or a scapular or parascapular axial flap can be used. When performing local tissue rearrangement around the axilla it is important to avoid moving hair-bearing tissue into an undesired area.

Elbow

Contracture of the elbow can occur secondary to scarring on the dorsal aspect of the forearm and upper arm or from scarring along the antecubital fossa – or both. Contracture release can be performed as described above with the resulting defects covered with thick split thickness skin grafts. For discrete bands local tissue rearrangement with Z-plasty or Y-V plasty can be considered, but as with the axilla, most significant defects are due to a deficiency of skin and require full release with subsequent grafting. Chronic ulcers over the elbow occur from deep burns over this area and likely represent failure to achieve adequate stable coverage. These ulcers often are difficult to close by skin grafting and may require flap coverage local fascial flaps from the forearm or upper arm (i.e., radial forearm fascial flap or lateral arm flap). Heterotopic ossification (HO) of the elbow is a severe complication of

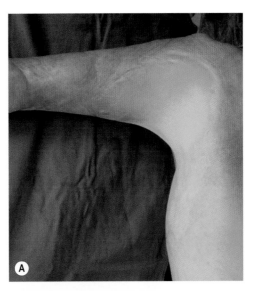
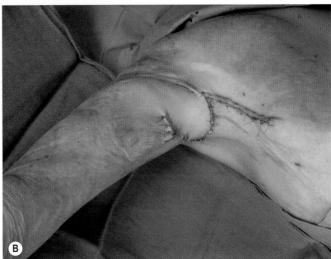

Fig. 22.7 (A) Axillary contracture prior to and **(B)** following release and closure with local transposition flap.

upper extremity injury and can be quite debilitating. HO results from the abnormal formation of lamellar bone around the elbow joint and has been associated with a prolonged time to elbow wound coverage. A number of pharmacologic agents have been used to treat HO but with variable results. Surgical correction is often required and may require extensive dissection of the elbow joint, including cubital tunnel release.[6] Aggressive postoperative range is then necessary so that operative gains can be maintained.

Wrist and hand

There are a number of burn injury complications that occur in the hand and wrist that can have substantial impact on function. Areas of hypertrophic scar can be excised and closed primarily or grafted as described above. Contractures that disrupt function can prove more challenging and often involve scarring and damage to underlying structures (*Fig. 22.8*).

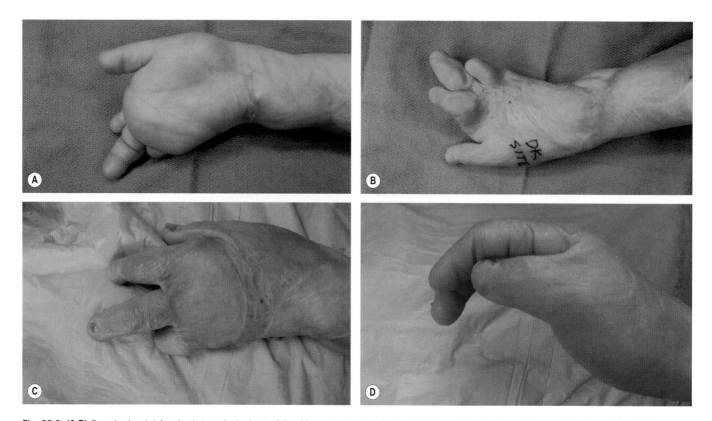

Fig. 22.8 (A,B) Complex hand deformity that required release of the skin contracture, tenolysis and joint capsulotomies in order to reposition the wrist and digits. **(C,D)** Patient is shown here 3 months following releases and skin graft.

Wrist

Wrist contractures occur more commonly on the wrist dorsum and are treated with release and skin grafting as described above for other joints. However, in cases of severe contracture, scarring of the extensor tendons may also be contributing to the defect. In these cases tenolysis is required. If the resulting defect is not able to be grafted (due to exposure of tendons or bone), then flap coverage is needed either with a local flap (radial forearm or posterior interosseus flap), pedicled flap (from abdominal wall or groin), or free flap.

Digit contractures

Flexion contractures of the digits require division (and in some cases excision) of the scar band and subsequent full thickness skin grafts. Long-standing digital contractures may also benefit from temporary (3–4 weeks) k-wire placement to maintain the digit in adequate position following release and graft placement. Again, it is important to avoid the temptation of performing only a Z-plasty or V-Y plasty on digital scar bands. If there is indeed a joint contracture, then there is likely a significant deficit in tissue that can only be addressed by the provision of additional tissue in the form of a graft. Flexion contractures of the PIP joints can occur from flexion contracture bands as well as from an initial injury to the extensor mechanism of the digit. The burn claw deformity results when the PIP joint flexion contracture leads to hyperextension of the metacarpophalangeal joints. These defects can be quite challenging to reconstruct given the lack of stable dorsal skin coverage. Tendon and joint reconstruction are therefore rarely feasible options. Rather, PIP joint arthrodesis should be considered as this would provide stable, durable joint positioning. If extensor tendon reconstruction or arthroplasty is to be carried out then flap coverage will likely be necessary. MP joint stiffness can often be treated by extensive capsulectomy.

Severe contractures may also warrant amputation. This is particularly true of the fifth digit where patients often feel the digit 'gets in the way' of performing daily tasks.

Web space contractures

Perhaps the most common burn reconstructive procedure performed is web space contracture release. All four web spaces are prone to contracture and when this occurs there can be a significant impact on range of motion and hand function. The thumb-index web is typically involved and usually most impacts hand function. This is another area where one may be tempted to perform a Z-plasty but typically if there is functional limitation (particularly for thumb-index webs), then the defect in skin is significant enough to require a skin graft. Contracture release requires an incision through the scar band and often several centimeters both palmar and dorsally. These defects are then closed using a full thickness skin graft usually from the inguinal region if available. Deformities of the other web spaces are typically less severe and can be addressed in mild cases with a Z-plasty or double opposing Z-plasty or, in more severe cases, with a full thickness skin graft.

Nail deformities

Deformities of the nail and nail bed are frequently seen in cases of very deep hand burns. Nail deformities can be unsightly and be quite painful. One of the most defects results from eponychial retraction and exposure of the proximal nail. Donelan and Garcia described a procedure wherein a bipedicled flap is created on the dorsum of the digit and advanced distally to recreate the fold and then the donor site is skin grafted.[7] This relatively technically simple procedure provides predictable positive results including pain relief.

Lower extremity

Lower extremity defects typically occur around the knee, foot, and ankle. Posterior thigh/leg scar bands and contracture can limit range of motion of the knee, impact ambulation and result in hip pain if gait is significantly affected. The most common contractures are due to posterior thigh/leg bands that extend across the popliteal fossa. These are best treated with release and skin grafting followed by at least one week of knee immobilization in the extended position.

Defects of the foot and ankle similarly often require scar release and grafting with thick split thickness skin grafts. Similar to the digits, the toe contractures are often difficult to correct particularly if they are longstanding. In order to restore the toes to proper position the extensor tendons may need to be sacrificed. If they are transected this typically does not interfere with ambulation. Consideration of temporary k-wire placement in the toes should be done in order to help keep the toes in the desired position and left in place for 3–4 weeks. Postoperatively, the toes should be maintained in slight plantar flexion.

Postoperative management: splints, pressure garments and rehabilitation

Regardless of the elegance and technical success of a reconstructive procedure a good ultimate outcome will be based on an effective postoperative plan that incorporates the principles of rehabilitation. Typically, following contracture release, immobilization occurs for the first 5–7 days postoperatively to allow for adequate healing to occur. During this period, patients are immobilized in a position that optimizes function which may or may not be a position that optimizes comfort. For example, the axilla will be splinted in ≥100° of shoulder abduction, the neck in mild hyperextension, and the eyelids will be kept on maximal stretch with traction sutures. Once graft/flap take has been achieved mobilization occurs. While physical and occupational therapists are of incredible value in helping patients achieve maximal function it is critical for patients to be instructed on range of motion exercises and be encouraged to perform them multiple times a day; not just when in therapy sessions. We will typically utilize splints for weeks to months following contracture release to minimize contracture recurrence. Patients are instructed to remove the splints for range of motion exercises but then to replace them. It is common that splints will need to be adjusted or remade during the scar maturation process and patients are therefore encouraged to bring splints with them to each clinic visit.

Custom-made pressure garments have long been used to minimize the risk of or to treat areas of scar hypertrophy. Garments are typically worn 23 h/day and removed only for cleaning of the patient and the garments. Garment wearing begins once wounds are closed and continues until scars are fully mature. Despite the widespread use of pressure garments over many years, their effectiveness in reducing scar formation has yet to be definitively demonstrated. In fact, there have been small-scale clinical studies which demonstrate little or no risk in scar formation.[8] However, patients do report that garments are helpful in providing vascular support, reducing itching as well as reducing pain. Garments can be uncomfortable for patients, particularly during times of warm weather. Silicon liners or inserts can be placed underneath garments to provide additional pressure over specific areas when needed.

Outcomes

The field of burn outcomes research remains in its embryonic stages. This is in part attributable to the traditional emphasis in burn care on survival alone. With the ongoing shift in emphasis in burn clinical care and research away from merely survival to psychosocial and functional outcomes, there is increasing attention to the development of suitable metrics for evaluating the results of reconstructive procedures. There is clearly a need for the development of patient reported outcome tools (PROs) that are validated in burn patient populations that are sensitive to changes that can occur over time following reconstructive procedures. Development of these instruments will mostly likely require a collaborative effort among several centers, as the number of burn reconstruction surgeries done at any one burn unit is quite small. Furthermore, improvements in burn outcome research will require the organization of multicenter studies with standardized definitions and measurements for assessment of baseline aesthetic and functional status and the use of PROs valid for persons with burn injury as described above. Finally, the development of instruments that can evaluate patient's preparedness and suitability for reconstructive procedures would also be of tremendous clinical benefit.

Conclusion

Burn reconstruction requires careful consideration of the clinical problem such that an accurate diagnosis and reconstructive procedure can be selected. It is also critical to assess the patient's emotional and psychological preparedness for surgery, including compliance with the potentially months' long period of aggressive physical therapy and splint wearing that may be needed. Furthermore, it is critical that the patient's expectations are appropriately aligned with the likely reality of surgical outcome. Given the increasing number of people surviving burn injury, the need for plastic surgeons' involvement in burn care will only increase. As plastic surgeons we possess the unique and necessary skills and creativity to improve the lives of those who survive burn injury.

References

1. Pereira C, Murphy K, Herndon D. Outcome measures in burn care. Is mortality dead? *Burns.* 2004;30: 761–771.2.

   This manuscript provides a thoughtful and rational foundation for the current goals of modern burn care. Given all of the advances in care it is quite clear that in the 21st century, survival alone is an inadequate end-point of care. Rather, ultimate successful outcome should be defined by the psychosocial and functional health.

2. Gangemi EN, Gregori D, Berchialla P, et al. Epidemiology and risk factors for pathologic scarring after burn wounds. *Arch Facial Plast Surg.* 2008;10: 93–102.

   This paper provides a good review of the current understanding of risk factors for scar formation following burn injury. Despite the incidence of scarring, little is still known about the epidemiology and risk factors for scarring.

3. Brent B. Reconstruction of the ear, eyebrow and sideburns in the burned patient. *Plast Reconstr Surg.* 1975;55:312–317.

4. Taylor HO, Carty M, Driscoll D, et al. Nasal reconstruction after severe facial burns using a local turndown flap. *Ann Plast Surg.* 2009;62:175–179.

   This paper provides a novel technique for a common and challenging problem of the burned nose. The paper is well written and the technique and evidence for its utility are clearly presented.

5. Spence RJ. An algorithm for total and subtotal facial reconstruction using an expanded transposition flap: a 20-year experience. *Plast Reconstr Surg.* 2008;121: 795–805.

   Dr Spence provides a useful algorithm for approaching reconstruction of the burned face based on his over two decades of experience. This paper provides a practical and useful approach to the management of both simple and complex facial scar problems.

6. Viola RW, Hanel DP. Early 'simple' release of posttraumatic elbow contracture associated with heterotopic ossification. *J Hand Surg.* 1999;24A:370–380.

7. Donelan MB, Garcia JA. Nailfold reconstruction for correction of burn fingernail deformity. *Plast Reconstr Surg.* 2006;117:2303–2308.

   This paper provides a technique for management of a common complication of burn injuries to the hands. The technique is well-defined and is quite easy to perform.

8. Chang P, Laubenthal KN, Lewis 2nd RW, et al. Prospective, randomized study of the efficacy of pressure garment therapy in patients with burns. *J Burn Care Rehabil.* 1995;16:473–475.

23

Management of patients with exfoliative disorders, epidermolysis bullosa, and TEN

Abdullah E. Kattan, Robert C. Cartotto, and Joel S. Fish

SYNOPSIS

Toxic epidermal necrolysis (TEN)

- Stevens–Johnson syndrome (SJS), SJS–TEN overlap, and TEN can be considered as a continuum of the same disease spectrum, with increased total body surface area and mucosal involvement.
- These exfoliative skin disorders are drug-induced in more than 50% of patients.
- Sulfonamides, anticonvulsants, some antibiotics as well as acetaminophen are some of the well-documented drugs associated with SJS and TEN.
- Detailed history of recent medications is essential.
- These conditions may have significant morbidity and mortality if not managed aggressively and early.
- The mainstay of management is early wound debridement, irrigation, and coverage with skin substitute.
- Contractures and hypertrophic scarring are frequent long-term complications that may need revisions.
- Ocular complications are also very common and early involvement of ophthalmology is crucial.

Epidermolysis bullosa

- Epidermolysis bullosa is a blistering skin condition resulting from defects in the anchoring system of epithelial tissue in the basement membrane.
- It is characterized by the development of fluid-filled blisters secondary to trauma.
- Skin biopsies, electron as well as immunofluorescent microscopy are essential for diagnosis.
- Adequate nutritional support is important to facilitate wound healing.
- Meticulous skin care is required to prevent further injuries to the skin.
- These patients present to the plastic surgeon with chronic nonhealing wounds, scar contractures, or syndactalysed digits from repeated scarring.
- Squamous cell carcinoma is a well-documented long-term complication in these patients with chronically healing wound.

Access the Historical Perspective section online at
http://www.expertconsult.com

Plastic surgeons encounter a variety of skin disorders apart from cancerous conditions and trauma for which extensive and difficult wound care is necessary. Other health practitioners will often diagnose these diseases, and the plastic surgeon is consulted for the wound care problems that follow. Knowledge of exfoliative disorders is helpful because they are often treated along with thermal injuries or as part of a wound care multidisciplinary approach. Although this chapter does not cover all dermatologic exfoliative disorders, it will discuss selected conditions that are more likely to be encountered by plastic surgeons with an emphasis on surgical treatments.

Toxic epidermal necrolysis

Basic science/disease process

Whereas the exact pathogenesis of SJS and TEN remains unknown, evidence has accumulated to suggest that the patients who develop SJS or TEN have aberrant metabolism of the culprit drug and altered detoxification of reactive drug metabolites. This has been most extensively studied in patients who developed TEN from sulfonamides or anticonvulsants.[10–15] It is believed that reactive drug metabolites then induce a cell-mediated cytotoxic immune response against the epidermis.[16–19] CD8+ T lymphocytes and macrophages appear within the epidermis[16–19] and are believed to mediate this autoimmune response. Cytokines such as tumor necrosis factor (which has been found in TEN blister fluid) probably contribute to epidermal cell injury as well.[4,20] Apoptosis, which is essentially an activation of a genetic program that leads to cell death, appears to be the final common pathway of keratinocyte death in TEN and SJS–TEN overlap.[21] The keratinocyte apoptosis in TEN appears to be activated by an interaction between the death receptor Fas (CD95), normally found on keratinocytes, and active Fas ligand (FasL or CD95L), abnormally produced by keratinocytes in patients with TEN.[22] This is a particularly exciting finding because the Fas–FasL interaction can be blocked by antibodies found in intravenous immune globulin,[22] leading to a potential therapeutic intervention for TEN.[22] In early SJS and TEN, patchy necrosis of keratinocytes is seen at the dermal–epidermal junction. Later, the necrosis extends throughout the epidermis, and detachment of the epidermis from the dermis is noted. The underlying dermis is essentially normal with only sparse dermal infiltrate of helper T lymphocytes.[20,23]

Patient presentation/diagnosis

Since Lyell's original description of the syndrome, substantial controversy and debate have surrounded the definition of TEN and the classification of the other severe related exfoliative diseases of the skin, such as erythema multiforme and SJS. A concise and clinically relevant classification system is essential because overlapping terminology and poor nomenclature plague the majority of published reports on TEN and the related disorders. This has arisen, in no small part, from the similarities between TEN and several of the related exfoliative skin disorders.

Erythema multiforme is a cutaneous hypersensitivity reaction usually associated with an infection, such as recurrent herpes simplex or *Mycoplasma pneumoniae* infection.[23,24] Erythema multiforme is subclassified as minor or major. Erythema multiforme minor is characterized by the appearance of dusky, erythematous "target" or "iris" lesions, sometimes with blisters or bullae, symmetrically distributed on the extensor surfaces of the limbs and on the palms and soles.[23,24] Erythema multiforme major features are a similar picture, but mucosal surfaces, usually the mouth, are involved with erosions as well.[24]

SJS was originally described in two children who presented with aggressive disseminated cutaneous eruptions, severe stomatitis, and conjunctivitis.[25] As a result of the apparent similarity with erythema multiforme major, SJS was thought to be a variant of it. However, SJS is distinct from erythema multiforme major and should be classified separately. Erythema multiforme major is caused by an infection, features characteristic target-like lesions in a symmetric acral distribution, and has low morbidity and no associated mortality. SJS is drug-induced, features more widespread and central areas of skin involvement with epidermal detachment, and has high morbidity and occasional mortality.[20]

TEN, like SJS, features mucosal involvement and is a severe drug-induced exfoliative disorder of the skin. Currently, SJS and TEN are considered to be variants of the same drug-induced process and probably exist on a spectrum, with TEN being the more severe form of the same process.[4,20,26,27] The current consensus is that the diagnosis of SJS is given to patients with mucosal involvement, widespread purpuric macules, and epidermal detachment involving less than 10% of the total body surface area. SJS–TEN overlap applies to patients with mucosal involvement, widespread purpuric macules, and epidermal detachment involving 10–30% of the total body surface area. The diagnosis of TEN is applied to those patients with widespread purpuric macules, mucosal involvement, and epidermal detachment involving more than 30% of the total body surface area (*Table 23.1*).[4,20,24,28]

Patients with SJS, SJS–TEN, and TEN are relatively rare. The incidence of SJS ranges from 1.2 to 6 patients per million per year.[4] The incidence of TEN is estimated to range from 0.4 to 1.9 patients per million per year.[29–33] However, it is recognized that TEN is probably an underreported disease entity. SJS and TEN have been observed worldwide in all human populations.[13] Whereas SJS is considered to be a drug-induced reaction, a causative drug is found in only about 50% of those patients with the disease.[4] This probably reflects erroneous diagnosis of SJS as erythema multiforme major. In TEN, a causative drug is identified in approximately 80% of patients, and less than 5% have no associated drug use.[34,35]

Table 23.1 Toxic epidermal necrolysis (TEN) and related exfoliative diseases of the skin[4,20,24]

	Erythema multiforme		SJS	SJS–TEN overlap	TEN
	Minor	Major			
Etiology	Infection	Infection	Drug-induced	Drug-induced	Drug-induced
Mucosal involvement	No	Yes (usually oral)	Yes (usually ≥2 sites)	Yes (usually ≥2 sites)	Yes (usually ≥2 sites)
Skin lesion	Iris or target lesions with dusky erythematous center Acral, symmetric distribution Lesions may blister		Irregular dusky purpuric macules Central distribution Atypical targets Confluence of lesions Lesions may blister	Irregular dusky purpuric macules Central distribution Atypical targets Confluence of lesions Lesions may blister	Extensive purpuric macules Central and acral distribution Rapid confluence of diffuse erythema
Epidermal detachment	None		<10% TBSA	10–30% TBSA	>30% TBSA
Mortality	0%		<5%		30%

SJS, Stevens–Johnson syndrome; TBSA, total body surface area.

The drugs most commonly implicated in SJS and TEN are the sulfonamides (co-trimoxazole), the anticonvulsants (phenobarbital, phenytoin, carbamazepine), some antibiotics (aminopenicillins, quinolones, cephalosporins), nonsteroidal anti-inflammatory drugs, and allopurinol.[36] However, many other drugs have been associated with the onset of SJS and TEN, including common antipyretics such as acetaminophen and acetylsalicylic acid.[26] Although no reliable test exists to prove the association between a specific drug and the onset of TEN,[26,37] the lymphocyte toxicity assay (LTA) shows promise. The LTA is based on the concept that reactive metabolites of certain drugs are implicated in TEN.[10] The LTA exposes the patient's lymphocytes *in vitro* to a drug in the presence of a metabolizing system. Cytotoxic effect is used as evidence of increased sensitivity to newly formed toxic metabolites from the drug.[38–40] The LTA has been used to confirm sensitivity to anticonvulsants in a patient with TEN treated at the authors' facility who had been receiving both anticonvulsants and cephalosporins.[41] The LTA has the potential to test not only the patient but also first-degree relatives of the patient for the likelihood of a similar adverse drug reaction. Hence, the LTA offers enormous possibilities in prevention of the disease in patients and their families. It has been shown that there is a very strong association of SJS–TEN with human leukocyte antigen (HLA)-B 5801 and allupurinol as well as HLA-B 1502 and carbamazepine in the Chinese population. This association was not as strong in the European population. The Food and Drug Administration has recommended genotyping all Asian Patients for HLA-B 1502 before starting carbamazepine.[42,43] However, at present, implication of a drug in the pathogenesis of SJS or TEN relies on obtaining a careful history of the patient's drug use with the recognition that most instances of TEN arise within 1–3 weeks of starting the causative drug.[20,44,45] Nonetheless, TEN may develop with use of a drug outside this range. For example, SJS and TEN have been significantly associated with up to 8 weeks of use of phenytoin, phenobarbital, and carbamazepine.[46] Some medical conditions may be associated with an increased risk of TEN. These include systemic lupus erythematosus,[31] recent bone marrow transplantation,[47,48] and the acquired immunodeficiency syndrome.[49–52] TEN is more common in the elderly, but this may only reflect greater use of medications in this group.[3,23]

The cutaneous manifestations of TEN are typically preceded by a 2–3-day prodrome of what appears to be influenza or an upper respiratory tract infection. Patients initially have fever and malaise, and they experience pharyngitis or conjunctivitis. The skin may become pruritic. After this prodrome, dusky erythematous macules appear on the skin, usually on the trunk and face initially and then spreading to the extremities. These macules may be target-like but more often are irregular and ill defined. Blisters or bullae may appear within these macules. Within 3 or 4 days (but occasionally within hours) of the onset of these skin lesions, confluence of the macules into diffuse erythema develops, large bullae appear, and extensive sheets of epidermis begin to detach *(Fig. 23.1)*, leaving raw areas of glistening bright red dermis exposed *(Fig. 23.2)*. The Nikolsky sign, although nonspecific, is present in the spectrum of SJS and TEN *(Fig. 23.3)*. This sign refers to the immediate detachment of the epidermis with lateral digital pressure on the skin in the areas where confluent erythema is present. Mucosal involvement is usually advanced

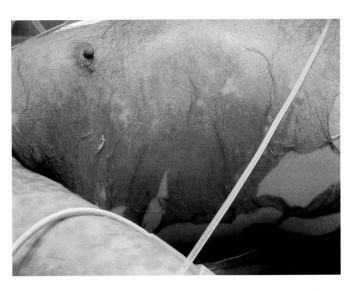

Fig. 23.1 Toxic epidermal necrolysis. Coalescence of macules with early blister formation (arm), with further progression to sheet-like epidermal detachment (chest).

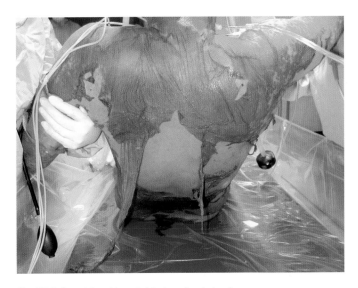

Fig. 23.2 Complete epidermal detachment and slough.

by this stage and involves blistering, slough, and erosion of mucosal surfaces *(Fig. 23.4)*. The lips and oral pharynx are most commonly involved, followed by the conjunctiva, genital mucosa, and anorectal mucosa. Mucosal sloughing may also involve the esophagus, the remainder of the gastrointestinal tract, and the tracheobronchial surfaces.[53,54]

Involvement of the lips and oropharynx can be particularly aggressive, with severe pain, dysphagia, odynophagia, and bleeding. The lips typically become crusted. Similarly, ocular involvement is also usually severe. Pseudomembranous conjunctival erosions may result in the formation of synechiae between the lids or between the conjunctiva and the eyelids.[8,45]

Laboratory abnormalities on presentation may include anemia, neutropenia, thrombocytopenia, and abnormal indices of renal and hepatic functions.[45] As a consequence of extensive areas of skin loss, the patient may develop problems related to fluid loss, hypothermia, and invasive infection.

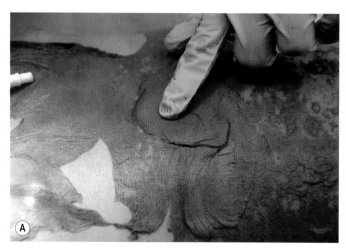

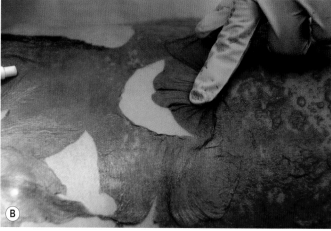

Fig. 23.3 **(A)** Area of involved skin. **(B)** Nikolsky sign, with detachment of epidermis with lateral digital pressure.

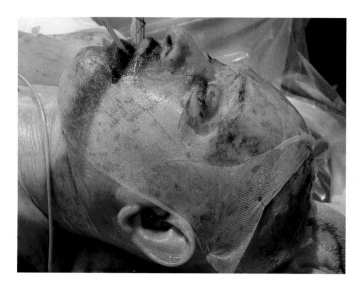

Fig. 23.4 Application of artificial skin substitute to raw dermal surface.

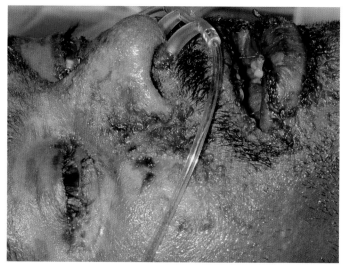

Fig. 23.5 Severe oral mucocutaneous involvement and conjunctivitis.

Prerenal azotemia, urosepsis, bronchopneumonia, and sepsis commonly occur.[9,23,45,55–58] The most common infective organisms appear to be *Staphylococcus aureus*, *Pseudomonas* species, and *Acinetobacter* species.[20,37,59] Mortality is most commonly the result of sepsis and multiple organ failure.[9,55,57–61]

Assuming the patient survives and the dermis is not secondarily injured by desiccation, infection, or mechanical trauma (e.g., pressure), re-epithelialization proceeds within a few days and is complete within 3 weeks.[8,20] Mucosal surfaces may remain eroded and crusted for several more weeks.

Although the diagnosis of SJS–TEN is usually clear, a biopsy should be performed to confirm the diagnosis (*Fig. 23.5*).[20,23,62] Important exfoliative disease entities to be distinguished from TEN include staphylococcal scalded-skin syndrome, pemphigus, pemphigoid, scarlet fever, acute generalized exanthematous pustulosis, toxic shock syndrome, and unrecognized scald injuries in comatose patients.[4,20,23]

Staphylococcal scalded-skin syndrome is probably the most common condition to masquerade as TEN. It is of interest that Lyell's 1956 description of TEN probably included a patient with staphylococcal scalded-skin syndrome.[1,20,62] Staphylococcal scalded-skin syndrome usually occurs in children and never has target lesions, and oropharyngeal involvement is uncommon. A biopsy easily differentiates the intraepidermal split within the granular layer in staphylococcal scalded-skin syndrome from the dermal–epidermal split in TEN.[62]

Patient selection

General

Burn units are ideally suited to the care of patients with large areas of skin loss. Thus, whereas patients with erythema multiforme or SJS may not qualify, those with more severe SJS–TEN overlap or TEN should be referred to a burn center.[6–9,55,59,60] Familiarity with the care of large open wounds, nursing expertise, and aggressive critical care are important advantages that a burn treatment facility can offer to a patient with

TEN. Early referral to a burn center (i.e., within 3–7 days of onset of skin slough) has been found to reduce mortality and hospital length of stay in patients with TEN.[9,57–60,63]

The main objective of treatment is to maintain a clean and healthy wound, and provide optimum conditions for re-epithelialization by removal of sloughed epidermis, irrigating the wound and temporary coverage.

Treatment/surgical technique

ABCs

In a prospective study of pulmonary complications in SJS–TEN overlap and TEN patients, significant involvement of the respiratory system at presentation was noted in 24% of patients.[64] Patients may be at risk for acute upper airway obstruction from excessive secretions, bleeding, or edema.[64,65] Alternatively, the patient may present with severe dyspnea or hypoxemia from bronchopulmonary desquamation, established bronchopneumonia, or evolving acute respiratory distress syndrome.[2,64] Therefore, careful consideration should be given to the need for intubation and mechanical ventilatory support. This must be counterbalanced with the recognition of the potential risk for ventilator-associated pneumonia in this group of patients.

Intubation of these patients may be extremely difficult because of mucosal sloughing, swelling, and bleeding in the upper airway. Intubation should be done by a physician experienced in dealing with the difficult airway. The airway is best secured with ties around the neck or by wiring the endotracheal tube to the dentition. Adhesive tape should not be used because it will not securely stick to the skin and may peel off facial and neck epidermis. If the endotracheal tube is wired, wire cutters must be immediately available at the bedside. It is recommended that TEN patients who are intubated undergo immediate fiberoptic bronchoscopy. This is done to assess the state of the tracheobronchial mucosa and to obtain bronchoalveolar lavage specimens for immediate Gram stain and then culture and sensitivity testing. Bronchial mucosal detachment identified at early fiberoptic bronchoscopy appears to indicate a poor prognosis.[64]

Although patients with TEN do not experience the massive fluid shifts that would occur in a patient with comparable second-degree burns, early attention must also be given to fluid and hemodynamic support. Peripheral intravenous access is preferred to avoid the infective risks associated with central access. However, the difficulty in finding and then securing a peripheral intravenous site in a patient with widespread exfoliation often necessitates a central line. Crystalloid fluid replacement may be necessary to reverse dehydration from inadequate oral intake due to severe stomatitis or from insensible fluid losses from open wounds. Some patients may present with established sepsis and may require more aggressive fluid and vasopressor support[58] and invasive monitoring.

Wound care

Dermal protection is the primary goal in the care of the wounds that result from exfoliation of the epidermis and is exactly analogous to the care of a superficial partial-thickness burn. Unimpeded re-epithelialization will occur as long as this goal is achieved. Desiccation, shear, pressure, and infection must be avoided. An early surgical approach is advocated in which the sloughing sheets of epidermis are removed, the raw dermal wounds are cleaned and irrigated, and the wound is covered with a temporary biologic or biosynthetic dressing.[8,9,55,57–60] Areas not involved with slough or imminent slough are left intact until such time as confluent epidermal detachment develops. During wound irrigation and debridement, caustic detergents should be avoided. Tap water from a hydrotherapy shower cart combined with chlorhexidine soap or, occasionally, bacitracin solution may be used. The choice of temporary skin substitute varies among institutions. In a multicenter survey of burn units that treat TEN patients,[57] Biobrane (Dow B Hickam, Sugarland, TX) was the most commonly used skin substitute, followed by porcine xenograft and cadaveric allograft.

Application of a skin substitute to the raw dermis provides protection, minimizes fluid electrolyte and heat loss from the wound, reduces exogenous bacterial invasion of the wound, reduces pain, and facilitates movement of the underlying parts *(Fig. 23.6)*. Regardless of the choice of substitute, the key principle is meticulous removal of the epidermis, irrigation and cleaning of the wound, and fixation of the substitute with sutures or staples. The substitute of choice is Biobrane.[66,67] Biobrane is preferable because it is inert, relatively inexpensive, available off the shelf, and transparent, which allows inspection of the wound through the material. Involved skin areas that have not yet begun to slough are treated with a nonadherent tulle gauze layer, covered with gauzes soaked in a topical antimicrobial solution, changed twice a day. Effective antimicrobial solutions include silver nitrate,[2,3,68] chlorhexidine gluconate solution,[3] and polymyxin-bacitracin.[69] Topical 5% mafenide acetate (Sulfamylon) and topical silver sulfadiazine cream (SSD) have been used,[57] but the unknown risk of sulfonamide cross-reactivity in a TEN patient makes the use of silver sulfadiazine cream a less suitable choice. A 5% mafenide acetate solution is preferred because it is clear and colorless and because of its broad-spectrum coverage abilities.

A second important goal of wound care in these patients is the separation of opposed mucosal surfaces. Erosion and subsequent fibrous synechiae formation can lead to adhesions and strictures between surfaces that should normally be mobile relative to each other. Examples of this include the vaginal labia, the external urethral meatus, and the conjunctivae. Daily perineal care with lubrication and frequent change of nonadherent materials (e.g., tulle gauze, Telfa) between the vaginal labia should be considered. A Foley catheter usually maintains patency of the urethral tract. Conjunctival care is discussed in the section on ocular care, below.

Other important principles of wound care include daily inspection and documentation of the skin involvement with use of a burn diagram, frequent turning and position changes, and use of specialty pressure reduction airbeds.

Drug withdrawal and the issue of corticosteroids

When the drug causing SJS or TEN is known, it should be immediately withdrawn. Evidence from a retrospective study involving 113 patients with SJS or TEN suggests that prognosis is improved by earlier withdrawal of the causative drug.[70]

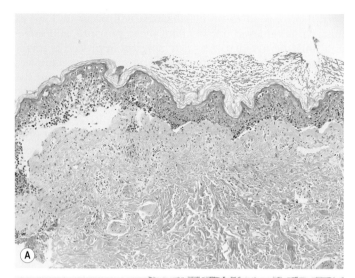

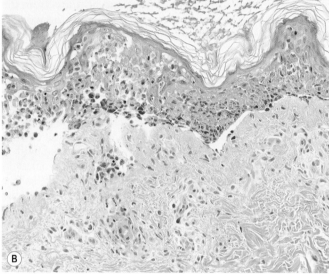

Fig. 23.6 (A) Hematoxylin and eosin (H&E) stain ×50, with epidermis showing necrosis of keratinocytes and subbasal separation. **(B)** H&E stain ×200 magnification of original slide. (Courtesy of Dr. G. Taylor, Toronto, Canada.)

The issue of corticosteroid therapy remains highly controversial. Use of corticosteroids has been recommended early in the course of the disease[71,72] in an effort to reverse inflammation and progression to skin sloughing. However, the effectiveness of this strategy has never been demonstrated in a clinical trial. TEN has developed in patients already receiving corticosteroids for other diseases,[73] suggesting that corticosteroids do not prevent or limit progression of TEN. A multicenter survey of TEN treated in US burn centers found that treatment with steroids before admission did not improve survival.[57] Retrospective data involving patients with SJS and TEN treated in burn centers revealed that survival rates were significantly lower in patients who received high-dose corticosteroids.[9,68] Although all of the evidence is retrospective, steroids do not appear to improve prognosis in SJS and TEN and may actually worsen morbidity and mortality. Hence, their use is not recommended, especially in patients who have significant skin slough (SJS–TEN overlap and TEN). A careful

drug use history should be obtained and the suspected inciting drugs should be immediately withdrawn. This may require substitution with an alternative drug, for example, when an anticonvulsant is implicated. If corticosteroids were started before admission, these should be stopped or rapidly tapered over 48–72 hours.

Postoperative care

General care issues

Attention should be given to fluid and electrolyte balance because there may be ongoing fluid losses from the wounds or evaporative losses when heated specialty airbeds are used. Aggressive pulmonary toilet, chest physiotherapy, and occasionally therapeutic fiberoptic bronchoscopy are essential for the removal of secretions and plugs of sloughed tracheobronchial mucosa. Oral care and hygiene are difficult and necessitate meticulous nursing care. Topical viscous lidocaine may alleviate some of the pain associated with severe stomatitis. Whereas skin substitutes may diminish some of the pain from the wounds, aggressive pain control with parenteral opioid analgesics is usually required. As with patients with major burn injuries, the ambient temperature should be raised to 30–32°C to reduce heat loss and hypermetabolism. Prophylaxis against deep venous thrombosis and gastric stress ulcers should be instituted.

Enteral nutrition is a mainstay of treatment and should be initiated as early as possible with a small orogastric or nasogastric feeding tube. Radiologic advancement of the feeding tube into the small bowel is ideal and may promote better tolerance of the feeding. Use of endoscopy to advance the feeding tube may not be advisable owing to the risks of perforating involved mucosal surfaces of the esophagus or gastrointestinal tract. Calorie and protein requirements may be initially calculated as for a burn of similar extent, but the estimated requirements should be adjusted on the basis of measured resting energy expenditure derived from a metabolic cart. Parenteral nutrition has been associated with increased mortality in TEN[57] and should be avoided whenever possible. A rehabilitation therapist should be involved early in the patient's care to reduce the risks of stiffness, weakness, and impaired mobility that frequently develop during this illness.[74]

Patients should be carefully monitored for evidence of infection. This usually includes regular documentation of temperature and leukocyte count and frequent microbiologic screening of the skin, urine, sputum, central lines, and blood for bacteria and fungus. Use of systemic prophylactic antibiotics is contraindicated, and antibiotics should be used only for documented infections and sepsis. Central line sites should be inspected daily, and central lines should be rotated to fresh sites every 3–5 days. A switch to peripheral intravenous access should be considered as soon as it is feasible.

Ocular care

An ophthalmologist should be consulted early and should observe the patient daily.[8] Antibiotic eye drops and lubricants are usually instilled every 2 hours, and synechiae must be carefully broken down with a glass rod on a daily basis.[75]

Novel pharmacologic therapy

At present, there are no definitive pharmacologic interventions that halt or reverse SJS or TEN. However, a number of novel approaches have been described. The use of any of these agents must be carefully considered and approached with caution; none has been evaluated in prospective randomized studies.

In small uncontrolled series, plasmapheresis[76,77] and cyclophosphamide[17] have been reported to have beneficial results in halting disease progression. Cyclosporine has anti-inflammatory and antiapoptotic properties and theoretically might be of use in SJS and TEN.[78] A number of reports have described favorable results in TEN patients treated with cyclosporine.[79–85] In an unblinded series of 11 TEN patients treated with cessation of steroids and cyclosporine compared with historical controls who had been treated with cyclophosphamide and varying doses of corticosteroids, therapy with cyclosporine was associated with faster arrest of disease and re-epithelialization and improved survival.[86] However, in the absence of a randomized prospective trial comparing cyclosporine with placebo that is not confounded by the use of corticosteroids, use of cyclosporine cannot be recommended, especially in view of its immunosuppressive effects in TEN patients, in whom there is a moderate to high risk of death from septic complications.

An interesting potential therapy is intravenous immune globulin (IVIG). Since the report of Viard et al.,[22] which described rapid reversal of TEN in 10 patients by blocking Fas-FasL-mediated apoptosis with IVIG, a number of reports and a small series have emerged seeming to confirm that IVIG successfully slows or halts TEN progression.[87–90] The authors' initial experience with IVIG in patients with TEN was similarly favorable.[43] However, in a retrospective study involving 16 TEN patients treated with IVIG and 16 TEN patients who did not receive IVIG, it was found that use of IVIG did not result in any reduction in length of stay, duration of mechanical ventilation, severity of multiple organ failure, or mortality rate, although there was a statistically insignificant trend toward less severe wound progression in the IVIG-treated patients.[91] Similarly, a study from the Loyola University Burn Center that compared 23 TEN patients treated with IVIG with 20 historical control patients found no improvement in hospital length of stay or survival with the use of IVIG.[92] Thus, although IVIG appears to be a promising therapy, its value must be assessed in a randomized double-blinded prospective trial against placebo. Current practice includes initiation of IVIG therapy immediately on admission in a dosage of approximately 0.7 g/kg per day for 4 days.

Outcomes, prognosis, and complications

The mortality rate for SJS is less than 5%.[4,35,37] The reported mortality rate for TEN is much more variable because this depends on the population of patients studied. For example, TEN patients treated at burn centers may represent the more severe end of the disease spectrum. The mortality rate from TEN reported in the larger series of patients (i.e., more than 30 patients) ranges from 4% to 83%[35,37,58–60]; however, the majority of these studies reported a mortality rate between 30% and 44%.[35,37,58,59] Factors that appear to worsen the prognosis are advanced age, extent of epidermal detachment, and serum urea level.[37] The multicenter review of TEN treated at US burn centers identified that increased mortality was also associated with an elevated score of the Acute Physiology and Chronic Health Evaluation (APACHE II) and parenteral nutrition before transfer to a burn center. In a study looking at the mortality of bullous skin disorders in the US from 1979 to 2002, Risser et al. reported that 5848 deaths were attributed to bullous disorders and 2387 were attributed to TENS. This corresponds to an age-adjusted mortality rate for TEN of 0.041 death per 100 000. Most of these deaths were in the elderly population.[93]

Survivors of TEN may experience a number of significant complications and permanent sequelae. As long as the epidermis regenerates within 2–3 weeks, the risk of cutaneous scarring is minimal.[94] However, in areas where delayed healing occurs (e.g., due to pressure, repetitive shear, or infection), hypertrophic scars may arise. Hyperpigmentation or mixed irregular pigmentation is common in healed areas. Nail deformities, phimosis, and vaginal synechiae have also been reported.[3,20,95] Ocular sequelae may be severe and can include entropion, ectropion, inverted eyelashes, corneal erosions or scarring, photophobia, visual impairment, and even blindness.[20,96] Some patients experience chronic tearing (due to tear duct obstruction from scar); others develop a chronic dry-eye "Sjögren-like" syndrome[36,96] with punctate keratitis. Long-term pulmonary dysfunction, even in patients who did not receive mechanical ventilation, has been reported.[97]

Secondary procedures

Most of the secondary procedures that these patients may require are related to release of abnormal scar tissue in the area of delayed healing or critical function in a manner very similar to burn patients. Massage, pressure garments, silicone sheets or steroid injections or a combination of these methods can be used to manage hypertrophic scars. Ultimately, they may require surgical excision and primary closure or skin grafting depending on the degree of impairment caused by the scar.

Ophthalmologic procedures such as release of synechiae, correction of ectropion or entropion, as well as procedures to deal with abnormal tearing may also be needed. Ensuring adequate and regular follow-up visits with an ophthalmologist is of paramount importance after discharge from the hospital.

Epidermolysis bullosa

Basic science/disease process

Epidermolysis bullosa is a group of inherited bullous disorders characterized by massive blistering of the skin developing in response to mechanical trauma.[98] Historically, epidermolysis bullosa subtypes have been classified according to morphologic features of the skin and the zone of the basement membrane that is involved. Three primary forms are seen: (1) epidermolysis bullosa simplex (intraepidermal skin separation); (2) recessive dystrophic epidermolysis bullosa (skin separation in lamina lucida or central basement

Table 23.2 Epidermolysis bullosa subtypes[105–110]

Morphologic type	Gross pathology	Molecular pathology
Epidermolysis bullosa simplex	Skin separation is at the mid basal cell	Mutation of the genes coding for keratins 5 and 14
Junctional epidermolysis bullosa	Blistering in the lamina lucida and variable hemidesmosomal abnormalities	Mutation in the genes coding for laminin 5 subunits, collagen XVII, 6 integrin and 4 integrin have been demonstrated
Dystrophic epidermolysis bullosa	Skin cleavage at the sublamina lucida	Mutations of the gene coding for type VII collagen

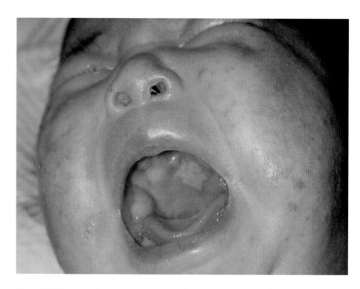

Fig. 23.7 Infant with palatal erosion from bottle-feeding, an indication of mucosal involvement in the gastrointestinal tract.

membrane zone); and (3) recessive junctional epidermolysis bullosa (sublamina densa basement membrane zone separation). A new category termed hemidesmosomal epidermolysis bullosa, which produces blistering at the hemidesmosomal level in the most superior aspect of the basement membrane zone, is also documented.[99–104]

The pathologic process is localized to the basement membrane zone of the skin and other surfaces lined by stratified squamous epithelial tissues. The underlying common mechanism is that defects in the anchoring system of the epithelial tissues allow detachment at a variable level of the skin with trauma *(Table 23.2).*[105–110]

Patient presentation/diagnosis

The hallmark of these conditions is the formation of large, fluid-filled blisters that develop in response to minor trauma. Some infants may have large blisters at birth *(Fig. 23.7)*. Others start shortly after birth. Minor degrees of chafing of the skin, rubbing, or even increased room temperature may cause blisters to form. The blister formation tends to be in anatomic areas of high wear and tear over the joints and on weight-bearing surfaces. Onset of epidermolysis bullosa is at birth or shortly after. The exception occurs in mild instances of epidermolysis bullosa simplex, which may remain undetected until adulthood or occasionally remain undiagnosed.

Epidermolysis bullosa simplex is usually associated with little or no extracutaneous involvement, whereas the more severe hemidesmosomal, junctional, and dystrophic forms of epidermolysis bullosa may produce significant multiorgan system involvement. This rare genetic disorder affects all ethnic and racial groups. Estimates indicate that as many as 100 000 Americans suffer from some form of epidermolysis bullosa. According to a National Epidermolysis Bullosa Registry report, 50 instances of epidermolysis bullosa occur per 1 million live births. Of these, approximately 92% are epidermolysis bullosa simplex, 5% are dystrophic epidermolysis bullosa, 1% are junctional epidermolysis bullosa, and 2% are unclassified.[99–102]

Infancy is an especially difficult time for patients with epidermolysis bullosa. Generalized blistering caused by any

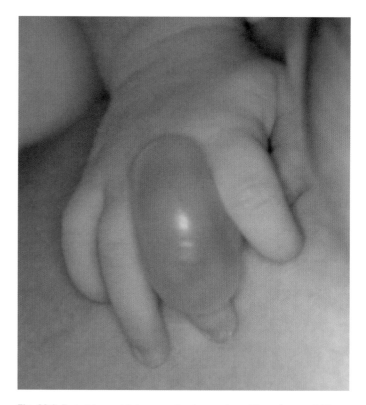

Fig. 23.8 Typical trauma blister presenting in a newborn. Biopsy is essential for diagnosis.

subtype may be complicated by infection, sepsis, and death. Severe forms of epidermolysis bullosa increase the mortality risk during infancy. Patients with junctional epidermolysis bullosa have the highest risk during infancy, with an estimated mortality rate of 87% during the first year of life, and have been cared for in burn units because of the large body surface area involved.[111,112]

In severe forms, the blistering process is followed by repeated cyclic scarring and healing resulting in severe

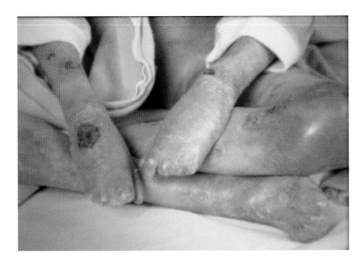

Fig. 23.9 Patient with dystrophic epidermolysis bullosa with characteristic syndactyly and contractures.

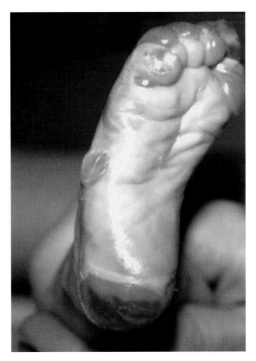

Fig. 23.10 Mild involvement of epidermolysis bullosa simplex, with blistering confined to the feet.

contractures and deformity *(Fig. 23.8)*. This is the point in time when plastic surgeons often become involved to help maintain or improve the function of hands and feet, particularly the fingers and toes. The oral and esophageal scarring that results from minor trauma of daily use also leads to feeding and swallowing difficulties resulting from the contracture and constriction rings. Severe malnutrition often results from an inability to handle solid foods *(Fig. 23.9)*.

Healing is of course delayed, and long-standing open areas can become colonized and secondarily infected.[111-115]

In patients with epidermolysis bullosa who survive childhood, the most common cause of death is metastatic squamous cell carcinoma. This skin cancer occurs specifically in patients with recessively inherited epidermolysis bullosa (recessive dystrophic epidermolysis bullosa), who most commonly are aged 15–35 years. In contrast, dominantly inherited epidermolysis bullosa simplex and dystrophic epidermolysis bullosa and milder forms of junctional epidermolysis bullosa may not affect a patient's life expectancy adversely.

Subtypes and clinical characteristics

Epidermolysis bullosa simplex is characterized by intraepidermal blistering with relatively mild internal involvement. Lesions typically heal without scarring. Most commonly, these diseases are dominantly inherited.

Mild epidermolysis bullosa simplex, or the Weber–Cockayne subtype, is the most common form. Blisters are usually precipitated by a known traumatic event. They can be mild to severe and most frequently occur on the palms and soles *(Fig. 23.10)*. Hyperhidrosis can accompany this disorder.

Severe epidermolysis bullosa simplex is usually characterized by a generalized onset of blisters at or shortly after birth. Hands, feet, and extremities are the most common sites of involvement. Hyperkeratosis and erosions of the hands and feet are common *(Fig. 23.11)*.

Junctional epidermolysis bullosa may be lethal or nonlethal. Lethal junctional epidermolysis bullosa is characterized by generalized blistering at birth and arises from an absence or a severe defect in expression of the anchoring filament

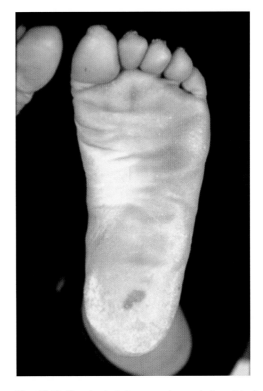

Fig. 23.11 Hyperkeratosis is commonly seen in the milder forms of epidermolysis bullosa simplex.

glycoprotein laminin 5.[115-117] Patients with lethal forms of junctional epidermolysis bullosa show characteristic involvement around the mouth, eyes, and nares, often accompanied by significant hypertrophic granulation tissue. Multisystemic involvement of the corneal, conjunctival, tracheobronchial,

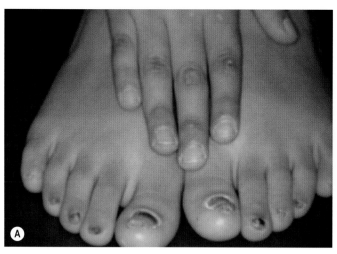

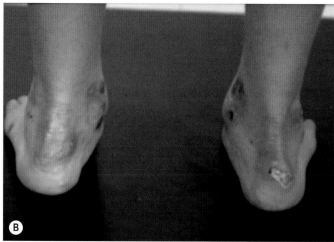

Fig. 23.12 (A) Patient with dystrophic epidermolysis bullosa diagnosed in adulthood after an orthopedic trauma admission to the hospital with acral involvement. **(B)** Limited blistering to the feet and hands, clinically present only during times of stress.

oral, pharyngeal, esophageal, rectal, and genitourinary mucosa is present. Patients usually do not survive past infancy.

Patients with nonlethal junctional epidermolysis bullosa manifesting generalized blistering who survive infancy and clinically improve with age have junctional epidermolysis bullosa mitis.[118] Scalp, nail, and tooth abnormalities may increasingly become apparent as patients age. Erosions and hypertrophic granulation tissue can be present. Mucous membranes are often affected by erosions, resulting in strictures. Some patients with junctional epidermolysis bullosa mitis can present with blistering localized to the intertriginous regions.

Dystrophic epidermolysis bullosa is a group of diseases caused by defects of anchoring fibrils.[118,119] Blisters heal followed by dystrophic scarring. Formation of milia (1–4-mm white papules) results as a consequence of damage to hair follicles.

Dominantly inherited dystrophic epidermolysis bullosa is characterized by the onset of disease usually at birth or during infancy, with generalized blistering as a common presentation. With increasing age, an evolution to localized blistering is present as well as changes in the nails.

Recessively inherited dystrophic epidermolysis bullosa ranges from mild to severe in presentation.[105,111,112,119,120] A mild form often involves acral areas and nails *(Fig. 23.12)* but shows little mucosal involvement. The severe form usually shows generalized blistering at birth and subsequent extensive dystrophic scarring that is most prominent on the acral surfaces. This is the form of the disease that may present to the plastic surgeon for pseudosyndactyly (mitten hand deformity) of the hands and feet *(see Fig. 23.15A, below).*[111,112,119] Flexion contractures of the extremities are increasingly common with age. Nails and teeth are also affected. Involvement of internal mucosa can result in esophageal strictures and webs, urethral and anal stenosis, phimosis, and corneal scarring.[120–122] Malabsorption commonly results in a mixed anemia from a lack of iron absorption, and overall malnutrition may cause failure to thrive.[113,119] Patients with

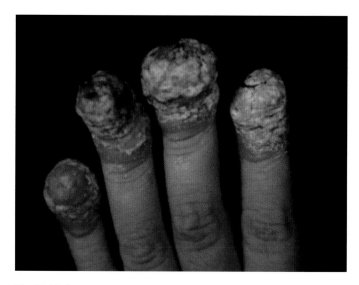

Fig. 23.13 Squamous cell carcinoma in severely involved terminal digits had been ignored until excessive keratinization was clinically evident. Open healing blistered areas more commonly form granulation tissue and not keratin because the keratinocytes are absent.

severe recessive dystrophic epidermolysis bullosa who survive to childhood are at significant risk for development of aggressive squamous cell carcinoma in areas of chronic erosions *(Fig. 23.13).*

Investigations

Skin biopsy is essential for the diagnosis *(Fig. 23.14)*; the specimen is sent for electron microscopy and immunofluorescent microscopy. Electron microscopy is the standard for determining the level of blistering. Immunomapping with antibodies can distinguish the different types of epidermolysis bullosa. If surgery is being contemplated, a nutritional evaluation is useful to aid in prediction of wound healing.[113]

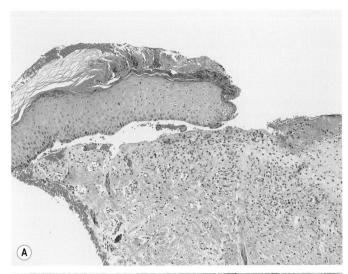

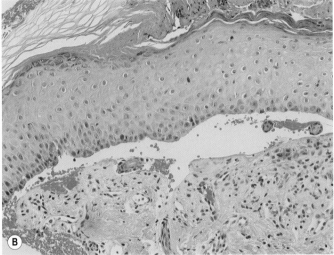

Fig. 23.14 (A) Hematoxylin and eosin (H&E) stain ×100, with epidermis showing subbasal separation. **(B)** H&E stain ×200 magnification of original slide. (Courtesy of Dr. G. Taylor, Toronto, Canada.)

Patient selection

The complete medical treatment of patients with epidermolysis bullosa involves many specialties. There are specific concerns of the respiratory, gastrointestinal, and urogenital systems that are vital to the overall treatment of patients with epidermolysis bullosa.[109] The manifestations of the disease resulting in wound care problems and physical deformities would be treated by a plastic surgeon. The patient should be evaluated by establishing the range of motion of limbs and digits to monitor contractures and effectiveness of physical therapy.

Optimizing wound healing in patients with epidermolysis bullosa involves controlling all of the factors that potentially delay wound healing, including foreign bodies, bacteria, nutritional deficiencies, tissue anoxia, and mechanical trauma. Extensive areas of denuded skin represent loss of the stratum corneum barrier to microbial penetration. Accumulation of serum and moisture on the surface enhances the growth of bacteria.

Extensive cutaneous injury is associated with marked alterations in both hemodynamic and metabolic responses, requiring increased calorie and protein intake for recovery. The development of nutritional deficiencies inhibits successful wound healing and the body's return to a normal hemodynamic and metabolic profile.

The nutritional well-being of patients with epidermolysis bullosa should be dealt with before any surgical intervention is considered.[109,112,113] Complications include oral blistering, abnormal esophageal motility, strictures, dysphagia, diarrhea, malabsorption, and dental problems. A nutritional assessment taking these factors into account is essential for replenishing the malnourished patient and improving wound healing.[110]

Treatment/surgical technique

Prevention of infection is the preferred strategy. With extensive areas of crusting and skin loss, a strict wound care regimen should be followed. Such a regimen entails regular whirlpool therapy followed by application of topical antibiotics. The wound should be covered with semiocclusive nonadherent dressings. Adhesive tape should not be applied directly to the skin. Self-adhering gauze or tape is a better choice for keeping dressings in place. Many adult patients will explore the use of multiple wound care products and often develop their own strategies to deal with recurrent areas of breakdown. Extensive areas of skin loss, particularly common in children who cannot avoid mechanical trauma, might require admission to a burn unit.

Squamous cell carcinoma often arises in chronic cutaneous lesions in patients with epidermolysis bullosa because of recurrent breakdown and repair; peak incidence begins to increase dramatically in the second and third decades of life.[119] Squamous cell carcinoma often occurs at multiple primary sites, which is especially true for patients with recessive dystrophic epidermolysis bullosa. The distribution of cutaneous squamous cell carcinoma in patients with recessive dystrophic epidermolysis bullosa is different and involves any area of nonhealing. Careful surveillance of nonhealing areas is important.

Chronic blepharitis can result in cicatricial ectropion and exposure keratitis.[122] Moisture chambers and ocular lubricants are commonly used for management. This disorder has also been treated with full-thickness skin grafting to the upper eyelid; however, complete correction is difficult to obtain because the oculofacial region will still continue to break down, and repeated scarring will often result in recurrence of the ectropion.

Potential future therapies include protein and gene therapies.[123–125] Protein therapy involves applying the missing or defective protein, which is produced *in vitro* by recombinant methods, directly to blistered skin. Protein therapy may be most useful in epidermolysis bullosa subtypes involving a defect or deficiency in laminin 5 because this protein does not require complex processing or transmembrane cellular anchorage. In gene therapy, the goal is to deliver genes targeted to restore normal protein production.

Surgical care

Surgical restoration of the hand involves treatment of the mitten deformity of the hand.[111] Repeated episodes of blistering and scarring eventually result in fusion of the web spaces. As a result, fine manipulative skills and digital prehension are lost. Surgical procedures can correct this deformity, but the rate of recurrence is high. The dominant hand has earlier recurrence. Recurrence appears to be delayed by the prolonged use of splinting in the interphalangeal spaces at night. The preferred method of release involves restoring the thumb opposition and separating the precision-based radial digits for fine motor skills. The surgical release involves fixation of grafts to the surgically formed clefts. Flaps have generally not been used because of the poor skin component.

Invasive aggressive squamous cell carcinoma is a particularly troubling complication of recessive dystrophic epidermolysis bullosa. When it is detected, excision of the carcinoma is indicated. Both Mohs and non-Mohs surgical approaches have been used. Skin graft harvesting can be difficult because of the total skin involvement in many patients. Split-thickness grafts should be harvested with a hand-held knife as opposed to electric or mechanical dermatomes, which have been reported to cause full-thickness wounds. Donor sites usually heal rapidly if they can be kept free of infection. The authors' experience suggests full examination of the integument in order to choose a donor site. Patients often have "spared" areas that are often dressing-free that do not have the adjacent open wounds that lead to secondary infection/contamination and donor site morbidity. Full-thickness grafts can be harvested from areas of intact skin with excellent healing of the donor site, but the thinning process of the full-thickness graft must be done with care because the epidermal layer will naturally fracture if it is overhandled.[111,112] A technique has been described in which the full-thickness graft is obtained by trying to cleave the dermis *in situ* with a large scalpel blade to minimize tissue handling.

The anesthetic care of patients with epidermolysis bullosa requires a presurgical consultation and is also beyond the scope of this chapter.[126] Consultation of an anesthesiologist experienced in the care of patients with epidermolysis bullosa is optimal. In general, endotracheal intubation is optimal as the large pharyngeal masks/stents cause surface abrasion and risk creating mucosal tears. Endotracheal tube fixation with gauze/cloth ties with adequate padding for the securing ties is recommended. Temporary fixation to the gingiva with wire or suture can be used to minimize contact to the face/neck.

Use of skin equivalents

It is safe to state that any new wound-healing product that has been produced has been used on this condition. An internet review reveals that the epidermolysis bullosa websites with interactive areas post numerous substances that have been tried with varying success. The literature includes reports of different products that are used to heal both open recurring wounds and donor sites for grafting procedures. None is known to be superior. Integra artificial skin has been tried, but the chronic nature of these wounds increases the rates of infection and loss of the dermal matrix while vascular ingrowth is awaited. Dermal replacement analogues and epithelial cell culture techniques have been used to treat patients with epidermolysis bullosa. Apligraf is a human allograft of fibroblasts and keratinocytes.[127] Whereas the short-term effects of Apligraf have been studied carefully, the long-term effects and the persistence of grafts remain in question *(Fig. 23.15)*. Apligraf may represent an effective short-term therapy for chronic nonhealing wounds in epidermolysis bullosa, but claims that Apligraf offers a long-term cure for epidermolysis bullosa remain unsubstantiated. This is not surprising given that Apligraf does not vascularize to the wound bed and the persistence of allografted cells is only temporary.

It is hoped that, in the future, tissue engineering will produce a product with characteristics that allow epithelial anchoring and a possible effective means of maintaining skin integrity for these patients.

Autografting procedures can now be accomplished with little or no suturing using cyanoacrylate adhesives for skin graft fixation. The wound can be covered with a nonadherent gauze to allow for fluid efflux and when the postoperative dressing is removed there is no need for suture removal allowing for minimal skin/wound contact. Owing to the contractures which might develop in hips, knees, shoulders, or elbows, particular attention at the onset of the operative procedure is recommended and can be accomplished with surgical foam or sheets *(Fig. 23.16)*, allowing the positioning such that intraoperative mechanical shear to the skin is avoided. Even gentle repeated limb repositioning will result in iatrogenic shearing. Patient placement on and off the operative table is a time when skin care is at greatest risk, necessitating many hands to allow for safe and gentle lifting as opposed to using any roller mechanisms which introduce shear forces.

Postoperative care

Patients with epidermolysis bullosa require specialized wound care pre-, intra-, and postoperatively. Careful and judicious padding and splinting are required to prevent the appearance of new areas of blistering. Minimizing dressing changes is another point to take into consideration in the postoperative period. The nutritional state of patients must be continuously monitored throughout the treatment process.

Outcomes, prognosis, and complications

Squamous cell carcinoma often arises in chronic cutaneous lesions in patients with epidermolysis bullosa because of recurrent breakdown and repair; peak incidence begins to increase dramatically in the second and third decades of life.[119] Squamous cell carcinoma often occurs at multiple primary sites, which is especially true for patients with recessive dystrophic epidermolysis bullosa. The distribution of cutaneous squamous cell carcinoma in patients with recessive dystrophic epidermolysis bullosa is different and involves any area of nonhealing. Careful surveillance of nonhealing areas is important.

Chronic blepharitis can result in cicatricial ectropion and exposure keratitis.[124] Moisture chambers and ocular lubricants are used commonly for management. This disorder has also been treated with full-thickness skin grafting to the upper eyelid; however, complete correction is difficult to obtain because the oculofacial region will still continue to break down, and repeated scarring will often result in recurrence of the ectropion.

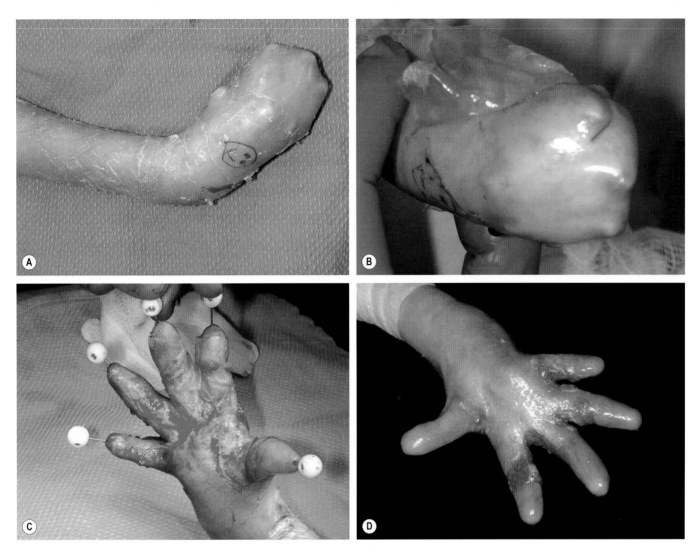

Fig. 23.15 (A) Classic mitten hand deformity with absent phalanges requires surgical release to restore function. **(B)** Intraoperatively, the epidermal "casting" due to minimal trauma of preparing the limb is common. It is for this reason that handling is gentle and the tourniquet cannot be used. **(C)** Apligraf used to cover index and middle fingers as donor sites that were judged to be poor for graft harvest. **(D)** Epithelialization eventually occurred after weeks of dressings. It was the authors' impression that the Apligraf provided a biologic dressing, allowing native epithelialization to occur. (Courtesy of Dr. R. Zuker, Toronto, Canada.)

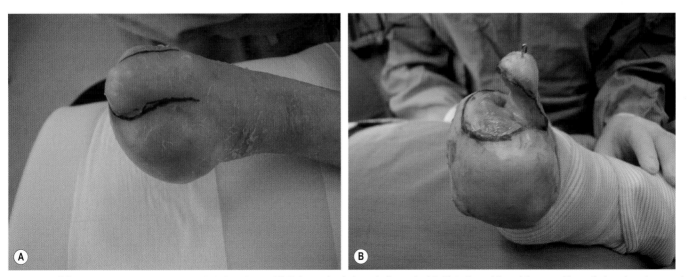

Fig. 23.16 (A) Mitten thumb marked intraoperatively for release. **(B)** Release of soft tissue in first web cleft. Note the padding of the arm with a soft sheer layer to prevent iatrogenic shearing of skin.

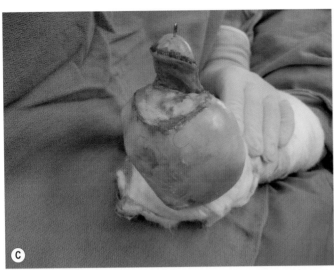

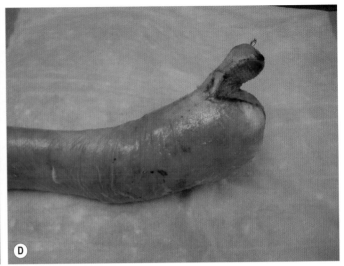

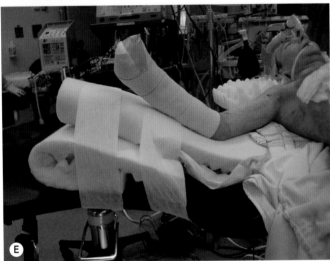

Fig. 23.16, cont'd (C) Partial-thickness graft using posterior trunk skin which is often preserved. Graft is glued in place as opposed to sutures for firm fixation. **(D)** Graft take at 10 days postoperatively. **(E)** Special care taken to position limbs intraoperatively with use of sponges so that minimal intraoperative manipulation is required to reduce shearing and damage from even gentle repositioning during surgery.

Access the complete references list online at **http://www.expertconsult.com**

4. Roujeau JC, Stern RS. Severe adverse cutaneous reactions to drugs. *N Engl J Med*. 1994;331:1272–1285.

This articles gives a very detailed description of the most common and severe drug-induced cutaneous reactions. The disorders discussed include SJS and TEN, hypersensitivity syndrome, vasculitis and serum sickness, anticoagulant-induced skin necrosis and angioedema. The review of each condition includes clinical presentation, differential diagnosis, pathophysiology, and treatment strategies.

8. Heimbach DM, Engrav LH, Marvin JA, et al. Toxic epidermal necrolysis. *JAMA*. 1987;257:2171–2175.

20. Wolkenstein P, Revuz J. Toxic epidermal necrolysis. *Dermatol Clin*. 2000;18:485–495.

This article gives a good overview of TEN. The authors discuss the history of the disease and differentiation between TEN and other exfoliative diseases. They also evaluate the pathophysiology and the most common culprit drugs and describe proposed mechanisms of action. They also give a detailed description of the clinical symptoms and presentation followed by a general overview on management.

23. Becker DS. Toxic epidermal necrolysis. *Lancet*. 1998; 351:1417–1420.

57. Palmieri TL, Greenhalgh DG, Saffle JR, et al. A multicenter review of toxic epidermal necrolysis treated in U.S. burn centers at the end of the twentieth century. *J Burn Care Rehabil*. 2002;23:87–96.

In this paper, the authors conduct a multicenter review of TEN patients in 15 US burn centers over a 5-year period. A total of 199 patients were included in their study. They outlined the different causative agents as well as management protocols. They were also able to identify factors that significantly affected mortality and morbidity. The factors that were found to affect outcome negatively included increased age and total body surface area involvement, duration before being transferred to a burn center if more than 7 days, pre-existing comorbidities as well as APACHE II and MOD scores.

72. Fine J. Management of acquired bullous skin diseases. *N Engl J Med*. 1995;133:1475–1484.

103. Uitto J, Eady R, Fine JD, et al. The DEBRA International Visioning/Consensus Meeting on Epidermolysis Bullosa: summary and recommendations. *J Invest Dermatol.* 2000;114:734–737.

111. Terrill PJ, Mayou BJ, Pemberton J. Experience in the surgical management of the hand in dystrophic epidermolysis bullosa. *Br J Plast Surg.* 1992;45:435–442.

    The authors report their experience operating on 45 patients with hand deformities secondary to epidermolysis bullosa over a 19-year period. They describe the different patterns of soft-tissue and bony deformities that were encountered and their approach to correct each deformity.

112. Terrill PJ, Mayou BJ, McKee PH, et al. The surgical management of dystrophic epidermolysis bullosa (excluding the hand). *Br J Plast Surg.* 1992;45:426–434.

    The authors review their experience with 50 epidermolysis bullosa patients over a course of 19 years. They describe different surgical procedures involving the feet and toes, elbow and axilla, oral cavity, anus, eyes, and penile area. They also report their experience with chronic ulcers as well as squamous cell carcinoma.

119. McGrath JA, Ishida-Yamamoto A, Tidman MJ, et al. Epidermolysis bullosa simplex (Dowling–Meara). A clinicopathological review. *Br J Dermatol.* 1992;126: 421–430.

Index

Note: **Boldface** *roman numerals indicate volume. Page numbers followed by f refer to figures; page numbers followed by t refer to tables; page numbers followed by b refer to boxes.*

Note: **Boldface** *roman numerals indicate volume. Page numbers followed by f refer to figures; page numbers followed by t refer to tables; page numbers followed by b refer to boxes.*

*Note: **Boldface** roman numerals indicate volume. Page numbers followed by f refer to figures; page numbers followed by t refer to tables; page numbers followed by b refer to boxes.*

*Note: **Boldface** roman numerals indicate volume. Page numbers followed by f refer to figures; page numbers followed by t refer to tables; page numbers followed by b refer to boxes.*

Note: **Boldface** *roman numerals indicate volume. Page numbers followed by f refer to figures; page numbers followed by t refer to tables; page numbers followed by b refer to boxes.*

*Note: **Boldface** roman numerals indicate volume. Page numbers followed by f refer to figures; page numbers followed by t refer to tables; page numbers followed by b refer to boxes.*

Note: **Boldface** *roman numerals indicate volume. Page numbers followed by f refer to figures; page numbers followed by t refer to tables; page numbers followed by b refer to boxes.*

Note: **Boldface** roman numerals indicate volume. Page numbers followed by f refer to figures; page numbers followed by t refer to tables; page numbers followed by b refer to boxes.

*Note: **Boldface** roman numerals indicate volume. Page numbers followed by f refer to figures; page numbers followed by t refer to tables; page numbers followed by b refer to boxes.*

*Note: **Boldface** roman numerals indicate volume. Page numbers followed by f refer to figures; page numbers followed by t refer to tables; page numbers followed by b refer to boxes.*

Note: **Boldface** roman numerals indicate volume. Page numbers followed by f refer to figures; page numbers followed by t refer to tables; page numbers followed by b refer to boxes.

Note: **Boldface** *roman numerals indicate volume. Page numbers followed by f refer to figures; page numbers followed by t refer to tables; page numbers followed by b refer to boxes.*

Note: **Boldface** *roman numerals indicate volume. Page numbers followed by f refer to figures; page numbers followed by t refer to tables; page numbers followed by b refer to boxes.*

Note: **Boldface** *roman numerals indicate volume. Page numbers followed by f refer to figures; page numbers followed by t refer to tables; page numbers followed by b refer to boxes.*

Note: **Boldface** roman numerals indicate volume. Page numbers followed by f refer to figures; page numbers followed by t refer to tables; page numbers followed by b refer to boxes.

*Note: **Boldface** roman numerals indicate volume. Page numbers followed by f refer to figures; page numbers followed by t refer to tables; page numbers followed by b refer to boxes.*

Note: **Boldface** *roman numerals indicate volume. Page numbers followed by f refer to figures; page numbers followed by t refer to tables; page numbers followed by b refer to boxes.*

Note: **Boldface** roman numerals indicate volume. Page numbers followed by f refer to figures; page numbers followed by t refer to tables; page numbers followed by b refer to boxes.

---

*Note: **Boldface** roman numerals indicate volume. Page numbers followed by f refer to figures; page numbers followed by t refer to tables; page numbers followed by b refer to boxes.*

Note: **Boldface** *roman numerals indicate volume. Page numbers followed by f refer to figures; page numbers followed by t refer to tables; page numbers followed by b refer to boxes.*

Note: **Boldface** *roman numerals indicate volume. Page numbers followed by f refer to figures; page numbers followed by t refer to tables; page numbers followed by b refer to boxes.*

Note: **Boldface** roman numerals indicate volume. Page numbers followed by f refer to figures; page numbers followed by t refer to tables; page numbers followed by b refer to boxes.

Note: **Boldface** roman numerals indicate volume. Page numbers followed by f refer to figures; page numbers followed by t refer to tables; page numbers followed by b refer to boxes.

Note: **Boldface** *roman numerals indicate volume. Page numbers followed by f refer to figures; page numbers followed by t refer to tables; page numbers followed by b refer to boxes.*

Note: **Boldface** *roman numerals indicate volume. Page numbers followed by f refer to figures; page numbers followed by t refer to tables; page numbers followed by b refer to boxes.*

*Note: **Boldface** roman numerals indicate volume. Page numbers followed by f refer to figures; page numbers followed by t refer to tables; page numbers followed by b refer to boxes.*

Note: **Boldface** *roman numerals indicate volume. Page numbers followed by f refer to figures; page numbers followed by t refer to tables; page numbers followed by b refer to boxes.*

Note: **Boldface** *roman numerals indicate volume. Page numbers followed by f refer to figures; page numbers followed by t refer to tables; page numbers followed by b refer to boxes.*

*Note: **Boldface** roman numerals indicate volume. Page numbers followed by f refer to figures; page numbers followed by t refer to tables; page numbers followed by b refer to boxes.*

*Note: **Boldface** roman numerals indicate volume. Page numbers followed by f refer to figures; page numbers followed by t refer to tables; page numbers followed by b refer to boxes.*

Note: **Boldface** *roman numerals indicate volume. Page numbers followed by f refer to figures; page numbers followed by t refer to tables; page numbers followed by b refer to boxes.*

*Note: **Boldface** roman numerals indicate volume. Page numbers followed by f refer to figures; page numbers followed by t refer to tables; page numbers followed by b refer to boxes.*

Note: **Boldface** *roman numerals indicate volume. Page numbers followed by f refer to figures; page numbers followed by t refer to tables; page numbers followed by b refer to boxes.*

Note: **Boldface** roman numerals indicate volume. Page numbers followed by f refer to figures; page numbers followed by t refer to tables; page numbers followed by b refer to boxes.

Note: **Boldface** roman numerals indicate volume. Page numbers followed by f refer to figures; page numbers followed by t refer to tables; page numbers followed by b refer to boxes.

Note: **Boldface** *roman numerals indicate volume. Page numbers followed by f refer to figures; page numbers followed by t refer to tables; page numbers followed by b refer to boxes.*

*Note: **Boldface** roman numerals indicate volume. Page numbers followed by f refer to figures; page numbers followed by t refer to tables; page numbers followed by b refer to boxes.*

Note: **Boldface** roman numerals indicate volume. Page numbers followed by f refer to figures; page numbers followed by t refer to tables; page numbers followed by b refer to boxes.

Note: **Boldface** roman numerals indicate volume. Page numbers followed by f refer to figures; page numbers followed by t refer to tables; page numbers followed by b refer to boxes.

Note: **Boldface** roman numerals indicate volume. Page numbers followed by f refer to figures; page numbers followed by t refer to tables; page numbers followed by b refer to boxes.

*Note: **Boldface** roman numerals indicate volume. Page numbers followed by f refer to figures; page numbers followed by t refer to tables; page numbers followed by b refer to boxes.*

Note: **Boldface** roman numerals indicate volume. Page numbers followed by f refer to figures; page numbers followed by t refer to tables; page numbers followed by b refer to boxes.

Note: **Boldface** roman numerals indicate volume. Page numbers followed by f refer to figures; page numbers followed by t refer to tables; page numbers followed by b refer to boxes.

Note: **Boldface** *roman numerals indicate volume. Page numbers followed by f refer to figures; page numbers followed by t refer to tables; page numbers followed by b refer to boxes.*

*Note: **Boldface** roman numerals indicate volume. Page numbers followed by f refer to figures; page numbers followed by t refer to tables; page numbers followed by b refer to boxes.*

*Note: **Boldface** roman numerals indicate volume. Page numbers followed by f refer to figures; page numbers followed by t refer to tables; page numbers followed by b refer to boxes.*

Note: **Boldface** *roman numerals indicate volume. Page numbers followed by f refer to figures; page numbers followed by t refer to tables; page numbers followed by b refer to boxes.*

*Note: **Boldface** roman numerals indicate volume. Page numbers followed by f refer to figures; page numbers followed by t refer to tables; page numbers followed by b refer to boxes.*

*Note: **Boldface** roman numerals indicate volume. Page numbers followed by f refer to figures; page numbers followed by t refer to tables; page numbers followed by b refer to boxes.*

*Note: **Boldface** roman numerals indicate volume. Page numbers followed by f refer to figures; page numbers followed by t refer to tables; page numbers followed by b refer to boxes.*

Note: **Boldface** *roman numerals indicate volume. Page numbers followed by f refer to figures; page numbers followed by t refer to tables; page numbers followed by b refer to boxes.*

Note: ***Boldface*** *roman numerals indicate volume. Page numbers followed by* f *refer to figures; page numbers followed by* t *refer to tables; page numbers followed by* b *refer to boxes.*

*Note: **Boldface** roman numerals indicate volume. Page numbers followed by f refer to figures; page numbers followed by t refer to tables; page numbers followed by b refer to boxes.*

Note: **Boldface** roman numerals indicate volume. Page numbers followed by f refer to figures; page numbers followed by t refer to tables; page numbers followed by b refer to boxes.

Note: **Boldface** roman numerals indicate volume. Page numbers followed by f refer to figures; page numbers followed by t refer to tables; page numbers followed by b refer to boxes.

Note: **Boldface** *roman numerals indicate volume. Page numbers followed by f refer to figures; page numbers followed by t refer to tables; page numbers followed by b refer to boxes.*

*Note: **Boldface** roman numerals indicate volume. Page numbers followed by f refer to figures; page numbers followed by t refer to tables; page numbers followed by b refer to boxes.*

Note: **Boldface** *roman numerals indicate volume. Page numbers followed by f refer to figures; page numbers followed by t refer to tables; page numbers followed by b refer to boxes.*

Note: **Boldface** *roman numerals indicate volume. Page numbers followed by f refer to figures; page numbers followed by t refer to tables; page numbers followed by b refer to boxes.*

Note: **Boldface** roman numerals indicate volume. Page numbers followed by f refer to figures; page numbers followed by t refer to tables; page numbers followed by b refer to boxes.

Note: **Boldface** roman numerals indicate volume. Page numbers followed by f refer to figures; page numbers followed by t refer to tables; page numbers followed by b refer to boxes.

*Note: **Boldface** roman numerals indicate volume. Page numbers followed by f refer to figures; page numbers followed by t refer to tables; page numbers followed by b refer to boxes.*

Note: **Boldface** *roman numerals indicate volume. Page numbers followed by f refer to figures; page numbers followed by t refer to tables; page numbers followed by b refer to boxes.*

*Note: **Boldface** roman numerals indicate volume. Page numbers followed by f refer to figures; page numbers followed by t refer to tables; page numbers followed by b refer to boxes.*